Textbook of
Pharmacology

Textbook of Pharmacology

W.C.BOWMAN

B.Pharm. Ph.D. D.Sc. M.P.S.

Professor of Pharmacology
University of Strathclyde

M.J.RAND

M.Sc. Ph.D.

Professor of Pharmacology
University of Melbourne

G.B.WEST

B.Pharm. Ph.D. D.Sc. F.P.S.

The British Industrial Biological
Research Association

REVISED SECOND PRINTING

BLACKWELL SCIENTIFIC PUBLICATIONS

OXFORD AND EDINBURGH

SBN: 632 04650 3

First Published 1968

Revised Reprint 1969

Printed in Great Britain by
SPOTTISWOODE, BALLANTYNE & CO LTD, COLCHESTER
and bound by
THE KEMP HALL BINDERY, OXFORD

Contents

v

Contents

Preface

When we decided to write this book we were members of the teaching staff of the Pharmacology Department of the School of Pharmacy, University of London. Each of us thought at the time that he had a clear idea of the kind of book needed by our students. The main problem was that our students needed pharmacology for a variety of reasons. Some became experimental pharmacologists in industry, research institutes and universities and to train these students adequately called for an emphasis on mechanisms of drug action and the theoretical aspects of pharmacology. At the other extreme, some students became retail pharmacists and needed a broad view of pharmacology with emphasis on the empirical aspects of therapeutically useful drugs. This volume represents a compromise between our different opinions about what was required. Now that we can view it as a whole we are all too aware of many of its shortcomings; there must be many more that will no doubt be pointed out to us soon. Nevertheless, we hope it will be useful, not only for students of science or pharmacy, but also for medical students and even as general reading for research workers in pharmacology and allied fields.

Part 1 deals with various aspects of physiology that we feel are necessary for understanding the actions of drugs: we have tried to emphasize, to a greater extent than is usual in most text-books, those physiological processes that are especially susceptible to modification by drugs.

The first three chapters in Part 2 deal with matters of general application in pharmacology; the remainder of the chapters deal with systematic pharmacology. We have chosen to group together drugs according to their actions on different systems of the body as far as this was practicable: in the numerous cases where the same drug acts on more than one system we have provided cross-references. We have also made extensive cross-references between the two parts of the book to emphasize the links between physiological processes and pharmacological actions.

We are grateful for the help given by many of our colleagues at London University, and wish to mention especially Professor G.A.H.Buttle, Drs Rosemary Cass, B.A.Callingham, A.W.Cuthbert and P.S.J.Spencer. We are especially indebted to Dr A.M.Barrett of Imperial Chemical Industry for contributing most of the material in chapters 14 and 33, and to Miss Alison Jowett and Dr Anne Stafford for their critical reading of most of the manuscript and the proofs. Mr Barrie Barber drew most of the diagrams and Mrs Lorna Solomon helped with the index; other acknowledgements are made in the text as they fall due. We are pleased to acknowledge our thanks to Per Saugman, Managing Director, and J.L.Robson, Production Manager, of Blackwell Scientific Publications for their almost limitless patience.

Physiological Basis for Drug Action

CHAPTER 1

Constituents of
Living Matter

The purpose of this book is to give an account of the science of pharmacology, and to do this a basis of those sciences underlying pharmacology must be provided. *Pharmacology* is the branch of medical science which relates to the actions and uses of drugs. The division of pharmacology which deals with the actions of drugs is *pharmacodynamics* and the science immediately underlying it is *physiology*, which is the study of the normal functions and phenomena of living things. The subjects which border on pharmacology are *therapeutics*, which is the application of drugs to the treatment of disease, and *toxicology*, which is the study of the effects of harmful doses of drugs. Drugs are chemicals which act upon the chemical systems of living matter, and hence a knowledge of *biochemistry* is also a prerequisite for the understanding of pharmacology. Biochemistry is one of the subjects basic to physiology, its old name being physiological chemistry. This chapter gives a brief outline of some aspects of biochemistry which are necessary to explain the actions of drugs on living matter. Living matter is highly organized, and the basic principles of cytology which is the study of living matter at the cellular level are outlined in Chapter 2.

The chemical constituents of living matter

Living matter contains fewer than one-third of the chemical elements (see Table 1.1). Only hydrogen, carbon, nitrogen and iodine are found in higher concentrations in the human body than in the earth's crust. Six other elements are found in roughly the same proportions: oxygen, phosphorus, sulphur, chlorine, potassium and calcium. The remaining elements are at least ten times more abundant in the earth than in the body. The unique nature of living matter is due to its organic constituents—that is, compounds based on a carbon skeleton. In fact, the word organic is derived from the outmoded idea that complex carbon-containing compounds required the vital processes of life for their formation.

About 72% of the adult human body is water. The remaining hydrogen and most of the oxygen is incorporated into organic compounds, as also are nitrogen, most of the sulphur, and about one-tenth of the phosphorus. Sodium, potassium and chlorine are present as the ions and so is part of the calcium and magnesium. Other important ions occurring in living matter, apart from organic acids and bases, are bicarbonate, phosphate and sulphate. Most of the solid matter of the bones is composed of calcium and magnesium phosphates: the teeth also contain lithium fluoride. The remaining elements are either incorporated into organic molecules or linked to them.

TABLE 1.1. Periodic table of the elements showing their relative abundance in the human body.

	I		II		III		IV		V		VI		VII		VIII	
	a	b	a	b	a	b	a	b	a	b	a	b	a	b	a	b
1	H															He
2	Li		Be		B				C		N		O		F	Ne
3	Na		Mg			Al		Si		P		S		Cl		A
4	K		Ca		Sc		Ti		V		Cr		Mn		Fe Co Ni	
		Cu		Zn		Ga		Ge	✳	As	✳	Se			Br		Kr
5	Rb		Sr	✳	Y		Zr		Nb		Mo		Tc		Ru Rh Pd	
		Ag		Cd		In		Sn	✳	Sb		Te		I		Xe
6	Cs		Ba	✳	Rare earths		Hf		Ta		W		Re		Os Ir Pt	
	✳	Au	✳	Hg		Tl	✳	Pb	✳	Bi		Po		At		Rn
7	Fr		Ra	✳	Unstable elements											

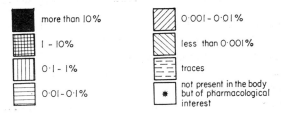

◼ more than 10%	▨ 0·001 - 0·01%
▦ 1 - 10%	◻ less than 0·001%
▥ 0·1 - 1%	⊟ traces
⊟ 0·01 - 0·1%	✳ not present in the body but of pharmacological interest

Living matter may therefore be considered as a matrix of insoluble organic compounds and minerals which supports and contains an aqueous medium containing organic colloids, dissolved organic compounds, gases and electrolytes. Living tissues may be isolated from the body and then maintained in simple solutions with many of their functions intact.

Physiological salt solutions. The composition of the solution that is usually used to maintain isolated frog tissues is given in Table 1.2; it is known as Ringer's solution, named after the man who first developed it. The concentrations of sodium, potassium, calcium and chloride which Ringer found most satisfactory are close to the amounts found in the blood plasma of the frog, although he worked out the composition of his solution empirically; that is, he used the solution which he found by experience to give the best results. Solutions which maintained the functioning of mammalian tissue were later determined by Locke and by Tyrode (Table 1.2). The solution evolved by Krebs was based on analyses of the constituents of mammalian plasma.

TABLE 1.2. The composition of some physiological salt solutions (g/litre).

Constituent	Frog Ringer	Locke	Tyrode	Krebs
NaCl	6·5	9·0	8·0	6·9
KCl	0·15	0·42	0·2	0·35
CaCl$_2$	0·12	0·24	0·2	0·28
MgCl$_2$	—	—	0·05	0·11
NaHCO$_3$	0·2	0·2	1·0	2·1
NaH$_2$PO$_4$	—	—	0·05	0·14
Glucose	0·5	1·0	1·0	2·0

Some of the requirements of a physiological salt solution are summarized below.

(a) OSMOTIC PRESSURE. Blood cells when placed in water swell up and burst, whereas when they are placed in a strong salt solution they lose water and shrivel. The cells are surrounded by a semipermeable membrane, and this allows the passage of water more freely than that of dissolved substances. When two solutions are separated by a semipermeable membrane, water tends to move through the membrane from the weaker solution to the stronger; this phenomenon is known as *osmosis*. The pressure applied in the opposite direction which is just sufficient to prevent osmosis is called the osmotic pressure. For Krebs solution at 37° C, the osmotic pressure is 8·2 atmospheres, whereas for human blood plasma it is 6·6 atmospheres. This is sufficiently good agreement to ensure that the red blood cells are not damaged by osmotic imbalance when they are suspended in Krebs solution. Solutions which have the same osmotic pressure (osmolarity) as blood plasma are *isotonic*, those with lower osmolarity are *hypotonic*, and those with higher values are *hypertonic*.

(b) IONIC COMPOSITION. The ratios between the amounts of the various ions in the physiological salt solutions are similar to those in plasma. Their roles are discussed later, particularly in relation to the electrical properties of cell membranes (Chapter 3) and the behaviour of muscles (Chapter 7).

(c) HYDROGEN ION CONCENTRATION (pH). The blood pH is maintained at 7·4 through an interplay of physiological mechanisms, but it largely depends on the buffering action of the bicarbonate ion/carbonic acid system. In most physiological salt solutions, this is the sole determinant of pH. The relationship between pH and bicarbonate is shown by the following equations:

$$HCO_3^- + H^+ \underset{}{\overset{(1)}{\rightleftharpoons}} H_2CO_3 \underset{}{\overset{(2)}{\rightleftharpoons}} H_2O + CO_2$$

Considering reaction (1):

$$\frac{[H_2CO_3]}{[HCO_3^-][H^+]} = \text{constant} = \frac{1}{K}$$

$$\therefore \quad \frac{1}{[H^+]} = \frac{1}{K} \times \frac{[HCO_3^-]}{[H_2CO_3]}$$

Rewriting in the pH notation:

$$pH = pK + \log_{10} \frac{[HCO_3^-]}{[H_2CO_3]}$$

The value of pK is about 3·1. At a pH of 7·4 the ratio of bicarbonate ion to carbonic acid is about 20,000 to 1. The buffering action of the system in reaction (1) is better at correcting acid than alkaline changes. Thus, on increasing $[H^+]$, the system is moved to the right—there is a large reserve of bicarbonate for this. However, on decreasing $[H^+]$ (increasing $[OH^-]$), there is little reserve of carbonic acid available to move the system to the left and reaction (2) then comes into play: carbon dioxide in solution combines with water to give carbonic acid thus increasing the alkaline buffering capacity of the solution. Taking this into account and adjusting the constant, pK, to include the overall reaction:

$$pH = 6·1 + \log_{10} \frac{[HCO_3^-]}{[CO_2]}$$

This is known as the Henderson-Hasselbalch equation. At pH 7·4, the ratio of concentrations of the bicarbonate ions to dissolved carbon dioxide is 20 to 1.

(d) AERATION OF THE SOLUTION. Isolated tissues need to be supplied with oxygen to maintain their function. Since oxygen is not very soluble in water, the usual practice is to bubble it continuously. The stream of gas, however, sweeps out carbon dioxide and the solution becomes alkaline. In physiological salt solutions which have a low sodium bicarbonate content, the pH after oxygenation may be as high as 8. Although such a high pH in the blood would be lethal to the organism, many isolated tissues still give satisfactory performances. It can be seen from the Henderson-Hasselbalch equation that the inclusion of carbon dioxide in the gas mixture reduces the pH, and aeration with a mixture of oxygen and carbon dioxide in the correct proportions therefore provides a closer control over pH. For example, a pH of 7·4 is maintained in Krebs solution if it is bubbled with the commercially available mixture of 5% CO_2 and 95% O_2.

(e) NUTRITIVE VALUE. The glucose in the solutions serves as a source of energy for the isolated tissues. This is discussed in more detail in Chapter 2.

Phosphate and organic phosphates. In the next pages, it is convenient to introduce the symbols ⓟ and ⓟ—ⓟ. The following examples show how the symbols are used:

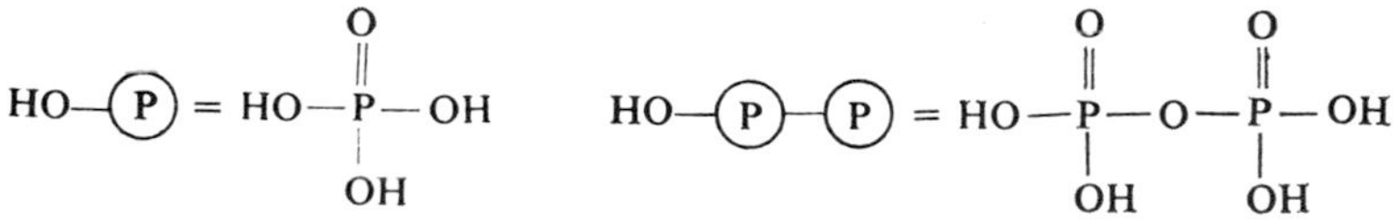

Orthophosphoric acid

Pyrophosphoric acid

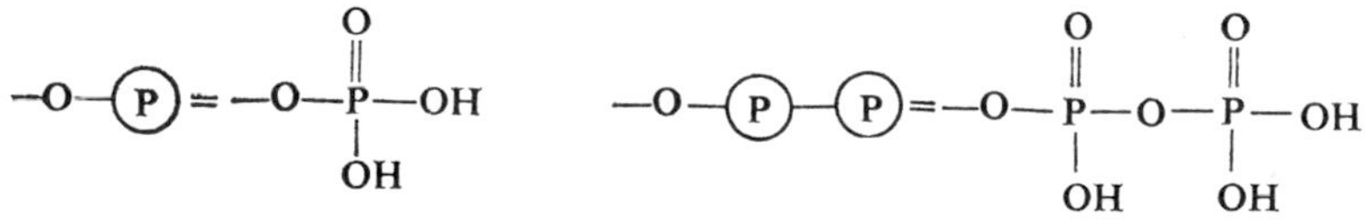

Orthophosphate

Pyrophosphate

The chemical bond attaching phosphate radicals to some organic compounds is referred to as an *energy-rich* bond, the free energy released when the bond is broken being about 10,000 cal/mole. There are four types of phosphate-organic compounds with energy-rich bonds.

Pyrophosphate esters with R—OH

$$ROH + \text{ⓟ} + 3{,}000\ cal \rightleftharpoons R—O—\text{ⓟ} + H_2O$$

The orthophosphate ester bond energy is about 3000 cal/mole. It is not considered as a high energy bond. The bonds attaching further phosphate radicals, however, require about 8000 cal/mole for their formation and are typical energy-rich bonds:

$$R-O-\boxed{P} + \boxed{P} + 8000\text{ cal} \rightleftharpoons R-O-\boxed{P}-\boxed{P} + H_2O$$

The bond attaching an additional phosphate to form triphosphates also requires 8000 cal/mole for its formation.

$$R-O-\boxed{P}-\boxed{P} + \boxed{P} + 8000\text{ cal} \rightleftharpoons R-O-\boxed{P}-\boxed{P}-\boxed{P} + H_2O$$

Acyl phosphates

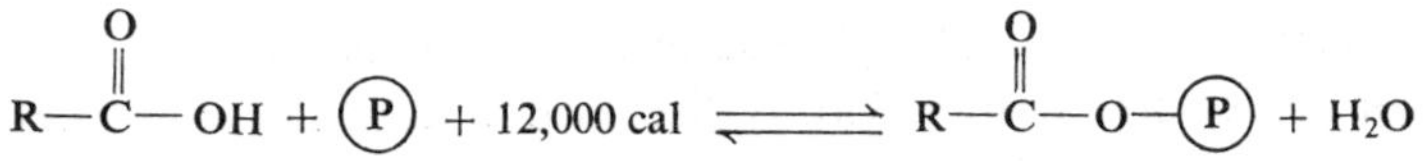

$$\underset{\displaystyle R-\overset{\displaystyle O}{\overset{\|}{C}}-OH}{} + \boxed{P} + 12{,}000\text{ cal} \rightleftharpoons R-\overset{O}{\overset{\|}{C}}-O-\boxed{P} + H_2O$$

Enol phosphates

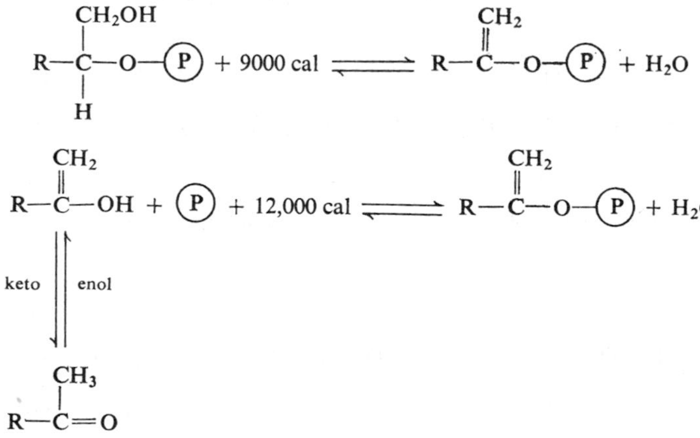

$$R-\overset{CH_2OH}{\underset{H}{\overset{|}{\underset{|}{C}}}}-O-\boxed{P} + 9000\text{ cal} \rightleftharpoons R-\overset{CH_2}{\overset{\|}{C}}-O-\boxed{P} + H_2O$$

$$R-\overset{CH_2}{\overset{\|}{C}}-OH + \boxed{P} + 12{,}000\text{ cal} \rightleftharpoons R-\overset{CH_2}{\overset{\|}{C}}-O-\boxed{P} + H_2O$$

keto $\updownarrow$ enol

$$R-\overset{CH_3}{\overset{|}{C}}=O$$

Guanidine phosphates

$$R-\overset{NH}{\overset{\|}{C}}-NH_2 + \boxed{P} + 10{,}000\text{ cal} \rightleftharpoons R-\overset{NH}{\overset{\|}{C}}-NH-\boxed{P} + H_2O$$

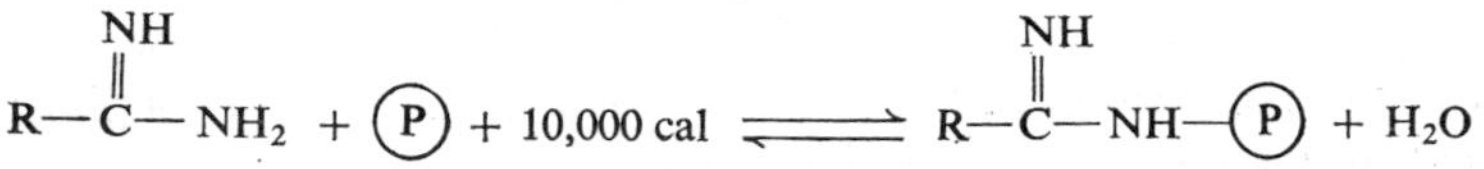

These four types of high energy compounds are involved in many biochemical reactions in which energy is transferred. Energy obtained from a reaction may be absorbed and temporarily stored as potential energy in a phosphate bond and energy required for driving a reaction may be obtained by disrupting a phosphate bond.

Organic constituents of tissues

The major divisions of organic substances in living matter are carbohydrates, lipids and proteins. These divisions by no means exhaust the variety of substances that are present in living matter, but they serve as a convenient starting point.

Carbohydrates. The simplest carbohydrates are the 3-carbon *triose* monosaccharides.

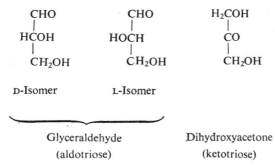

$$
\begin{array}{ccc}
\text{CHO} & \text{CHO} & \text{H}_2\text{COH} \\
| & | & | \\
\text{HCOH} & \text{HOCH} & \text{CO} \\
| & | & | \\
\text{CH}_2\text{OH} & \text{CH}_2\text{OH} & \text{CH}_2\text{OH} \\
\text{D-Isomer} & \text{L-Isomer} &
\end{array}
$$

Glyceraldehyde   Dihydroxyacetone

(aldotriose)   (ketotriose)

The longer chain monosaccharides (*tetroses, pentoses, hexoses* and *heptoses*) may be considered as derivatives of the trioses, formed by inserting

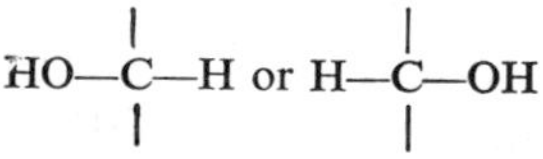

$$
\text{HO}-\overset{|}{\underset{|}{\text{C}}}-\text{H} \text{ or } \text{H}-\overset{|}{\underset{|}{\text{C}}}-\text{OH}
$$

before the terminal alcohol group. This gives rise to the two families; the aldoses and the ketoses. Glyceraldehyde contains one asymmetric carbon atom, and exists as two optically active isomers. Each additional group is asymmetric, so there are sixteen possible aldohexoses and eight ketohexoses. The only four hexoses that need be referred to at this stage are glucose, fructose, galactose and mannose. Their formulae are given below.

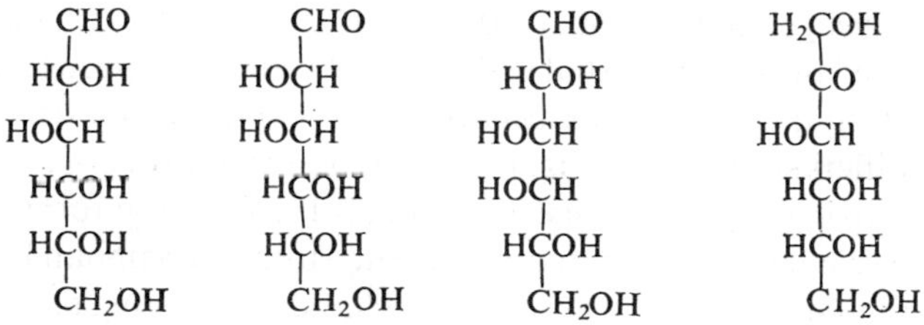

$$
\begin{array}{cccc}
\text{CHO} & \text{CHO} & \text{CHO} & \text{H}_2\text{COH} \\
| & | & | & | \\
\text{HCOH} & \text{HOCH} & \text{HCOH} & \text{CO} \\
| & | & | & | \\
\text{HOCH} & \text{HOCH} & \text{HOCH} & \text{HOCH} \\
| & | & | & | \\
\text{HCOH} & \text{HCOH} & \text{HOCH} & \text{HCOH} \\
| & | & | & | \\
\text{HCOH} & \text{HCOH} & \text{HCOH} & \text{HCOH} \\
| & | & | & | \\
\text{CH}_2\text{OH} & \text{CH}_2\text{OH} & \text{CH}_2\text{OH} & \text{CH}_2\text{OH} \\
\text{Glucose} & \text{Mannose} & \text{Galactose} & \text{Fructose}
\end{array}
$$

Aldohexoses   Ketohexose

1*

Formulae which correspond to the actual configurations of glucose and fructose are given in Fig. 1.1.

Glucose occupies a central position in biology, being the most important source of energy for animal tissues; it occurs free in many biological fluids (e.g. blood) and is combined into many polysaccharides. Most of the carbohydrate in the diet is in the form of the polysaccharide starch, which is a storage form of glucose in plants. The storage form of glucose in animals is glycogen. Glycogen

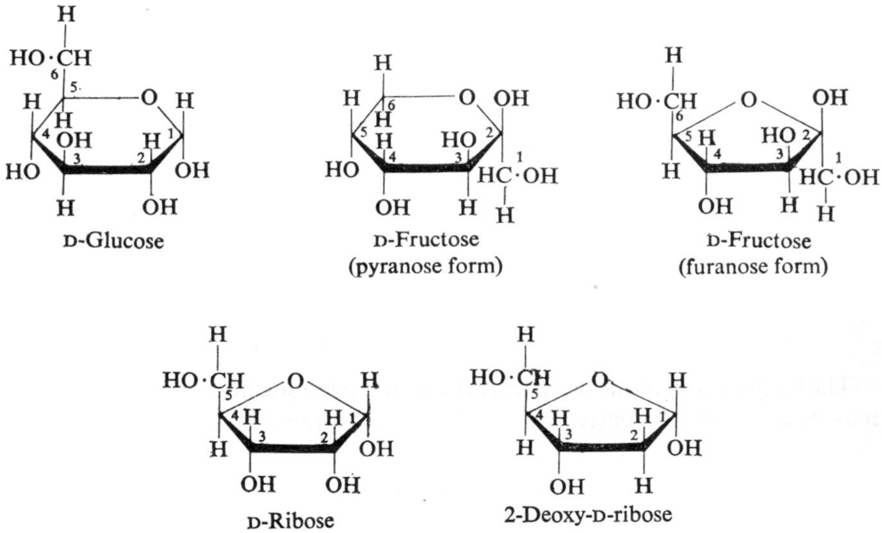

Fig. 1.1. Structural representation of some monosaccharides. The thickened portion of the ring indicates that it projects forward from the plane of the page; the thin portion projects behind the page. The vertical lines are in the plane of the page.

consists of chains of glucose molecules, linked through carbon atoms 1 and 4, and the chains are interlinked by bonds attached to carbons 1 and 6; each molecule of glycogen contains up to 10,000 glucose units. Dextrins are polysaccharides formed during the partial hydrolysis of starch and glycogen. Fructose, the sweetest tasting of the monosaccharides, has the same empirical formula as glucose but differs structurally (Fig. 1.1). Fructose exists in one of two forms, but naturally occurring compounds usually contain the furanose form. Fructofuranose units are combined into inulin, a plant storage compound resembling starch. Sucrose (sugar, cane sugar) is a disaccharide, consisting of one molecule of glucose and one of fructose. Maltose, a disaccharide containing two glucose units, occurs during digestion as a breakdown product of starch and glycogen. Lactose, a disaccharide of glucose and galactose, is present in milk. Ribose and deoxyribose are the most important of the pentoses (Fig. 1.1) and their occurrence as constituents of nucleosides and coenzymes is described later.

Lipids. Lipids (or lipoids) are substances containing a fatty acid combined into their molecule through an ester link. They may be divided into simple or compound lipids.

THE SIMPLE LIPIDS are of two types: triglycerides and waxes (Fig. 1.2). Triglycerides are usually referred to as *fats* if they are solid at room temperature, and as *oils* if they are liquid.

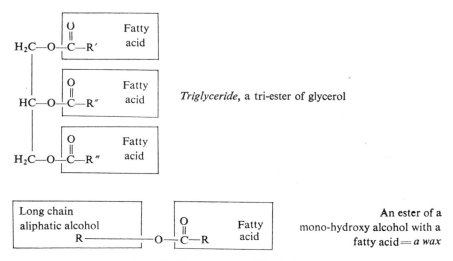

FIG. 1.2. The structure of simple lipids.

About seventy different fatty acids have been identified in animal and vegetable lipids. Most of them have a straight chain structure, which may be saturated or unsaturated, and a few contain a hydroxy or a keto group in the chain. Nearly all of the fatty acids contain even numbers of carbon atoms, which results from their synthesis in the tissues by the addition of 2-carbon units. In general, fats contain saturated fatty acids, and oils have many unsaturated fatty acids. The commonest fatty acids are: palmitic, $CH_3.(CH_2)_{14}.COOH$; stearic, $CH_3.(CH_2)_{16}.COOH$; oleic, $CH.(CH_2)_7.$ $CH:CH.(CH_2)_7.COOH$; and linoleic, $CH_3.(CH_2)_4.CH:CH.CH_2.CH:$ $CH(CH_2)_7.COOH$; but others containing 12 to 18 carbon atoms are widely distributed. Waxes contain longer chain (22 to 28 carbon atoms) saturated fatty acids. Unsaturated fatty acids exhibit geometrical isomerism, e.g.

$$\underset{\text{CH·(CH}_2\text{)}_7\text{·CH}_3}{\overset{\text{CH·(CH}_2\text{)}_7\text{·COOH}}{\|}}$$

$$\underset{\text{CH}_3\text{·(CH}_2\text{)}_7\text{·ĊH}}{\overset{\text{CH·(CH}_2\text{)}_7\text{·COOH}}{\|}}$$

Oleic acid   *trans*-form of oleic acid
cis-form   (= elaidic acid)

Almost all naturally occurring unsaturated fatty acids are the *cis*-isomers.

COMPOUND LIPIDS are subdivided into two groups, the glycerophosphatides and the sphingolipids. *Glycerophosphatides* are derivatives of phosphatidic acids which are diesters of fatty acids with α-glycerophosphoric acid.

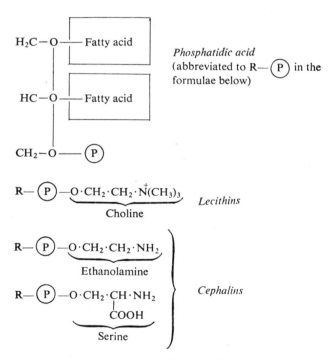

FIG. 1.3. The structure of glycerophosphatides.

The phosphoric acid group is commonly esterified with the alcoholic group of choline, ethanolamine or serine, giving compounds known as lecithins or cephalins (Fig. 1.3). *Sphingolipids* are found particularly in nervous tissue. Instead of glycerol they contain the amino-alcohol, sphingosine, to which the fatty acid is joined through the amino group as a peptide link. Some sphingolipids containing choline phosphate are known as sphingomyelins. Cerebrosides contain a hexose, usually galactose but sometimes glucose, in place of the choline phosphate. Gangliosides contain in addition a complex amino-alcohol, neuraminic acid, attached to the hexose. These substances are illustrated in Fig. 1.4.

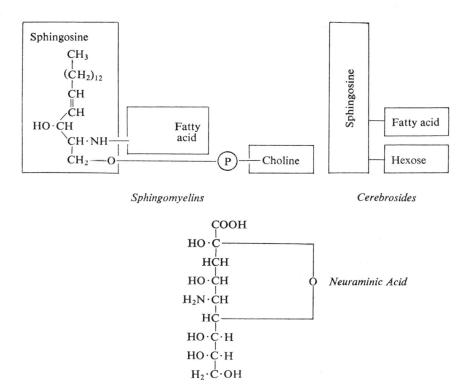

FIG. 1.4. The structure of sphingolipids and their components.

The hydrolysis of lipids under alkaline conditions yields the alkaline salts of the fatty acids. These are soaps and the process is known as saponification. Naturally occurring fats, oils and waxes contain a proportion of unsaponifiable matter, which consists chiefly of sterols and of fat-soluble vitamins.

STEROLS are alcohols of steroids, that is, compounds containing the cyclopentanophenanthrene nucleus, shown in Fig. 1.5. Cholesterol is the commonest sterol. Included amongst the steroids are certain hormones (Chapter 14), bile salts and many drugs.

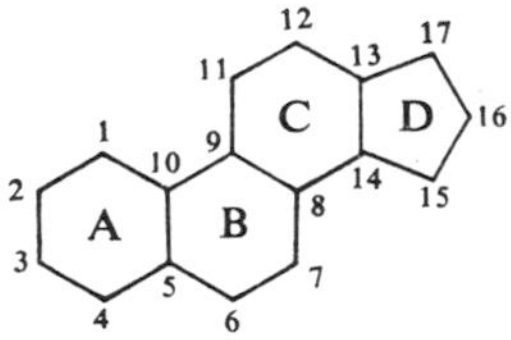

Cyclopentanophenanthrene
(showing the convention for
identifying the position
of substituents)

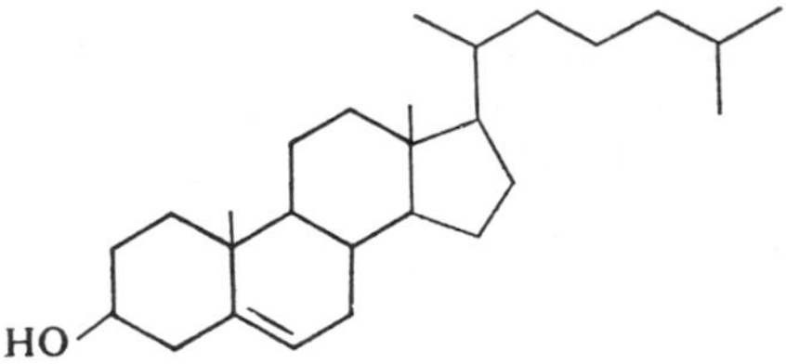

Cholesterol

Fig. 1.5. The steroid nucleus and the structure of cholesterol.

Proteins. Proteins are composed of amino acids, which have the general structure:

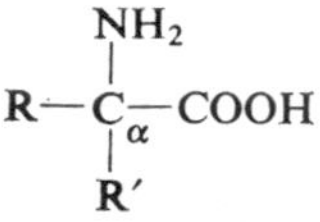

$$R-\underset{\underset{R'}{|}}{\overset{\overset{NH_2}{|}}{C}}{_\alpha}-COOH$$

The α-carbon atom of the amino acid usually has four different groups attached to it, and hence it is optically active. Only the L-amino acids are found in animal proteins; the D-amino acids occur in rare instances in bacterial and plant products.

Figure 1.6 gives the structure of the most common amino acids found in proteins. Some of the amino acids have to be taken in the diet to support life and growth of young animals; these so-called *essential* amino acids are underlined in Fig. 1.6. The other amino acids can be synthesized in sufficient amount in the body. Even some of the *essential* amino acids *can* be synthesized, but only from other essential amino acids; thus, cysteine is formed from methionine, and tyrosine is formed from phenylalanine. Many naturally occurring amino acids have been omitted from Fig. 1.6 for the following reasons: (1) they are not widely distributed; for example, hydroxyproline and hydroxylysine are found only in gelatine and in collagen, the tissue from which gelatine is obtained; however, some amino acids with a limited distribution are extremely important and will be dealt with later, for example, the iodo-tyrosine derivatives (page 370) dihydroxyphenylalanine (page 160) and 5-hydroxytryptophan (page 178); (2) they are closely related to amino acids included in Fig. 1.6 (e.g. glutamine and cystine) and may be derived during the hydrolysis of proteins; the formation of cystine from cysteine is shown on page 17; and (3) they are concerned with the chemical processes in living matter, but are not incorporated into proteins, for example, creatine and ornithine (see Fig. 2.11, page 51).

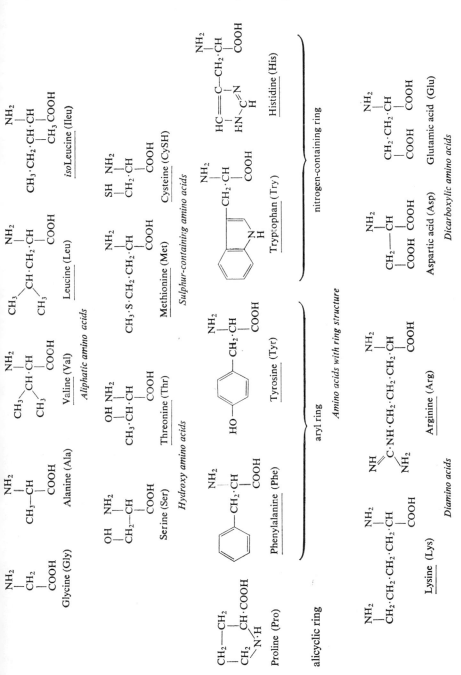

FIG. 1.6. The most common amino-acid constituents of protein. The essential amino acids are underlined. The abbreviations given in brackets are used as symbols for the amino acids.

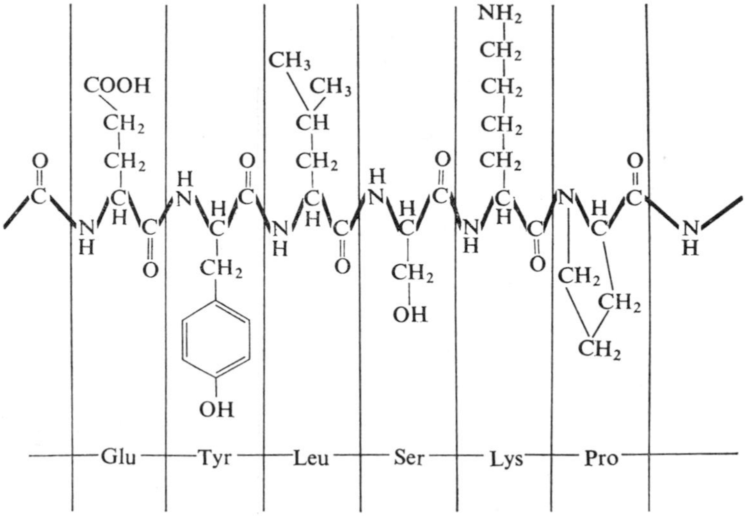

A polypeptide chain

FIG. 1.7. A chain of amino acids linked together by peptide bonds to form a polypeptide.

Amino acids are linked together by peptide bonds (Fig. 1.7), a chain of amino acids being called a polypeptide. The groups characterizing each amino acid stand out from the backbone of the polypeptide molecule, and the nature of these groups and their relationships to each other determine the special properties of each polypeptide. The backbone of the molecule is twisted and it may be coiled about itself to form a spiral. The spiral structure is particularly stable when cross-links are formed between the groups of amino acids which are brought near each other by the convolution of the backbone. Polypeptide chains are combined together to form proteins by similar cross-links.

Some of the types of cross-links between amino acids in polypeptide chains are shown below:

(a) 'Salt' link between free amino and free carboxylic groups:

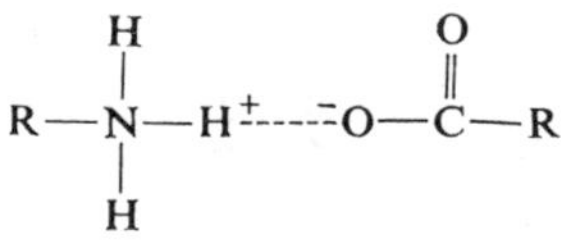

Lysine Arginine Any amino group of a terminal amino acid	Aspartic acid Glutamic acid Any carboxylic group of a terminal amino acid

(b) Peptide link between free amino and free carboxylic groups:

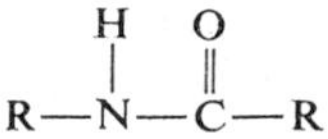

$$R-\underset{\underset{H}{|}}{N}-\underset{\overset{O}{\|}}{C}-R$$

(c) Ester link between hydroxyl group and free carboxylic group:

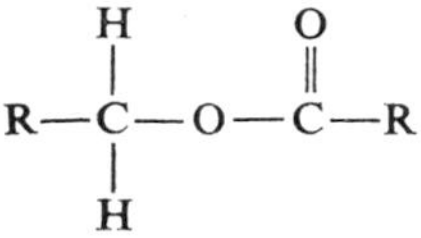

$$R-\underset{\underset{H}{|}}{\overset{\overset{H}{|}}{C}}-O-\underset{\overset{O}{\|}}{C}-R \qquad \left.\begin{array}{l}\text{Serine}\\\text{Threonine}\end{array}\right\} \left\{\begin{array}{l}\text{Aspartic acid}\\\text{Glutamic acid}\\\text{Terminal carboxyl group}\end{array}\right.$$

(d) Disulphide link between two thiol groups:

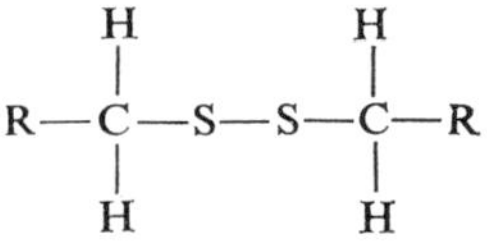

$$R-\underset{\underset{H}{|}}{\overset{\overset{H}{|}}{C}}-S-S-\underset{\underset{H}{|}}{\overset{\overset{H}{|}}{C}}-R \qquad \text{Cysteine}\Big\}\ \{\text{Cysteine}$$
$$= \text{Cystine}$$

(e) Hydrogen bonds between electronegative carbonyl oxygen and electropositive hydrogen of amino or hydroxyl groups:

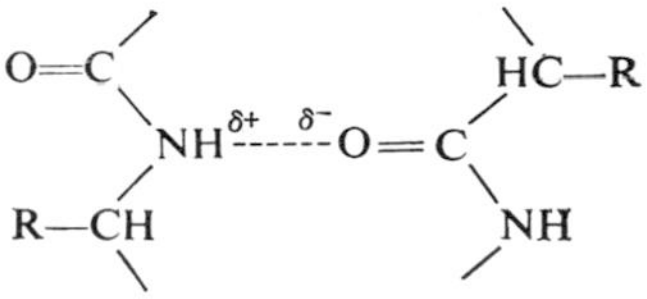

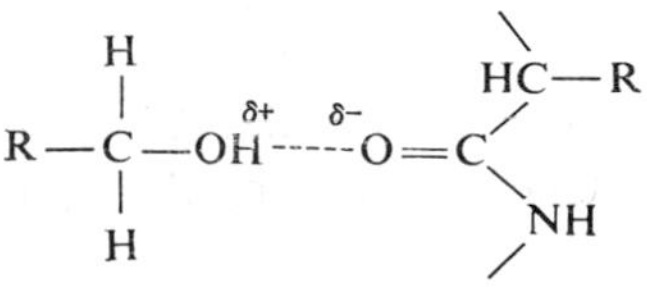

The hydrogen bonds are the weakest of the cross-links, but there are so many possibilities for hydrogen bonding between polypeptide chains that they are the most important.

Amino acids contain at least two dissociating groups. In acid solutions, they exist as cations and in alkaline solutions as anions:

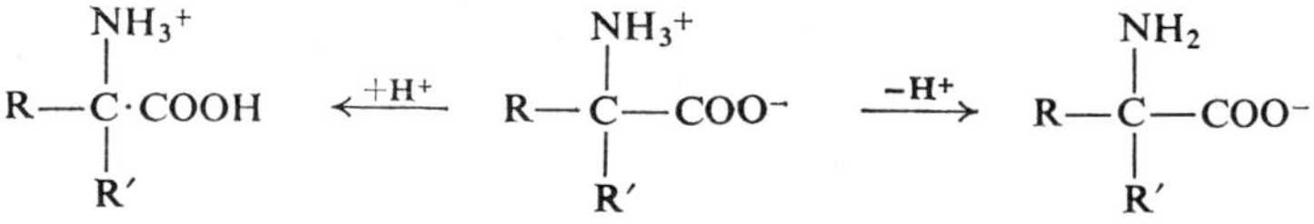

$$\underset{\text{Acid}}{R-\underset{\underset{R'}{|}}{\overset{\overset{NH_3^+}{|}}{C}}\cdot COOH} \quad\xleftarrow{+H^+}\quad \underset{\text{Isoelectric pH}}{R-\underset{\underset{R'}{|}}{\overset{\overset{NH_3^+}{|}}{C}}-COO^-} \quad\xrightarrow{-H^+}\quad \underset{\text{Alkaline}}{R-\underset{\underset{R'}{|}}{\overset{\overset{NH_2}{|}}{C}}-COO^-}$$

They have an isoelectric point, that is, a pH at which the charges on each molecule are exactly balanced, when they exist as the dipolar ion, 'zwitterion' or internal salt. The exact value of the isoelectric point depends on the nature of the substituent groups —R and —R'. The isoelectric point of polypeptides and proteins is determined by the numbers and strengths of the uncombined dissociating side groups. Many of the properties of proteins pass through a maximum or a minimum at the isoelectric point; for instance, their solubility is least and they do not migrate in an electric field.

Proteins are generally unstable chemical substances containing many reactive groups and they are held together by relatively weak bonds. The nature of a protein is changed by extremes of pH and by many chemical substances which combine with the reactive groups. For example, formaldehyde unites with free amino groups:

$$R-NH_2+HCHO \longrightarrow R-NH:CH_2+H_2O$$

Mercury and other heavy metals react with thiol groups:

$$Hg^++2(-SH) \longrightarrow (-S-Hg-S-)+2H^+$$

The weak bonds holding the polypeptide chains into the special form that characterizes a particular protein are easily broken when the energy is raised, for example, by heat, ultra-sonic vibration or radiation. An irreversible alteration of a protein, produced by chemicals, or by raising the energy, is termed *denaturation*.

Simple proteins are those containing only amino acids: *conjugated proteins* contain other groups in addition to polypeptide chains. Thus, glycoproteins contain carbohydrate groups, lipoproteins contain lipid groups, nucleo-proteins contain nucleic acids (page 52), and chromproteins contain highly coloured groups (haemoglobin, discussed in Chapter 8, is an example).

The simple proteins may be classified by their physical and chemical properties, as follows:

Class	*Basis of classification*
Albumins	soluble in water and dilute salt solutions; precipitated by full saturation with ammonium sulphate.
Globulins	insoluble in water, soluble in dilute salt solutions; precipitated by half saturation with ammonium sulphate.
Scleroproteins	insoluble in water and salt solutions (examples: *keratin* of hair and *collagen* and *elastin* from fibrous and elastic connective tissues).
Gliadins	plant proteins: insoluble in water but soluble in 70% alcohol.

Glutelins | plant proteins: insoluble in water, alcohol and salt solution, soluble in dilute alkali. The plant proteins are, in general, low in essential amino acids.

Protamines | small molecular weight; very basic as they contain a high proportion of arginine. Found in fish sperm.

Histones | incorporate a high proportion of ring-containing amino acids; slightly basic; often small molecular weight. Usually conjugated with nucleoprotein or chromprotein.

Points of special interest about certain proteins are listed in Table 1.3.

TABLE 1.3. Properties of some proteins.

Protein	Molecular weight	Points of special interest
Salmine	3000	A protamine isolated from salmon sperm.
Insulin	5700	Hormone. Contains 51 amino acid units; the complete amino acid sequence is known.
Ribonuclease	12,700	An enzyme isolated from pancreas. The amino acid sequence is known.
Cytochrome C	15,600	A chromprotein concerned with oxidation–reduction processes.
Pepsin	34,500	Enzyme, occurs in gastric juice.
Egg albumin	45,000	A storage protein present in egg-white.
Zein	40,000	A gliadin, occurs in maize. Contains no lysine or tryptophan.
Haemoglobin	68,000	A chromprotein concerned with oxygen transport. The protein portion, globin, is a histone; its complete amino acid sequence and structural configuration is known.
γ-Globulin	156,000	One of the globulins in the blood. Antibodies are usually γ-globulins.
Catalase	250,000	An enzyme, one of the most active known.
Fibrinogen	400,000	Occurs in the blood. It is a globulin; it is readily converted into a fibrous scleroprotein, fibrin.
Myosin	650,000	Occurs in muscle. It has enzyme activity.
Haemocyanin	More than 7,000,000	A copper-containing chromprotein concerned with oxygen transport; occurs in some invertebrates.

SEROLOGICAL PROPERTIES. The most sensitive way of distinguishing between proteins is to make use of their serological properties. If an animal is given an injection of a foreign protein, it generates another protein which is able to react with the foreign protein: the foreign protein is called an *antigen*, and the protein formed in response to it is called an *antibody*. As far as is known, antibodies are γ-globulins. The antigen may be disease-carrying bacteria, which are rendered harmless after reacting with antibodies; this is the basis of *immunity*, and is clearly beneficial to the host. On the other hand, the consequences of the reaction may be unpleasant and perhaps disastrous, when the tissues of the host are *sensitized* to the antigen and the antigen–antibody reaction produces *anaphylactic shock*. An allergy is a condition resulting from reactions between antigens present in some foodstuffs, pollens and a wide variety of other proteins, with antibodies formed by the allergic individual. Simple chemicals may become antigens by combining with proteins of the body, thereby forming foreign proteins. Animals do not usually generate antibodies to their own proteins, but, when they do, the reaction results in an *auto-immune* or *auto-sensitive* disease. Serological reactions distinguish between two similar proteins such as, for example, the serum albumin of cats and dogs. The specific antibody against cat albumin may be produced in a third animal, say, a rabbit, but the rabbit's γ-globulins, which then contain the antibodies to cat albumin, do not react with dog albumin. Some proteins are poor at eliciting antibody production: gelatin is an example. Some large carbohydrate molecules, on the other hand, have the capacity to act as antigens.

ENZYMATIC PROPERTIES. An important property of many proteins is their ability to act as enzymes. Enzymes have the general properties of catalysts; that is, they increase the rate of chemical reactions, they are unchanged at the end of the reaction, and they act in concentrations which are small compared with those of the substances undergoing reaction (the substrates). The special feature of enzyme catalysts is their specificity: some catalyse only one reaction and are said to have absolute specificity; the action of others may be confined to a narrow range of similar substrates or to a particular class of chemical reactions. Enzymes act only within certain media, and then often within narrow limits of pH, temperature and ionic composition. Some enzymes require the presence of an additional cofactor, called a coenzyme or a prosthetic group. The substrate attaches to a particular part of the enzyme protein, called the *active centre*. The goodness of fit between substrate and active centre, which is a prerequisite for the reaction to occur, is disturbed when the configuration of the enzyme protein is altered, or when the nature of the substrate molecule is modified.

Enzymes are now named according to their substrate and the reaction they catalyse; the tissue source of the enzyme may be included in the name. The name ends with -ase to denote that the substance is an enzyme. For example, *muscle acetylcholinesterase* hydrolyses acetylcholine at its ester link (to yield acetic acid and choline). However, the names of many enzymes (e.g. pepsin) were coined before a systematic nomenclature was proposed and have become established through long use.

Enzymes may be classified according to the type of chemical reaction which they catalyse.

(1) *Splitting or lytic enzymes.* In the simplest type of reaction, the substrate is split to yield two products, the enzymes being termed *lyases*.

$$H_2O_2 \xrightleftharpoons{\text{Catalase}} H_2O + \tfrac{1}{2}O_2$$

$$H_2CO_3 \xrightleftharpoons{\text{Carbonic anhydrase}} H_2O + CO_2$$

The most common splitting reaction is hydrolysis, in which water is used as a second reactant, the reaction being catalysed by *hydrolases*. The hydrolysis of acetylcholine is considered in detail on pages 156–158. All of the enzymes concerned with the digestion of food are hydrolases, the foodstuffs being broken down by hydrolytic reactions before they are assimilated. An example is *amylase*, which catalyses the hydrolysis of starch into maltose. The fat-splitting and protein-splitting digestive enzymes are called *lipases* and *peptidases* respectively.

$$\underbrace{Fat + H_2O}_{\text{Fatty acid esters of glycerol}} \xrightarrow{\text{Lipase}} \text{Fatty acids} + \text{glycerol}$$

$$\text{Polypeptide chain} + H_2O \xrightarrow{\text{Peptidase}} \text{Smaller polypeptide chains}$$

Splitting reactions involving substances other than water are known. For example, reactions in which the elements of phosphoric acid are added to the split product are catalysed by *phosphorylases*.

$$\underbrace{\text{Glycogen}}_{(\text{Glucose})_n} + H_3PO_4 \longrightarrow \text{Glucose phosphate} + H(\text{Glucose})_{n-1}$$

(2) *Oxidation-reduction enzymes.* The energy requirements for living processes are obtained principally from the oxidation of foodstuffs. The energy is released stepwise during a complex series of reversible oxidation–reduction reactions (Chapter 2), each reaction involving an enzyme. Not all oxidation–reduction reactions are concerned with the liberation of energy: some lead to the synthesis of new compounds or to the inactivation of toxic compounds.

(3) *Transferases.* The transfer of a radical from one molecule to another is catalysed by a transferase. The radicals that are transferred and the group name of the enzymes concerned are given below:

$-NH_2$	transaminase
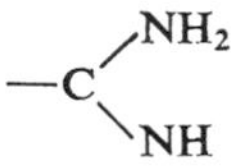 $-C{\Large\langle}^{NH_2}_{NH}$	transamidinase
$-CH_3$	transmethylase
$-SH$	transthiolase
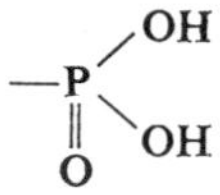 $-\overset{\underset{\parallel}{O}}{P}{\Large\langle}^{OH}_{OH}$	transphosphatase (= phosphokinase)

(4) *Isomerases.* The re-arrangement of the intramolecular structure of a substrate is catalysed by an isomerase, e.g.

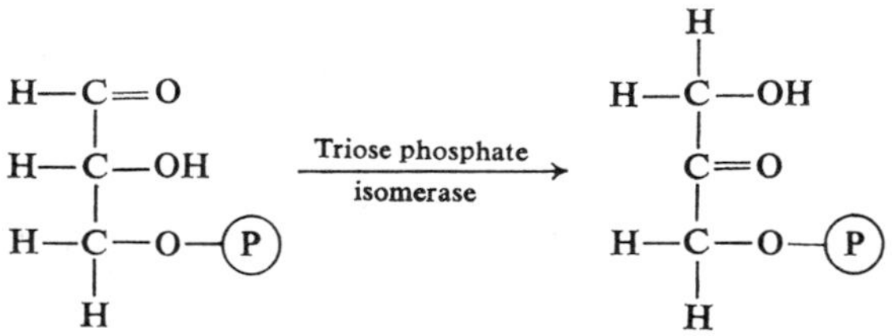

$$
\begin{array}{ccc}
\text{H}-\text{C}=\text{O} & & \text{H}-\overset{\underset{|}{\text{H}}}{\text{C}}-\text{OH} \\
\text{H}-\text{C}-\text{OH} & \xrightarrow[\text{isomerase}]{\text{Triose phosphate}} & \text{C}=\text{O} \\
\text{H}-\overset{\underset{|}{\text{H}}}{\text{C}}-\text{O}-\boxed{P} & & \text{H}-\overset{\underset{|}{\text{H}}}{\text{C}}-\text{O}-\boxed{P} \\
\end{array}
$$

Glyceraldehyde phosphate	Dihydroxyacetone phosphate

The name given to all the chemical reactions carried out during the life of an organism is *metabolism.* The incorporation of the synthesized products into living matter is called *anabolism. Catabolism* is the name given to the processes of degradation leading to the loss of substances from the body.

COENZYMES. Many enzymes require co-factors for their activity. Some enzymes require as co-factors the presence of metal ions such as Ca^{++} or Mg^{++}, or of metals such as Fe or Co contained in organic compounds. Other enzymes require as a co-factor a substance termed a coenzyme. The purine base, adenine, and the pyridine base, nicotinamide (shown in Fig. 1.8) are important constituents of many coenzymes. Adenine is usually linked with ribose to form adenosine, the combination being classed as a riboside or nucleoside. The addition of phosphate to the ribose then results in adenosine monophosphate (AMP; also known as adenylic acid), which is a nucleotide. The addition of further phosphate groups gives adenosine diphosphate (ADP) and adenosine triphosphate (ATP). Nicotinamide mononucleotide is formed from ribose phosphate.

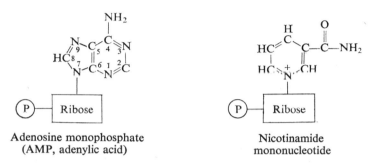

Adenosine monophosphate
(AMP, adenylic acid)

Nicotinamide
mononucleotide

Fig. 1.8. The structure of adenosine and nicotinamide nucleotides.

Coenzyme I, which is also called diphosphopyridine nucleotide (DPN) or nicotinamide adenine dinucleotide (NAD), may be represented as:

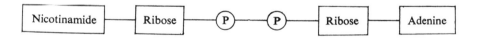

Coenzyme II, which is also called triphosphopyridine nucleotide (TPN) or nicotinamide adenine dinucleotide phosphate (NADP), may be represented as:

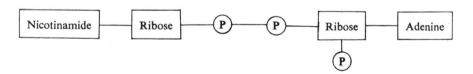

Coenzymes I and II serve with many dehydrogenating enzymes, the two hydrogen ions removed from the substrate being transferred on to the nicotinamide portion of the coenzyme (Fig. 1.9). The reduced forms of these coenzymes are indicated as NADH and NADPH, and they are regenerated by specific flavoprotein dehydrogenases.

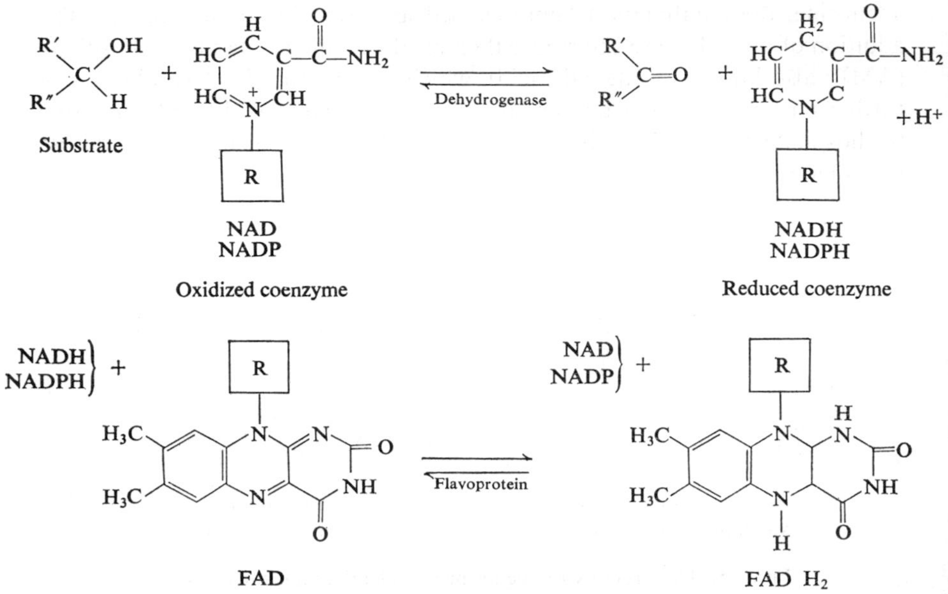

FIG. 1.9. Examples of the change in coenzymes occurring during dehydrogenation.

Flavin adenine dinucleotide (FAD) may be represented as:

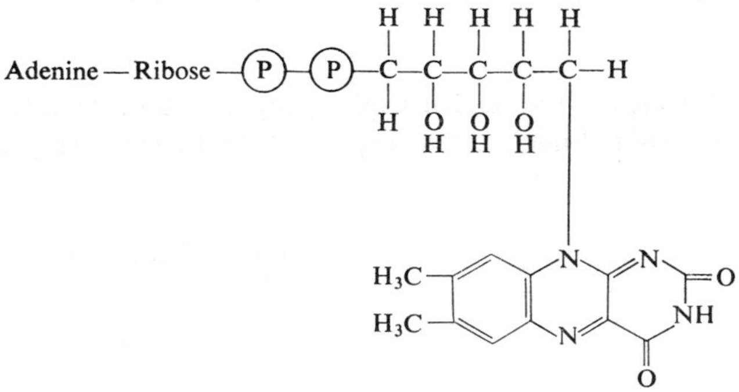

It may be considered as a dinucleotide containing adenosine monophosphate and flavin ribitol phosphate. FAD is firmly attached to the enzyme protein and for this reason it is described as a prosthetic group rather than as a coenzyme. The enzymes using FAD are termed flavoproteins and are yellow in colour as their name suggests. The reactions catalysed by flavoproteins are usually oxidation–reduction steps (see Fig. 1.9).

Glutathione is a tripeptide of glutamic acid, cysteine and glycine:

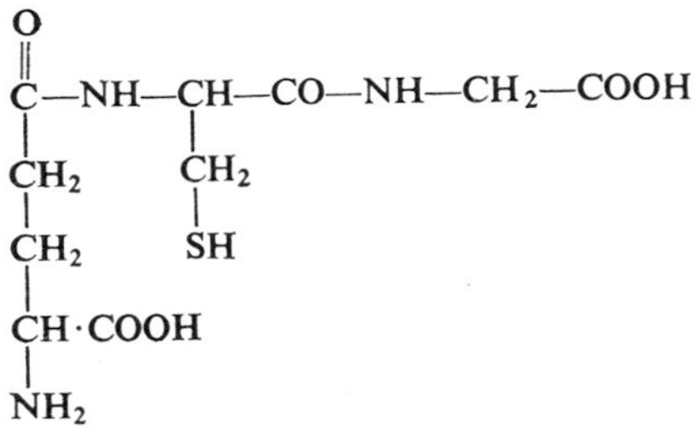

$$
\begin{array}{l}
\overset{\displaystyle O}{\overset{\|}{C}}\!-\!NH\!-\!\overset{\displaystyle |}{C}H\!-\!CO\!-\!NH\!-\!CH_2\!-\!COOH \\
\overset{\displaystyle |}{C}H_2 \qquad \overset{\displaystyle |}{C}H_2 \\
\overset{\displaystyle |}{C}H_2 \qquad SH \\
\overset{\displaystyle |}{C}H\cdot COOH \\
\overset{\displaystyle |}{N}H_2
\end{array}
$$

It is a coenzyme for some dehydrogenases and for some reactions of amino acids.

Coenzyme A may be considered as a derivative of ADP, pantothenic acid and cysteine (Fig. 1.10A). The role of coenzyme A is the transfer of acetyl groups and other longer chain fatty acid radicals (acyl groups), its reactive portion being the terminal —SH group which forms a thio-ester with the acid:

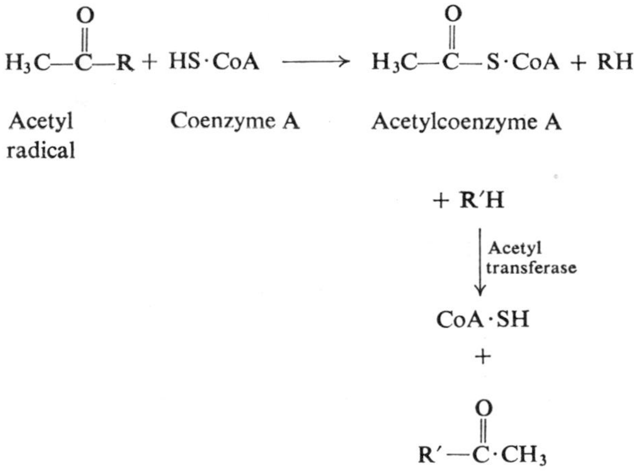

$$
\underset{\substack{\text{Acetyl}\\\text{radical}}}{H_3C\!-\!\overset{\displaystyle O}{\overset{\|}{C}}\!-\!R} + \underset{\text{Coenzyme A}}{HS\cdot CoA} \longrightarrow \underset{\text{Acetylcoenzyme A}}{H_3C\!-\!\overset{\displaystyle O}{\overset{\|}{C}}\!-\!S\cdot CoA} + RH
$$

$$+ R'H$$

Acetyl transferase

$$CoA\cdot SH$$

$$+$$

$$R'\!-\!\overset{\displaystyle O}{\overset{\|}{C}}\cdot CH_3$$

Another coenzyme provides the acetyl (or acyl) radicals for coenzyme A; it is acyladenosine monophosphate (Fig. 1.10B). Acetyl AMP may obtain the acetyl radical from S-acetyl-α-lipoic acid. The cycle of reactions for which α-lipoic acid is a coenzyme is shown in Fig. 1.10C. The cycle involves the reduction of a 2-carbon 'aldehyde' compound to yield an acetyl radical and reduced α-lipoic acid is re-oxidized by a dehydrogenase using NAD to complete

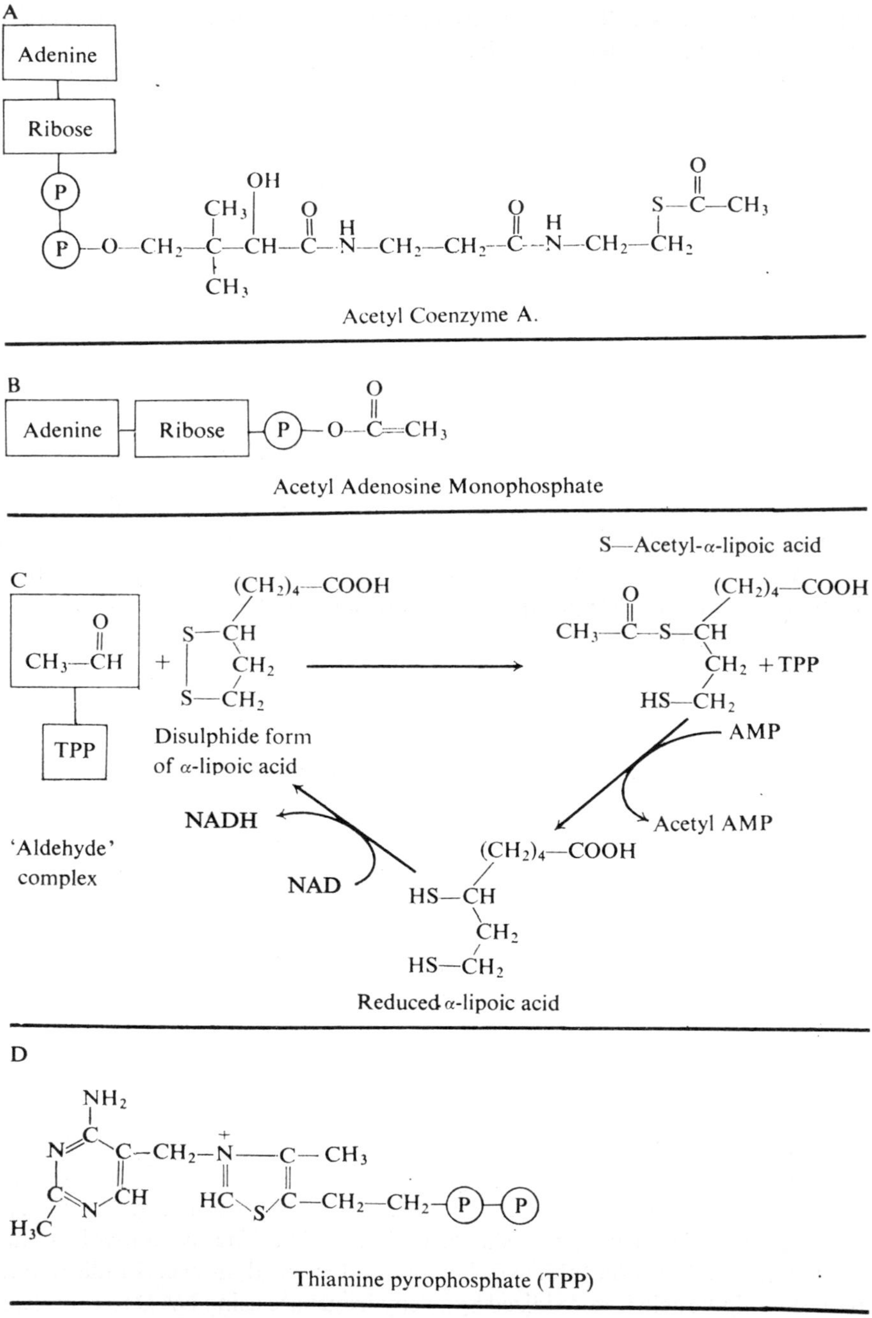

A

Adenine

Ribose

(P)

(P)—O—CH$_2$—C—CH—C—N—CH$_2$—CH$_2$—C—N—CH$_2$—CH$_2$

OH
CH$_3$ |
| CH$_3$

O   H
||
O   H

S—C—CH$_3$
||
O

Acetyl Coenzyme A.

B

| Adenine | Ribose | (P) —O—C=CH$_3$ |

Acetyl Adenosine Monophosphate

S—Acetyl-α-lipoic acid

C

CH$_3$—CH
||
O

TPP

'Aldehyde'
complex

+

S—CH
|
S—CH$_2$
CH$_2$

(CH$_2$)$_4$—COOH

Disulphide form
of α-lipoic acid

CH$_3$—C—S—CH
||
O

CH$_2$
HS—CH$_2$

(CH$_2$)$_4$—COOH

+TPP

AMP

NADH

NAD

HS—CH
CH$_2$
HS—CH$_2$

(CH$_2$)$_4$—COOH

Acetyl AMP

Reduced α-lipoic acid

D

NH$_2$
C

N   C—CH$_2$—N—C—CH$_3$
|| |
C   CH
N

HC   C—CH$_2$—CH$_2$—(P)—(P)
S

H$_3$C

Thiamine pyrophosphate (TPP)

FIG. 1.10. Coenzymes concerned with the transfer of acetyl radicals.

the cycle. The 2-carbon 'aldehyde' fragment is carried by thiamine pyro-phosphate (Fig. 1.10D), having been removed from pyruvic acid with the liberation of carbon dioxide:

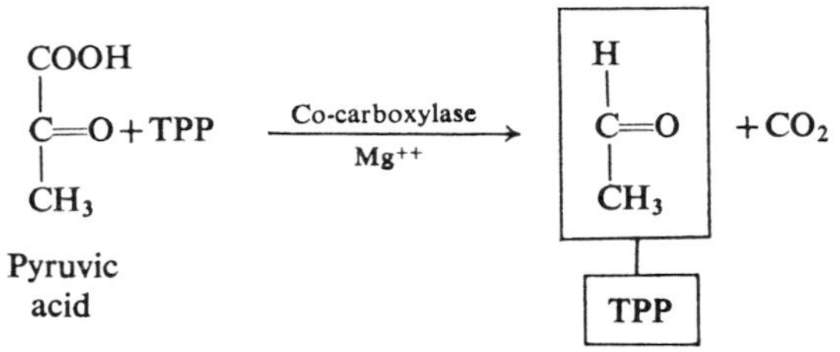

$$\begin{array}{c} COOH \\ | \\ C=O + TPP \\ | \\ CH_3 \end{array} \xrightarrow[\text{Mg}^{++}]{\text{Co-carboxylase}} \begin{array}{c} H \\ | \\ C=O \\ | \\ CH_3 \end{array} + CO_2$$

Pyruvic acid

TPP

The reaction is catalysed by the enzyme co-carboxylase, which needs Mg^{++} as an additional cofactor.

Uridine diphosphate (UDP, Fig. 1.11) is a coenzyme concerned with the transfer of saccharide units in the synthesis of polysaccharides, glycoproteins and related compounds. The saccharide groups being transferred form a glycoside link with the terminal phosphate of UDP. The role of UDP in the synthesis of glycogen is shown in Fig. 2.8, page 46.

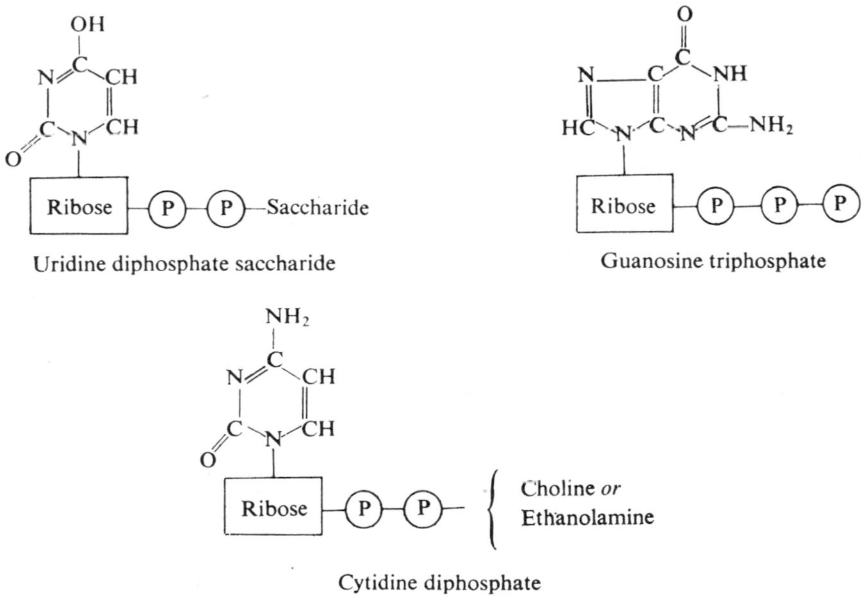

Uridine diphosphate saccharide

Guanosine triphosphate

Cytidine diphosphate

FIG. 1.11. Transfer coenzymes concerned with the syntheses of carbohydrate (uridine) and phosphatides (cytidine), and with the transfer of terminal phosphate groups (guanosine).

Cytidine phosphate (Fig. 1.11) transfers phosphorylcholine and phosphorylethanolamine for the synthesis of lecithins and cephalins (Fig. 1.3). *Adenosine monophosphate* (AMP, Fig. 1.8) and *adenosine diphosphate* (ADP) transfer amino acids, combined as phosphate esters, for the synthesis of protein. *Guanosine triphosphate* (GTP, Fig. 1.11) acts as a carrier for the transfer of high-energy phosphate groups to ADP. *Pyridoxal phosphate* and *pyridoxamine phosphate* (Fig. 1.12) are coenzymes for many enzymes concerned with the metabolism of amino acids, especially decarboxylation, deamination and transamination. These coenzymes are probably chelated with Fe^{++} or some other heavy metal ion.

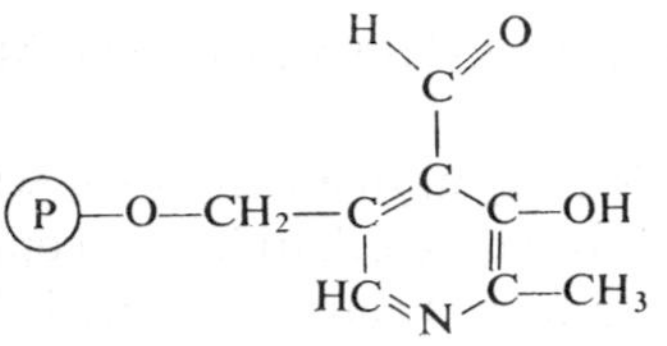

Pyridoxal phosphate 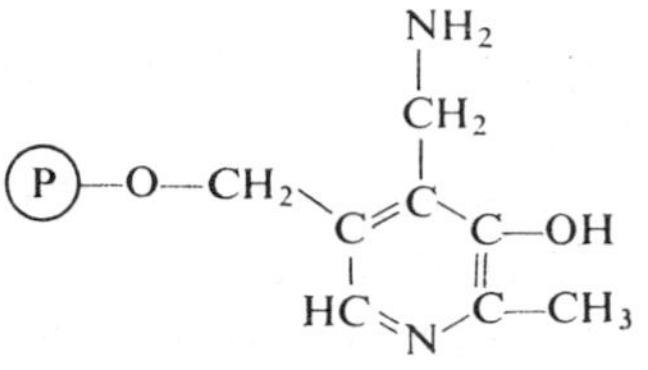   Pyridoxamine phosphate

FIG. 1.12. The structure of pyridoxal coenzymes.

The diet

The important constituents of diet are water, proteins, carbohydrates, fats, vitamins and mineral salts. These must be ingested in adequate proportions which vary according to the age, weight, health and activity of the individual. The dietary amounts required to maintain health are also dependent on the efficiency with which they are absorbed from the gastro-intestinal tract into the bloodstream, and on the efficiency with which the individual utilizes them once they are absorbed, the latter depending largely on the balance of secretions from some of the endocrine glands. Minimal amounts of constituents calculated to be essential can only be calculated for the 'average man'.

Water makes up 65–75% of the body weight of the human adult male and this amount must be maintained fairly constant, so that the water lost from the body is balanced by the water gained. Human life is possible for only a few days without water. In a temperate climate, about 3 litres per day are lost through the urine, the faeces, the breath and the sweat; a similar amount is gained from the diet and from many metabolic processes in which water is one of the products. The mechanisms concerned with the regulation of the body water are described in later chapters.

Dietary proteins are essential to provide the amino acids from which tissue protein is constructed during growth, to replace tissue lost by normal wear and tear, and for the synthesis of enzymes and some hormones.

The energy required for the maintenance of body temperature, for all forms of muscular movement and for synthetic processes occurring within the tissues is provided by the metabolism of carbohydrate, fat and surplus protein. It is convenient to express all forms of energy in terms of heat, the unit employed being the large Calorie, which is defined as the amount of heat required to raise the temperature of 1 kg of water from 14·5° C to 15·5° C. The Calorie is equal to 1000 small calories, i.e. 1 kcal. The number of Calories that a known weight of food gives is simply determined by burning it in a bomb calorimeter. However, the actual amount of energy derived by an individual after eating mixed foods is not known accurately since variable losses occur as a result of differing degrees of digestion and absorption. It is usual to subtract 10% from the theoretical Calorie value to allow for losses. It has been estimated, probably generously, that the average daily requirements of a man doing light work is 3000 Calories (i.e. equivalent to 3300 Calories as raw food). Children under 12 require less, while men doing heavy work require more. Women require slightly less than men engaged on similar work. Requirements are increased during pregnancy. A balanced daily diet supplying about 3000 Calories can be made up as follows:

protein, 100 g (410 Cals); fat, 100 g (930 Cals) and carbohydrate, 400 g (1640 Cals).

The recommended average protein intake for adults is not less than 1 g/kg body weight daily, some of it to be in the form of animal protein, which contains more of the essential amino acids than plant proteins. The minimum amount of fat recommended is 75 g/day. Weight for weight, fat has double the Calorie value of carbohydrate. Fat is also required as it is the vehicle for the fat soluble vitamins (A, D, E and K). Some unsaturated fatty acids—linoleic acid, linolenic acid, arachidonic acid and clupanodonic acid—have been found essential for the diet of rats, mice and dogs, since they cannot be synthesized in the body and their absence results in cessation of growth and a dry, scurfy skin. They are collectively referred to as vitamin F. However, it has not yet been established that these fatty acids are essential constituents of human diet.

Carbohydrate usually makes up most of the energy-providing food. Carbohydrate can be largely replaced by fat, but some carbohydrate is essential, as correct fat metabolism is dependent on one of the products of carbohydrate metabolism (Chapters 2 and 14). It is usually recommended that not more than about two-thirds of the total calorie intake be derived from carbohydrate.

The mineral constituents of the human body amount to about 4·3%, the bulk of this being present in the skeleton. The mineral constituents of diet and their functions in the body are indicated in Table 1.4.

TABLE 1.4. Important minerals of the diet.

Mineral	Source	Daily requirements in adult man	Specific functions
Sodium	Common salt (NaCl) and present in most foods	About 0·5 g. Average intake far exceeds need.	Present throughout extracellular fluids; necessary for excitable properties of nerve, muscle and gland cells, and for the regulation of pH and isotonicity
Potassium	Present in all plant and animal foodstuffs	About 2 g	Present mainly inside the cells. Necessary for excitable properties of the cell membrane and for the maintenance of pH and isotonicity
Calcium	Milk, cheese, flour	0·8 g	Necessary for the calcification of bones and teeth, for the clotting of blood, for the excitable properties of cell membranes, for the coupling mechanisms which enable an electrical change in a cell membrane to activate the cell, for the contractile process in all types of muscle, and as a co-factor in various enzyme reactions
Magnesium	Fruits, peas, beans, nuts, flour	0·4 g	Present in bone. Utilized in many of the functions in which calcium is concerned but often exerts the opposite effect. Some enzymes require Mg^{++} as a co-factor
Iron	Bread, meat, kidney, liver, potatoes, fruit, vegetables and cereals	12 mg	Formation of haemoglobin and the iron porphyrin enzymes
Copper	Liver, oysters, salmon, fruits and beans	1–2 mg	Essential for haemoglobin synthesis

TABLE 1.4.—*continued*

Mineral	Source	Daily requirements in adult man	Specific functions
Phosphorus (as phosphate)	Peas, beans, fruits, nuts, flour, milk, eggs and meat	0·88 g	Contained in bone in the form of calcium phosphate. Constituent of nucleic acids and phosphatides and forms high energy phosphate compounds. Phosphate ions are concerned in the regulation of pH
Fluorine	Fluorides in drinking water	1·5 mg	Bone and tooth formation especially the dentine of teeth
Iodine	Iodides in drinking water. Vegetables, fish and sea-weeds	0·15 mg	Synthesis of hormones of thyroid gland
Manganese, cobalt, molybdenum, zinc	Minute amounts present in various foods	Traces	Co-factors of some enzymes. Cobalt is a constituent of vitamin B_{12}

Vitamins are organic constituents of the diet which exert high biological activity in minute amounts. They are indispensable for certain bodily processes. Their mechanism of action in many metabolic processes is known, but it is difficult to ascribe all the symptoms of deficiency to inactivation of the particular metabolic cycles in which they are known to be concerned. Most of the deficiency symptoms can be reversed by administration of the appropriate vitamin. Vitamins were once thought to be amines and received the name 'vitamines' (amines essential to life). However, it is now known that many of them are not amines and the terminal 'e' has been omitted. The important vitamins in human diet are A, the B complex (thiamine, nicotinic acid, riboflavin, pantothenic acid, pyridoxine, cyanocobalamin, folic acid, para-aminobenzoic acid, biotin, choline, *meso*-inositol) C, D, E, K and P.

VITAMIN A. This is a fat-soluble vitamin found only in animal foods such as milk, eggs and liver fat, especially cod and halibut liver oils. Related substances, the *carotenes*, are widely distributed in vegetables and can be converted into vitamin A by the cells of the intestinal wall and liver.

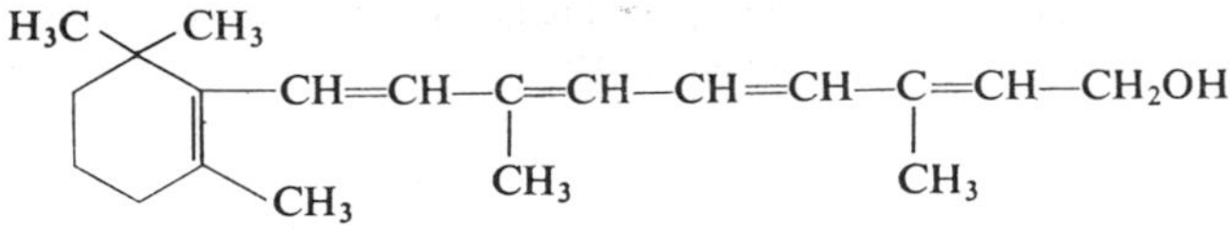

$$H_3C \quad CH_3$$
$$CH=CH-C=CH-CH=CH-C=CH-CH_2OH$$
$$CH_3 \qquad CH_3 \qquad\qquad CH_3$$

Vitamin A (alcohol)

The daily requirements of vitamin A are 2500 international units (1 i.u. = 0·3 μg crystalline vitamin A) or 5000 i.u. of carotene. Vitamin A is essential in the visual process (page 423). Deficiency of vitamin A results in poor vision in dim light. A thickened dry and wrinkled corneal epithelium (xerophthalmia) and impairment of epithelial tissues in the alimentary and upper respiratory tracts also occur.

VITAMIN B COMPLEX. The members of this group are water-soluble and generally found together in foods. Yeast is a good source and they also occur in meats, wholemeal flour, peas and beans. Since they occur together in foods, deficiency of single members is rarely encountered, although the effects of a single deficiency may predominate. Most of them can be synthesized by the intestinal bacteria.

THIAMINE (aneurine, vitamin B_1). The requirement of thiamine is related to the carbohydrate intake and is estimated at 0·66 mg per 1000 Calories obtained from non-fat sources. Thiamine forms part of the prosthetic group of various enzymes with a specific action on α-keto-fatty acids, particularly pyruvic acid. Acute deficiency causes weakness, fatiguability, nausea, fall in blood pressure, loss of appetite, loss of sensation, loss of reflexes and paralysis in the legs. Prolonged deficiency of the B-complex causes *beri-beri*, a disease characterized by polyneuritis and cardiac failure leading to raised venous pressure and oedema. Thiamine deficiency is responsible for most of the symptoms of beri-beri.

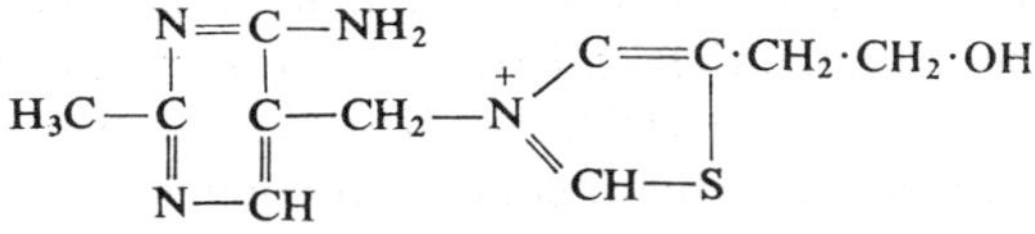

$$N=C-NH_2 \qquad\qquad C=C\cdot CH_2\cdot CH_2\cdot OH$$
$$H_3C-C \quad C-CH_2-\overset{+}{N}$$
$$N-CH \qquad\qquad CH-S$$

Thiamine

NICOTINIC ACID (niacin). NICOTINAMIDE (niacinamide). The main form is the amide. A daily intake of 10–15 mg/day is required. Nicotinamide forms part of coenzymes I and II (page 23) which are concerned in energy-producing metabolic reactions. Deficiency causes metabolic disturbances especially in the nervous system. Prolonged deficiency gives rise to *pellagra* characterized by inflamed and blistered skin, diarrhoea and impaired nervous function.

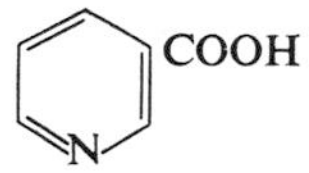

Nicotinic acid 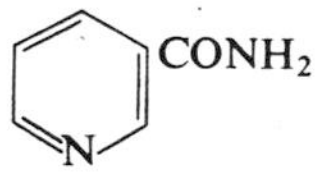   Nicotinamide

RIBOFLAVIN (Vitamin B_2). About 2 mg of riboflavin is required daily. It forms part of flavin–adenine–dinucleotide, a prosthetic group for a number of dehydrogenase enzymes. Deficiency causes inflammation of the mouth and tongue, dermatitis and defective vision but it is difficult to bring about vitamin B_2 deficiency in man probably because sufficient is synthesized by intestinal bacteria.

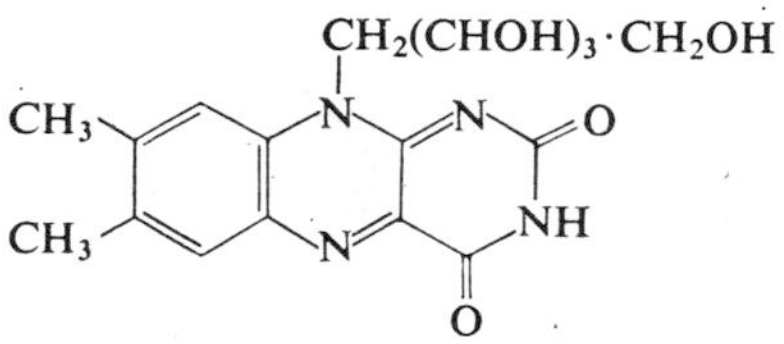

Riboflavin

PANTOTHENIC ACID. This vitamin occurs in food as the free acid. It is a component of coenzyme A which takes part in all acetylation processes (e.g. the tricarboxylic acid cycle, Fig. 2.5). Deficiency of dietary pantothenic acid has pronounced effects on animals but little is known about its effects in man, although lack of it contributes to the symptoms of beri-beri and pellagra.

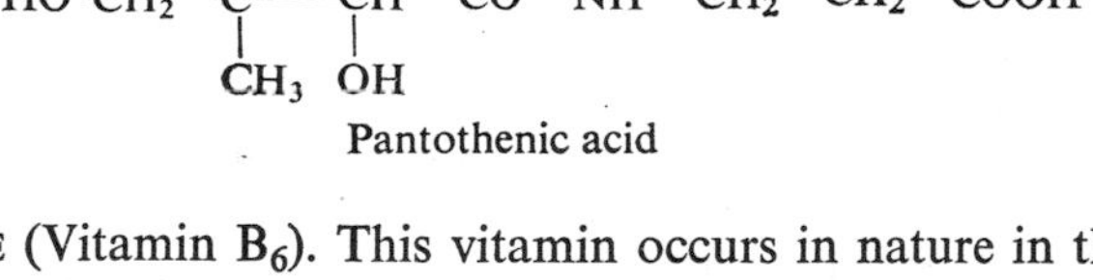

Pantothenic acid

PYRIDOXINE (Vitamin B_6). This vitamin occurs in nature in three forms— pyridoxine, pyridoxal and pyridoxamine. Pyridoxal, the aldehyde derivative of pyridoxine, is a coenzyme in decarboxylase and transaminase reactions, being important in fat and amino acid metabolism. It is essential in the diet of many animals but in man sufficient is synthesized by intestinal bacteria to overcome dietary deficiency. However, signs of deficiency in man (lesions on the skin of the face, and anaemia) are produced when anti-vitamins (deoxypyridoxine and isonicotinic acid hydrazide) are administered.

2

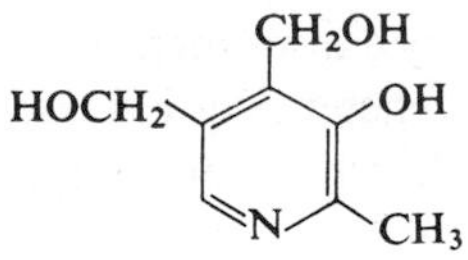

$$CH_2OH$$

HOCH$_2$ — OH

N — CH$_3$

Pyridoxine (Pyridoxol)

CYANOCOBALAMIN (Vitamin B$_{12}$, Fig. 1.13). This is the anti-pernicious anaemia vitamin originally extracted from liver but now obtained by large-scale fermentation procedures. Only minute daily amounts are required (1 μg) and deficiency is usually due to faulty absorption from the gut rather than to inadequate dietary intake. It is essential for the development of the red blood cells (pages 238–240) and is also involved, directly or indirectly, in the metabolism of nucleic acids, protein, fat and carbohydrate. Vitamin B$_{12}$ deficiency results in degenerative changes in the spinal cord, in addition to pernicious anaemia.

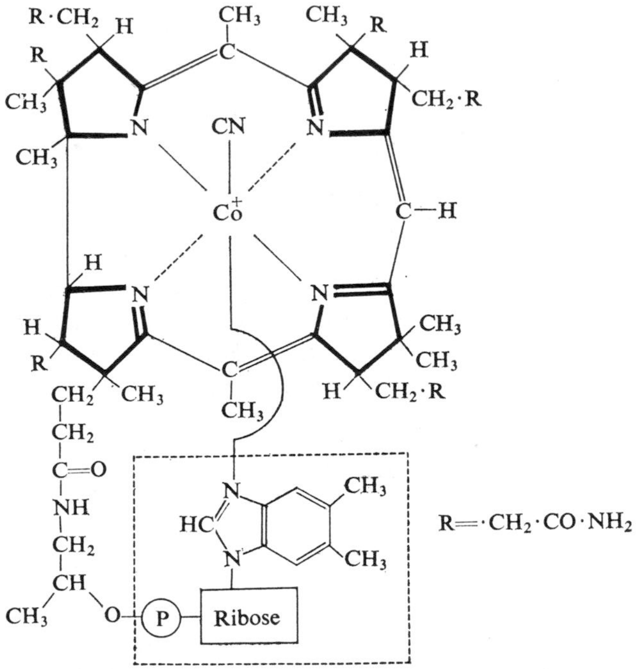

R = ·CH$_2$·CO·NH$_2$

FIG. 1.13. The formula of vitamin B$_{12}$. The thick lines indicate the tetra-pyrrole nucleus to which the —CoCN radical is attached by covalent bonds. The dotted lines enclose a nucleotide moiety of the molecule.

FOLIC ACID (pteroylglutamic acid). This vitamin occurs as the free acid and also conjugated with glutamic acid residues.

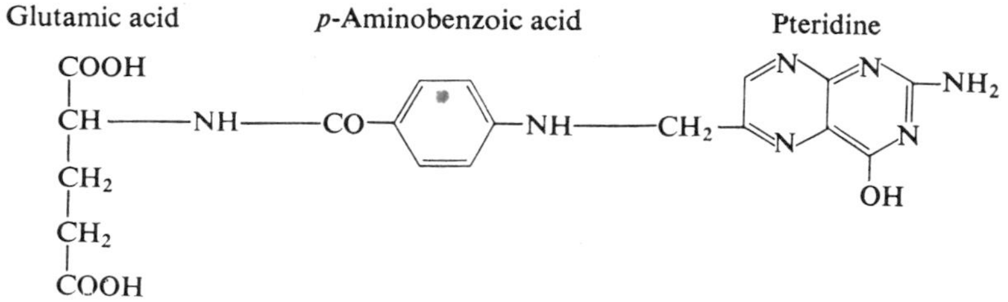

Glutamic acid   *p*-Aminobenzoic acid   Pteridine

$$
\begin{array}{l}
\text{COOH} \\
| \\
\text{CH}\text{---NH---CO---}\langle\text{ring}\rangle\text{---NH---CH}_2\text{---}\langle\text{pteridine}\rangle \\
| \\
\text{CH}_2 \\
| \\
\text{CH}_2 \\
| \\
\text{COOH}
\end{array}
$$

Folic acid

In health the gastric juice converts folic acid into another unknown conjugate which is absorbed. This capacity is lost in pernicious anaemia but the same conversion occurs in the blood if folic acid is injected. Folic acid is concerned, together with vitamin B_{12}, in the development of the red blood cells (pages 238–240). Folic acid improves the blood picture in pernicious anaemia but does not improve the associated degenerative changes in the spinal cord. Vitamin B_{12} can cure both conditions.

PARA-AMINOBENZOIC ACID. This acid is essential for normal pigmentation in chickens but little is known about its function in man.

BIOTIN. This acid, which used to be called vitamin H, is essential, although diseases of deficiency are rare. It is concerned in CO_2-fixation reactions in the formation of oxaloacetic acid and the synthesis of fat. Deficiency causes dermatitis, muscular pain, loss of appetite, depression and blood disorders.

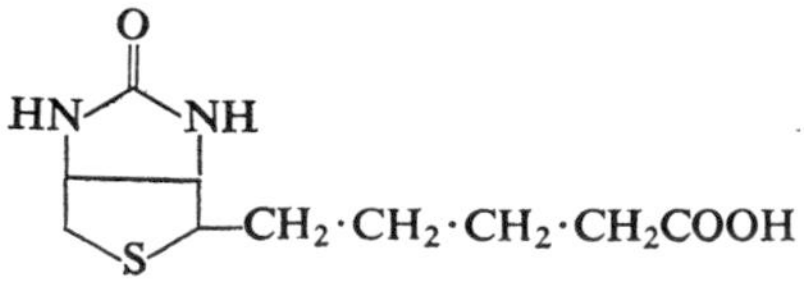

$$
\begin{array}{c}
\text{O} \\
\text{HN} \diagup \diagdown \text{NH} \\
| \\
\diagdown_{\text{S}} \diagup \text{---CH}_2\cdot\text{CH}_2\cdot\text{CH}_2\cdot\text{CH}_2\text{COOH}
\end{array}
$$

CHOLINE. The daily intake of choline is as much as 1 g per day. However, sufficient may be synthesized within the body, provided that other donors of methyl groups are available, and for this reason it is not always regarded as a vitamin.

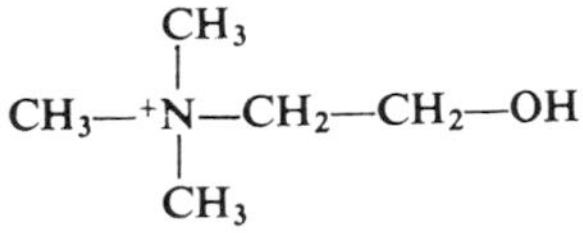

$$
\begin{array}{c}
\text{CH}_3 \\
| \\
\text{CH}_3\text{---}^+\text{N---CH}_2\text{---CH}_2\text{---OH} \\
| \\
\text{CH}_3
\end{array}
$$

The main function of choline is as a methyl donor. Its acetyl ester, acetylcholine, is the chemical transmitter at cholinergic nerve endings (Chapter 5). Deficiency of choline causes cirrhosis of the liver.

Meso-INOSITOL. This substance is present in muscle linked with protein, and in nervous tissue with the phospholipid, cephalin. The effects of deficiency in man are unknown. In rats deficiency causes loss of weight and loss of fur.

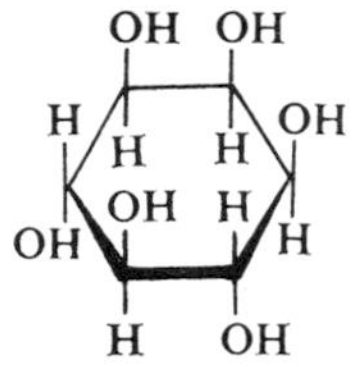

meso-Inositol

VITAMIN C. This is a water-soluble vitamin found in green plants and citrus fruits. It occurs in two forms—L-ascorbic acid and dehydroascorbic acid. The daily requirement is from 75–125 mg. At 125 mg/day, it increases resistance to infectious disease. Vitamin C is a factor in cell metabolism in all tissues but particularly bones and teeth.

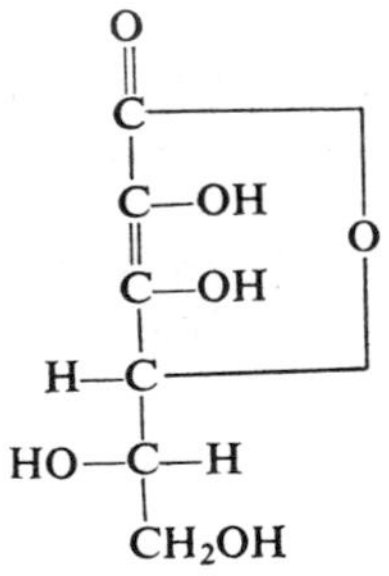

L-Ascorbic acid

Deficiency causes degenerative changes in skin and gums, reduced capillary resistance, diminished resistance to infections, slower healing of wounds, fatigue, anaemia and, in children, defects in bones and teeth. A combination of many of these symptoms is called *scurvy*. Vitamin C is synthesized by some species (see page 513).

VITAMIN D. This is a group of fat-soluble vitamins found in the fat of milk, fish liver oils and egg-yolk. The naturally occurring vitamin in man is vitamin D_3, formed by the action of sunlight on 7-dehydrocholesterol in the outermost layers of the skin. Other substances with vitamin D activity include vitamins D_2 (calciferol) and D_4 formed artificially by the action of ultra-violet light on ergosterol. Other potent D-vitamins are present in fish oils. The minimal daily requirements are not completely known but 250 i.u. (equivalent to 0·00625 mg crystalline vitamin D_3) are more than adequate.

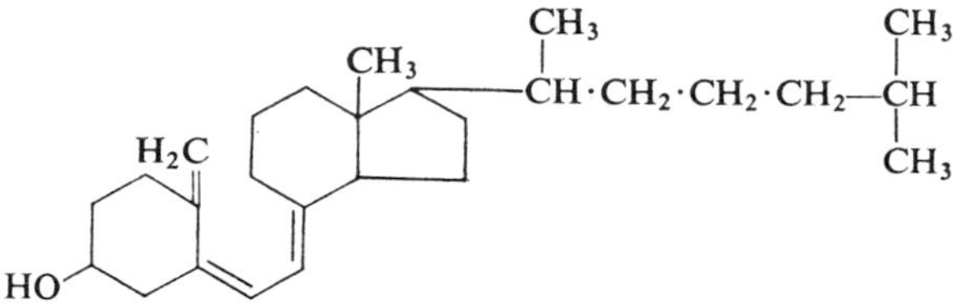

Vitamin D$_3$ (cholecalciferol)

Vitamin D acts on phosphorus metabolism and regulates the calcium and phosphorus balance. It mobilizes phosphorus from the soft tissues and aids the conversion of organic to inorganic phosphorus. It controls calcium metabolism indirectly through its action on phosphorus metabolism. Calcium phosphate, necessary for bone development, is formed as a result of the conversion of organic to inorganic phosphate. Calcium resorption is also enhanced. Vitamin D deficiency in children causes *rickets* due to insufficient calcification of bones which become soft. *Osteomalacia* is a similar condition in adults, occurring particularly during pregnancy and in old people.

VITAMIN E. Vitamin E is a fat-soluble vitamin occurring in three different forms, α-, β- and γ-tocopherol, of which the α-form is the most active. They are found in wheat-germ oil and in green plants.

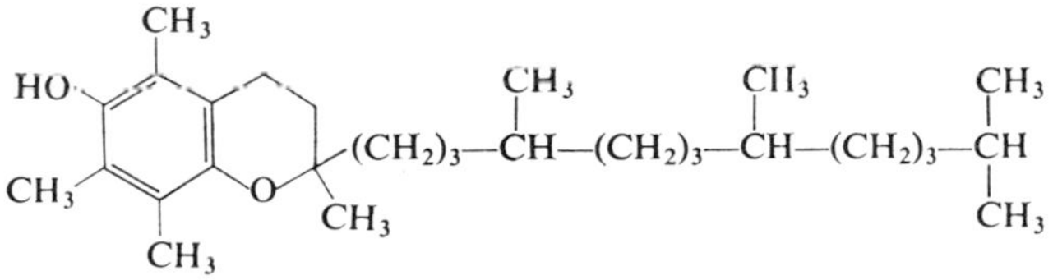

α-Tocopherol

Vitamin E plays important roles in various enzyme systems, particularly in protein metabolism, and it also influences the activity of vitamins A and C. Deficiency in animals causes degenerative changes in the muscles, nerves and enzymes but the significance of the vitamin in man is not yet established.

VITAMIN K. Vitamin K occurs naturally in at least two forms (K$_1$ and K$_2$) and many synthetic forms are known which have similar activity (e.g. menadione). The K-vitamins are fat-soluble and found in green vegetables, especially spinach, cabbage and Brussels sprouts. It is synthesized in adequate amounts by intestinal bacteria and its presence in food is probably not necessary. Deficiency may arise as a result of changes in the bacterial flora of the intestines or of impaired absorption.

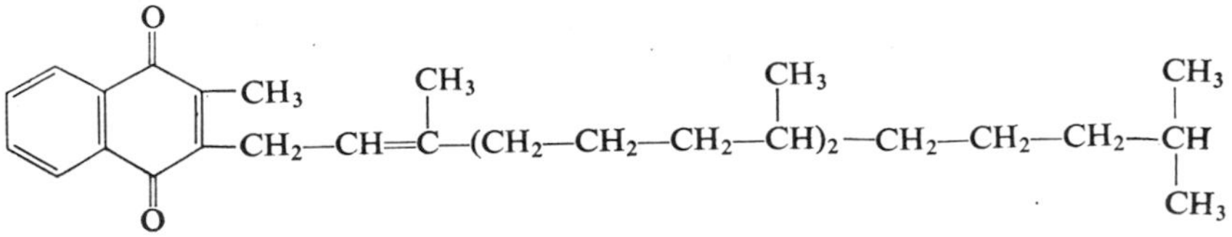

Vitamin K₁

Vitamin K is indispensable for normal blood coagulation (page 234).

VITAMIN P. This is a water-soluble vitamin present in citrus fruits and black currants. A series of compounds with similar activity is known; these include flavones, flavanones, flavanols, catechin, epicatechin and phloretin. Vitamin P, in addition to vitamin C, is necessary for normal capillary resistance and is used as a supplement in scurvy and similar diseases. The increase in capillary resistance produced by vitamin P may be a secondary effect brought about by inhibition of the metabolism of adrenaline.

CHAPTER 2

Cells and Tissues

The smallest unit of animal life is a single cell. Free-living unicellular animals require an equable medium containing plant products which supply their energy in the form of chemical substances that have been elaborated in sunlight. Multicellular organisms contain aggregates of cells which, with intercellular substances, form tissues and combinations of tissues, namely organs. In complex animals, the cells of various tissues and organs take on highly specialized functions, and accordingly they exhibit a wide diversity of form. A diagram of the general features of cellular structure is shown in Fig. 2.1.

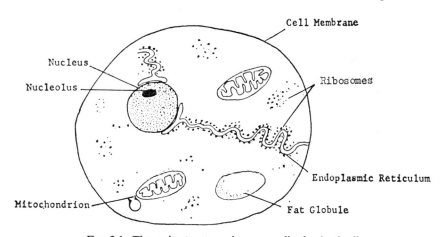

FIG. 2.1. The main structures in a generalized animal cell.

Cells are bounded by a *membrane* inside which is their *cytoplasm*. Most cells contain a nucleus. The cytoplasm also contains a variety of other structures, which include rod-shaped or spherical particles called *mitochondria*, present in numbers ranging from a dozen to hundreds in each cell. Other particles include *lysosomes* and *ribosomes*, and the cytoplasm is pierced by a system of canals and vesicles called the *endoplasmic reticulum*, which is often closely associated with ribosomes. Other inclusions are also present in amounts which depend on the function of the particular cell and its degree of activity: for example, protein fibres, globules of fat, deposits of carbohydrate and granules of secretion may be found in the cytoplasm. Subcellular particles may be isolated from gently homogenized tissues. Fractions containing nuclear, mitochondrial and the smaller *microsomal* particles may be separated by centrifugation.

39

The cell membrane

The cell membrane is a boundary zone through which substances enter and leave the cell. It consists of lipoprotein. There is an inner, bimolecular layer of lipid molecules, particularly lecithins and cephalins, arranged with the long tails of the fatty acids pointing together. This constitutes an inner lipid phase in which there is a considerable amount of cholesterol. The polar hydrophilic groups are presented to the outer surfaces and are attached to protein films, as represented diagrammatically in Fig. 2.2. The core of long non-polar fatty acid tails confers two properties on the membrane: first, it hinders the passage of water-soluble substances through the membrane, and second, it gives a high

100 Å

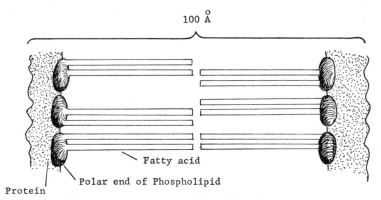

Fatty acid

Polar end of Phospholipid

Protein

Fig. 2.2. Diagram of the cell membrane.

electrical resistance. The protein surfaces incorporate a number of enzymes, and other substances such as carbohydrates or conjugated proteins. The antigen behaviour of the cell is determined by the nature of the outer layers of the membrane.

There are a number of ways in which substances traverse the cell membrane. Small non-polar molecules such as urea, cross the membrane by simple diffusion until they are in equilibrium on each side of the membrane. Their rate of diffusion depends upon their molecular weight and concentration differences. Molecules above a certain size do not penetrate, and the membrane is thus semi-permeable. The permeability of the membrane to polar molecules including ions depends not only on their size but also on their charge. The distribution of charged molecules across the membrane at equilibrium depends on the presence of other polar substances which are too large to cross the membrane, on the pH on each side of the membrane, and on the presence of a potential difference across the membrane. The unequal distribution of small ions across the membrane itself determines the potential difference across the membrane.

Water passes through the cell membrane and maintains an equal osmotic pressure across the membrane. Small lipid-soluble molecules cross the membrane by first being dissolved in the lipid layer, and their rate of diffusion depends on their partition coefficients between the lipid phase of the membrane and the aqueous phases on each side.

The permeabilities mentioned so far are due to the physical properties of the membrane, and the substances that move in accord with them are said to cross the membrane by *passive transfer*. However, certain substances cross cell membranes faster than one could predict or *against* a concentration gradient or a gradient of electrical potential, and they are said to cross by *active transport*. Active transport is an energy-requiring process and is inhibited by substances that interfere with the metabolism of the cell. The mechanism that is envisaged for active transport is that a 'carrier' moves across the membrane combining with the transported substance at one surface and releasing it at the other. Active transport mechanisms are sometimes called 'pumps'. They display some of the properties of enzyme reactions, and when two substances are transported by the same carrier, then a high concentration of one inhibits the transport of the other. Other properties of the cell membrane that distinguish it from an inert membrane are the special mechanisms that allow for the extrusion of the products of secretory cells, and for the engulfment of particles, as in *phagocytosis* and *pinocytosis*. Secretory cells contain a number of lipoidal structures called the Golgi complex, near which the secretory products are made. Before the secretion is discharged, it is surrounded by a temporary membrane which fuses with the outer membrane and then liberates the secretion. Phagocytosis is the reverse of this. Pinocytosis is the engulfment of smaller colloidal particle or of extracellular solution. Pinocytotic vesicles may unite with the endoplasmic reticulum, or if lipids have been ingested, they may fuse to form fat globules. The possible role of pinocytosis is to increase the effective membrane area during activity.

Mitochondria are present in almost every type of cell. They are between $0 \cdot 2$ and 3μ long, and contain a double lipo-protein membrane. The inner membrane is thrown into folds which give the mitochondria their striped appearance (Fig. 2.3). Their membranes have much the same properties as those of the cell membranes, and thus a portion of the cell interior is set apart for the special functions of the mitochondria; this is to contain the enzymes concerned with the oxidative catabolism of pyruvic acid, fatty acids and amino acid residues to yield chemical energy, water and carbon dioxide. The catabolism is carried out by a series of enzymatically controlled reactions and the energy produced is transferred to the terminal phosphate group of ATP. The whole process is termed *oxidative phosphorylation*.

2*

The first series of reactions which pyruvic acid undergoes yield acetyl coenzyme A and CO_2 (Fig. 2.4). These reactions involve the coenzymes shown in Fig. 1.10. The acetyl group is then transferred into the tricarboxylic acid cycle in which it is oxidized by a series of steps (Fig. 2.5).

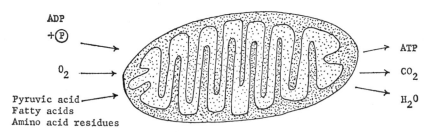

Fig. 2.3. Diagram of a mitochondrion showing the convoluted inner portion of membrane. The overall reactions of oxidative phosphorylation are catalysed by mitochondrial enzymes.

The coenzymes used in the tricarboxylic acid cycle are coenzyme A and TPP (Fig. 1.10), NAD, NADP and FAD (Fig. 1.9) and GTP (Fig. 1.11).

The net reactions of the oxidation of pyruvic acid to completion through the tricarboxylic acid cycle are: (*a*) from pyruvic acid; pyruvate + CoA + NAD

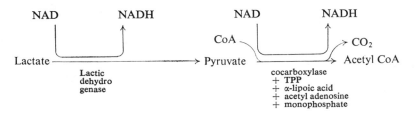

Fig. 2.4. Oxidation and decarboxylation of pyruvic acid to yield acetyl coenzyme A. This may be preceded by the oxidation of lactic acid.

→ acetyl CoA + NADH + CO_2: and (*b*) from acetyl CoA; acetyl CoA + 2NAD + NADP + FAD + (P) + $3H_2O$ → CoA + 2NADH + NADPH + $FADH_2$ + GTP + $2CO_2$.

The energy which has been released is contained in the reduced coenzymes and as the terminal phosphate of GTP. To make this energy available to the cell, it is passed into (P) attached as the terminal phosphate of ATP. These reactions, which complete the oxidative phosphorylation of pyruvate, are shown in Fig. 2.6.

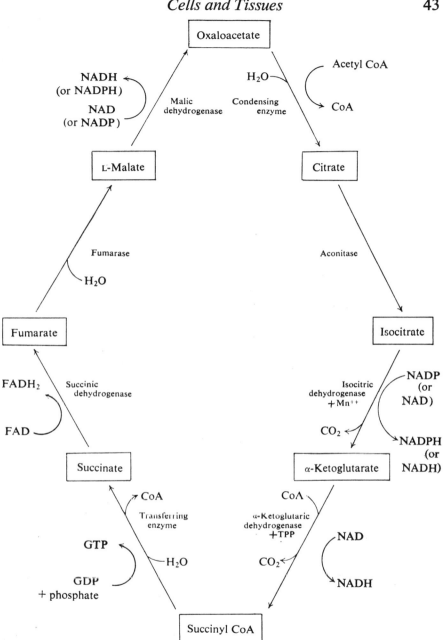

Fig. 2.5. The tricarboxylic acid cycle (also called the citric acid cycle, or the Krebs' cycle).

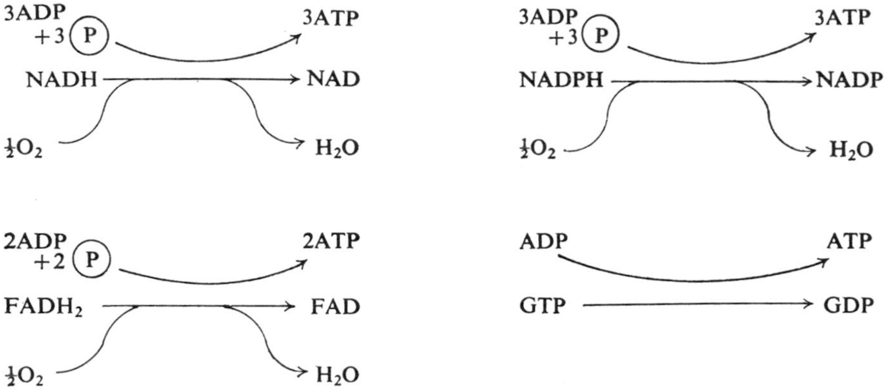

FIG. 2.6. Transfer of energy-rich products of pyruvic acid metabolism and of the tricarboxylic acid cycle to the terminal phosphate of ATP.

The enzymes that catalyse the oxidation of fatty acids are also located in the mitochondria. The oxidation of fatty acids is summarized in Fig. 2.7; it involves the removal of a 2-carbon fragment as acetylcoenzyme A with oxidation at the expense of reducing coenzymes. The reduced coenzymes are re-oxidized with the production of ATP as in Fig. 2.6 and the acetylcoenzyme A enters the tricarboxylic acid cycle (Fig. 2.5). The remainder of the fatty acid attached to coenzyme A is oxidized in another turn of the spiral shown in Fig. 2.7, and so on until the final product is acetylcoenzyme A if the original fatty acid had an even number of carbon atoms, or propionyl coenzyme A if it had an odd number. Propionyl coenzyme A is converted by a series of reactions to yield succinic acid:

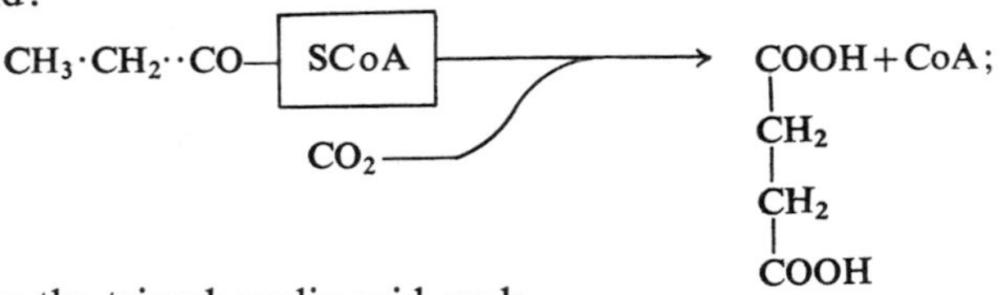

which enters the tricarboxylic acid cycle.

Lysosomes. These structures are somewhat smaller than mitochondria and more fragile. Like the mitochondria, they contain an organized system of enzymes within a semi-permeable membrane. Their enzymes are of the lytic type, such as lipases, phosphatases and peptidases. These intracellular peptidases are known as cathepsins. Materials ingested by the cell, particularly the pinocytotic vesicles, fuse with the lysosomes and the first stages of intracellular metabolism are carried out in these particles. The soluble products of metabolism in the lysosome diffuse into the cytoplasm where they become available to the remainder of the cell.

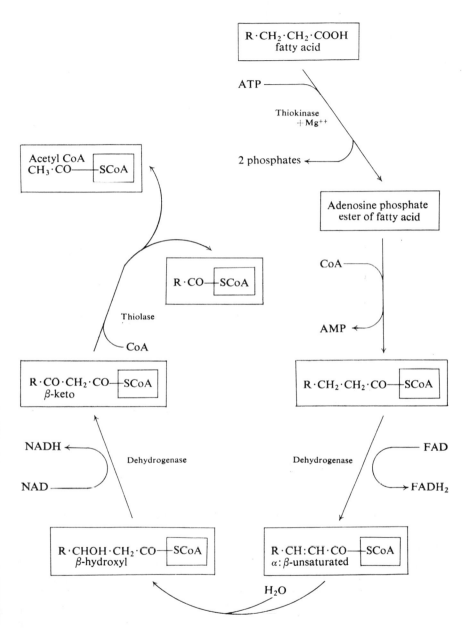

Fig. 2.7. Oxidation of a fatty acid with removal of an acetyl radical.

After death of a cell, the lytic enzymes escape from the lysosomes and break down the constituents of the cell itself, a process known as *autolysis*. It is probable that the continual reorganization and replacement of parts of the living cell are also carried out in the lysosomes.

Glycogen granules and glucose. The storage form of carbohydrate in animal cells is glycogen although carbohydrate is moved about the body as glucose. The reactions shown in Fig. 2.8 maintain the balance between glycogen and glucose. Glycogen is broken down by *phosphorylysis*, one glucose molecule at a time. The ester formed, glucose-1-phosphate, is isomerized into glucose-6-phosphate. In liver cells, which contain depots of glycogen, there is an enzyme which liberates free glucose.

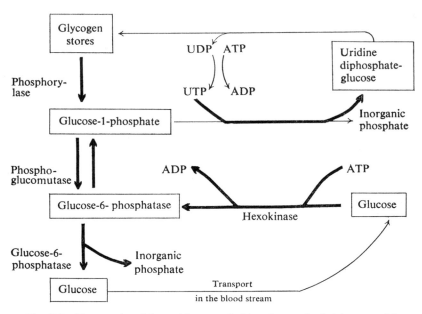

FIG. 2.8. Glycogen breakdown (glycogenolysis) and resynthesis (glycogenesis).

Glucose is able to pass the cell membrane, but phosphate esters of glucose do not. Glucose is taken up by cells and as fast as it diffuses across the cell membrane it is converted to glucose-6-phosphate by hexokinase, using the energy of the terminal phosphate of ATP (see Fig. 2.8). If glucose-6-phosphate accumulates, it is resynthesized into glycogen via an intermediary reaction with uridine triphosphate (UTP): the balance of these reactions is again in favour of synthesis of glycogen as ATP supplies energy for regenerating UTP.

Glycolysis (or glucolysis). If the cell as a whole is expending energy, then glucose-6-phosphate is metabolized to release its chemical energy, the principal pathway of metabolism being as in Fig. 2.9. When the oxygen supply is adequate, the end product is pyruvic acid which is metabolized to yield an acetyl radical (attached to coenzyme A) as shown in Fig. 2.4, and then further metabolized in the tricarboxylic acid cycle (Fig. 2.5). When there is an insufficient oxygen supply to the active cells, the breakdown of glucose (or fructose) gives lactic acid, with the release of some chemical energy as ATP. This process, known as anaerobic glycolysis, is traced in Fig. 2.9. The overall reaction (ignoring water) may be expressed as:

$$\text{Free glucose (or fructose)} + 2\text{ADP} + 2\,(\text{P}) \longrightarrow 2\text{ Lactic acid} + 2\text{ATP};$$

or, if the starting product is the glycogen store within the cell:

$$\text{Stored glucose} + 3\text{ADP} + 3\,(\text{P}) \longrightarrow 2\text{ Lactic acid} + 3\text{ATP}$$

There are other sources of chemically stored energy which come into play during periods when the energy demands of a cell temporarily exceed the rate of energy production by oxidative metabolism. (1) High energy phosphate groups are transferred from creatine phosphate to ADP:

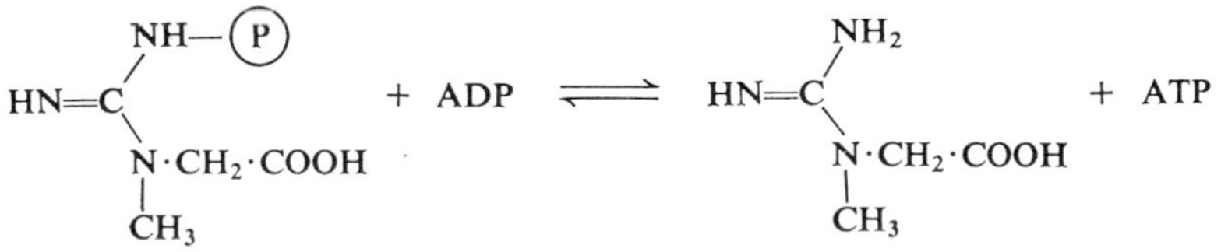

Creatine phosphate   Creatine
'phosphagen'

When the production of ATP exceeds its rate of consumption, that is, when the cell is relatively inactive, a reserve of energy is stored as creatine phosphate. (2) Two ADP molecules rearrange under the influence of the enzyme, myokinase:

$$2\text{ ADP} \xrightarrow{\text{Myokinase}} \text{ATP} + \text{AMP}$$

Amino acid metabolism. The range of reactions of amino acids is broad. Transamination is one important process and this is illustrated in Fig. 2.10.

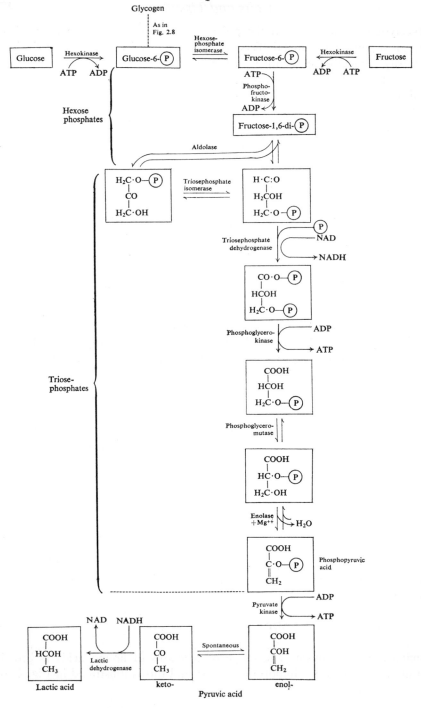

Fig. 2.9. The breakdown of glucose-6-phosphate by the triosephosphate route (the Embden-Meyerhoff route).

The first reaction is reversible, and, when the correct keto acid is available, the corresponding amino acid is formed by transamination with glutamic acid.

Glutamic acid is *formed* by transamination of α-ketoglutaric acid, the amino groups being obtained from amino acids which are surplus to the needs for

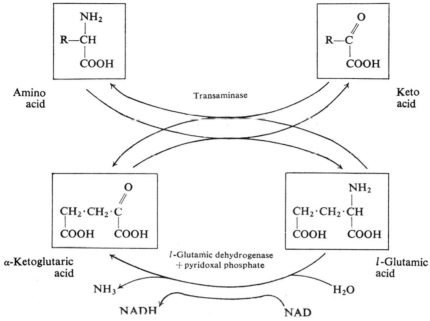

Fig. 2.10. Reactions of transamination and transdeamination of amino acids.

protein synthesis. Glutamic acid is oxidized by a dehydrogenase to regenerate α-ketoglutaric acid and yield ammonia. The net result is described as *trans-deamination*.

A few L-amino acids are directly deaminated as, for example, the following:

$$\text{L-Aspartic acid} \xrightleftharpoons{\text{Aspartase}} \text{Fumaric acid} + NH_3$$

$$\text{L-Serine} \xrightarrow{\text{Serine dehydrase}} \text{Pyruvic acid} + NH_3$$

$$\begin{array}{c}\text{L-Homoserine}\\ \updownarrow\\ \text{L-Threonine}\end{array} \longrightarrow \alpha\text{-Ketobutyric acid} + NH_3$$

The D-amino acids which occur in small amounts in plant and bacteria proteins give rise to spurious proteins if they are incorporated by animal cells, and are therefore potentially toxic. There are, however, enzymes which act rapidly to deaminate the D-amino acids, as illustrated below:

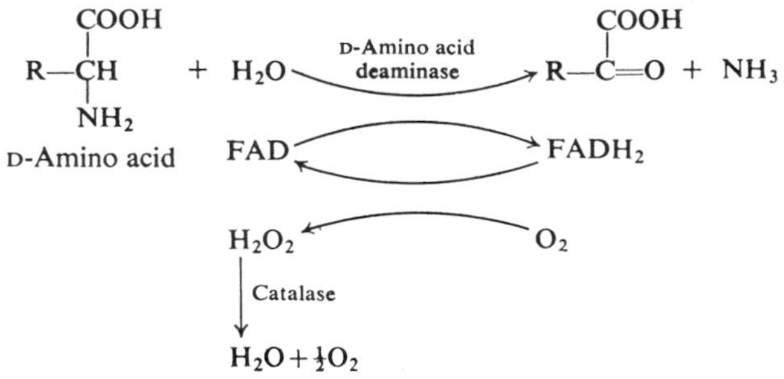

$$
\underset{\text{D-Amino acid}}{R-\underset{\underset{NH_2}{|}}{\overset{\overset{COOH}{|}}{CH}}} \;+\; H_2O \quad\xrightarrow[\text{deaminase}]{\text{D-Amino acid}}\quad R-\underset{\overset{COOH}{|}}{C}{=}O \;+\; NH_3
$$

$$FAD \rightleftarrows FADH_2$$

$$H_2O_2 \longleftarrow O_2$$

$$\Big\downarrow \text{Catalase}$$

$$H_2O + \tfrac{1}{2}O_2$$

The reduced FAD-flavoprotein is re-oxidized by molecular oxygen to give hydrogen peroxide which is rapidly split by catalase.

L-Amino acids may be decarboxylated using pyridoxal phosphate as a coenzyme, and the primary amine is then deaminated to the corresponding aldehyde:

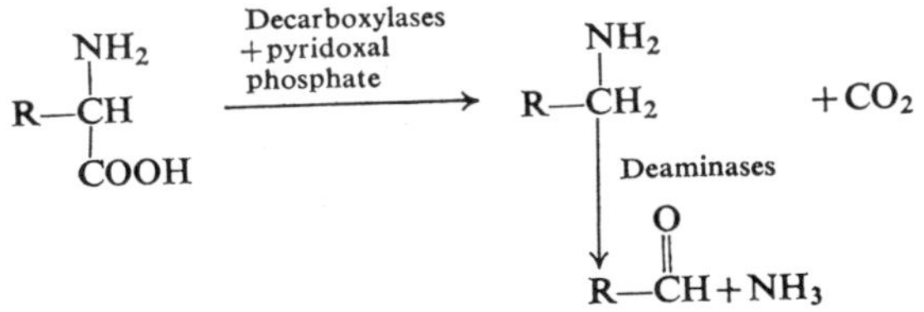

$$
R-\underset{\overset{COOH}{|}}{\overset{\overset{NH_2}{|}}{CH}} \quad\xrightarrow[\text{phosphate}]{\substack{\text{Decarboxylases}\\ +\text{pyridoxal}}}\quad R-\underset{\overset{NH_2}{|}}{CH_2} \quad + CO_2
$$

$$\Big\downarrow \text{Deaminases}$$

$$R-\overset{\overset{O}{\|}}{CH} + NH_3$$

A complex series of reactions of amino acids are shown as an example of the close interrelationship of their metabolic paths and products (Fig. 2.11). This scheme includes a number of reactions not dealt with elsewhere.

The terminal group of methionine, $-S-CH_3$, acts as a methyl donor, after activation by ATP. The enzyme responsible is a transmethylase, and the methyl group is transferred to an acceptor molecule, R. The resulting amino acid, homocysteine, does not occur as a constituent of proteins, and is converted into cysteine, the methylene group, $-CH_2-$ being transferred to convert serine to homoserine. Cysteine is broken down under the influence of desulphatase into pyruvic acid, liberating hydrogen sulphide and ammonia. Hydrogen sulphide is a toxic substance and is detoxified by oxidation to sulphate. Homoserine is another amino acid not found in proteins; it is isomeric with threonine and is converted into it. Threonine may then follow two paths: (1) an oxidative deamination to α-ketobutyric acid, followed by oxidation, loss of CO_2 and coupling of the remaining propionyl radical to coenzyme A, in a manner analogous to pyruvic acid in Fig. 2.4, and (2) a split into acetaldehyde and glycine, catalysed by an aldolase. Glycine may then follow a number of routes: (1) it may combine with 'active' formaldehyde to form serine; (2) it may combine with succinyl coenzyme A, the product being deaminated or

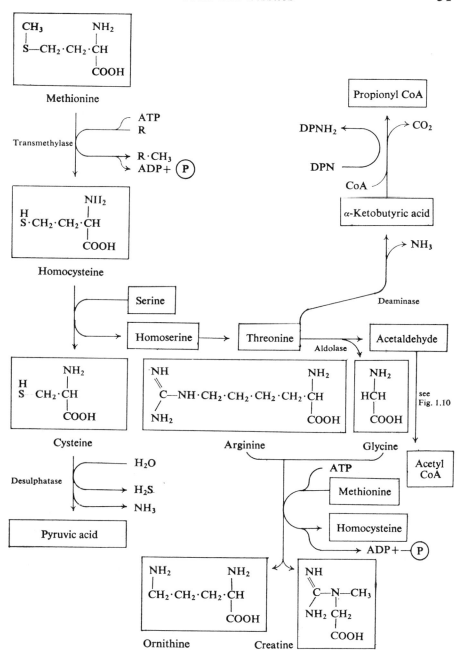

FIG. 2.11. Metabolic pathways of amino acids.

transdeaminated and oxidized to two CO_2 molecules and two molecules of reduced coenzyme, with regeneration of succinyl CoA; and (3) it may react with arginine and ATP-methionine complex, resulting in a double rearrangement, a transamidation of the amide group of arginine to glycine, and a transmethylation of the methyl group of methionine to glycine; the product, creatine, acts as a storage molecule for high energy Ⓟ groups. The other amino acid formed by loss of the amidine group of arginine is ornithine. This is not a constituent of proteins, but is important in cellular metabolism as an intermediary in the detoxification of ammonia (Fig. 12.9).

The nucleus

The cell nucleus, bounded by a nuclear membrane, contains structures, the most important of which are chromosomes. A normal human cell nucleus contains forty-six chromosomes, consisting of twenty-three pairs (Fig. 2.12). Chromosomes are elongated, sometimes branched structures, composed of *nucleoprotein*. The arrangement of nucleoprotein along each chromosome constitutes a store of information which determines the behaviour of the body cells and the hereditary content of the germ cells. Each item of information is located along the chromosome at a definite place called a *gene*.

Nucleoproteins are conjugates of protein with nucleic acids. The nucleic acids in chromosomes contain the bases adenine, thymine, guanine and cytosine (Fig. 2.13). These bases are combined with deoxyribose (Fig. 1.1) to form nucleosides (or deoxyribosides) and then with phosphate to form nucleotides (or deoxyribotides).

The unit structure of nucleic acid contains the nucleotide of each of the four bases, linked via their phosphate groups (Fig. 2.14). One molecule of deoxyribose nucleic acid (DNA) contains between 300 to 4000 such units.

The long chain nucleic acids are joined together by protein. A single thread of nucleic acid is linked to another thread in a definite way by hydrogen bonds between the bases: adenine–thymine and guanine–cytosine, as shown in Fig. 2.14. The two threads of nucleic acid are therefore precisely related to one another. Watson and Crick discovered that each chain of nucleic acid is coiled to form a spiral and the two adjacent complementary chains together form a double helix, as shown in Fig. 2.15. The conjugated protein is attached to the helical chains through the phosphate groups. During cell division leading to an increase in the number of body cells (i.e. mitotic division), each chromosome splits into two, and then each half acts as a template for regeneration of a complete chromosome. The way in which the chromosome is reformed by pairing of nucleotides in adjacent nucleic acid spirals is shown in Fig. 2.15.

The units of nucleic acid, each containing four different nucleotides, are

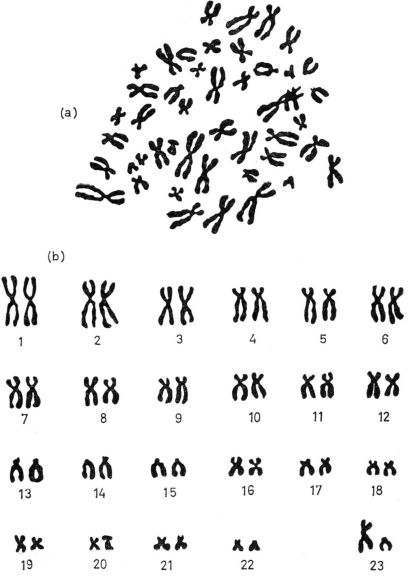

FIG. 2.12. Human male chromosomes. (*a*) A lymphocyte, cultured from peripheral blood, was treated with colchicine to prevent formation of the spindle metaphase (so that the chromosomes are widely dispersed), then treated with a hypotonic solution to make the cell swell, and fixed and spread on a slide; (*b*) The individual chromosomes from (*a*) have been identified and arranged in their pairs in order of size, the last of the twenty-three pairs being the sex chromosomes of the male—an X and a Y chromosome. In the female, there are two X chromosomes. The figure was copied from photomicrographs kindly supplied by Miss Rosemary Tanner.

believed to constitute genetic information in a code form. There are twenty-four possible combinations of four nucleotides, and upwards of 300 units in a chain of nucleic acid. It is believed that each chain spells out a distinctive message about a specific activity of the cell. In other words, these are the genes, the determinants of heredity; they determine the specific activities of cells.

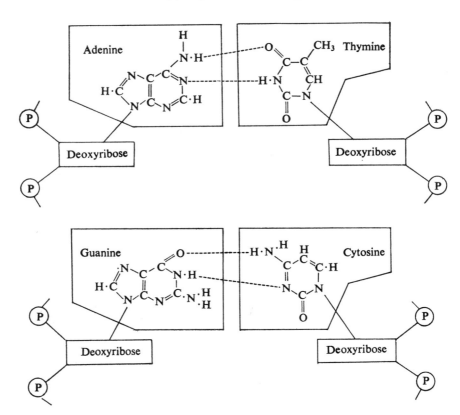

FIG. 2.13. The bases in DNA, showing how they are paired by hydrogen bonds (----).

Ribosomes are subcellular particles with a high content of ribose. They consist principally of nucleoproteins of ribonucleic acids (RNA). The unit structure of ribonucleic acid contains one of each of the nucleotides (ribosides) of adenine, guanine, cytosine and uracil (Fig. 2.16). The chain of RNA differs from DNA in that it has uracil in place of thymine, and it does not pair off with a complementary chain. The arrangement of the nucleotides in the molecules of RNA is determined in some way by the arrangement of nucleotides in DNA. The

RNA molecules then carry information corresponding to the genetic code. This information is believed to result in amino acids being assembled together in a specific sequence to form a particular protein. The code is actually a template against which the amino acids are laid down. Smaller molecules of RNA are present in the cytoplasm. They are sometimes called transfer RNA because they combine with the amino acids and transport them to the ribosomal template.

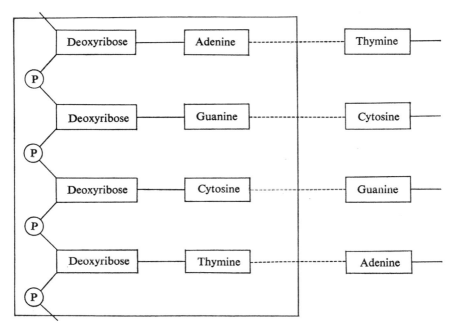

Fig. 2.14. Part of a long strand of deoxyribonucleic acid (DNA) showing the unit structure. The dotted lines indicate hydrogen bonds joining together two strands.

Specialized cells. In a single-celled animal (e.g. amoeba), that cell provides for all the functions of the animal. However, in more complex animals, groups of cells take over more or less specific functions; some cells becoming very highly specialized, other cells retaining the vestiges of more primitive characteristics. All animal bodies originate from a single cell formed by the union of the male and female gametes. Each gamete carries its share of the characteristic DNA nucleoprotein which determines the pattern of development of the animal. Then, after repeated cell divisions, the embryo consists essentially of a tube with an outer cell layer called the ectoderm, and an inner layer called the

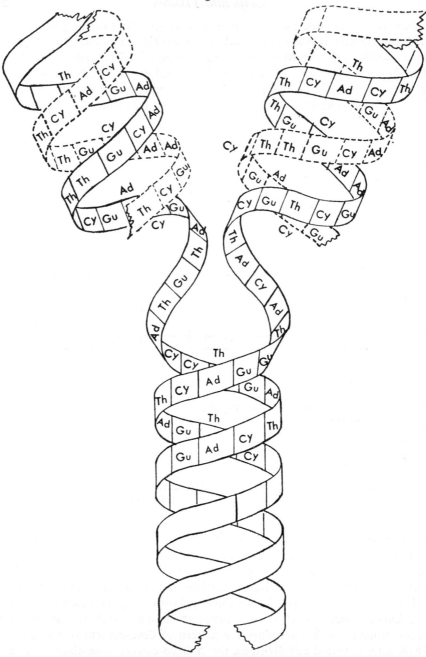

Fɪɢ. 2.15. Diagram of helices of nucleic acid, showing the relative positions of the bases in the chains. Adenine (Ad) is complementary to thymine (Th), and guanine (Gu) is complementary to cytosine (Cy). When the chromosome divides, a new complementary helix (shown dotted) is formed about each of the two helices as they separate. The nucleotide bases arranged into the spirals are shown on page 57 as straight chains; each sub-unit consists of the four nucleotides arranged in various orders.

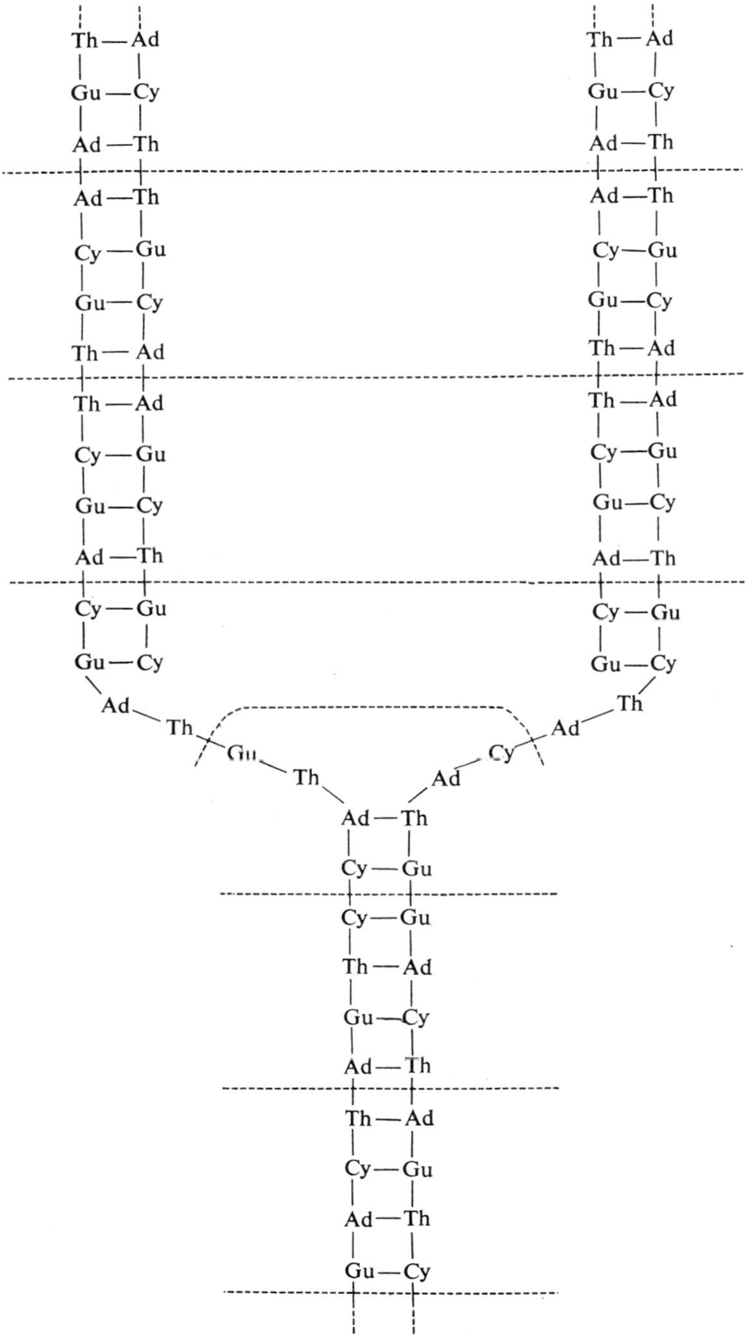

FIG. 2.15 (continued).

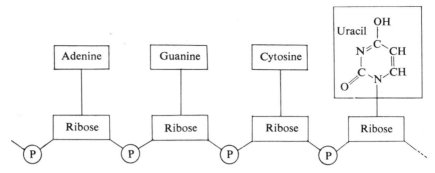

F‍ɪɢ. 2.16. Unit structure of RNA.

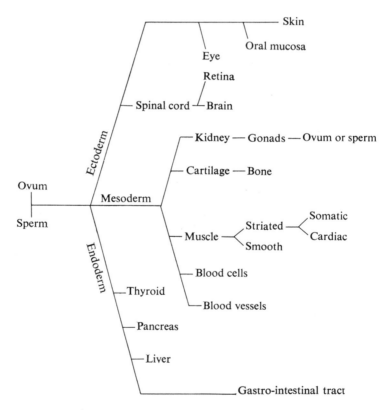

F‍ɪɢ. 2.17. Specialization of cells in terms of their development from the embryo.

endoderm, the cells between these two layers being the mesoderm. The degree of specialization of the embryonic cells is already largely determined at this stage. The three lines of cells then develop into the tissues and organs as shown in Fig. 2.17.

The classification of cells by their morphological characteristics is the particular field of study of the histologist. Four types of tissue are recognized: *epithelial* tissue, *connective* tissue, *nervous* tissue and *muscular* tissue. The cells

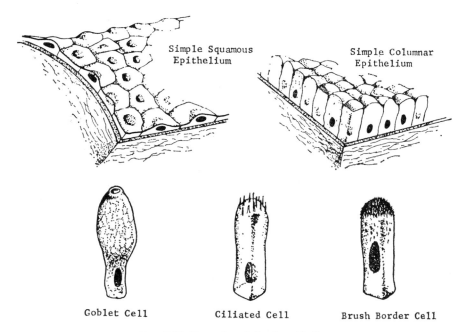

Fig. 2.18. Examples of simple epithelia.

of nervous tissue and muscular tissue undergo a high degree of specialization. Nerve cells exhibit conductivity whilst muscle cells exhibit contractility as their special properties, both types retaining the property of irritability but to rather special stimuli. Nervous tissue and muscular tissue are considered in more detail in Chapters 3, 4 and 7.

Epithelial tissues may be subdivided in the following way: (1) those covering surfaces and lining cavities (Fig. 2.18), usually classified as simple, pseudo-stratified, or stratified; and (2) those formed into glands—endocrine and exocrine.

Simple epithelial tissues are composed of a single layer of cells, which are squamous, cuboidal or columnar. Squamous cells are thin, flat cells, which line the smallest blood vessels allowing the free diffusion between the blood and the tissue fluids and which line the air spaces in the lungs, allowing diffusion of oxygen and carbon dioxide between the blood and the air. Cuboidal cells are rarely encountered.

Columnar cells are widely distributed on surfaces where they have a protective function. They exhibit the special properties of contractility, secretion and absorption. Some cells are ciliated, with protoplasmic processes projecting from their upper surface; each cilium is extremely fine, the number projecting from a single cell being either a few dozen or several hundred, depending on the location. The cilia on the surface move in rhythm (that is, they display contractility in a very specialized way) with the result that the layer of fluid over the surface is swept along. Some cells in ciliated columnar epithelia are modified into goblet cells, which contain *mucigen*, the precursor of mucin, the sticky or slimy secretion found on many surfaces. Mucin is a glycoprotein, the carbohydrate component consisting of amine derivatives of hexoses. The active role of these cells in forming mucigen is reflected in the presence of a well-formed Golgi complex and an abundance of RNA in ribosomes and free in the cytoplasm. Columnar epithelial cells with a brush border are specialized for absorption. The brush border is due to the appearance under the microscope of thousands of minute projections which have the effect of increasing the surface area of the cell membrane. Some columnar epithelia are described as pseudostratified as the nuclei of adjacent cells are on different levels.

Stratified epithelia contain layers of cells, which are specialized to resist damage. The lowest layer, containing many cells undergoing mitoses, is the germinal layer, and it is continually replacing the cells lost from the surface. In the skin, the outer layer is keratinized and the cells are fused together. Keratin is a scleroprotein characterized by a high content of the sulphur-containing amino acid, cysteine, which cross-links with cysteine in adjacent protein chains to form cystine (page 17) and so confers mechanical strength.

The property of secretion possessed by some epithelial cells is highly developed in glands. All glands develop from epithelial folds which form a tube. The cells at the bottom of the tube differentiate further until they become specialized as secretory units which produce a particular secretion. In endocrine glands, the tube separates from the original surface and the secretion is removed in the blood-stream. In exocrine glands, the tube persists and becomes the duct by which the secretion is delivered. The exocrine glands are classified morphologically into simple glands, which have an unbranched duct, and compound glands, in which the duct is branched. Each type is further designated as tubular, acinous or alveolar depending on whether the secretory unit takes the form of a tube, a sphere or a shape intermediate between these two. The nature of the secretion and the method of secreting are also used as a base for classification. Mucous glands contain cells resembling the goblet cells mentioned above. Serous glands contain the secretory product bound up as granules in the cytoplasm. The release of the secretory product through the cell membrane occurs in merocrine glands (salivary glands); in apocrine glands, some cytoplasm is lost with the secretion (mammary glands), whilst in holocrine glands the whole cell disintegrates to release the secretion (sebaceous glands).

CONNECTIVE TISSUE is especially distinguished by the relatively large amount of extracellular material in relation to the cells. Its functions are chiefly to support the other three tissues. Connective tissues are classified in the following way: (1) loose or areolar; (2) adipose; (3) dense fibrous; (4) cartilage; (5) bone; (6) dentine; (7) blood.

Loose connective tissues are found particularly beneath epithelial layers. The supporting layer of the epithelium, called the basement membrane, is formed from the connective tissue. The epithelial layers do not contain blood vessels and their nutrients come from blood vessels in the underlying connective tissue. The most numerous cells in loose connective tissue are fibroblasts, which lay down the extracellular fibres running through the tissue. The white collagen fibres are unbranched bundles of scleroprotein, and are extremely tough and resist extension and shearing. The fibres are orientated in such a way as to resist the stresses imposed on the tissue and it is probable that the stress stimulates their formation. The yellow elastic fibres are composed of finer branched bundles of a related scleroprotein, elastin. Both collagen and elastin are poor in the essential amino acids and have a high content of glycine and proline. The amino acid, hydroxyproline, is found only in collagen and elastin. Loose connective tissue contains phagocytic cells called histiocytes, and mast cells both of which are concerned with the local response of tissues to injury.

Adipose tissue is characterized by large numbers of fat-containing cells. The functions of adipose tissue are to give resilient support to structures, to provide insulation against heat loss since fat is a poor conductor of heat, and to act as a reservoir of energy-yielding material. The cytoplasm of the fat cells is almost entirely displaced by coalesced droplets of fatty acid triglycerides (Fig. 1.2). Under the appropriate condition, they release free fatty acids into the bloodstream and these serve as energy sources for other cells.

Dense connective tissue consists of closely packed bundles of collagen fibres. It forms the ligaments and tendons of bones and muscles, the tough capsules of the brain and of other organs, the pericardiac sac which encloses the heart and the valves of the heart.

Cartilage is an especially dense connective tissue. The cells, called chondrocytes, are embedded in a matrix or ground substance of extracellular material which may be of three types: hyaline, elastic or fibrous. Hyaline (or glass-like) cartilage which contains relatively few fibres consists of a firm amorphous mass of a sulphated mucopolysaccharide called chondroitin sulphate. Hyaline cartilage is present on the articulating jointed surfaces of bones where it forms a smooth surface. The union of the ribs with the sternum is made by hyaline cartilage and this allows some movement during respiration. Rings of hyaline cartilage in the larynx, trachea and bronchi hold open the passages without interfering with flexibility. Fibro-cartilage contains masses of collagen bundles and is stronger and more unyielding than hyaline cartilage. It forms more rigid junctions between certain bones (e.g. the vertebrae) and limits the range of freely movable joints (shoulder, hip) of the ball and socket type. Elastic cartilage contains a network of elastic fibres in the matrix. It is present in the ear and in parts of the larynx.

Bone and *dentine* are the hardest tissues of the body. They owe their hardness to deposits of mineral salts within the matrix. The cells, osteocytes, come to occupy cavities in the mineral matrix called lacunae. They are interconnected by protoplasmic processes running in channels called canaliculi. Not only does the skeleton provide structural support and protection for the soft tissues of the body, but the material of the bones, calcium and phosphate, acts as a reservoir from which these minerals may be drawn and replaced.

Organization and organisms

The metabolic activity of a cell is largely governed by the organization of its biochemical systems into structures, including the sub-cellular particles. The biochemical activity of intact cells cannot always be deduced from the activity of cell homogenates in which the cellular structure has been disintegrated. For example, it has long been known that the oxygen consumption of a tissue is considerably increased after homogenization. Loss of structure has removed a number of the constraints which normally play a part in regulating the activity of the cell. With the exception of single-celled organisms, the cells in turn are organized into structures and the nature of the organization provides constraints on activity. In higher animals, the cells are composed into tissues, organs and systems.

The increase in complexity which follows the transition from molecules to cells, and from cells to mammals may be appreciated by examination of Figs. 2.19 and 2.20. The first shows the differences in linear dimensions. The ratios of the lengths (or diameters) of a carbon atom, a typical protein, a typical cell and a small mammal are $1:100:100,000:1,000,000,000$. It is important to bear in mind that cubes of these numbers give the ratios of the volumes: $1:10^6:10^{15}:10^{27}$. A cell is about one thousand million times the volume of a protein molecule; assuming that only 10% of the cell consists of protein, there are still one hundred million protein molecules in each cell. This number is more than sufficient to account for all the enzymatic functions of cells, and for the proteins forming the cell structure including the nucleoprotein. In the human body, there are about one hundred million million (10^{14}) cells. The activity of each of these cells is integrated into the functioning of the whole organism.

One of the most striking and important properties of mammals is their ability to maintain their internal environment within narrow limits. This concept was first expounded by the French physiologist, Claude Bernard. He pointed out that animals can be regarded as living in two environments—the external environment and the internal environment (milieu interieur). The primitive forms of life which first evolved in the sea had a relatively constant external environment. But with the progress of evolution and the migration of living organisms to more unstable habitats various mechanisms developed to preserve the internal environment constant despite changes in the external environment. Thus there are mechanisms for regulating temperature, the amount of body water, and the chemical composition of tissues and fluids. Simple organisms are confined to a narrow range of habitats, but more highly developed forms are able to regulate their own internal environment and maintain it constant in the face of all but the most extreme of terrestial conditions. The American physiologist, W. B. Cannon, coined the term *homeostasis* to denote the maintenance of the constant internal environment. Physiology is largely concerned with the study of homeostatic mechanisms: these include the way in which a change is detected and the means by which it is counteracted. There are homeostatic mechanisms for regulating the body temperature, the blood pressure, the pH, the osmotic pressure and the volume of the blood and tissue fluids, the cell content and oxygen tension of the blood, the metabolic rates of cells, and so on. These factors are held fairly constant against changes in the external environment, and they are also integrated with the varying demands placed on them by varying levels of activity of different parts of the internal environment.

Many drugs are extremely powerful in their actions, amounts of only a few micrograms or milligrams being sufficient to produce marked changes in function in man. Pharmacologists who study the effects of drugs on various isolated tissues may sometimes use amounts as low as a few picograms per millilitre of solution. The relative magnitudes of these amounts may be realized by examining Fig. 2.20.

Health and disease. Health is the condition in which all of the bodily functions are integrated and are being maintained within the limits of optimal activity.

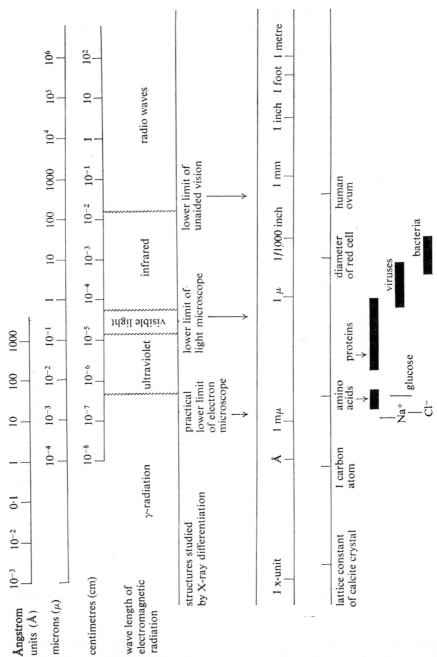

Fig. 2.19. Lengths and linear dimensions. A logarithmic scale has been used, each division representing a ten-fold change.

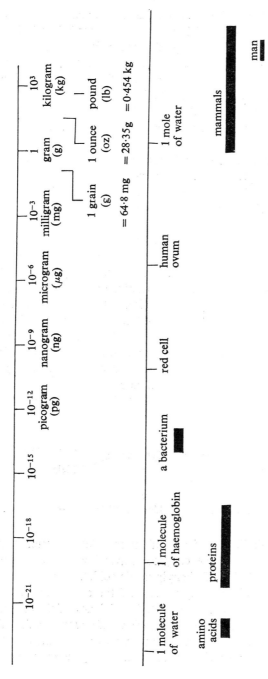

FIG. 2.20. Mass. The divisions of the logarithmic scale represent changes of one thousand-fold.

3

There is no sharp borderline between health and disease, but any wide divergence from optimal activity which results in an upset in bodily function may be considered as a disease. The study of disease is known as pathology, which is defined as the science concerned with abnormal states of the body, the functional disorders which accompany them, and the causes that bring them about. An understanding of the causes (or aetiology) of disease is valuable for therapeutics. There are two major categories of primary causes of disease: *congenital* and *environmental*, and these may be further subdivided as indicated in Fig. 2.21.

There are, in addition, contributory causes of disease which lead to an exacerbation of symptoms which might not have been produced by the primary cause acting alone. For example, an infectious disease like the common cold may occur in association with a contributory cause such as fatigue or a dietary deficiency which renders the subject more susceptible. Other contributory causes of disease include inherited susceptibilities, age and occupation.

Genetic (or hereditary) disease is due to the inheritance of an abnormal gene, and the occurrence of the disease follows Mendelian laws of inheritance. Haemophilia is probably the best known of the genetic diseases as it has occurred in some of the European royal families. In this disorder the clotting time of the blood is greatly prolonged (page 232). It is due to a recessive gene on an X (sex) chromosome, and hence it occurs in males where the presence of the gene is not masked by a second X chromosome. Another group of diseases caused by recessive genes are those in which there is a disturbance of metabolism of phenylalanine, but the genes are not on the sex chromosomes, so both sexes are affected equally. Some of the pathways of phenylalanine metabolism are:

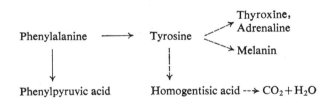

(the dotted lines indicate a series of intermediate reactions). A genetically determined deficiency of the enzyme converting phenylalanine to tyrosine leads to an accumulation of phenylpyruvic acid. This results in severe mental impairment (*imbecilitus phenylpyruvia*) and the appearance of unusual metabolites in the urine (*phenylketonuria*). A deficiency of the enzyme needed for the oxidation of homogentisic acid leads to *alcaptonuria*. A deficiency in the enzymes needed for formation of thyroxine or melanin results in *goitrous cretinism* or *albinism* respectively. The abnormal gene may be dominant, as in *achondroplasia,* in which there is a defect in the development of the skull and the long bones. The genetical abnormality, however, may be due to a mutation which leads to a defect, yet which confers some advantages. An example of this is *sickle-cell anaemia* in which the amino acid sequence of the haemoglobin molecule is altered. In this condition there is an increased resistance to malarial infection.

Congenital abnormalities due to visible defects in the chromosome pattern arise from defects in the cell divisions which produce the germ cells; usually

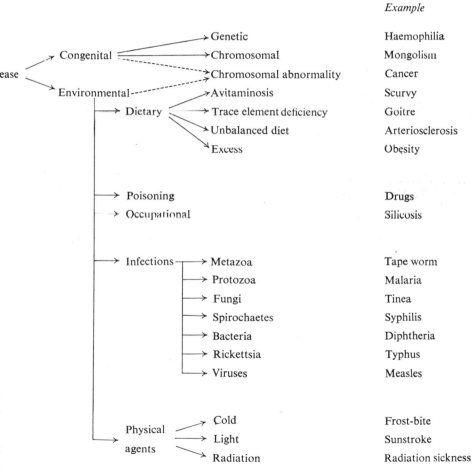

FIG. 2.21. Schematic diagram showing the relationships between some of the primary causes of diseases.

there is an extra chromosome or a missing chromosome. These are chance occurrences and are more common in pregnancies in older women. In *mongolism,* there is an extra number 21 chromosome (see Fig. 2.12).

Cancers are usually due to an altered chromosomal pattern which arises during cell division. There may be an inherited tendency or an environmental influence partly responsible for the abnormal growth. Chronic *myeloid leukaemia* is a cancerous increase in one type of blood cell. In this disorder there is a specific chromosal defect—both of the long arms on one of the number 21 chromosomes are reduced in length. This particular alteration is known as the Philadelaphia chromosome. In most cancer cells the chromosome pattern is grossly abnormal in number and shape.

In some diseases caused by environmental factors the site of action is on the chromosomal activity. For example, intense radiation leads to such a derangement of nucleoprotein that new cells cannot be formed, and some drugs inhibit cell division or cause other derangements in embryonic tissues which may lead to congenital malformations (*teratogenesis*).

Dietary deficiencies are many and varied. At the present time overeating and starvation are major contributory causes of disease. Vitamin deficiencies have been mentioned in Chapter 1. Deficiencies of mineral and trace elements are still important causes of disease, examples being deficiencies of iodine (goitre), iron (anaemia) and fluoride (dental caries).

Pathogenic organisms cause a wide range of diseases which are classified by the type of organism (as in Fig. 2.21). The treatment of this group of diseases by chemotherapeutic agents has been an outstanding contribution of pharmacology.

Physical injury, occupational hazards, and poisoning account for considerable ill health. Occupational hazards causing disease include dust, particularly in miners and quarrymen (silicosis), heat, high and low pressure, electric shock, toxic chemicals and venoms. Chemical agents which are occasionally responsible for disease, and of particular importance to pharmacologists, are the drugs themselves, some of which sometimes produce disorders which are worse than the disease being treated (*iatrogenic disease*).

CHAPTER 3

Properties of Neurones

The unit of the nervous system is the nerve cell or neurone which consists of a cell body and one or more slender protoplasmic outgrowths. A typical nerve cell is illustrated in the diagram of a motor unit in Chapter 4 (Fig. 4.6), but there are many different types which vary widely in shape and size and in the number, length and degree of branching of their processes. The cell body is from 5 to 100 μ in diameter, and contains a large spherical nucleus with a prominent nucleolus, mitochondria and the Golgi apparatus. The cytoplasm of the cell body contains ribonucleic acid which appears after staining as particles called Nissl granules. Each neurone has one main process known as the axon or nerve fibre, the protoplasm of which is continuous with the cytoplasm of the cell body. In man, nerve fibres vary in length in different types of nerve cell from a fraction of a millimetre to almost a metre. Axons may branch many times, the branches being known as collaterals. The dendrons, of which there may be many, branch into dendrites and, unlike the axons, contain Nissl granules. The direction of conduction in the dendrons is always towards the cell body. Sensory neurones with their cell bodies in the dorsal root ganglia (see page 105) possess an axon but no dendrons. The axon of these sensory neurones divides, soon after leaving the cell body, into peripheral and central components.

The axoplasm of nerve fibres contains many fine neurofibrils which run along the length of the fibre and pass through the cell body into the dendrons. Neurofibrils do not appear to play any part in the conductive activity of the neurone, although they are thought to play an important part in the regeneration of damaged nerve fibres.

The membrane surrounding the cell body is continuous with the membranes surrounding the axon and the dendrons. The structure of the membrane is such that it allows the diffusion of hydrated potassium ions (2·2 Å in diameter) but not of hydrated sodium ions (3·4 Å in diameter). Special lipid-soluble carrier molecules may be present which preferentially combine with certain ions and transport them across the membrane.

Nerve axons in vertebrates are classified as myelinated (or medullated) and non-myelinated (or non-medullated). Both types occur throughout the central nervous system (CNS) and in peripheral nerve trunks.

Myelinated fibres. Myelin is a white fatty substance made up of lipid and protein molecules. In peripheral nerves, myelin is formed from the much thickened surface membranes of the Schwann cells which lie next to the axons. The Schwann cells coil round the axon to form successive layers of myelin and create a laminated effect (Fig. 3.1a). The protoplasm of the Schwann cell forms an outer cylinder surrounding the myelin and containing the nucleus. The outer membrane of the Schwann cell is called the *neurilemma*. There are no Schwann cells in the brain and spinal cord where neuroglial cells are associated with the axons, and one type of neuroglial cell (oligodendroglial cells) lays down the myelin sheath and carries out functions similar to those of the Schwann cells in the peripheral nerves.

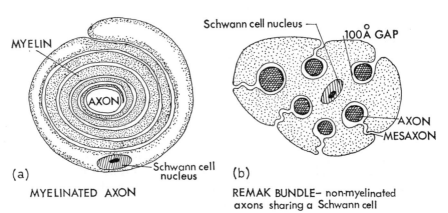

Fig. 3.1. Diagrammatic transverse sections of nerve fibres.

The myelin sheath does not extend continuously along the axon; it is interrupted at intervals by constrictions of the outer Schwann cell membrane. The constrictions are known as the nodes of Ranvier and there is one Schwann cell nucleus between each pair of nodes (Fig. 4.6). The internodal distance and the thickness of the myelin layer vary according to the diameter of the fibre. In a myelinated nerve fibre with an outside diameter of $10\,\mu$, the internodal distance is about 1 mm and the thickness of myelin about $1.3\,\mu$. Such a thickness of myelin corresponds to that built up from about eighty double layers of Schwann cell membrane. In larger fibres, the thickness of myelin and the internodal distance are proportionately greater. Vertebrate myelinated nerve fibres range in diameter from about 1 to $25\,\mu$, this dimension including the thickness of the covering sheaths. Nodes of Ranvier were once considered to be absent from myelinated nerve fibres in the CNS, but there is now evidence that similar node-like structures exist there.

The cell bodies, the dendrons and the fine branching endings of the axons are not covered with a myelin sheath and when seen in mass have a pinkish-grey appearance in contrast to the white colour of the myelinated fibres. Myelin plays an important part in the conductive ability of the neurone and some diseases of the central nervous system, in which progressive paralysis and loss of sensation are involved, are associated with degeneration of the myelin sheaths. An example of these demyelinating diseases is *disseminated sclerosis*.

Non-myelinated fibres. The axonal diameter of the non-myelinated fibres ranges from about 0·1 to 1 μ, the axons being enveloped in folds of the Schwann cells. The outer membrane of the axon is separated from the membrane of the Schwann cell by a distance of 100 to 200 Å, the space so formed being continuous with the extracellular space through the invagination (or mesaxon) of the Schwann cell. Some Schwann cells contain only a single non-myelinated fibre but the majority contain more. In a typical cutaneous nerve, up to 15 axons may be enveloped by a single Schwann cell and in the olfactory nerve the number may be several thousands. The Schwann cell, together with the axons running within it, is known as a *Remak bundle*. The size of most of the individual axons is below the limit of resolution of the light microscope and before the use of the electron microscope Remak bundles were often mistaken for single fibres. Consequently, the number of non-myelinated fibres present in a nerve trunk was considerably underestimated. The axons criss-cross from one Schwann cell to another along the course of a nerve trunk so that the companions of a particular fibre at one point in a Schwann cell may be quite different from those at another. Fig. 3.1b is a diagrammatic cross-section of non-myelinated nerve fibres sharing a Schwann cell.

Conduction velocity. Myelinated nerve fibres conduct very much faster than non-myelinated fibres; in general, speed of conduction and excitability increase with increase in fibre diameter. As already described, the dendrons, cell body and fine tapering nerve terminals are not myelinated. Excitability and conduction velocity therefore vary between one part of a nerve cell and another. Nerve fibres are classified into *A*, *B* and *C* fibres according to their diameter, conduction velocity and other properties: *A* fibres are the fastest of the myelinated fibres; *B* fibres are also myelinated but smaller than the *A* fibres and of slower conduction velocity, while *C* fibres are the non-myelinated fibres. The *A* fibres are further subdivided into α, β, γ and sometimes δ and ϵ fibres. Some of the characteristics and locations of the different types of fibre are presented in Table 3.1. A different classification is often used for afferent nerve fibres, that is, fibres conducting impulses towards the CNS. These are divided into groups denoted by a numeral and a letter. The numeral indicates the size range and therefore the conduction velocity of the fibre, while the letter indicates its function. For example, the Group IA afferents are large diameter fibres (12–21 μ) conducting at 60–120 m/sec and which transmit impulses from the

TABLE 3.1. Locations and properties of peripheral mammalian nerve fibres.

Fibre group	A			B	C	
	α	β	γ	Pre-ganglionic autonomic fibres	Sympathetic C	Dorsal root C
Location	Motor fibres to voluntary muscle and afferents from sensory receptors	Sensory afferents	Efferent fibres to muscle spindles and sensory afferents	Pre-ganglionic autonomic fibres	Post-ganglionic sympathetic fibres	Afferent sensory fibres
Fibre diameter in μ		1–22		3	3–5	1–1·3
Conduction velocity in metres/sec	100–120	60	40	10	50–80	1–2
Duration of spike in msec		0·4–0·5		1·2	1·5	2
Duration of absolute refractory period in msec		0·4–0·5		1·2		2
Negative after-potential { As per cent of spike amplitude		3–5		None		None
Negative after-potential { Duration in msec		12–20		—		—
Positive after-potential { As per cent of spike amplitude		0·2		1·5–4		Exhibit a large after-hyperpolarization of a different type from that of other fibres
Positive after-potential { Duration in msec		40–60		100–300	300–1000	

Note that fibre diameters overlap between groups. B fibres are distinguished from A fibres mainly by the absence of the negative after-potential in B fibres.

muscle spindles (see page 107). The Group IB afferents have the same size range and conduction velocity but transmit information from the Golgi tendon organs (see page 107). Group II have diameters of 6–12 μ, Group III, 1–6 μ and Group IV, less than 1 μ.

Nerve trunks. These are composed of bundles of both efferent and afferent nerve fibres, each bundle consisting of large numbers of both myelinated and non-myelinated axons. The connective tissue separating the individual fibres is known as *endoneurium,* that separating the bundles as *perineurium,* and that surrounding the whole nerve trunk as *epineurium.* The perineurium contains sheets of cells which prevent extracellular ions in the spaces between the fibres from mixing freely with those outside the nerve trunk. In the CNS, the nerve fibres are packed closely together. They run in tracts and are surrounded by neuroglial cells. The brain is composed of many thousands of millions of neurones making intricate connections with each other through their axons and dendrites.

Degeneration and regeneration of nerve fibres. When a nerve is cut, the parts of the fibres separated from the cell bodies degenerate. After about 24 h, the myelin and the axons break up and are gradually removed by macrophages. This process was first described by Waller in 1852 and is known as *Wallerian degeneration.* In peripheral nerves, the Schwann cells multiply and form tubes into which the central stumps of the severed axons grow at the rate of 1·5–2 mm/day. However, the growth of new fibres is random and the extent of re-innervation depends on the severity of the injury and the degree of scarring. Many axons reach the wrong terminations but the number of axons is so large that usually sufficient of them re-establish the correct functional connections. In the CNS, only very limited regeneration occurs and destruction of nerve tissue may lead to permanent loss of function.

Properties of nerve cell membranes

The information contained in this chapter applies to nerve cells and their membranes, but the membranes of all excitable cells (e.g. muscle cells) exhibit similar properties. Most of the important discoveries concerning the properties of nerve cell membranes were made with giant axons of the squid (*Loligo*) which have diameters of up to 1 mm.

The resting membrane potential. When a fine electrode is inserted inside a nerve fibre (with little damage to the cell membrane), a potential difference can be recorded between such an intracellular micro-electrode and a second electrode placed in the extracellular fluid; the interior is 60–100 mV negative with respect to the exterior. The extracellular fluid surrounding the nerve cells contains relatively high concentrations of sodium and chloride ions, while the intracellular fluid contains relatively high concentrations of potassium ions and of organic anions including phosphocreatinine, ATP, hexosemonophosphate, proteins and amino acids. The properties of the membrane are such that it is permeable to potassium and chloride ions, much less permeable to sodium ions, and almost completely impermeable to the organic anions. At the beginning of the century, Bernstein suggested that the resting potential arose from the existence of a concentration gradient for potassium (high inside, low outside) and a selective permeability of the cell membrane to this ion. Largely through the work of Hodgkin and Huxley in England and Curtis and Cole in the U.S.A., Bernstein's idea is now generally accepted by physiologists, although in a more elaborate form.

One widely accepted hypothesis to explain the membrane potential is as follows. Potassium ions tend to diffuse out of the cell along their concentration gradient carrying positive charges to the outside of the membrane. The organic anions, to which the membrane is impermeable, are left behind and thus the charges are separated by the membrane which is therefore polarized. At equilibrium, the positive charge on the outside of the membrane is strong enough to repel any further diffusion of potassium ions along their concentration gradient. Chloride ions which enter the membrane along their concentration gradient tend to be driven out again by the negative charges on the inside, and as a result there is little diffusion of chloride ion through the membrane. For sodium ion, the concentration gradient and the electrical forces are acting in the same direction and there is therefore a strong tendency for sodium ion to diffuse into the cell. However, in the resting state, the membrane is only slightly permeable to sodium ions. Furthermore, a metabolic process, known as the *sodium pump*, continually drives sodium out of the cell against its concentration gradient so that, in the resting cell, the net sodium gain is negligible. As the sodium ions are extruded by the sodium pump, they are replaced by potassium ions.

When a membrane separating two solutions is permeable to only one of the ions, the potential difference set up across the membrane may be calculated by the Nernst equation:

$$Em = \frac{RT}{Fn} \log_e \frac{\text{Inside concentration of penetrating ion}}{\text{Outside concentration of penetrating ion}}$$

where Em = potential difference across the membrane in volts, R = the thermodynamic gas constant (8·2 J/mol. deg. abs.), T = the absolute temperature, F = the Faraday (96,500 C/mol.) and n = the valency of the ion. At body temperature (37° C), for a univalent ion and for logarithms to the base 10, the equation simplifies to:

$$Em = 61 \log_{10} \frac{[\text{Penetrating ion inside}]}{[\text{Penetrating ion outside}]} \, mV$$

If the equilibrium potential for potassium ion (E_K) is calculated from the Nernst equation, the theoretical value obtained agrees fairly well with the membrane potential measured experimentally. The agreement is not exact, however, as sodium and chloride ions play a small part. A modified equation derived by Goldman takes the permeabilities of all the ions into account and enables more accurate values to be calculated.

One test of the theory that the resting membrane potential arises largely from the potassium concentration gradient is to alter the concentration of potassium ions in the fluid bathing isolated nerve cells. When the extracellular potassium concentration is increased, the concentration gradient is reduced and the potential difference across the membrane falls (i.e. the membrane is depolarized) to the expected value. When the outside potassium concentration is lowered below normal, the increase in membrane potential (i.e. the hyper-polarization) is slightly less than that arising solely from the potassium concentration gradient. However, this is to be expected since the small contributions of sodium and chloride ions become relatively more important when the outside potassium concentration is low.

Experiments with the giant axon of the squid have provided further convincing evidence that the membrane potential is the result of the potassium ion concentration gradient. The axoplasm from the nerve fibre was squeezed out and replaced by a solution of potassium sulphate. Despite the fact that the other normal constituents of the axoplasm were absent, the axon when placed in sea-water maintained a resting potential close to normal and continued to conduct nerve impulses.

The action potential. If two recording electrodes are placed on the surface of a nerve and connected to a sensitive galvanometer as illustrated in Fig. 3.2a, no current flows when the nerve is not conducting impulses since all points on the exterior of the nerve are at the same potential. A nerve impulse consists of a self propagated *reversal* in membrane potential which passes rapidly along the fibre. Thus when a nerve impulse reaches position 2 in the diagram of Fig. 3.2a, the electrode at this position is in contact with membrane surface which is negative with respect to that in contact with the other electrode and current flows through the galvanometer. If the electrodes are widely spaced, the membrane at position 2 may have returned to its normal state by the time the impulse reaches position 3. When the impulse reaches position 4, the conditions will be reversed and the galvanometer deflection will this time be in the opposite direction. When the two electrodes are placed closer together, the current flow is still diphasic but the two phases overlap one another as shown in Fig. 3.2b. If the membrane under the second electrode is destroyed by touching it with a hot wire or a piece of fused KCl, a steady current of injury (the *demarcation potential*) flows through the recording apparatus for a few hours. Under these conditions, nerve impulses cannot reach the second electrode and the recorded response is therefore monophasic (Fig. 3.2c). The advantage of such records is that they are more easily interpreted. By connecting the recording electrodes to a cathode ray oscilloscope in place of the galvanometer, the potential changes associated with the passage of the nerve impulse may be made

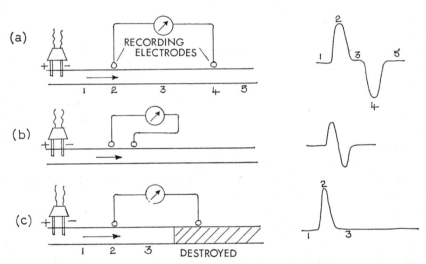

FIG. 3.2. The electrical changes accompanying the passage of a nerve impulse, as seen when external recording electrodes are used. The stimulating electrodes are shown on the left and the arrows show the direction of conduction. For further explanation, see text.

to deflect the electron beam of the cathode ray tube, giving records like those on the right of Fig. 3.2. The potential change, which constitutes the nerve impulse, is known as the *action potential.*

When the recording is made between an intracellular micro-electrode and a second electrode in the external fluid, the action potential or spike potential is superimposed on the resting potential to give records like that of Fig. 3.3a. This type of recording shows that at the peak of the spike the cell membrane is reversed in polarity for a short period.

The nerve axon may be stimulated by producing a localized reduction in the size of the potential across its membrane. The depolarization must reach a threshold level (about 15 mV smaller than the resting potential) before an

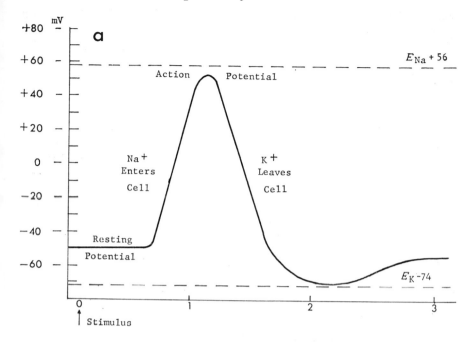

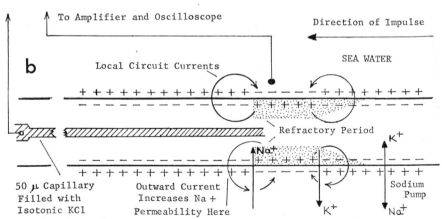

FIG. 3.3. (*a*) Diagram of the changes in membrane potential (in mV) occurring during the passage of an impulse along the squid giant axon when recorded between an intracellular electrode and an electrode in the external fluid, as illustrated in the lower half of the figure. The broken lines mark the equilibrium potentials (in mV) for sodium (E_{Na}) and potassium (E_K) calculated from the Nernst equation. The horizontal axis is calibrated in milliseconds. (*b*) Diagrammatic representation of the changes occurring during the passage of an impulse in the squid giant axon.

action potential is initiated. A sub-threshold stimulus does not initiate an action potential but briefly increases the excitability of the membrane. The depolarization produced by a second sub-threshold stimulus may therefore summate with that produced by the first so that the critical fall in membrane potential is reached and an action potential is initiated. The brief period during which the second sub-threshold stimulus may evoke an action potential is known as *the period of latent addition* (see Fig. 3.5).

The most effective experimental method of producing the necessary depolarization to excite the cell is to pass an electric current through a pair of electrodes in contact with the cell, but heat, pressure and some chemical agents may also produce depolarization. When an axon is stimulated at any point along its length, impulses are propagated in both directions away from the point of stimulation. In the living animal, the nerve fibre is stimulated at one end and conduction in a given fibre is therefore in one direction only. An impulse travelling in this direction is termed *orthodromic* while an *antidromic* impulse is one travelling in the opposite direction. Antidromic impulses take part in the axon reflex (page 177).

When stimulating electrodes are applied to the surface of a nerve cell and a brief pulse of current is passed, the voltage drop across the membrane resistance opposes the resting potential under the cathode of the stimulating electrodes and the membrane becomes partially depolarized at this point. The reverse occurs at the anode where the membrane becomes hyperpolarized and therefore less excitable. Depolarization of the membrane has two main effects. Initially it causes an abrupt but short-lasting selective increase in sodium permeability, but it also causes a delayed increase in potassium permeability over the resting value for this ion. A relatively small but critical degree of depolarization is all that is necessary to produce a large and sudden increase in *sodium* permeability. Consequently, in the partially depolarized region, sodium ions rapidly enter the cell along their concentration gradient and the membrane potential at this point becomes reversed, the inside then being positive with respect to the outside. The overshoot in the membrane potential is of the order of 30 to 60 mV and approaches the sodium equilibrium potential (E_{Na}) calculated from the Nernst equation. The increase in sodium permeability is only of very brief duration and decays with time from the moment when it is first triggered. The rapid reduction in sodium permeability is known as *inactivation*. This in itself gradually causes the membrane potential to return to its normal value, but the process is accelerated by the secondary increase in potassium permeability which becomes appreciable at the peak of the action potential. Potassium ions therefore leave the cell at a greatly increased rate and the membrane potential rapidly returns to its normal value, i.e. the membrane is repolarized. After activity, the sodium–potassium interchange is reversed to normal by an increase in the activity of the sodium pump.

The electrical resistance of the axoplasm and of the extracellular fluid is fairly low while that of the membrane is relatively high. Nerve fibres therefore have a structure resembling an underwater shielded electric cable, with a long central conducting core surrounded by insulation, outside which is another conducting layer. However, the resistance of the axoplasm is much higher, and that of the membrane much lower, than those of the materials used in an electric cable. As soon as the membrane potential is altered in one region, current starts to flow into it from adjacent regions of membrane still in the resting state. Thus an action potential set up at one point in the cell membrane causes a local circuit current to flow forwards in the axis cylinder, out through the membrane and back through the interstitial fluid to the active region. The resistance of the axoplasm rapidly attenuates the passive electrotonic spread of potential. In a non-myelinated nerve fibre, the resistance of the membrane is low and the local circuit current is therefore strongest in the region of membrane immediately adjacent to the active region. The outward flow of current at this new region acts like the outward flow of current produced by the cathode of the stimulating electrodes and depolarizes the membrane. Sodium ions therefore enter this new region and the whole process is repeated; each active region therefore excites that immediately ahead of it. In other words, once started the action potential is self-propagating. These changes are illustrated diagrammatically in Fig. 3.3b. The action potential obeys the *All-or-Nothing Law* which states that, if the tissue responds at all, it responds to the maximum of which it is capable under the prevailing conditions. Thus, all stimuli, of the threshold strength or above, initiate identical action potentials.

Tetrodotoxin, a poison obtained from the puffer fish, abolishes the action potential by preventing the rapid entry of sodium ions through the depolarized cell membrane.

Saltatory conduction in myelinated nerve fibres. Current knowledge of the function of myelin stems largely from the work of Kato and Tasaki and their colleagues, and of Huxley and Stämpfli. In myelinated fibres, the sodium and potassium interchange occurs only at the nodes of Ranvier. As already described, myelin is made up of large numbers of concentric layers of cell membrane and is therefore an insulating material which increases the electrical resistance of the nerve fibre membrane along the internodal stretches. The local circuit currents produced by the reversed membrane potential at one node of Ranvier cannot therefore flow through the internodal region of membrane but must flow forward through the axoplasm, out through the next node, and back in the extracellular fluid. The flow of local circuit currents is carried out by conduction in an electrolyte and is therefore nearly instantaneous. Delay occurs at the nodes of Ranvier due to the time necessary for the sodium ions to reverse the membrane potential. Conduction in myelinated nerves is known as saltatory conduction (from the Latin *saltare*—to dance) as the impulse appears to jump from node to node. One function of myelin is therefore to increase conduction velocity by forcing the currents produced during activity to act at a distance well ahead of the active region. In addition, myelination results in a reduced energy expenditure as the activity of the sodium pump is confined to the nodes of Ranvier. The greater the diameter of the axon, the lower is the resistance of the axoplasm and the further is the electrotonic spread of potential. Conduction is therefore more rapid in large fibres and in these the nodes are more widely spaced. There is a considerable margin of safety in conduction. If one or even two nodes are inactivated by painting them with a local anaesthetic, the local currents produced by the previous node are strong enough to excite

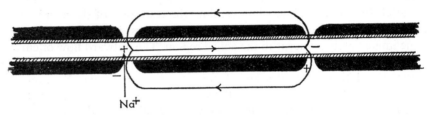

FIG. 3.4. Diagram of local circuit currents in a myelinated nerve fibre. The direction of conduction of the impulse is from left to right.

the next untreated node so that the impulse may pass an inactive region equal to as much as three internodes in length. Conduction in a myelinated nerve fibre is represented in Fig. 3.4.

The compound action potential. When recording electrodes are placed on the surface of a nerve trunk at some distance away from the stimulating electrodes, the monophasic record of the compound action potential of the whole nerve trunk consists of a series of potentials. This is because most nerve trunks contain fibres of all types and each type conducts at a different velocity (see Table 3.1); hence the impulses of each type arrive at the recording electrodes at different times. Each potential wave in the complex response represents the action potential of a different fibre group. The action potential travelling along the fast α-fibres reaches the recording electrodes first and this is followed by the β, γ, B and finally, C-fibre potentials. The thicker fibres are stimulated by weaker and briefer stimuli than are the fine fibres and it is therefore possible, by choosing the correct stimulus parameters, to excite the fast-conducting fibres preferentially. It is not possible to excite the slow-conducting fibres preferentially since stimuli strong enough to affect them are always well above threshold for the fast-conducting fibres.

Refractory period and after-potentials. For a brief period after a stimulus strong enough to excite an action potential has been applied, a second stimulus, no matter how strong it is, is incapable of re-exciting the cell. This period is known as the *absolute refractory period. The relative refractory period* occurs immediately afterwards and during this time the cell gradually regains its former excitability. During the relative refractory period, an extra-strong stimulus excites an action potential but its amplitude is usually smaller than normal and its velocity of propagation is reduced. The absolute refractory period is probably explained by the fact that after the peak of the action potential, sodium permeability is reduced below normal and potassium permeability increased above normal. Both changes act to prevent re-excitation. During the relative refractory period, the permeabilities to both ions are returning to normal. The duration of the absolute refractory period usually corresponds to the duration of the spike. Refractoriness limits the frequency at which the nerve conducts impulses. For example, the absolute refractory period of the largest *A* fibres of mammals is about 0·5 msec. Such a fibre can therefore conduct as many as, but no more than, 2000 impulses per sec, although it probably never approaches this rate in physiological circumstances.

After the action potential, the membrane potential undergoes further small and relatively slow variations known as *after-potentials*. These are seen in most fibres but are particularly well marked in sympathetic *C* fibres. After-potentials were named before the introduction of intracellular electrodes, so that a potential change in the same direction as the spike is called a *negative after-potential*, while the reverse, that is, a hyperpolarization relative to the resting potential, is called a *positive after-potential*.

The negative after-potential occurs immediately after the spike and usually appears as a small prolongation of the declining phase of the spike. It is followed by a more prolonged and smaller change in the opposite direction which is the positive after-potential. During the negative after-potential, excitability and conduction velocity are increased whereas the reverse holds during the positive after-potential. It is generally believed that the depressed excitability occurring during the positive after-potential is a late continuation of the relative refractory period. In fibres which exhibit after-potentials, therefore, the relative refractory period is temporarily interrupted soon after its onset by a period of enhanced excitability corresponding to the negative after-potential. These changes in membrane potential and excitability are represented in Fig. 3.5, and Table 3.1 shows some of the characteristics of the refractory period and after-potentials in different types of fibres.

The ionic changes giving rise to after-potentials are not fully understood although there is evidence that they arise through changes in the distribution of potassium ions. Repolarization after the spike is caused by the liberation of potassium ions into the interstitial fluid. The concentration of potassium ions outside the fibre is therefore temporarily higher than normal, especially in *C* fibres where the Schwann cells (see Fig. 3.1b) slow down diffusion into the main extracellular space. The fall in membrane potential caused by the reduced

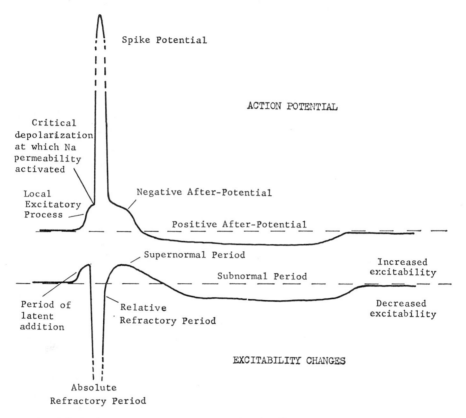

FIG. 3.5. Action potential (upper trace) and excitability changes (lower trace) during the passage of a nerve impulse. The durations of the first two phases of each trace have been exaggerated. (After Morgan, *Physiological Psychology*. McGraw-Hill, 1943.)

potassium concentration gradient across the cell membrane is probably sufficient to account for the negative after-potential.

After the action potential, there is an increase in the activity of the sodium pump. The extrusion of sodium ions is coupled with the uptake of potassium ions from the extracellular fluid immediately surrounding the axon. In non-myelinated fibres, this extracellular potassium is only slowly replaced from the main extracellular fluid because of the diffusion barriers imposed by the

Schwann cell. Thus the concentration of potassium ion in the fluid surrounding the axon falls below normal and the membrane is hyperpolarized during the positive after-potential. The positive after-potentials summate during repetitive stimulation resulting in a more pronounced hyperpolarization known as post-tetanic hyperpolarization. Post-tetanic hyperpolarization probably accounts for the phenomenon of post-tetanic potentiation described on pages 118 and 155.

After-potentials may be affected by pharmacological agents. For example, *veratrine* increases and prolongs the negative after-potential to the extent that it may re-excite the fibre and repetitive activity is produced in response to a single stimulus. *Yohimbine,* on the other hand, increases and prolongs the positive after-potential. *Tetraethylammonium* and, more recently, *neostigmine* have been shown to enhance both types of after-potential in the motor nerve terminals of isolated nerve-muscle preparations. Procedures which interfere with the active extrusion of sodium ions include bathing the fibres in potassium-free solutions, or exposing them to the cardiac glycoside, *ouabain,* or to the metabolic inhibitors, *sodium cyanide, dinitrophenol* or *antimycin A.* These have been shown to abolish the positive after-potential without initially affecting the spike potential.

Nerve metabolism. The immediate source of energy for the conduction of the nerve impulse is the pre-existing concentration gradients for Na^+ and K^+ ions; conduction does not derive energy directly from cell metabolism. Nerve metabolism is required, however, in order to drive the sodium pump which maintains the resting potential and restores the distribution of ions against their concentration gradients after the action potential has passed. This metabolism is oxidative and results in the production of CO_2 and a small amount of heat. The principal substrate is glucose which is metabolized to provide high energy phosphate bonded as phosphoprotein and ATP (see also page 811). In large nerve fibres, particularly those that are myelinated, the change in internal ionic concentration after an action potential is relatively small and many impulses continue to be conducted after inhibition of glucose metabolism. In small diameter fibres, on the other hand, where the volume is small in relation to the surface area of the membrane, even a single impulse appreciably lowers the internal potassium concentration so that, when the sodium pump is blocked, only a few nerve impulses are conducted. This explains the observation of Larabee and Bronk that post-ganglionic sympathetic fibres, which are non-myelinated *C* fibres, consume oxygen during activity very much faster than somatic myelinated nerves. It also explains why the central nervous system, with its vast numbers of non-myelinated cell bodies and dendrons, is so dependent on an adequate supply of glucose and oxygen in the blood, and why drugs which depress metabolic processes exert such pronounced effects on the brain, providing they can penetrate to the nervous tissue from the bloodstream.

Ephaptic transmission. The local circuit currents produced by an active nerve fibre flow through the surrounding tissues including adjacent resting nerve fibres, as illustrated in Fig. 3.6a. Remembering that outward flowing current opposes the resting membrane potential and tends to excite the cell, it can be seen from Fig. 3.6a that the excitability of the adjacent resting fibre is first lowered, then raised and then lowered again. Owing to the high impedence of the tissues between the nerve axons, local circuit currents produced by an active fibre are probably never large enough under normal conditions to initiate action potentials in adjacent fibres. However, the increased excitability produced in the resting fibre will facilitate any other activity in the fibre and this effect is probably important in the CNS where the nerve fibres are packed closely together. It has been suggested that a facilitating effect of this type is responsible for the synchronization of rhythmic activity in the CNS. The excitability of a resting nerve fibre may be raised by a constant sub-threshold cathodal current, by certain ionic changes in the extracellular medium, or by some drugs. Under these conditions, local circuit currents in an adjacent active fibre initiate action potentials in the resting fibre. This type of excitation of one nerve fibre by another is called *ephaptic transmission* and the region at which it occurs is called an *ephapse*. There are circumstances when transmission across the junction between two excitable cells is brought about by current flow from the active cell. It is not known whether ephaptic transmission ever occurs in the nervous system of mammals, where transmission from one cell to the next is chiefly brought about by chemical means (Chapter 5), but there is good evidence that it occurs at certain nerve junctions in invertebrates, and recent evidence suggests that it occurs in the ciliary ganglion of the chicken. Figure 3.6b is a diagrammatic representation of an ephaptic junction and shows how the spike of one cell provides a local circuit current which flows into the other cell where it initiates a propagating action potential. Such an arrangement may occur between the medial giant fibre of the crayfish nerve cord and the giant motor fibre. Ephaptic transmission may also play a part in conduction of the excitation wave from cell to cell in some smooth muscles (see Chapter 7) and some research workers believe that the intercalated discs of vertebrate cardiac muscle (page 210) are ephaptic junctions. The large action currents produced in mammalian skeletal muscle by synchronous stimulation of all of the constituent cells may ephaptically back-excite the nerve endings.

It is also possible for one cell to inhibit the activity of an adjacent cell through an ephaptic junction. A specifically inhibitory ephaptic junction occurs in the brains of fish between afferent fibres and the giant neurone or Mauthner cell. The complex anatomical arrangement and electrical properties of the fine afferent nerve endings allow them, when active, to become briefly positive with respect to the axon hillock of the Mauthner cell. Thus they act like an anode applied to the Mauthner cell and therefore inhibit any activity occurring in it.

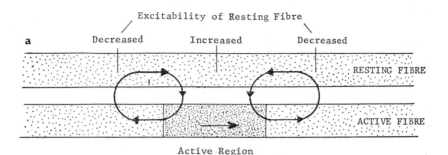

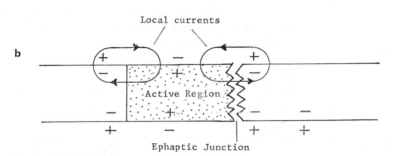

FIG. 3.6. (*a*) Excitability changes in a resting fibre produced by local currents flowing in a neighbouring active fibre. (*b*) Diagram of an ephaptic junction showing how the local current in an active cell flows into the post-junctional cell to initiate a propagating action potential (after Grundfest). This type of transmission can only occur when the adjacent area of the post-junctional cell membrane makes amplification unnecessary (see page. 137).

The effects of electric currents on nerve

(1) CATHODAL POLARIZATION. When a constant cathodal current of sufficient strength is first applied to a nerve, the membrane becomes depolarized and an action potential is initiated. However, vertebrate nerves do not continue to discharge repetitively during a constant application of current. As already described, depolarization initially acts to increase sodium permeability which therefore boosts the depolarization, but then the opposite occurs and sodium

permeability is reduced while potassium permeability is increased over its resting value. These delayed effects increase the threshold and oppose further excitation; they persist for a short time after removing the stimulus and give rise to *post-cathodal depression*.

When the strength of the current is made to increase slowly from a sub-threshold value, it is found that the strength of the stimulus required to excite the nerve is much greater than that necessary when its intensity is made to rise abruptly. This phenomenon is called *accommodation* and is explained by the increase in threshold almost keeping pace with the rise in current intensity. Motor nerves show the property of accommodation to a greater extent than sensory nerves. When the intensity of a cathodal current is made to rise very slowly, the increase in threshold may completely keep pace with the depolarization so that the nerve is not stimulated at all.

When a cathodal current too weak to excite is kept constant and continuously applied to part of a nerve, excitability is initially raised as the membrane is depolarized towards the critical firing level. Consequently, superimposed *brief* cathodal shocks, or other forms of stimulation, are then effective at a lower intensity. Action potentials travelling through a depolarized region are smaller in amplitude than normal because of the background depolarization already present. Eventually excitability is reduced on account of the threshold-raising mechanism already outlined and this occurs sooner or later depending upon the strength of the applied cathodal current. Conduction is blocked as soon as the threshold in the depolarized region is increased to the extent that the local circuit currents flowing ahead of the impulse in the normal region no longer excite the depolarized region. This *cathodal block* or *block by depolarization* is analogous to the block produced in excitable cells by some of the drugs described in later chapters. Strong evidence that the blocking effect of a drug is due to long-lasting depolarization may be obtained if it is shown to be reversed by anodal (hyperpolarizing) currents.

(2) ANODAL POLARIZATION. The passing of a continuous anodal current augments the membrane potential and the membrane becomes hyperpolarized and more stable. In the hyperpolarized region, a stronger stimulus is therefore required to depolarize the membrane to the critical level at which sodium permeability becomes rapidly increased. Action potentials travelling through a hyperpolarized region are larger in amplitude than normal and the after-potentials are exaggerated. Anodal block occurs if the increase in threshold is such that the local circuit currents produced by the normal length of nerve are too weak to depolarize the hyperpolarized region to the critical level for excitation.

Several pharmacological agents have been shown to cause hyperpolarization of the cell membranes of isolated nerves; among them are dyflos, adrenaline, 8-hydroxyquinoline and urethane. It is not suggested, however, that the main pharmacological effect of these agents necessarily depends upon this property as the concentration necessary to produce this effect is critical.

The effects of inorganic cations on nerve cell membranes. Physiological salt solutions (pages 4–7), like body fluids, contain the cations, sodium, potassium, calcium and sometimes magnesium. They are made isotonic with extra-cellular fluids of the body and adjusted to an optimal pH value; some of the anions present (e.g. bicarbonate and phosphate) serve to buffer the solution. In addition, they contain glucose and are bubbled with oxygen so that energy-yielding oxidative metabolic processes may continue. The concentrations of the ingredients of the physiological bathing solutions have mostly been determined empirically. That is, the particular solution used for a certain tissue is that in which the tissue happens to work best. However, a consideration of some of the effects of various cations indicates reasons for their presence in artificial media.

(1) SODIUM IONS. If the concentration of sodium ions is reduced, isotonicity being maintained by another ion such as choline, the amplitude of the action potential is reduced and its rate of rise is slowed. When all the sodium is removed, the resting membrane potential is adequately maintained but the cell is incapable of conducting an action potential. These effects would be expected from the previous account of the resting and action potentials; in fact, this observation forms part of the evidence in support of the theories about these potentials. Lithium appears to be the only cation capable of substituting for sodium in mammalian tissues, although barium ions have been found effective in crustacean muscle fibres, and certain quaternary ammonium ions, such as tetra-ethylammonium, can replace it in frog nerve and muscle fibres. These cations are not normally present in body fluids and it is a coincidence that their structures resemble that of the sodium ion sufficiently to enable them to penetrate some membranes.

(2) POTASSIUM IONS. The relationship between resting membrane potential and distribution of potassium ions across the membrane has already been described (page 74). Excess extracellular potassium depolarizes the membrane and may therefore stimulate or block the tissue according to the conditions. A small amount of extra potassium in the bathing fluid moves the resting membrane potential nearer to the firing level and therefore the threshold is initially lowered. Consequently, a weaker electrical stimulus or a smaller concentration of any drug which acts by depolarizing the membrane excites the tissue. However, prolonged immersion of the tissue in such a fluid eventually results

in a lowered excitability and block of conduction. The sustained depolarization leads to a type of block which is analogous to that already described for cathodal electric currents. Depolarization block occurs sooner, the greater the concentration of potassium ion. In physiological and pharmacological experiments, muscles are occasionally bathed in solutions containing high potassium concentrations in an attempt to remove the membrane potential and examine the effects of drugs on the contractile mechanism itself.

If a large excess of potassium ion is added to a tissue in a physiological salt solution, parts of the cell membranes are suddenly depolarized and action potentials are initiated. Uniform penetration does not occur as the connective tissue and Schwann cell diffusion barriers are uneven, and depolarization occurs in localized areas, thereby initiating repetitive discharges. Providing the tissue is washed with normal solution and time is allowed for re-equilibration, the stimulant effect of excess potassium ion may be repeatedly demonstrated.

(3) CALCIUM AND MAGNESIUM IONS. Calcium ions, which are present in all body fluids, have important effects on the excitability of cell membranes although their mechanism of action is not understood. Excess calcium ions raise the critical level of depolarization at which sodium permeability is increased, and therefore reduce excitability. A lowered calcium ion concentration has the opposite effect and increases excitability. If the calcium ion concentration outside nerve fibres is reduced, for example by chelation with citrate, excitability may be raised to the extent that action currents flowing in neighbouring fibres ephaptically stimulate them. When the calcium concentration is very low, the critical membrane potential at which sodium permeability is increased may come to equal the resting membrane potential and the nerve may begin to initiate repetitive action potentials in the absence of other forms of stimulation. This effect does not continue indefinitely; in the absence of calcium, the nerve gradually becomes inexcitable and conduction eventually fails completely. The effect of an *excess* calcium ion concentration is to stabilize the membrane so that stronger stimuli are required to excite it, but the resting membrane potential is not affected unless very large concentrations are used. In their actions on membranes, magnesium ions behave similarly to calcium ions but less powerfully.

However, calcium and magnesium ions are antagonistic to each other in their actions on transmitter release at cholinergic and adrenergic junctions, on the release of secretions from glands, and on excitation-contraction coupling and contractile mechanisms in muscle.

There are several drugs which, like excess calcium or magnesium ion, produce membrane stabilization. Among these are local anaesthetics, some general anaesthetics and alcohol. Drugs with the opposite type of action are known as *membrane labilizers*, and they produce effects like calcium lack. With these drugs also, resting membrane potential is unaffected, but the amount of depolarization necessary to increase sodium permeability is reduced so that excitability is increased. Membrane labilizers include substances such as veratrum alkaloids, calcium complexing agents, and calcium precipitants.

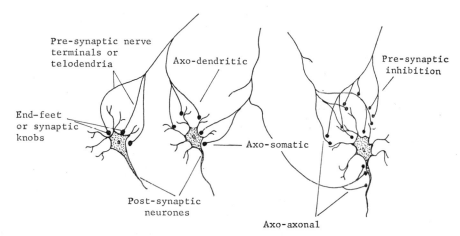

FIG. 3.7. Diagram of the various types of synapses between pre-synaptic nerve endings and the dendrites, cell body or axon of post-synaptic cells. The area of the post-synaptic cell membrane is much larger than that of the fine nerve endings in these types of junction (contrast Fig. 3.6(*b*)) and transmission requires a chemical amplification process.

Synapse and neuro-effector junction. The junction between two nerve cells is called a synapse, a term first used by Sherrington. The term synapse is also often used to describe the junction between a motor nerve fibre and a muscle or gland. However, 'neuro-effector junction' is a more appropriate description and the term synapse should be restricted to the junction between two neurones. In vertebrates there is no continuity of nervous tissue from one neurone to another or from a neurone to a muscle or gland cell and transmission of impulses is therefore across a gap. Near their endings, axons branch many times and the branches lose their myelin and other sheaths. At synapses, the fine naked branches, which frequently end in small swellings (the synaptic knobs, end-feet or *boutons terminaux*), make contact with the cell body (axosomatic), the dendrites (axodendritic) or the axon hillock (axo-axonal) of other neurones (Fig. 3.7). Transmission across a synapse is essentially in one direction only and is accompanied by a delay (synaptic delay) of the order of 0·5–3 msec in different synapses. A single fibre may make synaptic connections with many secondary neurones and similarly a single neurone may have pre-synaptic terminals from many axons impinging upon it. In the peripheral nervous system, the nerve impulses in the primary fibre are transmitted across the synaptic gap to initiate impulses in the secondary neurone. However, in the central nervous system, the nerve impulses in the primary neurone may serve to excite or to inhibit the secondary neurone. Synapses therefore act as valves, ensuring unidirectional transmission, and as relay and controlling stations. In the CNS, chains of neurones may be arranged in closed circuits which are self-re-exciting. Once activity is started in such circuits it may continue to reverberate around the loops for some time. Arrangements of this type may be the neuronal basis for some types of short-term learning and memory. The properties of synapses are described in more detail in Chapters 4 and 5 and neuro-effector junctions are discussed in Chapter 7.

In mammals, transmission of excitation at all synapses outside the central nervous system and at neuro-effector junctions is brought about chemically. Thus at peripheral synapses, the nerve impulse on reaching the pre-synaptic terminals causes the release of a chemical substance which diffuses across the minute gap to stimulate the post-synaptic cell and initiate nerve impulses in its axon. At neuro-effector junctions a chemical substance, released from the nerve endings, stimulates or inhibits the innervated muscle or gland. Although most research workers believe that transmission at central synapses is also chemical, the evidence for this is relatively scant and except in one case (the Renshaw cell, page 115) the identity of the central transmitters is unknown. Central transmitters in the CNS may excite or inhibit the post-synaptic neurone.

When an excitatory transmitter is released on to the cell body or dendrites of the secondary neurone at a synapse, it is believed to increase the ionic permeability of the receptive area of membrane. The post-synaptic membrane is therefore depolarized and a potential difference, known as the *excitatory post-synaptic potential* (EPSP) is set up between it and the rest of the neuronal membrane. The EPSP produced by a single pre-synaptic stimulus lasts for about 0·5 msec. It differs from an action potential in four ways: (1) it is a simple depolarization rather than a reversal in potential such as arises from a specific increase in sodium permeability; (2) it is a graded response and depends upon the amount of transmitter released; (3) it has no refractory period and therefore successive responses may summate; (4) it is non-propagated and quickly decays in intensity with distance from the receptive area. When the EPSP is large enough, or when it covers a great enough area of post-synaptic cell membrane, current flows into the depolarized area from the surrounding membrane and a self-propagating, all-or-nothing action potential is initiated and is conducted along the axon. An inhibitory transmitter has the opposite action and causes a localized hyperpolarization of the cell membrane known as the *inhibitory post-synaptic potential* (IPSP). According to Eccles, this is brought about by the inhibitory transmitter selectively increasing the permeability of the post-synaptic membrane to potassium and chloride ions. Hyperpolarization makes the cell less excitable by excitatory (depolarizing) transmitters and inhibits any activity of the cell already occurring. Similar effects occur at neuro-effector junctions, excitation of the muscle or gland cell being produced by depolarizing transmitters and inhibition by hyperpolarizing transmitters. An additional type of inhibitory synapse is present in the CNS. In these, synaptic contact is made between the axon terminals of two neurones as illustrated in Fig. 3.7. Inhibition of the excitatory neurone occurs when the other neurone releases its transmitter. This transmitter depolarizes the nerve endings of the excitatory neurone and therefore diminishes the size of action potentials travelling in them. The smaller action potentials cause a reduced release of excitatory chemical transmitter onto the post-synaptic cell. This type of inhibition is known as *pre-synaptic inhibition*. The evidence supporting chemical transmission and the identity and mechanisms of action of the transmitters are described in Chapters 5 and 7.

Many classes of drugs produce their characteristic effects either directly or indirectly by altering the electrical properties of the membranes of excitable cells. The chemical transmitters released from nerve endings themselves act in this way, and many drugs are believed to produce their effects by altering the release, synthesis or storage of the chemical transmitters, or by mimicking, potentiating or blocking their actions. Alternatively, drugs may affect the cell membrane at a site not acted upon by the natural chemical transmitters. The precise mechanisms of action of the large number of drugs which act on the CNS is not fully understood but it seems likely that most of these also act by altering the electrical properties of neurones. Further understanding of these drugs will probably be gained when the identity of the chemical transmitters at central synapses is discovered.

CHAPTER 4

The Nervous System

The nervous system is the main co-ordinator of body functions, being responsible for consciousness, behaviour, memory, recognition, learning and for the most highly developed attributes of man such as imagination, abstract reasoning and creative thought. The brain has been a favourite topic for philosophers. Descartes in his *Discourse on Method* wrote:

> All this I explained in the treatise it had once been my intention to publish....
> I had also shown what must occur in the brain to cause wakefulness, sleep and dreams; how, through the senses, it received the ideas of light, sound, smell, taste and warmth, and indeed of all the other qualities of external objects; how it is affected by hunger, thirst and the other internal feelings, and what there is in it which must be regarded as the common sense which receives all these ideas. [Common sense to Descartes was the co-ordination of all internal and external sensations.] Then there was the memory which preserved these ideas and the imagination which could change them in different ways and make up new ones, and which could, as the animal spirits are distributed through the muscles, cause the limbs of the body to move in as many different ways, according to the variety of sense perception and internal feelings, as our bodies can move automatically without the intervention of the will.

An understanding of the nervous system is important to the pharmacologist since its functions may be modified by drugs. Many drugs are used for their action on the nervous system, but some which act chiefly on other organs may produce side-effects by acting on the brain.

The central nervous system (CNS) consists of two parts—the brain lying within the skull and the spinal cord lying within the vertebral canal. In man, the CNS is composed of more than ten thousand million interconnecting neurones, all of which are formed before birth and none of which, if injured, is ever replaced. In addition to the neurones, there are a large number of cells of non-nervous origin which are collectively referred to as *neuroglial cells*. These are of three types: (1) *Astrocytes* are cells with many slender processes which are scattered throughout the CNS, particularly among the nerve cell bodies. Some of the processes are in contact with neurones and some are applied to the walls of capillary blood vessels. These cells are believed to be concerned with the transport of metabolites between the neurones and the blood-stream.

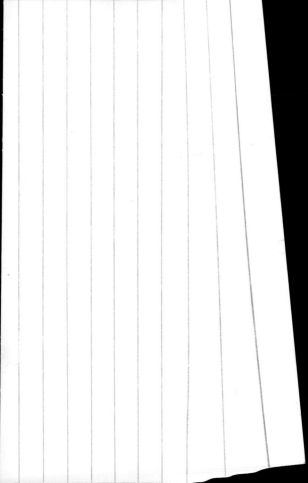

(2) *Oligodendrocytes* lie in rows between the nerve fibres and are believed to be concerned with the formation of myelin, like the Schwann cells of the peripheral nerve fibres. (3) *Microglia* are a type of wandering macrophage peculiar to the CNS. The CNS is richly supplied with blood vessels and, like their counterparts in peripheral tissues, the microglia may pass in and out of the capillaries in performing their scavenging function.

Many students are disconcerted by the confusing nomenclature used to describe parts of the CNS. This has arisen largely because the early anatomists were unaware of the functional significance of what they observed. All of the structures in the CNS consist simply of nerve cell bodies and neuroglia and their processes and the various terms therefore apply to different arrangements of these. Frequently, the name for a part of the brain was chosen when it was found that the gross shape of a group of neurones resembled that of some other object. For example, the *hippocampus* is a C-shaped mass of nerve cells with a fancied resemblance to a sea-horse. Confusion may also arise from the different terms that are used to describe similar structures in different parts of the CNS. For example, a group of associated nerve cell bodies, invariably described as a ganglion in the peripheral nervous system, may be referred to as a *ganglion*, a *nucleus* or simply as a *body* or *corpus* in the CNS. Groups of nerve fibres running together in a bundle may be called by any of a variety of names including a *column*, a *tract*, a *fasciculus* (a little bundle), a *funiculus* (a little cord) or, if they form a prominent stalk-like structure to a larger mass, a *peduncle* (a little foot).

The peripheral nervous system consists of twelve pairs of nerves which leave the brain stem (the cranial nerves) and thirty-one pairs which leave the spinal cord (the spinal nerves): these nerves serve all parts of the body. Each of the sixty-two spinal nerves arises from the spinal cord by two roots (Fig. 4.1); the *posterior, dorsal* or *sensory root* consists of *afferent* fibres which conduct nerve impulses towards the CNS, while the *anterior, ventral* or *motor root* is occupied by *efferent* fibres which conduct impulses from the CNS to the tissues. Each afferent fibre in the spinal nerves has its cell body outside the spinal cord in a *posterior* (or *dorsal*) *root ganglion*.

The cranial nerves differ from the spinal nerves in that they do not arise by such regular motor and sensory roots. The cranial nerves are denoted by numbers as well as names. Three of them are the afferent nerves for the special senses of smell (*olfactory*, I), sight (*optic*, II) and hearing (*auditory* or *stato-acoustic*, VIII). The VIIIth nerve also contains fibres from the organs of balance in the ears. Another three, the *oculomotor* (III), the *trochlear* (IV) and the *abducens* (VI, sometimes called the pathetic) are motor nerves supplying the muscles which move the eye-ball and alter the size of the pupil and the curvature of the lens. The *trigeminal* (V) consists of afferent fibres from the face and teeth, and of efferent fibres to the muscles concerned in mastication. The *facial* nerve (VII) is an efferent nerve supplying those muscles which alter the expression of the face, and the *hypoglossal* nerve (XII) is the efferent nerve to the tongue. The remaining cranial nerves—the *glossopharyngeal* (IX), the *vagus* (X) and the *accessory* (XI)—contain a mixture of

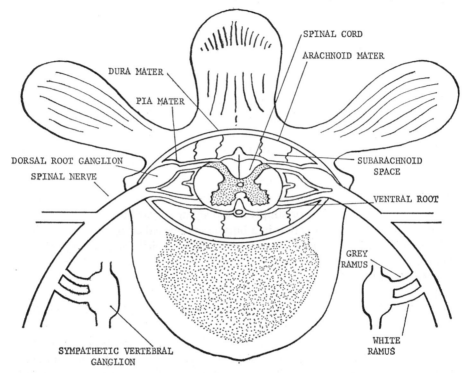

Fig. 4.1. Diagrammatic transverse section of the spine at the level of the thoracic vertebrae to show the arrangement of the spinal cord within the spinal column.

afferent and efferent fibres and form part of the nerve supply to the pharynx, the oesophagus, the larynx, the heart, the lungs and the abdominal organs.

The nervous system may also be divided into two anatomical and functional components, each made up of a central and a peripheral part and each consisting of both afferent and efferent fibres. These two components are: (i) the *somatic* or *cerebro-spinal* nervous system, which is concerned with the control of striated muscles; and (ii) the *autonomic* or *visceral* nervous system, which is mainly concerned with the regulation of the activity of the heart, the blood vessels, the alimentary canal, the bladder and the genitals. Although it is often convenient to think of these two as separate nervous systems, they are, in fact, closely interrelated and many body functions involve integrated activity of both.

The basic activity of the nervous system, through which it regulates the functioning of the body, depends on a mechanism of 'feed-back' control. Afferent nerves bring to the appropriate part of the CNS 'information' about the external world from sensory receptors sensitive to light, sound, smell, taste, temperature, touch, pressure and pain, distension in viscera, pressure in blood vessels, CO_2 level in blood and tension in muscles. The information is integrated in the CNS and results in 'instructions' being sent out along the efferent nerves. The instructions produce appropriate movements of muscles and secretions of glands, and these changes alter the information sent back to the CNS. Hence information and instructions constitute a feed-back control mechanism; they are coded into nerve impulses which vary in frequency and pattern according to the intensity of the sensory stimulus and the degree of activity required of the muscle or gland. During wakefulness, the brain is subjected to myriad patterns of nervous activity arriving from the periphery and from the internal organs, and these patterns are received, analysed and often stored by the appropriate group of central neurones. In a sense, therefore, the CNS behaves like an extremely complex computer which, after receiving its precisely coded information, feeds its results back into a control system.

Man's knowledge of the external world is limited to those objects and events which possess the necessary type of energy to excite his sense organs. The quality of a sensation depends upon the parts of the brain reached by the sensory nerve impulses. If, for example, the nerve fibres from the taste-buds in the tongue were cut and in some way grafted onto the nerve fibres leading from the ear to the part of the brain dealing with sound, the pattern of nerve impulses initiated from the taste-buds by applying acid to the tongue would be interpreted as sound, not as taste. The effects of numerous other 'cross-innervations' have been studied with nerves which are able to regenerate after being cut. Some examples have been produced experimentally in animals, or observed in man as an aftermath to surgery or disease. Cross-connection between the closely packed neurones within the CNS may be responsible for some types of hallucination.

Anatomy of the CNS

The nervous system, like the skin, is developed from the ectoderm of the embryo. A groove appears down the midline of the dorsal surface and this closes over to form the *neural tube* which becomes expanded at the head end into three dilatations: the fore-brain vesicle or *prosencephalon*, the mid-brain vesicle or *mesencephalon*, and the hind-brain vesicle or *rhombencephalon*. The remainder of the neural tube forms the spinal cord.

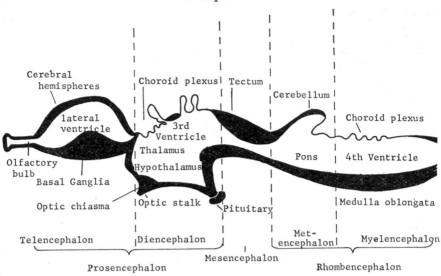

Fig. 4.2. The embryonic divisions of the brain.

The fore-brain vesicle becomes further divided to form (i) the *telencephalon* (the end-brain), which eventually develops into the *cerebral hemispheres* including the *rhinencephalon* (the 'nose-brain') and the *basal ganglia*, and (ii) the *diencephalon* (the 'between' brain) which forms the *thalamus* and the *hypothalamus* and is associated with the outgrowth of the optic nerve and the retina. The mid-brain vesicle forms the *corpora quadrigemina* and the *cerebral peduncle*. Further development of the hind-brain vesicle forms the *metencephalon*, which becomes the *cerebellum* and the *pons*, and the *myelencephalon* or *medulla oblongata*. The hollow centre of the neural tube persists as the inter-communicating ventricles of the brain and the spinal canal. The embryonic divisions of the CNS are illustrated in Fig. 4.2, and Figs. 4.3 and 4.4 illustrate the main parts of the mature brain and spinal cord. The peripheral nerves grow out from the brain stem and spinal cord and, in some way which is not yet understood, are attracted towards the tissue they eventually innervate. All nerve fibres are initially without a myelin sheath and the onset of their functional activity coincides with the laying down of myelin. In mammals, the maximal degree of myelination in the cerebral cortex does not occur until the completion of post-natal growth (i.e. about the age of 17 years in man).

Parts of the CNS

(1) **The spinal cord.** The spinal cord in man is about 45 cm long and extends from the base of the skull, where it is continuous with the brain stem, to the

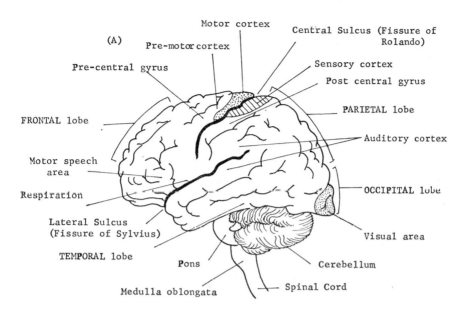

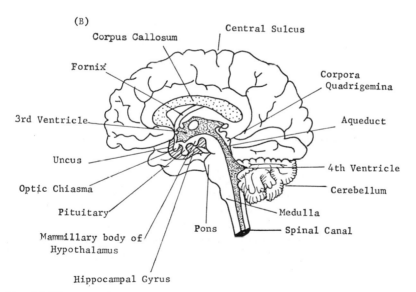

FIG. 4.3. The mature human brain viewed from the left side, (A) showing the surface, and (B) after medial longitudinal section.

level of the second lumbar vertebra. Over most of its length it is about 0·75 cm thick but there are enlargements in the neck and lumbar regions where the nerve supplies to the limbs arise. A transverse section of the cord reveals white matter almost surrounding an H-shaped mass of grey matter with the fine spinal canal in the centre (Figs. 4.1 and 4.4). The white matter is mainly nerve fibres of both myelinated and non-myelinated types grouped into 'ascending' and 'descending' tracts. Fibres in the ascending tracts convey sensory impulses to higher centres in the cord or brain. The terms used to

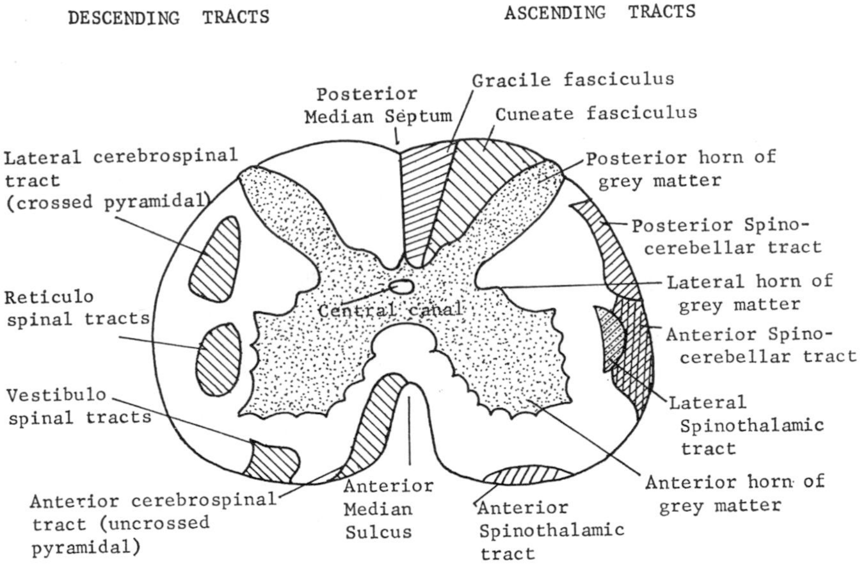

FIG. 4.4. Diagrammatic transverse section of the spinal cord in the thoracic region: for convenience, descending tracts are shown on the left, and ascending tracts on the right.

describe the direction of passage of nerve impulses in ascending fibres are *cranial, cephalic* or *rostral* (literally, towards the skull, head or beak). Fibres in the descending tracts convey impulses *caudally* (towards the tail) to lower centres in the cord. At various levels in the cord, some of the fibres of the white matter enter the grey matter where they synapse with other neurones. Figure 4.4 is a diagrammatic section through the cord in the thoracic region to show the position of the main tracts. The grey matter consists chiefly of nerve cell bodies, dendrons, and non-myelinated fibres. The synapses made by peripheral sensory nerve fibres with neurones of the ascending tracts of sensory fibres are in the posterior horns of grey matter. Some synaptic connections are made with interneurones; these are short fibres which begin and end within the grey matter and which connect sensory and motor neurones within the cord itself. The cell bodies in the anterior horns of grey matter are mainly those of the motor fibres which innervate skeletal muscles and the muscle spindles (see page 107): the cell bodies in the lateral horns of grey matter give rise to the pre-ganglionic fibres of the autonomic nervous system.

(2) **The medulla oblongata.** This region of the brain is continuous with the spinal cord (Figs. 4.3 and 4.5). Its grey matter contains a complex network of cell bodies and interlacing fibres which form part of the *brain stem reticular formation* (page 133). The medulla contains various important groups of synapses which are concerned with the reflex control of blood pressure (vasomotor centre), heart rate and force (cardiac centre), respiration (respiratory centre), vomiting (vomiting centre) and temperature. It also contains two groups of synapses, known as the *vestibular nuclei* (Fig. 4.5) which form relay stations for various fibres concerned with the equilibrium of the body. The white matter of the medulla is mainly a pathway for fibres conveying impulses to and from higher centres of the brain. The neural canal is expanded in the medulla into the diamond-shaped *fourth ventricle* (Figs. 4.3 and 4.5). The VIIIth to the XIIth cranial nerves leave the brain at the level of the medulla.

(3) **The pons.** The pons lies on the floor of the fourth ventricle and is mainly a pathway for ascending and descending tracts of fibres (Figs. 4.3 and 4.5). Descending fibres from the cerebral cortex synapse in the pons with neurones which enter the cerebellum. The reticular formation of the brain stem is also present in the grey matter of the pons. The Vth, VIth and VIIth cranial nerves leave the brain in this region.

(4) **The cerebellum.** The cerebellum lies on the dorsal side of the hind-brain (Figs. 4.3 and 4.5) and is attached to the brain stem by its peduncles which are formed of prominent tracts of nerve fibres. It has a folded outer layer of grey matter or *cortex*, and several small groups of ganglia are contained in the centrally placed white matter. The cerebellum forms part of the feed-back mechanisms concerned with the subconscious control of equilibrium, posture and movement.

(5) **The mid-brain.** This is a short segment largely concealed by the overhanging cerebral hemispheres (Fig. 4.5). The neural canal becomes narrow as it runs through the mid-brain and this segment of it is known as the *aqueduct*. The roof of the aqueduct has two pairs of rounded bodies known as the *corpora quadrigemina* or *colliculi*. The *superior colliculi* contain relay stations for fibres concerned with vision and the *inferior colliculi* are concerned with hearing.

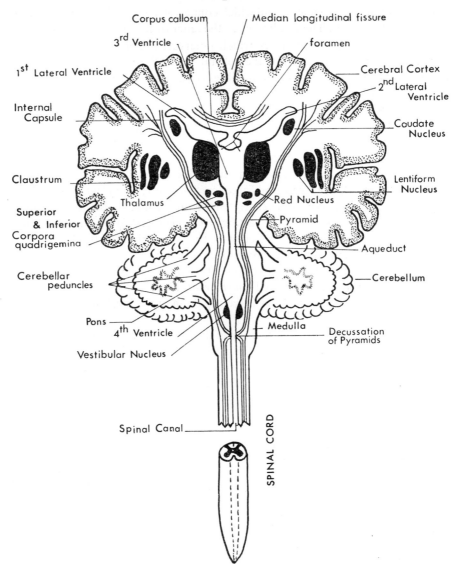

FIG. 4.5. Diagrammatic coronal section of the brain and spinal cord.

The two *red nuclei* and some melanin-pigmented grey matter known as the *substantia nigra* are also situated in the mid-brain. These form part of the extra-pyramidal system which is concerned with the control of skeletal muscle movement and tone. The cerebral penduncles occupy the ventral aspect of the mid-brain. The IIIrd and IVth cranial nerves leave the brain in this region.

(6) **The hypothalamus.** In this region the neural canal expands to form the third ventricle (Fig. 4.3 and 4.5) and the hypothalamus comprises its floor and part of its lateral walls. The hypothalamus is connected to an endocrine gland, the pituitary body (page 360), by a narrow stem, the infundibulum. The most important sub-cortical groups of cell bodies controlling the autonomic nervous system are situated in the hypothalamus. The hypothalamus also controls body temperature and, through its complex connections with other parts of the CNS, influences appetite, behaviour and sleep.

(7) **The thalamus.** The thalamus consists of right and left ovoid masses flanking the third ventricle (Fig. 4.5). It was once thought to be concerned mainly with vision and was then known as the optic thalamus. It is now known that, with the possible exception of impulses conveying the sense of smell, all sensory impulses from the surface of the body are conveyed to the thalamus. From there, most sensations are relayed on to the cerebral cortex, although the thalamus seems to be responsible for the conscious appreciation of pain. In birds, the thalamus is the highest sensory centre. The grey matter of the thalamus contains another complex network of nerve cells and fibres known as the *thalamic reticular formation.*

(8) **The cerebrum.** The cerebrum is by far the largest part of the brain of mammals and almost fills the skull (Figs. 4.3 and 4.5). It is incompletely separated into two halves, the *cerebral hemispheres,* by a median longitudinal fissure. At the bottom of the fissure, a band of fibres known as the *corpus callosum* bridges the two hemispheres. The outer layer of the cerebral hemispheres is composed of grey matter and is known as the *cerebral cortex.* Beneath this are the tracts of fibres comprising the white matter as well as numerous clumps of grey matter. The ventricles of the cerebrum are the *first and second lateral ventricles,* each of which communicates with the third ventricle via a narrow *intra-ventricular foramen.*

The deeper grey matter of the cerebral hemispheres is grouped into several masses which lie between the tracts of white fibres along the walls of the lateral ventricles. The more important masses of grey matter in each hemisphere are as follows: (i) *The corpus striatum.* The fibres conveying impulses between each cortex and lower centres in the CNS form narrow strips of white matter, known as the *internal capsules.* Each internal capsule divides the corpus striatum into a *caudate nucleus* and a *lentiform nucleus.* These nuclei are part of the extra-pyramidal system controlling muscular movement. (ii) The *claustrum* is a thin shield of grey matter lying between the lentiform nucleus and the cortex. (iii) The *amygdaloid nucleus* is a small globular mass of grey matter lying at the top of the lateral ventricle. The corpus striatum, the claustrum and the amygdaloid nucleus are collectively known as the *basal ganglia*. (iv) The *hippocampus* is a mass of grey matter lying close to the lateral ventricle. It is connected by a tract of fibres known as the *fornix* to the *mammillary bodies* in the hypothalamus. The hippocampus contains many large pyramidal cells like those in the motor cortex.

The hippocampus, the fornix, the amygdaloid nucleus, and those parts of the cortex of the rhinencephalon known as the *hippocampal gyrus* and the *uncus* are collectively referred to as the *limbic (border) system*; this system is believed to be concerned with the conscious experience of emotion.

THE CEREBRAL CORTEX. The outer layer of grey matter which covers each hemisphere varies in thickness from about 1·5 to 4·5 mm. It consists of closely packed cell bodies, dendrons, and synaptic terminals. The surface of the hemispheres is convoluted into ridges called *gyri*, and furrows called *fissures* or *sulci*. Each hemisphere is a continuous mass of nervous tissue but for descriptive purposes it is divided into four lobes which are named according to the bones of the skull under which they lie (Fig. 4.3A). These are: (i) the *frontal lobe* containing the motor cortex, the pre-motor cortex, the motor speech area and centres concerned with the co-ordination of autonomic and somatic activity, (ii) the *parietal lobe* containing the projection areas of the sensory cortex, (iii) the *occipital lobe* containing the visual cortex, and (iv) the *temporal lobe* containing the auditory cortex. In the neighbourhood of these motor and sensory areas lie other areas known as *association areas* which act in conjunction with them. Large parts of the cortex are often called the *silent areas* as no apparent effect follows electrical stimulation of them. It now appears that the so-called silent areas function as a whole, their neurones providing the anatomical basis for such mental attributes as recognition, memory, intelligence, imagination and creative thought. There does not seem to be localization of function in the silent areas but progressive damage leads to progressive impairment.

The fibres of the cerebral cortex are classified as (i) *commissural fibres* which link corresponding regions of the two hemispheres (the corpus callosum consists of about ten million commissural fibres), (ii) *association fibres* which make connections between the grey matter in different areas of the same hemisphere, and (iii) *projection fibres* which convey impulses in either direction between the cortex and other parts of the CNS.

Membranes and cerebrospinal fluid

The brain and spinal cord are covered by three membranes or *meninges*; a thick outer one, the *dura mater*, and two inner ones, the *arachnoid mater* and the *pia mater*. Figure 4.1 illustrates their arrangement in the spinal cord. The pia mater is very vascular and is closely applied to the outer surface of the brain and cord, while the arachnoid mater fits closely inside the dura. Inflammation of the membranes of the brain is called *meningitis* and usually affects the arachnoid and pia mater. The space between the arachnoid mater and the pia mater is known as the *sub-arachnoid space*. The fourth ventricle of the brain communicates with the sub-arachnoid space through three small channels.

The ventricles of the brain, the narrow spinal canal and the sub-arachnoid space are filled with *cerebrospinal fluid* (CSF). CSF therefore bathes both inner and outer surfaces of the brain and cord. It is a colourless liquid containing a few lymphocytes and is similar in composition to plasma but with a slightly different ionic composition and less protein. Most of the components of CSF are secreted by the vascular plexuses (the choroid plexuses) lining the ventricles, but some simply enter it by diffusion from the blood vessels. CSF is secreted at the rate of 50–400 ml/day. After circulating inside the brain and cord, the CSF escapes to the sub-arachnoid space and is finally reabsorbed into the venous blood leaving the cranium. The pressure of the CSF is usually equivalent to about 10 cm of water when lying down and to about 30 cm of water when sitting up. By variations in volume, the CSF serves to keep the intracranial pressure relatively constant. For example, if the blood content of the brain increases, there is a corresponding decrease in the amount of CSF. The CSF gives buoyancy to the brain inside the skull, and this fluid also acts as a shock absorber during head movement.

Each pair of spinal nerves passes out of the cord between different vertebrae. During growth, the lengthening of the cord fails to keep pace with the lengthening of the vertebral column with the result that, in adult man, the cord ends between the first and second lumbar vertebrae. Below the second lumbar vertebra, the spinal column contains only sub-arachnoid space and spinal nerves. This region therefore provides a convenient and safe place for making a lumbar puncture to obtain samples of CSF or to give intra-spinal injections. Another, although less safe, place from which CSF may be obtained is the *cisterna*, which is the angle between the cerebellum and the brain stem. A cisternal puncture is made between the occipital bone and the atlas.

Blood supply and blood-brain barrier

Nerve cells live for only a very short time without oxygen, and the CNS, particularly the grey matter, is richly supplied with blood vessels. Although the brain accounts for only 2% of the body weight, it receives nearly 17% of the total cardiac output and consumes 20% of the oxygen used by the whole body at rest. The brain is supplied by the two *internal carotid* and the two *vertebral arteries,* and the spinal cord by a single *anterior* and two *posterior spinal arteries.* All of the venous return from the CNS eventually drains into the superior vena cava.

The existence in the CNS of a mechanism capable of excluding many substances carried in the blood-stream has been realized ever since 1885 when Ehrlich showed that certain aniline dyes (e.g. trypan blue), injected into the blood-stream of animals, stained all the tissues of the body with the exception of the CNS and the CSF. This mechanism is generally referred to as '*the blood-brain barrier*' although it is unlikely that it consists of a single anatomical structure. It probably involves complex anatomical, physical and metabolic phenomena; which of these is effective in a particular instance depends upon the physico-chemical properties of the substance concerned. The barrier is selective: some substances such as water, glucose and sodium chloride readily penetrate it, while others, such as sodium nitrite, sodium iodide, sucrose and bile pigment do so with difficulty or not at all. Furthermore, some substances may penetrate into certain regions of the CNS but not into others. From a pharmacological point of view, the barrier is important since some drugs readily penetrate it while others do not. It should be realized, however, that some drugs which do not normally penetrate to the CNS may do so in disease.

Feldberg and his colleagues have recently developed a technique for inserting a cannula through the skull of cats so that its tip is placed in a lateral ventricle. The cannula may be left in position without discomfort to the cat and injections may therefore be made straight into the CSF of the conscious animal. The method provides a means of localizing the action of drugs to particular areas of the brain. Several drugs which do not penetrate the barrier from the blood-stream have been shown to produce pronounced effects when injected in this way. The barrier for such drugs is therefore probably located between the capillary or choroidal epithelium and the actual nervous tissue. However, other drugs do not penetrate the nervous tissue even when injected into the CSF. The cells of the CNS are very closely packed and the extracellular space is therefore extremely small so that free diffusion is difficult. It may be that the absence of penetration by some drugs, even from the CSF, is a consequence of the inability of carrier mechanisms (possibly involving the astrocytes) to transport them. In the tracts of white matter, the myelin sheaths may form yet another barrier to substances which are not lipid-soluble.

Sensory nerves

The peripheral sensory nerves are afferent nerves which conduct impulses towards the CNS from the sense organs or receptors in the tissues which are adapted to respond to different stimuli. The sensory nerve fibres in the peripheral nerves, which may be myelinated or non-myelinated, are called the *first-order sensory neurones*. The sensory input is classified as (i) *exteroceptive* when it originates in the skin or in the special sense organs for vision, hearing, smell and taste, (ii) *proprioceptive* when it originates in the muscles or joints or in the organs of balance in the ears, and (iii) *interoceptive* when it comes from the blood vessels and viscera such as the heart, the lungs and the gut. The interoceptive sensory system is responsible for the reflex control of the involuntary organs of the body. For example, receptors in the blood vessels and heart, sensitive to changes in pressure, osmotic pressure or CO_2 tension, bring about reflex adjustments of the circulatory and respiratory systems and usually operate below the level of consciousness. The reflexes served by interoceptive sensory nerves are dealt with later in the relevant chapters. Here, interoceptive nerves are considered only in so far as they convey impulses which give rise to the conscious experience of visceral pain.

Most of the sensory nerve fibres from the neck, trunk and limbs run in the spinal nerves. Their cell bodies lie outside the cord, but within the vertebral canal, in the dorsal root ganglia. They enter the cord by way of the dorsal roots (Fig. 4.1). The sensory nerve fibres from the face and from some of the viscera enter the brain stem in some of the cranial nerves.

Exteroceptive sensory system. The special senses of sight, hearing, smell and taste are discussed in Chapter 16; only the cutaneous sensations are considered here. The skin and subcutaneous layers contain large numbers of nerve endings organized into receptors which are stimulated by touch, pressure, pain, heat and cold. Itching may be a separate sensation or may be a combination of others. All other skin sensations are really combinations of these basic sensations. For example, 'wetness' is pressure plus cold, moisture itself not being necessary. This may be demonstrated by first covering the finger with a thin rubber sheath to protect it from moisture and then dipping the finger into water when the sensation of wetness is experienced. Variations in the degree of sensation arise from differences in the number of sensory receptors stimulated and in the frequency of nerve impulses discharged from them. The peripheral ends of sensory nerves terminate in a number of ways. Some are encased in fibrous capsules while others ramify as exposed, non-myelinated endings

4*

between the cells of the skin. The older histologists described distinct varieties of organized endings and classified them into touch receptors, cold receptors, pain receptors and so on. However, more recent work has shown that it is impossible to correlate a particular sense modality with a particular type of receptor.

The sensory stimulus in some way generates a local depolarization of the membrane of the nerve endings forming the receptor. This local potential resembles the synaptic potential described in Chapters 3 and 5. When it reaches a critical level, it initiates propagated action potentials which travel along the fibre to the CNS. After entering the spinal cord via the posterior roots, the first-order neurones branch and end in various ways. Some branches synapse with interneurones which in turn connect with the motoneurones innervating skeletal muscles. These provide the anatomical basis for the poly-synaptic spinal reflexes described later. Other branches synapse at different levels with *second-order neurones*, most of which, after crossing to the opposite side of the cord (sensory decussation), end in the thalamus. A few of the second-order neurones conveying the sensations of delicate touch and pressure remain on the same side of the cord and end in the cerebellum. Figure 4.4 illustrates a cross-section of the spinal cord and gives the names of the main ascending columns. At the level of the pons, the ascending second-order neurones are joined by the second-order neurones carrying sensory impulses from the face.

The thalamus receives impulses conveying all skin sensations. The sensation of pain is not experienced as a result of stimulation of the cerebral cortex and it is therefore believed that the thalamus is the area responsible for the perception of pain. From the thalamus, all skin sensations other than pain are relayed by *third-order neurones* to the parietal cortex. The parts of the body are repre-sented on the sensory cortex in inverted order, the feet above and the head below. As a result of the sensory decussation which occurs in the brain stem, most of the sensations from one side of the body are conveyed to the sensory cortex of the opposite side. Large areas of the parietal cortex appear to be concerned with correlating the sensory input with other events happening at the same time and with previously learned information. At this level of the brain, the nerve impulses may be passed into three-dimensional circuits of synapsing neurones which are self re-exciting so that impulses reverberate around them for some time.

Proprioceptive sensory system. Through the receptors and nerves of this system, the CNS receives information about movement and is able to appreciate the position of the body in relation to the force of gravity. Feed-back through this system enables the CNS to regulate movement and control posture auto-matically.

The proprioceptors are as follows:

(i) THE MUSCLE SPINDLES. These are embedded between, and parallel to, the fibres of voluntary muscles and consist of fibrous spindle-shaped capsules a few millimetres long containing several miniature contractile muscle fibres known as intrafusal fibres. They are supplied by fast-conducting myelinated *afferent* fibres and also by smaller myelinated motor fibres known as *fusimotor fibres* or *γ-efferents*. The muscle spindles are activated by stretch. Stretch, applied to a skeletal muscle, in turn stimulates the muscle spindles causing them to generate impulses which pass along the afferent nerves and enter the cord via the posterior roots. The sensitivity of the muscle spindles to stretch is greater when their intrafusal fibres are in a partially contracted state. This is brought about by the activity of the γ-efferents.

(ii) THE GOLGI TENDON ORGANS. These consist of a spiral winding of sensory nerve endings round the tendon fibres of skeletal muscles. They are also stimulated by stretch but their threshold is higher than that of the muscle spindles. The arrangement is such that both muscle stretch and muscle contraction result in stretch of the tendon organs.

(iii) DEEP CONNECTIVE TISSUE RECEPTORS. Encapsulated receptors, known as Paccinian corpuscles, and networks of fine naked fibres are found in the connective tissue of muscles, in the fascia around the joints and in the periosteum. These are activated by mechanical forces and convey to the CNS information about movement and position of joints. The pressure receptors found in the deeper layers of the skin are also Paccinian corpuscles.

(iv) THE VESTIBULAR SACS AND THE SEMI-CIRCULAR CANALS. These are the non-auditory parts of the labyrinths embedded within the skull. Their sensory fibres form the vestibular nerve which runs together with the cochlear nerve (page 429) to form the stato-acoustic or VIIIth cranial nerve. Information carried by these fibres to the CNS is the basis of awareness of the position and movement of the body. It is also fed back to muscles to maintain balance.

The semi-circular canals are sensitive to movement of the head (particularly rotation). There are three semi-circular canals on each side of the head, each being in a plane at right angles to the other two so that movement about any axis is detected. The receptor mechanism involves the displacement of a swinging, gelatinous tongue-shaped plate or *cupola* by the fluid inside the canals. The cupola contains the sensory nerve endings. On rotating the head, the fluid lags behind due to its inertia and swings the cupola to one side. When a brisk rotatory motion is suddenly stopped, the fluid continues to move for a short time, now swinging the cupola to the other side so that there is a sensation of movement in the reverse direction giving rise to a feeling of giddiness. The nerves from the semi-circular canals also help to co-ordinate eye movements so that the image remains in the correct position on the retina. At the start of rapid rotation, the eyes first move slowly in the opposite direction to the rotation and then flick back to the central position. These eye movements, which are known as *nystagmus*, are repeated until the rate of rotation becomes constant. When rotation is stopped, nystagmus occurs in the reverse direction for a short time and may also be accompanied by a feeling of giddiness. The vestibular sacs are sensitive to linear motion and to tilting the head. The sensory nerve endings are attached to small hairs lining the sacs, and these hairs are displaced by small crystals of calcium carbonate (otoliths) suspended in the fluid of the sacs. Motion sickness and Ménière's disease, both of which are characterized by giddiness and nausea, are the result of disturbance to the organs of balance.

Central connections of the proprioceptors. The first-order neurones from the proprioceptors, other than those from the labyrinths, enter the spinal cord through the posterior roots and give off branches which end in different ways. A branch of each sensory fibre from the muscle spindles passes to the anterior horn of grey matter on the same side of the cord where it synapses directly with the large motor cells innervating the *extra fusal* fibres (i.e. the ordinary muscle cells) of the same muscle. This is the monosynaptic pathway of the stretch reflex (page 114). Branches given off by the first-order neurones from all types of proprioceptor synapse with interneurones which in turn synapse with motor cells in the anterior horns of both sides of the cord. These pathways take part in the excitatory and inhibitory spinal reflexes described later. Some of the remaining branches of the first-order neurones are connected via second- and third-order neurones to the parietal cortex where they give rise to the sensation of movement termed *kinaesthesia*, and to the sense of joint position and muscle tension. These ascending fibres pass up the cord in the same tracts as those conveying the sense of light touch and pressure from the skin. The remaining branches synapse with second-order neurones some of which cross to the opposite side of the cord. These second-order neurones end in the cerebellum.

The vestibular nerve from the labyrinth apparatus enters the brain stem at the level of the pons. Some fibres pass straight to the cerebellum and some synapse in the vestibular nuclei. Second-order neurones connect the vestibular nuclei with the cerebellum, with the cells of the IIIrd, IVth and VIth cranial nerves supplying the muscles that move the eyeball (hence nystagmus), with the cell bodies of the nerves to skeletal muscles in the anterior horns of the spinal cord (descending vestibulo-spinal tracts, Fig. 4.4), and probably with the temporal lobe of the cortex.

All second-order sensory neurones from whatever source give off side branches into the reticular formation of the brain stem.

Pain

(1) **Cutaneous hyperalgesia.** In many pathological states of the skin, light innocuous stimuli, not normally painful, arouse pain. In *local* or *primary hyperalgesia*, the painful area is confined to the inflamed area. It is believed to be due to sensitization of the sensory nerve endings by some substance released during the inflammation process. In *secondary hyperalgesia*, the painful area extends well beyond the damaged area. Its cause is not known although it may depend upon a mechanism similar to that giving rise to referred visceral pain described below. The impulses conveying the sensation of itch are probably initiated in very superficial nerve endings and travel to the CNS along non-myelinated C fibres. Itching may be a consequence of the release of a chemical substance which stimulates the nerve endings. Naturally occurring chemical substances which produce pain or itch when released in the body are dealt with on pages 183–184.

(2) **Visceral pain.** The first-order afferent neurones conveying visceral pain are nearly all part of the sympathetic division of the autonomic nervous system (page 131) and therefore belong to the *interoceptive* sensory system. The viscera contain sensory receptors similar to some of those in the skin but their pain threshold in health is high. However, abnormal tension, for example in the gut, causes reflex spasms of the muscular walls and gives rise to the pain called colic. Inflammation of any of the internal organs lowers the pain threshold of their receptors and pain is experienced. After entering the cord via the posterior roots, the fibres branch. Some branches synapse with second-order neurones which pass to the thalamus in the same tracts as those conveying pain impulses originating from the exteroceptive receptors. The other branches are concerned with the reflex regulation of the viscera.

Nerve impulses conveying the sensation of pain from a diseased internal organ often give rise to an awareness of pain which appears to be located on the surface of the body. For example, pain impulses arising in the liver or gall-bladder may seem to be arising in the skin of the right shoulder; pain impulses arising in the heart are often perceived as pain in the inner surface of the arm, and pain impulses arising in the kidneys may seem to come from the groin. Sensations of pain so displaced are known as *referred* pain. The mechanism resulting in referred pain is probably that the first-order sensory neurones from the visceral organ and from the area of skin to which the pain is referred, form synapses in the cord with the same second-order neurones. Since the brain is unaccustomed to pain arriving from the viscera, it refers the sensation to the skin. Referred pain is always felt in the area of skin whose sensory neurones are in the same segment of the spinal cord as those of the affected organ. Referred pain is not the same as *projected pain*. Projected pain often appears to arise, for example, in a limb which has been amputated. Irritation of the severed sensory nerves sets up impulses which are perceived as sensation. This is also known as 'phantom pain'. 'Pins and needles' is an example of projected pain. Constriction of the blood supply to the sensory nerves in the region of the knee, caused by crossing the legs, initiates impulses in the trunk of the nerves. The sensation appears to arise in the foot where the peripheral receptors of these nerves are located.

(3) **Deep pain.** Deep pain originates in the receptors of muscles, tendons and joints. A powerful muscle contraction occludes the blood supply to the muscle and, if it is sustained, causes pain; but interrupted muscular activity does not cause pain unless the blood supply is inadequate, as when the vessels are damaged or obstructed by a blood clot. The pain occurring in ischaemic skeletal muscles is called *claudication*. In the heart, the severe pain of angina arises as a result of the ischaemia of the cardiac muscle. The pain may be caused by substances released during muscle contraction and which build up in concentration when the blood flow is poor. Sustained muscle contraction may arise reflexly through irritation of somatic or visceral afferents. The sustained contraction occludes the muscle blood supply and pain is experienced. Deep muscle pain, like visceral pain, is often referred to the surface of the body.

(4) **Headache.** Headache may arise in a number of ways. The headaches of anxiety states are often a consequence of tension in the neck and scalp muscles. Some headaches originate inside the skull and may arise from dilatation of, or traction on, intracranial arteries or to traction on the dura mater. Other headaches may be referred pains arising, for example, from the teeth. *Migraine* is characterized by paroxysmal pain on one side of the head associated with nausea and often preceded by disturbance of vision. The cause of migraine is not known but the headache is believed to arise from dilatation and increased pulsation of the arteries on the surface of the scalp. There is evidence to suggest that the formation or release of chemical substances may contribute to the symptoms (page 184).

Nervous control of voluntary muscle

Voluntary muscles are innervated by fast-conducting myelinated nerve fibres of the α-group which have their cell bodies in the motor nuclei of the cranial nerves in the brain stem, or in the anterior horn of the grey matter of the cord. These neurones are known as the *lower motoneurones*. They pass straight from the CNS to the muscle, where each fibre branches and loses its myelin sheath. Through its extensive branching, a single lower motoneurone innervates many muscle fibres. The lower motoneurone together with the muscle fibres it innervates is called a *motor unit* (Fig. 4.6). The lower motoneurones are the final common path for a vast number of nerve fibres originating from different centres in the CNS. It has been estimated that each lower motoneurone receives up to a thousand synaptic connections in the spinal cord.

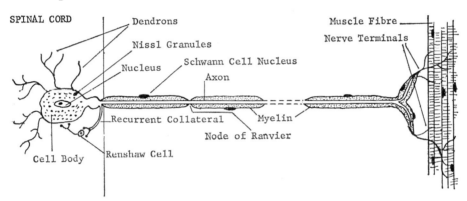

SPINAL CORD · Dendrons · Nissl Granules · Nucleus · Schwann Cell Nucleus · Axon · Muscle Fibre · Nerve Terminals · Recurrent Collateral · Myelin · Node of Ranvier · Cell Body · Renshaw Cell

FIG. 4.6. Diagram of a motor unit.

Spinal reflexes. Reflex action is the control mechanism whereby the routine working of the body is regulated. Nervous reflexes are involuntary acts which are set in motion by excitation of afferent nerves. Such actions occur at all levels of the CNS, in both the autonomic and the somatic nervous system, but here only the reflex control of skeletal muscle at spinal level is discussed. These reflexes were originally studied in detail by Sherrington. A familiar example of a spinal reflex is the rapid removal of the foot in response to painful stimulation or the quick regain of balance after tripping. The fact that the stimulus evoking a spinal reflex action is often perceived at conscious level is incidental, and in fact the response may occur before the cerebral cortex registers the stimulus.

When the CNS is intact, reflex activity of the spinal cord is modulated by descending fibres originating in higher centres. Consequently spinal reflexes may be studied in their simplest form only after destroying the brain. Such *spinal animals* 'survive' for many hours as long as the lungs are artificially ventilated and the body is kept warm. Spinal reflexes have also been studied in man where injury has caused complete transection of the cord (paraplegia). In the parts of the body supplied by nerves which leave the cord below the lesion, there is no feeling and no voluntary movement. However, some spinal reflexes may still be elicited and studied after recovery from *spinal shock*. In higher animals, transection of the cord at first causes a period of inhibition of all spinal reflexes below the transection known as spinal shock. The reflexes gradually reappear, first the flexor reflexes, then the extensor reflexes, and then the more complicated reflexes. In cats, the first reflexes reappear after about an hour and most reappear after a few days. In monkeys, the delay is considerably longer and in man recovery of reflexes is usually incomplete.

A convincing demonstration that spinal reflexes occur independently of higher centres may be shown in frogs. In this species, spinal shock is fleeting so that when the head of a live frog is cut off, the frog makes violent uncoordinated swimming movements when dropped into water a short time later. Here the water acts as a sensory stimulus to the skin and the afferent nerves, synapsing in the cord with the motor nerves to skeletal muscles, reflexly bring about swimming movements.

FLEXOR REFLEX. When a powerful stimulus is applied to the foot, the whole limb is withdrawn. This reflex may be elicited in a spinal animal and is an example of a *nociceptive* reflex (Latin: *noceo* = I injure), serving to protect the animal from injury. This type of reflex is termed *pre-potent* as it takes precedence over all other reflexes. The diagram of Fig. 4.7 illustrates the pathways involved in spinal reflexes. For simplification, only one afferent fibre and only one motor unit is illustrated in each reflex arc. The neurones labelled 1, 2 and 3 constitute the simplest reflex arc responsible for a flexor reflex. When the sensory receptor in the skin is stimulated, impulses are discharged along the afferent nerve fibres (neurone 1). In the cord, a branch of the afferent fibre synapses with an interneurone (2) which in turn synapses with the anterior horn cell (3) of the motor unit of a flexor muscle of the same (ipsilateral) limb. Since more than one synapse is involved in the cord, this reflex arc is termed *polysynaptic*. When a flexor reflex is evoked, the leg bends, and in order to allow this and to prevent damage to the muscle fibres, the antagonistic extensor muscles relax. This is brought about by the inhibitory interneurone (4) which impinges on the anterior horn cells of the motoneurone (5) supplying the extensor muscles of the same limb. The arrangement whereby a sensory nerve reflexly excites one muscle and inhibits its antagonist is known as *reciprocal inhibition*.

CROSSED EXTENSOR REFLEX. This reflex, which is also illustrated in Fig. 4.7, is part of the flexor reflex. When the sensory stimulus to one leg is severe, that

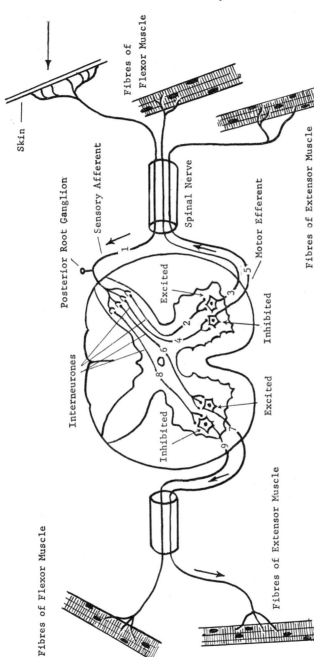

FIG. 4.7. Pathways involved in polysynaptic spinal reflexes. Neurones 1, 2 and 3 take part in the flexor reflex, the ipsilateral extensor muscles being inhibited through neurones 4 and 5. Neurones 1, 6 and 7 take part in the crossed extensor reflex, the flexor muscle being inhibited through neurones 8 and 9.

leg bends (flexor reflex) but the opposite leg extends to take the extra weight. This is brought about by interneurone (6) which crosses the cord and excites the motoneurone (7) supplying the extensor muscle of the contralateral limb. At the same time, interneurone (8) inhibits motoneurone (9) so that activity in the flexor muscle of this limb is depressed. The crossed extensor reflex may be readily elicited in cats and dogs but is less noticeable in man. In animal experiments designed to study the actions of drugs on the spinal cord, these reflexes may be repeatedly initiated, not by pinching or pricking the skin, but by applying constant electrical stimuli to the afferent nerves. The contractions of the muscle or the action potentials entering the cord in the dorsal roots and leaving the cord in the ventral roots may then be recorded.

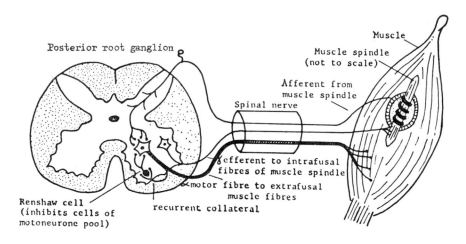

FIG. 4.8. Pathways involved in the monosynaptic stretch reflex.

THE STRETCH OR MYOTATIC REFLEXES. When a muscle is stretched, impulses are discharged along the afferent nerves from the muscle spindles (page 107). A branch of the afferent fibres carrying these impulses passes to the ipsilateral anterior horn and synapses directly with the motoneurone innervating the same muscle (monosynaptic reflex arc) which is quickly made to contract against the stretch (Fig. 4.8). The antagonistic muscles are reciprocally inhibited. The sensitivity of the stretch receptors is graded by the small motor nerves (γ-efferents) which supply the intrafusal fibres (page 107). The stretch reflex plays a part in the production of muscle tone (the slight state of contraction in which 'resting' muscles remain) and in the maintenance of posture. For example, if the body leans forward slightly, the muscles in the backs of the legs are slightly stretched. This induces a reflex contraction against the stretch and the body is smoothly pulled upright again. Stretch reflexes also take part in the rhythmic reflexes involved in running and walking. Thus, when the leg is flexed, the extensor muscles are stretched. Stretch of the extensors reflexly causes them to contract and also inhibits the flexors. Contraction of the extensors stretches the flexors and the cycle is repeated with the production of the rhythmic pattern of walking.

The fibres of the large anterior horn cells which innervate skeletal muscle give off side branches which pass back (recurrent collateral) into the grey matter of the cord. These side branches synapse with special interneurones known as *Renshaw cells* and they in turn make synaptic contact with the large anterior horn cells. The transmitter released by the Renshaw cell on to the motoneurone is inhibitory and this recurrent loop (Figs. 4.6 and 4.8) therefore forms a negative feed-back mechanism which damps down excessive activity in the motoneurones. Thus, whenever a burst of activity is induced in a motoneurone, the Renshaw cell is also excited and this in turn inhibits the motoneurone so that the muscle contraction is less vigorous than it would otherwise be, and it terminates sooner. This inhibitory mechanism is brought into play during strong stretch reflexes.

The Golgi tendon organs (page 107) are stretched, and therefore activated, not only when the muscle is stretched but also when it contracts. Unlike the muscle spindles, the Golgi organs are only excited by powerful degrees of stretch. The sensory fibres from the Golgi tendon organs form the afferent limb of an inhibitory spinal reflex which causes the muscle to relax when the stretching load against which it is contracting is very strong. This reflex therefore protects the muscle from overload which might otherwise damage it.

Several spinal reflexes may be tested during medical examinations as a means of diagnosing possible lesions in the CNS. Abnormalities are indicated by total absence of the reflex, by under-activity, by over-activity or by a change in the pattern of the response. Reflexes tested in this way include the following:

(i) *The knee* (*quadriceps*) *jerk* and (ii) *the ankle* (*triceps surae*) *jerk*. These reflexes are stretch reflexes and are elicited by sharply tapping the patellar and Achilles tendons respectively. The tap briefly stretches the appropriate muscle which contracts against the stretch. (iii) *The plantar reflex*. The normal response consists of a downward movement of the great toe when the skin of the sole is scratched. In certain diseases where there is injury to the corticospinal tracts, the great toe moves upwards (Babinski sign). (iv) *The cremasteric reflex*. The normal response is contraction of the cremaster muscle which causes elevation of the testicle when the inner and upper surface of the thigh is scratched. (v) *The abdominal reflex*. The abdominal muscles contract when the overlying skin is stroked. The last three reflexes are withdrawal reflexes similar to the flexor reflex previously described.

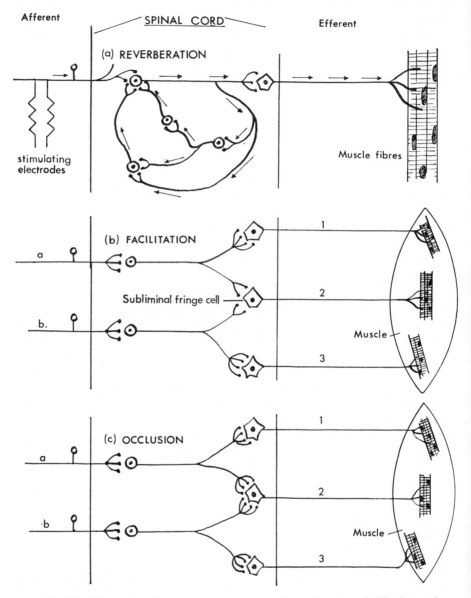

FIG. 4.9. Diagrams to illustrate the phenomena of reverberation, facilitation and occlusion in the spinal cord.

General characteristics of reflex activity. The action potential produced by a single stimulus applied to a sensory nerve fibre passes along all branches of that fibre inside the cord and therefore excites many interneurones. One afferent peripheral stimulus may give rise to many central impulses. Some of the interneurones may form closed-circuit chains like that illustrated in a simplified form in Fig. 4.9a. Reverberation of the impulses around these self re-exciting chains therefore results in the motoneurones being submitted to repeated synaptic stimulation. This relatively long-lasting activity in the spinal cord is known as a *central excitatory state* (CES) when the final synapse with the motoneurone is excitatory, and a *central inhibitory state* (CIS) when the final synapse acts to depress the excitability of the motoneurones. The CES produced by a single stimulus to the primary afferent may be too weak (subliminal) to depolarize the motoneurone to its critical firing level, but its excitability is raised and the CES produced by subsequent stimulation of the same sensory fibre, or of different sensory fibres with the same final common path, may summate with that produced by the first so that the motoneurone is activated. This may occur with stimulus intervals as long as 30 msec. In this way, preceding stimuli may *facilitate* the activity of subsequent stimuli so that *central summation* occurs. Central inhibitory state may be built up in a similar way. While the CES is being built up by a train of stimuli, activity spreads or *irradiates* through interneurones to more and more motoneurones so that the number excited gradually increases to a maximum. The addition of more and more units as time progresses is known as *recruitment*.

Facilitation, central summation, irradiation and recruitment are characteristic properties of polysynaptic reflex activity and may be demonstrated in the scratch reflex of the spinal dog. If the skin of the dog's abdomen is stroked, reflex scratching movements of the legs occur. However, if the area of skin stroked and the pressure of stroking are small, the reflex may not be initiated. Such weak stimuli may be applied at two different areas of skin and, although each is ineffective by itself, the reflex is evoked when both are applied together. Each stimulus therefore facilitates the other so that central summation occurs. If the stroking is continued, irradiation and recruitment cause an increase in the vigour of the scratching movement.

The production of CES also explains the occurrence of *after discharge*. Thus, when a sensory stimulus is terminated, the reflexly contracted muscles relax only slowly because reverberation continues for a short time (up to about 100 msec).

Many motoneurones receive synaptic connections from one interneurone. The group of motoneurones which may be activated by one interneurone is called the *motoneurone pool*. This arrangement explains two further properties of reflex activity, namely, *occlusion* and another type of *facilitation*. If two sensory nerves which reflexly excite the same muscle are stimulated together, the muscle tension produced may be greater (because of facilitation) or smaller (because of occlusion) than the sum of the tensions produced when each sensory nerve is stimulated separately. These effects may be explained with the aid of the simplified diagrams of Fig. 4.9b and 4.9c.

Figure 4.9b illustrates *facilitation*. Stimulation of the sensory neurone *a* activates only motoneurone 1 as the number of synaptic knobs supplied by the interneurone to motoneurone 2 is insufficient to produce an effective depolarization. For the same reason, stimulation of sensory *b* activates only motoneurone 3. Stimulation of either *a* or *b* alone therefore causes the contraction of only one group of muscle fibres. Cells such as motoneurone 2, whose excitability is raised but which are not made to discharge by stimulating a particular afferent, are known as *subliminal fringe* cells for that afferent. When both *a* and *b* are stimulated together, all three groups of muscle fibres contract since the combined effects of the two interneurones are sufficient to excite the subliminal fringe which is common to both. There is another mechanism which could account for facilitation even if motoneurone 2 of Fig. 4.9b did not receive boutons from either interneurone. The motoneurones of the anterior horn are closely packed and currents generated in some raise the excitability of adjacent ones by the process known as ephaptic transmission explained on pages 84–85. Thus when both *a* and *b* are stimulated together, the excitability of motoneurone 2 may be raised to the extent that it discharges. Probably both mechanisms contribute to facilitation in central synapses.

Figure 4.9c illustrates occlusion. Here the arrangement is such that both interneurones by themselves make sufficient synaptic connections to excite motoneurone 2. Thus stimulation of either *a* or *b* alone causes contraction of two groups of muscle cells. However, stimulation of both simultaneously causes the contraction, not of four, but of only three groups of muscle cells because of the overlapping of the interneurone connections.

Many synapses have been shown to exhibit the phenomenon of *post-tetanic potentiation* or *post-activation potentiation*. This was first described for the neuromuscular junction of skeletal muscle but has since been demonstrated in numerous different peripheral and central synapses of both excitatory and inhibitory types and may therefore be a general phenomenon. It may be briefly described as follows. After a short period of high-frequency (tetanic) stimulation of a pre-synaptic fibre, a single stimulus applied to the same fibre produces a greater response than formerly from the post-synaptic cell. The effect is due to a change induced in the pre-synaptic nerve endings and it is believed that a single nerve impulse causes a greater release of chemical transmitter after the burst of stimuli than before. High-frequency stimulation causes a prolonged after-hyperpolarization of nerve fibres and this may be the explanation of the increased transmitter release, as hyperpolarization of nerve endings by anodal electric currents also increases the release of transmitter in response to nerve impulses. Post-tetanic potentiation persists for minutes and sometimes for several hours after the high frequency stimulation. During the period of post-tetanic potentiation, the cells of the subliminal fringe may be excited by a single impulse in the interneurone. Post-tetanic potentiation in reverberating chains of neurones in the brain may contribute to the process of short-term memory and learning.

Upper motoneurones. The cell bodies of the upper motoneurones are scattered over a wide area of the cerebral cortex both in front and behind the central fissure of Rolando. About 3% of them are large and pyramid shaped (the giant cells of Betz) and are situated in the area known as the *motor cortex* immediately in front of the central fissure. The representation of the parts of the body in the motor cortex is similar to that in the sensory cortex with the feet above and the head below. The axons of the upper motoneurones pass down from each side via the *internal capsules* to the brain stem where they are known as the *pyramids* or *pyramidal tracts*. Some pyramidal fibres cross the brain stem and synapse with the cell bodies of the cranial motor nerves. At the level of the medulla, about three-quarters of the rest of the pyramidal fibres decussate and pass down the length of the cord on the opposite side in the lateral cortico-spinal tracts (Figs. 4.4 and 4.5). These tracts also contain a few uncrossed fibres. The remaining pyramidal fibres descend uncrossed as the anterior cerebro-spinal tracts (Fig. 4.4) which end in the thoracic region of the cord, but before terminating these fibres also cross to the grey matter of the opposite side. Throughout the length of the spinal cord, the upper motoneurones of the descending cerebro-spinal tracts synapse with interneurones which in turn synapse with the lower motoneurones. With few exceptions, the lower moto-neurones of one side are controlled by the motor cortex of the other. Injury to the motor cortex or internal capsule of one side therefore causes paralysis on the opposite side of the body, a condition known as *hemiplegia*.

Little is known of the neuronal pathways involved in planning a voluntary movement, but there are two-way connections between the motor cortex, its association areas, and other lobes of the cortex; these parts are presumably involved in the process. The performance of a voluntary movement is not carried out by the upper and lower motoneurone systems alone. Other central neuronal systems, collectively termed the *extra-pyramidal system*, serve to modulate and control movements initiated by the motor cortex. All of these systems converge on the lower motoneurones which therefore form the final common path.

The extra-pyramidal system. This system includes the basal ganglia, parts of the thalamus and the hypothalamus, the cerebellum, the red nucleus, the substantia nigra, the corpora quadrigemina, the vestibular nuclei, the reticular formation of the brain stem and some neurones of the motor association areas of the cortex. Some of the complex interconnections between these parts of the CNS are illustrated diagrammatically in Fig. 4.10. If the association area known as the pre-motor cortex is stimulated electrically, muscular movements occur which are much more complex than those elicited by stimulation of the motor cortex itself. Injury to the pre-motor cortex causes a condition known as *apraxia* in which the ability to co-ordinate muscular activity is lost. Although the individual movements necessary to perform a task may still be made, the person is incapable of co-ordinating them. Damage to other motor association areas may result, for example, in an inability to join words together into meaningful sentences although individual words may be spoken clearly. This condition is known as *aphasia*. *Parkinson's disease* (paralysis agitans) results from lesions in the corpus striatum and the substantia nigra. The characteristic signs of the disease are rigidity, tremor, involuntary movement and disturbance of voluntary movement (akinesia).

The cerebellum, receives sensory impulses originating from the skin, from the muscles and joints, from the organs of balance and from the ears and eyes. It also receives impulses from the motor areas of the cerebrum by way of fibres which synapse in the pons. The main efferent fibres leaving the cerebellum pass to the red nuclei in the mid-brain and to the thalamus where they synapse with other neurones passing to the motor cortex. In addition, efferent fibres pass to the reticular formation of the brain stem and to the vestibular nuclei. Through these connections, the cerebellum co-ordinates muscular activity and is concerned with equilibrium and the maintenance of posture. Damage to different parts of the cerebellum may cause disturbances of balance, choreiform (jerky) or atheloid (writhing) movements, tremor, nystagmus and an abnormal distribution of muscle tone.

Descending fibres from the vestibular nuclei (the vestibulo-spinal tracts, Figs. 4.4 and 4.10) and from the caudal part of the reticular formation (reticulo-spinal tracts, Figs. 4.4 and 4.10) act on the lower motoneurones and on the anterior horn cells of the γ-motor fibres which innervate the muscle spindles. Fibres of the vestibulo-spinal tracts, which are activated through the labyrinths, synapse directly with the lower motoneurones and the γ-efferents of extensor muscles, and facilitate their activity. Through reciprocal innervation, the flexors are inhibited. Over-activity of the vestibular nuclei is suppressed by inhibitory activity from higher centres. Stimulation of the medial nuclei of the descending reticular formation inhibits the lower motoneurones and the γ-efferents of extensor muscles, whereas stimulation of the lateral nuclei

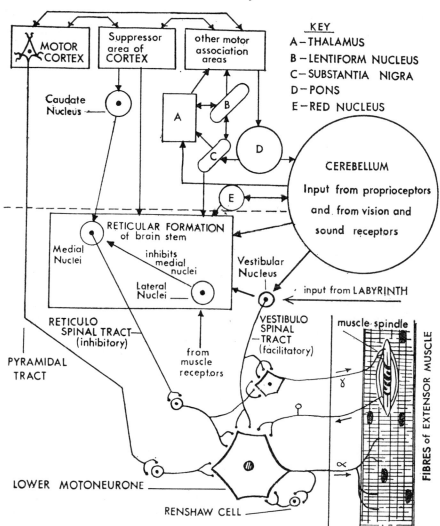

FIG. 4.10. Diagram to illustrate some of the interconnections involved in the control of skeletal muscles. Section of the brain along the position marked by the dotted line removes the inhibitory influence of the reticular formation and gives rise to decerebrate rigidity.

produces facilitation. In each case, reciprocal innervation causes the opposite action to be exerted on the flexor muscles. It appears likely that the facilitatory effect of the lateral nuclei on extensor muscles is brought about indirectly through an inhibitory action on the medial nuclei rather than by descending

. facilitatory fibres. The fibres in the descending reticulo-spinal tracts which pass to the lower motoneurones and γ-efferents of extensor muscles are therefore probably all inhibitory. The descending reticular formation receives its input partly from higher centres and partly by feed-back from the muscle proprioceptors.

The influence of both the vestibulo-spinal tracts and the reticulo-spinal tracts appears to be exerted mainly on the γ-efferents and only to a smaller extent on the lower motoneurones themselves. By sectioning the brain stem between the red nucleus and the vestibular nuclei, it is possible to cut off the inhibitory influence of the reticular formation on the extensor muscles (Fig. 4.10). However, the facilitatory influence of the vestibulo-spinal tracts is still present. The sensitivity of the muscle spindles to stretch is therefore greatly increased because of the unchecked facilitation of the γ-efferents. As a result, postural tone becomes exaggerated and the extensor muscles remain in strong contraction so that the legs are rigidly extended. This condition is known as *decerebrate rigidity*.

Autonomic nervous system

The autonomic nervous system consists of central neurones and both afferent and efferent peripheral neurones. It is largely concerned with the maintenance of homeostasis, that is, with the maintenance of a stable internal environment or *milieu interieur*. The organs innervated by the autonomic nervous system are shown in Table 4.1 and in Figs. 4.11 and 4.12. Through its control of these organs, the autonomic nervous system regulates circulation, respiration, excretion, secretion, body temperature, and the chemical constitution of the body fluids.

There are two divisions of the *efferent* side of the autonomic nervous system—the *sympathetic* and the *parasympathetic*. Figs. 4.11 and 4.12 are diagrammatic representations of the way in which these two systems innervate the various organs. The effects of separate stimulation of nerves of these two divisions are summarized in Table 4.1. General stimulation of the sympathetic produces responses which prepare the body for emergency while irrelevant activities are suppressed. Cannon described this as a 'fear—fright—flight' syndrome. Stimulation of the parasympathetic in general prepares the body for more sedentary activities.

Examination of Table 4.1 and Figs. 4.11 and 4.12 shows that most organs are innervated by both sympathetic and parasympathetic fibres and in many cases the responses evoked by the one are opposite to those evoked by the other. This led Gaskell in 1885 to the generalization that there is a reciprocal innervation by the two divisions of autonomic nerves. However, this generalization should not be extended too far as several tissues receive nerves from only

TABLE 4.1. Effects of autonomic nerve stimulation.

Tissue	Sympathetic nerves	Parasympathetic nerves
The eye		
Radial muscle, i.e. dilator pupillae of iris	Contraction giving dilated pupil, i.e. mydriasis	Not innervated
Circular muscle, i.e. constrictor pupillae of iris	Not innervated	Contraction giving constricted pupil, i.e. miosis
Smooth muscle of eye-lid	Contraction. Lid is elevated	Not innervated
Ciliary muscle	Not innervated	Contraction. Accommodation for near vision
Nictitating membrane	Contracted	Not innervated
Lacrimal glands and conjunctiva	Vasoconstriction	Secretion and vasodilatation
Salivary glands	Vasoconstriction. Sparse, thick, mucinous secretion of saliva	Vasodilatation. Profuse watery secretion
Thyroid gland	Increased secretion?	Not innervated?
Respiratory tract	Smooth muscle of bronchi relaxed. Vasoconstriction	Smooth muscle of bronchi contracted. Mucous glands stimulated
Heart	Rate and force increased. Coronaries dilated	Rate slowed. Refractory period reduced. Probably coronary constriction
Stomach	Motility and tone decreased. Sphincters contracted	Motility and tone increased. Sphincters relaxed. Secretion stimulated
Intestine	Motility and tone decreased. Sphincters contracted	Motility and tone increased. Sphincters relaxed. Secretions stimulated
Omentum and other fat depots	Fat and fatty acids released into blood	Not innervated
Liver	Glucose released into blood	Not innervated?
Gall bladder, bile duct	Contracted. Flow usually increased	Flow decreased
Spleen	Capsule contracted	Not innervated
Pancreas	Not innervated?	Increase in exocrine and endocrine secretion
Bladder		
Detrusor	Relaxed?	Contracted
Trigone and sphincters	Contracted	Relaxed
Ureter	Increased tone and motility	Not innervated

TABLE 4.1.—*continued*

Tissue	Sympathetic nerves	Parasympathetic nerves
Adrenal medulla	Discharges adrenaline and noradrenaline into blood-stream	Not innervated
Genital organs		
Uterus	Contraction or relaxation depending on species and state	Not innervated?
Vas deferens	Contraction	Not innervated
Erectile tissue	Loss of erection	Venous sphincters constricted: erection
Seminal vesicles	Contraction of internal vesicle sphincter	Not innervated?
Sweat glands		
Eccrine	Secretion of sweat	Not innervated
Apocrine	Not innervated	Not innervated
Pilomotor muscles	Contraction	Not innervated
Blood vessels		
Skin	Vasoconstriction	Mostly not innervated? Some areas vasodilatation
Skeletal muscle	Vasoconstrictor and vasodilator nerve fibres present	Not innervated?
Brain	Vasoconstriction	Not innervated?

one division (e.g. sweat glands, spleen and most blood vessels) and in the dually-innervated salivary glands the two systems are not opposed.

Under normal conditions, the influence of the two divisions of the autonomic nervous system on body functions are balanced and more or less continuous. Some visceral organs such as the heart and intestines have a rhythm of their own which is influenced, but not initiated, by nervous activity. Cannon found that survival was possible after complete surgical removal of the sympathetic ganglia and recently Levi-Montalcini found that young animals survived and grew to maturity after destruction of the sympathetic nerves with a specific antibody. Drugs which completely abolish the effects of stimulating sympathetic or parasympathetic nerves do not cause death by so doing. However, the capacity for coping with changes is impaired and life continues only in a controlled environment.

The anatomic existence of what is now known as the autonomic nervous

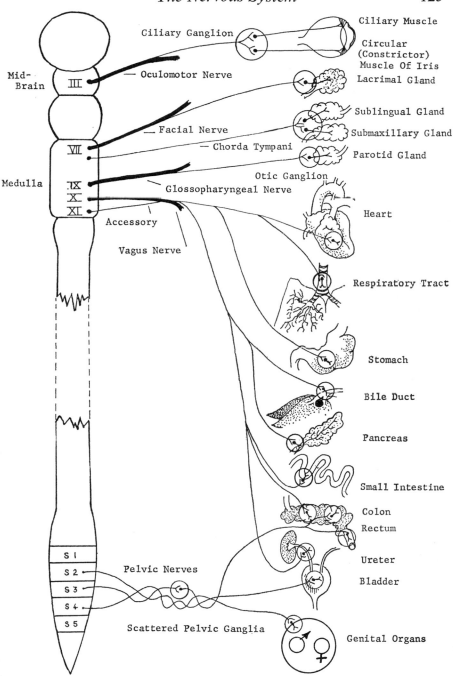

FIG. 4.11. Diagram of the parasympathetic nervous system and the organs innervated by it.

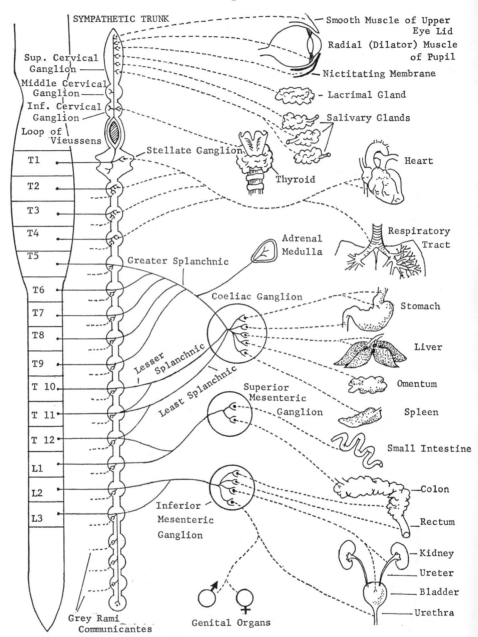

FIG. 4.12. Diagram of the sympathetic nervous system and the organs innervated by it.

system was an ancient discovery. The term 'sympathetic' applied to the peripheral nerves was introduced by the Danish anatomist Winslow in 1732. He believed that this system of nerves was responsible for regulating the 'sympathies' of the body, that is, the harmonious relationships between organs. In 1800, Bichat used the term 'vegetative', as he believed these nerves were concerned with the control of nutritive processes, the central nervous system being concerned with 'animalistic' processes. The term 'visceral' as opposed to 'somatic' has also been used. Langley, in 1898, first proposed the designation 'autonomic nervous system'. Gaskell, in 1916, suggested the term 'involuntary'. Cannon (1929) suggested that 'interofective' gave a better description of the regulation imposed by the autonomic nervous system, especially in relation to homeostasis, in contrast to the somatic system which he called 'exterofective'. The term autonomic nervous system has now been generally adopted, although many authors continue to use 'vegetative' and 'involuntary': it may be taken that these terms are synonymous, at least as far as the peripheral parts of the system are concerned.

Although Langley originated the term, he did state that the word 'autonomic' suggested a much greater degree of independence of the rest of the nervous system than in fact exists. Thus increased heart rate and respiration and alteration in the calibre of the blood vessels slightly precede and accompany increased activity of the skeletal muscles, and even thoughts and memories may be accompanied by autonomic responses such as flushing, pallor or sweating. Functional links between the autonomic and the somatic nervous systems have also been demonstrated by experiments involving Pavlovian conditioning (page 135). Thus responses mediated by somatic motoneurones may be conditioned to appear after excitation of sensory receptors normally concerned with unconditioned autonomic reflexes. The frontal areas of the cerebral cortex contain centres controlling autonomic activity, and co-ordination of autonomic and voluntary activity is probably brought about by association fibres at cortical level.

Respiration essentially involves co-ordinated activity of both autonomic and somatic nervous systems. Thus chemoreceptors and baroreceptors in the blood vessels, which are sensitive to CO_2 tension and to blood pressure respectively, are connected to the respiratory centre in the brain stem through sensory nerve fibres considered as part of the autonomic nervous system. Through synaptic connections in the CNS, efferent fibres are activated and these induce alterations in the calibre of the bronchi and the rate and depth of respiration. The smooth muscle of the bronchi is autonomically innervated but the intercostal muscles and the diaphragm, which control the rate and depth of inspiration, are skeletal muscles and are innervated by motoneurones of the somatic nervous system.

The physiological activities regulated by autonomic nerves are not entirely involuntary, although in general they proceed without volition and may take place without awareness. Focusing of the eye is brought about by alteration in the length of the parasympathetically innervated ciliary muscle, which in turn alters the focal length of the lens (page 418), and this is normally under voluntary control. A considerable degree of voluntary control may normally be exerted over the autonomically innervated sphincters of the anus and bladder, and some people can exercise voluntary control over functions such as heart rate and sweating.

Anatomy of the autonomic nervous system. All of the efferent neurones leaving the CNS, other than those innervating skeletal muscle, belong to the autonomic nervous system. The efferent autonomic fibres differ from the lower moto-neurones to skeletal muscle in that they do not run directly to an effector organ. Instead the fibres leaving the CNS terminate in synapses with the cell bodies or dendrons of other neurones which innervate the effector cells (Figs. 4.11, 4.12 and 4.13). The synapses outside the CNS generally occur in clusters called ganglia. The nerve fibres running from the CNS to the ganglion cells are called pre-ganglionic fibres, while the axons of the ganglion cells which terminate in the innervated tissue are called post-ganglionic fibres.

Sympathetic nerves. The pre-ganglionic fibres of the sympathetic division have their cell bodies in the lateral horn cells of the thoracic and the first and second lumbar segments of the spinal cord (Figs. 4.12 and 4.13). Their axons leave the cord in the anterior roots along with the lower motoneurones. These fibres are myelinated *B* fibres and after a short distance they branch off from the spinal nerves as the white *rami communicantes* and join the sympathetic chains (Fig. 4.12). The sympathetic chains consist of two chains of ganglia (the vertebral ganglia) which are anterior to, and one on each side of, the vertebral column (Figs. 4.1 and 4.12). Pre-ganglionic fibres in the white rami terminate in one of three main ways:

(1) Some fibres synapse with the post-ganglionic neurones in ganglia of the sympathetic chain. Many pre-ganglionic fibres do not synapse in the ganglion adjacent to the segment of cord from which they leave, but run up or down the sympathetic chain to synapse in a ganglion some distance away. Pre-ganglionic fibres which synapse in the cervical and sacral ganglia leave the cord in the thoracic and lumbar regions (Fig. 4.12). Some post-ganglionic fibres also run along the sympathetic chains before passing out to the periphery. Most post-ganglionic fibres of the sympathetic system are non-myelinated *C* fibres. After synapsing in the vertebral ganglia, many form grey rami communicantes which re-join the spinal nerves (Fig. 4.13) before passing out to the periphery to

innervate the blood vessels (vasomotor nerves), the sweat glands (sudomotor nerves) or the smooth muscles of the hair follicles (pilomotor nerves). Other post-ganglionic fibres do not join the spinal nerves but run to the organ which they innervate as discrete nerve bundles, or as plexuses accompanying the blood vessels.

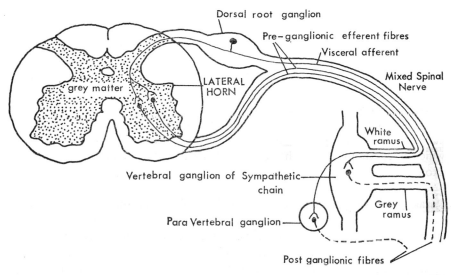

Fig. 4.13. Diagram of a reflex arc in the sympathetic nervous system.

(2) Many pre-ganglionic fibres pass straight through the vertebral ganglia to synapse in the paravertebral ganglia in the abdominal cavity (Figs. 4.12 and 4.13). The main paravertebral ganglia are: (*a*) *the coeliac ganglia*, which lie near the junction of the coeliac axis (or artery) with the aorta. The pre-ganglionic fibres synapsing in these ganglia are carried in the splanchnic nerves; (*b*) *the superior mesenteric ganglia*, and (*c*) *the inferior mesenteric ganglia*, both of which lie near the origins of the superior and inferior mesenteric arteries respectively.
(3) Some pre-ganglionic fibres leaving the middle thoracic segments of the spinal cord run in the greater splanchnic nerve and terminate in claw-like projections around cells of the medullae of the adrenal glands (Fig. 4.12). Like nervous tissue, the cells of the adrenal medullae are derived embryologically from ectodermal cells of the neural crest and are believed to be analogous to sympathetic ganglion cells.

Near the ganglion cells, each pre-ganglionic fibre divides into numerous fine terminal branches which lose their myelin and end in small swellings (the boutons terminaux, end-feet or synaptic knobs). The boutons are applied close to the surface of the cell bodies or the dendrites of the post-ganglionic fibres

5

and it has been estimated that about 70% of the surface of the cell body is covered by them. A pre-ganglionic fibre makes connection with many post-ganglionic cells and the latter may receive boutons from several pre-ganglionic fibres (Fig. 5.2). A post-ganglionic cell may therefore receive discharges of different frequencies simultaneously and its function is to modulate the patterns of nervous activity *en route* from the CNS to the effector cells. Sympathetic ganglia exhibit the properties of facilitation, occlusion, and recruitment already described for synapses in the CNS. Synaptic delay is many times longer than it is in central synapses. After the end of a brief repetitive stimulation of the pre-ganglionic fibres, the post-ganglionic fibres continue to discharge impulses for many seconds. This after-discharge is difficult to understand if sympathetic ganglia do not contain any interneurones, since these are believed to account for this phenomenon in the CNS. In most ganglia, each cell body is enveloped in a thin nucleated capsule of satellite cells which is continuous with the terminal Schwann cells of the pre-ganglionic axon.

Parasympathetic nerves. The pre-ganglionic fibres of the parasympathetic division are also myelinated *B* fibres. They issue from the cranial and sacral regions of the spinal cord (Fig. 4.11). In the sacral region, the cell bodies are in the lateral horns and the pre-ganglionic fibres are known as the pelvic nerves or *nervi erigentes*. The organs which they innervate are in the lower part of the abdominal cavity. Some pelvic nerve fibres relay with ganglion cells in the pelvic ganglia and post-ganglionic parasympathetic fibres then pass on to the organs; others continue to the organs as pre-ganglionic fibres and synapse with ganglion cells situated within the organs and in close proximity to the effector cells. Parasympathetic pre-ganglionic fibres from the cranial region are carried in the IIIrd (oculomotor), VIIth (facial), IXth (glossopharyngeal), Xth (vagus) and XIth (accessory) cranial nerves. As described at the beginning of this chapter, these cranial nerves carry many fibres other than efferent para-sympathetic fibres (see pages 93 and 94).

The pre-ganglionic fibres of the cranial parasympathetic nerves terminate in ganglion cells lying within or near the organs innervated. In the heart, most of the ganglion cells are situated in the vicinity of the sino-atrial and atrio-ventricular nodes (pages 213–214) and the post ganglionic axons are very short. In the intestine, the post-ganglionic neurones are possibly the nerve cells of Auerbach's plexus (page 314). The parasympathetic ganglion cells of the salivary glands and those of the eye are situated *outside* these organs (but very close to them), in discrete ganglia: the parasympathetic ganglion of the eye is the ciliary ganglion. The post-ganglionic fibres from the ciliary ganglion are myelinated. In contrast, the post-ganglionic fibres of parasympathetic ganglia within organs are non-myelinated, as are most sympathetic post-ganglionic fibres.

Sensory neurones and autonomic reflex arcs. Autonomic sensory neurones are often called *visceral afferents*. Outside the spinal cord they run in large numbers in the same nerve trunks as the efferent autonomic fibres. Like the somatic sensory neurones, the visceral afferents have their cell bodies in the posterior root ganglia (Fig. 4.13) or in the *sensory* ganglia of those cranial nerves which contain parasympathetic fibres.

Visceral afferents which enter the spinal cord branch in the posterior horns of grey matter. Some branches pass up the cord to synapse with second-order neurones which terminate in the brain stem. Other branches terminate in the lateral horns of the grey matter of the cord where they synapse with pre-ganglionic efferent fibres of the sympathetic or sacral parasympathetic systems. Visceral afferents in the cranial nerves have their cell bodies in the sensory ganglia of these nerves and terminate in the brain stem where branches synapse with the cell bodies of the pre-ganglionic parasympathetic fibres. Thus, the simple autonomic reflex arc (Fig. 4.13) resembles the three neurone spinal reflex arcs of the somatic system, the difference being that the second neurone in the autonomic arc is an efferent pre-ganglionic fibre which terminates outside the cord, and is not an interneurone. With the possible exception of the response of the pupil to light, probably all autonomic reflexes are influenced by control from higher centres; they are rarely entirely segmental in character. However, like the somatic spinal reflexes, they still take place when higher control is removed. For example, defaecation, micturition and ejaculation still occur reflexly after the spinal cord has been severed.

The peristaltic reflex (page 322) is an unusual reflex in that it may be observed in a segment of intestine completely isolated from the body. In this reflex, stretch of the walls of the gut stimulates sensory fibres. These, in turn, synapse either directly or through a local interneurone with post-ganglionic parasympathetic fibres. In the intact animal, however, this extra-spinal reflex arc is influenced by centres in the brain stem.

The interoceptive sensory receptors which activate the visceral afferents are distributed throughout the internal organs of the body. They consist of pressor receptors sensitive to pressure changes, chemoreceptors sensitive to CO_2 tension or to glucose concentration in the blood, and stretch receptors sensitive to stretch or tension in smooth muscle. Branches of the primary afferents from many of these receptors synapse in groups of cell bodies in various parts of the brain stem to form cardio-accelerator and inhibitory centres, a vasomotor centre, a vomiting centre, a respiratory centre and so on. The functioning of these centres is described more fully in the relevant chapters. Descending fibres from these centres synapse with the cell bodies of the pre-ganglionic para-sympathetic fibres of the cranial nerves or pass down the cord in the reticulo-spinal tracts to synapse in the lateral horns of the grey matter with the cell bodies of the pre-ganglionic sympathetic and sacral parasympathetic out-flow.

All the spinal and lower brain stem autonomic centres are controlled and co-ordinated by nuclei in the hypothalamus which is the most important sub-cortical autonomic centre. Stimulation of the posterior parts of the hypo-thalamus causes widespread sympathetic activity and stimulation of the anterior parts causes widespread parasympathetic activity. The hypothalamus also has connections with the frontal and orbital lobes of the cerebrum and with the pituitary gland (page 366) and through these connections autonomic activity is co-ordinated with somatic and endocrine activity.

The electroencephalogram

Electrical potential changes occurring in the brain may be detected by means of electrodes placed at various positions on the scalp and connected through amplifiers to an oscillograph. The record is known as the *electro-encephalogram* or EEG. A similar record obtained from the surface of the cortex itself is known as the *electrocorticogram*. The potentials occur in the form of waves of differing frequency and amplitude. They are believed to represent a rhythmic flow of current from the mass of dendrites in the cerebral cortex. Although the EEG arises in the cortex, it is strongly dependent on other parts of the brain. The dominant or α-rhythm (frequency, 10–14/sec; amplitude about 50 μV) is recorded best over the occipital area of cortex. Further forward, over the sensory and motor cortex, a more rapid lower-voltage rhythm called the β-rhythm (16–60/sec; 5–10 μV) is also recorded. During deep sleep or anaesthesia, the slow δ-rhythm (1–8/sec) of large amplitude is recorded. The δ-rhythm may be recorded in normal waking children, but in waking adults it is always indicative of some abnormality.

The α-rhythm has been called the rhythm of inattention because it is seen best when the subject is relaxed with the eyes closed. It appears to represent fluctuations in the excitability of the cortex and probably serves to maintain the optimal excitability of the cortical synapses, thus ensuring an effective response when the need arises. When the subject opens his eyes and concentrates on an object, when he performs some mental task, or when he is anxious or afraid, the relatively slow and synchronous α-rhythm is *desynchronized* into a rapid series of small waves. A similar change in the EEG may also be detected shortly before a voluntary movement is made. This desynchronization to a low-voltage fast rhythm is known as an *arousal* or *alerting reaction*.

The EEG has proved of value in the diagnosis of certain diseases, such as epilepsy, and in locating the area of brain affected by a tumour.

The reticular formations of the brain stem and thalamus

The role of the reticular formation of the brain stem in the extra-pyramidal system has already been briefly described. From its upper (rostral) end, the reticular formation also influences all sensory and psychological activity of the cortex. All sensory tracts conveying impulses to the thalamus and parietal cortex give off collaterals into the reticular formation which has connections with the whole of the cerebral cortex by way of the thalamus and hypothalamus. The ascending reticular formation is much more sensitive to metabolic changes and to some depressant drugs, such as barbiturates, than are the main ascending sensory pathways. If the fibres connecting the brain stem reticular formation to the cortex are severed, the EEG becomes synchronized and shows changes characteristic of deep sleep. This part of the brain stem is therefore believed to be concerned with maintaining wakefulness. Through the continual influence of the reticular formation on higher centres, impulses passing up the ascending sensory tracts spread into the cerebral cortex; thus it is placed in readiness to deal with the information. However, by means of descending fibres, the cortex itself influences this activity of the reticular formation. A desire to concentrate originates in some part of the cortex which then initiates increased facilitatory activity of the reticular formation.

The brain of an animal which is not constantly being submitted to a stream of sensory stimuli shows the EEG pattern typical of sleep. This may be produced either by anaesthetizing the animal or by interrupting the ascending sensory tracts by cutting the cord in the neck region. Under such conditions the slow waves are desynchronized to small fast waves (EEG arousal reaction) by electrical stimulation of the rostral end of the reticular formation itself or by strong stimulation of an intact sensory pathway. The effects of centrally acting drugs on the EEG arousal reaction have been studied in an attempt to determine their site of action.

Another reticular system communicating with the cortex is present in the thalamus. Electrical stimulation of this system at a low frequency brings the EEG rhythm of the cortex into step with the stimulation. The waves build up in amplitude during the first few seconds of stimulation; this is known as the *recruiting response*. The ascending thalamic reticular system is believed to mediate sudden brief shifts of attention in response to shades of sensory stimulation.

The ascending reticular formations also act to modulate those parts of the brain concerned with emotion, that is, the limbic system and the hypothalamus.

Sleep

Natural sleep is not fully understood but it involves a depression of the activity of the cerebral cortex by the brain stem reticular formations. Two types of ascending fibres are believed to originate in the reticular formation. One type activates the cortex, and this is reflected in a desynchronized EEG, and the other depresses the cortex and produces sleep which is reflected in a synchronized EEG. The latter action is facilitated by a reduction in the sensory input from the external environment such as is achieved in a quiet, darkened room. The hypothalamus may also be concerned in sleep since electrical stimulation of part of it has been shown to induce sleep in cats.

Emotion

Patients with hypothalamic disease often show changes in personality in which there are irrational outbursts of temper. In animals, electrical stimulation of the hypothalamus and the production of localized lesions produce changes resembling those seen in states of rage and fear. Working alone, the hypothalamus cannot initiate *directed* emotional behaviour which requires the cerebral cortex. De-corticate dogs exhibit the signs of fierce rage. This is called 'sham rage' as it is without any special target and presumably the dog cannot 'feel' enraged without a cortex.

Evidence is accumulating from animal experiments which indicates that the limbic system (pages 102 and 604) is concerned with the *conscious* experience of emotion. This is confirmed by electrical stimulation of the amygdaloid nuclei in man which results in subjective reports of fear and rage. It may be that sensations and thoughts which give rise to emotions, cause impulses to enter the hypothalamus from which impulses are discharged downwards to produce the bodily changes associated with emotion and upwards to produce subjective feelings.

Regulation of food intake

The hypothalamus in some way regulates appetite and food intake. Hypothalamic disorders may give rise to excessive appetite and obesity, or to the opposite when all food is refused and the patient starves unless force feeding is carried out. This latter condition is known as *anorexia nervosa*. In the ventromedial nucleus of the hypothalamus is the so called *satiety centre*. Destruction of this nucleus in animals produces excessive eating. Small doses of chloralose, insufficient to produce anaesthesia, produce a similar effect and possibly act by depressing this centre. In contrast, certain CNS stimulant drugs, such as amphetamine, depress appetite and may act by stimulating this centre. Slightly lateral to the satiety centre is a 'feeding centre', destruction of which causes fatal anorexia. An area in the anterior part of the hypothalamus is concerned with drinking and an area level with the mamillary bodies is concerned with both eating and drinking. When this area is stimulated electrically, animals eat and drink compulsively. Other aspects of the regulation of food and water intake are discussed on page 331.

Learning and memory

Conditioned reflexes are a form of learning. The reflexes described in previous pages are unconditioned and differ from conditioned reflexes in that they are independent of previous experience. When the mouth of a new-born animal is placed in contact with the nipple of the mammary glands, it begins to suck as the result of a simple unconditioned reflex. In more adult animals, the presence of food in the mouth excites taste receptors in the tongue and saliva is secreted. This is also an unconditioned reflex. As the animal gains experience, it associates the appearance of food with its taste, and saliva is secreted at the mere sight of food. This is a conditioned reflex.

The Russian physiologist, Pavlov, while studying the mechanism controlling salivation, made the first study of conditioned reflexes. Pavlov's experiments were carried out along the following lines. Each time a dog was given food, a neutral stimulus, such as the ringing of a bell, was applied at the same time. After repeating the combination of food and neutral stimulus several times, the neutral stimulus was given alone and caused a flow of saliva. A conditioned reflex to the previously neutral stimulus had therefore been established.

Conditioned reflexes have been established to many different kinds of stimuli and with many different unconditioned reflexes, such as vasomotor reactions, vomiting or the knee-jerk, as a basis. Great specificity is often shown to the stimulus. For example, dogs conditioned to respond to a certain musical note give a smaller response, or do not respond at all, to a note of a different pitch.

Nerve cells, once formed, never reproduce themselves and, in the mammal at least, there is no evidence that new neurones develop after birth. Learning and memory do not therefore depend upon the addition of new neurones but make use of the structures present from the beginning. The continual activity of the EEG indicates that neurones in the brain are in a state of continuous activity, so that it does not seem likely that additional memories and new learning involve the use of previously idle neurones. Furthermore, systematic removal of areas of cortex has shown that the ability of rats to remember behaviour learned before the lesion was made, diminishes only with the amount of cortex removed and not with the particular area selected for removal. While reverberating circuits may play a part in short-term learning and memory, it does not seem likely that continuously reverberating activity in the brain is responsible for the storage of long-established memories. Thus, once established, memories survive epileptic fits which are associated with violent electrical activity in the brain, and in hibernating animals learned patterns of behaviour persist despite the fact that during hibernation electrical activity in the brain is almost extinguished. Furthermore, established memories in rats have been found to be unimpaired after operations in which the cortex of the brain was criss-crossed with numerous cuts which must have destroyed many reverberating circuits.

It is now believed that nerve cells store memories by means of modifications in the structure of their RNA-protein complex. Part of the evidence in support of this hypothesis comes from experiments with 8-aza-guanine. This compound is sufficiently similar to guanine, one of the four bases of which RNA is composed (page 54), for the RNA-synthesizing enzymes to accept it in place of guanine. An artificial RNA containing 8-aza-guanine is therefore synthesized. Injection of 8-aza-guanine into rats does not impair their ability to recall established memories but reduces their ability to learn new behaviour, suggesting that when true RNA synthesis is blocked new memories cannot be stored. Although several possibilities have been suggested, it is not yet known how a particular pattern of nerve impulses, arriving in the brain as the result of a new experience, causes a modification of the structure of the RNA strand. A memory is recalled as the result either of a particular combination of sensory stimuli or of a conscious desire to remember, presumably because the modified RNA or the protein synthesized by it in some way recreates the pattern of electrical circuits that earlier specified the RNA.

Electrical stimulation of certain parts of the temporal lobes of the cortex in man produces auditory and visual memories of past experiences and it therefore appears that a mechanism for memory storage is present in this part of the brain.

CHAPTER 5

Humoral Transmission of Nervous Impulses

The existence of a gap at synaptic and neuroeffector junctions raises the question of how the nerve impulse is transmitted across the gap. In the past, there have been two principal theories about the transmission process: the *electrical theory* and the *humoral theory*.

The electrical theory holds that transmission is by action currents originating from the nerve endings. Accordingly, the mechanism of transmission beyond the nerve endings differs little from conduction along the axon. This theory had its early origin in the finding that nerves may be stimulated by bioelectric potentials. Thus, in Galvani's experiments on 'contraction without metals', a nerve-muscle preparation from a frog was stimulated to contract when the nerve was laid across the cut surface of another muscle; the current set up by the demarcation potential (page 76) of the cut muscle stimulated the nerve. Matteucci carried out similar experiments with what he called the 'rheoscopic preparation' (a rheoscope is a device for detecting an electric current); he laid the nerve of a nerve-muscle preparation across a beating heart, and the action currents spreading through the heart (page 214) stimulated the nerve so that the muscle contracted in time with the heart beats. These experiments show that the current from a large mass of muscle may excite a nerve. However, in the physiological process, excitation passes from nerve to muscle, but excitation of muscle does not occur when an active nerve is simply laid on it, because the current from the small mass of the nerve is too weak to excite the much larger muscle. Therefore, it is clear that a means of amplification of the nerve impulse is necessary in order to excite the muscle. Such an amplification takes place at the junction between nerve and muscle and is brought about chemically.

In most organs supplied with both sympathetic and parasympathetic nerves, stimulation of one nerve may cause excitation, whereas stimulation of the other may produce inhibition (Table 4.1). If transmission were due simply to spread of the nerve action currents to the organ, it would be difficult to explain how opposite effects could be produced; the theory that humoral transmitters with specific actions are released from each nerve to mediate the responses provides a satisfactory explanation.

Synapses and neuro-effector junctions possess at least four properties indicating that transmission across them differs from conduction along nerve fibres. Thus, (1) transmission across a junction takes place in one direction

137

only, (2) there is a delay in transmission across a junction, (3) fatigue occurs more readily at junctions, and (4) many drugs act selectively at junctions.

The classical work of Claude Bernard in 1851 showed that skeletal muscle poisoned with curare, a South American arrow poison, no longer contracted in response to electrical stimulation of its nerve, although the muscle still responded to direct electrical stimulation. He further showed that curare had no action on the nerve alone and concluded that the site of the paralysis was at the junction between the nerve and the muscle. Nicotine, too, has long been known to affect transmission at some synapses and neuro-effector junctions but to have no effect on conduction. Langley, in 1887, made use of the properties of nicotine to locate the precise site of ganglionic relays in various autonomic nerve pathways. He painted nicotine solution onto autonomic ganglia and observed that it first excited the ganglion cells and then blocked transmission through the ganglion.

In 1869, Schmiedeberg showed that the actions of the alkaloid, *muscarine*, extracted from the toadstool, *Amanita muscaria*, closely resembled the effects of stimulation of the vagus nerve; the explanation offered was that muscarine stimulated the vagus nerve endings. Then Dixon, in 1908, found that a muscarine-like substance was released from the frog's heart when the vagus nerve was stimulated and he suggested that excitation of a nerve induces the local liberation of a chemical mediator. Choline, a substance which is present in body tissues (pages 12 and 35), has actions like those of muscarine but it is much weaker. However, the acetyl ester of choline is about equi-potent with muscarine in lowering the blood pressure of the cat (Fig. 5.1).

$$CH_3-\overset{\overset{\displaystyle CH_3}{|+}}{\underset{\underset{\displaystyle CH_3}{|}}{N}}-CH_2-CH_2-O-\overset{\overset{\displaystyle O}{\|}}{C}-CH_3$$

Acetylcholine

Dale began his studies on acetylcholine in 1914 after it had been identified as the depressor substance present in an extract of ergot; he found that it resembled muscarine in being able to mimic the effects of parasympathetic nerve stimulation (Table 4.1). These actions of acetylcholine became known as *muscarinic* or *parasympathomimetic* actions. Dale further showed that after the injection of atropine the muscarinic actions of acetylcholine were abolished but larger doses of acetylcholine then produced a pronounced rise in blood pressure and in heart rate. The injection of nicotine also produced these effects by exciting sympathetic ganglion cells. After large doses of nicotine, the ganglion cells were blocked and this prevented the action of acetylcholine in the atropinized animal. These results suggested that acetylcholine, like nicotine, stimulated ganglion cells. The effects of acetylcholine, muscarine, atropine and nicotine on the blood pressure of an anaesthetized cat are shown in Fig. 5.1. Both acetylcholine and nicotine were also found to stimulate skeletal muscle and parasympathetic ganglia as well as sympathetic ganglia, and these actions of acetylcholine therefore became known as *nicotinic* actions.

Oliver and Schäfer reported in 1894 that the injection of an extract of adrenal glands raised the blood pressure of an animal, and then showed that

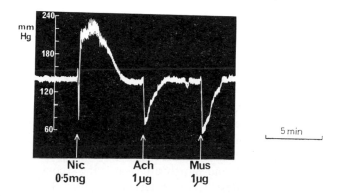

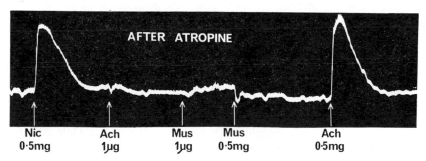

FIG. 5.1. The effects of acetylcholine (Ach), muscarine (Mus), and nicotine (Nic) on the blood pressure of an anaesthetized cat (weighing 3 kg) before and after atropine (2 mg/kg). All injections given into the femoral vein. Blood pressure recorded from the carotid artery. Note that atropine blocks the *muscarinic* action of acetylcholine and then larger doses of acetylcholine exert a *nicotinic* action.

the active principle was confined to the medulla. The chemical substance responsible for the activity was isolated and named adrenaline. Langley showed how closely the actions of an adrenal extract resembled the responses resulting from stimulation of sympathetic nerves (Table 4.1). The actions remained after the sympathetic nerves had been sectioned and allowed to degenerate; hence it was concluded that the extract acted on the effector cells and not on the nerves. Elliott was the first to suggest that adrenaline is liberated from sympathetic nerve endings when they are stimulated, and that the released adrenaline then acts on the responsive cells. However, in 1910 Dale emphasized that the responses to adrenaline were not always identical with those resulting from stimulation of sympathetic nerves, and he pointed out that noradrenaline mimicked the effects of sympathetic stimulation more closely, but this observation was ignored for many years.

Noradrenaline   Adrenaline

The first conclusive evidence that chemical transmission occurs was provided by Loewi in 1921. He perfused two isolated frog hearts so that the fluid flowed through one heart and then through the other. When the parasympathetic nerve (the vagus) to the first heart was stimulated, the heart slowed and its beats became weaker, and shortly afterwards the second heart responded in a similar manner. A substance, then termed Vagusstoff, was released from the nerve endings in the first heart and carried in the perfusion fluid to the second heart. When the sympathetic nerve (the nervus accelerans) to the first heart was stimulated, the heart beat faster and more powerfully and then the second heart responded in a similar way, indicating that another substance, then termed Acceleranstoff, was released from the sympathetic nerve endings. It seemed that acetylcholine was Vagusstoff and that adrenaline or nor-adrenaline was Acceleranstoff. Since then, a vast amount of evidence has been obtained to show that these compounds are responsible for chemical trans-mission at autonomic ganglia and at neuro-effector junctions. Dale classified those nerve fibres which release acetylcholine as *cholinergic*, and those which release an adrenaline-like substance as *adrenergic*.

Parasympathetic neuro-effector junctions

Loewi showed that Vagusstoff and acetylcholine had similar actions on the heart, and that atropine blocked, and physostigmine potentiated, the actions of both substances. Physostigmine, which is also known as eserine, acted by inhibiting cholinesterase, the enzyme which catalyses the hydrolysis of acetylcholine, and in fact Loewi's experiments with physostigmine were the first to show the action of a drug on an enzyme. Later, it was found that an acetylcholine-like substance was released into the coronary venous blood of mammals when the vagus nerve was stimulated. Since blood contains much cholinesterase, the acetylcholine-like substance was detected only when physostigmine was present. Stimulation of parasympathetic nerves to structures such as the stomach, intestine and salivary glands also resulted in the release of an acetylcholine-like substance into the bloodstream.

Besides electrical stimulation of the parasympathetic nerves, physiological stimuli were used. For example, shining a strong light into the eye causes a reflex contraction of the circularly arranged smooth muscle of the iris, and Engelhardt showed that the aqueous humour then contained an acetylcholine-like substance. Acetylcholine can be detected in extracts of the iris and ciliary muscle, but it is not present when the post-ganglionic fibres of the ciliary nerve have degenerated.

The amounts of acetylcholine released from tissues on stimulating para-sympathetic nerves, or contained in tissue extracts, are present in concentrations too low to allow chemical identification. Nevertheless, the presence of a substance which behaved in a similar way to acetylcholine in a variety of pharmacological tests was demonstrated, and its actions were prevented or potentiated by drugs which blocked or potentiated the actions of acetylcholine. When several pharmacological tests were used to estimate the amount present, all gave the same value; this procedure is commonly referred to as *parallel quantitative assay*.

Sympathetic neuro-effector junctions

ADRENERGIC TRANSMISSION. In 1930 Finkleman demonstrated that a humoral substance was released from the stimulated sympathetic nerves to the intestine. He employed a technique similar to that used by Loewi for the frog heart. One piece of rabbit intestine was suspended above another, and Locke's solution was allowed to run over the upper one and then on to the lower one. When the sympathetic nerves to the upper segment were stimulated, the spontaneous movements of the intestine were inhibited and the tissue relaxed; shortly afterwards a similar response was recorded in the lower segment. Adrenaline produced a response which resembled that to the substance released from the upper segment.

Cannon and his colleagues later carried out many experiments to show that an adrenaline-like substance was liberated as a result of stimulating sym-pathetic nerves. The substance released in one organ was carried in the blood-stream to produce a response in a remote effector organ, often called an 'auto-indicator'. The auto-indicating organ was made 10 to 100 times more sensitive to adrenaline by cutting the sympathetic nerves to it 2 weeks before-hand. Suitable auto-indicating tissues were the iris or the nictitating membrane after removing the superior cervical ganglion, the spleen after cutting the splenic nerves, and the heart after removing the stellate ganglion. In a typical experiment using the denervated nictitating membrane as an auto-indicator, stimulation of the sympathetic splenic nerve produced contraction of the spleen, and a few seconds later the adrenaline-like substance released in the spleen and carried by the blood-stream produced a contraction of the sensitive nictitating membrane. The actions of the substance liberated when the sympathetic nerves were stimulated did not always match those of adrenaline, and so Cannon coined the term *sympathin* to describe the sympathetic transmitter released by the adrenergic nerves. Finally, von Euler and his colleagues, in 1946, showed that noradrenaline and only a little adrenaline was present in sympathetically innervated tissues. After sectioning the sympathetic nerves and allowing them about 2 weeks to degenerate, the noradrenaline content of a tissue was reduced to very low levels; it was soon realized that sympathin was identical with noradrenaline. The sympathin obtained from the splenic vein when the splenic sympathetic nerves were stimulated behaved qualitatively and quantitatively like noradrenaline and was distinguished from other related substances. The evidence for noradrenaline being the transmitter at adrenergic sympathetic nerve endings thus rests on three main points: (i) the similarity in responses to nerve stimulation and to noradrenaline, (ii) the presence of noradrenaline in tissues and its disappearance after denervation, and (iii) the liberation of noradrenaline when the nerves are stimulated.

CHOLINERGIC SYMPATHETIC TRANSMISSION. The sweat glands are one of the structures in the skin innervated by the sympathetic nerves, and yet sweating may be evoked by an injection of acetylcholine. Atropine blocks this action of acetylcholine and prevents sweating produced by sympathetic nerve stimulation. These observations point to cholinergic transmission in sympathetic nerves innervating the sweat glands. Furthermore, Dale and Feldberg perfused the foot of a cat and found that acetylcholine appeared in the perfusion fluid when the sympathetic nerves to the sweat glands were stimulated. There are other cholinergic sympathetic fibres. Burn found that stimulation of sympathetic nerves to the blood vessels in skeletal muscle produced dilatation and an increased blood flow through the muscle; these sympathetic nerves are cholinergic, the effects being enhanced by physostigmine and blocked by atropine. Cholinergic sympathetic nerves may also be involved in vasodilatation of the blood vessels in the skin of the head and neck, which results in the emotional phenomena of flushing and blushing.

Autonomic ganglia

Transmission at synapses in peripheral ganglia has been investigated by comparing the responses of an organ to stimulation of the pre- and post-ganglionic fibres which innervate it. Langley's experiments to locate ganglionic synapses by applying nicotine have already been mentioned. These observations, together with those of Dale on the nicotinic action of acetylcholine, provided clues that transmission in ganglionic synapses was humoral. More elegant methods of studying ganglionic transmission were provided by the techniques made available by electrophysiologists.

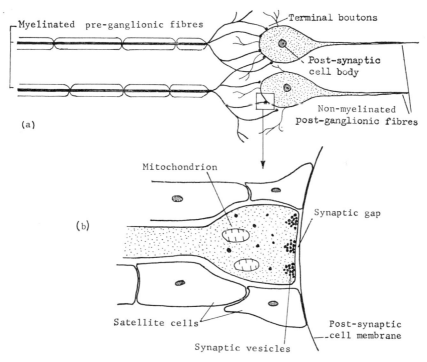

FIG. 5.2. General arrangement of nerve fibres entering and leaving a sympathetic ganglion. The lower part of the figure (*b*) is an enlargement of the nerve ending of a pre-ganglionic fibre to show the synaptic gap and vesicles, and the small satellite cells surrounding the synapse.

SYMPATHETIC GANGLIA. The superior cervical ganglion of the cat is the one which has been most thoroughly studied. Kibjakov, in 1933, perfused this ganglion through the carotid artery and collected the perfusate from the jugular vein. When the pre-ganglionic nerves were stimulated, the nictitating membrane contracted and the solution flowing from the ganglion contained a substance which stimulated the superior cervical ganglion of another cat. Feldberg and Gaddum showed that the substance liberated was acetylcholine. Experiments on other sympathetic ganglia have shown that the transmission process in them is similar to that in the superior cervical ganglion.

Noradrenaline has been detected in ganglia, and some of it has been shown to be present in adrenergic terminals impinging on the ganglion cells. Some noradrenaline is released from the ganglion on stimulation of the pre-ganglionic nerve and it may act to modulate cholinergic transmission. Small amounts of injected noradrenaline have been found to facilitate ganglionic transmission whereas larger amounts exert the opposite effect.

PARASYMPATHETIC GANGLIA. The ganglia of most parasympathetic nerves are situated within the tissues which they innervate and it is therefore difficult to study the transmission process. However, the ciliary ganglion (Fig. 4.11) is anatomically discrete and the experiments carried out on it have provided evidence that acetylcholine is the transmitter.

The adrenal medulla. The adrenal medulla is innervated by *pre-ganglionic sympathetic* fibres from the *splanchnic* nerves (Fig. 4.12). Stimulation of the nerves raises the blood pressure by releasing adrenaline and noradrenaline from the adrenal medulla into the blood-stream. Just before the rise in blood pressure, there is sometimes a slight fall which is greater after physostigmine and is abolished by atropine. These results suggest that acetylcholine is first liberated on stimulating the nerves, and it has been identified in the blood from the adrenal vein during stimulation. Small doses of acetylcholine injected into the arteries supplying the adrenal gland release adrenaline.

The neuromuscular junction in striated muscle

The short latency and brief contraction of a striated muscle in response to a single nerve impulse led many early investigators to doubt the possibility of a humoral mechanism at the neuromuscular junction. However, Dale, Feldberg and Vogt, in 1936, demonstrated the release of acetylcholine on stimulation of a somatic motor nerve. They perfused the blood vessels of the tongue of a cat and when they stimulated the hypoglossal nerve, producing contraction of the striated muscle in the tongue, acetylcholine was identified in the perfusion fluid leaving the tongue. In other experiments, the gastrocnemius muscle in the leg of the dog or the cat was perfused and the motor roots of the sciatic nerve were stimulated inside the spinal column, so as to avoid stimulating nerve fibres other than motoneurones. The substance appearing in the perfusate behaved qualitatively and quantitatively in the same way as a standard solution of acetylcholine, when tested on the dorsal muscle of the leech and on the cat's blood pressure. The presence of the substance was only detected when physostigmine was present in the perfusion fluid to inhibit the cholinesterase. Dale and his co-workers then showed that the release of acetylcholine was not due to the contraction of the muscle. Firstly, curare abolished the contractions although acetylcholine was still present in the perfusate after nerve stimulation. Secondly, direct electrical stimulation of the chronically denervated muscle elicited contractions, but no acetylcholine was detected in the perfusion fluid.

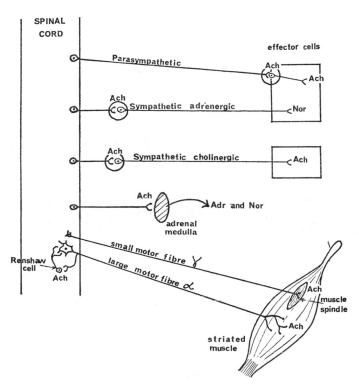

Fig. 5.3. General arrangement of nerve fibres leaving the spinal cord. The chemical transmitters at the different synapses are indicated as acetylcholine (Ach), noradrenaline (Nor) and adrenaline (Adr).

These experiments indicated that acetylcholine was released when the motor nerves were stimulated, and further work showed that it mimicked the effect of nerve stimulation in causing contraction. Some striated muscles, such as the frog's isolated rectus abdominis muscle, contract when acetylcholine is placed in the solution surrounding them. However, the contraction is slow, not in the least resembling the response to stimulation of a nerve (the reasons for this difference are discussed on page 207). Acetylcholine, injected intravenously into a cat (or any other mammal), produces profound effects on structures innervated by autonomic nerves, but has little effect on striated muscles, even after cholinesterase has been inactivated. However, Dale and his co-workers found that small doses of acetylcholine injected directly into the arteries supplying a skeletal muscle caused a quick contraction similar to that produced by nerve stimulation. Contractions produced by nerve stimulation and by 'close-arterially' injected acetylcholine were affected by drugs in a similar way. Thus curare blocked, and physostigmine potentiated, responses to both (Fig. 5.4).

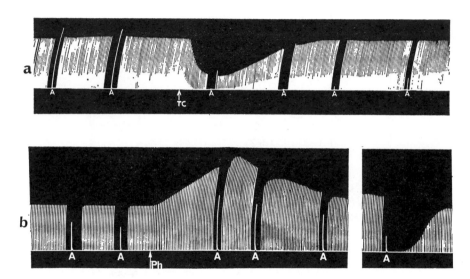

FIG. 5.4. Contractions of the anterior tibialis muscle of the cat when stimulated once every ten seconds through its motor nerve (unmarked contractions) and when stimulated by close arterial doses of acetylcholine (5 μg at points marked A). Tubo-curarine (0·3 mg/kg) injected intravenously at TC markedly reduced both contractions, whereas physostigmine (0·2 mg/kg) at Ph greatly potentiated both contractions. The last panel shows the block of transmission produced by a larger dose of acetylcholine (20 μg close-arterially) after a total of 0·5 mg/kg of physostigmine had been injected.

The failure of acetylcholine to produce a detectable contraction of striated muscle when given by intravenous injection is chiefly due to the extreme brevity of the contractions of the individual muscle fibres. The contractions of smooth muscle fibres are relatively prolonged and they therefore summate to produce a visible response when small amounts of acetylcholine are present in the blood-stream. For summation to occur in a striated muscle, a large number of muscle fibres must respond synchronously. This occurs only when the local concentration of acetylcholine is high, such as after a close-arterial injection. Recently a technique involving electrophoresis has been developed by which acetylcholine may be applied from a micro-pipette directly to the sensitive area of a striated muscle fibre. Using this technique, minute amounts of acetylcholine (much smaller than those effective by close-arterial injection) have been shown to stimulate the muscle.

Pharmacological evidence has indicated that the chemical transmitter released from the small motor nerve fibres (the γ-efferents) which innervate the muscle spindles (p. 107) is also acetylcholine.

Peripheral actions of chemical transmitters

Acetylcholine

MUSCARINIC ACTIONS. The muscarinic actions of acetylcholine correspond to those produced by the alkaloid, muscarine. Acetylcholine released from post-ganglionic parasympathetic nerves produces most of these effects, and the muscarinic actions of acetylcholine therefore include the responses produced by stimulation of parasympathetic nerves listed in Table 4.1. A few sympathetic post-ganglionic nerves are cholinergic, and actions of acetylcholine which mimic those of stimulation of cholinergic sympathetic nerves are also included among its muscarinic actions; these include secretion of sweat by the eccrine sweat glands, and vasodilatation in skeletal muscle and in some areas of skin. In addition, acetylcholine produces muscarinic effects on tissues which are innervated predominantly by adrenergic nerves; these effects include dilatation of peripheral arterioles, contraction of the nictitating membrane, contraction of the spleen in some species and contraction of smooth muscle in some parts of the urino-genital system. All of the muscarinic actions of injected acetylcholine, or of muscarine itself, are abolished by atropine.

Recent experiments on the superior cervical ganglion of the cat have shown that muscarine stimulates the ganglion cells and that this effect is blocked by atropine but not by drugs which block the nicotinic actions of acetylcholine; in addition, ganglion stimulation produced by acetylcholine is due not only to a nicotinic action but also has an atropine-sensitive component. It is not yet known if this muscarinic action of acetylcholine plays a physiological role in ganglionic transmission; in any case, the transmission of nerve impulses is completely prevented by drugs which block only the nicotinic actions of acetylcholine.

NICOTINIC ACTIONS. The main peripheral nicotinic actions of acetylcholine are to stimulate striated muscle, autonomic ganglion cells, and the adrenal medulla. The effect on muscle is contraction, and stimulation of the adrenal medulla releases adrenaline and noradrenaline into the blood-stream. The result of stimulation of ganglion cells depends on the conditions of the experiment and on whether sympathetic or parasympathetic ganglia are the more affected. The apparent insensitivity of striated muscle to intravenously injected acetylcholine has already been mentioned. Although more sensitive than muscle, autonomic ganglia respond only to relatively large intravenous doses of acetylcholine, since a large number of ganglion cells must be activated synchronously to produce a visible response from the effector organ. The brief duration of the response of each ganglion cell means that synchronous activity is produced only when the local concentration of acetylcholine is high.

Acetylcholine also possesses nicotinic actions which may not have any counterpart in physiological processes; thus it stimulates sensory nerve endings, and releases adrenaline and noradrenaline from chromaffin cells which are present in some tissues. Although there is no evidence that these chromaffin cells are innervated by cholinergic nerves, the action of injected acetylcholine upon them appears to be analogous to its action on the chromaffin tissue of the adrenal medulla.

All of the nicotinic actions of acetylcholine may be mimicked by the injection of nicotine. They are blocked by the previous injection either of large doses of nicotine itself or of tubocurarine. Large doses of acetylcholine itself, particularly in the presence of an anticholinesterase drug, block transmission at most, and possibly all sites at which acetylcholine exerts a nicotinic action. Thus transmission at the neuromuscular junction, at the ganglionic synapse and at the junction between the splanchnic nerves and the adrenal medulla is blocked by large doses of acetylcholine. Rapidly repeated stimulation of nerves may result in the accumulation of sufficient acetylcholine to block transmission at these sites, provided that cholinesterase has first been inactivated. This blocking effect of acetylcholine has particular significance for the neuromuscular junction, since drugs possessing the nicotinic action of acetylcholine at this site are used in medicine to produce muscle paralysis (pages 669–675).

Mechanism of action of acetylcholine. Acetylcholine is believed to exert its effects by combining and reacting with chemical groups on the external surface of the cell membranes. These groups are described as *receptors* but they must not be confused with the *sensory receptors* situated at the ends of first-order afferent nerves. The nature of acetylcholine receptors (sometimes called *cholinoceptive receptors*) has largely been deduced from pharmacological experiments and is therefore discussed on pages 710–712.

The combination of acetylcholine with its receptors produces a change in the permeability of the cell membrane. When the change is such that the permeability to small ions is increased, the ions move more freely down their concentration gradients and the membrane is depolarized. On the other hand, when acetylcholine induces a selective increase in permeability to some ions, such as K^+ and Cl^-, the membrane is hyperpolarized. In general, depolarization of the membrane increases activity of the cell. Thus depolarization of glandular cell membranes results in release of secretion, and depolarization of muscle and ganglion cell membranes initiates propagating action potentials, which in muscle cause contraction. Hyperpolarization of the cell membrane inhibits the production of propagating action potentials and therefore depresses activity. Acetylcholine may act to depolarize and therefore excite one effector cell, but to hyperpolarize and inhibit another. For example, it stimulates the gut but causes relaxation of the smooth muscle in many blood vessels and slows the heart.

The mechanisms of neuro-effector transmission in muscle are discussed more fully in Chapter 7 but it is convenient here to describe transmission in autonomic ganglia. Diagrams of the sympathetic ganglionic synapse are given in Fig. 5.2 and some of its properties are described in pp. 89–91. On the arrival of a nerve impulse at the pre-synaptic endings, acetylcholine is released from all of the synaptic knobs. The acetylcholine diffuses across the small synaptic gap and reacts with receptors on the dendrites or cell body of the post-ganglionic neurone to produce a localized, non-propagated, graded depolarization of the post-synaptic membrane. The external surface of the cell body or dendrite membrane therefore becomes negative with respect to the external surface of the post-ganglionic axon and this relative negativity is known as the *synaptic potential*. When the local depolarization reaches a critical value, which may represent a critical area or a critical degree of depolarization, or both, this part of the neurone acts as a current sink for regions immediately ahead of it. Local currents therefore flow into it and a propagating, all-or-nothing action potential is initiated and travels along the post-ganglionic fibre. Acetylcholinesterase (page 157) is present in ganglia and its role is presumably to destroy the transmitter. There is more than sufficient enzyme present to destroy all of the released transmitter within the refractory period of the ganglion cells. However, inhibition of cholinesterase by anti-cholinesterase drugs produces less striking effects on ganglionic transmission than it does at some other cholinergic transmission sites (e.g. the neuromuscular junction). It has been calculated that the small amount of acetylcholine released by a single impulse in a pre-ganglionic fibre (estimated to be about 1×10^{-10} g) would be diluted to a subeffective concentration by simple physical diffusion from the receptor sites within the refractory period of the ganglion cells. In some sympathetic ganglia, the cholinesterase is associated with the pre-synaptic nerve endings rather than with the ganglion cells, and it has been suggested that its function is to protect the nerve endings from depolarizing in the presence of the transmitter. It may be that in autonomic ganglia the acetylcholine is eliminated partly by enzyme action and partly by simple diffusion. The excess of enzyme present may therefore be a mechanism for the destruction of abnormally large accumulations of acetylcholine.

In the absence of nerve impulses, there is a spontaneous release of small amounts of acetylcholine from the pre-synaptic nerve endings. This gives rise to small potential changes known as *miniature synaptic potentials*, which are too small to initiate propagating action potentials in the post-synaptic neurone.

Detection of acetylcholine. Some tissues are particularly sensitive to the action of acetylcholine but most may be rendered more sensitive by inactivation of cholinesterase. The responses may then be used to identify and assay small quantities of acetylcholine present in tissue and perfusion fluids. Examples of preparations used in this way are given in Table 5.1.

Noradrenaline and adrenaline

Noradrenaline is released from most post-ganglionic sympathetic nerve endings, and an injection of noradrenaline produces responses which mimic most responses to sympathetic nerve stimulation listed in Table 4.1. Noradrenaline also causes secretion of sweat although the sympathetic innervation to the eccrine sweat glands is cholinergic. In most respects the actions of adrenaline are qualitatively similar to those of noradrenaline but there is one important difference. All effective doses of noradrenaline produce vasoconstriction in skeletal muscles, whereas adrenaline produces vasodilatation in small doses and vasoconstriction only when large doses are given. Small doses of adrenaline may lower the total peripheral resistance by producing vasodilatation in striated muscles. The diastolic blood pressure therefore falls but systolic blood pressure rises as adrenaline increases the force of the heart beat. Larger doses of adrenaline, and all effective doses of noradrenaline, increase the peripheral resistance by constricting most blood vessels, including those in striated muscle. The direct actions of both amines on the heart are qualitatively similar but in the whole animal reflexes initiated by the rise in blood pressure modify these effects. With noradrenaline, reflex slowing of the heart overcomes the relatively weak direct stimulant action and the net result is a slowing of the heart rate. With adrenaline, on the other hand, the direct action on the heart is greater so that the net effect usually remains as an increase in force and rate of the beat.

Both adrenaline and noradrenaline are released from the adrenal medullae into the blood-stream, and therefore the effects of splanchnic nerve stimulation are similar to those of injecting a mixture of the two amines. Adrenaline and noradrenaline stimulate some effector cells and inhibit others. In most cases, adrenaline is more potent than noradrenaline. As with acetylcholine, increased activity of a tissue results from a depolarizing action on the cell membranes while inhibition is associated with hyperpolarization. In some cases the change in membrane potential is believed to be a consequence of reaction of the amine with receptor sites on the external surface of the cell membranes, whereas in others it may be a consequence of an intracellular action arising from changes in the tissue metabolism, mediated through cyclic 3', 5' adenosine monophosphate (see page 738).

TABLE 5.1. Preparations used for the detection and assay of acetylcholine.

Tissue	Response	Sensitivity to acetylcholine after cholinesterase inhibition	Remarks
Blood pressure of anaesthetized eviscerated cat	Fall in blood pressure	1 to 2 ng	Blocked by atropine
Blood pressure of lightly anaesthetized rat	Fall in blood pressure	0·5 to 2 ng	Blocked by atropine
Isolated rectus abdominus muscle of frog	Contraction	5 to 20 ng/ml	Sensitized by ATP; blocked by tubocurarine
Isolated dorsal muscle of leech	Contraction	0·5 to 2 ng/ml	Blocked by tubocurarine
Isolated ileum of guinea-pig	Contraction	1 to 5 ng/ml	Blocked by atropine

Orbeli, in 1923, showed that stimulation of the lumbar sympathetic chain in the frog produced an increase in the contractions of the gastrocnemius muscle which had been fatigued by rapid stimulation of the motor roots (the Orbeli effect). A similar effect is produced in fatigued mammalian muscle and may be mimicked by injection of adrenaline or noradrenaline. It was once thought that the Orbeli effect was due to a direct adrenergic innervation of striated muscle fibres but this belief is no longer held; probably the effect is due to noradrenaline released from the nerves to the blood vessels diffusing to the muscle fibres. It is not known whether the defatiguing effect of adrenaline and noradrenaline plays any part in the normal functioning of muscle;

it is uncertain whether fatigue of the type produced by Orbeli has any physio-logical counterpart, and the frequencies of sympathetic stimulation required to produce the effect (10/sec and above) are probably higher than those occurring even in extreme conditions.

In non-fatigued muscles, adrenaline and noradrenaline exert two separate effects. They improve neuromuscular transmission, probably by increasing the release of acetylcholine in response to nerve impulses, and they affect contractions of the muscles by an action exerted directly on the muscle fibres. The direct effects on the muscle differ according to the type of muscle. The contractions of fast-contracting muscles are increased and prolonged, while the opposite effects are produced in slow-contracting muscles. The terms, fast- and slow-contracting, are explained on pages 206–207.

TABLE 5.2. Preparations used for the detection and assay of noradrenaline and adrenaline.

Preparation	Response	Sensitivity to	
		Noradrenaline	Adrenaline
Blood pressure of pithed rat	Rise in blood pressure	1 ng	5–10 ng
Rat's uterus contracted by carbachol	Inhibition of contraction	100 ng/ml	1 ng/ml
Fowl's rectal caecum	Relaxation	40 ng/ml	1 ng/ml

Detection of adrenaline and noradrenaline. Both amines may be identified and assayed chemically, the most sensitive method depending on the formation of compounds which fluoresce in ultra-violet light. Biological methods are often necessary when only small amounts are present, and some of these are tabulated above (Table 5.2).

Synthesis, storage, release and destruction of neurohormones

Acetylcholine

SYNTHESIS OF ACETYLCHOLINE. Acetylcholine is synthesized by a specific enzyme, *choline acetyltransferase* (choline acetylase), which transfers the acetyl radical from acetylcoenzyme A to choline (Fig. 5.5). Coenzyme A and choline are widely distributed and are found in most tissues. The choline acetyltransferase of cholinergic neurones is made in the cell body, probably by the ribosomes, and travels along the axon, being carried by the downward flow of axoplasm. When the trunk of a cholinergic nerve is cut, a high concentration of enzyme accumulates in the stump above the cut, while the enzyme is depleted from the nerve trunk below the cut. Choline acetyltransferase has not been isolated as a pure enzyme, but an extract of nerve tissue containing a high concentration of enzymatic activity has been prepared as a fairly stable dry powder. In the intact tissue, the acetylcholine-synthesizing system is contained in sub-cellular particles. The rate of synthesis of acetylcholine by extracts of nerve tissue is greatly increased when the sub-cellular particles are disrupted. The synthesis of acetylcholine by nervous tissue has been studied in slices of brain and in the perfused superior cervical ganglion. Synthesis occurs throughout the neurone, but it is most rapid at the nerve endings

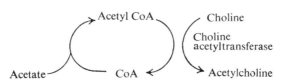

FIG. 5.5. Synthesis of acetylcholine from choline and acetyl groups.

where it provides the acetylcholine to replace that released by nerve impulses. Even after the release of considerable amounts of acetylcholine, the content is maintained or rapidly restored to the level in the resting state, suggesting that release stimulates resynthesis. In addition to the enzymes and substrate mentioned, glucose, oxygen and sodium ions are necessary for optimal acetylcholine synthesis.

The synthesis of acetylcholine in intact tissues, or in tissue extracts containing intact sub-cellular particles, is inhibited by a drug known as hemicholinium. However, choline acetyltransferase freed from the particles is not inhibited. Hemicholinium is believed to prevent the transport of choline across the cell membranes and into the sub-cellular particles. Repeated stimulation of a cholinergic nerve in the presence of hemicholinium results in the release of the stored acetylcholine, with no resynthesis of fresh stores. Ultimately the acetylcholine is exhausted and cholinergic transmission fails. Failure of transmission produced by hemicholinium may therefore be taken as evidence in support of acetylcholine being involved in the transmission process.

Chemical formula of hemicholinium: the two choline moieties in the molecule are indicated by the thick lines.

STORAGE OF ACETYLCHOLINE. Acetylcholine in tissues is bound in such a way that it does not exert its pharmacological action. In order to estimate the total quantity of acetylcholine in a tissue, it is necessary to disrupt the bonds by denaturing the tissue proteins (by heating, or with alcohol, trichloracetic acid or other protein precipitants). The bound acetylcholine is contained in sub-cellular particles which have a different density from other cell fractions and may therefore be separated by centrifugation. These particles have diameters of 300 to 600 Å and are termed *synaptic vesicles*. Electron microscopists have observed particles of this size in nerve terminals from the central nervous system, autonomic ganglia (Fig. 5.2) and the neuromuscular junction (Fig. 7.2).

RELEASE OF ACETYLCHOLINE. The release of acetylcholine by the nerve impulse has been studied using the cat's perfused superior cervical

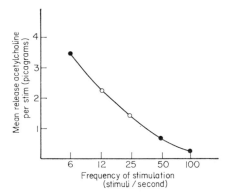

FIG. 5.6. Relationship between frequency of stimulation of phrenic nerve and the amount of acetylcholine released per stimulus from rat isolated hemi-diaphragms. At each frequency the stimulation was applied for 20 min. The acetylcholine in the fluid surrounding the diaphragm was assayed on the blood pressure of the rat. (Data calculated from Straughan (1960), *Brit. J. Pharmacol.*, **15**, 417.)

ganglion and the rat's isolated diaphragm. The amount released by each stimulus depends on the frequency of stimulation and at high frequencies it is diminished (Fig. 5.6). The rate of release declines to a constant value during the period of stimulation, but the reason for this is unknown. It may be that the store of preformed acetylcholine in the nerve endings becomes exhausted in a perfused organ so that the amount released becomes limited by the rate of resynthesis, or that, when the interval between stimuli is short, reserve acetylcholine is not mobilized fast enough. Another factor which contributes to the decline in transmitter output at high frequencies of stimulation is that not all the impulses reach the nerve ending: this is known as *pre-synaptic failure*. It is more pronounced the higher the frequency of stimulation and is more readily produced in isolated tissues than in muscles with intact circulation. Pre-synaptic failure is due to depolarization of the nerve endings and is abolished when the nerve endings are hyperpolarized by an anodal current.

After a brief period of high-frequency stimulation, a single nerve impulse releases a greater amount of transmitter than before. This occurs not only at cholinergic nerve endings but at all junctions, and probably accounts for the phenomenon of post-tetanic or post-activation potentiation (pp. 118–119). During the period of stimulation, the positive after-potentials summate so that the nerve endings remain hyperpolarized for a longer time than usual. This hyperpolarization probably accounts for the greater release of transmitter by subsequent single shocks, since hyperpolarization of the nerve endings produced by anodal currents also augments the release of transmitter in response to nerve impulses.

The temperature also affects the amount of acetylcholine released. In the ganglion, changing from 39°C to 20°C reduces the amount of acetylcholine released to one-tenth when the frequency of stimulation is 10/sec, but does not reduce the amount released at a frequency of 2/sec. At the lower temperature, resynthesis probably does not keep pace with the more rapid rate of release.

The mechanism of acetylcholine release involves the passage of calcium ions from the extracellular fluid into the axoplasm of the nerve endings. The amount of acetylcholine released by nerve impulses is proportional, over a wide range, to the concentration of calcium ion in the extracellular fluid. Calcium ions may in some way disrupt the synaptic vesicles causing them to spill their contents into the junctional gap. Calcium ions may also play a part in the increased release of transmitter in response to a single shock which occurs after a period of high-frequency stimulation. During the high-frequency stimulation, extra calcium ion enters the axoplasm and time is required for the excess calcium to be pumped out. An impulse arriving at the terminal during this time may therefore release more acetylcholine because more calcium ion is available to disrupt the vesicles. Magnesium ions have the opposite effect to calcium ions, increased magnesium concentrations depressing acetylcholine output. For the optimal release of acetylcholine, three other agents are necessary: bicarbonate ions, sodium ions, and an unidentified factor of low molecular weight present in plasma.

There is a slow spontaneous release of acetylcholine from somatic motor nerve endings and from pre-ganglionic autonomic fibres (page 150). Electro-physiological evidence indicates that the acetylcholine is released from small packets of constant size, believed to be the synaptic vesicles. Each contains the smallest releasable quantity of acetylcholine, which is therefore called a quantum of acetylcholine (estimated at between 1000 and 10,000 molecules).

The release of acetylcholine from cholinergic nerves is prevented by the toxin of the micro-organism *Clostridium botulinum*. Botulinum toxin may therefore be used in experiments to identify transmitter substances.

DESTRUCTION OF ACETYLCHOLINE. The presence of an enzyme capable of destroying acetylcholine was postulated by Dale in 1914, but it was not discovered until 1925 when it was demonstrated in the small intestine of the horse and pig. In 1932 a similar enzyme was found in horse serum and named *cholinesterase*. It is now known that there is a whole family of cholinesterases which differ in their substrate specificity and in other properties. Cholinesterases are often broadly classified into *true* or *specific cholinesterases* and *pseudo* or *non-specific cholinesterases*. True cholinesterases occur in red blood cells, in nervous tissue and in striated muscle. Where they are concentrated at the sites of cholinergic transmission, they are believed to be responsible for the destruction of the transmitter. Pseudocholinesterases occur in plasma, intestine, skin and many other tissues. Their function is uncertain except in the case of the intestine where they are believed to be responsible for controlling the effect of acetylcholine in increasing intrinsic rhythmic movements and tone of the gut.

Both types of enzyme destroy acetylcholine but only true cholinesterases destroy acetyl-β-methylcholine. In contrast, only pseudocholinesterases destroy benzoylcholine and succinyldicholine. High concentrations of acetylcholine inhibit true cholinesterases so that the enzyme shows its highest activity against an optimal concentration of substrate (about 2×10^{-3} M for acetylcholine). Pseudocholinesterases, on the other hand, increase in activity with increase in substrate concentration, no inhibition of the enzyme occurring with higher concentrations of substrate. Cholinesterases are now named according to the substrate against which they show the highest activity. Thus, *acetylcholinesterase* is more active against acetylcholine than against other choline esters and is the main true cholinesterase present in mammals. *Butyrylcholinesterase* shows its highest activity against butyrylcholine and is the main pseudocholinesterase present in mammals, although *propionylcholinesterase* has been found in rat brain and rat heart muscle and in the spleen of cattle. Propionylcholine is present in small amounts in the spleen of cattle, but the fact that a particular cholinesterase is most active against a certain substrate does not necessarily mean that its function in life is to destroy that substrate.

Extensive studies by Nachmansohn and his colleagues on the reaction of acetylcholinesterase with different substrates and inhibitors have demonstrated the presence of two active sites on the enzyme (Fig. 5.7). (1) *The anionic site* is negatively charged and stereospecific; it attracts the positively charged nitrogen atom of acetylcholine and binds the attached methyl groups by Van der Waals' forces. (2) *The esteratic site* combines with the carbonyl C-atom of the acetyl group.

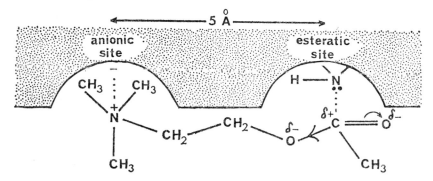

FIG. 5.7. The two active sites on the acetylcholinesterase enzyme by which acetylcholine is held.

The hydrolysis of acetylcholine, or of any other substrate, is believed to take place in three stages. The first stage consists of an equilibrium between the enzyme and acetylcholine and an adsorption complex of the two:

In the second stage, the complex reacts to release choline and leaves an acetylated enzyme:

In the third stage, the acetylenzyme reacts with water to give acetic acid and regenerated active enzyme:

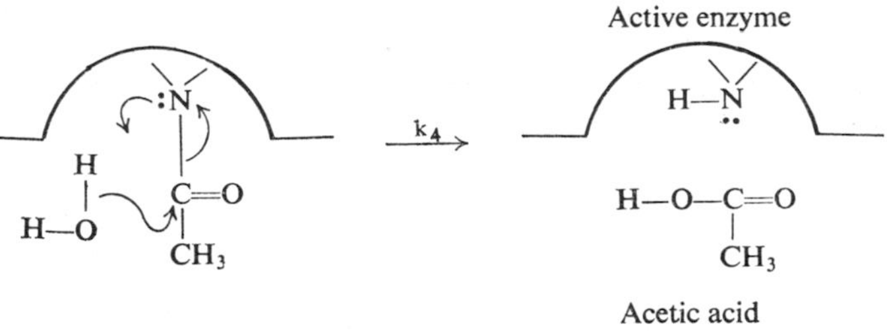

The hydrolysis of acetylcholine occurs extremely quickly. Each single active site in a purified sample of ox red cell acetylcholinesterase is capable of hydrolysing 3×10^5 molecules of acetylcholine per minute. Pseudocholinesterase also possesses two active sites, but that corresponding to the anionic site of acetylcholinesterase is probably not charged. Other esterases contain only an esteratic site.

ESTIMATION OF CHOLINESTERASE ACTIVITY. Methods for estimating cholinesterase activity usually depend on estimating the acid (acetic acid in the case of acetylcholine) released on hydrolysis of the ester. The most common is the *Warburg manometric technique* in which enzyme and substrate react in the presence of bicarbonate buffer. The volume of CO_2 released from the bicarbonate by the acid is measured with the manometer. Another method which is very sensitive but which requires great skill is to estimate the CO_2 in a Cartesian diver. Other methods involve measuring the change in pH using an indicator in a colorimeter or a glass electrode. Alternatively, the amount of alkali necessary to maintain constant pH may be continually titrated.

Histochemical methods for locating cholinesterase activity are also available. *Acetylthiocholine* is used as the substrate in the presence of a buffer containing copper glycinate. The hydrolysis of acetylthiocholine liberates thiocholine which is precipitated as the dark coloured copper thiocholine at the site of the enzyme.

The above methods may be adapted to study the activity of drugs which inhibit cholinesterases. In these studies, various concentrations of the drug are added to the enzyme-substrate mixture and the effect upon hydrolysis is determined.

Noradrenaline and adrenaline

SYNTHESIS. Noradrenaline and adrenaline are synthesized in sympathetic adrenergic neurones, in the adrenal medullae and other chromaffin tissues, and in parts of the central nervous system. These two catecholamines are optically active: only the *laevo*-isomers are present in the tissues. The main route of synthesis is shown in Fig. 5.8. The essential amino acids, phenylalanine and tyrosine, are derived from proteins in the diet. The oxidizing enzymes forming dopa from phenylalanine and tyrosine are found in adrenergic neurones and the adrenal medulla. They are also found in melanophore cells, which are specialized for the production of the dark brown pigment of the hair and skin known as melanin. Melanophore cells are derived embryologically from cells of the neural crest, as are sympathetic ganglion cells and the cells of the adrenal medulla. Melanins are formed from phenylalanine and tyrosine by a route which may involve the oxidation and condensation of dopamine, noradrenaline and adrenaline. The condition of albinism is due to an inborn failure of the enzymatic pathways concerned with the production of melanin. Another disorder due to lack of the enzyme oxidizing phenylalanine to tyrosine is phenylketonuria (pages 186–187). Phenylalanine and tyrosine are also the dietary precursors of the thyroid hormones (pages 368–374).

The formation of dopa is a relatively slow process and dopa does not accumulate in the tissues as it is rapidly converted to dopamine by *dopa decarboxylase*. This enzyme, first discovered in the kidney, resembles decarboxylases acting on other amino acids (p. 50). The pharmacological actions of dopamine resemble those of noradrenaline, but there are differences (see page 745). The amounts found in the tissues are probably a reserve of the precursor for the synthesis of noradrenaline. Dopamine is also found in the urine which suggests that an excess is always formed. The enzyme converting dopamine to noradrenaline is known as *ethylamine β-oxidase*. The reaction is energy-requiring and utilizes ATP, with either NAD or NADP as co-factors and an oxygen donor such as ascorbic acid. The enzyme is not specific for dopamine and catalyses a similar oxidation of the side-chains of tyramine and epinine to yield octopamine and adrenaline respectively (Fig. 5.9).

The formation of adrenaline from noradrenaline by the enzyme *phenyl-ethanolamine N-methyl transferase* requires a methyl donor such as methionine, choline or creatine. This enzyme also is not specific, and the substances formed by the *N*-methylation of octopamine (yielding synephrine), of dopamine (yielding epinine) and of adrenaline (yielding dimethylnoradrenaline) have been demonstrated in tissues (Fig. 5.9). The rate of synthesis of noradrenaline in adrenergic nerves and of noradrenaline and adrenaline in the adrenal medulla depends on the rate of release of these substances, and there is rapid replacement when some is lost as a result of nerve stimulation.

STORAGE OF CATECHOLAMINES (noradrenaline, adrenaline and dopamine). The largest stores of catecholamines are in the adrenal medulla where the mean

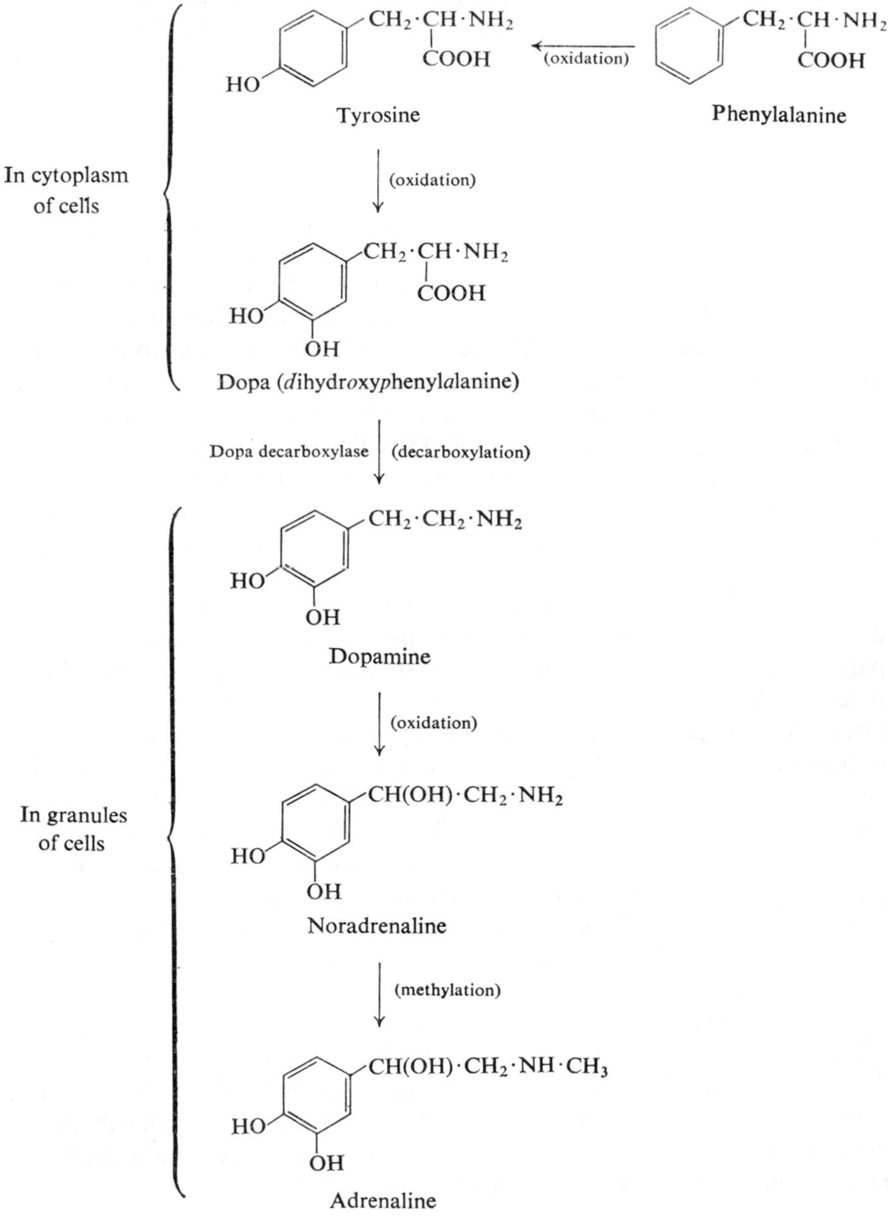

FIG. 5.8. Biosynthesis of catecholamines.

content, depending on the species, ranges from 0·3 to 10 milligrams per gram of tissue. Usually more adrenaline than noradrenaline is present, the two adrenal glands from one animal having similar contents. After depleting the stores of catecholamine in the adrenals, noradrenaline is reformed rapidly and in excess, and then it is more slowly converted to adrenaline. In the embryo and in young animals, there is more noradrenaline than adrenaline.

Noradrenaline, adrenaline and dopamine present in the adrenal medulla are contained in granules within the cells. These granules have diameters of 0·1 to 0·6 μ; their density differs from that of other sub-cellular particles such as mitochondria, fragments of cell membranes, and nuclei, and this allows their separation from homogenized tissues by differential centrifugation. Particles containing only one of the catecholamines (noradrenaline, adrenaline or dopamine) have been isolated. Histochemically, two different medullary cell types have been distinguished. The histochemical reaction which reveals the catecholamine-containing granules in the adrenal medulla was discovered in 1865 by Henle, who found that solutions of dichromate salts stained them brown, the reaction being due to the oxidation of catechols to give melanin-like substances. Staining by dichromate is known as the chromaffin reaction, and cells so stained are called chromaffin cells. Clumps of chromaffin cells, called paraganglia, are situated along the length of the aorta, the most conspicuous being a pair of bodies, known as the *organs of Zuckerkandl,* located on either side of the abdominal aorta near the origin of the inferior mesenteric artery. The organs of Zuckerkandl are present in the foetus and achieve their greatest size soon after birth, thereafter gradually regressing. They contain principally noradrenaline, but the proportion of noradrenaline to adrenaline diminishes with age, as in the adrenals. Groups of chromaffin cells are also found in the carotid bodies and the aortic bodies, structures which are considered elsewhere as sites containing the endings of sensory nerves subserving respiratory reflexes (page 289) and cardiovascular reflexes (page 274). The principal catecholamine in these bodies is noradrenaline. Scattered chromaffin cells occur in sympathetic ganglia, along the trunks of sympathetic nerves, and in some sympathetically innervated tissues. These cells contain the small amounts of adrenaline present in tissues. Tumours of chromaffin cells may contain large amounts of one of the catecholamines or a mixture of them, and are usually of adrenal origin although other tumours may occur in the chromaffin cells of the paraganglia. Dopamine-containing chromaffin cells have been found in the lungs and in parts of the intestine. Accumulation of dopamine is not the result of a deficiency in the activity of the enzyme converting dopamine to noradrenaline; the dopamine is bound, presumably at specific storage sites in the granules, and is not accessible to the enzyme.

The adrenergic nerves principally contain noradrenaline. The nerves do not

6

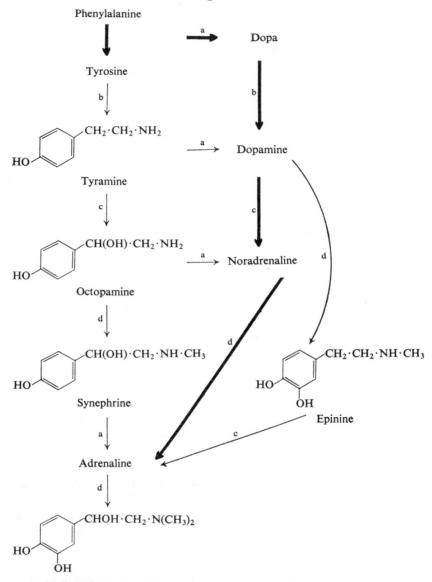

Fig. 5.9. Inter-relationships of metabolic pathways concerned in the biosynthesis of catecholamines and related pharmacologically active amines occurring in some tissues. The heavy arrows show the principal route of formation (see Fig. 5.8). The enzymes acting on more than one substrate in this scheme are: a, phenyl oxidase; b, decarboxylase; c, β-oxidase; d, N-methyl transferase.

give a chromaffin reaction, but recently developed histochemical techniques make it possible to detect their noradrenaline content microscopically. Small noradrenaline-containing granules are present, about 0·1 to 0·5 μ in diameter. Some of the noradrenaline may be free in the cytoplasm or distributed in more diffuse structures than the granules. After cutting a post-ganglionic sympathetic nerve trunk, the fibres beyond the cut degenerate and the content of noradrenaline disappears from the tissues they formerly supplied. The small amount of adrenaline found in the tissues persists as it is contained in the scattered chromaffin cells which are unaffected by the denervation. Cutting the pre-ganglionic fibres does not affect the content of noradrenaline in the innervated effector tissue. The chromaffin cells of the adrenal medulla are innervated by pre-ganglionic sympathetic nerve fibres of the splanchnic nerve, and the ability of these cells to synthesize and store catecholamines is also unaffected by denervation. Little is known about the innervation of other chromaffin cells. Parts of the central nervous system also contain appreciable stores of the catecholamines, and the related substance, tyramine, has also been detected, particularly in the spinal cord.

The catecholamine-containing granules isolated from the cells of the adrenal medulla and from sympathetic nerve trunks contain ATP, and the amount of catecholamine bound is related to the amount of ATP. The isolated granules take up and bind catecholamines from the surrounding medium, the uptake being activated by ATP and by magnesium ions. Infusions of catecholamines, or of precursors of catecholamines, into isolated tissues or intact animals, leads to an increase in the amounts bound in the tissues. The ability of an organ to take up noradrenaline is lost after degeneration of the sympathetic nerve supply. However, some non-innervated cells, for example, erythrocytes and platelets, take up small amounts of catecholamines.

The stores of catecholamines in tissues, including the central nervous system, are depleted after giving drugs such as reserpine. The mechanism of action of reserpine, however, is not fully explained. It does not impair the synthesis of catecholamines (thus its mechanism of action differs from that of hemicholinium in depleting stores of acetylcholine from cholinergic nerves), and the tissue content of noradrenaline (except that in the brain) may be temporarily restored by giving an infusion of noradrenaline. The most likely explanation is that reserpine weakens the strength of the attachment between catecholamines and the binding site.

RELEASE OF CATECHOLAMINES. The release of catecholamines from the cells of the adrenal medulla in response to stimulation of the splanchnic nerve fibres is mediated by acetylcholine. The granules may disrupt through the cell membrane and empty their contents extracellularly (this would be analogous to the discharge of acetylcholine from synaptic vesicles), or they may release the catecholamines from the granules intracellularly, in which case the amines would then have to pass across the cell membrane. In the cat, the maximum rate of secretion of catecholamine from one adrenal gland is sufficient to produce considerable (but not maximal) excitation of tissues which respond to catecholamines. The content of adrenaline in the plasma is derived mainly from that released by the adrenal glands. In man under resting conditions, the average is about 0·1 ng/ml, corresponding to a total amount of 0·3 μg. When there are conditions of stress, excitement or heavy muscular activity, the amount increases tenfold or more. The spontaneous release of catecholamines from a chromaffin cell tumour (phaeochromocytoma) may be sufficient to elevate the blood pressure. Prolonged stimulation of adrenergic nerves does not cause any significant depletion of noradrenaline from them, and hence the rate of replacement is as rapid as the release. This suggests that, as in cholinergic nerves, the process of release provides the stimulus for resynthesis. Some of the noradrenaline released by nerve impulses re-enters storage sites in the nerve endings. There is evidence that the release of adrenaline and noradrenaline from the adrenal medullae and from adrenergic nerve endings, like that of acetylcholine from cholinergic nerve endings, is dependent on the extracellular calcium concentration.

Burn and Rand in 1959 suggested that acetylcholine is involved as an intermediary in the release of noradrenaline at adrenergic nerve endings. Their evidence depended, at first, on the fact that acetylcholine is released from many sympathetic nerve trunks which contain predominantly adrenergic fibres, and that acetylcholine (in the presence of atropine to block its muscarinic actions) has a similar effect to that of sympathetic nerve stimulation. For example, the effect of acetylcholine in mimicking sympathetic nerve stimulation occurs in the isolated heart, which is accelerated by acetylcholine in the presence of atropine. Further, the injection of acetylcholine into the skin produces pilo-erection and into the atropinized rabbit ear causes vasoconstriction. The adrenergic effects of acetylcholine are blocked by anti-adrenaline drugs and are absent after depleting tissue stores of noradrenaline, either with reserpine or by sympathetic denervation. The liberation by acetylcholine of an adrenaline-like substances from the heart and spleen has also been demonstrated. Responses to stimulation of some sympathetic nerves are blocked by hemicholinium which interferes with the synthesis of acetylcholine and by botulinum toxin which interferes with the release of acetylcholine. Section and degeneration of the sympathetic nerves to the spleen leads to a parallel loss of noradrenaline and of acetylcholine. At the present time, there is controversy over the hypothesis that acetylcholine is involved at adrenergic nerve endings as an intermediary transmitter which in turn releases noradrenaline.

INACTIVATION OF CATECHOLAMINES. The action of catecholamines on effector cells is terminated when the concentrations are reduced below a critical level. One way in which this is brought about is by enzymatic action. The enzymes principally concerned in reducing the activity of catecholamines by metabolizing them are *monoamine oxidase* and *catechol O-methyl transferase*.

Monoamine oxidase (*MAO*) is an oxidative deaminase; the amine is oxidized to yield the corresponding aldehyde and ammonia (or methylamine in the case of adrenaline); the aldehyde is then oxidized to the acid. Dopamine and tyramine are better substrates (i.e. they are converted more rapidly) than adrenaline and noradrenaline. The reactions are as follows:

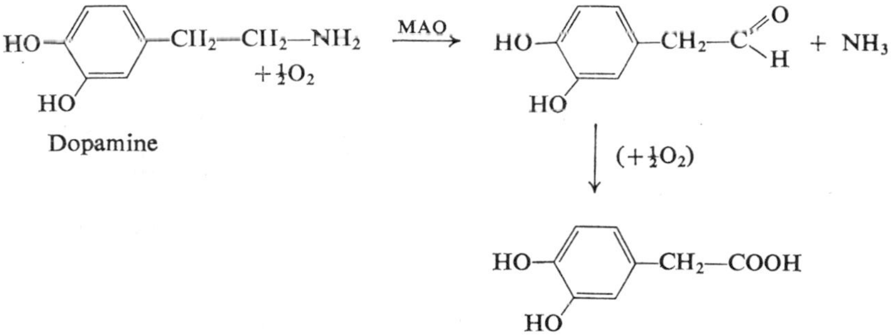

Dopamine

(homoprotocatechuic acid)
dihydroxyphenylacetic acid

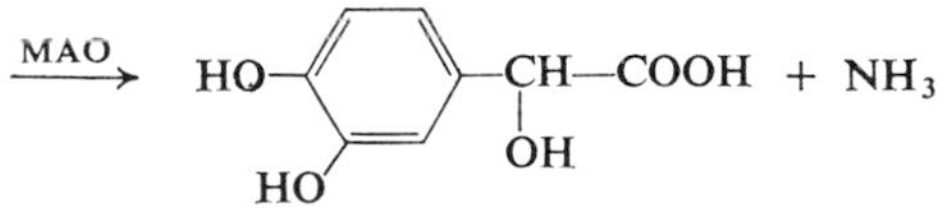

3,4-Dihydroxymandelic acid

$$\text{adrenaline} \xrightarrow{\text{MAO}} \text{3,4-dihydroxymandelic acid} + CH_3NH_2$$

$$\text{tyramine} \xrightarrow{\text{MAO}} \text{4-hydroxyphenylacetic acid} + NH_3$$

Catechol O-methyl transferase (*COMT*) catalyses the transfer of methyl groups (from a methyl donor) to the *meta*-hydroxyl group of catechols. The reaction is shown below.

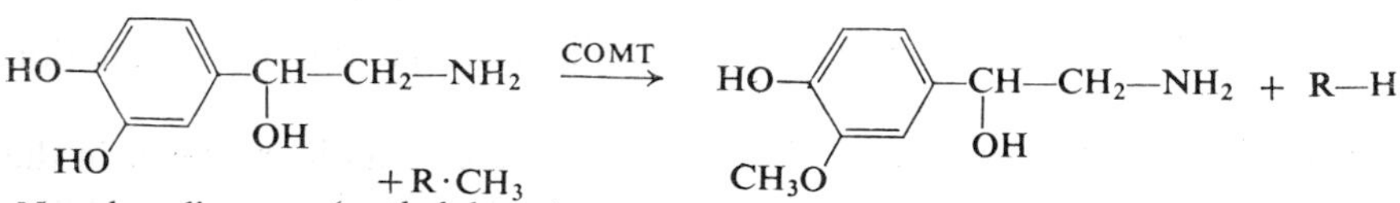

Noradrenaline (norepinephrine)   + R·CH₃ (methyl donor)

Normetanephrine

The end products of metabolism of catecholamines appearing in the urine are the result of actions by both enzymes, as shown below.

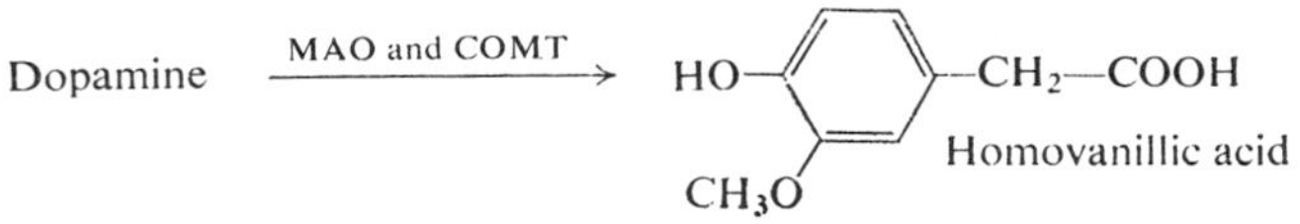

Dopamine $\xrightarrow{\text{MAO and COMT}}$ HO—⟨benzene ring⟩—CH_2—COOH
CH₃O
Homovanillic acid

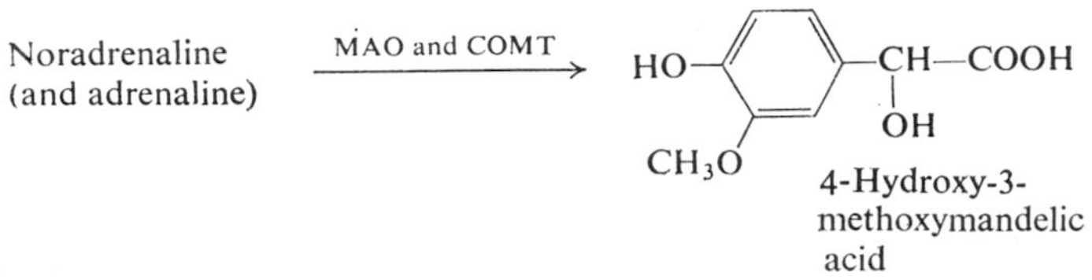

Noradrenaline $\xrightarrow{\text{MAO and COMT}}$ HO—⟨benzene ring⟩—CH—COOH
(and adrenaline)
OH
CH₃O
4-Hydroxy-3-
methoxymandelic
acid

When there are considerable amounts of catecholamines in the plasma, they are excreted as such into the urine. This occurs in patients with chromaffin cell tumours (phaeochromocytoma). The adrenaline and noradrenaline appearing in the urine of these patients may be detected by its pharmacological activity on various test preparations.

There are other enzymatic routes of metabolism for catecholamines. In common with other phenolic substances, they are subject to conjugation with sulphuric or glucuronic acids: this is a general detoxification route for phenols. The catechol nucleus may be oxidized, and the product then undergoes ring closure (this is a similar change to that occurring in the formation of melanins).

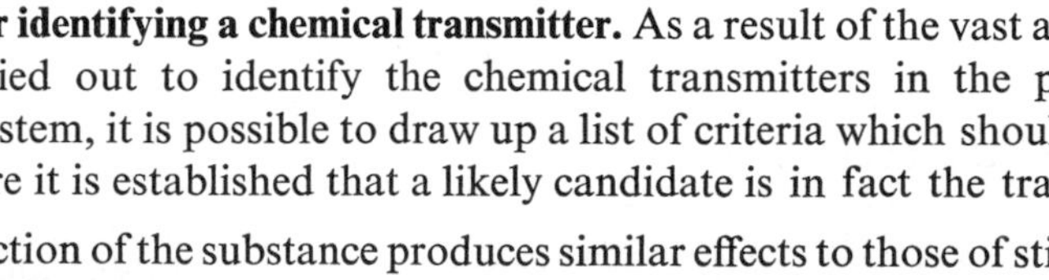

HO—⟨ring⟩—CHOH
HO—⟨ring⟩—CH_2
H—N—CH_3
$\xrightarrow[\text{(ring closure)}]{\text{Phenol oxidase}}$
O=⟨ring⟩—OH, N—CH_3

Adrenaline   Adrenochrome

Criteria for identifying a chemical transmitter. As a result of the vast amount of work carried out to identify the chemical transmitters in the peripheral nervous system, it is possible to draw up a list of criteria which should be fulfilled before it is established that a likely candidate is in fact the transmitter:

(1) Injection of the substance produces similar effects to those of stimulation of the nerve.

(2) Stimulation of the nerve releases the substance, and its presence in the blood or fluid perfusing the organ is shown by its actions on at least two pharmacological preparations.

(3) The tissue which is innervated contains the substance. After section and degeneration of the nerves, the content in the tissue is diminished.
(4) Drugs which block the effect of the proposed transmitter also block the effect of nerve stimulation. Similarly, drugs which prevent the destruction of the proposed transmitter and so potentiate its action, also potentiate the response to nerve stimulation.
(5) Enzyme systems synthesizing the substance are present, and drugs which interfere with these enzymes produce the appropriate effects on the responses to nerve stimulation.

Synaptic transmission in the central nervous system

There is considerable evidence that transmission at synapses in the CNS is humoral. Many pharmacologically active substances have been detected in various areas of the CNS. Electron-microscopy has demonstrated the presence of synaptic vesicles and granules in central pre-synaptic nerve endings. According to Grundfest, the synaptic regions of many central neurones differ from other regions of the same cells in being inexcitable by electrical stimulation. If this is shown to be a general property of central synapses, there will be little doubt that transmission is mediated chemically. However, with few exceptions, the identities of the transmitters at central synapses are unknown, and proof of humoral transmission as rigorous as that for peripheral junctions is still wanting. The main problem in demonstrating humoral transmission at synapses in the brain and spinal cord is the inaccessibility of central synapses to the experimenter. Another difficulty is that the blood-brain barrier prevents many drugs from reaching the brain; this has been overcome by injecting the proposed transmitter, or other drugs, directly into the CSF (Feldberg's method using an indwelling cannula inserted into a cerebral ventricle has already been mentioned on page 104). However, the drug may still be incapable of penetrating from the CSF into the nervous tissue. The most precise information has been obtained by a technique developed by Eccles and his colleagues in which a multiple barrel micropipette is applied to a single cell in the CNS. The electrical activity of the cell is recorded from one barrel while drugs are applied by electrophoresis through the others. In the future, the most convincing evidence for the identity and function of central transmitters will probably come from comparison of the effects of micro-application of substances found in the CNS with the effects of stimulation of pre-synaptic neurones.

Most nerve cells in the CNS have boutons of both excitatory and inhibitory neurones impinging upon them. Eccles and his colleagues have impaled the cell bodies of individual motoneurones in the spinal cord with micro-electrodes and recorded the changes in membrane potential which result from stimulation of pre-synaptic fibres. Stimulation of excitatory fibres causes depolarization of the motoneurone cell membrane (i.e. an excitatory post-synaptic potential), while stimulation of inhibitory fibres does not simply prevent depolarization, but actively causes hyperpolarization (i.e. an inhibitory post-synaptic potential) (pp. 90–91). The synaptic delay and the time course and other properties of the excitatory and inhibitory post-synaptic potentials in the CNS are most convincingly explained on the basis of changes in ionic permeability of the post-synaptic cell membrane produced by chemical transmitters released from the pre-synaptic nerve endings.

Inhibition in the CNS also occurs through the mechanism known as *pre-synaptic inhibition* (page 91) in which a depolarizing transmitter is believed to be released on to the nerve endings of an excitatory neurone. The transmitter responsible for pre-synaptic inhibition reduces the size of the post-synaptic excitatory potential, but it has no effect on the *resting* membrane potential of the post-synaptic cell body and it therefore differs from the transmitter responsible for producing a post-synaptic inhibitory potential.

Thus it appears that there are at least three types of chemical transmitter in the CNS: (1) excitatory transmitters which depolarize the post-synaptic cell membranes, (2) inhibitory transmitters which hyperpolarize the post-synaptic cell membranes, and (3) a transmitter which depolarizes nerve endings of excitatory neurones giving rise to pre-synaptic inhibition. It is possible that, as at peripheral neuro-effector junctions, a transmitter which is inhibitory at one central synapse may be excitatory at others.

The nature of inhibitory synaptic transmission in the spinal cord of all vertebrates so far studied is similar, suggesting that there may be only one inhibitory transmitter. Several substances with an inhibitory action on nervous tissue have been extracted from the CNS but none of those yet found possesses the same mechanism of action as the actual transmitter. The functions of most of the inhibitory substances found in the CNS may be to act as local hormones rather than as transmitters, and they are therefore dealt with in Chapter 6, pages 184–189.

Although the chemical nature of the post-synaptic inhibitory transmitter is unknown, there is good evidence that its action in the spinal cord is blocked by the powerful convulsant drug, strychnine. The toxin of the micro-organism *Clostridium tetani* produces symptoms very like those of strychnine poisoning. Tetanus toxin is believed to prevent the release of inhibitory transmitter from the endings of inhibitory neurones; its action therefore resembles that of botulinum toxin on peripheral cholinergic neurones. Pre-synaptic inhibition in the CNS is prevented by another convulsant drug, picrotoxin. The pharmacology of these substances is discussed on pages 628–629. Their use in the elucidation of the nature of CNS transmitters is analogous to the use of atropine, tubocurarine and botulinum toxin in experiments on peripheral transmission.

Acetylcholine. Some parts of the CNS contain acetylcholine, choline acetyltransferase and acetylcholinesterase, and are thus equipped for cholinergic transmission. Homogenates prepared by gently grinding the nervous tissue can be fractionated by centrifugation. The fraction containing the bulk of the acetylcholine and of the choline acetyltransferase consists of pinched-off nerve endings associated with a fragment of post-synaptic membrane. The nerve endings are packed with synaptic vesicles, just like those seen in peripheral cholinergic nerves. The parts of the CNS particularly rich in the components of the cholinergic apparatus are the motor cortex, the thalamus and hypothalamus, the geniculate bodies and the anterior spinal roots. However, other parts of the CNS do not contain the components of a cholinergic mechanism. The first-order sensory neurones are not cholinergic. The next neurone (second-order neurone) in the chain is equipped for cholinergic transmission, but the final neurone in the three-neurone pathway is not. From these observations, Feldberg and Vogt suggested that the neurones in the chain are alternately non-cholinergic and cholinergic. The presence of cholinesterase by itself is not evidence for cholinergic transmission. For example, the cerebellum contains cholinesterase but the other components of the cholinergic apparatus are absent.

Acetylcholine has been collected from the outer surface of the brain after diffusion into saline-filled cups placed in contact with the exposed cerebral cortex of the anaesthetized cat. The rate of accumulation diminishes as anaesthesia deepens. Acetylcholine has also been detected after diffusion into the CSF of the ventricles and has been found in the CSF of patients after epileptic fits. In animals, the content of acetylcholine in the CSF is high if convulsions precede death, and at the same time the content of acetylcholine in the brain cells is decreased.

Intravenous injections of acetylcholine have no direct effect on the brain or spinal cord because the drug penetrates the blood-brain barrier with difficulty and is destroyed rapidly in the blood. Intra-arterial injections of acetylcholine have been reported to affect the activity of the cells in the reticular formation. Injections into the cerebral ventricles produce rather complex responses, many functions of the body being altered. For example, there are changes in respiratory movements like those produced by stimulating the sensory fibres in the vagus nerves, nausea, vomiting, increased intestinal movements, sweating, flushing and sometimes sleep. Small doses of acetylcholine injected into the ventricles of the cat cause excitement, tremor and convulsions. Tubocurarine, which blocks the peripheral nicotinic actions of acetylcholine, produces

6*

similar effects to those of acetylcholine when injected into the ventricles. Atropine blocks many of the actions of acetylcholine in the central nervous system. For example, atropine-like drugs are used to treat some of the symptoms of Parkinson's disease and this effect is probably the result of a central anti-acetylcholine action (Chapter 28).

Many symptoms of poisoning with anticholinestase agents resemble the effects produced by acetylcholine injected into the cerebral ventricles. This resemblance suggests that acetylcholine is continually being released in the CNS and accumulates after inhibition of cholinesterase. Atropine prevents the central as well as the peripheral (muscarinic) actions of anticholinesterase drugs.

The disorientation and states of mental confusion produced by anticholinesterase drugs resemble the symptoms reported by schizophrenic patients; there may be nightmares and hallucinations. Anticholinesterase drugs aggravate the symptons of schizophrenics. Feldberg observed that injection of acetylcholine or anticholinesterase drugs into the lateral ventricles of cats produced a state of immobility (catatonia), resembling the catatonic stupor seen in schizophrenic patients. In this connection it is interesting to note that injection of purified cholinesterase into the lateral ventricles of patients with catatonia has been reported to produce a dramatic relief of the stupor. Acetylcholine may stimulate or block synaptic transmission according to its concentration, and which of these actions contributes to its effects on behaviour is not known.

The recurrent axon collaterals of the lower motoneurons synapse with the Renshaw cells (page 115). The motoneurones release acetylcholine at the neuromuscular junction and the recurrent branches of the same motoneurone also release acetylcholine (Fig. 5.3). Eccles and his colleagues have shown that excitation of the Renshaw cell, produced by stimulation of the axon collateral, is potentiated by anticholinesterase drugs and blocked by dihydro-β-erythroidine, a drug which blocks the peripheral nicotinic actions of acetylcholine and which is capable of penetrating the blood-brain barrier. Furthermore, the Renshaw cell is stimulated by the micro-application of acetylcholine. Receptors sensitive to the muscarinic action of acetylcholine are also present on the Renshaw cell, as in autonomic ganglion cells (page 147); their role in physiological transmission is unknown. Stimulation of a Renshaw cell causes it to inhibit the motoneurone, but the nature of the inhibitory transmitter is unknown. Acetylcholine and anticholinesterase drugs applied to the spinal cord depress the knee jerk reflex. When the cells in the spinal cord have been partly denervated by severing the cord, there is an increased sensitivity to acetylcholine.

The Betz cells in the cerebral cortex (page 119) can be stimulated by the micro-application of acetylcholine, and it is probable that some of the synaptic endings on the Betz cells are cholinergic. The neurones whose cell bodies are in the supra-optic nucleus and whose axons terminate in the posterior lobe of the pituitary gland are also stimulated by acetylcholine and by anticholinesterase drugs. There is a high content of choline acetyltransferase in the supra-optic nucleus. These observations suggest that cholinergic nerve endings synapse with cells of the supra-optic nucleus.

CHAPTER 6

Local Hormones

The term hormone is usually applied to substances elaborated in endocrine glands and released from them into the blood-stream to exert their actions on certain cells in other tissues; the endocrine hormones are described in Chapter 14. The chemical transmitters which mediate the nervous impulse are often called neurohormones (Chapter 5). A number of substances concerned with the regulation of the activity of the digestive system have the characteristics of hormones; they are released by specific stimuli from parts of the alimentary canal and produce effects on other parts of the digestive system, being conveyed by the blood to their site of action (Chapter 12). There are other pharmacologically active substances in tissues which have been termed *local hormones*. However, the precise site of formation and of action is not known for all substances which may be classed as local hormones, nor is it known which physiological function each serves. Some pathological conditions are associated with, and may be due to, changes in the amounts of local hormones released in the tissues. The presence in a tissue of a substance with a powerful pharmacological action does not itself constitute proof that it normally exerts such an action; it may be the by-product of metabolism, being held in the tissues in an inactive form until further metabolized or excreted.

Local hormones in peripheral tissues

Acetylcholine. There is much evidence to show that acetylcholine, acting independently of nervous structures, is responsible for automaticity in a number of tissues. Firstly, acetylcholine, together with the enzymes necessary for its synthesis and breakdown, has been found in these tissues, and secondly, drugs which potentiate or inhibit the actions of acetylcholine modify the activity of the tissues.

The following examples serve to illustrate these points. (i) The smooth muscle cells of the nerve-free amniotic membrane of the chick embryo exhibit rhythmic contractions. The amnion contains choline acetyltransferase, and acetylcholine has been shown to be released from the tissue during contraction. The rhythmic contractions are enhanced when cholinesterase is inhibited by physostigmine. (ii) The placenta is another nerve-free tissue and it contains even more choline acetyltransferase and acetylcholine than are found in most cholinergic nerves. The role of acetylcholine in this location

172

may be to dilate the blood vessels of the placenta and adjacent tissues so as to facilitate nutrition of the embryo. (iii) The rhythmic beating of the cilia of epithelial cells may be influenced by acetylcholine acting as a local hormone. The ciliated cells lining the trachea, oesophagus, and the gill-plates of mussels contain choline acetyltransferase and cholinesterase, and the beating of the cilia is accelerated by physostigmine. (iv) Acetylcholine may play a part in maintaining the heart beat. For example, atria which have been dissected from an animal and suspended in a physiological salt solution stop beating after 24 to 48 hours. At this stage, the membrane potential has fallen and the choline acetyltransferase activity has been reduced. Then, the addition of acetylcholine usually restores the beat, and at the same time both the membrane potential and the enzyme activity are increased. (v) The ventricles of the heart receive no cholinergic innervation yet they produce acetylcholine, especially in the region of the conducting tissue; this suggests that acetylcholine may be involved in conduction of the cardiac impulses. (vi) Acetylcholine is released from the intestinal tissues where it is not solely derived from cholinergic nerves; the non-nervous tissue contains choline acetyltransferase and cholinesterase, and in the presence of physostigmine acetylcholine accumulates and produces spasm of the smooth muscle.

According to Nachmansohn, acetylcholine plays an essential role not only in the transmission process at synapses and neuro-effector junctions but also in the generation of the action potential in all nerve- and muscle-cell membranes. He believes that the local circuit currents moving in advance of the propagated action potential (Fig. 3.3b) release acetylcholine from an inactive bound form present in the cell membranes and that this acetylcholine, rather than the local currents themselves, increases the permeability of the membrane to sodium ions. The membrane potential is restored when the cholinesterase present in the membrane hydrolyses the acetylcholine, and then the impermeability to sodium returns. Nachmansohn's hypothesis is not accepted by all physiologists, chiefly as there are large variations in the quantities of the enzymes which synthesize and destroy acetylcholine in different membranes, and as cholinesterase is completely absent from some nerve fibres. Furthermore, the actions of anticholinesterase drugs on the membrane potential are not what would be predicted from his hypothesis.

Pharmacological evidence suggests that some components of the cholinergic system, particularly cholinesterase, are involved in active ion transport across cell membranes. For example, inhibition of cholinesterase in frog skin and muscle and in crab gills, has been found to prevent active sodium transport. Although such an effect has not been demonstrated in mammalian tissues, it is possible that acetylcholinesterase in red blood cells is concerned with ion transport.

Noradrenaline and adrenaline. There is a widespread distribution of chromaffin cells in the body (page 161), but the physiological role of their catecholamine stores has not been fully elucidated. In some lower animals, such as cyclostomal fish, there is no nerve supply to the heart and yet the tissue is rich in noradrenaline; this is contained in branched chromaffin cells which form a plexus-like network throughout the heart, and may represent a primitive stage in the development of adrenergic nerves; the release of this noradrenaline produces an increase in the force of beat. In mammals, the atria beat more slowly when their stores of noradrenaline have been depleted, and so noradrenaline may be continually released from the stores to modify the activity of the pacemaker. The noradrenaline released from stores in ganglia may act as a moderator of ganglionic transmission (page 144).

Histamine. Histamine is found in nearly every tissue of the body. It also occurs in some foodstuffs. It is formed from the amino acid, histidine, by the action of the enzyme, *histidine decarboxylase* (Fig. 6.1). This enzyme is found in many tissues and it also occurs in the intestinal bacteria of many mammals. The relative amounts of histamine formed in the gut and in other tissues can be determined by estimating the urinary excretion of histamine before and after sterilization of the gut contents by treatment with antibiotics. A meat diet is generally richer in histidine than a vegetable diet. Much histamine is formed from it by bacterial decarboxylation in carnivores (dog, cat and man) but less histamine is formed in the gut of herbivores (rabbit and guinea-pig).

The lungs and intestines of most mammals contain large amounts of histamine, but the histamine content of other tissues differs from species to species. For example, dog liver contains much histamine but rat liver has almost none; rat skin is rich in histamine but guinea-pig skin has very little. There is no simple relationship between the content of histamine in a tissue and the ability of that tissue to form histamine. Tissue mast cells and blood basophils contain histamine bound in their cytoplasmic granules, which also contain heparin (page 231), and mast cell tumours have a high content both of histamine and of heparin. In most tissues the histamine is chiefly contained in the mast cells, although in the intestine much is located elsewhere.

The urine contains free histamine and also its metabolic products. The routes of metabolism of histamine are deamination of the side-chain amino group, methyl substitution on an imidazolyl nitrogen, and acetylation of the side-chain amino group (Fig. 6.1). Deamination of histamine is catalysed by the enzyme *histaminase*, which acts on diamines and so differs from monoamine oxidase. The end-product of histamine deamination is imidazolylacetic acid, which is excreted in the urine conjugated with ribose. Histaminase is found in the kidneys of most species (the rat is an exception). It is of interest that there is a high histaminase content of the blood plasma during pregnancy and of the placenta in some species (e.g. man, guinea-pig and rat). The increase in these histaminase levels suggests that histamine is involved in the process of pregnancy in these species. Both histamine and histaminase are present in some tissues, but the bound histamine is not available to the enzyme. It is believed that the function of the histaminase in the intestinal mucosa is to destroy histamine and some other toxic diamines formed by putrefactive bacteria in

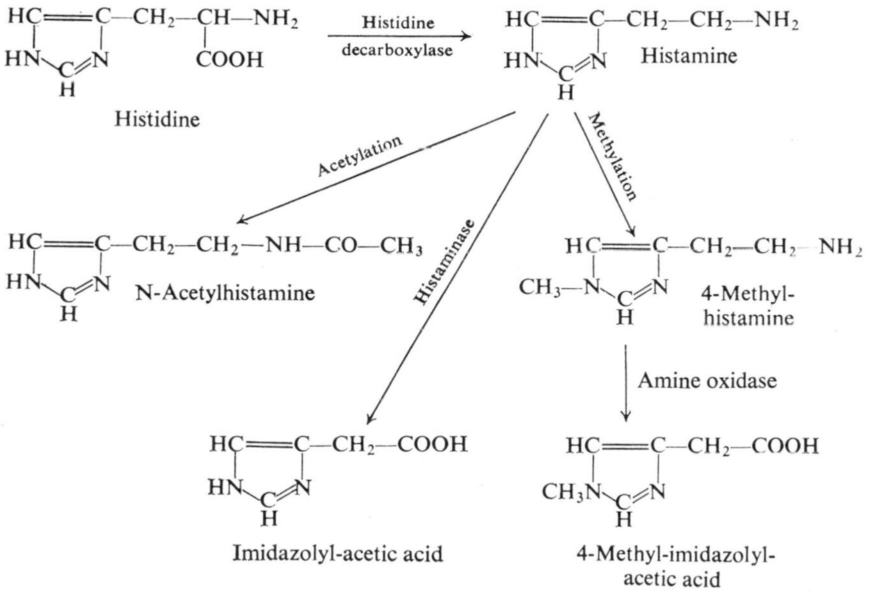

FIG. 6.1. Main pathways in the biosynthesis and metabolism of histamine.

the gut. Histaminase is the principal enzyme inactivating histamine in man, whereas methylation is the principal route of inactivation in the cat and dog. Both methylation and deamination occur in rodents. In addition, female rats and mice excrete much free histamine. In most species, histamine present in the blood stream is metabolized to a greater extent by methylation than by deamination; part of the 4-methylhistamine formed is then deaminated before excretion. Acetylhistamine is pharmacologically inactive. It is excreted in the urine and can be estimated biologically after hydrolysis. Ingestion of meat leads to a considerable increase in the proportion of acetylhistamine excreted. After ingestion of histamine itself, only about 5% of the amount administered appears as the acetyl conjugate. The amount of conjugated histamine in the urine depends largely on the diet, whereas free histamine in the urine is derived principally from histamine released in the body.

Histamine has pronounced pharmacological activity. It dilates blood vessels and increases the permeability of the capillary walls. Smooth muscle in other tissues is, in general, contracted by histamine. However, smooth muscle from the rat, mouse and rabbit is relatively insensitive to histamine. Histamine stimulates the secretion of acid into the gastric juice. A fuller account of the pharmacology of histamine is given on pages 776–777.

The pharmacological effects of histamine are used for its detection and estimation. The contractions of the guinea-pig's isolated intestine and the fall of blood pressure in the cat are particularly useful for this purpose. Similar responses are also produced by acetylcholine, but the two substances are readily distinguished by using atropine to block responses to acetylcholine. Sensitive and specific chemical methods are also available for the estimation of histamine.

The physiological role of histamine is still a matter for investigation. Some physiologists believe that histamine mediates the secretion of gastric acid. Stimulation of the vagus nerve releases acetylcholine and this in turn may release histamine, which then stimulates the oxyntic (acid-secreting) cells of the gastric mucosa. Moreover, histamine is present in the gastric secretion. The mechanisms for the control of gastric secretion are described more fully on page 311. Histamine is used in medical practice to test the functional capacity of the oxyntic cells of the gastric mucosa.

Histamine is present in a bound form in the skin of many animals in amounts sufficient to produce profound effects, should it all be released. The intra-dermal injection of histamine causes a series of events termed the 'triple response' (Fig. 6.2). The blood vessels immediately affected by the histamine dilate and produce a flush. Then the surrounding blood vessels dilate, and a flare is produced. The flare is probably due to an axon reflex, the histamine stimulating sensory nerves which send impulses orthodromically and then antidromically down the other branches of the sensory nerve fibres to produce dilatation. The secondary dilatation may be caused by the release of a chemical substance from the sensory nerve endings supplying the blood vessels. There is evidence that ATP or substance P (page 188) may be the vasodilator substance released. The increased permeability of the widely dilated blood vessels in the flushed area results in accumulation of tissue fluid, the local oedema being termed a wheal. These three components of the triple response—flush, flare and wheal—are produced by mechanical injury to the skin, by injurious chemicals and histamine-liberating drugs (page 779), and by animal venoms, toxins and plant poisons. The response is due to histamine released from the damaged skin. Some venoms and plant poisons themselves contain histamine. The functional significance of the triple response is in the mobilization of the body's protective mechanism at the site of injury: these include the increased passage of plasma proteins and white blood cells into the tissue spaces.

Histamine is released in anaphylactic reactions and in allergic conditions including asthma. Some of the symptoms of these conditions are due to the released histamine, but other pharmacologically active substances are also released.

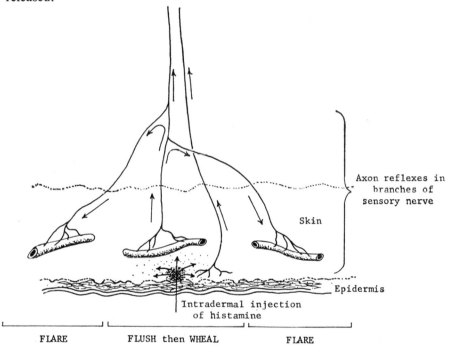

Fig. 6.2. The triple response produced by histamine (for explanation, see text). The impulses travelling centrally in the sensory nerves give rise to the feelings of itch and pain.

Histamine liberates adrenaline from the adrenals. After severe stress, particularly when there has been widespread tissue damage, both histamine and adrenaline are released in appreciable amounts.

5-Hydroxytryptamine (Serotonin). It has been known for many years that when blood clots a substance which constricts blood vessels appears in the serum. It comes from platelets which are broken down in the clotting process. Originally it was called 'vasoconstrictine', 'vasotonin', or 'serotonin', but it has now been isolated and identified as 5-hydroxytryptamine (5-HT). Enteramine, a substance first detected in the walls of the mammalian intestine and in the salivary glands of the octopus, is identical with 5-hydroxytryptamine.

5-Hydroxytryptamine acts on most smooth muscle, although there are wide differences in sensitivity. The veins are contracted relatively more than the arterioles, so that blood may be dammed back in the capillaries and cause flushing. The pulmonary blood vessels are considerably more sensitive to the constrictor action than are the systemic vessels. 5-Hydroxytryptamine also stimulates ganglion cells and releases adrenaline from the adrenal medulla.

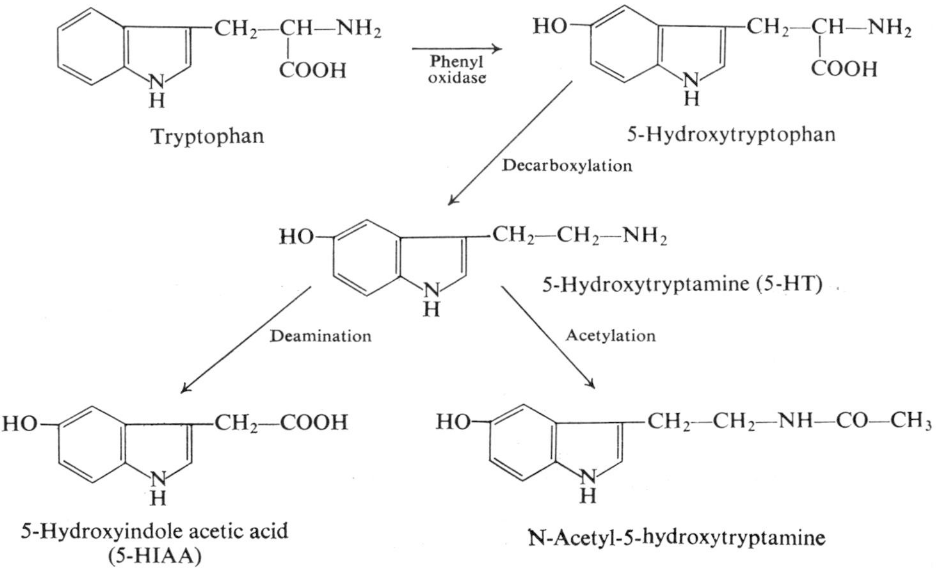

FIG. 6.3. Main pathways in the biosynthesis and metabolism of 5-HT.

5-Hydroxytryptamine may be identified and estimated using sensitive tissues such as the rat colon, stomach wall and uterus (in oestrus), all of which have the advantage of being insensitive to histamine. The heart of the mollusc *Venus mercenaria* is also extremely sensitive but rather unspecific in that it also responds to histamine, adrenaline and other pharmacologically active substances in tissues.

The biological synthesis of 5-hydroxytryptamine (Fig. 6.3) begins with the amino acid, tryptophan. This is hydroxylated to 5-hydroxytryptophan by *phenyl oxidase* (the same enzyme that converts phenylalanine to tyrosine), and then decarboxylated by the same enzyme which decarboxylates dopa to dopamine (compare Fig. 5.8, page 160).

Most of the 5-hydroxytryptamine in the body is found in the gastro-intestinal tract, particularly in the pylorus of the stomach and in the upper part of the small intestine. It is confined to the mucosa where it is contained in the enterochromaffin cells (also called argentaffin cells as they have an affinity for silver stains). The addition of antibiotics to the diet of mice and rats increases the 5-hydroxytryptamine content in the intestinal wall, showing that the amount stored may be modified by changes in the intestinal flora.

5-Hydroxytryptamine in the blood is contained in platelets where the concentration is as much as 1000 times that in the surrounding plasma. There is a considerable species variation. In man, 10^8 platelets contain about 60 ng, whereas the same number of rabbit platelets contain about fifteen times as much. Considerable amounts are also found in the spleen and lungs in association with platelets entrapped in these organs. The only other peripheral tissue containing much 5-hydroxytryptamine is the skin of rats and mice, where some is contained in mast cells.

In lower animals and plants, 5-hydroxytryptamine is widely distributed. It is found in the gastro-intestinal tract of all vertebrates and in the skin of some but not all amphibia. In invertebrates, it is found in the salivary glands of the octopus, and in the venom of the scorpion and wasp (but not that of the bee). It is also present in the stinging fluid of the common nettle and in the trichomes of cowhage (itching powder), as well as in some fruits such as the banana and tomato.

The structures in which 5-hydroxytryptamine is stored, namely, the platelets and the granules of enterochromaffin cells and mast cells, are able to take up considerable amounts against a concentration gradient. Since all these structures contain ATP, it is probable that 5-hydroxytryptamine, like the catecholamines, is bound in association with ATP. 5-Hydroxytryptamine is more strongly bound in platelets where the half-life is about 30 h, than in enterochromaffin cells where the half-life is about 10 h.

The main routes of inactivation of 5-hydroxytryptamine are shown in Fig. 6.3. Oxidation by monoamine oxidase yields 5-hydroxyindoleacetic acid (5-HIAA), which is excreted in the urine. Another metabolic route is acetylation of the amino group. The administration of amine oxidase inhibitors leads to the accumulation of 5-hydroxytryptamine (and of noradrenaline) in some tissues.

5-Hydroxytryptamine placed in the lumen of the intestine stimulates peristaltic movements by lowering the threshold of intraluminal pressure necessary to initiate the reflex. It has been suggested that 5-hydroxytryptamine has a physiological function in peristalsis since it is released from the enterochromaffin cells into the lumen when the intraluminal pressure is raised. It is thought to act by stimulating the sensory nerve endings involved in the peristaltic reflex. Tumours of the enterochromaffin cells of the intestine are called carcinoid. The symptoms of carcinoid crises are largely due to the pharmacological effects of 5-hydroxytryptamine released from the tumour, and include diarrhoea, flushing of the skin and spasm of the bronchioles. Large amounts of the amine, its metabolites, and sometimes 5-hydroxytryptophan, appear in the urine in carcinoid cases.

When platelets are disrupted at the site of damage to the wall of a blood vessel or during the clotting process, the 5-hydroxytryptamine released may constrict the blood vessels, so contributing to the haemostatic mechanisms. The blood vessels in the kidney are markedly constricted by 5-hydroxytryptamine and urine formation is inhibited. In rats and mice (but not in other species), there is evidence that this is a physiological function.

Adenyl compounds. Derivatives of adenosine are present in all cells where they are concerned with the transfer and storage of chemical energy (pages 41–48). Some coenzymes contain adenosine and it is one of the constituents of the nucleic acids (Fig. 6.4). Adenosine and adenosine nucleotides are pharmacologically active. They relax most smooth muscle, although that of the guinea-pig uterus is contracted. Their actions on the heart and blood vessels resemble those of acetylcholine, but differ in that they are not blocked by atropine. ATP stimulates ganglion cells. The biochemical properties of adenyl compounds are usually exploited to detect and measure their presence in tissues. However, their pharmacological activity in relaxing the fowl's rectal caecum and slowing the rate of the guinea-pig's heart also provide sensitive tests. Adenosine in tissue extracts is not destroyed by boiling in alkali, but this treatment hydrolyses the phosphate groups from its nucleotides and also destroys most other pharmacologically active constituents of tissue.

Most tissues contain adenosine deaminase; striated muscle contains adenylic acid deaminase. The deaminated products, inosine and its derivatives (Fig. 6.4), are pharmacologically inert. It is presumed that the role of the deaminating enzymes is to curtail the pharmacological action of adenyl compounds, should they be released. It is not known whether adenyl compounds exert their pharmacological actions as local hormones in physiological processes. However, their actions have been detected after tissue damage, when considerable amounts may be released. For example, intravenous injections of solutions which disrupt the red blood cells release adenyl compounds (principally ATP) from them: these substances then produce vasodilatation and slowing of the heart. The nucleic acids and their breakdown products stimulate the production of white blood cells, and their release may provide a signal for the rapid regeneration of leucocytes used up at the site of cell damage.

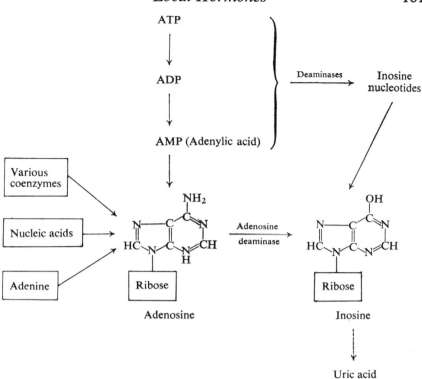

FIG. 6.4. Metabolic relationships of adenyl compounds and their degradation products.

Bradykinin. This is a nonapeptide split off from a plasma globulin (an α_2-globulin called *bradykininogen*) by proteolytic enzymes such as trypsin. It was originally discovered after treating plasma with a snake venom. Plasma itself contains an enzyme capable of forming bradykinin, and this is activated by various procedures (such as diluting the plasma) and in some pathological states (after severe trauma, or when clots form in the blood vessels). Enzymes present in saliva, pancreatic juice and sweat are also capable of producing a bradykinin-like substance from plasma.

Bradykinin causes a slow contraction of most intestinal smooth muscle, except that of the rat duodenum which is relaxed. It contracts uterine and bronchial smooth muscle, but relaxes that of the blood vessels. Thus, bradykinin produces vasodilatation and a fall in blood pressure. It increases capillary permeability, and stimulates some sensory nerve endings. There is an enzyme in plasma and in kidney which acts on bradykinin to destroy its pharmacological activity. A small fraction of the total amount of bradykinin that could be released from its globulin-precursor would have profound effects in the body. Bradykinin is released in anaphylactic and allergic reactions, and is partly responsible for the symptoms. Physiological roles have also been suggested for bradykinin. During secretion of saliva, pancreatic juice or sweat, enzymes released from gland cells convert the precursor into bradykinin which may then produce a local vasodilatation and an increased blood flow to the active tissues. The presence of a bradykinin-like substance in urine suggests that local blood flow in the kidney may be regulated by a kinin. *Kallidin* is formed from plasma globulin by an enzyme called kallikrein present in urine. It closely resembles bradykinin and may be identical with it. *Kinins*, or the kinin-forming enzymes, are found in some animal venoms. They are often given a name to indicate their source, for example, vespakinin from wasp venom and scorpiokinin from scorpion venom.

Substance P is a polypeptide first found in extracts of intestine. In tissues, it is preformed and loosely bound in subcellular particles. Its actions resemble those of acetylcholine but they are not blocked by atropine. It differs from bradykinin in that it causes contraction of the rat duodenum (relaxed by bradykinin) and the fowl rectal caecum (insensitive to bradykinin). It stimulates peristaltic movements by an action on the intestinal nerve plexus, and it may play a physiological role as a local hormone regulating peristalsis.

Angiotensin is an octapeptide formed from a plasma globulin by the enzyme, *renin*, present in the kidneys. The precursor (angiotensinogen) is an α_2-globulin similar to bradykininogen. Angiotensin causes constriction of blood vessels by a direct action and raises the blood pressure. In addition, it releases catecholamines from the adrenal medulla. Smooth muscle in the gastro-intestinal tract, the urino-genital system and the bronchi is contracted by angiotensin. Angiotensin has been implicated in one form of high blood pressure and in the control of the calibre of kidney blood vessels (page 276). It stimulates the release of aldosterone (pages 380 and 833).

Prostaglandins are unsaturated fatty acids containing one or more hydroxyl groups. They are found in the semen of man, sheep and goats, but are absent from the semen and the accessory genital glands of other species. The main source of prostaglandins is the seminal vesicles (and *not* the prostate gland). Their pharmacological actions include contraction of most smooth muscle, but they cause dilatation of the blood vessels. The physiological role of prostaglandin may be to aid the transport and nutrition of the sperm in both the male and the female genital tracts.

Darmstoff is a mixture of phosphorylated derivatives of glycerol-fatty acid esters present in intestine (Darm is the German word for intestine). Some is present preformed and may be released by gentle extraction but more vigorous methods of extraction yield greater amounts of activity, probably by breaking down otherwise inert constituents of the intestinal tissues. Darmstoff causes contraction of the intestine, largely by an action on the intestinal nerves. Phospholipids like Darmstoff may be concerned in the transport of cations across cell membranes.

Irin is a long-chain unsaturated fatty acid containing one or more hydroxyl groups, and is extractable from the iris of rabbits and man. Irin causes contraction of the iris of several species and contraction of intestinal and uterine smooth muscle. Damage to the rabbit's eye results in an atropine-resistant constriction of the pupil which may be due to irin released into the aqueous humor.

Menstrual fluid contains substances that stimulate smooth muscle. They are fatty acids that cause powerful contractions of uterine and intestinal smooth muscle. They may be responsible for the uterine spasms and other signs of smooth muscle activity occurring during menstruation.

Slow-reacting substances (SRS) are so named because they produce a slowly developing contraction of smooth muscle of the guinea-pig ileum. Incubation of egg yolk or of various mammalian tissues with cobra venom hydrolyses lecithin to yield an unsaturated fatty acid (SRS-C). The other product of the reaction, lysolecithin, is an extremely active haemolysing agent. Another fatty acid substance (SRS-A) is released from the lungs during anaphylactic shock. It may be identical with neuraminic acid (page 13).

LOCAL HORMONES AS MEDIATORS OF PAINFUL STIMULI. Several of the pharmacologically active substances present in tissues have the property of stimulating sensory nerve endings or of lowering their threshold for excitation, and some, released or formed as a result of tissue damage, may play a part in the production of pain and itching. In the skin, the agents which may be responsible for the prolonged pain of injury and inflammation include potassium ions, histamine, 5-hydroxytryptamine, lactic acid, substance P, an irin-like substance, and plasma kinins such as bradykinin. Most of these also participate in the vascular reactions to injury, producing vasodilatation and increased capillary or venular permeability, and have been shown to produce pain and hyperalgesia when applied to exposed sensory nerve endings in concentrations which may be produced in injury. The juice of stinging nettle hairs contains acetylcholine, histamine and 5-hydroxytryptamine in sufficient quantity to cause pain, and wasp venom contains histamine, 5-hydroxy-tryptamine and a kinin-like polypeptide.

Ischaemic pain in striated muscles (claudication, page 110) and in the heart (angina, page 263) may also be attributed to the action of a chemical mediator, probably a metabolite produced by muscular activity which accumulates as a result of the impaired blood flow. Potassium ions or the plasma kinins are possible candidates. The pain-producing substance released from ischaemic muscle may also serve to dilate the blood vessels.

The severe headache of migraine is believed to be caused by: (i) vasodilatation of the arteries of the scalp, with increased amplitude of pulsation, (ii) lowered pain threshold of the sensory nerve endings, and (iii) oedema of the affected region. A fluid collected from the subsurface tissues of the affected part of the head during a migraine attack contains substances which produce the above-mentioned effects when injected into the skin of other persons. The chief active principle appears to be a polypeptide which has been named 'neurokinin', as it differs slightly from other known kinins. Acetylcholine, histamine, 5-hydroxytryptamine, ATP and potassium ions are also present in small amounts in the fluid.

Local hormones of the central nervous system

The tissues of the central nervous system (CNS) contain many pharmacologically active substances. In Chapter 5 it was pointed out that only one of these substances, acetylcholine, has been identified as a neurotransmitter at central synapses. This does not imply that the other substances are not neurotransmitters, but rather it is a statement about the incomplete knowledge of the physiology of central synaptic transmission and ignorance of the exact role of these substances.

Noradrenaline. Noradrenaline is found in parts of the CNS, the highest concentrations being in the hypothalamus and the medulla. The injection of noradrenaline into the cerebral ventricles causes drowsiness and a sleep-like state, differing from true sleep in that the EEG is desynchronized, just as it is in the alert state. On the other hand, noradrenaline causes awakening from sleep when injected intravenously. This is probably because the peripheral actions of noradrenaline induce secondary changes in the CNS via the afferent nerves.

Adrenaline occurs in association with noradrenaline in the brain but in only one-tenth or less of the concentration. The central actions of adrenaline are similar to those of noradrenaline but an intravenous injection of adrenaline produces feelings of excitement and apprehension, an action not shared by noradrenaline.

When injected into the cerebral ventricles or directly into the anterior hypothalamus of a cat, both adrenaline and noradrenaline cause a fall in body temperature.

Dopamine is found in the brain, localized in definite regions. The highest concentration is in the caudate nucleus which contains little noradrenaline. In some regions, dopamine probably exists as a precursor of noradrenaline but it has actions of its own which it produces more powerfully than noradrenaline. Thus, small concentrations painted directly on to the spinal cord produce inhibition of the monosynaptic stretch reflex, and the substance may therefore serve a physiological role in controlling these reflexes. Dopamine is deficient in the brain of Parkinsonian patients and this may be responsible for some of the symptoms (page 120).

Tyramine has also been detected in the CNS, particularly in the spinal cord. It has the same action on reflexes as dopamine and may serve a similar function.

5-Hydroxytryptamine occurs in the CNS with about the same distribution as noradrenaline, but in addition it has been found in the rhinencephalic structures and in the hippocampus, cerebellum and the pineal gland. 5-Hydroxytryptamine does not penetrate the blood-brain barrier, but its precursor amino acid, 5-hydroxytryptophan, does. It is synthesized in the brain and then stored in sub-cellular particles. Alteration in the level of 5-hydroxytrypamine in the nervous system is associated with changes in behaviour and in the EEG. Many drugs which either mimic or block the pharmacological actions of 5-hydroxytryptamine on peripheral tissues, produce changes in behaviour or mood, suggesting that they interfere with the actions of 5-hydroxytryptamine in the brain.

5-Hydroxytryptamine may serve as the central neurohormone for the trophotropic system whilst noradrenaline may be the transmitter for the opposing ergotropic system. These systems were first designated by Hess. The trophotropic system consists of the centres regulating the activity of the parasympathetic nerves and their integration with sensory and motor centres and the limbic system (page 102). Activation of the trophotropic system results in diminished motor activity and relaxation leading to drowsiness and sleep and an increased activity of parasympathetically innervated structures; the general picture has been described as ruminative. The ergotrophic system consists of the centres regulating sympathetic outflow and their integration with the reticular activating system and the sensory and motor centres,

Activation of the ergotrophic system leads to increased motor activity and alertness and increased activity of sympathetically innervated structures.

When injected into the cerebral ventricles or into the anterior hypothalamus, 5-hydroxytryptamine raises the body temperature. Feldberg has suggested that temperature control by the hypothalamus is brought about by the release of catecholamines and 5-hydroxytryptamine which are present in this region.

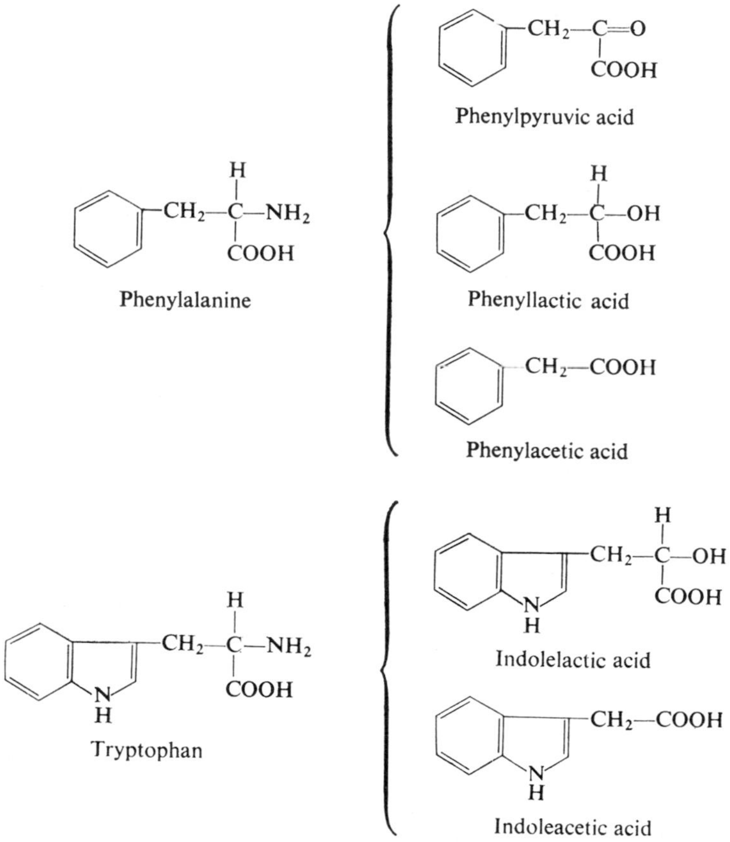

Fig. 6.5. Some of the abnormal constituents of blood and urine found in phenyl-ketonurics.

Phenylketonuria is a disease resulting from the absence of the enzyme phenyl oxidase which converts phenylalanine to tyrosine and tryptophan to 5-hydroxy-tryptophan. It is a rare inherited condition caused by a recessive gene, the incidence in the population being about 25 per million. Almost all phenylketon-urics are mentally deficient. At birth they appear normal, but signs of mental deficiency appear within a few weeks. The disease derives its name from the abnormal appearance of *phenylpyruvic acid* in the urine. The urine and blood contain a number of substances derived from phenylalanine and tryptophan (Fig. 6.5). Most phenylketonurics have fair hair and complexion, as part of the metabolic route leading to melanin is missing. The exact relationship between the lack of the enzyme and the mental deficiency is not known. Patients fed on a diet from which phenylalanine has been removed lose the abnormal constituents of blood and urine, and when this is begun at an early age the mental condition is improved.

Schizophrenia is a large and ill-defined group of psychotic disorders. The common symptoms include hallucinations and a trance-like state of immobility termed catatonia. The discovery of drugs with pronounced hallucinogenic activity has led to the suggestion that this symptom of the disease is caused by hallucinogenic substances produced in the body. One of these may be adrenochrome, which can be formed from adrenaline (page 166).

Histamine is present in some parts of the CNS and, in general, is distributed with noradrenaline and 5-hydroxytryptamine. The concentrations are low compared with those found in some peripheral tissues. It is one of the few substances acting on the cerebellum. Injection of histamine into the cerebral ventricles stimulates sympathetic centres, which produces a rise in blood pressure.

Factor I is an extract of mammalian brain which inhibits the stretch reflex in the cat when applied to the spinal cord. The substances known to be constituents of factor I include derivatives of glutamic acid (γ-aminobutyric acid, γ-amino-β-hydroxybutyric acid, γ-aminobutyrylcholine, see Fig. 6.6), imidazoleacetic acid and catecholamines, particularly dopamine. The relative concentrations of these substances in factor I vary with the area of CNS chosen for extraction. The action of dopamine itself on the stretch reflex of the cat corresponds most closely to the action of factor I, and dopamine may therefore be the important constituent producing this action. None of the constituents of factor I produces exactly the same effects as the chemical transmitter released at inhibitory synapses, and it therefore appears that the constituents of factor I may serve, not as inhibitory transmitters, but as local hormones to moderate the activity of parts of the nervous system.

Bradykinin may possess central functions since amounts less than those obtained from 1 ml of plasma injected into the cerebral ventricles produce a long lasting fall of blood pressure and catatonia or tranquillization.

Substance P occurs in all parts of the brain and spinal cord, the substantia nigra containing the largest concentration. The posterior roots and columns of the spinal cord contain considerable quantities of substance P, but only traces of other pharmacologically active substances. It may be that substance P serves as a neuro-transmitter at the endings of first-order sensory neurones. Substance P is also present in the retina of the eye, a structure which, from the embryological point of view, is part of the CNS. Its concentration is highest in darkness and diminishes on exposure to light. Substance P inhibits many polysynaptic reflex pathways in the CNS but has no effect on monosynaptic reflex arcs.

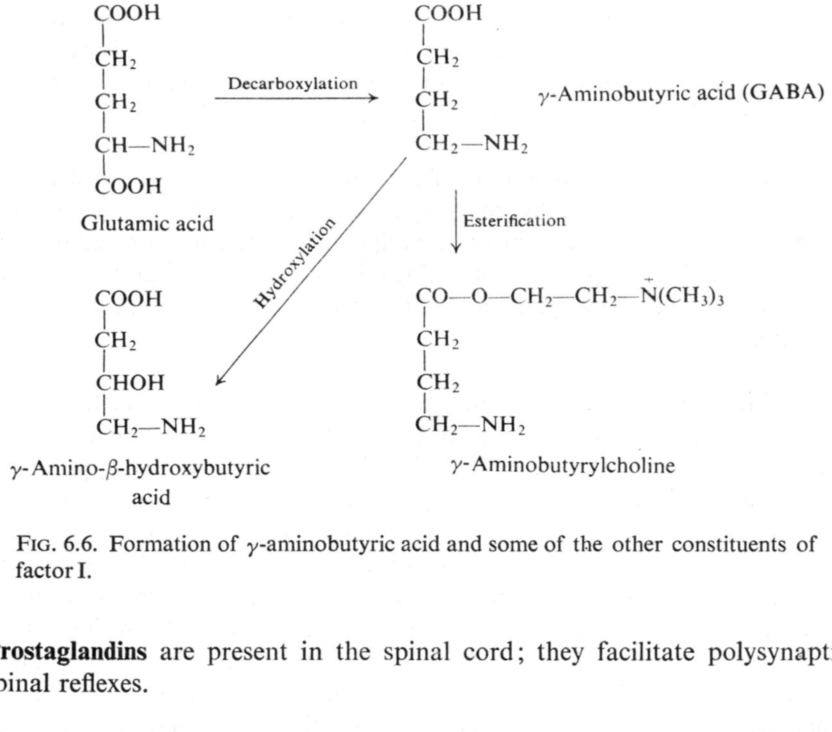

$$
\begin{array}{l}
\text{COOH} \\
|\\
\text{CH}_2 \\
|\\
\text{CH}_2 \\
|\\
\text{CH—NH}_2 \\
|\\
\text{COOH}
\end{array}
\xrightarrow{\text{Decarboxylation}}
\begin{array}{l}
\text{COOH} \\
|\\
\text{CH}_2 \\
|\\
\text{CH}_2 \\
|\\
\text{CH}_2\text{—NH}_2
\end{array}
\quad \gamma\text{-Aminobutyric acid (GABA)}
$$

Glutamic acid

Esterification

$$
\begin{array}{l}
\text{COOH} \\
|\\
\text{CH}_2 \\
|\\
\text{CHOH} \\
|\\
\text{CH}_2\text{—NH}_2
\end{array}
\qquad
\begin{array}{l}
\text{CO—O—CH}_2\text{—CH}_2\text{—}\overset{+}{\text{N}}(\text{CH}_3)_3 \\
|\\
\text{CH}_2 \\
|\\
\text{CH}_2 \\
|\\
\text{CH}_2\text{—NH}_2
\end{array}
$$

Hydroxylation

γ-Amino-β-hydroxybutyric acid

γ-Aminobutyrylcholine

Fig. 6.6. Formation of γ-aminobutyric acid and some of the other constituents of factor I.

Prostaglandins are present in the spinal cord; they facilitate polysynaptic spinal reflexes.

Cerebellar factor. The cerebellum is concerned with the co-ordination of muscular activity, and is richly endowed with nervous connections to other parts of the CNS. The pharmacologically active substances found elsewhere in the brain are absent, or occur only in very low concentrations, despite the high density of neurones and synaptic connections. The effects of cerebellar extracts have been studied and a factor which increased the electrical activity recorded from the cerebellum was found to be present. The cerebellar factor has been identified as *ergothioneine* which may be an excitatory transmitter in this region.

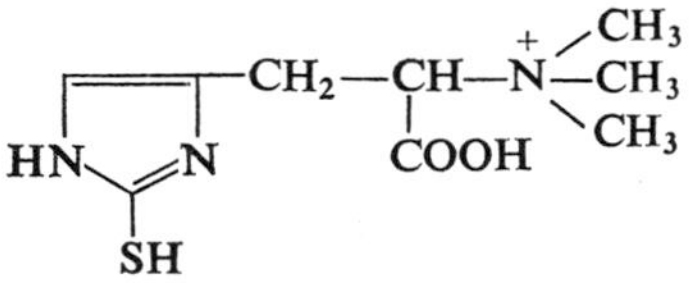

$$HN\diagdown\diagup N \text{ ring} -CH_2-CH-N^+(CH_3)(CH_3)(CH_3)$$

Ergothioneine

CHAPTER 7

Properties of Muscle

The special property of muscle cells is their contractility which is exhibited as movement or force. They contain mechanisms for converting energy derived from chemical reactions into mechanical energy. The functions of muscles are: (i) to produce movements of the body, (ii) to maintain the position of the body against the force of gravity, (iii) to produce movements of structures within the body, and (iv) to alter pressures or tensions in structures within the body.

One way of classifying muscle is according to its anatomical arrangement. Thus, *skeletal muscle* is attached to the skeleton (*somatic muscle* is an alternative name), *cardiac muscle* is contained in the walls of the heart, and *visceral* or *splanchnic muscle* is present in other viscera. Another classification depends on the histological appearance of the muscle fibres; those which show cross-striations are termed *striated* or *striped*, and those in which cross-striations are absent are termed *smooth, plain* or *non-striated*. A third system of classification depends on the nature of the nervous control over the activity of the muscle, so that the terms *voluntary* and *involuntary* are also used. These classifications have often been combined. Thus: skeletal = striated, voluntary muscle; cardiac = striated, involuntary muscle, and visceral = smooth, involuntary muscle. However, this is not entirely satisfactory as there are many exceptions. For instance, the striated muscle in the oesophagus is under involuntary control, and in fact the oesophagus is a viscus. Many striated voluntary muscles are not skeletal, since they are attached to skin, cartilage, ligaments or to other muscles, and not to bone. The striated muscles concerned in respiratory movements are usually under involuntary control, yet they are skeletal muscles. Indeed, most of the information being fed to striated muscle is not derived voluntarily, i.e. from acts of will. The ciliary muscle of the eye, which alters the focal length of the lens, consists of smooth muscle, but it can be controlled voluntarily. Many people can learn to exercise some degree of voluntary control over various other smooth muscles. Not all smooth muscle is visceral, an important exception being the smooth muscle of blood vessels. The heart is, strictly speaking, a viscus, but custom has sanctioned the term visceral muscle to exclude the muscle of the heart. Although the heart is composed of striated fibres, their histological features enable them to be readily distinguished from the fibres of striated muscles elsewhere in the body. The terms *striated muscle*,

190

cardiac muscle and *smooth muscle* provide an adequate classification for practical purposes, particularly from the point of view of pharmacology.

Striated muscle

The function of most striated muscles is to move one part of the skeleton in relation to another. At one end (the origin) the muscle is anchored, often by a tendon, to a bone which is more or less stationary. At the other end of the muscle, the tendon of insertion is attached to an adjacent bone which moves upon a joint between the two bones when the muscle shortens. Muscles which bend a limb at a joint are called *flexor muscles,* and those which straighten the limb are called *extensor muscles. Abductor muscles* are those which move the limbs in a direction away from the mid-line while *adductor muscles* move the limb towards the mid-line. *Fixation muscles* hold a bone stationary so that muscles anchored to it have their origins fixed and are able to move the bone into which their tendons are inserted. A voluntary movement calls into play the integrated activity of a number of muscles. Those producing movement are termed *prime movers,* and while they are contracting, the muscles having the opposite action (*the antagonists*) relax. Integration of a voluntary movement is brought about in the central nervous system which relies on continuous feedback from the proprioceptors and the special sense receptors in order to produce the correct degree of excitation or inhibition of the motoneurones.

Striated muscles are composed of a large number of muscle cells or fibres which range in size, in different muscles of man, from a few millimetres to over 30 cm in length and from about 10 to 100 μ in diameter. In most muscles, each fibre blends with a tendon fibre. Tendons are strong, inelastic fibrous cords, which, in different muscles, vary in length over a range similar to that for muscle fibres. The fibres within a muscle are arranged in bundles. Each fibre is embedded in fine connective tissue called *endomysium,* each bundle is sheathed in *perimysium,* and the whole muscle is enclosed in *epimysium.* The cell membrane of the muscle fibre is called the *sarcolemma.* Each fibre has one or more nuclei lying just beneath the sarcolemma. The cytoplasm of muscle cells, the *sarcoplasm,* contains numerous *myofibrils,* each of the order of 1 μ in diameter. The fibril is composed of myofilaments which are about 50–100 Å in diameter. A single muscle fibre may contain as many as 10^7 myofilaments. All the units and sub-units of the muscle fibre, including the long protein molecules within each myofilament, are orientated longitudinally. The muscle fibres appear cross-striated under the microscope, owing to the presence in the fibrils of alternating bands of high and low refractive index (Fig. 7.1a). The darker bands are called the A (anisotropic) bands and the narrower lighter ones, the I (isotropic) bands. These terms are derived from the optical properties of the

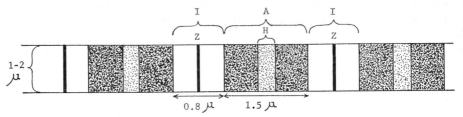

(a) Myofibril showing band pattern at rest

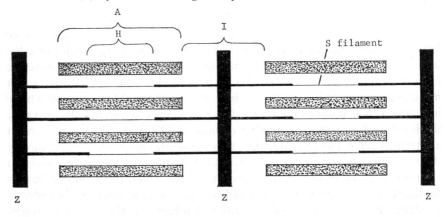

(b) Probable arrangement of filaments within a myofibril (2 Sarcomeres)

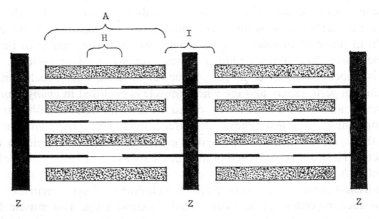

(c) Contracted fibril showing increased interpenetration of filaments. The A band is unchanged in width but the I and H bands become narrower.

Fig. 7.1. Diagrams of the myofibrils of striated muscle.

bands, the A bands being birefringent (doubly refracting) owing to the orientation of the long molecules. The electron microscope shows that the I band is divided by a strip of higher density called the Z line. Some workers believe that the Z line is continuous between myofibrils and consists of a membrane attached to the sarcolemma. The A band contains a paler central region, the H band. The region between two Z lines is called a *sarcomere* and is regarded as the smallest contractile unit in muscle.

The two main proteins of muscle, known as *actin* and *myosin*, make up more than half of the total protein content. Myosin has enzymatic properties and is capable of catalysing the breakdown of ATP to ADP and inorganic phosphate. This reaction is enhanced by calcium ions and inhibited by magnesium ions. When solutions of actin and myosin are mixed, they combine to form a very viscous complex known as *actomyosin*. Szent-Györgyi showed that artificial threads of actomyosin contract and are capable of lifting weights when placed in a suitable solution containing ATP, the energy for contraction being liberated by the enzymic breakdown of ATP. When more ATP is added to the system in the presence of mersalyl, a mercurial diuretic (pages 875–878) which has the property of inhibiting the breakdown of ATP, the actomyosin thread passively relaxes to its original length, and this suggests that ATP also plays a part in the relaxation process. The relaxation is due to actomyosin dissociating into actin and myosin. These reactions may underly the process of contraction in the living muscle. In the resting muscle, the enzymatic activity of myosin is suppressed. When the muscle is stimulated an activating substance, which may be calcium ions, is released and allows the breakdown of ATP which produces a sudden liberation energy for contraction. Subsequently the re-generation of ATP and the re-binding of calcium ions makes the contractile proteins extensible again.

According to H. E. Huxley, actin and myosin in the living muscle are organized into two sets of filaments, as illustrated in Fig. 7.1b. The separate organization of actin and myosin gives the fibres their striated appearance. The ends of corresponding actin filaments are thought to be joined by a fine extensible connection known as the S filament. During passive stretch or active contraction, the width of the A band remains constant, the change in length arising from a change in the widths of the H and I bands. H. E. Huxley and A. F. Huxley and their colleagues have developed a theory of contraction which takes into account much of the current knowledge of muscle structure and function. According to this scheme, contraction is the result of an increase in the number of cross-linkages between the actin and myosin, so that the two sets of filaments slide past one another.

The immediate source of energy for muscle contraction is released by the breakdown of ATP to ADP. In the resting muscle, the energy derived from

7

oxidative metabolism in the tricarboxylic acid cycle is transferred to ATP and to creatine phosphate, which acts as reserve of stored energy. During exercise, the work done by the muscle may exceed the energy available as ATP. During continued exercise, the lungs and circulation may be incapable of supplying oxygen at a sufficient rate for the energy released during oxidative phosphorylation to keep pace with the energy expended. The energy stored as creatine phosphate then comes into play, and additional supplies of ATP are generated by glycolysis with the accumulation of lactic acid, and by the rearrangement of ADP by myokinase with the accumulation of AMP. The difference between the energy expended by the muscle and that produced by oxidative processes represents an *oxygen debt*. The extra oxygen required for metabolism of the accumulated lactic acid and rephosphorylation of ADP and AMP and creatine is taken in over a longer period. Further details of these biochemical processes are given on pages 41–48.

Excitation of striated muscle. Figure 7.2 is a diagram of a mammalian neuro-muscular junction as it appears under an electron microscope. The motoneurone branches as it approaches the muscle fibres and the branches lose their myelin sheaths (Fig. 4.6). A branch makes contact with the sarcolemma of each fibre. The terminal Schwann cells (teloglia) of the nerve endings fuse with the sarcolemma to enclose the neuro-muscular junction. The ending of each branch of the neurone occupies a hollow indentation of the surface of the muscle fibre. The specialized part of the muscle fibre membrane which lies in close apposition to the nerve ending is known as the *motor end-plate*. (Note that an older terminology described the nerve ending as the 'nerve end-plate' and the motor end-plate as the 'muscle sole plate'.) The surface of the motor end-plate is expanded by numerous convolutions and it is at this site that the enzyme acetylcholinesterase is concentrated. The nerve endings contain the synaptic vesicles which are believed to contain the stores of pre-formed acetylcholine.

   The potential difference across the muscle membrane is measured by inserting an intracellular micro-electrode and by having a second electrode in the external fluid, whereas the potential difference between the end-plate region and the rest of the muscle fibre membrane is measured with external electrodes as shown in the diagram of Fig. 7.3. The membrane of the muscle fibre, like that of the nerve fibre, is polarized, the interior being about 90 mV negative with respect to the exterior. As in nerve fibres, the potential difference arises largely from the potassium ion concentration gradient (high inside, low outside). In the resting state, the potential difference across the motor end-plate is the same as that across the rest of the muscle cell membrane (Fig. 7.3a). The motor end-plate differs from the rest of the muscle cell membrane in that it is extremely sensitive to the action of acetylcholine, but, according to Grundfest, it is electrically inexcitable. In contrast, the rest of the muscle fibre membrane is readily excited by electrical currents but acetylcholine is without effect. When a single stimulus is applied to a motor nerve fibre, an impulse passes along the fibre and, after a short junctional delay (about 0·5 msec), the potential difference between the inside and the outside of the motor end-plate membrane becomes reduced (that is, the end-plate is depolarized), but there is no reversal in potential like that constituting an action potential. The depolarization occurs as a result of the acetylcholine, released from the nerve ending, making

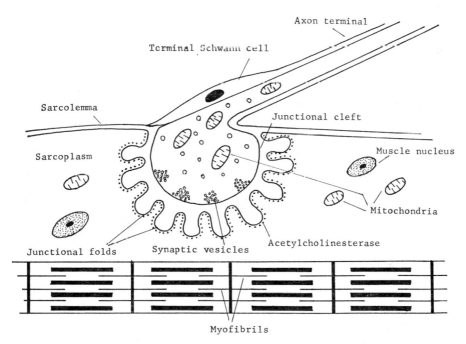

Axon terminal

Terminal Schwann cell

Sarcolemma

Junctional cleft

Sarcoplasm

Muscle nucleus

Mitochondria

Junctional folds   Synaptic vesicles   Acetylcholinesterase

Myofibrils

Fig. 7.2. Diagram of the neuromuscular junction, as seen under the electron microscope.

the end-plate membrane permeable to several small anions and cations, rather than making it selectively permeable to sodium ions as occurs during an action potential. The reduced potential difference across the end-plate membrane means that its external surface is negative with respect to that of the muscle cell membrane elsewhere (Fig. 7.3b). This localized negativity of the external surface of the motor end-plate is known as the *end-plate potential*, (e.p.p.); it constitutes the amplification process which must take place so that excitation may be transferred from the fine nerve ending to the enormously

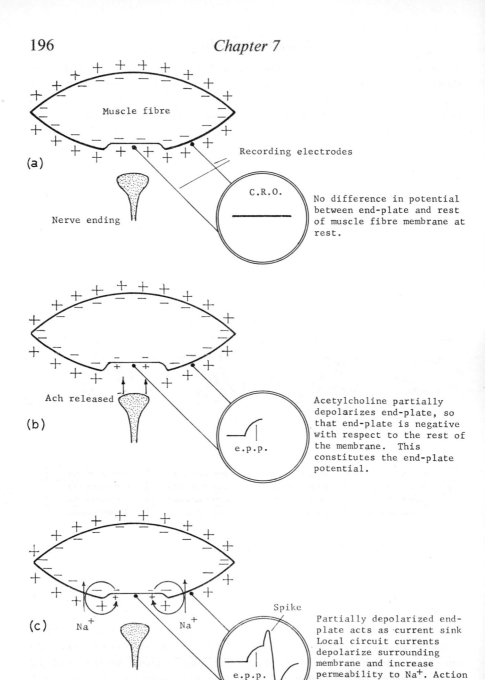

FIG. 7.3. Diagrams to illustrate the electrical changes during excitation of striated muscle, as recorded on a cathode ray oscilloscope (CRO) with external electrodes.

greater surface of the muscle fibre. The end-plate potential is graded, non-propagating and without a refractory period; it resembles the synaptic potential described on pages 90 and 149. When the external surface of the motor end-plate becomes sufficiently negative with respect to the surrounding membrane, it acts as a current sink and local circuit currents flow into it from the surrounding muscle membrane (Fig. 7.3b). This critical level of end-plate potential is usually about half of its resting potential; it is not necessary for full depolarization to zero potential to occur. The local circuit currents flowing outwards through adjacent areas of muscle fibre membrane increase sodium permeability in these regions. Sodium ions therefore rapidly penetrate the muscle fibre membrane and *reverse* the potential difference. In this way a self-propagating 'all-or-nothing' action potential passes rapidly around the muscle fibre membrane (Fig. 7.3c) in a manner similar to that described for non-myelinated nerve fibres on page 78. The propagating muscle action potential is associated with a refractory period of the order of 2 msec in mammalian muscle.

Although the amount of acetylcholine released by a single nerve impulse is probably considerably in excess of that required to produce the critical degree of end-plate depolarization, it is hydrolysed within the refractory period of the muscle cell membrane. The motor end-plate is therefore allowed to repolarize quickly and is ready to respond to a further release of acetylcholine. A single nerve impulse therefore gives rise to a single muscle action potential and this in turn results in a single muscle contraction.

In the absence of nerve impulses, there is a random release of quanta of acetylcholine giving rise to minute voltage fluctuations at the motor end-plate. These are known as *miniature end-plate potentials* and occur at a frequency of 1 to 2/sec. They are about one hundredth of the size of the full-sized end-plate potential and do not therefore give rise to muscle contractions. It has been suggested that each miniature end-plate potential is due to the release of the acetylcholine contained in one synaptic vesicle when the random movement of the vesicle results in its collision with the inside of the nerve membrane.

Similar effects to those of nerve stimulation are produced when acetylcholine is applied to the end-plate from a micro-pipette by electrophoresis. Acetylcholine is without effect when applied intracellularly to the inside surface of the motor end-plate membrane, and this shows that the receptor sites with which it reacts are located on the external surface. Drugs which inhibit cholinesterase, and so prevent the destruction of acetylcholine, increase the size and duration of the end-plate potential produced either in response to a nerve shock or by the application of a small amount of acetylcholine from a micro-pipette. As a result the end-plate potential persists beyond the refractory period of the muscle fibre membrane and so initiates more than one propagating muscle action potential. In these circumstances, the muscle fibre is said to fire repetitively.

When a large amount of acetylcholine is applied to a striated muscle in the presence of an anticholinesterase drug, the large and prolonged end-plate potential leads to an initial stimulation which is followed by block of conduction in the surrounding muscle fibre membrane, so that the muscle fails to contract (Fig. 5.4b). Excess acetylcholine may also accumulate as a result of frequent motor nerve stimulation in the presence of an anticholinesterase drug. Transmission failure produced in this way is known as *block by depolarization* and is also produced by other drugs with an acetylcholine-like action (see pages 669–674). The underlying mechanism is similar to that of cathodal block of nerve conduction (page 86). Block by depolarization may be overcome by applying an anodal (hyperpolarizing) electrode to the motor end-plate of the muscle fibres. Prolonged depolarization produces secondary changes in ionic permeability which oppose further excitation. Because the acetylcholine-sensitive area in mammalian muscle is localized, the inexcitability occurs only at the motor end-plates and in the region of the membrane immediately surrounding them. The muscle fibre action potential cannot therefore propagate away from the end-plate region and so contraction does not occur.

The muscle fibre action potential activates the contractile mechanism, but the events taking part in the process of *excitation-contraction coupling*, as it is called, are not understood, although it appears that the Z line is involved. Huxley and Taylor stimulated a muscle fibre by means of current from a micro-electrode. When the micro-electrode tip was placed on the membrane adjacent to a Z line, a moderate depolarization of the underlying membrane produced a localized contraction. But when stimulation was applied mid-way between two Z lines, a much larger depolarization was without effect. The Z line may therefore be responsible for carrying the electrical charge into the interior of the fibre where it releases the activating substance which allows the breakdown of ATP by myosin. The process of excitation-contraction coupling in muscle is analogous to the coupling process at nerve endings through which the action potential releases the chemical transmitter.

EFFECTS OF INORGANIC CATIONS ON STRIATED MUSCLE. Potassium, sodium, calcium and magnesium ions exert effects on striated muscle similar to those described for nerve on page 87. Potassium and sodium ions are necessary for the maintenance of the resting potential and for the production of action potentials. Calcium and magnesium ions play an important part in regulating the excitable properties of the membrane; they are concerned in the coupling process through which excitation of the membrane leads to contraction; and they are involved in the contractile process itself. The first effect of calcium deficiency in the external solution is that the membrane of the muscle fibre becomes unstable and repetitive action potentials are discharged. The muscle fibres contract in response to these action potentials as there is usually sufficient calcium bound within the muscle to maintain coupling and contractility. The labilizing effect of lack of calcium on nerve and muscle is responsible for the tetany of parathyroid deficiency (Chapter 14). In continued calcium lack, inexcitability of the membrane develops. Excess calcium stabilizes the membrane and in this respect magnesium ions behave similarly but less powerfully. Excess calcium ions facilitate coupling and contractility but magnesium ions exert the opposite effects. To demonstrate the effect of calcium lack on coupling and contractility in striated muscle, it is usually necessary to use a calcium complexing agent (such as sodium ethylenediaminetetra-acetate) to remove the bound calcium from the muscle. Some drugs (e.g., caffeine) may affect striated muscle contractions by influencing the binding or movement of calcium ions within the muscle.

Characteristics of striated muscle contraction

TWITCH AND TETANUS. The contraction of a muscle in response to a single brief stimulus applied either to its motor nerve or to the muscle itself, is called a *twitch*. The functional unit of a muscle is not the single fibre but the motor unit (page 111). Weak stimulation applied to a motor nerve trunk may excite only one nerve fibre and give rise to a twitch of only one motor unit. As the strength of the stimulus is increased, more and more motor units are excited until a strength is reached at which a twitch of the whole muscle results. A single synchronous contraction of all the fibres in a muscle is called a *maximal twitch*; further increase in the strength of the stimulus does not produce a greater twitch. The electrical and mechanical changes produced in the tibialis anterior muscle of an anaesthetized cat in response to a single stimulus applied to the motor nerve are illustrated in Fig. 7.4a. The action potential in this record is the summed effect of all the action potentials in the individual muscle fibres; it was recorded with external electrodes, one on the belly of the muscle and one on the tendon.

The twitch is triggered by the action potential, and both obey the *all-or-nothing-law*. However, the amplitude of the maximal twitch depends on the prevailing conditions. For example, the size of the twitch varies with the resting length of the muscle and is greatest at an optimal resting length.

When a series of stimuli is applied to a muscle, or its nerve, each stimulus produces a discrete action potential but the mechanical responses fuse and summate, as shown in Fig. 7.5. At a sufficiently high frequency of stimulation, there is complete fusion and this is called a *tetanus*. The action potentials do not summate because of the refractory period of the membrane (about 2 msec).

Therefore, at frequencies above 500/sec the muscle does not respond to all stimuli, and high-frequency inhibition occurs (sometimes called Wedensky inhibition after the physiologist who first described it), the tension rapidly returning to the base-line. Low rates of stimulation produce an incomplete tetanus or *clonus*.

After a tetanus, the maximal twitch is increased in tension by as much as 100% over the pretetanic level (Fig. 7.5). The effect gradually wanes so that 10–15 min after the tetanus, the twitches have returned to their initial amplitude. This type of post-tetanic potentiation is due to a change in the con-

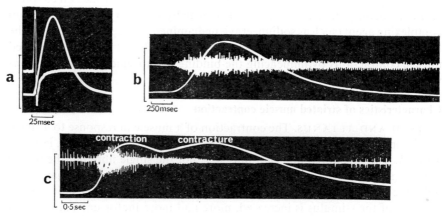

FIG. 7.4. Isometric tension (lower trace) and muscle action potential (upper trace) simultaneously recorded on a cathode ray oscilloscope from the tibialis anterior muscle of anaesthetized cats. The tension calibrations on the left are equal to 0·5 kg. (a) The maximal twitch in response to stimulation of the motor nerve with a single electric pulse (50 μsec) (b) The responses to close-arterial injection of 5 μg acetylcholine; note that the burst of electrical activity continues throughout the tension change. (c) The biphasic response of a chronically denervated muscle to close-arterial injection of 0·1 μg acetylcholine; note that action potentials are present before the injection, and that propagated action potentials cease during the second part of the tension response (the contracture).

tractility of the muscle fibre and not to an effect on neuromuscular transmission. (A facilitatory effect on neuro-muscular transmission, similar to that described for synaptic transmission on page 155, occurs simultaneously but is not detected when *maximal* twitches are being recorded.) The increased contractility resulting from previous activity may also be seen with single twitches providing the interval between successive twitches is not too long. For example, if a muscle is stimulated once every second, each twitch during the first 1 to 2 min of stimulation is greater than its predecessor. The twitches then become constant at an

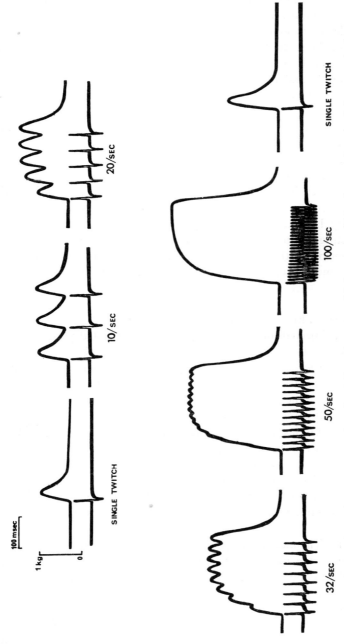

FIG. 7.5. Isometric tension (upper trace) and muscle action potential (lower trace) simultaneously recorded on a cathode ray oscilloscope from the tibialis anterior muscle of an anaesthetized cat in response to stimulation of the motor nerve. Repetitive stimulation of the nerve was applied at the frequencies shown for periods of 250 msec. At a frequency of 100/sec, complete fusion of the twitches occurred but the action potentials remained discrete. Note that the single twitch after the repetitive stimulation is greater than that recorded first.

7*

amplitude 30–50% greater than the first twitch. This type of increasing response with successive stimuli is known as a *staircase or Treppe effect*; it also occurs in cardiac muscle and in some smooth muscles. It is due partly to a reduction in the viscosity of the sarcoplasm and partly to prolongation of the *active state* (described below). Repetitive muscle activity mobilizes bound calcium ions within the muscle and the effect of these calcium ions on the contractile mechanism probably also plays a part in the enhanced contractions to single stimuli.

To a physiologist, the term *contraction* does not always imply shortening. An *isotonic* contraction is one in which the muscle shortens under constant load. This occurs in muscles used during walking, running or lifting. An *isometric* contraction is one in which the muscle develops tension but does not alter in length. Tension developed during isometric contractions is used to oppose other forces, for example, in the maintenance of posture against the force of gravity. If the tension exerted by a muscle is less than the force against which it is acting, the muscle increases in length; this occurs during walking when the extensors of the hip begin to check the forward swing of the leg. Many types of muscle activity involve a mixture of both isotonic and isometric contraction.

CONTRACTION PRODUCED BY INJECTED ACETYLCHOLINE. When acetylcholine is injected into the artery supplying a striated muscle, the contraction of the muscle which it produces is not a twitch but a brief asynchronous tetanus. It is *asynchronous* because the acetylcholine stimulates the motor end-plates one after the other as it is carried along by the blood-stream; in contrast, acetylcholine released from the nerve endings stimulates them simultaneously. It is *repetitive* because no matter how quickly the injection is made, it is bound to last longer than the refractory period of the muscle fibre membrane (about 2 msec). Consequently, fibres which are stimulated at the beginning of the injection are stimulated many more times as the injection continues. Figure 7.4b illustrates the electrical and mechanical responses of the tibialis anterior muscle of a cat to a close-arterial injection of acetylcholine, and shows that action potentials continue throughout the contraction.

ACTIVE STATE. The mechanical properties of striated muscle indicate that it consists of *contractile* and *elastic components* arranged in series. Shortening of the contractile component stretches the elastic component (Fig. 7.6a). The elastic component has the effect of smoothing out abrupt changes in tension. When a muscle is stimulated, the contractile component shortens abruptly and its maximal contraction is known as the *active state*. Before the muscle itself develops tension, the elastic component must be stretched by the contractile component and time is required for this process. The development of tension by the muscle as a whole is therefore relatively slow. These effects are illustrated diagrammatically in Fig. 7.6b. In frog muscle at 0°C, the active state remains at full intensity for only 25 msec after a single stimulus and in the warmer mammalian muscles the period is even shorter. Thus, in a maximal isometric twitch, the duration of the active state is insufficient to allow the muscle to reach the full tension of which it is capable. At the peak of the twitch, the active state has already decayed to a fraction of its maximal value. When the muscle is stimulated tetanically, the active state is maintained at full activity by the successive stimuli and the muscle has time to develop its maximal tension. The maximal tetanic tension of a muscle is therefore equal to the maximal tension exerted by its contractile components.

Several substances which increase the maximal isometric twitch tension of striated muscle are believed to do so by prolonging the plateau of the active state of the stimulated muscle, thereby allowing the muscle more time to develop tension. Among these are the drugs adrenaline, noradrenaline, isoprenaline, caffeine and quinidine, and nitrate ions. These substances increase the tension of single maximal twitches and of incomplete tetani but do not affect the tension of a maximal *tetanus*, since in this case the active state is already fully maintained by the repeated stimuli. The enhancement of twitch tension brought about in this way is not accompanied by repetitive firing and therefore differs from the effect of anticholinesterases (see page 681). Cooling the muscle has also been shown to prolong the active state. However, cooling slows down metabolic processes and increases the viscosity of the sarcoplasm so that, except under special conditions, these effects of cooling are usually sufficient to mask or reverse the increase in twitch tension which would otherwise arise from prolongation of the active state.

When isotonic contractions are recorded, there is no change in tension and consequently the series elastic component is not stretched during the contraction. The contraction is therefore shorter in duration and directly reflects the shortening of the contractile component.

Chronically denervated muscle. When the motor nerve to a striated muscle is cut and a few days are allowed to elapse for full degeneration of the peripheral portion of the nerve, the membrane potential of the muscle fibres begins to undergo rhythmic oscillations which trigger propagated action potentials whenever the depolarizations reach a critical value. The propagating action potentials in the individual fibres give rise to asynchronous contractions termed *fibrillations* which are visible to the naked eye. Figure 7.7 illustrates the spontaneous electrical and mechanical changes in a denervated muscle; their cause is as yet unknown.

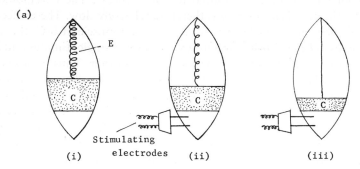

(i) A muscle is composed of a contractile component (C) and a series elastic component (E).

(ii) On stimulation the contractile component shortens, but in an isometric contraction, the maximum external tension is not produced until the series elastic component is fully extended, as in (iii).

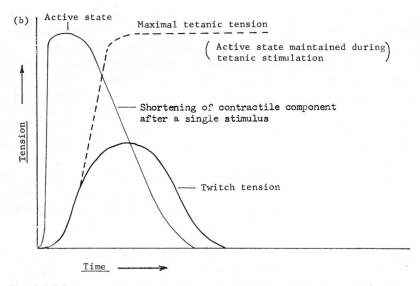

FIG. 7.6. Diagrams to illustrate the changes in striated muscle during excitation. The *active state* corresponds to the shortened state of the contractile component.

It was once thought that there was an increase in the cholinesterase content of a denervated muscle. However, muscle decreases in weight after denervation, and it is now realized that the absolute amount of cholinesterase does not increase, but gradually decreases. Histochemical methods have shown that, after denervation, cholinesterase persists at the motor end-plate long after complete degeneration of the nerve has occurred. The time during which it persists varies with the animal species. For example, in guinea-pig muscle the enzyme disappears within 4 to 5 days, whereas in rat muscle some is still present up to 6 months after denervation. The nerve appears to induce the presence of cholinesterase at the motor end-plate. When a nerve is allowed to regenerate after the cholinesterase has disappeared, the re-innervated end-plates almost immediately acquire their original quantities of enzyme. Furthermore, in frog muscle a functional connection may be

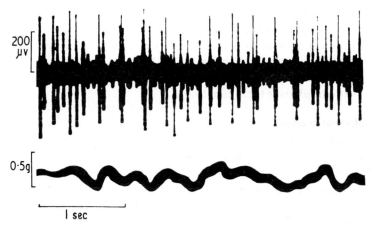

FIG. 7.7. Spontaneous activity recorded on a cathode ray oscilloscope from a chronically denervated soleus muscle in an anaesthetized cat. Upper trace, fibrillary potentials; lower trace, isometric tension. (From Bowman & Raper (1964), *Nature, Lond.*, **201**, 160.)

induced when a sectioned motor nerve is made to innervate part of a muscle fibre which was formerly without an end-plate, and the new junction quickly acquires cholinesterase. In a chronically denervated muscle, the whole of the muscle fibre membrane, and not just the motor end-plate region, is sensitive to acetylcholine (and to drugs with a similar action). Consequently, quantities of such drugs much smaller than those necessary to excite an innervated muscle, stimulate a denervated muscle; supersensitivity to acetylcholine is particularly well developed, probably because it then acts at parts of the membrane not protected by cholinesterase. Denervation may increase the sensitivity to acetylcholine as much as 1000 times.

When acetylcholine or a similar drug acts on a denervated muscle, propagated action potentials may be initiated from any point on the fibre membranes and the muscle contracts. Gradually, however, the whole fibre membrane becomes depolarized by the drug and the contractile mechanism is continuously activated so that the muscle remains contracted until the concentration of the drug diminishes. As the membrane is already depolarized, all propagated action potentials disappear. This type of contraction, which is unaccompanied by propagated electrical activity, is known as a *contracture*. Figure 7.4c illustrates the biphasic mechanical and electrical responses of the chronically denervated tibialis anterior muscle of a cat to acetylcholine. This record should be compared with that of a response of innervated muscle to the same drug (Fig. 7.4b). Chronically denervated muscles provide sensitive preparations for the detection of a depolarizing or nicotinic drug action.

All of the changes induced by denervation revert to normal when functional re-innervation is allowed to occur. In many respects, chronically denervated muscles resemble embryo striated muscle fibres at a time before innervation has taken place. These, too, exhibit spontaneous fibrillations and are sensitive to acetylcholine all over their membranes.

Types of striated muscle

FAST- AND SLOW-CONTRACTING MUSCLE FIBRES. Muscles differ in their speed of contraction and are classified as fast- and slow-contracting muscles. The time from the start of the contraction to the tension crest in an isometric twitch of a fast-contracting muscle in the mammal is 30 msec or less. The fastest mammalian muscle studied is the internal rectus of the eye with a contraction time of 7·5 msec. Slow-contracting mammalian muscles have a contraction time in an isometric twitch of 70 msec or more, and therefore tetanic fusion occurs with lower frequencies of stimulation than those necessary in fast-contracting muscles. Flexor muscles (such as tibialis anterior) and superficial extensor muscles (such as gastrocnemius) are usually fast-contracting muscles, whereas deep extensors (such as soleus and crureus) are slow-contracting muscles in most mammalian species. In some respects, slow-contracting muscles differ from fast-contracting muscles in their responses to drugs. At birth, all limb muscles in mammals are slow-contracting and differentiation into fast and slow types occurs during the first few weeks. The speed of contraction of a muscle appears to be determined either by the type of motoneurone which innervates it or by the pattern of nerve impulses discharged to it from the CNS. If the nerves to a fast- and a slow-contracting muscle are severed and each central portion is joined to the peripheral stump of the opposite type of muscle, the fast muscle becomes slow and the slow muscle becomes fast when functional cross-innervation is established. The changes in cholinesterase and muscle speed are striking examples of the trophic influence of the nervous system on the properties of peripheral effector organs.

Usually, but not invariably, slow-contracting muscles contain more myoglobin than fast-contracting muscles and are therefore of a deeper red colour. Owing to their high oxygen storing capacity and their large content of cytochrome oxidase, red muscles are less liable to accumulate an oxygen debt than are pale muscles. Red muscles are usually concerned in functions requiring prolonged activity such as the maintenance of posture. In man, the differentiation of muscles into fast or slow, and red or pale, types is less marked than it is in many species.

FOCALLY- AND MULTIPLY-INNERVATED MUSCLE FIBRES. In most of the muscles of mammals, each fibre is innervated by only one branch of a nerve fibre and it is termed a *focally-innervated* or twitch fibre. However, in many of the muscles of birds and amphibia, *multiply-innervated* muscle fibres occur in large numbers. For example, about half of the fibres in the chicken's gastrocnemius muscle have been shown to possess about eighty motor end-plates each. The end-plates may be supplied by different branches of a single nerve fibre or by branches derived from several nerve fibres (polyneuronal innervation). Multiply-innervated fibres are sensitive to acetylcholine at many points on their membranes. The nerve fibres innervating these muscles do not appear to release an excess of acetylcholine; that is, the *safety factor* in transmitter release is less than it is in focally-innervated muscles. If the areas of membrane sensitive to acetylcholine are extensive, the contractile mechanism is activated without the production of propagating action potentials. In their reaction to injected acetylcholine and drugs with a similar 'nicotinic' action, these muscles therefore behave in many respects like chronically denervated muscles, exhibiting, in their electrical and mechanical responses both contraction and contracture. The effects of depolarizing drugs on the chicken's gastrocnemius muscle are illustrated in Fig. 26.6. This muscle, having a mixture of focally and multiply-innervated fibres, exhibits the properties of both types, although the multiply-innervated fibres are more sensitive to depolarizing drugs. The frog's rectus abdominis muscle also contains many multiply-innervated fibres and responds to acetylcholine-like drugs by a sustained depolarization and contracture. Since propagating action potentials are not involved, conduction block does not affect the response, and there is therefore no real counterpart to the muscle paralysis which results from prolonged end-plate depolarization in focally-innervated muscles. However, when a large amount of depolarizing drug is left in contact with the frog's rectus abdominis muscle preparation for a long time, the contracture does gradually wane, possibly due to an ionic imbalance arising from the sustained depolarization. As paralysis due to depolarization block does not occur, the isolated rectus abdominis muscle of the frog continues to respond to repeated additions of acetylcholine-like drugs, and the muscle therefore serves as a useful assay preparation. In mammals, including man, there is evidence that the intrafusal fibres of the muscle spindles (page 107) and some of the fibres of the external ocular muscles are multiply-innervated.

Voluntary movements. Voluntary contractions do not consist of maximal twitches nor of synchronous tetanic contractions of the whole muscle. The value of experimentally produced twitches and tetani of the muscle as a whole is simply that they represent, on a larger scale, the responses of the individual motor units occurring during a voluntary contraction. A smooth voluntary contraction is the algebraic sum of the asynchronous contractions of the motor units which may discharge at rates from about 5 to 100/sec. The strength of a voluntary contraction is graded by alterations both in the frequency of motor nerve impulses and in the number of motor units contributing.

During a sustained sub-maximal contraction, motor units undergo periods of rest and activity so that fatigue is less evident than it is during sustained electrically produced tetani. Fatigue of a maintained voluntary contraction has been shown to be due to a peripheral phenomenon occurring in the muscle itself. During severe exercise, however, when many muscles are involved, fatigue is experienced as a result of a protective mechanism occurring at the synapses in the CNS. This type of fatigue occurs before the muscles themselves lose their ability to contract. A feeling of fatigue may also be experienced if the subject is bored by the task being performed.

Some diseases of striated muscle

MYASTHENIA GRAVIS. The main symptoms of this disease are weakness, fatigue and rapid exhaustion during activity, with partial recovery during rest. These symptoms may affect any muscle and may remain localized or become generalized. Disturbances involving the extraocular muscles and the extremities are most common. The disease is relatively rare, there being about 25,000 cases in the U.S.A.; slightly more females than males are affected. Death from respiratory paralysis occurs in about 20% of patients, usually within the first 3 years of contracting the disease. The site of the lesion appears to be the neuro-muscular junction and histologists have described both pre- and post-junctional abnormalities. The cause of the disease is unknown but several possibilities have been put forward: (i) A circulating neuro-muscular blocking agent may be present, although, so far, extensive tests have failed to detect such a substance. The symptoms of the disease are in many respects similar to the effects of an injection of hemicholinium (page 662), and it has been found that the spontaneous release of acetylcholine from the nerve endings in myasthenic muscle is less than that in normal muscle. (ii) The motor end-plates in myasthenic muscle may react abnormally to acetylcholine. Myasthenics are resistant to decamethonium (a depolarizing drug); this suggests that they may also be less able to respond to acetylcholine. (iii) The lesions at the junctional region may be the result of an auto-immune disease in which an antibody to the motor end-plate receptor proteins is produced by the reticulo-endothelial system including the thymus gland. In many cases of myasthenia gravis, the thymus gland is enlarged, and thymectomy may be of benefit, particularly in young female patients.

FAMILIAL PERIODIC PARALYSIS. The main symptom of this rare disease is irregular attacks of paralysis. The site of the paralysis is peripheral; stimulation of the motor nerve or of the muscle itself during an attack fails to elicit muscle contractions. The attacks appear to result from a fall in plasma potassium, since the administration of KCl usually produces recovery.

MYOTONIA CONGENITA. This is a rare congenital disease in which the patient's muscles are thrown into violent spasm when the attempt to perform a voluntary movement is first made. For example, if the patient yawns, the mouth remains open for some time. As movements are repeated, however, they become more normal. The condition appears to be due to a change in the excitability of the muscle fibres themselves since direct stimulation of the fully-curarized muscles produces a contraction which persists long after the stimulation is stopped. In some respects, the diseased muscle resembles muscle poisoned with veratrine. In each case, a single stimulus produces a train of action potentials and a tetanic contraction. One species of goat in the U.S.A. suffers from a condition indistinguishable from that of human myotonia, and these animals are used to study the disease.

Cardiac muscle

Cardiac muscle (or *myocardial*) fibres contain structural elements similar to those in striated muscle fibres. Their sarcoplasm contains longitudinally arranged myofibrils with A, I and Z bands which appear as cross-striations of the cell. In cardiac muscle, the cross-striations are not as well marked as they are in striated muscle cells because the sarcoplasm is granular. Mitochondria and inclusions of fat and glycogen are also present in the sarcoplasm.

The histological features which particularly distinguish cardiac muscle are the centrally situated nucleus, the branching of the fibres and the occurrence of transverse markings known as *intercalated* discs (Fig. 7.8). It was believed at one time that the myofibrils of cardiac muscle continued through the intercalated discs, and that intercalated discs were absent from the hearts of embryos and the young, so that the fibres were composed into a network or a *structural syncytium*. However, recent work with the electron-microscope indicates that cardiac muscle consists of large numbers of separate cells abutting at intercalated discs. At the abutments the membranes interdigitate, thus increasing the mechanical strength of the junctions between the cells and perhaps facilitating conduction of excitation from one cell to the next. Cardiac muscle first appears in the embryo as fusiform cells arranged in a plexus. The cell membranes between adjacent cells become the intercalated discs. Cardiac muscle *functions* as if the fibres were composed of two syncytia, all the muscle

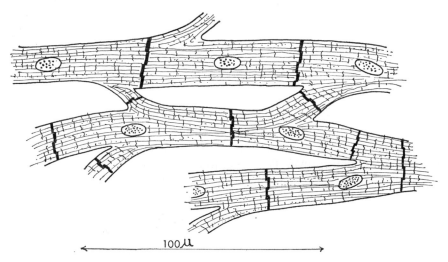

Fig. 7.8. Diagram of cardiac muscle cells. The nuclei are situated centrally within the fibres. The fibres branch and interconnect. There are longitudinal myofibrils and cross-striations. Intercalated discs cross the fibres between adjacent nuclei.

fibres of the atria behaving as one syncytium and all those of the ventricles as another.

Some cardiac muscle cells take on specialized functions and are responsible for the initiation of the heart's beat and for the conduction of the impulse through various parts of the heart. William Harvey, in 1686, observing the slowly beating hearts of snakes and frogs, noticed that the heart beat arose first in the atria and then passed to the ventricle. Later it was found that the rate of beating of the frog's heart was increased or decreased by warming or cooling a small part of the heart at the junction of the sinus venosus and the right atrium. Stannius (1852) tied a ligature between the sinus venosus and the atrium of the frog heart and noted that the sinus continued to beat although the atria and ventricle stopped. These observations showed that the normal beat of the frog's heart originated in the sinus. In the mammalian heart, distinctive structures are present in the wall of the right atrium adjacent to the orifice of the superior vena cava (Fig. 7.9). The fibres here are about one-third the size of other atrial fibres and resemble embryonic heart cells. These cells are richly supplied with blood vessels and with nerves. By analogy with the frog's heart, this region is called the *sino-atrial node* (S-A node). Because it initiates the heart's beat and governs the rate of beating, it is called the *pacemaker*. The sino-atrial pacemaker cells are in direct contact with other atrial cells. The impulse, originating in the pacemaker cells, excites the surrounding atrial cells and is then conducted throughout the right and left atria.

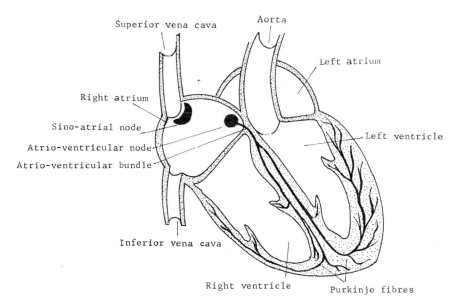

FIG. 7.9. Diagram of the pacemaker and conducting tissues of the heart.

In the right side of the septum between the two atria, the myocardial fibres converge on another structure resembling the sino-atrial node; this is the *atrio-ventricular node* (A-V node) discovered by Tawara in 1906 (Fig. 7.9). The cells of the atrio-ventricular node are somewhat larger than those of the sino-atrial node, but otherwise are similar in being richly supplied with blood vessels and autonomic nerve endings.

In 1845, the physiologist Purkinje described bundles of modified cardiac fibres in the ventricles. These *Purkinje fibres* are larger than contractile cells, have less dense myofibrils, and commonly contain two or more nuclei between a pair of intercalated discs. A bundle of Purkinje fibres begins at the atrio-ventricular node and runs in a connective tissue sheath across the junction between the atria and ventricles and into the ventricular septum (Fig. 7.9). This is called the *atrio-ventricular bundle* (A-V bundle) or *bundle of His*, after the Swiss who discovered it. In mammalian hearts, there is no other connection between cardiac fibres of the atria and the ventricles, the junction consisting of fibrous tissue; the cardiac impulses pass from the atria into the ventricles via the bundle of His. In the ventricular septum the bundle divides into two branches, one to each ventricle, and then breaks up into branches which penetrate the myocardium. The function of the Purkinje tissue is to conduct the cardiac impulse rapidly throughout the mass of ventricular muscle so that the ventricular fibres contract almost synchronously. The Purkinje cells at the termination of the conducting fibres are continuous with the ordinary myocardial cells, one type merging into the other.

In the heart of the frog there is continuity between the muscle fibres of the atria and the ventricle, and there is no specially distinguishable conducting tissue corresponding to the bundle of His.

Mechanical properties of cardiac muscle. The contraction of heart muscle is called *systole* and relaxation is called *diastole*. These are the Greek words for contraction and relaxation of the heart. Excitation of cardiac muscle fibres at one point is conducted throughout the heart and all the fibres contract. In mammals the atria function as one syncytium and the ventricles as another, these two syncytia being connected by the atrio-ventricular bundle. Therefore the heart as a whole obeys the *all-or-none-law*, functioning as one unit. It was in cardiac muscle that Bowditch in 1871 first demonstrated the all-or-none law. As pointed out earlier (page 79), the all-or-none law states that the weakest stimulus which evokes a response evokes a maximal response, but this has to be reconciled with two variables: the sensitivity to stimuli may change with time and the magnitude of the maximal response may change. These changes may be caused by alterations in the environment or by preceding events. Cardiac muscle exhibits a 'staircase' effect, also discovered by Bowditch. When successive stimuli are given with a suitable interval between them, the contractions elicited by the first few stimuli increase and then they continue at a steady level.

Cardiac muscle has a *refractory period* considerably longer than that of striated muscle. In fact, the absolute refractory period lasts for almost as long as the contraction. Therefore heart muscle cannot be thrown into a tetanic contraction by rapid stimuli.

The work output from cardiac muscle, measured during isotonic contraction, increases with increasing initial lengths of the fibres up to a critical length, beyond which it decreases. If measurements are made during isometric contraction, the tension developed is related to the resting tension, the energy appearing as heat. Stating both these observations in one form, *the energy of contraction increases with increasing resting length (or tension)*. This generalization is related to the *law of the heart*, which deals with the output of blood from the heart in relationship to the amount of blood returning to the heart in the veins (page 261).

Rhythmicity. The pacemaker cells in the sino-atrial node discharge at a rhythm which depends on the particular conditions operating in their immediate environment. Factors known to influence their rate include temperature, electrolytes and neurohormones. The property of rhythmicity is inherent in cardiac muscle cells and does not depend on the nerves. It is said to be *myogenic* (that is, in contrast to neurogenic). In the early embryo, the first recognizable cardiac cells contract rhythmically long before the nerves grow out to the heart. The heart isolated from the body and kept in a suitable medium (for example, oxygenated Locke's solution) continues to beat for hours. Separate heart muscle cells grown in tissue culture exhibit rhythmic contractions. If the impulses from the sino-atrial pacemaker are prevented from spreading over the heart, the heart remains quiescent for a while and then begins to beat again, but at a slower rate. This is because another part of the heart has taken over the role of pacemaker. Stannius occluded the sino-atrial pacemaker by fastening a tight ligature between the sinus venosus and the atria in the frog's heart; the sinus continued to beat at its original rhythm. After a pause of some minutes, the atria and the ventricle began to beat again, but at a slower rate. Such a ligature is known as *Stannius's first ligature*. A second Stannius ligature, tied between the atria and the ventricle, resulted in cessation of ventricular contractions although the atria continued to beat at their own rate. After a longer pause the ventricle again began to beat, but at a still slower rhythm, in response to a ventricular pacemaker. In isolated turtle heart, the pacemaker cells may be cut away, beginning with the pacemaker in the sinus and proceeding throughout the heart until last of all only a piece of the apex of the ventricle remains; this beats at the slowest rate. Pacemakers may therefore arise in any part of the myocardium, but the sino-atrial pacemaker dominates the rate of the normal heart beat because its rhythm is the fastest. In some diseases, the excitability of other parts of the heart is increased, and the beats arising from the so-called *ectopic foci* result in disorders of the heart's rhythm.

Nerve supply of cardiac muscle. There is an abundant supply of myelinated sensory nerve fibres in the heart, and some of these end in close relationship to the myocardial fibres. *Parasympathetic pre-ganglionic fibres* from the vagus synapse with ganglion cells which are thickly distributed in the vicinity of the

S-A and A-V nodes and in the A-V bundles. The post-ganglionic fibres terminate amongst the pacemaker and conducting (Purkinje) cells in these regions, but the rest of the atrial myocardium also receives parasympathetic innervation. The vagus does not innervate the ventricular myocardium. Stimulation of the vagus nerves results in slowing of the rate of the pacemaker, a decrease in the rate of conduction along the atrio-ventricular bundle and a reduction in the force of atrial contraction. *Sympathetic post-ganglionic fibres* from the stellate ganglia and the second and third thoracic ganglia innervate both the atrial and the ventricular myocardium, as well as the pacemaker and the conducting tissue of the heart. Stimulation of the sympathetic nerves to the heart increases the rate and force of contraction of the atrial and ventricular myocardium.

Membrane potentials in cardiac tissue. The value of the resting potential and the configuration of the action potential depends not only on the species, but also on the type of cardiac tissue (whether atrial or ventricular myocardial fibres, pacemaker cells or Purkinje fibres). The potential difference across the membrane of a cardiac muscle fibre at rest is 60 to 90 mV, the inside of the fibre being negative. An action potential has an amplitude of 90 to 120 mV, the 'overshoot' being 20 to 30 mV. The phase of depolarization takes about 0·5 msec. The total duration of the action potential is 100–500 msec. Action potentials from various types of cardiac tissue are shown in Fig. 7.10. The relationship of the membrane potentials to the electrolyte concentration gradients and permeabilities of the cell membrane established for nerve and striated muscle holds, in general, for cardiac tissue. The resting membrane potential of cardiac muscle is in reasonable agreement with that predicted by the Nernst equation (page 74). The depolarization phase of the action potential is due to a sudden increase in permeability to sodium ions.

The prolonged action potential of cardiac muscle is maintained by metabolic processes. It has been observed in isolated cardiac muscle that metabolic inhibitors (such as dinitrophenol, azide, monoiodoacetate and fluoride) decrease the duration of the action potential; lack of oxygen or of metabolic substrates (e.g. glucose) has the same effect.

The refractory period for cardiac muscle coincides approximately with the duration of the action potential. The absolute refractory period lasts until repolarization has proceeded to about 40–60 mV. Thereafter, the tissue is relatively refractory until repolarization is complete. Excitation of the tissue during the relative refractory period depends on the rate of passage of current through the membrane. An action potential being propagated through the heart excites the tissue during the relative refractory period in normal circumstances, i.e. the rate of current change in advance of the action potential is

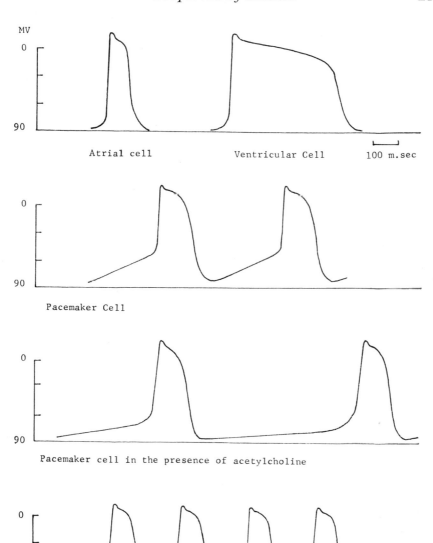

MV

Atrial cell   Ventricular Cell   100 m.sec

Pacemaker Cell

Pacemaker cell in the presence of acetylcholine

Pacemaker cell in the presence of noradrenaline

FIG. 7.10. Cardiac action potentials. (Redrawn from Trautwein, 1963.)

sufficient to excite. But if the rate of rise of the action potential is slowed, then the rate of current change in advance of the more slowly forming action potential may be insufficient and the impulse is not propagated.

The membrane potentials recorded from fibres in pacemaker tissue differ from those in myocardial fibres in that there is no steady value for the membrane potential of pacemaker tissue between successive action potentials. The membrane potential gradually declines because the K^+ permeability gradually decreases. When a critical value is reached (40 to 60 mV), sodium permeability abruptly increases and the action potential is initiated (Fig. 7.10), and propagates through the surrounding myocardial cells. Pacemaker cells are more permeable to Na^+ than quiescent cells, and this tends to make the membrane less stable.

THE EFFECTS OF ACETYLCHOLINE. The action potential of atrial (but not of ventricular) myocardial cells is altered by acetylcholine: the membrane repolarizes more rapidly and the refractory period is therefore decreased. Acetylcholine decreases the rate of the heart beat, and its effects on the membrane potential of pacemaker fibres explain this. The rate of depolarization of the membrane of pacemaker cells during diastole is slowed by acetylcholine, so that a longer time elapses before the critical potential for discharge of the action potential is reached (Fig. 7.10). Acetylcholine produces this effect by making the membrane less permeable to sodium. Noradrenaline has the opposite effect; the membrane is rendered more permeable to sodium, so that the rate of depolarization during diastole is more rapid, and the critical potential is reached more quickly.

Conduction. The rate at which the action potentials are propagated through the heart varies in different cardiac tissues. For example, in the atrial myocardium, it is 1 m/sec; in the atrio-ventricular bundle it is 0·2 m/sec; in the ventricular conducting system it is 4 m/sec; and in ventricular myocardium it is 0·4 m/sec. The action potential is conducted rapidly throughout the atria, and then there is a distinct pause before ventricular excitation occurs, because of the slow rate of conduction through the A-V bundle. Action potentials are conveyed rapidly to all parts of the ventricles, and therefore the contraction of the mass of ventricular muscle is almost synchronous.

Effects of Ionic Milieu on Cardiac Muscle. The actions of sodium, potassium and calcium ions on cardiac cells are similar to their actions on other excitable cells but they are complicated by the fact that the heart is spontaneously active and not all parts of the heart are equally sensitive. Ringer, in 1880–1883, studied the effects of various ions on the beat of isolated frog hearts.

His main findings were (1) that during perfusion with isotonic sodium chloride solution the beats weakened and the ventricle stopped in diastole, (2) that addition of calcium salts to the solution restored the beats, although in the presence of excess calcium the ventricle failed to relax and stopped in systole, and (3) that addition of potassium salts to the solution already containing sodium and calcium ions, enabled the ventricle to relax, although in the presence of excess potassium the ventricle stopped in diastole.

The salts used by Ringer were $NaCl$, KCl, $CaCl_2$ and $NaHCO_3$. A solution containing the optimal concentrations of these salts is known as Ringer's solution (page 5) and is used to perfuse isolated frog tissues. Frog plasma has an ionic composition similar to that of Ringer's solution. The salts exert similar effects on mammalian heart muscle although the optimal concentrations are different.

When calcium is removed from the solution perfusing a heart, the cardiac action potentials remain unchanged for some time but the contractions rapidly become weaker and fail completely. The initial effect of calcium deficiency therefore appears to be concerned with the contractile process. Recent work has shown that lack of potassium or sodium increases the uptake of calcium by the heart, while excess potassium or sodium has the opposite effect. Thus, in addition to their action on the membrane, potassium and sodium affect contractility indirectly by influencing the uptake of calcium, and the observations made by Ringer with these ions may largely be explained in this way. Cardiac muscle differs from striated muscle in that coupling and contractility are more susceptible to calcium deficiency in the external medium.

As in other excitable tissues, calcium ions are also responsible for regulating the selective permeability of the cardiac cell membranes to other ions, and they therefore play a part in maintaining excitability. The effects of calcium administration on the heart *in situ* are complex. The first effects resemble those of vagal stimulation, consisting of a slowed heart rate, sinus arrhythmia, shifting pacemaker and some heart block. Higher concentrations stimulate the ventricle muscle and produce ectopic pacemakers which give rise to large ventricular extrasystoles and sometimes to ventricular fibrillation. Still larger concentrations produce systolic arrest. In many respects, deficiency of potassium produces effects resembling those of calcium excess.

These effects of ions on the heart are of pharmacological importance since they emphasize the caution which is necessary when solutions of potassium or calcium salts have to be administered, especially to patients receiving other drugs which may synergize with or antagonize their action. Solutions of potassium or calcium salts are occasionally used to stop the heart temporarily during cardiac operations. Circulation is then maintained by a mechanically operated pump for the duration of the operation.

Metabolism of cardiac muscle. Isolated heart tissue can metabolize carbo-hydrates, fatty acids and amino acids, and the intact heart extracts these substances from the blood in proportion to their concentrations. However, the principal energy-yielding metabolites used by cardiac tissue are lactate and succinate. These substances are metabolized via the tricarboxylic acid cycle, yielding ATP for the immediate supply of energy for contraction and also for building a reserve of creatine phosphate. In anoxia, the heart beats continue only as long as the reserve of creatine phosphate lasts, that is, for 2 or 3 min. The glycogen in cardiac muscle cannot be utilized rapidly enough by anaerobic pathways to supply sufficient energy for the work of the heart. Therefore the heart, unlike striated muscle, cannot accumulate an oxygen debt. Thiamine (vitamin B) is required as a co-factor by enzymes in the tricarboxylic acid cycle, and in thiamine deficiency (*beri-beri*) there is a myocardial failure.

The oxygen consumption of cardiac muscle depends on the work output of the heart. When the supply of oxygen is inadequate, the excruciating pain of angina pectoris is precipitated. The use of drugs to relieve angina is dealt with on pages 821–829.

The heart, like skeletal muscle, increases in size (hypertrophies) when subjected to an increased work load. The hypertrophy is due solely to an increase in the size of individual fibres and not to the generation of new fibres. Cardiac muscle does not have the capacity for regeneration, so that damaged fibres atrophy and are replaced by fibrous scar tissue.

Smooth muscle

Smooth muscle is present in the walls of the hollow organs of the abdominal viscera (the gastro-intestinal and the urino-genital systems), in the walls of vascular structures (blood vessels other than capillaries, and in the spleen), in the walls of the bronchi, in the capsules and ducts of exocrine glands, in structures associated with the eye, and in the skin. There are marked species differences among smooth muscles and their properties in any one species depend on the organ in which they occur: the diversity of properties probably represents their adaptation to their particular functions.

Smooth muscle cells are fusiform or spindle shaped, with a centrally placed nucleus. Their dimensions vary considerably; in the intestine, they are 5–6 μ in diameter and 30–40 μ long, whereas in the uterus they may be as long as 0·5 mm. The smallest smooth muscle cells are in the walls of blood vessels where they are 2–3 μ in diameter and 15–20 μ long. The cytoplasm of each smooth muscle cell is completely bounded by the cell membrane. At one time it was thought that myofibrils connected adjacent cells so as to form a structural syncytium, but it is now realized that this appearance is due to artifacts arising during the preparation of the tissue.

The terms 'smooth' and 'plain' imply that no cross-striations are seen in the whole cell. Nevertheless, the individual myofibrils are cross-striated, but their striations are not orientated as regularly as they are in striated muscle cells. The myofibrils of vertebrate smooth muscle cells are thin straight filaments. Myofibrils from other species may consist of spirals or ribbons. The contractile proteins of smooth muscle are similar to those of striated muscle but differ in the relative concentrations of actin and myosin.

Bundles and layers of smooth muscle cells always contain numerous elastic fibres which are continuous with those in the surrounding connective tissue. This arrangement gives a uniform transmission of tension throughout the tissue. In most locations, smooth muscle cells are arranged in layers with the fibres orientated parallel to one another. The direction of the cells in adjacent layers varies. The smooth muscle layers in tubular organs are usually arranged in such a way that the cells form a spiral around the tube. If the spiral has a tight pitch, contraction of the cells constricts the tube. If the spiral is loosely pitched, contraction of the cells results in longitudinal shortening of the tube. In the intestine and in certain other organs (e.g. ureter and vas deferens) in which the function of the smooth muscle is to promote movement of the contents, there is an inner layer orientated in a close spiral and an outer layer forming a long spiral: these layers are usually described as *circularly* arranged and *longitudinally* arranged smooth muscle. In parts of the large intestine the longitudinally arranged muscle is grouped into bands, called taeniae. Circularly arranged smooth muscle is especially dense or powerful in the sphincters which completely close off one segment of the tube from another when the muscle cells contract.

The smooth muscle cells in the skin are scattered singly or in small groups and are associated with collagen and elastic fibres. When they contract the skin is thrown into folds. This is well marked in the skin of the scrotum and in the nipple and areola of the breast. The muscle attached to the base of a hair consists of parallel smooth muscle cells arranged in a bundle (Fig. 17.2).

According to Bozler, mammalian smooth muscle may be classified into two types termed *multi-unit* and *single-unit* (unitary) depending on the relationship between the cells. Multi-unit smooth muscle is found in the walls of blood vessels, the arrector pili and in the structures associated with the eye. In these tissues the smooth muscle cells are separated by gaps of about 1μ, without any points of close apposition. It is believed that in these muscles there is no transmission of excitation from cell to cell and that each cell is separately innervated. Unitary or single-unit smooth muscle is found in the walls of the organs of the gastro-intestinal and urino-genital systems, and hence it is sometimes called visceral smooth muscle. The cells are separated by gaps of less that 1 μ. At various points of juxtaposition of adjacent cells the membranes appear thickened and closer together. In structure these points resemble those seen at the junction between adjacent cardiac muscle cells (the intercalated discs), and may be concerned with transmission from one cell to another. The junction between adjacent cells may be more elaborate and consist of a protuberance from one cell inserted into a pocket in the other. In unitary smooth muscle, excitation can be transmitted from one cell to another and only 'key' cells may be innervated. Conduction of excitation through a mass of unitary smooth muscle spreads decrementally, that is, the tissue as a whole does not give an all-or-none response. The distance for which the excitation spreads depends on the number of cells excited initially, that is, it depends on the strength of the stimulus. The velocity of conduction ranges from 0·03–0·1 m/sec.

There are three hypotheses about the mechanism of transmission between smooth muscle cells in unitary muscles; they depend on electrical, chemical or mechanical processes. The most favoured hypothesis is that action currents originating in active cells excite adjacent resting cells ephaptically (see page 84), the points of close apposition of the membranes of adjacent cells may be low resistance pathways through each membrane, and may therefore be ephaptic junctions. The evidence for chemical transmission is two-fold: various smooth muscle-stimulating substances have been extracted from tissues containing smooth muscle, and structures resembling synaptic vesicles have been observed in electron-micrographs of the closest junctions between smooth muscle cell membranes. However, the various tests which have been employed to provide evidence for chemical transmission at nerve endings do not, in general, support the hypothesis of chemical transmission between smooth smooth cells. The hypothesis favouring mechanical transmission envisages that the contraction of a group of cells stretches an adjacent group, causing depolarization followed by contraction; however, it has been shown that action potentials are propagated through some unitary smooth muscles even when contraction waves are absent as a result of treatment with metabolic inhibitors (dinitrophenol or sodium azide) or of removing glucose from the medium. It is possible that different unitary smooth muscles possess different conduction mechanisms.

Multi-unit smooth muscle responds to a single stimulus applied to the nerve, although the response is small. As in other muscles, trains of stimuli are required to produce maximal responses. Every cell in a multi-unit muscle may be separately innervated but stimulation of only part of the nerve supply can elicit a maximal response, probably because of diffusion of chemical transmitter through the tissue. Cells in unitary smooth muscle respond to a single stimulus applied to an excitatory nerve with a small depolarization, but without a mechanical response. When trains of stimuli are given the depolarizations summate, until finally an action potential is discharged, followed by a mechanical response.

The speed of contraction of smooth muscle is slow compared with that of striated muscle and the persistence of contraction is long. Striking contrasts can be drawn from examples in invertebrates: the smooth adductor muscle which closes the shell of molluscs takes several seconds to develop its maximal tension which is then maintained for several hours, but the striated muscle fibres driving the wings of insects may contract and relax a thousand times a second.

The tone of a smooth muscle is an expression of the amount of background activity exhibited. Tone may be due to a steady arrival of nerve impulses (neurogenic) or it may be myogenic. When a degree of contraction pre-exists in the tissue, smooth muscle can respond with relaxation. However, increases in length of smooth muscle cells are not always due to relaxation. In certain circumstances, the change may be the result of contraction of another smooth muscle layer arranged antagonistically. For example, in the iris, contraction of the circular muscle increases the length of the radial muscle, and vice versa (see page 417).

Many smooth muscle-containing tissues exhibit fluctuations in length or tension due to rhythmic contractions and relaxations of the smooth muscle cells. This is seen more usually in unitary smooth muscle than in multi-unit muscle, although not all unitary smooth muscles exhibit spontaneous activity. The rhythmic movements are due to properties inherent in the muscle cells, that is, they are *myogenic*. The phenomenon is described as auto-rhythmicity. A group of cells spontaneously depolarizes in a rhythmic manner, and each time an action potential is generated it propagates and is conducted through the tissue. Thus the rhythmicity is governed by the activity of a pacemaker, as is the rate of the heart beat. In some tissues the pacemaker is fixed, for example, the rhythmic movements of the ureter are dominated by a pacemaker at the end nearest the kidney. In other tissues the site of the pacemaker changes, first one group of cells and then another group dominating. The position of the pacemaker group and its rate of discharge may be related to acetylcholine, acting as a local hormone (page 172).

The membranes of smooth muscle cells, like those of other excitable cells, are polarized, the inside of the cell being negative with respect to the outside. The membrane potential is approximately that expected from the potassium concentration gradient, as calculated from the Nernst equation. The values of the membrane potential, determined experimentally in different smooth muscles, range from 30 to 70 mV.

On account of the smallness of the cells, the measurement of membrane potentials and action potentials in smooth muscle is more difficult than in striated muscle. It has been done with extremely fine micro-electrodes with tip diameter of 0·5 μ or less. Another method which has been particularly useful with smooth muscle is the 'sucrose-gap' technique. The apparatus is shown diagrammatically in Fig. 7.11: it is similar to the use of extracellular electrodes in other excitable tissues. The sucrose solution fills the gap between the electrodes and permeates the extracellular space of the smooth muscle tissue. The sucrose solution presents a very high electrical resistance relative to the electrical resistance through the chain of smooth muscle cells. The effect of this is that potential differences can be measured between the end bathed in a

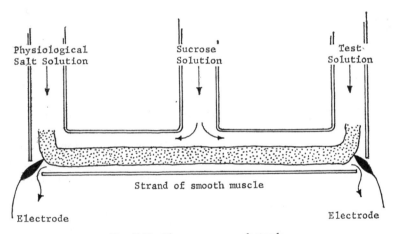

Fig. 7.11. The sucrose-gap electrode.

standard physiological salt solution, where the cells have a resting membrane, and the other end, which is stimulated by drugs or electrically, so that the cells have an active membrane. The full value of the membrane potential can be obtained by using potassium sulphate in the test solution, so that the cells nearest to one electrode are completely depolarized.

As in other excitable cells, reduction of the membrane potential to a critical level generates a conducted action potential and this is followed by contraction. The form of the action potential recorded from smooth muscle cells in different tissues varies considerably (Fig. 7.12). The membrane potential of smooth muscle cells is affected by a variety of physical and chemical factors. Stretch produces depolarization and so moves the membrane potential closer to the critical firing potential. The frequency of rhythmic action potentials is higher when the tissue is stretched. Many tissues containing smooth muscle respond to a quick stretch with one or more conducted waves of contraction. Stretching beyond a certain point may reduce the membrane potential so much that action potentials cannot be generated and a state resembling depolarization block ensues.

Depolarization may be brought about by raising the concentration of extracellular potassium ions, or by the passage of electric current, which depolarizes the membrane adjacent to the cathode. A sufficient depolarization initiates an action potential and a smaller depolarization increases the ex-

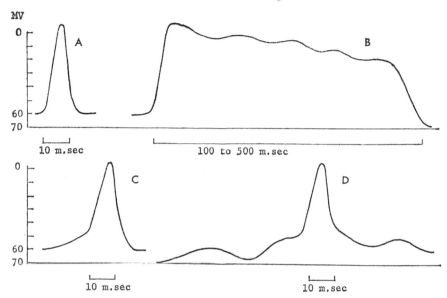

FIG. 7.12. Smooth muscle action potentials. A. A spike (common). B. A plateau (rare). C. Spike with a prepotential (from a pacemaker region). D. Slow oscillation of membrane potential with an action potential occurring at a peak of depolarization. (Data derived from Burnstock, Holman & Prosser, 1963.)

citability. The membrane adjacent to the anode is hyperpolarized and is less excitable. The neurotransmitters released from autonomic nerve endings impinging on the smooth muscle cells may cause excitation by depolarizing or inhibition by hyperpolarizing the cell membrane. Other factors influencing smooth muscle include pH, the ionic composition of the surrounding fluid and the temperature. Slightly acid solutions produce relaxation of smooth muscle and raising the pH causes contraction. Calcium ions exert effects on smooth muscle similar to those produced in other excitable tissues. Lack of calcium initially labilizes the membrane and propagated spikes are initiated or increased in frequency. The spikes may or may not be accompanied by contractions depending upon the availability, in the particular tissue, of sufficient intracellular calcium to support the coupling and contractile processes. In all types of smooth muscle, membrane excitability is eventually depressed by lack of calcium, and contraction is diminished because of the effect on the coupling and contractile processes. Physiological salt solutions containing a deficiency of calcium and an excess of magnesium are sometimes used to depress spontaneous activity in smooth muscles. However, sufficient calcium is included to support contractions evoked by strong stimuli such as drugs or electric currents.

The excitability of some smooth muscle is influenced by hormones. Thus, the cells of the uterus of an immature rat have a membrane potential of 30 mV and are relatively inexcitable. After treatment with oestrogen the membrane potential is increased to 40 mV, and the excitability is increased. Then, progesterone produces a further hyperpolarization to 60 mV and the excitability is again decreased.

The study of smooth muscle is complicated because ganglion cells, nerve plexuses and nerve endings are in close association to the muscle cells. Electrical stimulation of tissues containing smooth muscle cells may cause excitation by stimulating nerve fibres within the tissue. Smooth muscle cells in nerve-free tissues can be stimulated electrically, but direct currents lasting for 0·01–0·1 sec are required. Contractions of smooth muscle can also be induced by passing alternating currents through the tissue. However, it is not clear how the contraction is brought about, since it can still be obtained in the presence of a concentration of potassium ions in the extracellular fluid which is sufficient to depolarize the membrane: possibly it is an effect of an alternating electric current on the contractile proteins. Contractions of smooth muscle cells which have been depolarized by immersion in a potassium-rich solution can also be elicited by drugs such as acetylcholine and histamine.

Tissues containing smooth muscle are innervated by post-ganglionic fibres of the autonomic nervous system. The responses of organs containing smooth muscle to stimulation of these nerves are listed in Table 4.1 on page 123. Some smooth muscles are not innervated; for example, some of the structures associated with the growth and development of the foetus (the foetal membranes and the umbilical blood vessels) contain smooth muscle cells but receive no nerves.

The junction between autonomic nerve endings and smooth muscle cells does not appear to be as specialized as the neuro-muscular junction of striated muscle. Single, fine nerve fibres, unaccompanied by a Schwann cell, run in close apposition to the membrane of the muscle cell, and may lie within a fold of the muscle cell membrane. Structures resembling synaptic vesicles and granules are present in the nerve fibres.

Smooth muscle cells exhibit miniature potentials which are believed to be analogous to the miniature end-plate potentials of striated muscle. The miniature potentials occur at irregular intervals and although they vary in size, they appear to be due to the release of one quantum of transmitter, or to an integer multiple of a quantum.

Damaged smooth muscle cells can be replaced, although it is not established whether they are replaced by mitoses of surviving cells, or by differentiation from fibroblast cells. Some smooth muscle organs exhibit marked hypertrophy. The increase in size of the uterus during pregnancy is due partly to increases in the size of each cell and partly to the formation of new cells (hyperplasia).

There are sensory nerve endings in smooth muscle. Most of them respond to tension or pressure. Unusually high tensions or pressures give rise to pain often described as colic (e.g. biliary colic, intestinal colic). The cause may be a mechanical obstruction opposing the work of the smooth muscle, or it may be due to a powerful contraction (spasm) of the smooth muscle. The contractions of uterine smooth muscle during childbirth give rise to labour pains. Local spasms of smooth muscle are sometimes relieved by sectioning its autonomic supply or by destroying the nerve with an injection of alcohol or phenol. Such treatment is used particularly for spasms of the blood vessels which result in an insufficient blood flow to the extremities. If the post-ganglionic nerve fibres are destroyed, the denervated state persists until the nerve fibres grow out again. However, if the ganglion cells are removed (ganglionectomy), there is no re-innervation. The denervated blood vessels become hypersensitive to adrenaline and noradrenaline circulating in the blood-stream.

Smooth muscle receives a smaller blood supply than does an equal bulk of striated or cardiac muscle. In experiments with isolated tissues, it is a commonplace observation that less attention need be paid to the oxygenation of smooth muscle than of other muscle.

8

Blood and Tissue Fluids

Blood

Blood circulates through the tissues of the body, its chief function being that of transport. It carries oxygen from the lungs to the tissues where the oxygen is exchanged for carbon dioxide which it returns to the lungs. It links together the metabolic activities of the organs by carrying nutrients from the gastro-intestinal tract to the liver, intermediary metabolites from one tissue to another tissue, and waste products of metabolism to the organs of excretion. In addition, the blood carries hormones from the endocrine glands to the various tissues whose activities are regulated by them. Another function of the blood is to help protect the organism; blood contains both antibodies which combine with foreign proteins including micro-organisms, so rendering them innocuous, and special cells which are phagocytic and ingest bacteria and other particulate matter. Some of the constituents of blood are also concerned with local reactions to injury and with the repair of tissue damage.

Blood may be considered as one of the connective tissues: it consists of cells suspended in a fluid matrix called plasma. The constituents of blood are shown in Fig. 8.1.

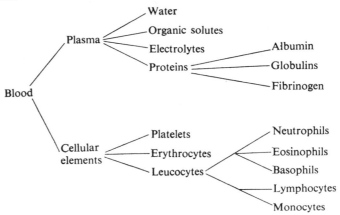

FIG. 8.1. The composition of blood.

Organic constituents. The nutrient substances present in plasma include amino acids, carbohydrate (principally as glucose) and lipids. Part of the lipid is

226

present in minute globules of fat called microchyla, which give a milky appearance to the plasma, particularly noticeable after a fatty meal. Free fatty acids, triglycerides, phospholipids and cholesterol are present, partly in solution and partly in association with protein. Intermediary metabolites in blood include lactic and pyruvic acids and some of the constituents of the tricarboxylic acid cycle. The principal catabolic products in plasma are the end products of amino acid metabolism (urea, ammonia, creatinine), purine metabolism (uric acid is the end product of degradation of adenine and guanine in man) and porphyrin metabolism (bilirubin, Fig. 8.4, gives a pale yellow colour to the plasma): these substances are removed from the plasma in the kidneys (Chapter 13, page 348).

Electrolytes. Plasma contains about 0·75 g of dissolved inorganic salts per 100 ml. The amounts of some of the ions present are given in Table 8.1.

TABLE 8.1. Plasma electrolytes.

Cations	Concentration		Anions	Concentration	
	mg %	mE/litre		mg %	mE/litre
Na^+	300–330	130–144	Cl^-	360–390	100–110
K^+	16–20	4–5	HCO_3^-	120–144	20–24
Ca^{++}	8–12	4–6	$H_2PO_4^-$	3–5	1–1·5
Mg^{++}	2	1	SO_4^{--}	2–3	1–2
Total		140–155	Total		125–135

The molar concentration of cation exceeds that of the inorganic anion, the discrepancy being accounted for by organic anions and by the ionization of the free carboxylic acid groups of the protein. Plasma electrolyte levels are closely maintained within narrow limits. The sodium and potassium ion levels are regulated by the cells of the renal tubules acting under the influence of the adrenal cortical hormones. Failure of kidney function results in a rise in the plasma potassium concentration; an increase to 10 mE/litre severely impairs the action of the heart. Heart failure is the cause of death in anuria. Depletion of sodium may occur through excessive sweating or vomiting, and results in headache, cramp and muscular weakness. The plasma levels of calcium and phosphate are controlled by the parathyroid hormone (pages 374–375). A severe decrease of the plasma calcium to 2 mE/litre results in the muscular spasms of tetany (page 199).

Some of the anions in the plasma contribute to the maintenance of the plasma pH by acting as buffers. The principal anion is the bicarbonate ion although phosphate ions and the carboxyl groups of proteins also contribute. The electrolyte shift across the membranes of red blood cells, which accompanies the exchange of oxygen for the carbon dioxide attached to haemoglobin, is of particular importance for maintaining the pH of blood (page 296). Plasma pH remains very close to 7·36. Deviations from this give rise to conditions termed *acidosis* and *alkalosis*. A change of pH of more than 0·2 endangers life. In diabetes, the abnormal metabolism leads to the accumulation of organic acids with the result that acidosis prevails. Acidosis may also result from metabolic formation of sulphate or phosphate from foodstuffs containing sulphur or phosphorus in organic (non-ionized) forms. Alkalosis results from the ingestion of foodstuffs containing salts of cations (sodium, potassium, calcium) with organic acids. The organic acids are metabolized so that there is a net loss of anion.

Plasma proteins. There is about 6·7 g of protein per 100 ml of plasma. The proteins can be divided into three groups—albumin, the globulins and fibrinogen—depending on differences in their physico-chemical properties. Thus they may be 'salted out' by the addition of different amounts of ammonium sulphate and by adjusting the pH to their different iso-electric points (albumin, 4·9; fibrinogen, 5·2; the globulins, 5·2 to 6·3). The electrophoretic separation of the plasma proteins depends on their different rates of movement in an electric field. The estimation of their relative amounts is of value in the diagnosis of disease. Average values for the plasma proteins are given in Table 8.2.

TABLE 8.2. The plasma proteins.

Protein	Average content g/100 ml	Relative proportion (%)	Molecular weight
Albumin	4·0	60	69,000
α-globulins	0·8 ⎫		250,000 ⎧
β-globulins	0·8 ⎬	35	120,000 ⎨
γ-globulins	0·7 ⎭		156,000 ⎩
Fibrinogen	0·4	5	400,000

Plasma albumin is the protein present in highest concentration but it has the lowest molecular weight. It is thus responsible for almost all of the colloidal osmotic pressure of the plasma, which is about 25 mmHg. Albumin is synthesized in the liver from the amino-acid pool which is maintained by dietary proteins. During protein starvation, plasma albumin is formed at the expense of tissue proteins. In disease, the plasma albumin content often falls whilst that of globulin increases.

Plasma globulins comprise a number of distinct proteins. They are grouped together as they are soluble in water, whereas albumins are not; both albumins and globulins are soluble in dilute salt solutions. By this test fibrinogen is a member of the globulin group, but it is convenient to consider it separately. Many of the plasma globulins have specific physiological functions. The γ-globulins include the antibodies, which are formed in the cells of the reticulo-endothelial system in response to foreign proteins (antigens) such as bacteria and bacterial toxins. An antibody is able to combine with the antigen that has stimulated its production, and thus immobilize it. During the course of an infectious disease the plasma γ-globulin content gradually increases, and the level of activity of the specific antibody against the invading organism or its exotoxins increases. Thereafter there is a gradual decline in the activity of the specific antibody. However, on a subsequent exposure to the antigen the plasma antibody titre rises rapidly; the reticulo-endothelial cells have retained the RNA molecules which synthesize that particular antibody. Thus the γ-globulins are responsible for the development of resistance to infection and immunity. Active immunization against disease can be produced by injecting suitable preparations of killed or attenuated bacteria, viruses or bacterial toxins. These preparations cause little or no ill effects, but stimulate the formation of specific antibodies.

Passive immunity against infection may be obtained by injecting serum, or purified γ-globulins containing the required antibody. Suitable antisera may be obtained either from animals in which production of the required antibody has been stimulated by injecting the antigen, or from humans who have recently recovered from the infection. Passive immunity persists for only as long as the administered antibody is present.

Closely related to the antibodies formed in response to foreign protein are the so-called auto-immune bodies; they include the plasma agglutinins which cause haemolysis of incompatible red blood cells. An individual's particular agglutinins are determined genetically.

The protein hormones of the anterior pituitary and many enzymes, particularly those concerned in the coagulation of the blood, are also included among the globulins.

Fibrinogen is the protein responsible for the coagulation of the blood which begins when blood comes into contact with damaged tissue (or wettable surfaces such as glass). The clot is formed by fibrinogen polymerizing into a network of long fibres of fibrin which bind the blood into a jelly-like mass. Then the fibrin threads retract, thus increasing the strength of the clot.

PLATELETS. These are the smallest of the formed elements of the blood, being about 2 μ in diameter. They are formed in bone marrow by the budding-off of portions of cytoplasm from large cells called megokaryocytes. The platelet count is usually between 250,000 and 500,000/mm^3 of blood. In smears of blood they frequently occur in clumps. The platelets play an important part in haemostasis, the cessation of bleeding. Minute lesions in the walls of blood vessels are plugged by the deposition of a fused mass of platelets. In more extensive damage the platelets accumulate at the severed ends of the blood vessels, where they liberate their contents. These include 5-hydroxytryptamine (which may aid haemostasis by causing a local vasoconstriction), a factor concerned in coagulation, and a factor necessary for retraction of fibrin.

COAGULATION. The last stages of the coagulatory process can be summarized as:

$$\text{Prothrombin} \xrightarrow{\text{thromboplastin} + Ca^{++}} \text{Thrombin}$$

$$\text{Fibrinogen} \xrightarrow{\text{thrombin}} \text{Fibrin}$$

The conversion of fibrinogen to fibrin is catalysed by thrombin; it is a rapid reaction taking about 4 sec. The formation of thrombin from an inactive precursor, prothrombin (a β-globulin), is catalysed by thromboplastin and calcium ions. Thromboplastin is produced from platelets or from damaged tissue. In either case a number of factors are concerned.

The formation of thromboplastin in blood shed without contact with damaged tissue is brought about in the following way: The total time for these reactions to occur is 4 to 8 min (the *in vitro* clotting time).

$$\text{Factor VIII} \xrightarrow{\text{Factor IX} + Ca^{++}} \text{Product I}$$

$$\text{Platelets} \xrightarrow{\text{Product I}} \text{Platelet factor}$$

$$\text{Platelet factor} + \text{Factor V} \longrightarrow \text{Platelet thromboplastin}$$

When blood comes into contact with damaged tissues, as in a wound, thromboplastin is produced more rapidly (12 to 20 sec) by the following reaction:

$$\text{Tissue factor} + \text{Factor V} \xrightarrow{\text{Factor VII} + Ca^{++}} \text{Tissue thromboplastin}$$

The fibrin formed influences the coagulatory processes in two ways: it increases the rate of disintegration of platelets, thus accelerating the production of thromboplastin and coagulation, and it adsorbs thrombin, thereby limiting clot formation.

Factors concerned in coagulation have been designated with Roman numerals, as shown in Table 8.3.

TABLE 8.3. Factors in blood coagulation.

Name	Factor
Fibrinogen	I
Prothrombin	II
Thromboplastin	III
Calcium	IV
Labile factor, or proaccelerin	V
Existence of Factor VI is disputed	
Stable factor, or provertin	VII
Antihaemophilic globulin	VIII
Christmas factor	IX

Heparin prevents coagulation by acting at three sites: its main effect is to prevent the action of thrombin in catalysing the conversion of fibrinogen into fibrin: in addition, heparin slows down the conversion of prothrombin to thrombin, and it acts to stabilize the platelets against clumping and disintegrating. Heparin is found in the intimal layer of blood vessels and in the granules of basophils and tissue mast cells. Heparin is a mucopolysaccharide built up of units of glucosamine, glucuronic acid and sulphuric acid. Being acidic, it stains deeply with basic dyes. It is closely related chemically to chondroitin, the principal constituent of cartilages (see also pages 907–908).

Fibrinolysin (*or plasmin*) is an enzyme formed from an inactive precursor, fibrinolysinogen, in response to the products of coagulation in the bloodstream. It breaks down fibrin and renders the clotted blood liquid again. A recent medical use of fibrinolysin is in the removal of fibrin layers formed around cancerous growths, so that the defences of the host may gain access to the actively proliferating cells on the periphery of the tumour.

DISORDERS OF COAGULATION. In health, there is a balance between the many factors concerned with blood coagulation, but disorders may occur—

intravascular clotting which is treated by anti-coagulant drugs, and impaired coagulation which can be treated when the coagulation defect has been identified. Drugs affecting coagulation are dealt with in Chapter 36.

INTRAVASCULAR CLOTTING. A clot being swept along with the blood is called an *embolus*. A *thrombus* is a clot remaining attached to the vascular endothelium or an embolus which has become lodged. Intravascular clotting occurs in vessels when the flow is impaired in varicose veins or in vascular spasm, and in the atrial appendages during atrial fibrillation. An injury to the vascular endothelium promotes intravascular clotting; for example, the lesions on the cardiac valves caused by bacterial endocarditis are a site of clot formation. Some bacterial toxins and animal venoms cause intravascular clotting. Russell's viper venom contains a potent thromboplastin.

IMPAIRED COAGULATION. An *in vitro* clotting time of more than 10 min indicates a defect in coagulation. The defect is more precisely located by carrying out an additional test, the *accelerated clotting time*. The patient's blood is collected in sodium oxalate solution (to remove calcium ions) and then, under carefully controlled conditions, the clotting time is measured after the addition of an excess of calcium ions and of thromboplastin. Usually, the accelerated clotting time does not exceed 13 sec. When this is normal but the simple clotting time is prolonged, the defect in coagulation resides in one of the

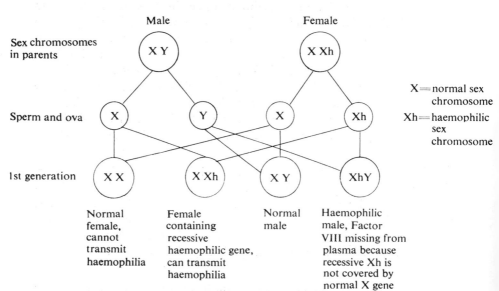

FIG. 8.2. Inheritance of haemophilia.

reactions leading to the formation of thromboplastin; it is usually a deficiency of factor VIII or IX.

Patients who have the bleeding disease *haemophilia* are deficient in Factor VIII (anti-haemophilic globulin). This deficiency is due to an inherited defect of a recessive gene on the sex chromosome as shown in Fig. 8.2, from which it can be seen that female carriers transmit the disease to male offspring. The gene is rare, and the chance of a cross between a haemophilic male and a female carrier of haemophilia, thereby producing a haemophilic female, is extremely unlikely. Another coagulation defect resulting in excessive bleeding

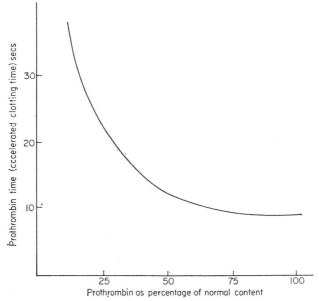

FIG. 8.3. Prothrombin time determinations.

resembling haemophilia occurs from lack of Factor IX. This disorder is called Christmas disease, after the surname of the patient in whom this defect was first identified. Bleeding in haemophilics may be controlled by applying a thrombin or thromboplastin preparation locally. The missing factors can be temporarily restored by injection of purified factor or by transfusion of normal blood.

A prolonged accelerated clotting time may indicate that the fibrinogen has been completely exhausted, but the more usual cause is that insufficient prothrombin is available: hence it is also known as the *prothrombin time* which provides an index of the amount of prothrombin present, as shown in Fig. 8.3.

Reduction in the amount of prothrombin in the plasma occurs as a result

8*

of extensive liver damage, of an impairment in the absorption of vitamin K which is essential for the production of prothrombin, or of blockade of the action of vitamin K by anti-vitamins belonging to the coumarin and indandione group of *in vitro* anti-coagulants (see pages 908–911).

Vitamin K

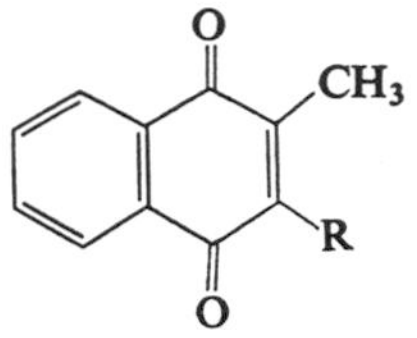

2-Methyl-3-R-naphthoquinone

In vitamin K_1, R is phytyl:

$$-CH_2-CH=\overset{\overset{\displaystyle CH_3}{|}}{C}-(CH_2)_3-[\overset{\overset{\displaystyle CH_3}{|}}{CH}-(CH_2)_3]_2-\overset{\overset{\displaystyle CH_3}{|}}{CH}-CH_3$$

In vitamin K_2, R is difarnesyl:

$$-CH_2-CH=[\overset{\overset{\displaystyle CH_3}{|}}{C}-(CH_2)_2-CH]_5=\overset{\overset{\displaystyle CH_3}{|}}{C}-CH_3$$

Vitamin K_1 occurs in green plants. The diet provides only part of the human vitamin K requirements, the chief source being vitamin K_2 which is synthesized by intestinal bacteria, including *Escherichia coli*. A deficiency may occur when the intestinal flora are severely disturbed as in chronic diarrhoea or after sterilization of the gut contents. New-born infants are dependent on stores of vitamin K reaching them from the mother and so additional supplies of the vitamin may be required by the expectant mother. Vitamin K is a fat-soluble vitamin, requiring the presence of bile salts for its absorption from the intestine. In obstructive jaundice, the bile cannot pass through the bile duct into the intestine and so hypoprothrombinaemia results; it is treated by injections of vitamin K. The action of vitamin K in the synthesis of prothrombin is probably that of a coenzyme necessary for a synthesizing enzyme; it is not incorporated into the prothrombin molecule.

Erythrocytes. In most mammals, including man, the red blood cells are non-nucleated, circular, biconcave discs: they are sufficiently flexible to be deformed during their passage through small capillaries. The erythrocytes in some mammals are ellipsoidal, and in lower vertebrates they contain a nucleus. In man they have a mean diameter of $7 \cdot 3 \, \mu$, and a thickness of about $2 \, \mu$. Their mean volume is 86 μ^3 and their surface area is about 138 μ^2. The average content of erythrocytes in blood is 5·5 million/mm^3 in men and 4·8 million/mm^3 in women. The packed red cells occupy about 40% of the volume of the blood, a value which is called the *haematocrit* or packed cell volume (PVC). The specific gravity of erythrocytes is slightly greater than that of plasma and hence they can be readily deposited by centrifugation. The rate of settling of cells under gravity in a stationary column of blood is called the *erythrocyte sedimentation rate* (ESR). In health it averages 4 to 6 mm/h; rates of more than 10 mm/h are considered to be significantly high in the diagnosis of disease, but the factors involved in the ESR are complex. The erythrocyte membrane is relatively more permeable to water than to solutes. When erythrocytes are placed in hypotonic salt solutions they swell and burst; conversely in hypertonic solutions they shrink and buckle. The limits of tonicity which the cells can resist without being disrupted is a measure of their fragility.

The chief function of the erythrocytes is the transport of oxygen and carbon dioxide in combination with the haemoglobin they contain. In addition they help to maintain blood pH and they carry certain enzymes, notably phosphatases, esterases and catalase, which are probably concerned with the detoxification of some metabolites.

Haemoglobin is a conjugated protein, consisting of a histone, globin, to which is attached a prosthetic group, haem. One molecule of haemoglobin (MW, 68,000) consists of four polypeptide chains and four haems. Haem is an iron-containing tetrapyrrole; its structure is shown in Fig. 8.4. One molecule of oxygen or of carbon dioxide combines with each haem.

Erythropoiesis is the term used to describe the formation of the red blood cells. In the first 3 months of the human foetus, the red cells are produced in the foetal membranes. Later they are formed in the liver and spleen, and from the fifth month they are produced in the red bone marrow. At birth, all the bones contain red marrow but with increasing age yellow marrow replaces most of the red. Yellow marrow consists chiefly of fat cells and it is laid down first in the distal bones of the limbs (tarsus and carpus), then in the intermediate bones (tibia and fibula, radius and ulna), and finally in the proximal bones (femur and humerus). At 20 years of age, red marrow persists only at the uppermost ends of the femur and humerus, and in the vertebrae, sternum, ribs and bones of the skull and pelvis. Samples of bone marrow are usually obtained by puncturing the sternum.

In the red bone marrow, the blood vessels consist of thin-walled sacs called sinusoids. Erythrocytes are formed after repeated sub-division of certain of the endothelial cells lining the sinusoids. A summary of the process of erythropoiesis is shown in Table 8.4.

The cell types which form erythrocytes become more and more specialized for their ultimate function as each successive division occurs. The first major change is the appearance of haemoglobin in the cytoplasm, as demonstrated by the affinity for the acid stain eosin (eosinophilia), which is present in the intermediate normoblast. In the late normoblastic stage, the nucleus is

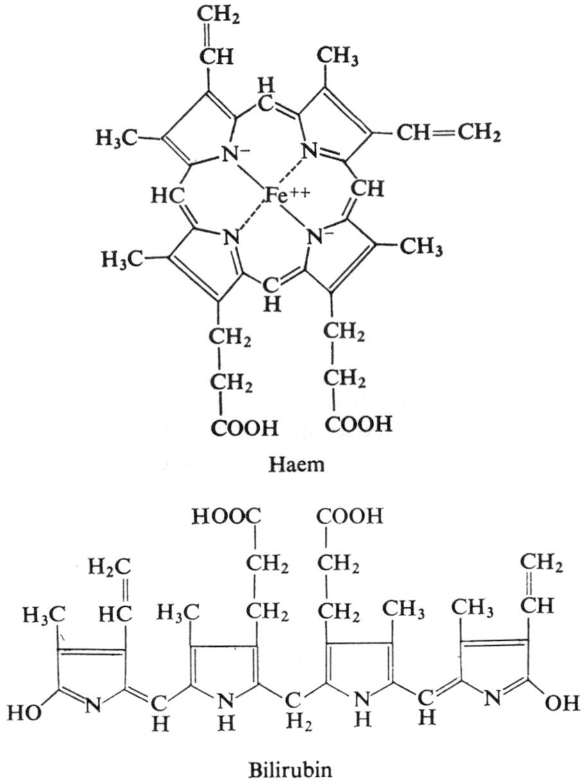

Haem

Bilirubin

FIG. 8.4. Structure of haem and one of its breakdown products, bilirubin.

degenerating, and later, after extrusion of the remains of the nuclear mass, the cytoplasm contains a network of fine threads of chromatin material, hence the name reticulocyte. Reticulocytes usually remain in the marrow sinusoids until they lose their chromatin, but they can be found in the circulation, particularly after a period of anoxia.

The rate of erythropoiesis is governed by the oxygen tension of the blood. Oxygen lack (anoxia) leads to the production of a humoral factor called erythropoietin; its chemical nature has not yet been elucidated. Erythropoietin stimulates the division of the parent cells of erythrocytes in the bone marrow and the rate of maturation and release of erythrocytes. Anoxia may arise because of a low oxygen tension in the inspired air, for example, in people living at high altitudes; tissue anoxia may be due to inadequate oxygenation of the circulating blood, for example, in congenital heart disease, or to a reduced oxygen-carrying capacity of the blood, for example, after severe haemorrhage or in anaemic conditions. Whatever the cause, the rate of red-cell production is increased and part of the yellow marrow is replaced by red marrow. Erythropoiesis is suppressed by high oxygen tensions.

The life time of an erythrocyte is about 120 days. Old erythrocytes are continually being removed from the circulation and are replaced through the process of erythropoiesis.

TABLE 8.4. Stages in erythropoiesis.

Cell type	Characteristic features	
	Nucleus	Cytoplasm
Endothelial cell	Occasional mitoses	Basophilic; mitochondria present
Proerythroblast	Occasional mitoses	Basophilic; mitochondria present
Early normoblast	Many cells in mitotic division	Basophilic; mitochondria present
Intermediate normoblast	Many cells in mitotic division	Eosinophilia appears; mitochondria present
Late normoblast	Degenerating	Eosinophilic; few mitochondria
Reticulocyte	Absent	Eosinophilic; chromatin threads present
Erythrocyte	Absent	Eosinophilic; undifferentiated cytoplasm

Old erythrocytes are destroyed by cells of the *reticulo-endothelial system.* This term refers to a broad group of large phagocytic cells found in various organs. They are identified by their property of engulfing particulate matter, such as carmine particles or colloidal carbon. Reticulo-endothelial cells are found particularly in the spleen, lymph nodes and other lymphoid tissues. In some diseases the spleen becomes grossly enlarged when there is an excessive breakdown of erythrocytes. The protein of the red cell is returned to the body's amino-acid pool; the porphyrin from haem is converted into bilirubin (Fig. 8.4), removed from the blood by the liver and secreted into the bile; most of the iron is retained.

Iron is required for incorporation into haem, and copper, manganese and cobalt in trace amounts must be present for this to occur. The human body contains about 5 g of iron, of which about half is bound up in haemoglobin of the circulating erythrocytes. About 0·5 g of iron is bound up in myoglobin, the oxygen-carrying protein of muscle. A number of enzymes concerned with oxidation–reduction systems (for example, the cytochromes, catalase and peroxidase) contain iron, again linked with a porphyrin and attached to a protein. The remainder of the iron is stored as a compound called *ferritin* in the walls of the intestine and in liver, spleen and bone marrow.

The daily intake of iron by a man on an average diet is about 15 mg, although about one third of this amount ensures that enough is absorbed to replace the iron lost by the excretion of that released from old erythrocytes. It is absorbed from the intestine as the ferrous ion and taken up in the ferritin stores. Iron ingested in the ferric form can be absorbed only after reduction. In growing children, the bodily demands for iron are somewhat greater than in adults and anaemia due to an inadequate intake of iron may occur. Loss of haemoglobin through haemorrhage or during menstruation may also impose the need for an increased intake. A strain is thrown on the mother's iron reserves during pregnancy and childbirth. An iron deficiency anaemia is characterized by hypochromic, microcytic erythrocytes; the red cells are deficient in haemoglobin and smaller than normal red cells. It is treated with preparations containing iron given by mouth or by injection (see pages 913–916).

Vitamin deficiency anaemias. Cyanocobalamin (vitamin B_{12}) and folic acid (also a B vitamin) are necessary for the synthesis of the nucleoproteins made during cell division. (The formulae of these vitamins are given on pp. 34–35.)

In the adult, erythropoiesis exerts the greatest call on the synthesis of new nucleoproteins for cell divisions, since about 20 g of cells are formed per day. If the necessary vitamins are not available, cell division becomes faulty at the stage when intermediate normoblasts are formed, and the production of normal erythrocytes is blocked. However, the stimulus to produce new cells, brought about by the formation of erythropoietin when the tissues become slightly anoxic, increases cell division. The red marrow advances through the shafts of the bones and large numbers of the early cell forms found in erythropoiesis develop. The early normoblasts form abnormal cells called megaloblasts which develop into non-nucleated cells containing haemoglobin. These are called macrocytes since they are larger than normal erythrocytes; the haemoglobin content per cell is high. The macrocytes are rapidly destroyed by the cells of the reticulo-endothelial system, the plasma bilirubin concentration rises, and the iron storage tissues become saturated. Despite the rapid production of macrocytes, the number of circulating cells is low, often as low as 1 million/mm^3.

Cyanocobalamin is a complex molecule containing the radical —CoCN⁻—

linked by covalent bonds into a porphyrin and containing ribose and phosphoric acid. It occurs in most foodstuffs of animal origin and it is synthesized by bacteria in the colon. The daily requirement for adequate erythropoiesis is very low (about 1 μg), and anaemias due to dietary defects are rare. During pregnancy the requirements of the foetus for cyanocobalamin and folic acid are

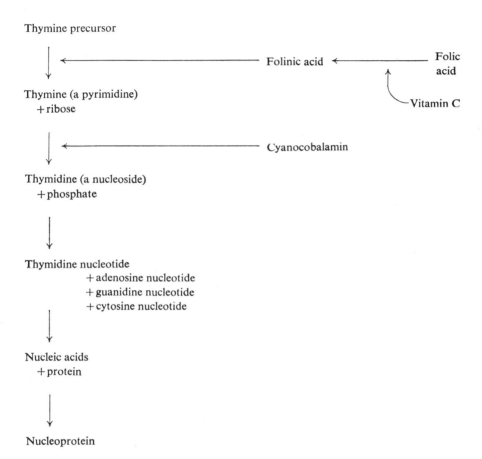

Thymine precursor

Thymine (a pyrimidine)
  + ribose

Thymidine (a nucleoside)
  + phosphate

Thymidine nucleotide
        + adenosine nucleotide
        + guanidine nucleotide
        + cytosine nucleotide

Nucleic acids
  + protein

Nucleoprotein

Folinic acid ← Folic acid

Vitamin C

Cyanocobalamin

high because of the large number of dividing cells. Since this requirement can only be met from the mother's diet, the net amount of the vitamins for erythropoiesis in the mother may be insufficient. A macrocytic anaemia occurring in pregnancy is usually rapidly corrected by vitamin supplements to the diet. A tapeworm infestation can lead to a macrocytic anaemia in the host: apparently the worm gets the vitamins first.

Pernicious anaemia is a macrocytic anaemia caused by the inability to absorb cyanocobalamin. Associated with the anaemia there are degenerative changes in the brain, spinal cord and peripheral nerves, and there are defects in epithelial tissues leading to such symptoms as soreness of the mouth and tongue. Before the identification of cyanocobalamin, the dietary factor essential for normal erythropoiesis was called the *extrinsic factor*. The mucosa of the stomach contains a substance which is essential for the absorption of cyanocobalamin; this is usually referred to as the *intrinsic factor*. It is missing when the gastric mucosa is atrophied or damaged, after gastrectomy, and in many cases of cancer of the stomach. Evidence that the defect is due to failure of absorption has been obtained by giving cyanocobalamin labelled with radioactive cobalt. In normal people, 30 to 40% is excreted in the faeces, whereas in pernicious anaemia more than 90% is lost in this way, and the plasma level of cyanocobalamin is very low. Cyanocobalamin given by mouth is almost ineffective in relieving the anaemia, but it may be given together with an extract of gastric mucosa containing intrinsic factor. Injection of cyanocobalamin is a simpler treatment; only 50 μg every other week is usually sufficient to prevent anaemia and to cure the nervous and epithelial symptoms.

Folic acid is found in many foodstuffs of animal and vegetable origin. Liver and spinach are particularly rich sources. The daily requirement is about 0·2 mg. Dietary deficiencies of folic acid are rare. Folic acid may improve the blood picture of pernicious anaemia, but it has no effect on the associated lesions of the nervous and epithelial tissues. Therefore it is never given without cyanocobalamin, and usually cyanocobalamin alone is sufficient.

Haemorrhagic anaemias result from excessive, persistent bleeding. The plasma is rapidly replaced from the body's reserves of water and protein. The red cells are hypochromic as the stored iron is released rather more slowly than is necessary to meet the capacity of the erythropoietic tissue to form new cells.

Haemolytic anaemias occur in conditions in which there is an increased rate of destruction of erythrocytes. (1) In sickle-cell disease, the deformed erythrocytes are rapidly broken down by the reticulo-endothelial cells. This is a hereditary disease associated with resistance to malarial infections. The sickle cells contain abnormal forms of haemoglobin, called C and S haemoglobins which differ from normal haemoglobin in that one amino acid is replaced in the polypeptide chain:

Haemoglobin A (normal)	—thr—pro—glu—glu—
Haemoglobin S	—thr—pro—val—glu—
Haemoglobin C	—thr—pro—lys—glu—

The disease is thought to be due to the inheritance of a mutation in a single gene. (2) In some people the production of abnormal *haemolysins* is stimulated by cold and in others by a slight acidosis, such as that occurring in sleep owing to the accumulation of carbon dioxide. The products of intravascular haemolysis appear in the urine, giving rise to the names paroxysmal (cold) and nocturnal haemoglobinurias respectively. (3) Intravascular haemolysis may be caused by some snake venoms, and bacterial toxins, or by transfusion of incompatible blood. It also occurs during bouts of malaria. If there is recovery from the immediate deleterious effects a secondary anaemia follows.

BLOOD GROUPS. Early attempts to transfuse blood from one person to another were often unsuccessful and dangerous because the plasma of some individuals contains factors which result in agglutination and haemolysis of the erythrocytes of others. This phenomenon is produced by processes akin

TABLE 8.5. The blood groups.

Plasma or Serum agglutinin	Blood group	Red cell agglutinogen			
		A	B	AB	O
β(anti-B)	A	42%	+	+	−
α(anti-A)	B	+	9%	+	−
None	AB	−	−	3%	−
$\alpha\beta$(anti-AB)	O	+	+	+	46%

+ = agglutination; − = no agglutination

to antigen–antibody reactions. The erythrocytes have an antigen-like component called an *agglutinogen* whilst the plasma contains an antibody-like γ-globulin called an *agglutinin*. Individuals may be divided into four groups on the basis of the reactions between the plasma (or serum) of one group with the erythrocytes of another (see Table 8.5). Persons with the A-agglutinogen on their erythrocytes have the β-agglutinin in their plasma, whilst those with the B-agglutinogen have the α-agglutinin. Those with both the A- and the B-agglutinogens have neither type of agglutinin in their plasma, and lastly those with no agglutinogen in their red cells have both α- and β-agglutinins.

The approximate proportions of the Western European populations having each blood group is also shown in the table. Eighty-eight per cent of the population belong to either the A group or the O group. The table also shows where agglutination and haemolysis occurs; thus cells of group A agglutinate with plasma of groups B and O (which contain the α-agglutinin); cells of group B agglutinate with plasma of groups A and O; cells of group AB agglutinate with plasma of groups A, B or O; cells of group O do not agglutinate with plasma of any group. Blood transfusions are usually given only when the donor and the recipient are of the same group. However, in emergencies blood from a group O donor may be given to a recipient of any other group as the donor cells contain no agglutinogens. Usually, only small volumes of blood are transfused relative to the circulating blood volume of the recipient, and the agglutinins in the donor's plasma are diluted so that the recipient's own red cells are not agglutinated. Individuals of blood group O are known as universal donors, whereas those of group AB are universal recipients. Severe haemolysis after transfusion of incompatible blood results in a marked fall of blood pressure (due to the vasodilator action of released adenosine nucleotides), hyperkalaemia (often sufficient to impair the heart), haemoglobinuria (often leading to fatal anuria) and intravascular embolus formation.

The agglutinogenic components of the erythrocyte responsible for the ABO grouping are glycoproteins and these are genetically controlled. The genes concerned are designated A, B and O, giving the genotypes AA, AB, AO, BB, BO and OO; the corresponding phenotypes belong to groups A, AB, A, B, B, and O. Thus, A or B is dominant to O, and A and B together contribute equally. The agglutinogens first appear just after birth and persist unchanged throughout life. Recent work suggests that if the foetus is exposed to erythrocytes of a group other than its own before its own agglutinogens are formed, the agglutins against that group do not develop.

The ABO agglutinogens are present in colostrum as well as in serum. In some persons, known as *secretors*, they are also found in saliva, semen and other secretions: there are about 80% secretors in the population and 20% *non-secretors*. This trait is hereditary and controlled by a dominant (secretor) and recessive (non-secretor) gene.

The erythrocytes of the *Macacus rhesus* monkey contains an antigenic lipoprotein which is also present in the erythrocytes of 85% of people of Western European extraction. People carrying the rhesus antigen are termed Rh-positive. The serum from animals injected with Rh-positive blood is used to test for Rh antigens in the blood of human subjects. In the ABO-grouping the absence of an antigen dictates the presence of the complementary antibody, but the Rh-grouping differs. Persons without Rh-antigen, that is Rh-negative, only produce an anti-Rh γ-globulin after they have been injected with Rh-positive blood. The presence of Rh-antigen is genetically determined. If the plasma of an Rh-negative individual contains an antibody against Rh-antigen because of a previous exposure to Rh-positive blood, then a later transfusion of Rh-positive blood produces agglutination and haemolysis of the transfused erythrocytes. Particular attention must be given to the Rh-factor in pregnancy when a Rh-negative woman has a Rh-positive foetus. If the woman has previously been given a blood transfusion from a Rh-positive donor, she will have developed Rh-antibodies. The antibody may cross the placenta and haemolyse the foetal erythrocytes causing death of the foetus *in utero* or soon after birth. A Rh-negative woman who has not received a transfusion of Rh-positive blood can develop Rh-antibodies when she has a Rh-positive foetus, as the foetal red cells may penetrate into the maternal circulation; in this case, the first Rh-positive baby is usually healthy, but subsequent Rh-positive babies are usually erythroblastic. The only treatment then is to exchange completely the blood of the newly-born baby for Rh-negative blood in order to eliminate both the Rh-antibody which has passed through the placenta from the mother and the Rh-positive foetal cells already damaged. If the mother has a history of death *in utero* of Rh-positive foetuses, then a premature delivery by Caesarian section, followed by exchange transfusion, may save the life of the child.

There are several additional blood groups. The most important, after the ABO and Rh groups, are MNS and Pp. They may become significant in patients who are given a long series of transfusions. The main reasons for studying them is their application to forensic medicine and the data that they provide in human genetics.

Leucocytes. The white blood cells (or leucocytes) are divided into two groups: the granulocytes and the lymphoid leucocytes.

The three types of granulocytes are distinguished by the affinity of the granules in their cytoplasm for various dyes. The most common cell is the *neutrophil* in which the granules take up both acid and basic dyes and usually appear purple in colour; the other types are the *eosinophil* (the granules staining with acid dyes) and the *basophil* (the granules staining with basic dyes). Granulocytes are formed in the red bone marrow from sinusoidal cells and are sometimes termed myeloid cells (Greek: *myelos* = marrow). As the age of the neutrophil increases, its nucleus becomes horse-shoe shaped and then develops lobes. A study of the distribution of the number of lobes in the circulating neutrophils (called an Arneth index) gives information about the relative ages of the neutrophils and indicates indirectly their rate of formation. When formation is rapid (as a result of leukaemia or infection) there is a high proportion of young forms with a spherical or indented nucleus. However, if formation is impaired (for example, in pernicious anaemia) there is a high proportion of old forms whose nuclei contain up to five lobes.

The two types of lymphoid leucocytes are the *lymphocytes* and *monocytes*, neither of which has granular inclusions in the cytoplasm. Both types are formed chiefly in the lymph nodes, spleen, thymus, tonsils and Peyer's patches, and pass into the blood-stream via the lymphatic system. The red marrow may also be the source of a few lymphoid cells.

The total leucocyte count of adult human blood varies from 4000 to 11,000 per mm^3. The distribution of leucocytes is shown in Table 8.6. The condition in which the total leucocyte count is elevated is termed *leucocytosis*. Gross leucocytosis as a result of a neoplasm (tumour) of the tissues producing the

TABLE 8.6. The leucocytes.

Cell type	Number per mm^3		Percentage of total
	Range	Mean	
Neutrophil	3000–7000	4500	66
Eosinophil	50–400	100	1·5
Basophil	0–50	25	0·5
Lymphocyte	1000–3000	1800	26
Monocyte	100–600	450	6

leucocytes is called *leukaemia*. A marked reduction in the number of leucocytes is called *leucopenia*. The contribution of the various types of leucocytes to the change in the total count is described by various specialized terms. For example, *agranulocytosis* is a specific diminution in the numbers of the granulocytes: one of the untoward side-effects of many drugs is to produce an agranulocytosis by depressing the capacity of the bone marrow to form new cells. *Neutrophilia*, or an increase in the number of neutrophils, occurs in many inflammatory conditions. In patients suffering from parasitic infections (such as tapeworm) and in allergic conditions, there is usually an *eosinophilia*. Stress produces an *eosinopenia*.

The leucocytes are concerned with the body's reaction to infection. Neutrophils engulf bacteria and completely digest them. Monocytes are also phagocytic; they inactivate bacteria but do not completely digest them. The lymphocytes contain γ-globulins. Susceptibility to infection is increased when the leucocyte count is greatly reduced.

Tissue fluids

The water content of the body can be divided into the extracellular and intra-cellular compartments. About one-quarter of the extracellular water is in the plasma and smaller amounts are accounted for by other fluids, such as cerebro-spinal fluid, aqueous humor, freshly formed urine, intestinal contents and glandular secretions. The remainder of the extracellular water, which amounts

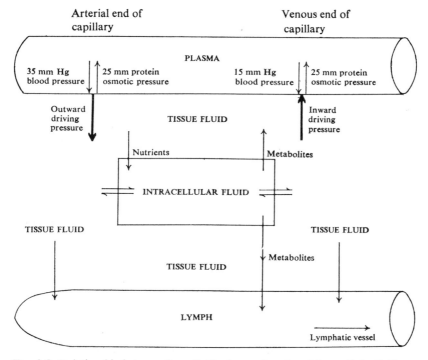

FIG. 8.5. Relationship between tissue fluid, plasma, lymph and intracellular fluid.

to about 18% of the body weight, constitutes the tissue fluid and lymph. Tissue fluid permeates the interstices between the cells and is in immediate contact with the cells. The volume of extracellular space differs considerably in different tissues. Average values are 15% for striated muscle, 30% for cardiac and smooth muscle, and 50% or more for connective tissues. The exchange of metabolites and of oxygen and carbon dioxide between the blood and the body cells involves diffusion through the tissue fluid. The exchange between plasma and tissue fluid occurs through the capillary walls, which act as a semi-permeable membrane, being relatively impermeable to protein but freely permeable to water and solutes of low molecular weight. Thus tissue fluid contains the same constituents in the same proportions as plasma, with the exception of protein, and it is described as an *ultra-filtrate* of plasma. A little protein usually escapes through the capillary wall but in some conditions a considerable proportion of the plasma protein and even the blood cells pass into the extra-vascular spaces.

The dynamics of the exchange are summarized in Fig. 8.5. The forces acting to move fluid across the capillary endothelium are the blood pressure in the capillary and the osmotic pressure of the plasma proteins. At the arterial end of the capillary, the difference in these forces is a driving pressure which forms tissue fluid. At the venous end, the blood pressure is lower, and the resultant pressure difference favours the resorption of tissue fluid. Thus there is a continual exchange of water and the freely permeable solutes between plasma and tissue fluid; about 75% of the plasma water and 60% of the plasma sodium are exchanged each minute. When the rate of resorption of tissue fluid is faster than the rate of formation, fluid moves from the tissue spaces into the blood-stream. This is of particular importance in restoring the blood volume after haemorrhage: the loss of blood results in lower capillary blood pressures and the force due to the plasma protein osmotic pressure favours the uptake of water. The rate of formation of tissue fluid is increased when the blood pressure in the capillaries is increased, when the osmotic pressure is reduced, or when the permeability of the capillary endothelium is increased. The increased amounts of tissue fluid are then removed from the tissues by the lymphatic system. The lymph, therefore, is formed mainly by the overflow of tissue fluids. In health, the total daily lymph flow amounts to about 20% of the body weight per day. Substances that increase the flow of lymph, by increasing capillary permeability or by diminishing plasma protein osmotic pressure, are termed *lymphagogues*.

An increase in tissue activity results in an increased rate of formation of tissue fluid and of lymph flow. There are several factors involved. (*a*) The capillary blood pressure is raised because of dilatation of the arterioles in response to reflexes conveyed by vasomotor nerves. (*b*) Capillary dilatation is produced by various substances, including metabolites, released from the active tissue cells—such substances include histamine, bradykinin, lactic acid, carbon dioxide and hydrogen ions. (*c*) The osmotic pressure of the tissue fluid is increased because of the low molecular-weight metabolites released from the cells. (*d*) The changes in the tissue fluid which are the result of increased cellular activity (increased pH, decrease in calcium ion concentration, release of histamine and bradykinin) increase capillary permeability thus increasing the rate of formation of tissue fluid. In addition a greater amount of protein escapes into the tissue fluid and this retards resorption into the blood at the venous end of the capillary. (*e*) Some of the substances released from active tissues produce vasodilatation by axon reflexes.

Lymphatic system. The lymphatic capillaries begin in the tissues as thin-walled endothelial tubes with closed ends. Tissue fluid, protein and even particulate matter and cells can pass through the lymphatic endothelium and enter the lumen of the tube. Lymphatic capillaries beginning in the intestinal villi take in a large proportion of the fat absorbed from the intestines: the opaque lymph they contain after a meal rich in fats is called *chyle*. The lymphatic capillaries unite to form lymphatic ducts which convey the lymph to lymph nodes. Other lymphatic ducts take lymph from the nodes to the main lymphatic vessel, the thoracic duct, which discharges into the subclavian vein. The ducts have endothelial flaps at intervals along their length which act as valves, permitting movement of lymph only away from the tissues.

The movement of lymph towards the lymph nodes and then to the thoracic duct is aided by pressures applied to the ducts during contractions of skeletal muscle, respiratory movements, the heart beats and intestinal movements. Lymph nodes (or glands) are usually bean-shaped structures about 1 cm in diameter. They are surrounded by a fibrous connective tissue capsule which penetrates the interior dividing it into compartments. Each compartment receives an afferent lymphatic vessel and an artery and vein. Lymph percolates through the masses of lymphocytes, lymphoblasts and reticulo-endothelial cells which are packed into each compartment, it becomes enriched with lymphocytes, and leaves the node in the efferent lymphatic vessel arising from the hilus. Lymph nodes are situated at the proximal ends of the limbs, in the neck and in the abdomen and thorax; lymphoid tissue is also contained in the Peyer's patches of the intestine, the spleen, the thymus gland and the tonsils and adenoids. The lymph nodes exercise a protective function: thus bacteria and particulate matter, picked up from the tissues in the lymphatic vessels, are taken in by the phagocytic cells; and antigenic material arriving at the lymph node stimulates the production of antibody by the dividing lymphoblasts. A severely infected lymph node is swollen and tender.

Oedema. A gross increase in the volume of the extracellular fluid is described as oedema. This may arise because of prolonged tissue activity: the swelling of severely fatigued muscles is a manifestation of this. An increase in the venous pressure, which may be caused by a mechanical restriction of venous blood flow or by heart failure, results in oedema owing to diminished capillary resorption of tissue fluid. Restriction of lymph flow also causes oedema, the most striking example of this is in the condition of elephantitis, caused by the obstruction of lymphatic vessels by filaria parasites. In severe starvation, there is ultimately a reduction in plasma protein and the diminished plasma protein osmotic pressure results in an increased rate of formation and decreased rate of resorption of tissue fluid. Furthermore, there may be an increased capillary permeability due to the lack of certain dietary factors. In oedema of the liver, mesentery, omentum and intestine, fluid passes from the tissue spaces into the peritoneal cavity: this fluid is known as *ascites*.

Inflammation. The redness of inflamed tissues is due to dilatation of the capillaries: this may be caused by the administration of vasodilator substances, such as occur in stinging nettles and certain venoms and toxins, or it may be caused by the liberation of vasodilator substances, including histamine, from the damaged tissues by a variety of damaging stimuli such as mechanical trauma, heat and chemical irritants. Capillary dilatation, together with an increase in capillary permeability, results in the formation of copious protein-rich tissue fluid which gives rise to the swelling of the inflamed area. Leucocytes tend to adhere to the damaged capillary endothelium and pass through into the tissue spaces by amoeboid movements. In damaged tissues, particularly when there is an infection, the leucocytes migrate through the tissue spaces to the seat of the damage: it is believed that their migration is influenced by chemical substances, and their directed movements are described as positive *chemotropism*. A polypeptide which can be extracted from inflammatory exudate and which has the property of attracting leucocytes has been called *leucotaxine*. The phagocytic leucocytes (neutrophils and monocytes) invade the damaged areas in large numbers and ingest cell debris and infecting bacteria. The mass of leucocytes, both dead and alive, together with the tissue debris and inflammatory exudate form *pus*.

CHAPTER 9

Cardiovascular System : The Heart

The cardiovascular system is concerned with the circulation of the blood. It consists essentially of a pump, namely the heart, and a system of tubes, the blood vessels. A general scheme of the circulatory system is shown in Fig. 9.1.

The mammalian heart contains four chambers, the right and left atria, and the right and left ventricles. The walls of each chamber consist of cardiac muscle cells (page 209), and the pumping action of the heart is a result of their contractions. The atria are relatively thin walled chambers which receive blood from veins and pass blood into the ventricles. The ventricles are thicker walled, the walls of the left ventricle being thicker than those of the right. Blood is pumped from the ventricles into arteries.

The position of the heart in the thorax is shown in Fig. 9.2. The atria and the arteries and veins are at the *base* of the heart. The tip of the ventricles is called the *apex* of the heart. The left atrium and left ventricle face the anterior surface of the thorax and the right atrium and right ventricle face the posterior surface of the thorax. The *axis* of the heart is orientated with the base pointing towards the right shoulder and the apex towards the lower left side of the thorax.

The valves. The forward flow of blood through the heart is the result of the action of eleven flaps, arranged in sets at the outlets of the chambers (Fig. 9.3). The three triangular flaps of the *tricuspid valve* offer no resistance to the passage of blood from the right atrium into the right ventricle, but when the pressure in the right ventricle increases, as it does during ventricular systole, the sides and tips of the flaps make contact and prevent the reflux of blood into the atrium. Attached to the tips of each flap are fibres known as *chordae tendineae*; these fibres are inserted into *papillary muscles*, which are muscular projections of the wall inside the ventricle. The function of the chordae tendineae is to prevent the flaps of the valve from being forced backward into the atrium. Blood pumped from the right ventricle passes through three *semilunar valves* situated at the entrance to the pulmonary artery. At the completion of ventricular systole, the pressure in the ventricle is similar to that in the pulmonary artery; as the ventricle relaxes, the pressure in it falls and the higher pressure in the artery forces out the semilunar valves which close the orifice and prevent the back-flow of blood. Blood flowing from the left atrium into the left ventricle passes through the *bicuspid valve*, which consists of two triangular flaps; it is also known as the *mitral valve* from its fancied resemblance to a

249

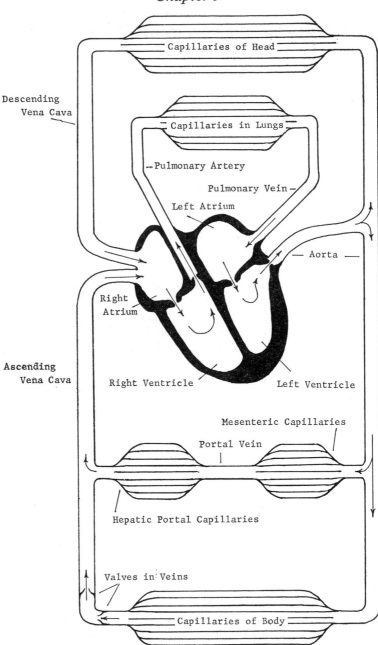

FIG. 9.1. Schematic diagram of circulation.

bishop's mitre. Contraction of the left ventricle forces the two flaps together, preventing the regurgitation of blood into the left atrium. As with the tricuspid valve, the tips of the bicuspid valve are attached to chordae tendineae and papillary muscles. The orifice of the aorta is guarded by three *semilunar valves*

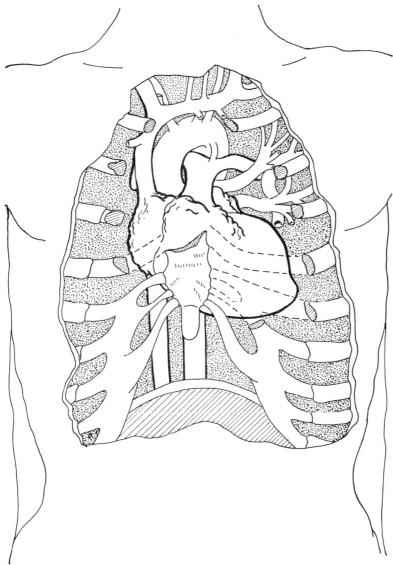

FIG. 9.2. The heart in the thorax.

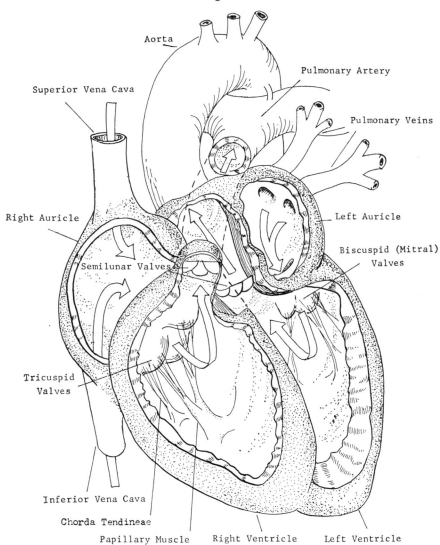

FIG. 9.3. The valves of the heart.

(the *aortic valves*) arranged like those in the orifice of the pulmonary artery. There are no valves at the orifices of the great veins where they enter the atria, but regurgitation of blood in the veins during atrial systole is hindered by the contractions of rings of atrial muscle which surround the orifices and act as sphincters.

In addition to the valves of the heart, the one-way movement of blood within the cardiovascular system is aided by pocket-shaped valves in some of the veins, particularly in the limbs.

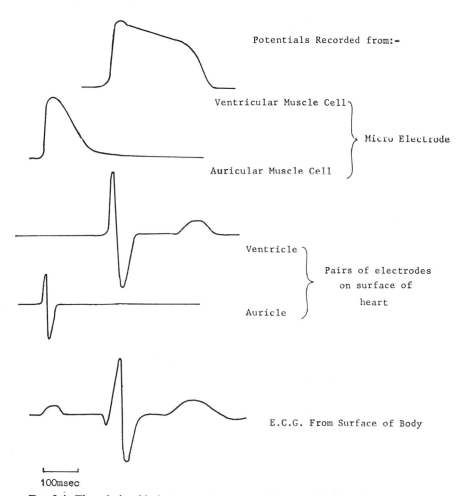

Potentials Recorded from:-

Ventricular Muscle Cell

Micro Electrode

Auricular Muscle Cell

Ventricle

Pairs of electrodes on surface of heart

Auricle

E.C.G. From Surface of Body

100msec

FIG. 9.4. The relationship between action potentials recorded with microelectrodes inserted into single cells, the action potentials recorded from the surface of the heart, and the electrocardiograph recorded at the surface of the body.

The electrocardiogram. With each beat of the heart, the action potentials of cardiac muscle fibres are propagated throughout the heart (page 214), and can be detected with electrodes placed on the heart's surface. Records obtained in this way are exactly analogous to the action potentials recorded from pairs of electrodes placed in contact with a nerve trunk (page 75) or skeletal muscle (page 199). The relationship between an action potential recorded with a single intracellular electrode and that recorded with a pair of electrodes on the surface of cardiac muscle is shown in Fig. 9.4.

The tissues of the body are sufficiently good conductors for the electrical activity of the heart to be detected at the surface of the body, provided steps are taken to reduce the electrical resistance of the skin. Thus pairs of electrodes attached to the skin at suitable points detect the resultant electrical potentials produced by action potentials as they sweep through the heart; a record obtained in this way is called an electrocardiogram (ECG). The first observer to detect the electrical activity accompanying the heart beat at the surface of the body was Waller in 1887, using a capillary electrometer. In 1903, the Dutch physician, Einthoven used a more versatile instrument, the string galvanometer, and established the technique of electrocardiography by determining the form of the normal ECG and by showing that it detected abnormal cardiac activity. Lewis later correlated the pattern of the ECG waves with various disorders of the heart.

Various conventions have been adopted as to the placing of the electrodes on the surface of the body. In Einthoven's system, electrodes were placed on each wrist and on the left ankle. The electrocardiogram was recorded taking these electrodes in pairs, that from the right arm and left arm being known as lead I, that between the right arm and left leg as lead II, and that between the left arm and left leg as lead III. These constitute the so-called 'limb-leads', typical records being shown in Fig. 9.5.

The deflections of the ECG record have been named as the P-wave, the Q-, R- and S-waves, which are usually considered together as the QRS complex, and the T-wave (Fig. 9.6). The P-wave is caused by depolarization of the atrial muscle, the QRS complex is caused by depolarization of the ventricles, and the T-wave reflects the rate of spread of repolarization of the ventricular muscle cells. The P-wave in lead I is upright when the beats originate in the pacemaker or sino-auricular node. If the beats arise in another part of the atrial muscle (an ectopic focus), the P-wave may be inverted. An increased mass of muscle contributes a larger component to the electrical activity recorded from the surface of the body. Thus, as a result of stenosis (or narrowing) of the mitral valve the left atrium develops a higher pressure in pumping blood into the ventricle, hypertrophies, and contributes an additional peak to the P-wave.

The interval between the P-wave and the start of the QRS complex is an index of the time needed for the impulse to be conducted through the atria and along the atrio-ventricular bundle. For convenience, the P–R interval is measured, the usual time being 0·12 to 0·18 sec. A longer interval denotes an impairment of conduction, whereas a shorter interval suggests that the atrial impulse is originating in the atrial muscle closer to the atrio-ventricular node than the usual pacemaker, the sino-atrial node. A P–R interval which varies from beat to beat is interpreted as the pacemaker moving to different parts of the atrial tissue instead of remaining in the sino-atrial node. Lack of correlation between the P-waves and the QRST components suggests that the atria are being driven by one pacemaker and the ventricles by another, perhaps located in the atrio-ventricular bundle. The P-wave may be completely hidden in the QRS-waves if the impulse is propagated from a bundle pacemaker so that it reaches atrial and ventricular muscle simultaneously.

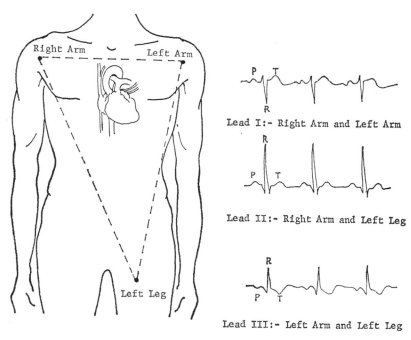

Lead I:- Right Arm and Left Arm

Lead II:- Right Arm and Left Leg

Lead III:- Left Arm and Left Leg

FIG. 9.5. ECG records from the limb leads.

The duration of the ventricular complex, from the start of the QRS-waves to the end of the T-wave, gives an index of the time during which the ventricular muscle is depolarized and approximately equals the refractory period of the ventricles. The duration of the QRS-waves is determined by the rate of spread of the action potentials throughout the ventricular muscle; usually it is 0·06 to 0·09 sec. If conduction is impaired or if the action potentials are conducted asynchronously it is longer. If part of the ventricular conducting system is injured (as in bundle branch block), excitation of the muscle served by that part is delayed and notches appear in the QRS deflection. Excitation arising in the ventricles from an ectopic focus is conducted more slowly than usual, and the waves are wider and altered in form as the direction of travel of the potentials is different from that in normal beating.

The orientation of the heart in the chest, or more properly the orientation of the *electrical axis* of the heart, may be interpreted from the relative sizes of the Q-, R- and S-waves in the various leads. Hypertrophy of the left ventricle, resulting fron an increased work load, as in hypertension or aortic stenosis, results in a larger current from it, and an alteration in the electrical axis. During respiratory movements, the position of the heart in the thorax alters slightly, producing cyclic changes in the electrical axis. The presence of damaged areas in heart caused by blockage of part of the coronary circulation with consequent anoxia of the muscle, leads to a form of damage known as an *infarct*. The resultant disturbances in the ECG consist of elevation of the T-wave and alteration of the S–T segment. Elevation of the T-wave also occurs when the work output of the heart exceeds the supply of oxygen available for a corresponding output of energy from metabolism. The effect of adrenaline in elevating the T-wave may be due to the raised work output of the heart. The T-wave is also higher when there is hyperkalaemia (a raised level of plasma potassium).

The frequency at which a part of the ECG wave pattern recurs is a measure of the rate at which the impulses are arriving at that part of the heart giving rise to the wave. The regular rhythm of the heart, with the impulse initiated at the sino-atrial node, may be disturbed in a number of ways. The normal rate of beating in adults is between 60 and 90/min, whilst in children it is higher. Rates below 60 or above 90/min are termed *bradycardia* and *tachycardia* respectively. There is a cyclic change in heart rate accompanying respiratory movement; this is called *respiratory arrhythmia*, the rate increasing during inspiration and decreasing in expiration.

When the rate of beating of the atria exceeds 250/min, not all the impulses are conducted down the atrio-ventricular bundle, since some of them fall in the refractory period of the conducting tissue. The ventricles may receive only two out of every three impulses, and there is a 3 to 2 heart block, or they may receive every second impulse, and there is a 2 to 1 block. Increasing the rate of atrial beating leads to higher degrees of block. In heart block, the atrial beats appear as P-waves on the ECG, but the QRST complex is absent after occasional P-waves. When the tachycardia is 400/min or more, the atria are said to be in *flutter*; the ECG then shows runs of P-waves between the ventricular complexes. In atrial *fibrillation*, the atria as a whole are not beating, but contractions are occurring irregularly and asynchronously at rapid rates throughout the atrial muscle. No P-waves are distinguishable, and the ECG shows fluctuations of the record between the ventricular complexes. The atrio-ventricular node is being bombarded by rapid but irregular impulses but most of them are blocked; the occasional impulse which is conducted leads to a ventricular beat and a QRST complex.

Tachycardia may occur as a result of an ectopic pacemaker in the ventricles. In ventricular tachycardia, the P-waves and the QRST complexes are not synchronized and the QRS may be deformed in shape. In ventricular fibrillation, different parts of the ventricular muscle are contracting asynchronously, and the ECG shows large random fluctuations. In the absence of co-ordinated contractions no blood is pumped, the blood pressure falls to zero and death ensues rapidly. The circulation may be maintained by direct massage of the heart and survival is possible if the heart is defibrillated so that regular contractions return.

Other conventions of recording the ECG are used. A method popular with clinicians uses a so-called unipolar lead. One terminal of the measuring apparatus is connected to the right arm, left arm and left leg simultaneously. This is the indifferent electrode, and it remains at zero potential because of the vector relationships of the action potentials recorded from these three points. The other electrode, called the exploring or recording electrode, is placed at various positions on the chest. The records obtained in this way are known as precordial unipolar electrocardiograms. The convention adopted for designating the various positions of the recording electrode are:

V_1: on the right margin of the sternum in the 4th intra-costal space (*ics*);
V_2: left sternal margin, 4th ics;
V_3: between V_2 and V_4;
V_4: below the middle of the left clavicle in the 5th ics;
V_5: below the anterior margin of the left axilla in the 5th ics.

The unipolar chest leads record primarily the electrical activity of that part of the heart nearest to the electrode: the thicker walled left ventricle has a predominant influence. The relationships between the precordial electrodes and the parts of the heart can be worked out by reference to Fig. 9.2.

The heart sounds and murmurs. The first heart sound results from the cusps of the atrio-ventricular valves snapping together, the intensity depending on the vigour with which they shut, and on how close together the cusps are at the start of ventricular systole. When ventricular filling is complete, as happens when the heart is beating slowly, the valves float up until they almost touch, and the final closure is quiet. The first sound is loudest during tachycardia, particularly after exercise. Asynchronous contraction of the right and left ventricles may result in the sound being split into two components.

The second heart sound occurs when the semilunar valves are snapped shut

9

by the back pressure in the aorta, and it signals the end of ventricular systole. The momentary check in the forward movement of the blood through the arteries may be detected in the pulse as a flexion in the pressure curve known as the *dicrotic notch*.

In the normal heart the flow of blood is streamlined. Turbulence may be detected as a murmur, part of the energy of flow appearing as noise. Murmurs from the heart occur when the cardiac output is very high, or when there is a defect in the heart. Stenosis (or narrowing) of the semilunar valves at the orifice of the aorta or pulmonary artery results in a murmur during systole. If these valves areincom petent (that is, leaking), the blood flowing backwards results in a murmur during diastole. Stenosis of mitral or tricuspid valves results in a murmur during ventricular diastole and especially during atrial systole (that is, just before the first heart sound). Incompetence of the atrio-ventricular valves results in a murmur during systole. Persistence of parts of the foetal mode of circulation (see page 277), such as a patent ductus arteriosus, patent foramen ovale, or an open passage between the ventricles, also results in murmurs.

The venous pulse. The venous pulse may be detected in the external jugular vein in a recumbent subject. By lifting the head it may also be made visible in the neck just above the clavicle. It has two components: the respiratory movements impose a slow pulsation, whereas the cardiac movements impose faster pulsations. The cardiac venous pulse may be recorded by placing a capsule over the jugular vein and connecting it to a sensitive membrane recorder. Accompanying each heart beat, there are three changes in venous pressure: the a-wave caused by atrial systole, the c-wave caused by ventricular systole and the v-wave occurring at the end of ventricular systole (see Fig. 9.6).

The cardiac cycle

At the start of diastole, the pressures in the right atrium and right ventricle are equal, as are those in the left atrium and ventricle. Blood flows into the chambers of the heart from the veins; the atrio-ventricular valves are open. The semilunar valves were closed as soon as the diastolic blood pressures in the pulmonary artery and in the aorta exceeded the pressures in the right and left ventricles respectively. The discharge from the sino-atrial pacemaker marks the beginning of the cardiac cycle, and the spread of the action potential through the atrial musculature results in the P-wave on the ECG. Atrial systole causes a rise in pressure in the atria, and this is transmitted backwards through the veins to produce the a-wave in the jugular pulse. Blood is driven into the ventricles, the amount depending on the duration of the previous diastole, the strength of atrial contraction, the venous pressure, and the amount of blood already present in the ventricle.

The cardiac action potential is conducted down the atrio-ventricular bundle and through the Purkinje tissue of the ventricles. When it reaches the ventricular contractile tissue, ventricular systole begins. The QRS-complex wave shows, in the ECG, the pressures in the ventricles increasing between the R and S waves. Immediately the pressures are above those in the atria, the atrio-ventricular valves shut. The first heart sound is the noise of the surfaces of the valves slapping together. The valves bulge upwards into the atrial cavities, and on the right side this results in a second peak in the jugular pulse curve, the c-wave. The pressures in the ventricles increase until they equal those in the arteries and, as there is no change in ventricular volume, this part of ventricular systole is known as the isometric contraction phase. As soon as the pressures exceed those in the arteries, the semilunar valves open and blood is ejected from the heart. Contraction continues and the pressures reach their systolic peaks.

Meanwhile, atrial diastole has begun and venous blood passively enters the atria. During the rapid ejection phase of ventricular systole, the heart recoils against the blood, and the atria are pulled down at the atrio-ventricular junction, while the parts near the orifices of the veins remain stationary. The enlargement of the atrial cavities results in an inrushing of blood and a fall in the jugular pulse pressure. The ventricles remain contracted with little further decrease in volume, and then the T-wave appears in the ECG and ventricular diastole commences. As soon as the relaxation of the ventricles reduces the pressures below those in the arteries, the semi-lunar valves snap shut and the second heart sound results. The ventricles relax further and, when their pressures equal those in the atria, the atrio-ventricular valves open and blood flows from the now distended atria into the ventricles. This completes one cardiac cycle. The events are shown graphically in Fig. 9.6.

Cardiac output. The *cardiac output* in man at rest is 4 to 6 litres/min. When this value is divided by the number of beats per minute, the volume of blood emerging from the heart at each beat is obtained. This is the *stroke volume*, the value of which is usually between 40 and 70 ml. As the heart is a double pump driving blood through two circuits arranged in series, the output through the two circuits must be equal. The cardiac output is always given as the output from one side of the heart; in fact the heart pumps twice this amount of blood.

The cardiac output depends on three factors—the extent to which the ventricles expel the blood they contain during each contraction, the rate of the heart, and the degree of venous filling. Ventricular systole does not empty the blood from the cavities of the heart, the amount of blood remaining being called the end-systolic volume. When the heart contracts more vigorously, as during sympathetic nerve stimulation or after adrenaline or noradrenaline administration, the end-systolic volume is reduced (i.e. the stroke volume increases) and the systolic blood pressure increases. When the contractions are weak, as in heart failure, the end-systolic volume is larger. Stenosis (or narrowing) of the semilunar valves in the aorta or pulmonary artery prevents the proper emptying of the ventricles.

Changes in the heart rate, between normal limits, has little effect on cardiac

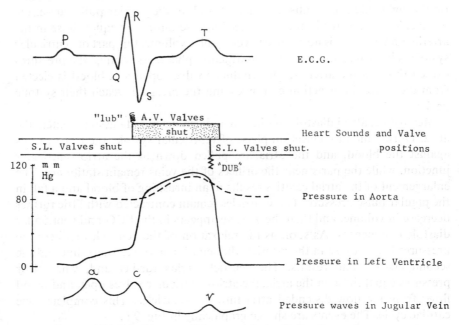

FIG. 9.6. Diagram of the events during the cardiac cycle.

output, but when it is very slow or very fast the cardiac output decreases. In severe bradycardia, even with maximum stroke volume, the cardiac output falls. As bradycardia is usually the result of disease, and as the force of contractions then is also weak, the circulation is inadequate. Circulatory failure due to this combination of circumstances occurs in beri-beri (a dietary deficiency of vitamin B complex). If the heart rate increases without alteration in the stroke volume, the systolic and diastolic blood pressures increase. But in severe tachycardia there is insufficient time for the ventricles to fill during the short diastolic intervals. When the rate at which impulses arising from the atria impinge on the atrio-ventricular bundle is above about 250/min there is a degree of heart block (page 256) and a decrease in ventricular rate. This results in an improvement of cardiac output, and may be considered as a protective function of the atrio-ventricular bundle.

The amount of blood returning to the heart in the veins is important in determining the cardiac output. Increased venous return causes a rise in pressure in the great veins and the atria, so that more blood is forced into the heart during diastole and more blood is expelled by the contraction of the ventricles. This phenomenon was discovered by Starling in experiments on the *heart-lung* preparation of the dog. In this preparation, a branch of the aorta close to the heart is cannulated, and the blood expelled from the left ventricle is then passed through a resistance and returned to the heart through a cannula inserted in the vena cava. The resistance in the circuit is adjusted so that a suitable blood pressure is maintained. The height of the blood in the venous reservoir above the level of the right atrium determines the filling pressure, and thus the volume of blood entering the atrium. The volume of blood pumped from the heart is measured. The pulmonary circulation is left intact and the lungs are rhythmically inflated by a respiration pump to oxygenate the blood. The heart functions for several hours under these conditions, and its behaviour can be studied without the influence of the nervous system. Starling expressed the results from his experiments as the 'Law of the Heart'. Briefly, when the venous pressure is raised, the output of blood from the heart increases to keep pace with the increased input until, at high venous filling pressures, the output decreases. The rate of the heart beat does not change, and therefore it is the stroke volume which alters.

THE MEASUREMENT OF CARDIAC OUTPUT. In Starling's experiments with the dog's heart-lung preparation, the volume of blood pumped by the heart was measured directly. In man the cardiac output is measured indirectly by one of the following methods.

Fick's method. The volume of carbon dioxide removed from the blood during its passage through the lungs in a given period can be measured by analysing the expired air. The amount of carbon dioxide in deoxygenated (venous) blood and in blood after passage through the lungs (arterial blood) can also be determined in samples of blood taken during the time in which the expired air is collected. The cardiac output can be obtained from these measurements, thus:

Cardiac output (in ml/min)

$$= \frac{\text{ml of } CO_2 \text{ in expired air in 1 min} \times 100}{(\text{ml of } CO_2/100 \text{ ml venous blood}) - (\text{ml of } CO_2/100 \text{ ml arterial blood})}$$

the difference in the concentration of carbon dioxide in arterial and venous blood multiplied by the volume of blood passing through the lungs in a fixed period of time is equal to the amount of carbon dioxide expired in the same period. The measurement of cardiac output by Fick's principle may employ gases other than expired carbon dioxide. It may be applied to oxygen taken up from inspired air, or to other gases, notably acetylene and nitrous oxide, which are readily detected in the blood. These gases simply dissolve in the plasma.

Dye-dilution method. In this method a known amount of a dyestuff (e.g. azovan blue) is injected rapidly into a vein. At suitable intervals, the concentration of dye in an artery is measured. The amount of blood pumped through the heart can then be determined from the formula: $F = I/ct$, where F is the flow in litres/sec, I is the total amount of dye injected, c is the mean concentration of dye in the arterial blood, and t is the duration in seconds of the first passage of dye through the artery. In a modification of this technique, a radioisotope has been injected and its transit measured with counters mounted over an artery. Recently a heat-dilution technique has also been used. A small volume of hot or cold saline is injected and the change in temperature of the blood flowing in an artery is measured with a delicate instrument called a thermistor.

The coronary vessels. In amphibia, the heart cells exchange metabolites directly with the blood in the chambers of the heart, but in mammalia the heart contains its own system of blood vessels, the coronary circulation. The coronary arteries arise from the first part of the aorta and penetrate through the mass of the cardiac muscle breaking up into arterioles and capillaries. Some of the coronary blood is discharged directly into the ventricular cavities via the Thebesian vessels, but the bulk of it passes into coronary veins which empty into the coronary sinus lying in the wall of the right auricle, from whence it is discharged into the auricle. Blood flow in the coronary circulation is complicated by the rhythmic changes in tension in the walls of the beating heart. About 5% of the cardiac output (i.e. 200 to 300 ml/min) passes through the coronary circulation, but during severe exercise the coronary flow may increase to 1 to 1·5 litres/min.

ANGINA PECTORIS. The main symptom of this disorder is pain referred to the chest wall, shoulder or arm. The attacks are usually precipitated by states in which the work performed by the heart is relatively greater than the energy made available by oxidative metabolism of the cardiac muscle, which in turn depends on the efficiency of the coronary blood flow. Sympathetic stimulation produced by exertion or by an emotional disturbance is often to blame for an anginal attack. Although there is an increased coronary blood flow resulting from the raised blood pressure, this may not be sufficient to compensate for the increased work done in pumping against the raised pressure. In most patients with a predisposition to angina the coronary arteries are narrowed by arteriosclerotic lesions (see page 280). The pain is thought to be due to metabolites from the active muscle cells stimulating sensory nerve endings, with which the coronary blood vessels are richly endowed. The metabolites accumulate because the rate of coronary blood flow is not sufficiently rapid to remove them as fast as they are formed. Angina is treated by giving drugs which dilate the coronary blood vessels or reduce the oxygen consumption of the heart (see pages 821–829).

Nerves of the heart. The heart is supplied with nerves from both divisions of the autonomic nervous system and it also contains a rich network of sensory nerves. Their function is uncertain, but a number of substances stimulate these nerves which may therefore be linked with chemoreceptors. The parasympathetic innervation of the heart is provided by pre-ganglionic fibres running in the vagus nerves. The ganglia are in the atria, chiefly in the vicinity of the sino-auricular node and the atrio-ventricular node. Stimulation of the vagus nerves results in an immediate slowing of the heart rate, a weaker force of contraction of the atria, and prolongation of atrio-ventricular conduction time. Stimulation of some small twigs of the vagus may produce only a decrease in rate, while stimulation of others may produce only a decrease in force of contraction. Presumably these effects are due to fibres innervating exclusively the sino-atrial node and the atrial musculature respectively. With intense stimulation, atrio-ventricular conduction is completely blocked, but if stimulation is continued the ventricle recommences to beat at a slower rate than the original sinus rhythm. The heart is said to have 'escaped' from the effects of the vagus. This beating is due to the setting up of a pacemaker below the atrio-ventricular node. If stimulation of the vagus nerve is then stopped, the rhythm almost immediately returns to normal, the beat then originating from the sino-auricular node. These effects of vagus nerve stimulation are mimicked by acetylcholine.

The sympathetic nerve supply to the heart comes from fibres arising in the upper thoracic segments. Most of these fibres synapse at ganglion cells in the 1st thoracic vertebral ganglia (the stellate ganglia) or in the inferior cervical ganglia. The post-ganglionic fibres run to the heart in a number of strands known as the *nervi accelerantes*. Stimulation of the sympathetic supply to the heart results in an increase in rate and in the force of contractions. There is also an increase in oxygen consumption which is proportionately greater than the increase in work done, that is, the efficiency of the heart is decreased.

The nerves to the heart are never completely at rest, but are always exerting a slight 'tonic' influence. If the vagus nerves are cut, the heart is released from their influence and the rate increases, often to twice the initial rate. When the sympathetic nerves are cut, the rate decreases by 15 to 25%.

The activities of the nerves to the heart are integrated by centres in the medulla oblongata, the cardio-inhibitory or vagal centre, and the cardio-excitatory centre.

BAINBRIDGE REFLEX. At the junctions between the venae cavae and the right atrium, there are also baroreceptors which reflexly produce changes in heart rate (the so-called Bainbridge reflex). A rise in the venous pressure increases the heart rate by diminishing vagal tone and by raising sympathetic tone to the heart. The Bainbridge reflex only operates when the heart rate is slow.

A rise in arterial blood pressure stimulates baroreceptors in blood vessels (page 274) and causes a reflex slowing of the heart rate. The slowing is due in part to increase in vagal tone and in part to decrease in sympathetic tone.

In addition, there are receptors in the abdominal viscera which reflexly reduce the heart rate by increasing vagal tone. The boxer's blow to the solar (coeliac) plexus produces unconsciousness as the heart is temporarily stopped. Sudden exposure to cold may also result in profound vagal inhibition.

Responses of the heart. *A positive chronotropic response* is the term used when there is an increase in rate, whilst a *negative chronotropic response* is a decrease in rate. Changes in the force of contraction are termed *inotropic responses* (*inos* is the Greek word for force). Changes in excitability are termed *bathmotropic*, whilst changes in conduction are termed *dromotropic* (from *dromos*, a race-track).

CHAPTER 10

Cardiovascular System: Blood Vessels and Circulation

Blood is conveyed between the heart and the organs of the body by the large arteries and veins, which generally offer little resistance to the blood flow. Figure 10.1 shows a diagram of the aorta and venae cavae with the principal blood vessels arising from them. The arrangement of the large vessels is similar in most mammals and the same names are used.

Blood vessels

ARTERIES. The histological structure of an artery is shown diagrammatically in Fig. 10.2. Three layers of tissue are distinguished in the walls: the inner or intimal layer consists of a smooth endothelial lining containing elastic fibres; the middle layer or media consists of circularly or spirally arranged smooth muscle; and the outer or adventitial layer consists of collagenous connective tissue.

The intimal elastic layer is highly developed in the parts of the aorta and of the pulmonary artery nearest the heart, while the muscle fibres are less in evidence. The elastic tissue stretches and the vessels accommodate more blood during the rise of pressure caused by ventricular systole. This elastic buffering action results in a flattening of the pressure peaks and provides a smoother onward flow of blood. The smaller arteries contain relatively larger medial smooth muscle layers.

The arterial pulse. The pressure wave produced by systole of the left ventricle travels through the large arteries at 6 to 12 m/sec, that is, six to ten times faster than the speed of blood flow. The delay between cardiac systole and the arrival of the pulse at the radial (wrist) artery is 0·04–0·08 sec. If the walls of the arteries are rigid, as in diseases such as arteriosclerosis, the pressure wave travels more rapidly. In healthy arteries, the blood flow is streamlined, but when the flow is disturbed, as a result of a thrombus or an aneurysm, the flow is turbulent and murmurs may be detected.

ARTERIOLES. In the final arterial element called the arteriole, the intimal layer consists of an endothelial lining and a single membraneous layer of elastic tissue, the medial layer is richly supplied with nerves running to the smooth

9*

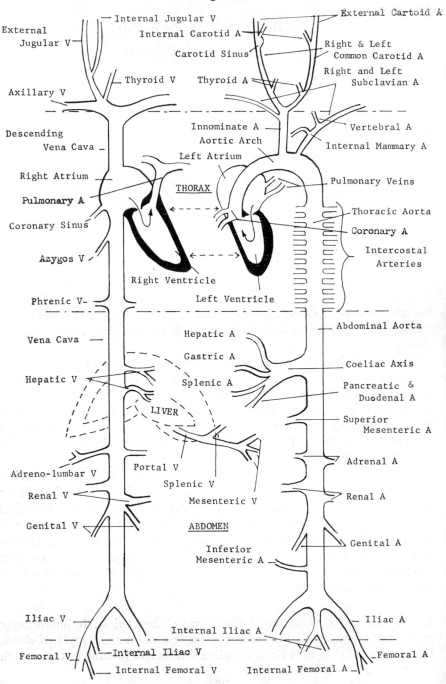

FIG. 10.1. The principal blood vessels in a mammal.

muscle, and the outer adventitial layer merges with the connective tissue of surrounding structures. The arterioles, owing to their small calibre and muscular walls, present the greatest component of resistance to blood flow. Thus, regulation of the blood pressure is accomplished mainly by alterations in the tone of the smooth muscle in the arteriolar wall. When the arterioles in one part of the body are dilated, more blood flows through the tissue which they serve; conversely, when the arterioles are constricted, more blood is shunted to other parts.

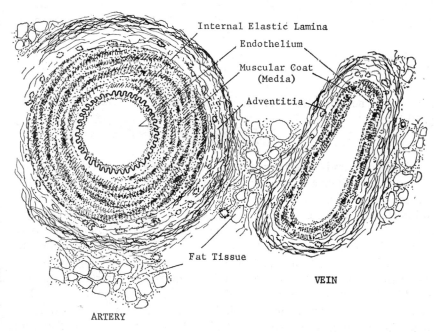

FIG. 10.2. Transverse sections of an artery (left) and a vein (right).

CAPILLARIES. The smallest arterioles merge into capillaries which contain only an endothelial layer. The exchange between blood constituents and those of the tissues takes place through the capillary walls. Each capillary runs a tortuous path of about 200 to 400 μ in length through the tissues. The narrowest capillaries continuously involved in circulation are about 7 μ in diameter, and smaller vessels are probably disengaged from the circulation of a tissue at rest. Krogh has estimated that there are 100 to 200 open capillaries in 1 mm^3 of resting tissue whereas there are as many as 3000 open in 1 mm^3 of active tissue. The diameter of the capillary depends on the pressure of the blood entering it and on the rate at which the blood leaves. The capillary walls in mammals do not contain smooth muscle but in amphibia they contain contractile cells called Rouget cells.

VENULES. The termination of a capillary on the venous side of the circulation is marked by the reappearance of smooth muscle cells in the media and a thick layer of collagenous tissue in the adventitia.

VEINS. The venules reunite to form veins. The walls of veins have three layers (Fig. 10.2): a tunica intima consisting of endothelial cells and a loose network of thin elastic fibres; a tunica media consisting of circularly arranged smooth muscle cells separated by collagenous fibres; and a tunica adventitia of loose connective tissue. In some larger veins, the tunica media is not well developed and some bundles of longitudinally arranged smooth muscle appear in the adventitia. In comparison with the diameter of the lumen, the walls of veins are much thinner than those of arteries. The principal veins are shown in Fig. 10.1.

Blood pressure

Blood in the arteries is under pressure, as is well known from the observation that blood spurts from a severed vessel. The first measurement of the pressure was made by Stephen Hales, an English clergyman in the eighteenth century, who inserted a catheter connected to a glass tube into the carotid artery of a horse and found that the blood rose to a height of 6 to 8 ft. The specific gravity of mercury is about 13·5 times that of blood, so Hale's figures are equivalent to pressures of 110 to 150 mmHg. Physiologists and pharmacologists usually measure the blood pressure in anaesthetized animals by inserting a cannula into a blood vessel and connecting it directly to a mercury manometer. The mercury column possesses considerable inertia, so it does not follow rapid changes in pressure. The systolic and diastolic pressures cannot therefore be determined accurately with a mercury manometer. The mercury column also has a natural frequency of oscillation, and any changes in pressure of about this frequency appear disproportionately larger. For instance, respiratory movements cause fluctuations in blood pressure, and in some animals the rate of respiration is similar to the natural rate of oscillation of the mercury column; this explains why the records obtained show a wide fluctuation coincident with respiratory movements and only narrow fluctuations corresponding to the systolic and diastolic peaks. Nevertheless, the mercury manometer provides a convenient means of measuring the mean pressure. To record the blood pressure precisely, it is necessary to use instruments with low inertia (to ensure a rapid response) and a high natural frequency (to eliminate resonance effects). The first accurate measurements were made using a mirror fastened to a membrane which yielded only slightly to changes in pressure, the movements being magnified by a light beam. More recently, the small movements of the membrane have been recorded electrically.

The blood pressure may also be measured indirectly without cannulating blood vessels. The principle is to apply pressure to a limb by inflating a cuff and to determine at what inflation pressure the pulse wave disappears at a point distal to the cuff. This device is called a *sphygmomanometer*. The arterial pulse wave below the cuff is detected by palpation or with a stethoscope; more recently, sensitive instruments incorporating a strain gauge or a piezzo-electric crystal have been used. The sounds heard in a stethoscope when an artery is almost occluded by a sphygmomanometer cuff between the stethoscope and the heart are called Korotkov's sounds, after their discoverer. They are caused by spurts of blood impinging on a stationary column of blood below the point of occlusion. The sounds are first heard when the peaks of systolic pressure just exceed the pressure with which the artery is occluded, and they cease when the occlusion pressure is lower than the diastolic pressure.

The blood pressure in man varies with age, the state of health, and the conditions under which it is measured. *Average* values for the systolic and diastolic blood pressures at various ages are given in Fig. 10.3, but at any given age there is a considerable range of pressures in random samples of healthy subjects. The blood pressure depends on the cardiac output (which is discussed on pages 259–262) and on the resistance to flow in the small blood vessels. This interrelationship may be expressed as

$$\text{cardiac output} = \frac{\text{blood pressure}}{\text{peripheral resistance}}$$

PERIPHERAL RESISTANCE. The repeated branching of the vessels from the aorta into large and then small arteries and finally into arterioles and capillaries leads to a decrease in the diameter of each vessel and to an increase in the total cross-sectional area. The pressure and the rate of flow of the blood decrease as the cross-sectional area increases, as shown in Fig. 10.4. The most important component of the peripheral resistance is provided by the arterioles which are maintained in a state of partial constriction (the vascular tone). The extent of the tone can be gauged from the calculation that more than three-quarters of all the blood in the body could be accommodated in the blood vessels of the abdominal viscera if the arterioles supplying these organs were fully relaxed.

VISCOSITY OF THE BLOOD. This is of less importance than the cardiac output or the peripheral resistance as a determinant of blood pressure. However, the blood viscosity may change markedly in some disorders. For example,

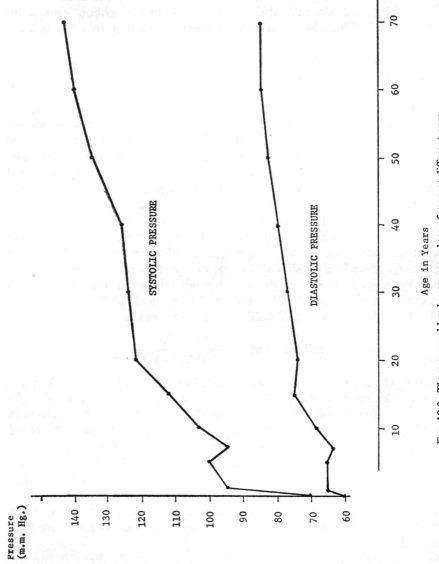

FIG. 10.3. The average blood pressure values of man at different ages.

the number of red blood corpuscles in pernicious anaemia may amount to only about one-fifth the average count, and the viscosity is then only about one-half of the average value so that the blood pressure is lowered. On the other hand, the increase in the red cell count in polycythemia results in a higher viscosity of the blood and a higher blood pressure.

MEASUREMENT OF VASCULAR CHANGES. Variations in the amount of blood in an organ may be detected by inserting it into a hollow chamber called a *plethysmograph,* which measures the volume of the organ. The artery and

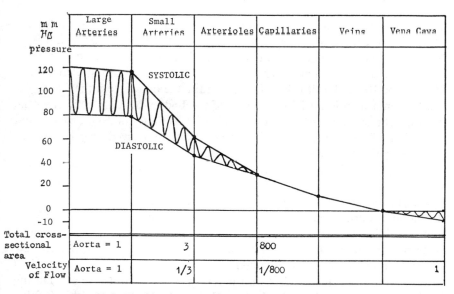

m m Hg pressure	Large Arteries	Small Arteries	Arterioles	Capillaries	Veins	Vena Cava
Total cross-sectional area	Aorta = 1	3		800		
Velocity of Flow	Aorta = 1	1/3		1/800		1

FIG. 10.4. The blood pressure in various parts of the circulation.

vein pass through an air-tight seal which does not impede the blood flow through them. Constriction of the blood vessels produces a decrease in volume and, conversely, the volume increases when there is vasodilatation. The rate of flow of blood through an organ can be determined using the techniques of venous occlusion plethysmography. If the vein is occluded for a brief period of time, the blood entering the organ cannot escape and the volume increases. The rate of increase in volume is therefore a measure of the rate of arrival of blood. More direct measurements may be obtained by cannulating the blood vessels and interposing suitable instruments for measuring flow.

Measurement of the *circulation time* also gives a measure of the rate of blood flow. The principle of the method is to inject a substance at one site and to measure the time at which it arrives at another site. Non-toxic dyestuffs and substances labelled with a radioactive tracer have been used (compare the dye-dilution method for estimating cardiac output). Another method is to inject substances which produce a specific effect when they arrive in the blood-stream; thus saccharine, injected intravenously, gives rise to the sensation of a sweet taste when it reaches the tongue, and small doses of lobeline or cyanide cause a gasping intake of breath when they arrive at the carotid body (page 289): the circulation time from a large vein, through the pulmonary circulation, then to the carotid bodies is about 12 sec.

Venous return. The driving pressure of the blood at the venous end of the capillaries is reduced to about 15 mmHg and is one of the factors comprising the forces driving the blood back to the heart. It is sometimes called *vis a tergo*, a force acting from behind. Such a pressure is capable of lifting a column of blood some 10 cm, but it is insufficient to raise the blood from the feet to the heart when a man is upright. In parts of the body which are subject to the highest hydrostatic pressure (for example, the feet and ankles), oedema and distension of the superficial veins is commonly observed, particularly in people standing for long periods.

The large veins in the limbs are equipped at intervals with pocket-shaped valves which allow passage of the blood only in one direction towards the heart. The movement of muscles in the limbs compresses the veins, so forcing the blood onwards, and this muscle pump is extremely important for venous return. Soldiers who are kept rigidly at attention may faint as, without muscular movement, insufficient blood returns to the heart and an adequate cerebral circulation is not maintained.

Respiratory movements also aid the return of blood to the heart. During inspiration, the thoracic cavity is expanded and the pressure within it falls; this change of pressure is relayed through the relatively thin walls of the vena cava, and the venous pressure, at the level of the heart during inspiration, reaches a minimum of 4 to 7 mmHg below atmospheric pressure. The downward movement of the diaphragm increases the pressure in the abdominal vena cava. As a result of this differential application of pressure, the movement of blood towards the heart is facilitated. This force is sometimes called a *vis a fronte*, a force acting from in front.

Nervous control of blood pressure

Vasomotor nerves. The efferent nerves supplying the cardiovascular system belong to the autonomic nervous system. Those to the heart, the cardiac nerves, are described on page 263. The nerves to the blood vessels, the vasomotor nerves, are *principally* from the sympathetic division of the autonomic nervous system. Blood vessels in the head and neck are supplied by post-ganglionic fibres from the superior cervical ganglia, those in the arms and the upper part of the body by fibres from the stellate ganglia and the upper thoracic ganglia, those in the abdominal viscera by fibres from the coeliac and mesenteric ganglia, and those in the lower part of the trunk and the legs by fibres from the lumbar ganglia. Excitation of the sympathetic nerves to the blood vessels of the skin and the abdominal viscera produces vasoconstriction, these nerves being adrenergic and releasing noradrenaline. In some species, sympathetic cholinergic dilator nerves supply the blood vessels of skeletal muscle. The sympathetic nerves to the coronary blood vessels contain both adrenergic and cholinergic fibres; the effects produced by stimulating these nerves are thus complex and may be influenced by changes in the contraction and metabolism of ventricular muscle. Blood vessels, in general, do not receive fibres from the parasympathetic nervous system; an exception is the nerve supply to the erectile tissues in which stimulation of the sacral parasympathetic *nervi erigentes* produces dilatation of the arterioles and constriction of the veins so that the tissues become engorged with blood. Stimulation of the nerves to the salivary and sweat glands also produces vasodilatation but this may be in part due to the release of bradykinin which is formed as an accompaniment to activity of the glands (page 182).

Antidromic stimulation of sensory nerves produces vasodilatation of the area of skin from which the sensory nerves arise, but it is unlikely that this plays a physiological role in regulating the calibre of blood vessels; it may explain, however, the flushing observed in some abnormal conditions.

Central control of vasomotor activity. The activity of the vasomotor nerves, and hence the regulation of the circulation, is integrated at various levels in the central nervous system. The sympathetic pre-ganglionic neurones in the lateral horns of the spinal cord are connected with other nerve fibres to form spinal vasomotor centres. The spinal centres are usually controlled by impulses descending from the brain, but in spinal animals and in paraplegic patients a few reflexively induced responses of blood vessels persist, including local vascular changes associated with the control of body temperature (pages 435–436) and of erection. The main vasomotor centre is in the medulla oblongata in the floor of the fourth ventricle; a section through the brain stem below this centre results in a fall of blood pressure and loss of most vasomotor reflexes. A higher section (leaving the centre intact), does not greatly alter the blood pressure and the vasomotor reflexes may be readily elicited. The medullary vasomotor centre is in turn under the control of the cerebral cortex. During sleep, the blood pressure is lower than during wakefulness.

CAROTID SINUS PRESSOR REFLEX. At the origin of the internal carotid artery in the neck, the common carotid trunk is enlarged to form the *carotid sinus*. The walls of the carotid sinus contain baroreceptors, that is, receptors sensitive to pressure. The sensory nerve running from these receptors is called the nerve of Hering or simply the carotid sinus nerve. It enters the skull with the glossopharyngeal (IXth cranial) nerve and runs to the medulla oblongata. The mechanism by which pressures in the carotid sinus reflexly alter the blood pressure was elucidated by Heymans, a Belgian physiologist. He supplied the carotid sinus of one dog, termed the recipient, with blood from another dog, termed the donor. The nervous connections between the carotid sinus and brain of the recipient were left intact. When the blood pressure of the donor dog was increased, that of the recipient decreased and, conversely, when the donor's pressure decreased, that of the recipient increased. A rise in the pressure in the carotid sinus increases the rate at which impulses are discharged along the carotid sinus nerve, and this results in a reciprocal decrease in the impulses passing along vasoconstrictor nerves from the vasomotor centre. Conversely, a fall in the carotid sinus pressure leads to fewer impulses travelling to the vasomotor centre, and the output from the vasoconstrictor nerves increases. Thus, impulses in the carotid sinus nerves inhibit the vasomotor centre.

There are additional baroreceptors in other parts of the cardiovascular system. In the walls of the aortic arch, for example, there are aggregates of receptors known as aortic bodies. Baroreceptors also occur in the endothelium of the heart, and the sensory fibres from them join the *depressor* nerve. In some species this nerve runs adjacent to the vagus, whereas in others (man) its fibres run in the vagus trunk. Stimulation of the depressor nerve causes a fall in blood pressure.

Moderation of the output of the vasomotor centre by that of the baro-receptors forms an example of a feed-back control loop. A slight change in blood pressure automatically sets up signals, the effects of which are to oppose the change in pressure.

There are chemoreceptors throughout the vascular system. Those in the carotid body are concerned principally with respiratory reflexes. Chemoreceptors in other parts of the body may have the function of detecting metabolites formed locally so that circulatory adjustments may be made to suit local demands. Stimulation of chemoreceptors in the heart and aorta elicits a reflex, known as the Jarish-Bezold reflex, in which the heart is slowed and the peripheral blood vessels are dilated, giving a fall in blood pressure.

VARIATIONS IN BLOOD PRESSURE. The blood pressure fluctuates rhythmically with respiration, giving rise to the so-called Traube-Hering waves. The variations in venous return due to the respiratory movements partly explain these waves, but if the chest is opened and the lungs inflated by a pump the waves persist although there is then no mechanical cause. The explanation is that the vasomotor centre is excited rhythmically by impulses irradiated from the nearby respiratory centre in the medulla. There may be other rhythmic variations of the blood pressure unrelated to respiratory movements. For example, Mayer's waves are slower than the respiratory rate. They may result from a periodic excitation of the vasomotor centre, but another possibility is that part of the cardiovascular system is undergoing rhythmic variations in tone. Thus, rhythmic changes in the volume of the spleen alternately holds back blood and discharges it, and this may cause synchronous changes in the blood pressure.

POSTURE. On changing from the lying position to the standing position there is an accumulation of blood in the distensible vessels of the lower part of the body which become engorged with blood, because of the increase in hydrostatic pressure. Consequently, there is a drop in pressure in the carotid sinus which results in a reflex constriction of blood vessels, and so the circulation is restored. This control over the blood vessels is exerted by sympathetic vasoconstrictor nerves. In patients being treated with drugs which prevent the sympathetic nerve impulses from reaching the blood vessels (e.g. ganglion blocking drugs, or adrenergic neurone blocking drugs), moving from the supine to the erect position does not result in readjustment of the tone of the blood vessels, so that less blood returns to the heart, and the blood pressure falls. This condition is known as orthostatic hypotension. In some patients the cardiac output may fall below the level necessary to maintain an adequate flow through the brain, and syncope (fainting) occurs.

EXERCISE. During pronounced muscular exertion, the cardiac output rises to 20 to 35 litre/min, the heart rate increases to 180 to 240 beats/min, and the stroke volume rises to 100 to 180 ml. Blood flow through the coronary circulation and through skeletal muscle is increased, while the flow through the splanchnic vascular bed is diminished. These changes are brought about by the activity of sympathetic nerves under the control of the hypothalamic centres. In turn, the hypothalamus is dominated by influences from the cerebral cortex so that the cardiovascular changes may occur in anticipation of exercise.

HUMORAL FACTORS ACTING ON THE CIRCULATION. Carbon dioxide dilates peripheral blood vessels by a direct action, but it also releases adrenaline from the adrenal medulla, and acts centrally to increase vasomotor tone. The vascular responses to increased levels of carbon dioxide are therefore complex, and depend on whether the raised levels are due to breathing air with a high partial pressure of carbon dioxide, to asphyxia, or to increased metabolism.

The adrenal glands also play an important role in influencing the blood pressure. The adrenal medulla secretes adrenaline which acts on the heart and blood vessels. The hormones of the adrenal cortex also have an effect on blood pressure by altering the sensitivity of the cardiovascular system to other agents.

The secretion of the posterior pituitary has marked effects on the blood pressure. Antidiuretic hormone (ADH) causes constriction of blood vessels and an increase in blood pressure. The coronary blood vessels are also constricted, and ADH may precipitate attacks of angina by decreasing the blood supply to cardiac muscle. The physiological role of ADH is probably confined to its effects on the kidney.

ANGIOTENSIN. The observation that the injection of a saline extract of the kidney produces a rise in blood pressure was made by Tigerstedt and Bergman in 1898. Later workers showed that the kidney contains an enzyme, renin, which acts on an α-globulin in the plasma to give a polypeptide containing ten amino acids (angiotensin I). Another enzyme present in plasma converts this to an octapeptide called angiotensin II. These angiotensins have now been synthesized. Renin is located in cells (juxta-glomerular cells) near the glomerular apparatus in the kidney (page 339). When the kidney is anoxic, renin is released, angiotensin is formed and the blood pressure is increased. The experimental production of renal hypertension was first carried out by Goldblatt in 1934, who removed one kidney from a dog and partially occluded the other renal artery by placing a clip on it. Obstruction of renal blood flow by a tumour or by kidney disease leads to a condition in which the blood pressure is at an abnormally high level; this is called *renal hypertension*. It has been suggested that renal hypertension is a physiological adjustment to ensure an adequate blood flow through the kidney. In addition to this effect on blood vessels, angiotensin stimulates the secretion of aldosterone.

Regional circulations

THE PULMONARY CIRCULATION. The pulmonary arterial pressure is about one-fifth of the pressure in the aorta, the systolic pressure being 20 to 40 mmHg, with the diastolic between 5 and 15 mmHg. Since the output of blood from the right ventricle is the same as that from the left ventricle, the resistance to blood flow in the pulmonary circulation is about one-fifth of that in the systemic circulation. A slight difference in output from the two ventricles during a few beats is rapidly readjusted as a result of the dependence of the output of the ventricles on the amount of blood entering them. Thus, a larger stroke volume of the right ventricle increases the amount of blood in the pulmonary circulation, the pressure in the pulmonary veins increases, and the raised filling pressure of the left ventricle results in a larger stroke volume of the left ventricles so that the output from both sides of the heart is restored to balance.

The pulmonary blood vessels are innervated by sympathetic nerve fibres. These, on stimulation, produce vasoconstriction, as does the injection of noradrenaline. There are also cholinergic dilator nerves but it has not been established if they are fibres from the vagus nerve or if they are sympathetic cholinergic nerves.

In addition to the nervous control, the pulmonary blood vessels respond to changes in oxygen tension of the inspired air, e.g. they constrict when the oxygen tension is decreased. The physiological role of this phenomenon may be to divert blood away from a portion of the lungs which is not adequately served with air because of obstruction of the airways, the diverted blood being shunted through other parts of the lungs.

CEREBRAL CIRCULATION. The skull is a rigid container, and thus changes in the volume of blood contained in the cerebral blood vessels may only occur if there is an opposite change in the content of cerebro-spinal fluid. The cerebral blood vessels are innervated by sympathetic nerve fibres arising from the superior cervical ganglia, and stimulation of these nerves results in vasoconstriction.

There appears to be some connection between the calibre of cerebral blood vessels and headache. Both amyl nitrite and histamine cause vasodilatation, and in man these drugs often precipitate headache. Furthermore, attacks of migraine may be relieved by ergotamine, a drug which constricts cerebral blood vessels.

FOETAL CIRCULATION. The exchange of nutrients, oxygen and excretory products between the embryo and the mother takes place between the blood vessels of the placenta and the uterus. A diagram of the foetal circulation is shown in Fig. 10.5. The arterial blood supply of the placenta is derived from the abdominal aorta and carries deoxygenated blood. Oxygenated blood returns in the umbilical vein; part of it passes to the inferior vena cava *via* the *ductus venosus*, the remainder passes through the liver and thence into the inferior vena cava. Part of the blood arriving at the right atrium then passes into the left atrium via the *foramen ovale*, which is an opening in the septum between the two atria. Blood from each atrium enters the corresponding ventricle and is pumped into the pulmonary artery and the aorta. Then most

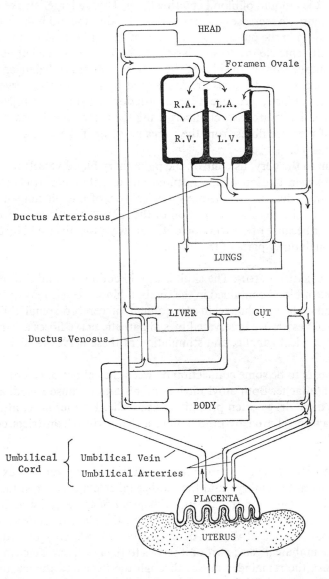

Artery and Vein of Maternal Circulation

FIG. 10.5. Diagram of the foetal circulation.

of the blood in the pulmonary artery joins that in the aorta via the *ductus arteriosus*. Only a small proportion of the blood continues along the pulmonary artery and through the lungs. After delivery the umbilical vessels constrict down and the infant is separated from the placenta. The first few breaths of the new-born infant expand the lungs and the blood flows more readily through the pulmonary blood vessels. The increased return of blood in the pulmonary veins produces a higher pressure in the left atrium and the foramen ovale is occluded by a flap of tissue which projects into the left atrium. This flap becomes firmly attached, so permanently closing the foramen. The ductus arteriosus constricts down, and the course of the blood pumped into the pulmonary artery is entirely through the lungs.

PORTAL CIRCULATIONS. A portal circulation is one in which the course of the blood is as follows: artery→capillaries→veins→capillaries→vein. The blood supply to the abdominal viscera which originates from the superior mesenteric and coeliac arteries divides into capillaries which reunite to form the hepatic portal vein. This vein runs to the liver and again divides into capillaries. In addition, the liver receives an arterial blood supply from the hepatic artery which is a separate branch of the coeliac artery. All the venous blood from the liver rejoins the vena cava via the hepatic vein. Another portal circulation supplies blood to the pituitary gland: capillaries in the hypothalamus reunite to form veins which run to the anterior lobe of the pituitary where they again divide into capillaries.

Rete mirabile. In this, the arrangement of vessels is as follows: artery→capillaries→artery. In the kidney, the smallest divisions of the renal artery running to a glomerulus, the vasa afferentia, divide into the looped glomerular capillaries, which reunite to form another artery, the vasa efferentia. This arrangement allows a degree of control of the pressure of blood in the glomerular capillaries. Constriction of the vasa afferentia diminishes the pressure, but constriction of the vasa efferentia increases the pressure beyond that usually encountered in a capillary.

Vasa vasorum. The walls of the large and medium sized blood vessels are themselves supplied with blood vessels which divide into capillaries in the adventitia and the outer part of the media.

Blood sinuses and the spleen. In some tissues of the body, particularly in those concerned with the formation and destruction of blood cells (the bone marrow, the liver and the spleen), the capillaries widen into larger vascular sacs termed sinusoids. These constitute a reservoir of blood which may be discharged into the circulation during exercise or after haemorrhage. For example, the capsule of the spleen in many species contains smooth muscle which is innervated by sympathetic nerves, and on contraction it forces stored blood into the circulation. In the dog, some 15% of the total blood cells are held in the spleen; in man it is less.

Anastomoses. Arterial anastomoses are passages from one main artery to another. They occur in various parts of the body where their function is to maintain an adequate supply of blood in the event of blockage of one arterial channel. Thus, they occur in the vicinity of joints where bending of the joint may occlude an artery. The arteries supplying the brain, the two internal carotid arteries and the two vertebral arteries, unite to form an anastomotic channel called the *Circle of Willis*. When the arterial supply does not anastomose, it is spoken of as an end artery. Blockage of an end artery leads to profound damage in the tissue, such as blindness when the retinal artery is blocked.

Arterio-venous anastomoses occur in some organs:

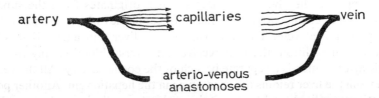

the anastomotic channel offers less resistance to the passage of blood. The smooth muscle in the walls of the anastomosis is under the control of the vasomotor nerves. When the channel is constricted, blood flows through the multitude of small capillary vessels and a greater surface of slowly moving blood is exposed. When the anastomotic channel is dilated, the blood flows rapidly through it and only a small surface area is exposed. Arterio-venous anastomoses occur particularly in tissue concerned with temperature regulation such as human skin, the rabbit's ear, and the dog's tongue.

Some disorders of blood vessels and circulation

ARTERIOSCLEROSIS. This is the most common cause of death in old age, the arteries becoming hardened. There are three main changes in blood vessels with advancing years: (1) The elasticity of the vessels decreases owing to calcification of the elastic fibres and of the medial layers; the sudden rise of pressure in ventricular systole cannot be accommodated by expansion of the arteries and this results in an increase in systolic blood pressure, calling for additional work by the heart in expelling blood. (2) The intima proliferates, deposits of cholesterol-containing lipoid material being laid down in it, and later these deposits become calcified; these changes are usually termed *atheroma*; the lumen of the vessel is partly occluded and the blood flow is impaired. (3) The walls of the blood vessels become so weak that they have a tendency to rupture. A rupture in the intima and media of the aorta or other large artery is known as an *aneurysm*, and escaping blood collects beneath the adventitia which becomes grossly distended. A rupture in a blood vessel in the brain causes the disorder known as a *stroke*.

PERIPHERAL VASCULAR SPASMS. These are disorders in which there is a prolonged and powerful contraction of the smooth muscle of arteries, leading to ischaemia of the tissues and, in extreme cases, to gangrene. The most common form is *Raynaud's disease* in which arteries of the arms or legs are affected; the cause is not known, but vasodilator drugs and anti-adrenaline drugs give some relief. Other conditions in which there is a spasm of peripheral blood vessels include frostbite and ergotism (p. 758). In *Buerger's disease* or thrombo-angitis obliterans, there is an arterial spasm which is complicated by other defects of the vessel walls.

VARICOSE VEINS. Obstruction of venous blood flows over long periods of time may lead to failure of the valves in the walls of the veins and to gross and persistent distension of the vessels.

SHOCK AND CIRCULATORY COLLAPSE. In shock, insufficient blood is returned to the heart to maintain an adequate circulation. There are three causes for this: peripheral vasodilatation may be so great that the blood collects in the distended blood vessels; blood may be lost in haemorrhage; plasma may be lost into the tissue fluid. Depending on the nature of the shock, one or two or all three of these factors may operate.

Severe pain or fright or mechanical pressure on the carotid sinus causes reflex vasodilatation. The subject may faint as blood accumulates in the dilated vessels and insufficient is pumped to the brain to maintain consciousness. In the supine position, the blood returns more easily to the heart, the circulation improves and the patient recovers. In severe injuries, blood loss as well as pain contributes to shock. Loss of plasma occurs after severe burning and after poisoning with various venoms and toxins, and also after anaphylactoid reactions.

When the state of shock persists, the poor circulation to the tissue results in a further vasodilatation and the loss of additional fluid into the tissue spaces. Thus, a vicious cycle is established. The blood pressure may fall too low to permit the formation of urine or to support an adequate coronary circulation.

The treatment consists of restoring the blood volume by giving an intra-venous infusion of plasma or blood or a suitable fluid containing a blood substitute such as dextran (page 917). In addition, drugs are sometimes given to improve the circulation (pages 845–850).

HYPERTENSION. The blood pressure is usually considered to be abnormally high when the resting systolic pressure exceeds 140 mmHg and the diastolic pressure exceeds 90 mmHg. However, there are individuals in whom such pressures have apparently no ill-effects. When the cause of the elevated pressure is known, the condition is referred to as a *secondary hypertension*. Examples of this abnormality are the hypertensive states resulting from phaeochromo-cytoma (page 166) and from obstruction of the renal blood flow (page 276). In most subjects with abnormally raised blood pressures, there is no known cause and the condition is termed *essential* or *primary hypertension*. The condition may persist for many years or it may rapidly become worse, when it is then described as *malignant hypertension*. The complications that ensue from the raised blood pressure are heart failure, rupture of blood vessels particularly when atherosclerotic changes are present, disturbances in the retinal circulation giving rise to blurred vision, and degenerative changes in the kidneys. The degree of hypertension is judged not only from the measurement of the blood pressure but also from the appearance of the retina, observed with the ophthal-moscope, and the presence of plasma protein in the urine. The drugs which have been most useful in the treatment of hypertension are those which interfere with the function of the sympathetic vasomotor nerves. Drugs used in the treatment of hypertension are dealt with on pages 831–845.

CHAPTER 11

The Respiratory System

Respiration is the exchange of gases between the tissues of the body and the outside environment. It entails the breathing in of air through the respiratory tract, the uptake of oxygen from the lungs, the transport of oxygen through the body in the blood-stream and its utilization in the metabolic activities of the cells; the carbon dioxide produced is carried in the blood back to the lungs where it is eliminated from the body in the breath.

The respiratory tract. The air passages start at the nostrils, or nares, which lead into the nasal cavity, and then comes the pharynx which communicates with the buccal cavity. The airway through the neck is the trachea, with the larynx at its upper end. The walls of the trachea contain a series of incomplete rings of cartilage which hold it open but allow movements of the head and neck. The open segments of the rings are in the posterior wall of the trachea, adjacent to the oesophagus. The lower end of the trachea divides into the two main bronchi which lead to each lung and these again divide into smaller bronchi. The walls of the bronchi contain irregularly shaped pieces of cartilage. The last portion of the respiratory tract is the bronchiole which terminates in the alveolar sac. The structure of the tract in man is shown diagrammatically in Fig. 11.1.

The lining of most of the respiratory tract is a mucus-secreting ciliated columnar epithelium. Fine particles of dust in the air are trapped by the mucus and swept away from the lungs by the beating of the cilia. In the terminal bronchioles and the alveolar sacs, the epithelial lining is composed of a single layer of extremely flat cells forming a membrane which allows the free diffusion of gases. Gaseous exchange is facilitated by the enormous area of the alveolar surfaces. The lungs of an adult man contain about 700 million alveoli, each about 190 μ in diameter, giving a surface which has been estimated to be at least 80 square metres.

The open segments of the C-shaped rings of cartilage in the trachea contain bands of smooth muscle. The walls of the smaller respiratory passages contain a layer of smooth muscle beneath the mucosa. The smooth muscle in the respiratory tract is innervated by both parasympathetic and sympathetic fibres. The parasympathetic fibres are carried in the vagus and impulses travelling in them give rise to bronchoconstriction. The sympathetic fibres are adrenergic and, when these are active, bronchodilatation is produced.

283

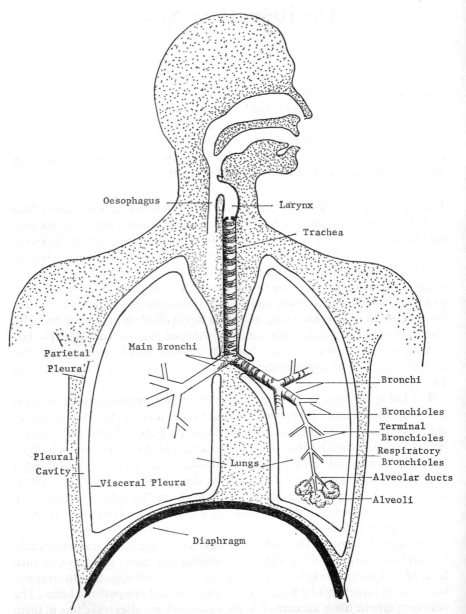

FIG. 11.1. The structure of the respiratory tract. The bronchioles and alveoli are not to scale.

The outer surfaces of the lungs are covered with a connective tissue membrane, the visceral pleura, which is continuous with the lining of the thoracic cavity, the parietal pleura (Fig. 11.1). A film of serous fluid lubricates the two surfaces as they slide over one another during breathing. Inflammation of the pleura is called pleurisy. The space between the two pleura is not normally evident, because it is at a sub-atmospheric pressure which varies during quiet breathing from about 2 to 8 mmHg below atmospheric pressure. If air is introduced between the two layers of pleura, the lung collapses by virtue of its own elasticity and the pleural cavity becomes apparent. This is known as a *pneumothorax* and may arise from injury or from disease, or may be produced intentionally in order to collapse one lung as a therapeutic measure.

Lung circulation. The pulmonary artery originates from the right ventricle of the heart and carries deoxygenated blood. The blood in the extensive capillary bed in the alveolar walls gives up carbon dioxide and is enriched with oxygen. The pulmonary veins return the oxygenated blood to the left atrium. Most of the blood flowing through the lungs is in the pulmonary vessels and is involved in the respiratory function of the lungs, but, in addition, the bronchial arteries, which are branches of the aorta, carry blood to the bronchi and other non-alveolar parts of the lung. This blood is returned chiefly to the right atrium by the bronchial veins, but some drains into the pulmonary vein.

The lungs are supplied with an abundant network of lymphatic vessels. Dust particles which adhere to the walls of the alveoli are engulfed by phagocytic cells termed free macrophages, since they move through the tissue by amoeboid movement. Some macrophages reach the ciliated bronchial mucosa and are swept upwards by ciliary action and then removed together with mucus by coughing. Others enter the lymphatics and are carried to the lymph nodes at the roots of the lungs; these nodes become quite black in coal miners and even in city dwellers who inhale air laden with carbon particles.

Respiratory movements. The chief muscles used in breathing are the diaphragm and the intercostal muscles, the diaphragm being the most important. The diaphragm is a sheet of striated muscle innervated by the two phrenic nerves which arise from the third, fourth and fifth cervical roots of the spinal cord. The muscle fibres run from the edges of the diaphragm to a central tendinous sheet. The outer edge of the diaphragm is attached to the sternum, the inner surface of the lower ribs, and the upper lumbar vertebrae. The diaphragm is domed upwards into the thorax; contraction of its muscles draws the central tendon downwards, thereby flattening the diaphragm and increasing the volume of the thorax. During quiet breathing, the vertical movement of the central tendon is about 1·5 cm, whereas in deep breathing it may increase to about 7 cm. Although diaphragmatic movement is normally responsible for about 70% of the volume of inspired air, it is not essential to breathing as other auxiliary muscles may be used. The intercostal muscles occupy the spaces between the ribs. Some of the intercostal muscles are arranged in such a way that the chest wall moves upwards and outwards when they contract.

The increase in thoracic volume produced by contraction of the diaphragm and intercostal muscles results in a fall of pressure in the thoracic cavity, and air then flows into the lungs to equalize external and internal pressures. Expiration during quiet breathing is largely a passive process brought about by the recoil of the diaphragm and chest wall when the muscles relax; it is assisted by contraction of other intercostal muscles which move the chest wall inwards and downwards. In forced expiration the muscles of the abdominal wall also take part. On contraction, they decrease the thoracic volume by drawing the lower ribs downwards and inwards and compressing the abdominal contents, thus forcing the diaphragm upwards.

Respiratory volumes. The volume of air breathed in and out in a single quiet respiration is called the *resting tidal volume* and amounts to about 500 ml. Adults at rest breath 12 to 15 times/min, giving a volume of 6–10 litres/min. During exercise, the increased rate and depth of respiratory movements increases the volume to as much as 70 litres/min.

After a maximal inspiration, the maximal volume of air which can then be expelled from the lungs by forceful effort is called the *vital capacity* (about 3·4 litres in adults). Even after the most forcible expiration, the lungs still contain about 1600 ml of air, which constitutes the *residual volume*. The total lung volume equals the sum of the vital capacity and residual volume and is of the order of 5–6 litres. These lung capacities are expressed diagrammatically in Fig. 11.2.

The volume of air entering the lungs in a given time is referred to as the pulmonary ventilation volume. The greatest volume of air that can be ventilated during a given time is the maximum ventilation volume. In the standard test the subject breathes as rapidly and deeply as possible for 15 sec. In young healthy adults the volume ranges from 82 to 169 litres/min.

REGULATION OF BREATHING. Respiratory movements are controlled and co-ordinated involuntarily by centres in the medulla oblongata, but considerable voluntary control may be superimposed. Until recently it was thought that an inspiratory centre in the medulla discharged continuously when isolated from its connections with other parts of the CNS, and that inspiratory activity was rhythmically inhibited by an expiratory centre in the medulla; the periodic activity of the expiratory centre was in turn influenced by a pneumotaxic centre in the pons which discharged intermittently, acting as a pacemaker for breathing movements. Recent work has led to some modifications of the concepts of central respiratory control. The main factors which are now believed to contribute to the central control of breathing are illustrated in Fig. 11.3. The respiratory centre is located in the lateral reticular formation of the medulla and its neurones may be divided into two groups, one concerned with inspiration and the other with expiration. The neurones in each group are arranged into separate self re-exciting chains so that once activity starts, it persists for a short time because repetitive firing reverberates

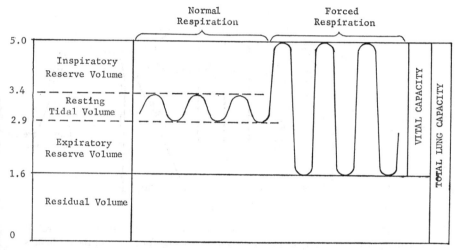

Fig. 11.2. Lung capacities.

round the chains. The two groups of neurones are interconnected by inhibitory fibres which ensure that, when one group is maximally active, the antagonistic group is inhibited. Thus activity in the inspiratory group causes a discharge of impulses downwards to the motoneurones supplying the inspiratory muscles of the thorax, and at the same time, a discharge laterally which inhibits activity in the expiratory group of neurones. As soon as the reverberation in the inspiratory group dies down, inhibition of the expiratory group is reduced. Activity then spreads through the expiratory neurones and impulses are discharged downwards to the expiratory muscles and at the same time they inhibit activity in the inspiratory neurones. In this way excitation oscillates from one group of neurones to the other bringing about the rhythmic movements of breathing.

When the respiratory centre is isolated from other neurones in the brain

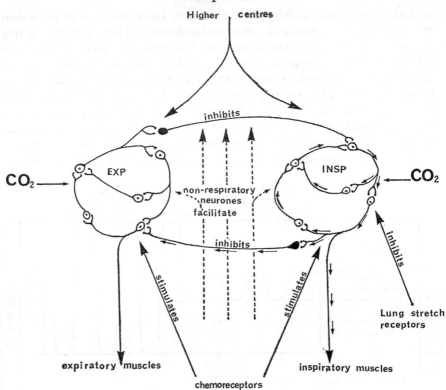

Higher centres

inhibits

CO_2 ⟶   ⟵ CO_2

EXP   INSP

non-respiratory
neurones
facilitate

inhibits

stimulates   stimulates   inhibits

Lung stretch
receptors

expiratory muscles   inspiratory muscles

chemoreceptors

FIG. 11.3. Diagram summarizing the main mechanisms involved in the control of breathing. The respiratory centre in the lateral reticular formation of the medulla is divided into an expiratory and an inspiratory group of self re-exciting neurones. Activity oscillates between these two groups because at the height of its activity, each group completely inhibits the other. The excitability of the centre is dependent on activity in adjacent non-respiratory systems and is under the control of higher centres. Excess CO_2 in the blood passing through the centre raises the excitability of its neurones and therefore stimulates breathing. Oxygen-lack stimulates breathing reflexly via the chemoreceptors. Activation of stretch receptors in the lungs reflexly inhibits inspiration.

stem it becomes quiescent. This is because its level of excitability is influenced by activity in other neurones, and it is capable of spontaneous discharge only when surrounded by a sufficient traffic of action potentials in non-respiratory systems. The mechanism through which activity in closely packed neurones influences the excitability of adjacent neurones is described on page 84. This dependence of the respiratory centre on activity in other neuronal systems may explain the respiratory stimulation produced by many forms of sensory stimuli, especially when respiration is depressed as, for example, by an anaesthetic. It also explains the onset of breathing in the new-born, in which the sensory input is suddenly increased at the moment of birth, and it provides a rational basis for the practice of slapping the baby to start it breathing, since this stimulus augments the sensory input.

The respiratory centre is influenced by higher centres of the brain. The cerebral cortex contains centres which both facilitate and inhibit breathing; these are probably concerned in the degree of voluntary control which can be exerted. A centre in the lateral hypothalamus also exerts a facilitating action on the respiratory centre. Connections between the vasomotor centre and the respiratory centre result in inhibition of breathing when the blood pressure rises.

Breathing is also influenced by reflex mechanisms initiated in the lungs and by the clinical constitution of blood and CSF. Inflation of the lungs stimulates stretch receptors in the airways and this causes a discharge of impulses in afferent fibres in the vagus nerves which builds up during each breath until, at a sufficient intensity, it inhibits inspiration. If the vagi are cut, inspiration is deeper; conversely, stimulation of the central end of the vagus inhibits inspiratory movements. The inhibition of inspiration by the stimulation of stretch receptors in the lungs is known as the Hering-Breuer reflex. Deflation of the lungs increases the rate and force of inspiratory efforts.

Chemoreceptors which respond to decreased oxygen in the blood are situated in the carotid and aortic bodies. The carotid body lies in the bifurcation of the common carotid artery; it is richly supplied with blood vessels and sensory nerve endings which run with the carotid sinus nerve. The aortic bodies are similar structures found at the root of the subclavian artery and scattered around the transverse part of the aortic arch. They contain the endings of sensory nerves which run in the vagi. When the oxygen supplied by the blood to the cells of the carotid and aortic bodies is inadequate, they metabolize anaerobically and it is believed that the metabolites so formed stimulate the chemosensory nerve endings. Whether an anaerobic metabolite itself is responsible for exciting the nerve endings, or whether it, in turn, causes the release of another humoral agent remains a matter of controversy. Acetylcholine causes a pronounced stimulation of the chemosensory nerves and the bodies are rich in cholinesterase, which suggests that a cholinergic mechanism may be involved. There are also chemoreceptors in the medulla which are affected by increased CO_2 and decreased pH of blood and CSF. Carbon dioxide diffuses rapidly into CSF where it lowers the pH because of the low buffering capacity of this fluid. This is probably the most important stimulus for central chemoreceptors.

10

CARBON DIOXIDE. An increase in the CO_2 tension of the blood increases the excitability of both the inspiratory and the expiratory centres in the medulla, and the rate and depth of breathing increase. This effect of CO_2 excess occurs even when the tension of O_2 in the arterial blood is normal. Lack of oxygen enhances the stimulant actions of CO_2 on the respiratory centre. The CO_2 tension may rise because of diminished respiratory movements or of increased metabolic activity, or as the result of acid production (when the ratio of CO_2 to HCO_3^- increases).

After a period of forced breathing (hyperpnoea), the tension of carbon dioxide in the blood falls but the oxygen tension barely changes because the blood is normally almost completely saturated with oxygen. As a result of the low carbon dioxide tension, the breath can be held (voluntary apnoea) for longer than normal because the blood does not possess its normal stimulating effect on the respiratory centre. If hyperpnoea is carried to excess, so much CO_2 is blown off that the pH-regulating mechanism of the blood is impaired, and a state of alkalaemia may occur.

The blood pH is determined mainly by the ratio of bicarbonate ion to carbon dioxide in solution according to Henderson-Hasselbalch equation (page 6). Respiration is therefore an important mechanism for regulating the pH of the blood, by altering the CO_2 tension in the blood.

OXYGEN. Oxygen-lack stimulates the chemoreceptors in the carotid and aortic bodies and thus induces a reflex stimulation of breathing. This effect of oxygen-lack is enhanced by the presence of excess carbon dioxide.

Although respiratory movements are very sensitive to small increases in the tension of carbon dioxide in the blood, they are not very sensitive to oxygen-lack, which is without any stimulant effect until the percentage of oxygen in the inspired air falls from the normal 21% to below 14%. The only direct effect of oxygen-lack on the respiratory centre is a depressant one due to decreased metabolic activity of the neurones at dangerously low O_2 tensions.

Pure oxygen may be breathed by man for several hours without ill-effect providing it is at atmospheric pressure. However, high oxygen pressures (3–4 atmospheres) cause toxic symptoms including faintness, fall in blood pressure and convulsions. High oxygen pressures have been found to poison many of the enzymes concerned with tissue oxidation and this effect, occurring in the central nervous system, probably gives rise to the toxic symptoms.

Respiratory movements are also influenced by stimuli arising from the baroreceptors of the carotid sinus and aortic arch (page 274). In experimental animals it can be demonstrated that a rise in blood pressure depresses breathing, and a fall in blood pressure stimulates it. However, this is probably of little significance for the physiological control of respiratory movements. Painful stimuli cause an initial apnoea followed by hyperpnoea.

CHEYNE-STOKES BREATHING. This is a form of periodic breathing in which groups of breaths are separated by periods of apnoea lasting up to 1 min. The breaths in each group may be of similar size, may gradually diminish in size, or may build up to a maximum and then decline. Cheyne-Stokes breathing occasionally occurs in man at high altitudes or during sleep, and is not uncommon in healthy babies. However, it is often a sign of serious depression of the respiratory centre and the periods of apnoea may be accompanied by loss of consciousness. The insensitivity of the respiratory centre is such that O_2 lack and an excessive accumulation of CO_2 are necessary to stimulate respiration. After a few breaths, the CO_2 tension of the arterial blood is reduced to a level too low to stimulate the centre and a period of apnoea follows until the CO_2 tension builds up again to a high level. The depression of the respiratory centre may arise from ischaemia of the medulla oblongata as a result either of heart failure or of a cerebral tumour or haemorrhage. The vasomotor centre responds to the reduced blood flow by inducing a rise in blood pressure which improves the blood supply to the medullary centres. The stimulus evoking the high blood pressure is thus diminished and the blood pressure falls again. The periodic breathing may therefore be accompanied by reciprocal variations in blood pressure. Cheyne-Stokes breathing may also occur in uraemia where the disturbed acid-base balance and accumulated metabolic products impair the activity of the respiratory centre.

COUGH. An accumulation of mucus or the presence of an irritant substance in the upper parts of the bronchi or trachea stimulates sensory receptors and this reflexly initiates coughing. The afferent fibres run in the vagus nerves. A preliminary deep inspiration is followed by a strong expiratory effort against a closed glottis, which results in a considerable rise in pressure in the airways. When the glottis is suddenly relaxed and the mouth opened, the air is released at high velocity and drives out the irritant material.

SNEEZE. Stimulation of the mucosa of the nasal passages or upper pharynx by chemical irritants or mechanical stimulation initiates a sneeze. Sneezing during bouts of hay fever or other allergic complaints is due to a combination of mechanical and chemical stimulations. The antigen (e.g. pollen) causes inflammation of the mucosa in sensitive subjects with increased secretion of mucus, and the threshold for stimulation of the sensory nerve endings is lowered, as it is in inflammatory conditions elsewhere. The sensory fibres run in the trigeminal nerves. A sneeze is preceded by a deep inspiration and this is followed by a rapid and powerful forced expiration with the mouth partly or completely closed.

HICCUP. This is an involuntary rapid inspiratory movement of the diaphragm during which the air flow is impeded by closure of the glottis. Persistent hiccup is often associated with inflammatory conditions of the thorax and abdomen. It may follow abdominal surgery, and often occurs in uraemia and in some diseases of the central nervous system. The treatments of hiccup—holding the breath, drinking cold water, rebreathing into a paper bag or inhaling CO_2, —probably work by altering the pattern of respiratory movements. In persistent hiccup it is sometimes necessary to destroy part of the phrenic nerve to lessen the severity of the spasms. Chlorpromazine (pages 595–598) has been used with success in some cases.

YAWN. A yawn is a prolonged inspiration during which the mouth is stretched wide open and the pharynx is widely dilated. It is usually part of a larger yawn-stretch reflex. The yawn is accompanied by a transient reflex vaso-constriction in the skin, as is any deep breath, and by a slight increase in heart rate. There is no evidence of any circulatory alteration elsewhere. Yawning may be induced by psychological influences or by fatigue but its cause and function are unknown. There is usually no overall increase in oxygenation as the yawn is followed by a short apnoeic period which cancels out any initial increase.

Exchange and transport of gases. Dry air contains about 21% oxygen and 79% nitrogen (by volume). The air in the alveoli is saturated with water vapour and differs in composition from the outside air because of the exchange of gases with the blood passing through the lungs. Samples of alveolar air, when dry contain about 14% oxygen, 80% nitrogen and 6% carbon dioxide.

The partial pressure of a constituent in a gas mixture is a more useful measure than percentage volume, since the amount of gas dissolving in a liquid is proportional to the partial pressure. The pressure of a gas mixture is equal to the sum of the partial pressure of its constituents. In alveolar air at baro-metric pressure and at the body temperature of 37° C the vapour pressure of water is 47 mmHg. The partial pressure of oxygen (P_{O_2}) is 100 mmHg and of carbon dioxide (P_{CO_2}) is 40 mmHg.

In the tissues at rest the amounts of dissolved oxygen and carbon dioxide are proportional to partial pressures of 35 mmHg (P_{O_2}) and about 46 mmHg (P_{CO_2}). The term 'tension' is sometimes used to express the amount dissolved; thus, the oxygen tension of the resting tissues is 35 mmHg. The rate of diffusion of oxygen and carbon dioxide across the alveolar and pulmonary capillary membranes and across the capillary membranes in the tissues is proportional to the partial pressure gradients. Oxygen passes from the alveolar air into the the blood because the partial pressure of oxygen in the alveolar air is higher than that in the blood arriving at the lungs. Carbon dioxide passes in the opposite direction because its partial pressure is highest in the blood arriving at the lungs. In the tissues, the situation is reversed; oxygen passes from blood to tissues and carbon dioxide enters the blood.

CARRIAGE OF OXYGEN. At a partial pressure of 100 mmHg, 0·3 ml oxygen dissolves in every 100 ml blood (0·3 vol.%). The amount of oxygen in simple solution in the blood is inadequate for complex forms of animal life and the evolutionary adaptation has been the development of respiratory pigments which bind larger amounts of oxygen in a loose complex. In the blood, these pigments allow the transport of more oxygen per unit volume. The best known respiratory pigment is the iron-containing haemoglobin, which is present in all vertebrates and many invertebrates. Other respiratory pigments are known; for example, haemocyanin, which is a blue copper-containing pigment, is present in molluscs and arthropods, and some marine worms have a green iron-containing pigment called chlorocruorin. In these lower animals the respiratory pigment is in free solution, but in vertebrates the haemoglobin is contained entirely in the erythrocytes.

Haemoglobin consists of the iron-containing porphyrin, haem, united with globin. The iron is in the ferrous form and each atom is attached to four pyrrole groups by valency bonds. A fifth bond is attached to globin and the sixth is available for combination with oxygen. The molecule of haemoglobin consists of four haemoglobin units and has a molecular weight of 67,000. Each of the four iron atoms in the molecule can combine with a molecule of oxygen, and the reversible reaction, which really occurs in four stages, may be written:

$$Hb_4 + 4O_2 \rightleftharpoons Hb_4O_8$$

The process is not one of *oxidation* but of *oxygenation*; the iron is present in the ferrous form in both haemoglobin and oxyhaemoglobin.

The amount of oxygen combined with haemoglobin in the erythrocytes depends on the oxygen tension in the surrounding plasma, the relationship being expressed as an S-shaped curve called the oxygen dissociation curve (Fig. 11.4). At O_2-partial pressures sufficient to saturate the haemoglobin completely, 20 ml of oxygen combines with the amount of haemoglobin normally present in 100 ml blood (14·6 g haemoglobin per 100 ml blood). At an O_2-partial pressure of 100 mmHg in the alveoli, each 100 ml of blood in the pulmonary vein contains 19 ml of oxygen in combination with haemoglobin (i.e. the haemoglobin is 95% saturated) and 0·3 ml oxygen in simple solution in the plasma. The rate of combination and dissociation of oxygen with haemoglobin is extremely rapid, and although the blood takes only about 0·5 sec to traverse a capillary in the lungs, this is more than sufficient time for equilibrium to be reached.

The oxygen tension in resting tissue cells is only about 35 mmHg. Oxygen in simple solution in the capillary plasma therefore rapidly diffuses out through the capillary wall and interstitial fluid to the tissue cell. As a result the oxygen tension in the blood falls to about 40 mmHg (complete equilibrium with the

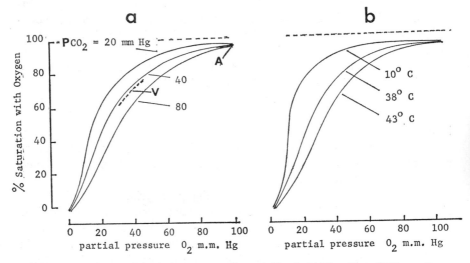

FIG. 11.4. Oxygen dissociation curves of human blood. (*a*) The effect of CO_2 on the oxygen dissociation curve at 38° C. With an increase in CO_2 the curve is shifted to the right (The Bohr Shift). A is the arterial point ($P_{O_2} = 100$ mmHg, $P_{CO_2} = 40$ mmHg), V is the venous point ($P_{O_2} = 40$ mmHg, $P_{CO_2} = 46$ mmHg). (*b*) The effect of temperature on the oxygen dissociation curve determined at a constant P_{CO_2} of 40 mmHg.

tissues is not reached). The amount of oxygen combined with haemoglobin at an oxygen tension of 40 mmHg is about 14 ml/100 ml of blood with a normal haemoglobin content, and the amount of oxygen in solution falls to 0·13 ml %. About 5 ml oxygen/100 ml is liberated from the erythrocytes. The venous blood therefore returns to the lungs with an oxygen tension of 40 mmHg and haemoglobin only 70% saturated. The oxygen given up to the tissues is then replaced in the lungs.

The oxygen content of the blood is influenced not only by the oxygen tension and haemoglobin content, but also by the amount of carbon dioxide carried simultaneously, and by the temperature. With an increase in carbon dioxide, less oxygen is carried, that is, the oxygen dissociation curve is shifted to the right (the Bohr Shift, Fig. 11.4a). Thus more oxygen is given up to tissues rich in carbon dioxide. An increase in temperature also shifts the oxygen dissociation curve to the right (Fig. 11.4b) and this effect is important when oxygen dissociation curves are being determined; the blood must be held at constant temperature.

CARRIAGE OF CARBON DIOXIDE. The P_{CO_2} of resting tissues is about 46 mmHg and carbon dioxide diffuses rapidly into the blood to reach equilibrium. Carbon dioxide is carried in three ways in the blood: in simple solution, as bicarbonate ion, and combined with protein including haemoglobin. Carbon dioxide is a more soluble gas than oxygen and at a P_{CO_2} of 46 mmHg about 3·5 vol.% is carried in simple solution. The carbon dioxide in solution is in equilibrium with carbonic acid. This equilibrium is achieved relatively slowly, but it is accelerated by carbonic anhydrase, which is present in the red cells, but not in the plasma. The carbonic acid is, in turn, in equilibrium with bicarbonate and hydrogen ions. The amount dissociated depends on the pH and on the demand made on the bicarbonate buffering capacity of the plasma.

Carbon dioxide reacts with the amino groups of the plasma proteins and of haemoglobin to form carbamino compounds:

$$-NH_2 + CO_2 \underset{\text{lungs}}{\overset{\text{tissues}}{\rightleftharpoons}} -NH.COOH$$

The amount combined with haemoglobin depends upon the oxygenation of haemoglobin. When haemoglobin is 100% oxygenated, all the combined CO_2 (3 ml%) is in the form of carbamino compounds with the plasma proteins, whereas with haemoglobin completely free of oxygen, an additional 5 ml% of CO_2 is combined as carbamino-haemoglobin. The blood from resting tissues is 70% saturated with oxygen and under these circumstances 0·7 ml% of CO_2 is carried as carbaminohaemoglobin, making the total carried as carbamino compounds equal to 3·7 ml%. More can be carried in this way during exercise because the haemoglobin gives up more oxygen.

The amounts of carbon dioxide in simple solution and as carbamino compounds together account for only 15–20% of that transported in the blood. By far the most important mechanism depends on the erythrocytes and their ability to form bicarbonate, and 80–85% of the CO_2 is carried in this way. The enzyme, carbonic anhydrase, is present in the blood only within the erythrocytes. Dissolved CO_2 in the plasma diffuses readily into the erythrocytes, where it is rapidly hydrated to form carbonic acid. The blood pH of 7·4 is on the alkaline side of the isoelectric point of haemoglobin, which therefore exists as a weak acid and can act as a hydrogen ion acceptor. The carbonic acid in the erythrocytes dissociates into hydrogen ions and bicarbonate ions. The hydrogen ions are mopped up by the haemoglobin molecules; bicarbonate ions accumulate and diffuse into the plasma under their concentration gradient.

The erythrocyte membrane is impermeable to the haemoglobin anion which remains within the cell, and the cations Na^+ and K^+ are restricted to the outside and inside of the cell respectively by metabolic processes similar to the 'sodium pump' described for nerve cells on page 74. However, some of the anions can diffuse across the erythrocyte membrane, the most important of

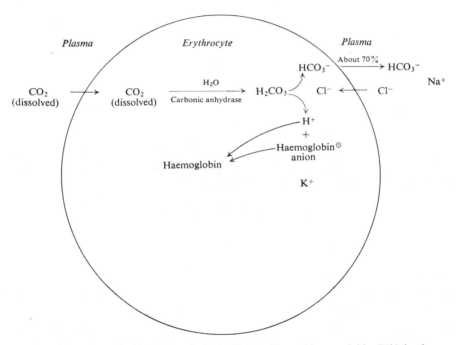

FIG. 11.5. The chloride shift and the buffering effect of haemoglobin (Hb) in the tissue capillaries.

these being HCO_3^- and Cl^-. These ions are therefore distributed across the erythrocyte membrane according to a Donnan equilibrium, thus:

$$\frac{[Cl^-]_{inside}}{[Cl^-]_{outside}} = \frac{[HCO_3^-]_{inside}}{[HCO_3^-]_{outside}}$$

The departure of each bicarbonate ion from the erythrocyte is therefore accompanied by the uptake of a chloride ion so that electro-chemical equilibrium is maintained. This mechanism is known as the *chloride shift* (or Hamburger shift). About 70% of the bicarbonate formed within the erythrocyte diffuses into the plasma, the rest remaining within the erythrocyte. The chloride shift across the erythrocyte membrane, and its relationship to the buffering action of haemoglobin, are illustrated in Fig. 11.5. The chloride shift from the plasma into the erythrocytes occurs in the tissue capillaries. The whole process is reversed when the blood reaches the lungs: chloride leaves the erythrocytes and bicarbonate enters; the bicarbonate is converted by carbonic anhydrase to CO_2 which passes into the plasma and diffuses through into the alveoli. The haemoglobin is simultaneously being oxygenated to oxyhaemoglobin.

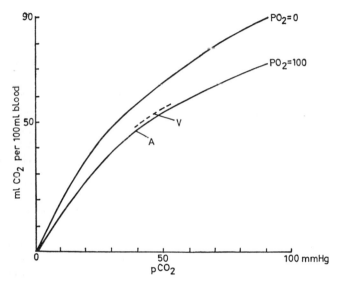

FIG. 11.6. The carbon dioxide dissociation curves of human blood at 37° C. A is the arterial point ($P_{O_2} = 100$ mmHg, $P_{CO_2} = 40$ mmHg and the blood contains 48 ml $CO_2\%$). V is the venous point ($P_{O_2} = 40$ mmHg, $P_{CO_2} = 46$ mmHg and the blood contains 52 ml $CO_2\%$).

The amount of carbon dioxide carried by venous blood is about 52 ml%. In the lungs it gives up about 4 ml leaving 48 ml%. The relationship between total carbon dioxide content and tension is given by the carbon dioxide dissociation curve (Fig. 11.6). Since saturation does not occur, percentage saturation is not employed and the ordinate in Fig. 11.6 is millilitres of CO_2 per 100 ml blood. The curve is affected by oxygenation of the blood, being moved to the right by an increase in oxygenation.

Table 11.1 gives the amounts of oxygen and carbon dioxide carried by the blood at the tensions existing in arterial blood and in venous blood leaving resting tissues.

10*

CARRIAGE OF NITROGEN. At atmospheric pressure, the partial pressure of nitrogen in the alveolar air is 573 mmHg. It is about half as soluble as oxygen and each 100 ml of blood therefore contains about 0·85 ml of nitrogen in simple solution. At high atmospheric pressures, such as are necessary in diving bells, more nitrogen is dissolved. If the pressure is released too suddenly, the excess nitrogen quickly comes out of solution and forms bubbles throughout the body. The pain produced by bubbles forming in the synovial fluid of the joints is known as the 'bends'. Bubbles may also form in the CNS and lead to damage of the nerve cells. Decompression must therefore be brought about gradually.

TABLE 11.1.

Gas	Carried:	Arterial blood $P_{CO_2} = 40$ mmHg	Venous blood $P_{CO_2} = 46$ mmHg
CO_2	In solution	3 ml%	3·5 ml%
	As carbamino compounds	3 ml%	3·7 ml%
	As bicarbonate	42 ml%	44·8 ml%
	TOTAL	48 ml%	52 ml%
		$P_{O_2} = 100$ mmHg	$P_{O_2} = 40$ mmHg
O_2	In solution	0·3 ml%	0·13 ml%
	Combined with haemoglobin	19 ml%	14 ml%
	TOTAL	19·3 ml%	14·13 ml%

Anoxia. Oxygen lack in the body is termed anoxia; four types of anoxia can be recognized: (1) anoxic anoxia, (2) anaemic anoxia, (3) stagnant anoxia, and (4) histotoxic anoxia.

ANOXIC ANOXIA. In this condition the oxygen tension in the arterial blood is low. This may be caused by a low partial pressure of oxygen in the air (the proportion of oxygen may be low, or the air pressure may be low as at high altitudes), or there may be an alteration in the alveolar epithelium so that oxygen transfer is reduced; some war gases have this latter effect.

ANAEMIC ANOXIA. In this condition the oxygen-carrying capacity of the blood is low. It may result from severe anaemia, from a massive blood loss, or from impairment of the formation of oxyhaemoglobin.

Carbon monoxide poisoning results in an anaemic anoxia. Carbon monoxide combines with haemoglobin in the same manner as does oxygen, occupying the free linkage of the iron atoms to form carboxyhaemoglobin. The affinity of haemoglobin for carbon monoxide is about 250 times that for oxygen, and carboxyhaemoglobin is a more stable compound than oxyhaemoglobin. In carbon monoxide poisoning, therefore, some of the haemoglobin is no longer available for combination with oxygen. A carbon monoxide tension of only 0·4 mmHg causes a dangerous degree of carboxyhaemoglobinaemia. The symptoms of carbon monoxide poisoning are headache, vomiting, dizziness, mental confusion and shooting pains in the muscles. The chemoreceptors of the carotid and aortic bodies are sensitive to a fall in the P_{O_2} of the blood, but in carbon monoxide poisoning the usual amount of oxygen is dissolved in the plasma and therefore the oxygen tension is normal. Consequently, there is no oxygen-lack stimulus to breathing.

Anaemic anoxia also occurs if the ferrous iron of haemoglobin is oxidized to the ferric condition in which form it combines firmly with oxygen to form the stable *methaemoglobin* from which the oxygen is not released in the tissues. Methaemoglobin formation results from poisoning with nitrites and is a side-effect of treatment with some sulphonamide drugs.

STAGNANT ANOXIA. The circulation is at fault in this condition. It occurs as a result of cardiac failure, haemorrhage and shock. The oxygen tension of the arterial blood is normal but the rate of flow of blood through the tissues is too low to maintain adequate tissue respiration.

HISTOTOXIC ANOXIA. After large doses of many drugs, the dehydrogenase systems of the body are depressed and the tissues cannot utilize the oxygen.

Tissue respiration. During vigorous exercise, muscle requires as much as forty-eight times more oxygen than when at rest. This is achieved by circulatory adjustments as well as by an increase in the oxygen uptake by the muscles from a given volume of blood. Cardiac output, and hence lung blood-flow, increases about six times to 30 litres/min. At the same time, vasoconstriction in the skin and splanchnic region and vasodilatation in muscle cause a redistribution of blood so that, if cardiac output had remained constant, muscle blood flow would have increased about three-fold. This effect, coupled with a six-fold increase in cardiac output, means that muscle blood-flow is increased by about eighteen times. The oxygen tension in the interstitial fluid surrounding the active muscle cells is very low and the blood gives up a correspondingly greater amount of oxygen. Instead of the 5 ml of O_2 usually given up by 100 ml of blood the amount may be as high as 15 ml O_2/100 ml. This three-fold increase, together with the eighteen-fold increase in blood flow, means that fifty-four times the amount of oxygen required at rest is available for the active muscles. Breathing is correspondingly increased so that the blood is adequately re-oxygenated.

Muscles, particularly red muscles (page 207), contain the respiratory pigment *myoglobin* which resembles haemoglobin except that its molecule consists of only one haem unit combined with one molecule of globin. Each molecule of myoglobin therefore contains one iron atom and consequently combines

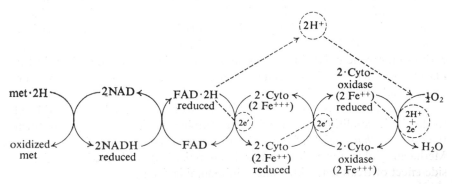

FIG. 11.7. Oxidation through the respiratory chain. NAD (nicotinic acid dinucleotide or coenzyme I, page 23) oxidizes the metabolite (met. 2H) by removing hydrogen atoms, itself becoming reduced. The reduced form of NAD is re-oxidized by FAD (flavin adenine dinucleotide, page 24) which takes up the hydrogen atoms. These reactions are catalysed by dehydrogenase enzymes. Cytochrome (Cyto) re-oxidizes FAD by taking up electrons (e′) and liberating hydrogen ions. The iron in the porphyrin of the cytochrome is reduced from the ferric to the ferrous form. Oxidation is continued by electron transfer along the cytochrome chain. The final stage involves cytochrome oxidase (Cyto-oxidase), the reduced form of which gives up its electrons and these recombine with hydrogen ions and oxygen to form water.

with only one molecule of oxygen. Myoglobin has a greater affinity for oxygen than does haemoglobin, and at a P_{O_2} of 40 mmHg it is 95% saturated. Hence myoglobin can extract oxygen from the blood haemoglobin. The oxygen dissociation curve of myoglobin is not shifted to the right by an increase in P_{CO_2}. When a muscle is in contraction, its blood vessels are temporarily occluded and the blood supply is reduced. Myoglobin then acts as an oxygen store during the period of ischaemia, and can hand over adequate oxygen for oxidative metabolism to continue even at a P_{O_2} as low as 5 mmHg.

The haemoglobin in the blood of the foetus differs from that in the adult in that it has a greater affinity for oxygen; therefore it becomes fully oxygenated in the placenta, while the maternal blood is de-oxygenated. The foetal form of haemoglobin is replaced by the adult type in the first few days after parturition.

The energy-yielding metabolic processes in the tissues are, for the most part, oxidative (pages 41–45). However, the reactions usually do not utilize molecular oxygen directly. The metabolites are oxidized by dehydrogenation, the hydrogens being transferred to various hydrogen acceptors by reactions catalysed by dehydrogenases. The hydrogen acceptors are coenzymes which are converted to the reduced form. They are re-oxidized by transferring hydrogen to the cytochrome system.

The cytochromes, or tissue respiratory pigments, are conjugated proteins containing iron–porphyrin prosthetic groups (allied to haem). The iron is reduced to the ferrous form by taking up an electron from the hydrogen of the reduced coenzyme (flavin) which is therefore re-oxidized, and hydrogen ion is released. The cytochrome then passes on the electron to the iron of cytochrome oxidase and itself returns to the oxidized ferric state. *Reduced cytochrome oxidase* differs from the other participants in the chain of substances involved in tissue oxidations in that it is readily oxidized by molecular oxygen. In the presence of molecular oxygen, reduced cytochrome oxidase gives up its electrons which recombine with hydrogen ions to form atomic hydrogen and this forms water with molecular oxygen. Some of the links in the chain of reactions involved in the oxidation of a metabolite in mitochondria are shown in Fig. 11.7. The main function of respiratory oxygen can be considered as keeping the cytochromes in the oxidized condition.

CHAPTER 12

The Digestive System and the Liver

The digestive system consists of the alimentary canal and the accessory digestive glands. It is concerned with the digestion and absorption of food. The food passing along the alimentary canal is digested by hydrolase enzymes, which split proteins, most carbohydrates and fats into smaller molecules suitable for absorption. Some substances in the diet—water, mineral salts, vitamins and glucose—are already in a suitable form for absorption. The main constituents which are necessary for the nutritional requirements of the body are described on pages 28–38. Some constituents of foodstuffs are not digested in man as the appropriate enzymes are absent from the digestive tract; these constituents have no nutritive value and pass through the small intestine to be expelled in the faeces. The inclusion of some of these substances (e.g. cellulose and pectin) in the diet may be advantageous since they confer bulk to the intestinal contents and so improve propulsion.

The alimentary canal

The major divisions of the human alimentary canal are the mouth, pharynx, oesophagus, stomach, small intestine, large intestine and anus. The abdominal portion of the alimentary canal—the lower end of the oesophagus, the stomach and the intestines—is sometimes referred to as the gastro-intestinal tract or as the splanchnic viscera.

The mouth. The epithelial lining of the mouth is composed of stratified squamous cells. Embryologically, it is derived from ectoderm, but it differs from the epithelium of the skin in that the outer layers of cells are not keratinized. The surface of the epithelium is continually renewed, the dislodged cells being found in the saliva. The first preparation of food ready for the digestive processes takes place in the mouth. Pieces of food may be taken in by biting and these are further reduced in size by chewing. The jaws are closed by contraction of the powerful masseter muscles, the force exerted by the teeth during biting being as much as 90 kg. The rhythmic movements of chewing take place without volition; the presence of food in the mouth causes a reflex closure of the jaw by contraction of the masseter muscles, and then the increase in tension detected by spindle receptors in the masseters reflexly produces relaxation of the jaw. Mastication of the food with saliva aids the first of the

302

digestive processes by the salivary enzymes. Movements of the tongue place the food in position between the teeth and form the masticated food into a bolus of a suitable size for swallowing. The muscle in the tongue is composed of striated fibres arranged in bundles running in several directions, thus giving mobility of movement. This muscle is under voluntary control. The surface of

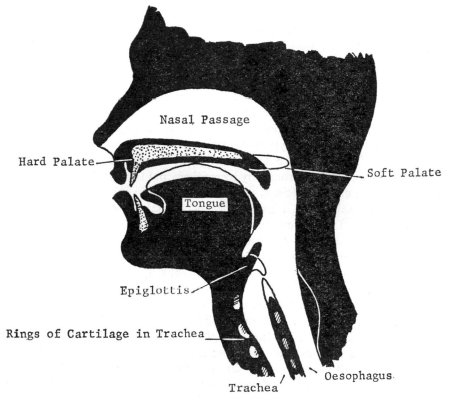

Nasal Passage

Hard Palate

Soft Palate

Tongue

Epiglottis

Rings of Cartilage in Trachea

Oesophagus

Trachea

FIG. 12.1. The upper part of the alimentary canal. The change in position of some of the structures during deglutition is indicated.

the tongue is covered with a mucous membrane in which lie the sensory receptors subserving taste (pages 426–428) and also receptors sensitive to touch, temperature and pain. In the first part of the act of swallowing (or deglutition), the mouth is closed and the tongue is raised against the hard palate so that the food bolus is forced back against the pharynx, causing stimulation of stretch receptors in the pharyngeal wall and initiating a number of reflexes. The nasal passages are closed by the elevation of the soft palate, the entrance to the trachea is closed by the downward movement of the epiglottis and the upward movement of the trachea, and the pharyngeal end of the oesophagus relaxes to admit the bolus: the mechanisms may be understood by reference to Fig. 12.1. Respiratory movements are inhibited during swallowing (deglutition apnoea).

SALIVA. In man, 1 to 2 litres of saliva are secreted each day from the three pairs of salivary glands as well as from secretory cells in the mucous membrane. The first stage of carbohydrate digestion begins in the mouth. Saliva contains an enzyme, salivary amylase (or ptyalin), which catalyses the hydrolysis of starch to yield first dextrins and then maltose. Ptyalin requires the presence of chloride ions and a pH of about 6 for its optimal activity. Digestion by ptyalin continues for about $\frac{1}{2}$ h after the food enters the stomach and then the enzyme is inhibited by the increase in acidity of the stomach contents. Saliva contains inorganic ions including chloride, and has a pH of about 6, being buffered by bicarbonate. The electrolyte composition of salivary secretion differs from that of plasma, and therefore it is formed by active processes. Thiocyanate is secreted into the saliva, particularly by smokers, but the significance of this is not known. The mucin present in saliva lubricates the food bolus, thus assisting its passage in swallowing; it also lubricates the oral mucosa so assisting the free movements of the tongue in the mouth which are necessary for speech. An enzyme called lysozyme secreted with the mucus attacks a bacterial mucopolysaccharide and so may help to prevent infection. Freely diffusible substances occurring in the plasma (e.g. urea) also appear in the saliva.

THE SALIVARY GLANDS. In man the three pairs of salivary glands are the parotid, the submaxillary and the sublingual. The parotid contains only serous cells, and the secretion is rich in ptyalin. The other two glands contain both serous and mucous secreting cells; their secretion is rich in mucin and contains only a little ptyalin. The serous cells contain granules of zymogen which is the precursor form of ptyalin, and the mucous cells contain larger granules of mucinogen. The secretory portions of the glands are composed of alveoli which are connected to the oral cavity by ducts. In the mixed alveoli, the serous cells often appear as crescents (demi-lune cells), peripheral to the mucous cells: the secretion from them runs through fine canaliculi between the mucous cells. Diagrams of the alveoli are shown in Fig. 12.2.

The salivary glands are innervated by both sympathetic and parasympathetic fibres. Sympathetic stimulation elicits a small quantity of viscid saliva rich in enzymes (with degranulation of the serous cells), and parasympathetic stimulation produces a copious flow of saliva poor in ptyalin (with degranulation of the mucous cells). Secretion is stimulated reflexly, the composition of the saliva depending on the stimulus; for example, stimulation of the taste buds by food calls forth a secretion rich in ptyalin and mucin, but secretion stimulated by acid or bitter substances elicits a more copious thinner saliva containing less ptyalin. The reflex for salivary secretion may be conditioned (page 135), and probably the conditioned reflexes predominate in initiating secretion. The nervous pathways involved in salivation are illustrated in Fig. 12.3.

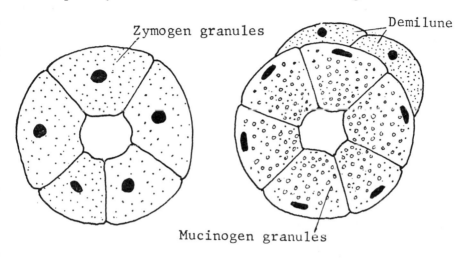

FIG. 12.2. Salivary gland alveoli.

Oesophagus. The oesophagus begins in the neck where it connects with the pharynx, runs through the thorax and enters the abdomen where it joins with the stomach. In man, it is about 1 ft long. Four layers may be distinguished in the wall of the oesophagus. They are an outer adventitial layer of connective tissue, a muscular layer containing circularly and longitudinally arranged fibres, a submucosa of loose connective tissue containing mucous glands and smooth muscle fibres (the muscularis mucosae), and an inner epithelial layer of stratified squamous cells. In the upper part of the oesophagus most of the muscle fibres are striated, in the middle portion both striated and smooth fibres are present, and in the lower part smooth muscle predominates. The principal innervation of the oesophagus is by the vagus nerves, which supply both motoneurones to the striated muscle and parasympathetic fibres to the smooth muscle. Sensory fibres from the oesophagus also run in the vagi; they are activated by distension of the lumen. In the act of swallowing, the presence of the bolus in the oesophageal lumen reflexly causes relaxation of the circular muscle below the bolus and contraction of that above the bolus, thus driving it along the tube into the stomach. These reflex movements are coordinated by a swallowing centre in the medulla oblongata. The rate of passage of materials along the oesophagus depends on their consistency. Liquids are conveyed rapidly in aliquots, each corresponding to the amount forced into the pharynx in the first stage of swallowing. Viscous fluids are conveyed more slowly, and a

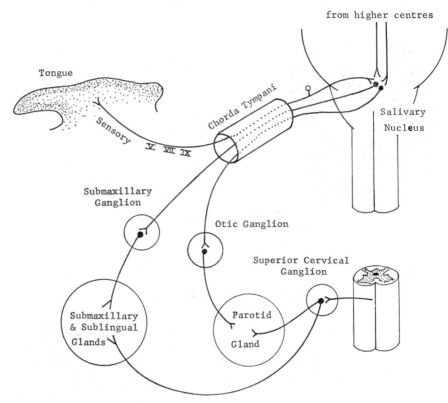

FIG. 12.3. Nerve pathways involved in salivation.

solid mass formed into a bolus moves more slowly still. In normal circumstances in man, gravity aids the movements of the oesophageal contents, and an oesophagus which is occluded by a carcinoma or which has been severely damaged by corrosive poisons can be replaced by an inert tube. But with a normal oesophagus, swallowing is possible without gravity (e.g. in space flight) and even against gravity, in which case the contraction waves are more powerful. Contractions of the oesophagus which are ineffective in moving a swallowed mass give rise to a painful sensation; this may occur when a swallowed mass becomes lodged, or when the circular muscle in advance of the mass fails to relax. The rings of circular smooth muscle at the upper and lower ends of the oesophagus are more powerful than elsewhere along its length, and, except during swallowing, they remain in a state of tonic contraction: these regions are described as the pharyngeal and cardiac sphincters, respectively.

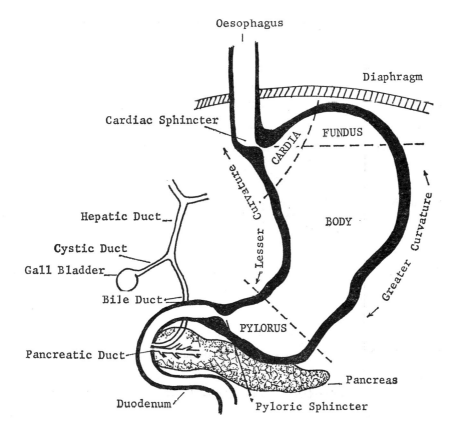

FIG. 12.4. Diagram of the stomach from its anterior aspect showing its relation with other structures.

Muscle fibres of the muscularis mucosae are especially abundant at the lower end of the oesophagus and are thought to be the major contribution of muscle to the cardiac sphincter. When this sphincter is incompetent and admits a reflux of gastric contents, the resultant stimulation of the lower end of the oesophagus gives rise to a painful sensation referred to the wall of the thorax; this is one of the causes of the pain described as 'heartburn'.

Stomach. The entrance to the stomach is through the cardiac sphincter. The size and shape of the stomach varies considerably in different people, and in any one person from time to time depending on its contents, on the other abdominal contents and on the posture. The stomach is distensible, its capacity being 1 to 2 litres. The parts of the stomach are shown in Fig. 12.4. The cardia

TABLE 12.1. The structure of the regions of the stomach wall.

Layer	Region of stomach			
	Cardia	Fundus	Body	Pylorus
Serosa (outer)	Connective tissue membrane, continuous with the peritoneum and omentum			
Muscularis	Outer longitudinal layer and inner circular layer	Outer longitudinal layer, middle circular layer and inner oblique layer		
Submucosa	――――――――――――――――Connective tissue――――――――――――――			
				Some mucous glands
Mucosa (inner)	―――――――――――――Simple columnar epithelium―――――――――――			
	Cardiac glands	Gastric glands―――――――		Pyloric glands

is immediately adjacent to the junction with the oesophagus: the line of demarcation shows clearly from the mucosal surface because of the change in the type of epithelium from stratified squamous to simple columnar. The fundus is that part of the stomach above the insertion of the oesophagus: it contains swallowed air. The pylorus has thicker sheets of muscle in its walls than the other parts of the stomach and its junction with the thin-walled duodenum is usually quite abrupt. The body of the stomach is that part between the fundus and the pylorus. The wall of the stomach contains four layers

(Table 12.1); the variations in structure in different parts of the stomach are not abrupt and can only be identified histologically.

The epithelium of the stomach is principally concerned with secretion, but water, alcohol and other non-ionized substances of low molecular weight and some drugs (see pages 486 and 492) are absorbed.

The glands in the cardia and the pylorus secrete an alkaline viscid mucus, whose function is principally that of protecting the epithelium. The gastric glands consist of infoldings of the mucosa which form deep pits lined by secretory epithelium containing three types of cells. Goblet cells secrete mucin; these cells are mostly near the mouths of the gastric pits. Peptic (or chief) cells secrete pepsinogen (the inactive precursor of the proteolytic enzyme, pepsin); pepsinogen is present in the cells as granules. Oxyntic (or parietal) cells secrete hydrochloric acid; these cells lie slightly behind the peptic cells and their secretion passes into the gastric pit through canaliculi between the other cells.

GASTRIC JUICE. There is a continuous resting secretion from the glands of the stomach, but the secretion of most of the gastric juice is stimulated by eating and by the presence of food in the stomach. In man, 2 to 3 litres of gastric juice are secreted each day. It contains mucin, electrolytes and enzymes, and has a pH of 1 to 2 due to the hydrochloric acid it contains. The principal enzyme is pepsin, for which the optimum pH is between 2 and 4. Pepsinogen (MW, 42,000) is converted to pepsin (MW, 36,000) by the loss of part of the molecule known as 'pepsin inhibitor'; this loss begins in acid media and is autocatalytic. The particular peptide link which is hydrolysed by pepsin is that between the amino group of tyrosine or phenylalanine and the carboxylic group of a dibasic amino acid (lysine or arginine):

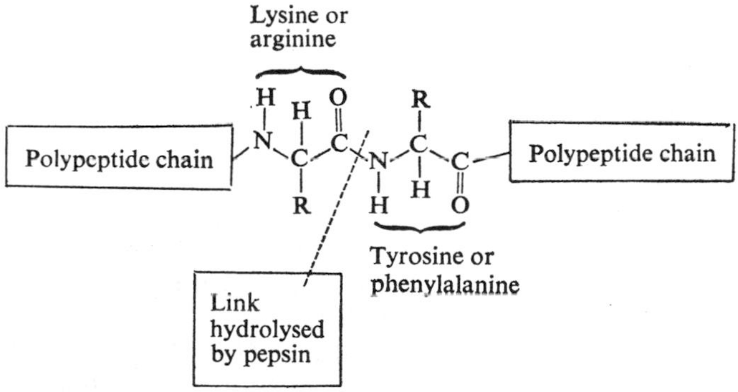

In vitro, gastric juice hydrolyses proteins completely to amino acids, but during digestion in the stomach it only acts so far as to convert proteins into smaller polypeptides called peptones.

In young animals the gastric juice contains another enzyme called rennin. This enzyme coagulates milk by converting the milk protein, caseinogen, to an insoluble form, casein. In addition, rennin is proteolytic and liberates peptones from the coagulum. The oxyntic cells are not fully functional in infants and the gastric juice is less acid. The optimal pH for rennin is about 4 to 5.

Gastric juice also contains a factor (intrinsic factor) whose presence is necessary for the absorption of vitamin B_{12} in the intestine. The exact nature of intrinsic factor is not known, but the absorption of vitamin B_{12} is impaired when the oxyntic glands are absent or not functional, and the symptoms of deficiency then occur (pages 34 and 238–240).

The electrolyte composition of the secretion of the oxyntic cells closely resembles that of plasma, with the difference that it contains H^+ in place of some of the sodium: it can be considered as containing hydrochloric acid with a strength of 0·1 to 0·15N. The secretion is formed by the exchange of chloride ions from the plasma with bicarbonate ions produced by the metabolic activity of the oxyntic cells, as illustrated below.

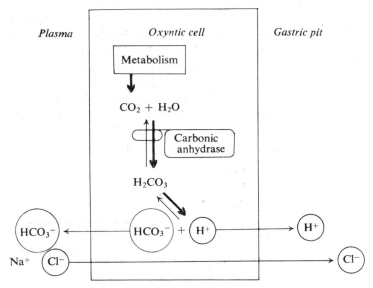

In the absence of carbonic anhydrase, these changes do not occur fast enough to form the usual amounts of acid secretion.

The determination of the content of acid and of chloride in gastric juice is an important diagnostic procedure. The juice is collected after stimulating secretion either by eating a specially prepared gruel 'test meal', by drinking a dose of 7% alcohol, or by the subcutaneous injection of histamine. The functions of gastric acid include activation of pepsin, inhibition of salivary amylase, the swelling of collagen fibres in food masses and stimulation of pancreatic secretion: the nature of the bacterial population of the stomach is affected by the predominant pH of gastric secretion.

The food remains in the stomach for 2 to 6 h, during which time gastric digestion converts the food masses into a smooth fluid called chyme.

Control of gastric secretion. Samples of stomach contents and secretions may be removed for examination by withdrawal through a stomach tube. The tip of the tube is introduced into the mouth or through the nostrils and is then swallowed until it rests in the stomach. A closer examination may be made when there is a hole from the exterior of the body through to the interior of the stomach. Such a hole, known as a gastric fistula, is sometimes formed in man as a result of injury or is made surgically in man and in experimental animals. A convenient preparation for studying gastric secretion in experimental animals may be made by cutting out a segment of the stomach and transferring it to the surface of the body with the mucosal side outwards. The blood vessels and nerves supplying the transferred portion are left intact. A structure formed in this way is known as a Pavlov pouch. A similar preparation, but without the nerve supply, is known as a Heidenhain pouch. The remainder of the stomach is closed and it continues to function normally. The secretions formed in response to stimulation of the nerves to the stomach, to the ingestion of food, or to other stimuli may be examined by these means.

Food taken into the mouth serves as a stimulus for the formation of gastric juice. Stimulation of the taste buds causes a reflex excitation via a centre in the medulla oblongata. This reflex is readily conditioned so that the sight, smell or thought of food, or even of other stimuli originally unrelated to food, become effective stimuli for secretion (page 135). A fall in blood sugar stimulates the nuclei of the vagal secretory fibres in the medulla. During the nervous or primary phase of gastric secretion the gastric juice is rich in both pepsin and acid.

The secondary phase of secretion is initiated by the presence of food in the stomach, which causes the release from the pyloric region of a polypeptide known as *gastrin*. Proteins, and particularly peptones, are most effective in causing the release of gastrin, which then passes into the venous blood leaving the pylorus and reaches the gastric glands after passing through the general circulation. Secretion into a Heidenhain pouch after food enters the main stomach is mediated by gastrin. The secretion is rich in acid but low in pepsin, and it is thought that gastrin acts specifically on the oxyntic cells. Mechanical distension of the stomach, particularly of the pylorus, causes the release of gastrin. Maximal secretion of gastric juice requires excitation both by the vagus and by gastrin. Histamine also stimulates the secretion of oxyntic cells and histamine is present in considerable amounts in the gastric mucosa but it has not been established that it plays a physiological role in the control of gastric secretion.

Gastric activity is also controlled by the inhibiting hormone, enterogastrone, which is released into the blood-stream from the duodenal mucosa when fat is present in the duodenum. Enterogastrone inhibits the secretion of acid and of pepsin, depresses stomach movements and delays emptying time. A substance extracted from urine, called *urogastrone*, produces similar effects.

Peptic ulcer. The secretion of mucin normally protects the mucosa itself from being digested by the gastric juices. However, should erosion of the mucosa occur, the damaged area is liable to further attack as it lacks the usual protection and a peptic ulcer is formed. Vagal overactivity appears to be an important causal factor. Thus, peptic ulcer may arise from stimulation of hypothalamic vagal centres either resulting from lesions or induced by drugs. Ulcers commonly occur in the stomach and duodenum or more rarely in the oesophagus. Duodenal ulcers are formed when there is an overabundant gastric secretion and a too rapid emptying of the stomach with the result that a large volume of acid gastric juice enters the duodenum; the excess of acid is not neutralized by duodenal secretions, and the active pepsin erodes the duodenal mucosa. Duodenal ulcer is commonly seen in patients with a worrying disposition. Gastric ulcers occur when there is excessive secretion of gastric juice into the empty stomach. They tend to occur in patients given to anxiety or emotional outbursts. Oesophageal ulcers result from reflux of gastric contents caused by spasms of the stomach and an incompetent cardiac sphincter. A peptic ulcer sometimes follows severe injury, particularly by burning. The excessive secretion of gastric juice under these circumstances is probably due to the liberation of histamine from the damaged tissues.

Movements of the stomach. The muscular walls of the empty stomach are in a state of tonic contraction and they relax to accommodate the stomach contents. The movement of chyme towards the pylorus is produced by peristaltic waves of contraction of circular muscle which begin at about the middle of the stomach body. They occur at intervals of 20 sec and take about 20 sec to travel to the pylorus. The pyloric sphincter contracts when the wave is moving towards it, and relaxes in the intervals. This arrangement allows the outflow of the most fluid portion of the chyme, while retaining the thicker portions in the stomach. The rate and intensity of the movements are decreased by enterogastrone. During fasting, bouts of powerful contractions give rise to the sensation described as hunger pangs.

The movements of the stomach are coordinated by the plexus of nerve fibres and ganglia lying between the longitudinal and circular muscle layers. Stimulation of the extrinsic nerves to the stomach muscles produces complex effects.

Stimulation of the vagi causes contraction and increases peristaltic movements, but the response to stimulation of the sympathetic nerves may be relaxation or contraction depending on the pre-existing conditions and experimental circumstances.

VOMITING. The complex series of movements which occur during vomiting are as follows: (1) The epiglottis closes and remains so till the vomited material is expelled. (2) The pylorus of the stomach contracts, forcing the gastric contents into the relaxed body of the stomach. (3) The flaccid stomach is compressed by descent of the diaphragm and contraction of the abdominal wall. (4) The cardiac sphincter and oesophagus are relaxed, so that the stomach contents are driven into the dilated oesophagus. (5) The diaphragm ascends (relaxes) and the intercostal muscles and abdominal wall contract resulting in compression of the oesophagus, which also may exhibit anti-peristalsis and longitudinal contraction with the result that its contents are forced into the mouth. (6) At the same time the soft palate is raised, so preventing vomit entering the nasal cavity.

These movement are controlled and coordinated through a vomiting centre in the reticular formation of the medulla oblongata. Vomiting may arise reflexly as a result of afferent impulses passing to the vomiting centre from the stomach and other parts of the alimentary canal, from the vestibular apparatus (e.g. motion sickness), from the heart and from other organs. It may also result from emotional disturbances such as fear. The vomiting centre is sensitized by another centre in the medulla, called the chemoreceptive trigger zone, which has neuronal connections with the vomiting centre. Certain drugs (e.g. apomorphine) or local damage to the brain may stimulate the chemoreceptive trigger zone which in turn activates the vomiting centre.

The small intestine. This part of the alimentary canal extends from the pylorus of the stomach to the proximal end of the large intestine: in man, it is about 20 ft long when fully relaxed, but in life its smooth muscle is in a state of tonic contraction and the length is usually about 7 ft. The processes of digestion, which are started in the mouth and stomach, are carried to completion in the small intestine with the aid of secretions from its epithelium and from accessory glands. The absorption of most of the nutrients takes place through the epithelium of the small intestine: they are carried away in the blood and lymphatic vessels.

The small intestine is divided into three regions, the *duodenum*, the *jejunum* and the *ileum*. There are slight differences between these regions with a gradual transition between them, but the general arrangement of the tissues comprising the wall is, in principle, the same throughout its length; it is shown diagrammatically in Fig. 12.5. There are four layers, the *serosa*, the *muscularis*, the *submucosa* and the *mucosa*.

The outer serous layer (or serosa) consists of a membrane of connective tissue which is continuous with the mesentery and the lining of the abdominal cavity. These membranes, collectively known as *peritoneum*, enclose the peritoneal cavity. The mesentery is a double membrane of connective tissue

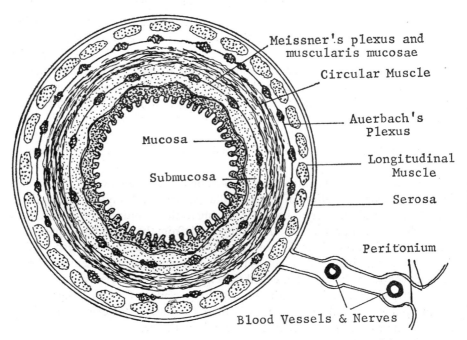

Fig. 12.5. Generalized arrangement of tissues in a transverse section of the gastro-intestinal tract.

attached at the midline of the posterior abdominal wall. It supports the intestines but at the same time allows them considerable freedom of movement.

The muscularis contains two layers of smooth muscle; the outer layer, lying immediately beneath the serosa, has longitudinally arranged fibres, and the inner layer has circularly arranged fibres. Between the two muscle layers there are many ganglion cells and a network of nerve fibres, termed the *myenteric plexus of Auerbach*. Nerve fibres from the plexus innervate both muscle layers.

The next layer, the submucosa, consists of adipose connective tissue. In the duodenum the submucosa contains the secretory alveoli of glands. Another network of nerve fibres and ganglion cells in the submucosa is known as the *submucous plexus of Meissner*. The *lamina propria* divides the submucosa from the mucosa. This is a fibro-elastic connective tissue containing loosely arranged smooth muscle fibres of the *muscularis mucosae*; these muscle cells are innervated by axons from Meissner's plexus. The lamina propria also contains

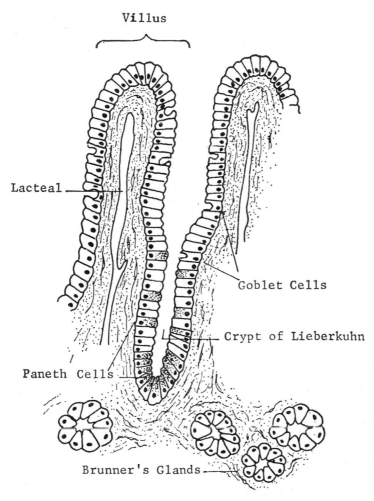

Villus

Lacteal

Goblet Cells

Crypt of Lieberkuhn

Paneth Cells

Brunner's Glands

FIG. 12.6. Mucosa and submucosa of the duodenum.

many blood vessels and lymphatics. The basement membrane of the epithelial cells of the mucosa is formed by fibres of the lamina propria. Many of the epithelial cells are adapted for special functions: some are absorptive and have a brush border; others are secretory and contain granules or appear as goblet cells (see pages 60–61); the *enterochromaffin cells*, which contain 5-hydroxytryptamine (page 179), are also present in the mucosa.

The mucosa is thrown into folds arranged circularly, and has vast numbers of fine projections known as *villi*. The villi are from 0·5 to 1·5 mm high and there are from 10 to 40/mm². These structures have the effect of increasing the surface area of the mucosa. The folds and villi have a core of submucosa or lamina propria. Each villus contains a central, blind-ended lymphatic vessel known as a *lacteal*, blood vessels connected with an extensive capillary network, and muscle fibres of the muscularis mucosae. Most of the epithelial cells of the villi have a brush border. Between the villi there are tubes of epithelium which penetrate about 0·5 mm into the submucosa; these are called the crypts of Lieberkühn. The cells at the bottom of the crypts are packed with a dense mass of acidophil secretory granules; these are known as the *cells of Paneth*. There are also scattered goblet cells. A diagram of villi and a crypt is shown in Fig. 12.6.

Duodenum. The submucosa of the duodenum contains many branched and coiled secretory tubules with excretory ducts emptying into the crypts; they are known as Brunner's glands (Fig. 12.6). Their secretion is an alkaline mucin resembling that from the cardia and the pylorus. It contains the precursor of an enzyme that resembles trypsin in its actions (see Table 12.2). It is activated by hyrochloric acid and acts specifically to hydrolyse peptide links made by lysine. Since this amino acid occurs particularly in collagen, the fibrous framework of adipose tissue in the diet is destroyed and the fat is set free.

The ducts of two other glands also discharge into the duodenum. These glands, the liver and the pancreas, are formed embryologically as outgrowths of the gut. The bile duct and the pancreatic duct, which carry their secretions, usually have a common orifice into the duodenum (Fig. 12.4). The smooth muscle in the wall of the terminal portions of the ducts is enlarged into sphincters: the one around the terminal bile duct is known as the choledochal (or Oddi's) sphincter; it is more highly developed than the pancreatic sphincter. In some people, Oddi's sphincter surrounds both ducts.

The bile. Bile is produced in the liver at the rate of 500 to 1000 ml/day and is stored and concentrated in the gall bladder from which it is discharged through the common bile duct at intervals into the duodenum. Bile is an alkaline, bitter fluid, containing bile salts (sodium taurocholate and sodium glycocholate), bile pigments (bilirubin and biliverdin), cholesterol, mucin and diffusible plasma constituents. The bile salts reduce surface tension and emulsify fats. They promote the lipolytic activity of pancreatic juice in the duodenum by increasing the surface area of the fat exposed to the lipase. They also facilitate absorption from the intestine of neutral fat, fatty acids, fat soluble vitamins (A,

D and K) and cholesterol. In the bile, the bile salts solubilize cholesterol; when bile salts are deficient, bile stones consisting chiefly of cholesterol are deposited in the gall bladder. Bile salts are absorbed from the small intestine, carried in the blood to the hepatic portal system, and reabsorbed by the liver from whence they are re-secreted.

Control of biliary secretion. The dilute bile from the liver is concentrated in the gall bladder by absorption of water and electrolytes. The continuous secretion from the liver is converted into an intermittent flow coinciding with the entry of food into the duodenum. Bile is forced into the duodenum by contraction of the gall bladder and relaxation of the sphincter of Oddi. Contractions of the gall bladder may be studied following injections of radio-opaque substances such as tetra-iodophenolphthalein, which are secreted into the bile (see pages 524–526) and enter the gall bladder in which they become concentrated. Stimulation of the vagus nerve causes contraction of the gall bladder, but a contraction also occurs after vagotomy when fats are placed in the duodenum. This is due to the release from the duodenal mucosa of a hormone, cholecystokinin, which contracts the gall bladder when carried to it in the blood-stream.

The pancreas. The relationship of the pancreas to the duodenum and stomach is shown in Fig. 12.4. It is a mixed gland, producing both endocrine and exocrine secretions. The endocrine activity of the pancreas is dealt with on pages 381–383. The exocrine secretion of pancreatic juice is formed in alveoli lined with serous cells. The secretion from a group of alveoli is discharged into an intercalated duct, several of which unite to form an intralobular duct. Ducts from different lobes of the pancreas then unite to form interlobular ducts, which finally discharge into the pancreatic duct.

Pancreatic juice. In man, about 1 litre is secreted per day. It contains enzymes, enzyme precursors and electrolytes. The electrolyte composition differs from that of plasma in that there is relatively more HCO_3^- and less Cl^-, hence there is an active secretion of some electrolytes. The pH is about 8 owing to the high bicarbonate concentration; this provides buffering capacity for neutralizing the acidity of the chyme entering the duodenum from the pylorus, and the optimal pH for the digestive enzymes secreted from the pancreas (Table 12.2) and from the epithelial secretory cells of the intestine.

Enzymes which hydrolyse nucleic acids, carbohydrates and simple and compound lipids are secreted by the pancreas. The essential data about them are summarized in Table 12.2.

The three proteolytic enzymes derived from the pancreatic juice are secreted as inactive precursors. The first stage in their activation is the removal by enzymatic hydrolysis of a 'masking' portion from trypsinogen: the enzyme that accomplishes this is enterokinase which is secreted by the duodenal mucosa. The optimal pH for the reaction is about 6, so it can be started before the gastric chyme has been fully neutralized. Then, as the pH becomes more alkaline, trypsin continues the activation of trypsinogen, and also activates chymotrypsinogen and procarboxypeptidase.

In the event of the pancreatic pro-enzymes becoming activated within the gland, the enzymes attack the pancreas itself, causing necrosis and severe pain. The condition is known as pancreatitis. The cause of the disorder has been variously ascribed to activation of pancreatic juice by a reflux of bile into the pancreatic duct, and to rupture of the walls of the duct because of a high pressure developing in it, followed by the activation of the pro-enzymes by tissue cathepsins, which are intracellular enzymes resembling trypsin.

The proteolytic enzymes from the pancreas, like pepsin, are highly specific in the reactions that they catalyse (Table 12.2). Trypsin and chymotrypsin are endopeptidases, that is, they act for the most part on peptide bonds in polypeptide chains to form proteoses and only a few free amino acids. Carboxypeptidase, on the other hand is an exopeptidase, and removes terminal amino acids one at a time.

An insufficiency of pancreatic secretion results in incomplete digestion and the faeces contain undigested muscle fibres (creatorrhea) from ingested meats. There may also be undigested fat in the faeces (steatorrhea) if there is a large fat intake, but pancreatic secretion is not the sole source of digestive lipase. These digestive disorders may be relieved by oral administration of pancreatin, a preparation of animal pancreas containing active enzymes together with sodium bicarbonate.

Control of pancreatic secretion. The pancreatic secretory cells are innervated by fibres from the vagus nerves. Stimulation of the vagus produces a secretion rich in enzymes, and this is associated with depletion of zymogen granules from the alveolar cells. The passage of chyme through the pylorus causes a reflex secretion of pancreatic juice. However, secretion in response to the presence of gastric chyme in the duodenum still occurs after the pancreas has been denervated. This is because of the release of humoral agents, known as *secretin* and *pancreozymin*, from the duodenal wall; these substances are carried in the blood-stream to the pancreas, where they stimulate secretion. The pancreatic juice formed in response to secretin is relatively low in enzyme content but has a high pH, while that stimulated by pancreozymin is rich in enzymes. The relative importance of the nervous and humoral mechanisms for controlling pancreatic secretion is difficult to assess; probably both are involved, the nervous excitation being more rapid in onset but shorter lasting and the humoral mechanism maintaining the secretion for as long as there is acid chyme in the duodenum.

TABLE 12.2. Enzymes and enzyme precursors secreted by the pancreas.

Constituent of pancreatic juice	Active enzyme	Reaction catalysed and conditions
Trypsinogen	Trypsin (activated by enterokinase, and then autocatalytically)	Hydrolysis of peptide bonds formed by carboxylic group of dibasic amino acids (lysine or arginine). Optimal pH, 7 to 8. Activity increased by Ca^{++}
α-Chymotrypsinogen. Chymotrypsinogen-B	α-Chymotrypsin. Chymotrypsin-B (activated by trypsin)	Hydrolysis of peptide bonds formed by carboxylic group of tyrosine, phenylalanine, tryptophan or methionine. Optimal pH, about 8. The two types differ slightly in physical properties and in the rate at which they attack certain proteins
Procarboxypeptidase	Carboxypeptidase (activated by trypsin)	Hydrolysis of peptide bond formed by amino group of a terminal amino acid (i.e. with the carboxyl group free). The activity depends on the amino acid: Tyr > Try > Leu > Met > isoLeu > Ala > Gly. Optimal pH, 7·5 to 8·5. Requires Zn^{++} as an essential co-factor
Ribonuclease and deoxyribonuclease		Specific to RNA and DNA respectively. Hydrolysis of link between the phosphate of a pyrimidine nucleotide and the 5-carbon of the next pentose:

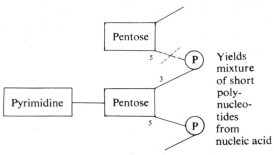

Lipase		Hydrolysis of fats to yield fatty acids and glycerol. Optimal pH, about 8. Activity increased by bile salts and other surface active agents
Phospholipase A Phospholipase B		Hydrolysis of phospholipids to yield fatty acids and glycerophosphates. A splits only saturated fatty acids
Amylase		Hydrolysis of starch, glycogen and dextrins to yield shorter polysaccharides and maltose. Optimal pH, 6·9. Identical with salivary amylase, p. 304
Maltase		Hydrolysis of maltose to glucose. Optimal pH, 6·6

INTESTINAL JUICE (succus entericus). This is formed by secretory cells, principally in the crypts of Lieberkühn, along the whole length of the small intestine. It contains a large number of enzymes, not all of which have been characterized. Enterokinase has already been mentioned above; it is secreted only by the duodenal mucosa. The proteolytic enzymes in succus entericus were once known by the name *erepsin*. This is actually a mixture of exopeptidases which hydrolyse very short-chain peptides; each of them has considerable specificity and the better known ones are given in Table 12.3. The optimal pH for all of them is about 8. The glycosidases in succus entericus include an amylase, like that in saliva and pancreatic juice, and also enzymes which hydrolyse maltose and other utilizable disaccharides: the disaccharides most common in the diet are sucrose and lactose. A lipase is secreted in the jejunum, but not in the ileum. The intestinal juice contains mucin, secreted from goblet cells, and also the debris of cells detached from the epithelium. New epithelial cells are continually being generated by mitotic division. The discarded cells and the mucus become constituents of the faeces, which continue to be formed even in starvation.

Control of intestinal secretion. It is doubtful whether the nerve fibres to the intestine stimulate secretion. A substance which does stimulate secretion has been extracted from the mucosa and named *enterocrinin*. In transplanted segments of intestine with an intact innervation, neither enterocrinin nor the presence of chyme in the intestine stimulate secretion. However, if the transplant is denervated, both of these become effective stimuli for secretion, suggesting that there is a humoral stimulant mechanism and a nervous inhibitory mechanism.

NERVES OF THE SMALL INTESTINE. There are afferent nerve fibres from the intestine, usually arising from receptors which respond to distension of the walls. Parasympathetic fibres to the small intestine are in the vagus nerves. The post-ganglionic sympathetic fibres arise in the coeliac and mesenteric ganglia. They run to the intestinal wall in the mesentery, usually accompanying the blood vessels. These nerves together comprise the extrinsic innervation: the nerves in Auerbach's and Meissner's plexuses are the intrinsic nerves. The ganglion cells of the post-ganglionic vagal fibres are believed to be included in Auerbach's plexus. It is commonly stated that the nerves of Auerbach's plexus are motor in function, whereas Meissner's plexus contains sensory fibres; however, the evidence for a strict division into motor and sensory plexuses is scanty.

Movements of the small intestine. These serve to mix the chyme with the secretions, to promote absorption, and to move the chyme along the intestine. The movements may be myogenic (page 221) or neurogenic. The latter may

TABLE 12.3. Peptidase in succus entericus

Enzyme	Reaction catalysed	Co-factor
Glycylglycine dipeptidase	Hydrolyses only the dipeptide 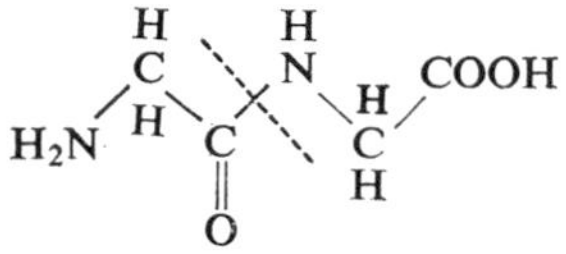	Contains Co^{++}

Iminopeptidase	Hydrolyses only dipeptides made with the carboxylic group of proline or hydroxyproline 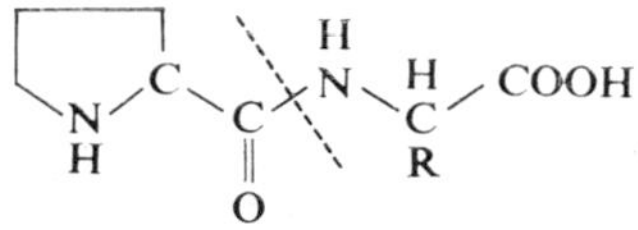	Activated by Mn^{++}

Imidodipeptidase	Hydrolyses only dipeptides made with the imino group of proline and hydroxyproline 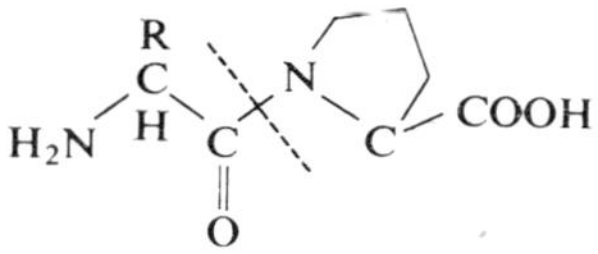	Activated by Mn^{++}

Leucine aminodipeptidase	Hydrolyses polypeptides more slowly than dipeptidases	Requires Mg^{++} or Mn^{++}

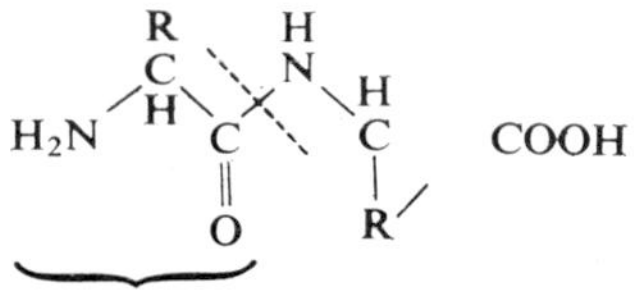

MOST active when this is leucine

Aminotripeptidase	Acts *only* on tripeptides to hydrolyse the amino acid from the end with the free amino group 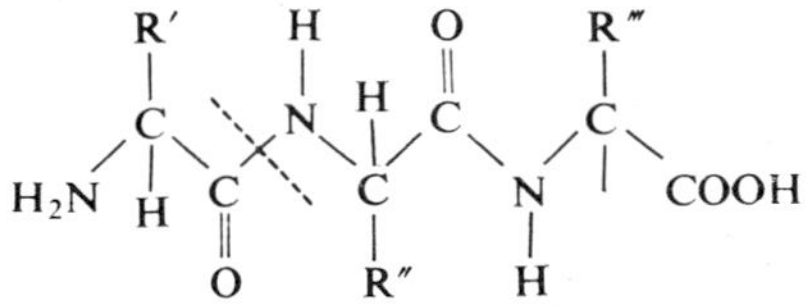

11

be due to impulses from extrinsic or intrinsic nerves. The two myogenic movements, which aid mixing and absorption, are segmentation and pendular movements. Segmentation is produced by contractions of rings of circular muscle which appear from place to place and persist for varying lengths of time. Pendular movement results from rhythmic contractions of longitudinal muscle. The villi change in length and diameter as a result of contractions of fibres of the muscularis mucosae; these movements also promote absorption and express chyle from the lacteals (chyle is described on page 247). Smooth muscle-stimulating substances in the chyme can stimulate the movements of the villi. Such substances include histamine and a polypeptide called villikinin which is liberated from the mucosa of the duodenum by gastric chyme.

The onward movement of chyme is produced by waves of activity called peristalsis. The movements are complex and involve a wave of contraction of the circular muscle which moves along the intestine; the longitudinal muscle ahead of the wave relaxes and in its wake the longitudinal muscle contracts: these movements are coordinated by the intrinsic nerve plexuses. Peristalsis is initiated by an increase in pressure in the intestinal lumen. This stimulates sensory nerve endings, either by activating stretch receptors or indirectly by releasing chemical mediators which stimulate the sensory endings (5-hydroxytryptamine and substance P have been suggested as possible candidates, pages 179 and 182). The sensory nerves reflexly excite efferent nerves also contained in the intrinsic plexuses. Thus the peristaltic reflex occurs in isolated segments of intestine, but in the body it is dominated by impulses from the central nervous system. Peristaltic waves advance at varying rates and may commence anywhere in the small intestine. They may travel only a few inches or they may move rapidly for many feet, in which case the movement is called a peristaltic rush.

Large intestine. The divisions of the large intestine are shown in Fig. 12.7. They are the caecum and appendix, the colon, and the rectum which terminates in the anal canal. The functions of the large intestine are the formation, transport and evacuation of faeces. The structure of the wall differs in some respects from that in the small intestine; villi are completely absent. The mucosa contains deep crypts lined with goblet cells and simple epithelial cells. The secretion is mucin, which serves to bind together the faecal mass and to lubricate its passage. The absorption of water from the colon consolidates the faecal masses. If the faeces are retained too long they become dry and mucin is ineffective in lubricating it, thus giving rise to discomfort from constipation.

The special features of the *appendix* are the many enterochromaffin cells in the mucosa, and the mass of lymphoid tissue in the lamina propria. Distension of the appendix or spasm of its smooth muscle causes pain, which is more acute when the tissue is inflamed.

The outer longitudinal muscle in the colon and caecum is gathered into three bundles, the *taeniae coli*. The local movements of the colon brought about by contractions of segments of circular muscle and taeniae coli produce folds of

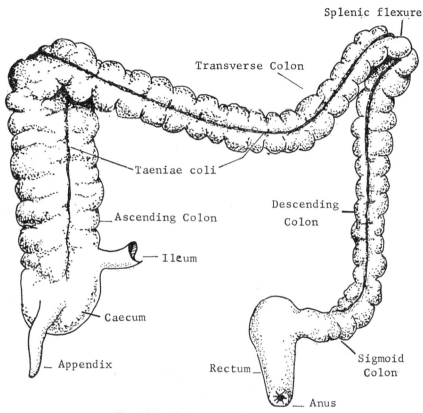

FIG. 12.7. Divisions of the large intestine.

the wall known as *sacculations* or *haustra*. It is thought that this movement aids the absorption of water by kneading the faecal mass.

The contents of the ileum are transferred to the caecum by peristaltic movements. The ileocaecal junction is guarded by a fold of tissue which is sometimes described as a valve, but no true sphincter is present as the contents of an enema readily pass retrogradely into the terminal ileum. The caecum and colon relax to accommodate the exhausted chyme from the ileum. At infrequent intervals the faecal masses are transferred to the sigmoid colon by peristalsis. This occurs as a 'mass movement' involving almost the whole of the colon. In a disorder known as *megacolon* (or Hirschsprung's disease), the colon becomes grossly distended. The defect is attributable to the absence of ganglion cells from the intrinsic nerve plexuses.

The extrinsic parasympathetic nerves to the proximal portions of the large intestine (as far as the splenic flexure) come from the vagi, those to the distal end are from the sacral division. Parasympathetic nerve stimulation increases movements. Sympathetic fibres arise in the superior and inferior mesenteric ganglia and innervate the proximal and distal portions respectively. Stimulation of the sympathetic nerves inhibits movements.

Distension of the sigmoid colon gives rise to an awareness of the need for defaecation, but the sensation can be held in abeyance by the conscious wish to suppress defaecation. The presence of faeces in the rectum gives a feeling of urgency, and defaecation can only be prevented by voluntarily maintaining the contraction of the external anal sphincter. The first voluntary act of defaecation is relaxation of the external sphincter. Other voluntary acts which help to evacuate the faeces are contraction of the abdominal rectus muscles and forcible expiration against a closed glottis. After transection of the spinal cord, dcfaccation is carried out entirely under the control of a reflex centre in the spinal cord. The defaecation reflex is initiated by distension of the sigmoid colon and the rectum and is reinforced by relaxation of the external sphincter. Evacuation is accomplished by a series of peristaltic mass movements in the sigmoid colon and the rectum, and by relaxation of the internal anal sphincter.

In the anal canal, columnar epithelium gives way to stratified squamous epithelium which is continuous with that of the skin. The lamina propria of the anus contains loops of large veins which appear as haemorrhoids (piles) when they become overdistended and varicosed.

The faeces consist of the indigestible constituents of the food, cell debris from the intestinal mucosa, mucin, and both dead and living bacteria which may amount to 50% of the mass of the faeces. The colour is due to stercobilin, which is derived from the bile pigments.

Absorption from the gastro-intestinal tract. Water is absorbed from all parts of the tract, but more particularly from the stomach and the large intestine. Absorption from the stomach reduces the volume of the liquid taken with a meal, thus allowing a higher concentration of digestive enzymes. Absorption from the large intestine results in a firmer consistency of the faecal material.

Carbohydrates are completely hydrolysed to *monosaccharides*, most of which are absorbed by active transport through the mucosal epithelium of the small intestine and pass into the portal vein blood.

Proteins are completely hydrolysed to *l*-amino acids, most of which are absorbed by active transport and pass into the blood. Peptide bonds made by *d*-amino acids (the so-called unnatural amino acids) are usually not attacked by the digestive enzymes; furthermore, *d*-amino acids are not absorbed by active transport. In the new-born infant, some protein can be absorbed intact and passes into the lymph. The importance of this is that the first milk (the colostrum) secreted by the mother after childbirth contains γ-globulins which confer immunity to some diseases (page 229).

Fats are hydrolysed to *fatty acids* and *glycerol* and are absorbed from the small intestine. No fat or fatty acid is absorbed from the large intestine. Some fatty acids may appear in the blood, but a considerable proportion is resynthesized to fat which passes into the lymph. After ingesting a meal rich in fats, the lacteals and the lymphatic collecting vessels contain a milky white fluid called *chyle*; this appearance is due to the presence in the lymph of *chylomicra*, which are minute globules of fat. The long-chain fatty acids and perhaps some unchanged fat are absorbed by pinocytosis (page 41). The presence of bile salts is essential for the absorption of long-chain fatty acids and fat-soluble vitamins.

Blood and lymphatic vessels. The arterial supply to the gastrointestinal tract comes from the coeliac artery and the superior and inferior mesenteric arteries. The arteries run in the mesentery, and after branching several times they join the segment of intestine which they serve. The venous blood from the stomach, small intestine and most of the large intestine is conveyed in the mesenteric veins which finally flow into the hepatic portal vein; venous blood from the pancreas, gall bladder and spleen also runs into the portal vein. The venous blood from the rectum is carried to the vena cava by the rectal veins and does not enter the hepatic portal system. The lacteals and other lymphatic capillaries join into collecting ducts which pass through lymph nodes. In the ileum the nodes are in the lamina propria, where they form swellings known as Peyer's patches. The afferent lymph vessels accompany the blood vessels through the mesentery before they join the thoracic duct (page 247).

The liver

The liver is composed of several lobes, each of which is subdivided into *lobules*. The connective tissue capsule surrounding the liver gives off septa which envelope each lobule in a connective tissue sheath known as *Glisson's capsule*. The blood vessels, bile canals, lymphatic vessels and nerves traverse the liver in the septa. The liver receives 80% of its blood from the portal vein and 20% from the hepatic artery. Interlobular branches of the hepatic artery and portal vein empty into sinusoids whose walls are made up of columns of hepatic cells. The sinusoids are arranged more or less radially in the lobule, the blood from them collecting in the central intralobular vein. The intralobular veins unite to form hepatic veins, which drain into the vena cava. The *sinusoid* is the unit structure of the liver. Figure 12.8 gives a diagrammatic representation of a sinusoid and a bile canaliculus. The hepatic cells form bile (page 316) which is secreted into the *bile canaliculus*. The biliary vessels collect to form the hepatic duct which runs to the gall bladder and common bile duct (Fig. 12.4). The walls of the sinusoids also contain occasional phagocytic *Küpffer cells* which belong to the reticulo-endothelial system.

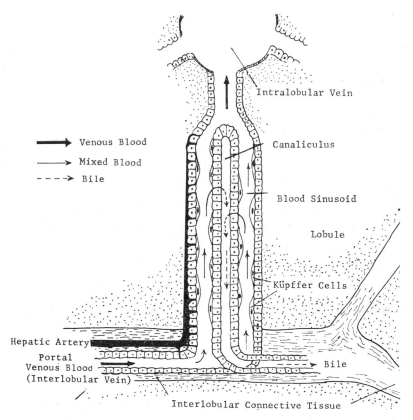

FIG. 12.8. Blood and bile flow in a liver lobule.

Apart from the formation of bile, the liver has other functions. They include processes concerned with the blood, with the storage and release of nutrients, and with detoxification. Many of these functions are described in other chapters, but it is useful to collect them together here.

Functions concerned with blood. *Storage of blood.* The liver contains a considerable amount of blood in its sinusoids and veins. Some of this blood is discharged into the circulation to replace blood lost in haemorrhage so helping to maintain the blood pressure. Thus the liver, like the spleen, acts as a blood reservoir.

Formation of blood constituents. Of the plasma proteins, all of the albumin, the fibrinogen and some of the globulins (e.g. prothrombin) are formed in the liver. In the foetus, the liver is one of the sites of erythropoiesis, and in the adult some erythropoietic factors are stored in the liver.

Destruction of blood constituents. Old erythrocytes may be trapped and destroyed in the liver as well as in the spleen; the products of red cell destruction in the spleen reach the liver in the portal vein. The porphyrin derived from haemoglobin is metabolized in the liver to *bilirubin* (Fig. 8.4, page 236). Most of the bilirubin appears in the bile, but a little is absorbed into the blood where it is bound with an α-globulin. An excess of bilirubin in the plasma and tissue fluids imparts a yellow colour to the skin; the condition is known as *jaundice*. Jaundice may be due either to an excessive breakdown of erythrocytes (haemolytic), to damage to the liver (hepatic), or to obstruction of the bile ducts (obstructive). In the bile, part of the bilirubin is oxidized to *biliverdin*. In adults the main bile pigment is bilirubin, but in infants and in herbivorous animals biliverdin predominates. After being excreted into the intestines, bilirubin is converted into *stercobilinogen* by bacterial enzymes in the colon and part of it is further oxidized to *stercobilin*. Some stercobilinogen is re-absorbed and either re-excreted in the bile or filtered off in the kidney, from which it appears in the urine and is called *urobilinogen*. Porphyrins as such are also excreted in the urine and faeces; they may be derived in part from the body's own haemoglobin, but the most important source is from the diet, where they are derived from animal and plant porphyrins (including chlorophyll). Increased amounts of porphyrin are excreted after liver damage. This may result from disease, in the conditions known as *porphyrias*, or after poisoning with heavy metals; it may occur as a toxic side-effect of some drugs.

Functions concerned with nutrients and intermediary metabolism. *Heat production.* The liver produces a considerable proportion of the body heat as a result of its pronounced and continuous metabolic activities.

Vitamins. Some of the vitamins are stored in the liver, particularly vitamins A, D and K.

Carbohydrate synthesis and storage. Monosaccharides absorbed from the intestine are carried in the portal venous blood and removed in the liver where they are synthesized into glycogen which is stored there. This process is known as *glycogenesis*; the metabolic paths involved are shown in Fig. 2.8, page 46. The liver is also the site of *neoglycogenesis*, by which glycogen is synthesized from non-carbohydrates sources, including amino acids (which are first broken down to acetyl radicals.)

The blood glucose level is held at an approximately constant level by the balance of *glycogenesis* and *glycogenolysis*. The breakdown of glycogen is stimulated by a low glucose content of the blood within the liver itself, and also by the effects of hypoglycaemia on the central nervous system. These result in the liberation of adrenaline from the adrenals and of diabetogenic factor from the anterior pituitary, both of which stimulate liver glycogenolysis.

Fat metabolism. The liver is the most important site for the β-oxidation of fatty acids (Fig. 2.7, page 45) and for maintaining the balance of the metabolic conversions of fatty acids and carbohydrates. The acetylcoenzyme A produced by the breakdown of fatty acids may enter the tricarboxylic acid cycle where it is completely oxidized (Fig. 2.5, page 43). However, this depends on the availability of oxaloacetic acid which is derived from carbohydrate metabolism. If insufficient carbohydrate is metabolized there is a deficiency of oxaloacetic acid. This may occur as a result of carbohydrate starvation, or when carbohydrate metabolism is disturbed in diabetes mellitus (pages 384–386). Excess acetyl coenzyme A forms acetoacetic acid:

$$2CH_3CO \cdot S \cdot CoA \longrightarrow CH_3CO \cdot CH_2COOH + 2CoA \cdot SH$$
$$\text{acetoacetic acid}$$

Acetoacetic acid can be partly metabolized, but the end products include a number of ketones, the so-called acetone bodies, which give rise to the condition known as ketosis. They accumulate in the blood, appear in the urine, and can be detected on the breath. Ketosis finally results in coma and death.

Cholesterol. The structure of cholesterol is given in Fig. 1.5, page 14. It is a constituent of the diet and is also synthesized in the body, mainly in the liver. It is an intermediate in the synthesis of adrenal corticoids (pages 377–378), sex hormones (pages 394 and 398), bile acids (cholic acid and deoxycholic acid), bile salts, and vitamin D. The bile salts, taurocholate and glycocholate, are formed by the conjugation of cholic acid with taurine (derived from cystine) and glycine, respectively. A precursor of vitamin D_3, 7-dehydrocholesterol, is formed from cholesterol in the skin under the influence of ultra-violet light.

The blood cholesterol level is of some significance in arteriosclerotic diseases, in which cholesterol is deposited in the blood vessels (pages 280–281). In these conditions the high blood cholesterol level is associated with a diet rich in saturated fatty acids, usually from animal fats. The plasma cholesterol level may be lowered by taking fats containing unsaturated fatty acids in the diet, and by restricting the intake of animal fat. High blood cholesterol levels also result from some hormonal imbalance such as thyroid deficiency.

Amino acid metabolism. Amino acids which are surplus to the requirements for protein synthesis are deaminated by a number of metabolic routes
(pages 47–52). The ammonia that is formed is rapidly detoxified; should any
accumulate, it produces severe toxic signs and death. A study of the mechanisms for the elimination of ammonia from an evolutionary point of
view gives an insight into biochemical and physiological adaptations. In some

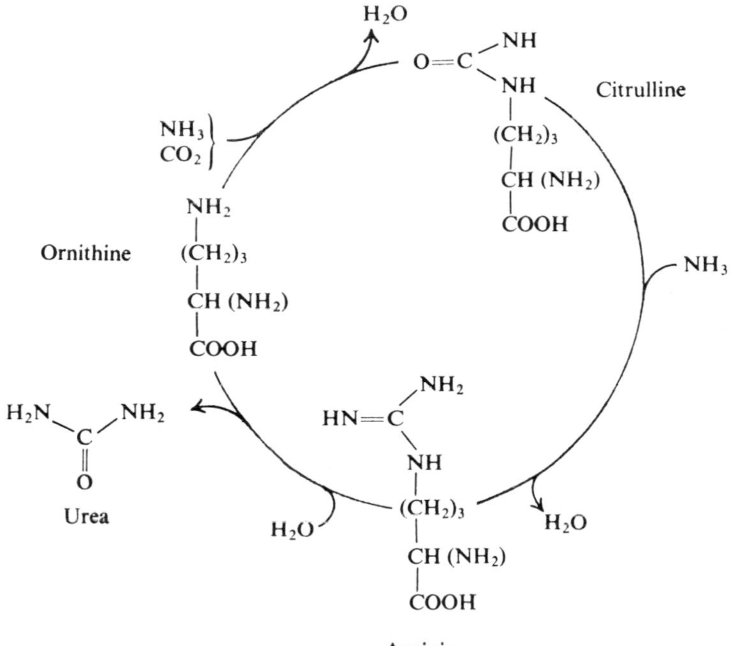

FIG. 12.9. Ureogenesis. A simplified version of the reactions involved in the formation
of urea from ammonia in the ornithine cycle.

aquatic animals ammonia is excreted as such and their environment allows it
to be rapidly diluted and carried away. Land animals have evolved a mechanism
for detoxifying ammonia: this is the ornithine cycle (Fig. 12.9); the process it
carries out is known as *ureogenesis*. Ornithine combines with ammonia and
carbon dioxide to form citrulline, which incorporates a further molecule of
ammonia to make arginine. Arginase hydrolyses arginine to yield urea and
regenerates ornithine. The urea is excreted in the urine (page 348).

A further development of detoxification involves the synthesis of *uric acid*
(Fig. 12.10). Uric acid is almost completely insoluble and, molecule for

11*

molecule, it eliminates more of the ammonia than does urea; thus it requires less water for its excretion. Birds and reptiles lack arginase, and ammonia from amino acids is eliminated entirely as uric acid. It is postulated that their mechanism for the entrapment of the toxic ammonia as the insoluble, non-toxic uric acid allowed the development of the embryo in an egg completely sealed off from the environment.

The uric acid secreted by man is mainly derived from the oxidation of purines (adenine and guanine) which are constituents of coenzymes (pages

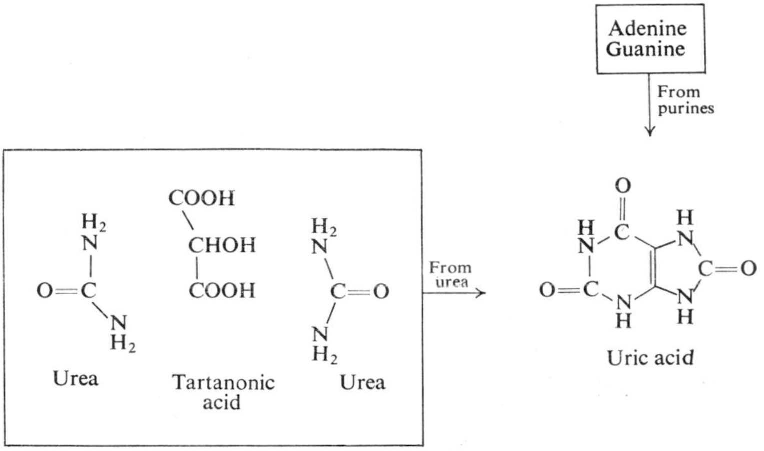

FIG. 12.10. Sources of uric acid.

22–28) and nucleic acid (page 52). In most mammals, but *not* man or the other primates, uric acid is further metabolized to allantoin which appears in the urine.

Detoxification in the liver. The formation of urea is only one of the many detoxifying mechanisms of the liver. Other potentially toxic products of metabolism are further metabolized to non-toxic substances in the liver prior to excretion. Many of these detoxifying mechanisms involve conjugations; for example, phenolic compounds are conjugated with sulphate, alcoholic and phenolic compounds are conjugated with glucuronic acid, aromatic acids are conjugated with glycine or glutamic acid, and aromatic amines are conjugated with acetic acid. A knowledge of these metabolic pathways is essential for the pharmacologist because drugs may be metabolized in a similar way. Amongst drugs, the metabolite may have less pharmacological activity than the substance originally administered, but there are instances when the metabolite is more active. Drug metabolism is dealt with in more detail on pages 503–521.

The detoxifying mechanisms of the liver are impaired as a result of liver disease, and particularly care must be taken in giving drugs to such patients. For example, the very short acting barbiturates (page 590) are normally destroyed in the liver by oxidation, but in liver disease they are metabolized less rapidly with the result that the normal dose produces an effect which is too intense and persists for too long.

Regulation of food and water intake

The physiological mechanisms underlying the urges to eat and drink have been studied in man and in animals. Many factors have been shown to affect the regulation of food and water intake but, as yet, the mechanisms are incompletely understood.

The locations of the hypothalamic centres concerned with feeding and satiety are described on page 134. Higher centres have been found to influence the hypothalamic centres. Thus, lesions in parts of the frontal lobes of the cortex cause a decreased food intake while temporal lobe lesions lead to an increased food intake; the limbic system (page 102) also exerts some control over eating. Habit and conditioning influence the control by the higher centres which form a discriminating mechanism (appetite) that modifies the urge to eat (hunger) originating in the hypothalamus.

Several factors together appear to form the stimulus for feeding; the important ones so far discovered are as follows. (1) Contractions of the empty stomach (hunger pangs, page 312) are believed to stimulate the feeding centre giving rise to a desire to eat. Passage of food through the mouth and oesophagus and distension of the stomach exert the opposite effect. However, afferent impulses arising from the alimentary canal are not a very important mechanism, as patients with complete gastrectomy or vagotomy still experience hunger. (2) A fall in blood glucose (hypoglycaemia) has a powerful stimulant effect on the hunger drive and an intravenous injection of glucose will depress hunger. The stimulus is the rate of glucose utilization rather than the absolute amount of glucose; when the difference in the glucose contents of the carotid artery and jugular vein blood approaches zero, hunger is experienced. It is postulated that the satiety centre contains 'glucoreceptors' sensitive to the rate of glucose utilization. As long as the glucoreceptors are adequately stimulated, the satiety centre acts as a brake on the otherwise continuously-active feeding centre. When glucose utilization is low, hunger is experienced because the satiety centre is no longer stimulated and inhibition of the feeding centre ceases. (3) The amount of fat stored in the body influences hunger and it appears that the hypothalamus is sensitive to some circulating metabolite which is in equilibrium with the stored fat, and which depresses the hunger urge. (4) The hunger urge is influenced by the heat content of the body and therefore by increased metabolism. Foods, especially protein, stimulate metabolism (specific dynamic action, page 434) and depress hunger. As well as being concerned with feeding, the hypothalamus regulates body temperature and it appears that these two functions are integrated at this level.

Hunger for specific foods is largely the result of changes in the internal environment, produced, for example, by pregnancy, dietary deficiencies or endocrine disturbances. There is a tendency to choose nutritionally wise diets. For example, during pregnancy and lactation there is increased hunger for protein and fat but little change in carbohydrate appetite, and a specific salt hunger is exhibited when the diet is deficient in salt or after adrenalectomy which leads to an increased urinary excretion of sodium. The mechanisms underlying specific hungers are not understood.

An increased food intake over a long period of time results in obesity which may in turn lead to diseases of the circulation or to diabetes mellitus. Obesity may arise through an imbalance in the nervous mechanisms regulating feeding. Nervous imbalance may be congenital, may be caused by hypothalamic lesions or, more commonly, may result from habit and conditioning. On the other hand, obesity may arise from endocrine disorders (e.g. deficiency of pituitary gonadotrophin, Chapter 14). Obesity is an important health problem in some countries and many pharmacological studies have been directed towards the discovery of appetite suppressant drugs. Amphetamine and phenmetrazine (page 619) are commonly used to suppress appetite. They stimulate the satiety centre indirectly through an action on the frontal lobes of the cortex; their anorexigenic action in dogs disappears after prefrontal lobotomy.

The sensation of thirst is an important adjuvant to the regulation of body water. It is an expression of a general bodily need for water and is not simply the result of a dry mouth. The mouth is the normal route for ingestion of water and the fact that the sensation of thirst is felt in the mouth may be the result of a conditioned reflex.

Water deprivation results in a decrease in extra- and intracellular fluid volumes and an increased tonicity in both fluid compartments. Of these, the main stimulus giving rise to the sensation of thirst has been shown to be a decreased intracellular fluid volume. In animal experiments, the direct injection of minute amounts of hypertonic saline into a specific area of the anterior hypothalamus elicits drinking, and it has been postulated that receptors sensitive to cellular dehydration are located there. These receptors appear to resemble the osmoreceptors which cause the release of the antidiuretic hormone (vasopressin, page 368).

The ingestion of food and water are closely related and the sensation of thirst occurs as a result of eating (post-prandial thirst). During eating, large quantities of fluid, comprising the digestive juices, move into the gastro-intestinal tract. As a result, extracellular fluid volume is reduced and this, in turn, mobilizes intracellular water. Thus food intake temporarily causes the same effects on water balance as does deprivation of water, and thirst therefore follows upon eating.

Amphetamine and phenmetrazine inhibit drinking partly as a secondary effect to hunger depression, and partly by an action on the thirst centres.

CHAPTER 13

The Urinary System

The urinary system comprises the two kidneys, the ureters, the bladder and the urethra; its functions are to form, store and void the urine. Essentially, the urine is an aqueous solution of the waste products of metabolism other than the gaseous end-product, carbon dioxide, which is eliminated from the lungs (Chapter 11); the faeces are a relatively unimportant route of elimination of metabolic products. The homeostatic mechanisms for maintaining constant the volume, pH and ionic composition of the body fluids depend mainly on kidney function.

The kidneys

The kidneys lie against the posterior wall of the abdominal cavity, one on each side of the vertebral column. They are described as retroperitoneal, that is, they lie between the peritoneum and the abdominal wall. Each kidney is enclosed in a tough fibrous connective tissue capsule, outside which there is often a considerable amount of adipose tissue. The attachments of the kidney with the renal artery, vein and nerves, and with the ureter are in its concave medial border, at the hilum (Fig. 13.1).

Structure of the kidney. The kidney contains an outer zone or cortex, an inner zone or medulla, and a pelvis which is just inside the hilum (Fig. 13.1).

THE NEPHRON. The functional unit of the kidney is the nephron, which consists of the glomerular (or Bowman's) capsule and the renal tubule (Fig. 13.2). Each human kidney contains approximately one million nephrons, although probably not all of these are active at any one time. The glomerular capsule is the blind terminal dilatation of the tubule which is indented and envelops a tuft of capillary vessels called the glomerulus. The glomerular capsule and the capillary tuft together constitute the Malpighian or renal corpuscle.

The epithelium of the glomerular capsule is of the simple squamous type. On the interior surface of the capsule it forms a membrane which is in close apposition to the endothelium of the capillary loops. The elucidation of this structure led to the suggestion that filtration of the blood took place in the glomeruli, and this was subsequently confirmed by direct experiment. The tubule proper emerges from the capsule. The first part, known as the proximal convoluted tubule, is lined with cuboid epithelial cells which have a 'brush border' consisting of microvilli, suggesting that the epithelium is adapted for absorption. The next part of the tubule is the loop of Henle (Fig. 13.2). These straight portions of the tubule penetrate into the medulla. The wall of the descending limb has flatter cells than that of the ascending limb. The final

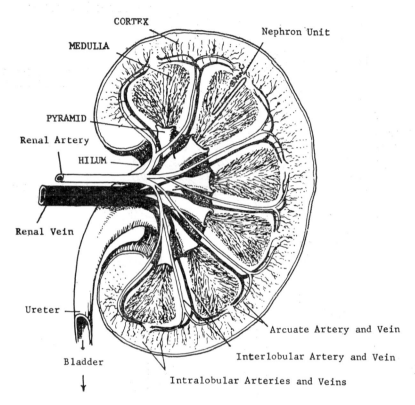

FIG. 13.1. The kidney. Vertical median section.

portion of the tubule, the distal convoluted tubule, is lined with cuboid epithelial cells (without a brush border). The distal tubules of the nephrons empty into collecting ducts lined with columnar epithelium. The collecting ducts run through the medulla, uniting with each other at an acute angle. This arrangement produces the ray-like medullary striations. The collecting ducts empty into the renal pelvis at the apices of the renal pyramids (Fig. 13.1).

The length of a human nephron is about 4 cm, and the total length of all the tubules from both kidneys is about 80 km (50 miles).

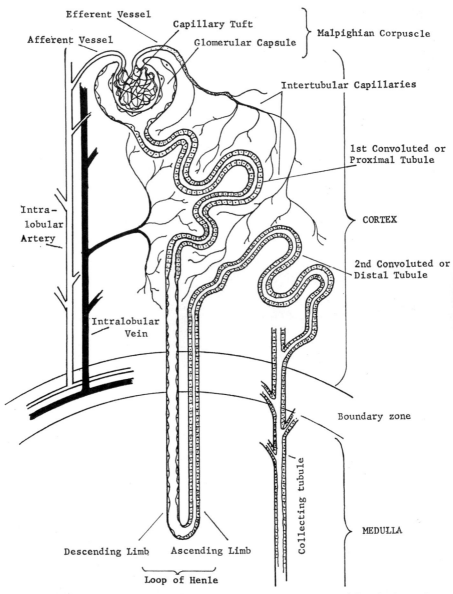

Fig. 13.2. The nephron and its blood supply. The vasa recta supplying the loop of Henle have been omitted from the diagram.

RENAL BLOOD VESSELS. The renal artery divides into interlobular arteries which fan out radially between the pyramids (Fig. 13.1). At the boundary between the medulla and the cortex they divide again into the arcuate arteries which run in the boundary zone. These give off the intralobular arteries which penetrate radially into the cortex, where they give off an afferent vessel (vas afferens) to each glomerulus. The vasa afferentia are arterioles which are shorter and have a wider diameter than arterioles in most other organs. Each glomerular tuft consists of about fifty capillary loops which arise directly from the vas afferens. The capillaries reunite to form a single vas efferens which has about one-half of the diameter of the vas afferens. The vas efferens also has the structure of an arteriole. This unusual arrangement of the blood vessels is known as a *rete mirabile*. The vasa efferentia from glomeruli in the outer zone of the cortex divide into a second set of capillaries which supply the convoluted tubules, while vasa efferentia from glomeruli near the medullary border divide into a number of parallel vessels, the vasa recta, which penetrate into the medulla and then give off capillary branches to the loops of Henle. The second set of capillaries reunite to form intralobular veins, then arcuate veins, interlobular veins and a renal vein, each accompanying the corresponding arteries.

The kidneys have a large blood flow: their weight is about 0·5% of the total body weight, yet they receive about 25% of the whole cardiac output which amounts to some 1300 ml of blood or 700 ml of plasma per min.

RENAL NERVES. The sympathetic nerve fibres to the kidney originate from the coeliac and superior mesenteric ganglia. They accompany the renal arteries as a plexus and terminate amongst the smooth muscle of the renal blood vessels, particularly of the vasa afferentia and efferentia. Stimulation of the renal nerve plexus, or the injection of noradrenaline, causes a reduction in renal blood flow by general vasoconstriction and consequently a reduction in the rate of urine formation. However, nerve impulses arising physiologically can produce an increased rate of urine formation by selective constriction of the vasa efferentia. Sensory nerve fibres, probably subserving pain sensations, arise mostly from the renal pelvis, the proximal end of the ureter and from the adventitia of the blood vessels. Urine formation continues without impairment in the completely denervated kidney.

The functioning of the kidney. There are three processes involved in the formation of urine. Firstly, an ultra-filtrate of plasma is collected in the glomerular capsule; secondly, some of the solutes and water are reabsorbed from various parts of the tubule; and thirdly, some solutes are actively secreted by epithelial cells of the tubule. The composition of urine is given in Table 13.1. The normal range of pH is 5 to 7 with a mean of 6·25; the extreme range is 4·5 to 8.

Glomerular filtration. The formation of tissue fluid (discussed on pages 245–246) and the formation of glomerular filtrate are similar processes. The composition of the ultra-filtrate of plasma depends on the permeability of the membrane separating the plasma and the capsular space. This membrane consists of the endothelium of the capillary loop and the epithelium of the inner wall of the glomerular capsule. It is freely permeable to water, electrolytes and to other constituents of plasma with a small molecular weight; consequently these are present in the glomerular filtrate in the same proportions as in plasma. Under normal circumstances the plasma proteins do not pass into the glomerular filtrate, but if there is free haemoglobin in the plasma (as the result of intra-vascular haemolysis) it does do so and appears in the urine. From these data the effective pore size of the glomerular membrane can be judged as allowing the passage of molecules with a molecular weight of 68,000 (haemoglobin) but not of 69,000 (plasma albumin). However, this should not be taken as a definite criterion of pore size since a small amount of plasma albumin may occur in urine (for example, when the blood pressure is high) and only a small proportion of any free haemoglobin passes through. Owing to the semi-permeable nature of the glomerular membrane, which retains the plasma proteins but allows free diffusion of water and solutes of low molecular weight, the plasma proteins exert an osmotic pressure which acts to return water to the plasma.

The composition of glomerular filtrate in the frog has been determined in samples collected by puncturing the capsule with a micropipette; it was shown by direct comparison that it differed from the plasma only in the absence of proteins and fats. This technique was possible in the frog because in amphibia there are two separate structures corresponding to the glomerular and tubular portions of the mammalian kidney. It is much more difficult to perform in mammalian kidneys; nevertheless, there is abundant evidence that glomerular function is the same in mammals as in frogs.

The rate of formation of glomerular filtrate is proportional to the pressure at which it is formed. There are three factors determining the filtration pressure: (*a*) the blood pressure in the glomerular capillaries, which supplies the driving pressure; (*b*) the pressure within the glomerular capsule, and (*c*) the osmotic pressure of the plasma proteins, both of which oppose the driving pressure. The factors can be summarized in the formula:

$$P_F = P_B - (P_O + P_C)$$

where, P_F is the net filtration pressure;

P_B is the glomerular capillary pressure;

P_O is the osmotic pressure of the plasma proteins;

P_C is the back pressure in the glomerular capsule.

Approximate values (in mmHg pressure) give: $35 = 65 - (25 + 5)$.

The pressure in the glomerular capillaries is considerably higher than in capillaries elsewhere in the body, and may amount to more than 60% of the arterial blood pressure (c.f. Fig. 10.4, page 271). The arrangement of the glomerular capillaries in a rete mirabile with a muscular walled vas afferens and vas efferens provides a considerable scope for regulation of capillary pressure. Constriction of the vas afferens and dilatation of the vas efferens results in a reduction of the amount and pressure of blood in the glomerulus. If the driving pressure falls below the opposing pressures (that is, if $(P_O + P_C)$ is more than P_B), then filtration ceases in that glomerulus. On the other hand, if the vas afferens is fully dilated and the vas efferens is constricted, blood is dammed back in the glomerulus and the capillaries are fully expanded with blood at a pressure approaching the arterial blood pressure. Under these circumstances the rate of glomerular filtration is high. However, as a corollary of this, the pressure in the capillaries supplying the tubules is low, and the rate of re-absorption of fluid from the tubules into the capillaries is increased. When the systemic arterial pressure falls, or when the pressure in the renal arteries is low, the enzyme *renin* is released from specialized cells surrounding the afferent arterioles near their entry into the glomeruli. Renin catalyses the formation of angiotensin (pages 182 and 276) which may act to constrict the efferent arterioles, thereby tending to maintain the glomerular filtration pressure.

The total osmotic pressure of the plasma is lower after drinking, and the protein osmotic pressure is lower after the intravenous infusion of isotonic solutions which do not contain high molecular weight constituents to provide a colloid osmotic pressure; consequently the rate of glomerular filtration is increased. The loss of plasma dialysate through the glomerular membrane raises the protein osmotic pressure of the plasma in the efferent vessel which consequently has an increased tendency to resorb water by osmosis.

The pressure in the glomerular capsule depends only slightly on the back pressure of the fluid within the tubules because the tubule has a comparatively wide diameter offering only a slight resistance to flow; furthermore, the re-absorption of fluid in the proximal tubule reduces the volume of the filtrate. The pressure in the capsule, usually amounting to about 5 mmHg, is chiefly due to the tension of the kidney tissues within its inelastic connective tissue coat. However, if the urinary ducts are blocked, glomerular filtration ceases when the pressure in the tubules rises to equal the glomerular capillary blood pressure less the plasma protein osmotic pressure, that is, at about 50 mmHg.

The total filtration surface of the glomeruli in both kidneys has been estimated to be about 2 square metres. From the 700 ml of plasma passing over the glomerular surfaces per min, about 125 ml appears as the filtrate. The amounts of solute present in the filtrate are given in Table 13.1.

TUBULAR REABSORPTION. The volume and composition of the urine differ considerably from those of the glomerular filtrate (Table 13.1), because reabsorption and secretion by the epithelial cells of the tubule modify its composition as it passes through the nephron. The exchange of water and solutes between the fluid in the tubules and the plasma in the capillaries takes place through the epithelial cells of the tubule, the extracellular space and the capillary endothelium. The extracellular space is occupied by loose connective

TABLE 13.1. Important constituents of glomerular filtrate and of urine.

Constituent	Glomerular filtrate		Urine	
	Amount in 24 h	Concentration % W/V	Amount in 24 h	Concentration % W/V
Water	180 litres	—	1·5 litres	—
Glucose	180 g	0·1	Trace	—
HCO_3^-	255 g	0·14	None	—
Cl^-	620 g	0·3	9 g	0·6
Phosphate (as P)	5 g	0·003	1·5 g	0·1
SO_4^{2-} (as H_2SO_4)	5·4 g	0·003	2·7 g	0·18
Na^+	580 g	0·31	6 g	0·4
K^+	30 g	0·017	2 g	0·13
Ca^{++}	17 g	0·01	0·2 g	0·013
Mg^{++}	4·5 g	0·0025	0·15 g	0·01
Urea	50 g	0·028	30 g	2
Uric acid	3·6 g	0·002	0·5 g	0·03
Creatinine	1·8 g	0·001	1·5 g	0·1
Ammonia	0·18 g	0·0001	0·75 g	0·05

tissue which is continuous with the adventitia of the capillaries and the basement membrane of the tubular epithelium, and contains interstitial fluid. Certain constituents of the fluid in the tubule are reabsorbed by active transport (active reabsorption). This implies that they are moved against concentration or electrochemical gradients and that the movement requires expenditure of metabolic energy. When a particular ionic species is actively transported, electrochemical equilibrium is maintained, either by the exchange of an equivalent amount of ion of the same charge which moves passively in the opposite direction, or by the passive movement of an equivalent amount of ion with the opposite charge in the same direction. A net change in the concentration of solute alters the tonicity of the solution and water moves passively to restore osmotic equilibrium. In every case, passive movements occur only for substances to which the membranes are permeable.

The amount of a solute appearing in the glomerular filtrate depends on its concentration in the plasma and on the filtration rate; the amount is described as the 'load'. There is a maximal rate at which any particular constituent of the glomerular filtrate can be actively transported across the tubular epithelium; for each constituent there is a maximal reabsorptive capacity. For example, all of the glucose appearing in the glomerular filtrate is normally reabsorbed from the tubules. However, if the glucose concentration of the blood is gradually raised by an intravenous infusion, the concentration of glucose in the glomerular filtrate eventually reaches a level at which the capacity of the tubules to reabsorb it is exceeded and the glucose appears in the urine: the blood concentration of glucose above which glucose appears in the urine is normally about 180 mg/100 ml and this is termed the *renal threshold* for glucose. However, when the rate of glomerular filtration is reduced, for example because of a low blood pressure, a high plasma protein osmotic pressure, or tubular obstruction, then glucose may not appear in the urine even though the blood glucose concentration exceeds 180 mg/100 ml. The normal blood glucose concentration is about 100 mg/ml and glucose is not present in the urine.

The differences in the epithelial wall in different parts of the tubule suggest that the functions of the tubule vary along its length. This has been studied directly by withdrawing samples of fluid from micropunctures of the proximal and distal tubules and the tip of the loop of Henle, and comparing their composition. Samples have also been taken from the distal tubule and the renal pelvis and found to differ, thus indicating that further modifications take place in the collecting ducts. Another method for studying tubular function is described as the 'stop-flow' technique. The ureter is clamped so that the pressure in the tubules rises until glomerular filtration ceases, usually within 90 sec. The stagnation of the tubular contents is allowed to continue for several minutes, during which time each segment of the tubule produces its characteristic changes on the static tubular fluid. A substance which will appear in the glomerular filtrate is then injected; it is called a 'marker', since it will be used to determine the end of the static column of fluid. The clamp is removed and the fluid is withdrawn rapidly from the renal pelvis; the first sample contains the fluid which had been held in the collecting ducts, and then come samples from the distal tubules, the loops of Henle and the proximal tubules.

The differences in composition of the various samples reveal the changes produced in different segments of the tubule.

Proximal convoluted tubule. In this part of the tubule, as much as 80% of the glomerular filtrate is reabsorbed (i.e. about 100 ml/min), water being reabsorbed passively to restore the osmotic imbalance caused by the active absorption of solutes. The epithelium of the proximal tubule is freely permeable to water and its permeability is not influenced by anti-diuretic hormone.

Glucose is completely reabsorbed from the proximal tubule, provided that the load does not exceed the maximal reabsorptive capacity. The active transport of glucose is blocked by phloridzin or cyanide. These substances interfere with the metabolic energy-yielding processes which are necessary for active transport; phloridzin acts probably by depressing the synthesis of ATP, and cyanide interferes with cytochrome oxidase.

Sodium ions are also reabsorbed by active transport across the tubular epithelium. There is normally no difference between the concentrations of Na^+ in the proximal tubule fluid and in the surrounding interstitial fluid, but there is an electrochemical gradient, the lumen of the tubule being about 20 mV negative with respect to the interstitial fluid. If the tubule fluid contains a large amount of a solute which is not reabsorbed, water is retained in the tubule and the active removal of Na^+ creates a concentration gradient in addition to the electrochemical gradient. Under these conditions active reabsorption of Na^+ continues until the tubular concentration is reduced to about 60% of that in the glomerular filtrate, at which point the rate of passive back-diffusion down the concentration and electrochemical gradients equals the rate of active transport.

The proximal tubule is highly permeable to chloride ions and the electrochemical gradient favours reabsorption. About 80% of the Cl^- in glomerular filtrate is passively reabsorbed in the proximal tubule and accompanies some of the actively transported Na^+. About 70% of the phosphate ions in the filtrate are passively reabsorbed, and this occurs only from the proximal tubule, where they accompany Na^+.

Bicarbonate in the filtrate is reabsorbed chiefly from the proximal tubule. The mechanism depends on hydrogen secretion by the tubular epithelium and makes use of active sodium transport. The mechanism is illustrated in Fig. 13.3. In the lumen, bicarbonate ions and hydrogen ions are in equilibrium with carbonic acid and carbon dioxide. The carbon dioxide diffuses freely into the epithelial cells and again it is in equilibrium with carbonic acid and bicarbonate and hydrogen ions. The bicarbonate ions accompany the sodium ions into the interstitial fluid, so that the net effect is that $NaHCO_3$ is reabsorbed from the tubule. The rate at which equilibrium is reached in the reaction $H_2CO_3 \rightleftharpoons H_2O + CO_2$ is increased by carbonic anhydrase present in the walls of the tubular epithelium. The exchange of hydrogen ions for sodium completes the mechanism for the reabsorption of filtered bicarbonate. Normally little bicarbonate appears in the urine which is slightly acid. The bicarbonate reabsorbed from the tubule carries water with it and tends to make the urine more acid: it does not correct an acidosis, since the amount of bicarbonate returned to the plasma from the tubule is the same as that which originally left it. Correction of acidosis requires the return to the plasma of more bicarbonate than that lost by glomerular filtration and this occurs in the distal tubule.

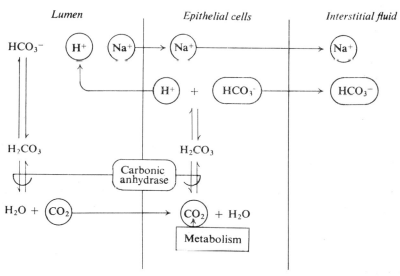

Fig. 13.3. Reabsorption of bicarbonate in the proximal tubule. Hydrogen ions are secreted by the tubule cells in exchange for sodium ions.

If the amount of bicarbonate filtered is excessive, as, for example, after ingestion of sodium bicarbonate, or if the rate of hydrogen ion secretion is depressed as a result of a low P_{CO_2} or because of the effect of a drug which inhibits carbonic anhydrase, then filtered bicarbonate is still present in the tubule when more distant segments are reached. If there is more bicarbonate than the total amount of hydrogen ion secreted, then the excess bicarbonate is not reabsorbed but is excreted in an alkaline urine.

The fluid reaching the end of the proximal tubule differs from the glomerular filtrate in that its volume has been reduced to about one-fifth, the concentrations of the sulphate ion and of the nitrogenous constituents is greater, there is no glucose, and about 80% of the sodium ion has been reabsorbed in company with chloride, bicarbonate and phosphate. The amount of sodium ion appearing in the glomerular filtrate in 24 h is about 580 g, of which 460 g are reabsorbed in the proximal tubule. But only about 6 g of sodium ion are eliminated in the urine in 24 h, therefore about 110 g of sodium ion must be reabsorbed from the remainder of the nephron.

Potassium ions are probably reabsorbed by similar mechanisms to those accounting for sodium ions. The precise site of K^+ absorption is not known, but all of that filtered has been removed from the tubular fluid by the time it reaches the beginning of the distal segment. However, K^+ is present in the urine, hence it must be secreted into the tubule at a later stage.

The loop of Henle. Further reabsorption of solute (mainly NaCl) and water takes place in the loop of Henle. The two limbs of the loop have different properties: the descending limb is freely permeable to water, while the ascending limb is relatively impermeable to water. The epithelium of the ascending limb actively transports Na^+ from within the tubule into the interstitial fluid, the cation being passively accompanied by anions (mainly Cl^-). The net outward movement of solute renders the interstitial fluid hypertonic and water moves out from the descending limb under the osmotic gradient, which in turn makes the fluid in the descending limb hypertonic. This hypertonicity reaches a peak in the fluid at the tip of the loop, after which the reabsorption of solute from the ascending limb is sufficiently pronounced to render its contents hypotonic by the time the distal convoluted tubule is reached. These processes are facilitated by the parallel arrangement of the two limbs of the loop; by making the interstitia hypertonic, the ascending limb facilitates water reabsorption from the descending limb; in turn, water reabsorption from the descending limb facilitates active Na^+ reabsorption from the ascending limb by increasing the intraluminal concentration of Na^+ and by diluting the interstitial fluid, thus lowering the concentration gradient against which Na^+ is transported. The overall mechanism is described as a 'counter current multiplier'. The hypertonic fluid from the interstices of the renal medulla is taken up in the capillaries branching off the vasa recta because the protein osmotic pressure of their plasma is high owing to the fluid lost in forming the glomerular filtrate. The net gain of solute by the plasma carried away by the veins leaving the renal medulla results in it being hypertonic with respect to plasma elsewhere.

The mechanism of active transport of Na^+ in the ascending limb of the loop of Henle is not known; it does not involve carbonic anhydrase and exchange with H^+.

The distal convoluted tubule. The distal tubule receives about one-eighth of the volume of the original glomerular filtrate containing, in 24 h, about 70 g of Na^+ out of the 560 g originally filtered. About 64 g of Na^+ is reabsorbed from the distal tubules, and to some extent from the collecting ducts. About 110 g of chloride is reabsorbed from the distal tubule in company with some of the actively transported sodium. The remainder of the reabsorbed Na^+ is exchanged for H+ or K+. This mechanism is under the influence of *aldosterone*, a steroid hormone secreted from the adrenal cortex (page 378), which specifically promotes the reabsorption of Na+ in exchange for other cations. The stimulus for aldosterone release is an increase in the circulating level of angiotensin. The tubular fluid is normally acidified in the distal tubule so that the secretion of hydrogen ion is against a concentration gradient. However, it is not known for certain which of the inter-linked processes is active and requires metabolic energy; one of them must be active and this will drive the others. The

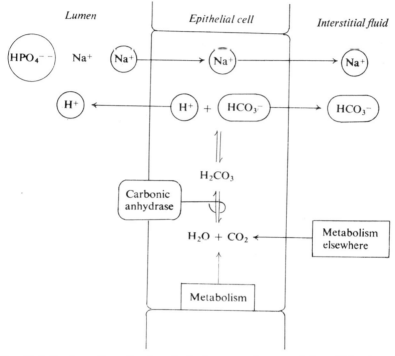

FIG. 13.4. Reabsorption of sodium by hydrogen exchange and the acidification of urinary buffers in the distal tubule.

mechanism for the reabsorption of Na+ in exchange for H+ in the distal tubule is illustrated in Fig. 13.4. By the time the fluid reaches the distal tubule there is usually no bicarbonate remaining and the sodium ions are present along with other anions such as phosphate. The concentration of phosphate ions has been increased by reabsorption of the filtrate to the extent that the system $HPO_4^{--}/H_2PO_4^-$ now has considerable buffering power. The secretion of hydrogen ions by the cells of the distal tubule depends on carbonic acid formed by the hydration of carbon dioxide produced by cellular metabolism. Although no bicarbonate is present in the tubular fluid, the secretion of each hydrogen ion into the lumen is accompanied by the uptake of a bicarbonate ion into the plasma. This mechanism therefore forms part of the kidney's share in eliminating acid from the body to preserve the alkaline reaction of the plasma.

If the pH of the urine falls to 6 or below, the ammonium mechanism is

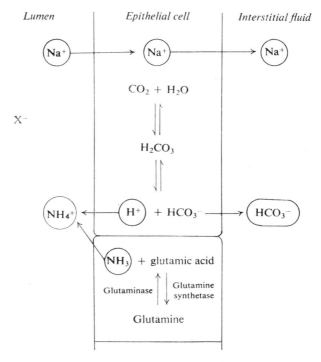

FIG. 13.5. The ammonium mechanism.

stimulated. This mechanism permits the secretion of hydrogen ions in exchange for sodium ions to continue without further lowering the pH of the urine. As a result, additional bicarbonate is added to the plasma. The ammonium mechanism is illustrated in Fig. 13.5.

Ammonia is produced in the cells of the distal tubule and of the collecting ducts. The principal source of ammonia is from hydrolysis of the amide group of glutamine, the reaction being catalysed by glutaminase. Glutamine synthetase occurs in the liver and the kidney. Glutamine accounts for about 60% of the ammonia produced, the remainder being derived from the oxidative deamination of other amino acids. The epithelial cells are freely permeable to ammonia in solution which therefore diffuses into the lumen where it combines with protons to form ammonium ions. Ammonium ions cannot penetrate the epithelial cells and therefore remain in the lumen and appear in the urine. The removal of hydrogen ions from the lumen in this way prevents the concentration gradient for these ions from increasing any further so that secretion of hydrogen ions by the tubular cells is not inhibited.

Potassium ions as well as hydrogen ions may be secreted by the distal tubule in exchange for sodium ions. Potassium and hydrogen ions appear to compete for a common pathway of secretion and the amounts of each excreted depend on their relative availabilities in the tubular epithelium. A large intake of potassium with the diet raises the plasma potassium. At first, the increase is partly offset by an increase in intracellular potassium so that the extracellular/ intracellular K^+ ratio is held constant, but, subsequently, the secretion of K^+ into the urine gradually restores the potassium balance. The secretion of K^+ does not result in the uptake of a bicarbonate ion into the plasma and the reabsorbed Na^+ therefore enters the plasma in company with another anion such as Cl^-.

About 16 ml of fluid per min enter the distal tubule from the loop of Henle. The normal rate of urine formation is about 1 ml/min, therefore about 15 ml of water are absorbed per min from the distal tubules and collecting ducts. Water is reabsorbed passively in company with solute. However, the permeability of the tubular epithelium to water is influenced by anti-diuretic hormone released from the posterior lobe of the pituitary gland (page 365). In the presence of anti-diuretic hormone, the distal tubule is impermeable to water. Anti-diuretic hormone therefore facilitates the reabsorption of water by increasing the permeability of the distal tubule. The stimulus for the secretion of anti-diuretic hormone is an increase in the osmotic pressure of the blood, or a decrease in blood volume. The tubular fluid regains isotonicity in the last third of the distal tubule, and remains isotonic until it reaches the collecting ducts.

The collecting ducts. Further passive reabsorption of water occurs from the collecting ducts, the permeability of which is also influenced by anti-diuretic hormone. The ducts run through the renal medulla in which the interstitial fluid is hypertonic. Reabsorption of water in the ducts therefore renders the urine hypertonic.

The urine contains calcium and magnesium ions and these may precipitate as the sparingly soluble alkaline phosphates when the urine is alkaline. When urine is allowed to stand it becomes alkaline because urea is converted to ammonia by bacterial action. When this occurs these insoluble phosphates are precipitated together with ammonium magnesium phosphate making the urine cloudy.

NITROGENOUS CONSTITUENTS OF URINE. The principal nitrogen containing substances in urine are urea, creatinine, uric acid, ammonia and small amounts of amino acids. The production of ammonia has been described previously.

Urea is formed in the liver from ammonia released by the deamination of amino acids (page 329). It is dissolved in the plasma, from which it is filtered in the glomerulus and passes through the proximal tubule which is impermeable to it. However, the loop of Henle is permeable to urea, and some urea is actively reabsorbed from the ascending limb. The interstitial fluid of the renal medulla therefore contains a high concentration of urea which helps to keep it hypertonic as part of the mechanism described previously for reabsorbing water. Urea is lost from this interstitial fluid into the blood and some may re-enter the urine by diffusion into the collecting ducts.

Creatinine is a metabolite formed from creatine via creatine phosphate (a high energy storage compound, page 47).

$$
\begin{array}{ccc}
\underset{\displaystyle NH=C}{\overset{\displaystyle NH_2}{|}} & \underset{\displaystyle HN=C}{\overset{\displaystyle NH-\textcircled{P}}{|}} & \underset{\displaystyle HN=C}{\overset{\displaystyle NH-CO}{|}} \\
| & \longrightarrow \quad | & \longrightarrow \quad | \quad | \\
CH_3-N-CH_2-COOH & CH_3-N-CH_2-COOH & CH_3-N-CH_2 \\
\text{Creatine} & \text{Creatine phosphate} & \text{Creatinine}
\end{array}
$$

Creatinine passes into the glomerular filtrate and it is also secreted by the tubules; only negligible amounts are reabsorbed.

Uric acid arises chiefly from the breakdown of purine bases from nucleic acids which are both released during cell destruction and replacement and ingested in the diet; a little is synthesized from glycine. Uric acid is excreted as such in man, but in most mammals it is further oxidized to allantoin. Uric acid appears in the glomerular filtrate, but much of it is reabsorbed from the tubules. Certain drugs (e.g. probenecid and salicylates) diminish the reabsorption of uric acid, so more appears in the urine. An excess of uric acid in the blood leads to the deposition of sodium mono-urate in the joints, which causes attacks of acute pain called gout. Urates are also deposited under the skin and form swellings. Chronic gout is a metabolic disorder associated with an increased production of uric acid from amino acids.

The yellow colour of urine is due mainly to the pigment urochrome, the chemical structure of which is unknown. It probably arises as a metabolic product since its concentration is increased when metabolic activity, including destruction of protein, is increased. Traces of other pigments, such as urobilinogen (page 327), are also present.

ABNORMAL CONSTITUENTS OF URINE. Examination of the urine forms an important part of diagnosis of disease. A few of the abnormal substances which may be found in urine are given in Table 13.2, together with the conditions which may give rise to them.

TABLE 13.2. Some abnormal constituents of urine and their causes.

Abnormal constituent	Possible underlying disorders
Protein (proteinuria, albuminuria)	Kidney disease, high blood pressure
Haemoglobin (haemoglobinuria)	Intravascular haemolysis
Glucose (glycosuria)	High blood glucose, especially diabetes mellitus
Keto-acids and acetone (ketosis)	Abnormal metabolism, especially in diabetes mellitus
Bile pigments	Haemolytic or hepatic jaundice
Bile salts	Obstructive jaundice
Phenylpyruvic acid (phenylketonuria)	Inherited metabolic disorder (page 186)
Homogentisic acid (alcaptonuria)	Inherited metabolic disorder due to absence of enzyme oxidizing dihydroxyphenylacetic acid

Methods of studying renal function

CLEARANCE VALUE. The rate at which a substance is eliminated in the urine is often expressed as a clearance value, which relates rate of elimination to plasma concentration. Thus, if the rate of elimination of urea in urine is 20 mg/min and the concentration of urea in plasma is 0·3 mg/ml the clearance value is expressed as 67 ml/min. This value is *equivalent* to the volume of plasma that has been cleared of urea per min. Urea is filtered into the glomerulus, but some is reabsorbed in the tubule, so the measurement of urea clearance by itself does not give any specific information about either one of these kidney functions.

GLOMERULAR FILTRATION RATE. A clearance value of a substance which is filtered but not reabsorbed will give a measure of the rate of formation of glomerular filtrate. Inulin is such a substance. It is a water-soluble polysaccharide of fructose with a molecular weight of 5200; it is non-toxic and is not metabolized; it is not adsorbed on plasma proteins and it does not penetrate cell membranes. If inulin is eliminated into the urine at a rate of 125 mg/min when the plasma concentration of inulin has been raised to 1 mg/ml by giving an intravenous infusion of inulin, then the clearance value for inulin is 125 ml/min, and this is also the rate of formation of glomerular filtrate. The ability of the kidneys to reabsorb water can be determined if the rate of formation of urine is known. The rate of absorption of urea can also be determined now that the volume of glomerular filtrate is known; the concentration of urea in plasma (0·3 mg/ml) and in glomerular filtrate is the same, and 125 ml of filtrate are formed per min; therefore, 37·5 mg of urea enter the tubules each minute; since 20 mg leave the tubules each minute (i.e. appear in the urine), the difference, 17·5 mg, is the amount reabsorbed from the tubules each minute.

The glomerular filtration rate has also been measured with potassium ferrocyanide. Creatinine was used at one time for this purpose but, in man, some is reabsorbed and the clearance values were lower than for inulin or ferrocyanide. In the dog, creatinine is not reabsorbed and the clearance value is the same for all three compounds. Cyanocobalamin is also used (see page 916).

MAXIMAL TUBULAR REABSORPTION. The reabsorptive power of the tubules may be determined in the following way. When the plasma concentration of glucose is progressively raised, a point is reached at which the tubular reabsorptive capacity is exceeded and glucose appears in the urine. For example, at a plasma glucose level of 4 mg/ml, the rate at which glucose appears in the urine may be 150 mg/min. Now the volume of the glomerular filtrate formed in 1 min (determined by simultaneous inulin clearance) is, say, 125 ml/min. Since the concentration of glucose in the filtrate is the same as in plasma (4 mg/ml), 500 mg of glucose is present to the tubules each minute, of which 150 mg escapes reabsorption and appears in the urine. Therefore the amount reabsorbed is 350 mg/min. The term, maximal tubular reabsorption, is often abbreviated to T_m, and in the example given above, the result would be expressed: glucose $- T_m = 350$ mg/min.

It has already been mentioned that glucose is completely reabsorbed from the glomerular filtrate when the blood concentration is less than 180 mg/ml, but when tubular reabsorption is blocked by phloridzin, glucose clearance values approach those for inulin. Expressed in another way, phloridzin decreases the glucose-T_m, and when T_m reaches zero, glucose clearance equals inulin clearance.

MAXIMAL TUBULAR SECRETION. Some organic compounds injected into the blood-stream (e.g. diodone and para-aminohippuric acid) are actively secreted by the distal tubules, and the method for measurement of maximal tubular secretion makes use of such a substance. When the plasma concentration of diodone or para-aminohippuric acid is progressively raised, a point is reached at which the tubules are secreting at their maximal capacity. At this point, a further increase in plasma concentration causes an increased rate of excretion which is due only to glomerular filtration. If the excretion rate and plasma concentration are expressed graphically, there is an abrupt change in the slope of the graph at the point at which tubular secretion reaches its maximal capacity. The maximal tubular secretion (also abbreviated to T_m) is determined in a similar way to tubular reabsorption. The T_m for secretion of para-aminohippuric acid is about 70 mg/min.

RENAL BLOOD FLOW. Provided that the tubular secretory capacity for diodone or para-aminohippuric acid is not exceeded, either of these substances is completely extracted from the plasma during its passage through the glomerular and tubular capillaries. If the plasma concentration of diodone is 1 mg/100 ml and the rate of urinary excretion is 7 mg/min, then the clearance value is 700 ml/min, but, since the plasma is completely cleared, this is also the rate of plasma flow through the excretory portion of the kidney. Direct measurement of renal blood flow (in animal experiments) gives a figure only slightly higher, and it is known that about 80% of the blood entering the renal arteries enters the excretory portion of the kidney.

FILTRATION FRACTION. If the rate of glomerular filtration (from inulin clearance) is 125 ml/min, and the rate of renal plasma flow (from diodone clearance) is 700 ml/min, then the fraction of plasma passing through the glomerular membrane is 0·18, or 18%.

DIODONE AND PARA-AMINOHIPPURIC ACID. Diodone, and other similar iodine-containing organic compounds, may sometimes produce unpleasant side-effects when injected; they have been largely replaced by para-amino-hippuric acid for clearance studies. However, the iodine compounds do have another advantage in that they are radio-opaque, that is, they block the passage of X-rays. Since they accumulate in the kidneys and in the urinary passages, these structures can be made to stand out clearly (see pages 525).

Kidney failure, nephrectomy, and the artificial kidney

The power of the kidney to do osmotic work is approximately gauged by the specific gravity of the urine. If, after a 12-h abstinence from food and water, the subject passes a morning sample of urine with a specific gravity below 1·025 (about 1000 milliosmoles per litre), there is a loss of concentrating power.

The kidney is very sensitive to damage by ischaemia; arrest of the blood supply to the kidney for only a few minutes leads to a proteinuria caused by increased glomerular capillary permeability. Complete arrest of blood flow for 8 h causes severe tubular damage which is generally irreversible.

The detailed processes carried out by the kidney are many and it is unlikely in disease that all these functions are disturbed simultaneously, or to the same degree. Any one of the following indicates renal failure of some degree: (1) failure to excrete nitrogenous waste products, such as urea, (2) acidaemia, (3) raised serum K^+ levels, and (4) cellular dehydration. Symptoms of complete kidney failure are vomiting, diarrhoea, later breathlessness, and finally a CNS depression. This starts as a listlessness and confusion, progressing to drowsiness and eventual coma. Death ensues in about 5 to 7 days unless remedial measures are started. The true cause of these symptoms is not understood. It is not solely due to the high blood concentrations of urea or uric acid, as these substances alone when administered experimentally in very high doses are not toxic. However, a high blood urea concentration is a sign of impending renal failure.

The removal of a diseased kidney (partial or unilateral nephrectomy) may preserve function in the remaining kidney. Previously inactive glomeruli in the remaining kidney become active, and the kidney hypertrophies and takes over the functional capacity of the two. An artificial kidney may be used to overcome acute crises where one or both kidneys do not function efficiently.

The artificial kidney consists of about 45 m of cellophane tubing, wound round a cylinder rotating in a tank of physiological saline. Heparinized blood from the patient is led from a suitable artery (the femoral or radial) through the cellophane tubing and returned to the body in a suitable vein. Diffusable crystalloids exchange between the plasma and the saline, and by suitable renewal, replenishment, and control of the saline constituents, urea and other nitrogenous wastes are lost from the blood, and the blood may be made to lose or take up water, Na^+, K^+, Cl^- or H^+.

Micturition

The urine is conveyed from the kidneys to the bladder along the ureters by peristaltic waves which travel down to the bladder about every 10 sec. The junction of each ureter with the bladder acts like a valve preventing urine from being forced back into the ureter when the pressure in the bladder is raised. The ureters receive both motor and inhibitory fibres from the sympathetic; there is no parasympathetic innervation.

The emptying of the bladder (micturition) is under both autonomic and voluntary control, although it becomes a purely involuntary spinal reflex after section of the spinal cord above the lumbar region. The smooth muscle of the bladder walls (detrusor muscle) and the internal sphincter receive both sympathetic (adrenergic) and parasympathetic innervation. The external sphincter receives motoneurones of the somatic nervous system which leave the spinal column at the level of the second, third and fourth sacral vertebrae and which are carried in the pudendal nerve. The sympathetic fibres arise in the first and second lumbar segments and run in the two hypogastric nerves. In man these fibres relay in the hypogastric ganglia on the lateral aspects of the rectum. In many animals most of the fibres relay in the inferior mesenteric ganglia which are rarely present in man. The parasympathetic fibres arise in the second and third sacral segments and run in the nervi erigentes. These fibres also relay in the hypogastric ganglia. Afferent fibres run together with both sympathetic and parasympathetic supplies. These fibres terminate in receptors sensitive to distension of the bladder and to painful stimuli.

When the bladder is full (about 500 ml urine) contraction waves appear which stimulate the pressure receptors in the bladder wall. Afferent impulses discharged to the spinal cord and to the cerebral cortex give rise to the desire to micturate. If it is convenient to micturate, internal and external sphincters are relaxed by inhibition of their motor supply (sympathetic and somatic respectively), and the bladder is contracted by increased parasympathetic activity and by increased intra-abdominal pressure caused by descent of the diaphragm and contraction of the abdominal muscles. If it is inconvenient to micturate, the cerebral cortex can cause elongation of the bladder wall by inhibiting parasympathetic activity and probably by increasing sympathetic activity so that the pressure in the bladder is reduced and the afferent discharge is temporarily depressed. Voluntary emptying of the bladder can also be initiated by the cerebral cortex before the afferent nerves signal that the bladder is full.

Regulation of the pH of the body fluids

The regulation of body fluid pH involves the blood buffers, the lungs and the kidneys. The blood and the lungs have been dealt with in previous chapters and it is therefore convenient at this point to summarize the body's reaction to excess acid or alkali.

The pH of the plasma of arterial blood is normally maintained between 7·36 and 7·44, the extreme range compatible with life being 7·0 to 7·8. A change of 1 unit of pH would denote a ten-fold change in hydrogen ion concentration so that, in terms of relative hydrogen ion concentration, these extremes correspond to a range of from 2·5 times the normal to two-fifths the normal. At body temperature, the pH of a neutral solution is 6·8, and the reaction of the plasma is therefore always alkaline. The pH of the intracellular fluid is less alkaline than that of plasma and approaches neutrality (pH 6·8 to 6·9). An increase in the alkaline reaction of the body fluids to pH 7·8 and above leads to headache, nausea, mental confusion, lassitude, tetany of striated muscles and

12

death; reduced alkalinity to pH 7·0 and below leads to breathlessness, stupor, coma and death.

Changes in pH tend to occur through the production of large amounts of acid during metabolism and through the ingestion of both acids and alkalis in the diet. When the total concentration of available buffer is less than normal, as a result of its being used up in buffering excess hydrogen ions, the condition is called *acidosis*. Providing the pH is held above the normal lower limit of 7·36, the acidosis is not accompanied by *acidaemia*. Acidaemia may be defined as a condition in which the blood pH is less than 7·36. *Alkalosis* is a condition in which the total concentration of buffers is greater than normal, and *alkalaemia* is an abnormally alkaline reaction of the blood (pH greater than 7·4).

Excess acid. Metabolic processes yield greater quantities of carbonic acid than of any other acid (about 13,000 mmoles of CO_2 are produced in a day). Hydrogen ions derived from this carbonic acid are adequately buffered by haemoglobin and the plasma proteins, and carbonic acid is readily converted to water and carbon dioxide which is removed by the lungs. Furthermore, carbonic acid is a weak acid and the system HCO_3^-/H_2CO_3 forms the principal buffer system of the body fluids.

The pH of the blood will fall when there is an increased P_{CO_2} in the plasma as a result of hypoventilation of the lungs. The increase in carbonic acid concentration causes an increase in bicarbonate. There is then a redistribution between bicarbonate and the other buffers but the total amount of buffer is not changed (i.e. there is a tendency to acidaemia but no acidosis). A high P_{CO_2} favours the secretion of H^+ by the kidney tubules so that the urine is acidified and even more bicarbonate is added to the plasma. The acid urine removes acid from the body and corrects the acidaemia; the imbalance in bicarbonate is corrected by a subsequent increase in ventilation of the lungs.

A few strong acids are produced by metabolism, and the most important of these is the non-volatile sulphuric acid formed from the oxidation of sulphur ingested chiefly in the amino acids, methionine and cysteine. It has been estimated that the metabolism of 100 g of protein produces 60 m-equiv. of sulphuric acid. The ingestion of ammonium chloride as a diuretic (pages 887–888) provides another example of acid production, since the NH_3 is converted to urea by the liver, leaving HCl. These acids, which are produced in localized regions, are rapidly diluted throughout the body fluids and this itself has some effect in raising the pH (a ten-fold dilution of a strong acid raises the pH by 1 unit). Most of the hydrogen ions are instantly buffered by the buffering systems of the blood so that there is an acidosis but the fall in pH is slight: in order of importance the blood buffers are bicarbonate, haemoglobin, plasma protein and phosphate. Some of the hydrogen ions are removed by exchanging for metallic cations (Na^+, Ca^{++}, Mg^{++}) in the skeleton. Consequently, prolonged acidosis may lead to decalcification of bone as the calcium is excreted in the urine.

When the bicarbonate buffer takes up hydrogen ions it is converted to water and CO_2 which is removed from the lungs; breathing is stimulated by a rise in P_{CO_2} (page 290). The respiratory mechanism therefore reduces the tendency to acidaemia, but the acidosis remains because the body has lost bicarbonate buffer in the form of CO_2, and some of the other buffers have combined with hydrogen ions and have therefore lost their buffering capacity. In the examples quoted, the body fluids now contain excess sulphates and chlorides. Some of the sulphate is conjugated in the liver with phenolic compounds to form neutral ethereal sulphates which are excreted in the urine. The final correction of the acidosis is accomplished by the kidneys. The glomerular filtrate contains sulphate and chloride in the same concentration as in the plasma, together with an equivalent amount of cation which is mainly Na^+. The cells of the distal tubule manufacture and secrete hydrogen ions in exchange for sodium ions which re-enter the plasma in company with bicarbonate. In this way, the excess acid is removed and the bicarbonate buffer and sodium ions are restored to the plasma. Reabsorption of sodium ions reverses any exchange which occurred with cations in the skeleton, and reabsorption of bicarbonate regenerates other buffers by removing the hydrogen ions which they had taken up.

The hydrogen ion in the urine is buffered by the phosphate buffers until the pH of the urine falls to about 6 when the ammonium mechanism is stimulated. The ammonium mechanism allows additional secretion of hydrogen ions, and reabsorption of bicarbonate and sodium ions, without further significant fall in urinary pH. The normal quantity of acid secreted in the urine is 20–30 m-equiv. of titratable acid and 30–50 m-equiv. of ammonium each day, and this corresponds to the 50–80 m-equiv. of strong acid produced daily by metabolism.

In severe untreated diabetes mellitus, β-hydroxybutyric acid and acetoacetic acid are produced as a result of impaired fat metabolism (page 328) in amounts up to 1000 m-equiv./day. These acids are partly buffered in the plasma and partly undissociated. They pass into the kidney tubules as undissociated acid and as anions in company with metallic cations. In a sustained acidosis arising from this and other causes, the urine may contain as much as 500 m-equiv. of ammonium daily.

Excess alkali. The amount of alkali in the plasma may increase as a result of the ingestion of sodium bicarbonate, of alkalizing salts such as potassium citrate and sodium lactate, or of vegetable diets which contain large amounts of the potassium salts of organic acids. Metabolism of organic anions results in the formation of bicarbonate so that the ingestion of these substances is equivalent to ingestion of bicarbonate. An increased plasma concentration of bicarbonate means that buffering capacity is increased, thereby giving an alkalosis. The tendency of excess buffer to produce alkalaemia by removing hydrogen ions is offset by a decrease in ventilation of the lungs so that CO_2 is retained. The bicarbonate, accompanied by metallic cations, is filtered at the glomerulus. Because of the alkalosis the rate at which the tubules can form hydrogen ions is depressed. The increased load of bicarbonate delivered to the tubules exceeds the capacity of the tubular epithelium to secrete H^+ ion in exchange for Na^+, so that bicarbonate remains in the urine which is alkaline. A diet rich in potassium salts favours the excretion of K^+ in exchange for Na^+ in the distal tubule, and this mechanism acts to return Na^+ to the plasma accompanied by anions other than bicarbonate which remains in the urine.

Overbreathing causes a rise in blood pH by removing carbonic acid. The fall in P_{CO_2} reduces the concentration of bicarbonate in the plasma and this is exaggerated by the kidneys. There is no change in the total blood concentration of buffer, but only a redistribution between bicarbonate and other buffers. Because of the low P_{CO_2}, the ability of the kidney tubule to manufacture hydrogen ions is reduced and bicarbonate remains in the urine which is alkaline. By removing alkali, the kidneys restore the normal reaction of the plasma but the concentration of bicarbonate buffer can only be restored by subsequent hypoventilation.

Alkalaemia may arise from excessive vomiting and the consequent loss of gastric acid from the body. The main gastric glands secrete a large volume of HCl and water but the pyloric glands secrete an alkaline fluid containing Na^+ so that the alkalaemia may be accompanied by sodium deficiency. The pH of the blood may be compensated by the respiratory mechanism but the alkalosis, which is normally corrected by the excretion of $NaHCO_3$ in the urine, does not occur because of the sodium deficiency. The kidneys in fact reabsorb Na^+ in exchange for H^+ and so secrete an acid urine in spite of the alkalosis. If NaCl is given to such patients, the sodium deficiency is corrected and a highly alkaline urine is excreted with the result that the alkalosis is quickly corrected.

CHAPTER 14

The Endocrine System

The endocrine system consists of ductless glands which form hormones and secrete them directly into the blood-stream. The term *hormone* (derived from the Greek word meaning 'to urge on') denotes a specific chemical entity that is secreted into the blood by a well-defined group of cells and is then transported via the vascular system to a site distant from its point of origin, where its action takes place. Compounds which exhibit hormonal action may be found in many molecular sizes and shapes. On the basis of chemical structure, however, three main groups may be classified: *amino acids* or their derivatives (from the adrenal medulla and the thyroid gland), *steroids* related to cholesterol (from the sex glands and the adrenal cortex), and *polypeptides* and proteins (from the pituitary gland and pancreas). All hormones act in trace amounts, are not sources of energy for biological reactions but regulate rates of chemical reactions, require a latent period before an effect is apparent, and appear to be active only in particular sensitive tissues.

The actions of hormones may be classified under the following three headings: *morphogenesis*, involving the growth, differentiation and maturation of the organism; *homeostasis*, maintaining a steady but dynamic equilibrium of the components of the internal environment of an animal; and *functional integration*, whereby the endocrine and nervous systems depend upon one another and complement each other in many of their actions.

The methods of regulating the secretion of an endocrine gland are varied, and a number of mechanisms may be involved in an individual instance. If the hormone is rapidly lost from the circulation either through utilization, degradation or excretion, then the level drops rapidly; this, in turn, excites the pituitary gland to secrete more trophic or stimulating hormone into the blood to act on the target endocrine gland. This *feedback system* is a relatively simple one involving mutual control of secretion rates of the trophic hormone and the target gland hormone by the level of these substances in circulation. For example, the thyroid-stimulating hormone of the pituitary gland stimulates the release of the thyroid hormone from the thyroid gland, and this in turn acts back on the pituitary gland to inhibit the further release of thyroid-stimulating hormone. Comparable systems control the secretions of the adrenal cortex and of the sex glands. A modified type of feedback mechanism involves a blood constituent such as glucose; the blood concentration of glucose is controlled by insulin, the hormone secreted by the pancreas, and this in turn influences the rate of release of insulin.

357

A list of the source and chief physiological actions of the main hormones found in mammals is given in Table 14.1.

TABLE 14.1. The source and chief actions of mammalian hormones.

Source	Hormone	Chief actions
Pituitary gland (anterior lobe) = adenohypophysis	Growth hormone	Stimulates growth
	Thyrotrophic hormone	Stimulates release of thyroid hormone
	Adrenocorticotrophic hormone	Stimulates release of adrenal cortical hormones
	Follicle-stimulating hormone	Stimulates maturation of sex cells and synthesis of sex hormones
	Luteinizing hormone	Stimulates release of sex hormones and development of corpus luteum
	Lactogenic hormone	Stimulates milk production
Pituitary gland (posterior lobe) = neurohypophysis	Oxytocin	Stimulates uterine movement
	Vasopressin	Exerts an anti-diuretic action
Thyroid gland	Thyroxine, Tri-iodothyronine	Cause increased oxygen utilization
	Thyrocalcitonin	Controls calcium metabolism
Parathyroid gland	Parathormone	Controls calcium and phosphorus metabolism
Adrenal gland (medulla)	Adrenaline, Noradrenaline	Influence blood pressure and blood sugar
Adrenal gland (cortex)	Glucocorticoids	Influence carbohydrate and nitrogen metabolism
	Mineralocorticoids	Influence salt and water balance
Pancreas	Insulin, glucagon	Control carbohydrate metabolism
Ovary (follicle)	Oestrogens	Stimulate growth and development of female reproductive tract
Ovary (corpus luteum)	Progestins	Maintain pregnancy and stimulate growth and development of uterus and mammary gland
Testis	Androgens	Stimulate both general protein synthesis and the growth and development of the male reproductive tract

The hormones of the pituitary gland stimulate the release of a number of other hormones and therefore they will be considered first.

The pituitary gland (hypophysis)

The pituitary is situated in a hollow, called the sella turcica, at the base of the skull. It is attached to the brain below the floor of the third ventricle and behind the optic chiasma. The gland is composed of two parts which are fused together but are of separate embryological origin and function. The adenohypophysis (or anterior lobe) arises from the ectodermal layer of the roof of the buccal cavity from which a blind pouch grows upwards (the pouch of Rathke). The neurohypophysis (or posterior lobe) is derived from a downward projection of the floor of the third ventricle and is composed of neural tissue. The top of the pouch from the ectodermal layer becomes pushed in and wrapped around the tip of the neural downgrowth. The anterior wall of the pouch then thickens and the central cavity is reduced to a narrow cleft (see Fig. 14.1). The adult pituitary is readily separated into anterior and posterior portions along a natural line of cleavage, the original embryonic cavity of Rathke's pouch.

The adenohypophysis. There are three distinct parts of the adenohypophysis (see Fig. 14.1). By far the largest is the *pars distalis*, arising from the thickened anterior wall of the pouch of Rathke; the *pars intermedia* is the flattened posterior wall; and the uppermost portion surrounding the pituitary stalk is called the *pars tuberalis*. The pars distalis is composed of cords of cells between which are numerous vascular sinusoids supported by connective tissue. The cells are of two main types which are differentiated by their affinity for various dyes. About half of the cells stain lightly, possess no granules, and are not engaged in secretion. The other half are granule-containing chromophilic cells in which the adenohypophysial hormones are elaborated. About 80% of the chromophils are acidophilic (the alpha cells) and the rest are basophilic (the beta cells). The pars intermedia contains basophil cells which have vesicles containing a colloid material. The pars tuberalis is composed only of agranular cells. There is no nerve supply to the adenohypophysis, apart from a few sympathetic fibres which innervate the larger blood vessels.

The trophic hormones of the adenohypophysis influence a variety of physiological functions related to general metabolism and the complex processes of growth and reproduction. Six such hormones are listed in Table 14.2. All are protein in nature but they vary considerably in composition.

GROWTH HORMONE (SOMATOTROPHIC HORMONE, STH). Human growth hormone has a molecular weight of about 29,000 and is formed in acidophil cells of the adenohypophysis. Repeated injections increase the rate of growth of the long bones of animals, and it is possible in this way to produce rats which are twice the weight of their untreated littermates. Conversely,

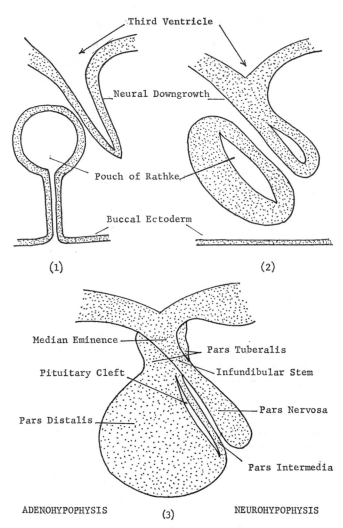

FIG. 14.1. Stages in the development of the pituitary gland.

hypophysectomy (the removal of the hypophysis) leads to the arrest of growth and development. Treatment of hypophysectomized animals with growth hormone restores growth but, in the absence of other pituitary hormones, the effects are less spectacular than those found in intact animals. Some organs such as the thymus and liver increase in weight, and there is an increase in nitrogen retention. Growth hormone also enhances the utilization of fatty acids for protein synthesis. Growth hormone is capable of inducing diabetes in normal animals probably by exhaustion of pancreatic supplies of insulin.

Both over- and under-production of growth hormone result in deformities in man, but the clinical condition is dependent on the time at which the

TABLE 14.2. The adenohypophysial hormones.

Name of hormone	Abbreviation	Target organ	Chief actions
Growth hormone (somatotrophic hormone)	STH	Skeleton	Anabolism
Thyrotrophic hormone (thyroid-stimulating hormone)	TSH	Thyroid gland	Release of thyroid hormones
Adrenocorticotrophic hormone (corticotrophin)	ACTH	Adrenal cortex	Release of adrenocortical steroids
Follicle-stimulating hormone (prolan A)	FSH	Ovary	Growth of ovum. Release of oestrogen (in association with LH)
		Testis	Growth of sperm
Luteinizing hormone (interstitial cell-stimulating hormone, prolan B)	LH (ICSH)	Ovary	Development of corpus luteum. Release of progesterone (in association with FSH)
		Testis	Release of testosterone
Lactogenic hormone, prolactin (luteotrophic hormone)	LTH	Mammary gland (and ovary in some species)	Milk production

derangement occurs. Before puberty, over-production leads to *gigantism* when height may exceed 7 feet. In the adult, hypersecretion is frequently associated with an acidophilic pituitary tumour and produces the condition called *acromegaly*. Hyposecretion of growth hormone in the child may result in a pituitary dwarf who may be completely normal, apart from size. Encouraging results in the treatment of pituitary dwarfs with purified human growth hormone have been reported. Hyposecretion of only growth hormone rarely occurs in the adult, as there is usually a depression of all adenohypophysial secretions; this condition is known as panhypopituitarism. The potency of a growth hormone preparation is assessed either by its effect on the body weight of normal or hypophysectomized rats or by its action in increasing the width of the proximal cartilage of the tibia in immature hypophysectomized rats.

THYROTROPHIC HORMONE (THYROID-STIMULATING HORMONE, TSH). Thyrotrophic hormone (molecular weight about 28,000) is formed in basophil cells of the adenohypophysis. Atrophy of the thyroid gland which follows hypophysectomy is reversed by treatment with thyrotrophic hormone. Administration of TSH to an intact animal leads to an increased production of the thyroid hormones and a consequent increase in metabolic rate. There is thyroid hypertrophy but these effects diminish after further dosage. Thus, the primary defects in TSH production lead to symptoms of hypo- or hyperthyroidism. Deposition of adipose tissue behind the eyes leading to *exophthalmos* (i.e. protrusion of the eyes) in thyrotoxicosis is probably associated with hypersecretion of the thyrotrophic hormone. Thyrotrophic hormone may be assayed by its ability to increase the thyroidal uptake of radioactive iodine, or by its effect on plasma thyroid hormone levels or on basal metabolic rate.

ADRENOCORTICOTROPHIC HORMONE (CORTICOTROPHIN, ACTH). ACTH is contained in the pituitary in a protein of molecular weight about 4,500. The corticortrophins from beef, sheep and swine pituitary glands have recently been purified sufficiently to permit the determination of the sequences of amino acids in the protein molecule; the first twenty-four amino acids residues in the three species are identical and only minor differences occur in the order of the remaining fifteen amino acids. A synthetic active peptide has been prepared in which the first twenty-three amino acids are identical with those found naturally.

After hypophysectomy, the adrenal glands are reduced in size. Histological examination shows that this is due to atrophy of one layer in the cortex, namely the zona fasciculata. There is a consequent reduction in adrenal cortical secretion. Administration of adrenocorticotrophic hormone to such animals increases the weight of the adrenal glands and restores the zona fasciculata to its original histological appearance. When given to intact animals, ACTH induces a rapid increase in the level of corticosteroids (predominantly glucocorticoids) in adrenal venous blood and then in peripheral blood, and finally a marked adrenal hypertrophy results. Cholesterol is a precursor of the adrenal steroids and its concentration in the adrenal gland is reduced after ACTH, presumably reflecting increased steroid synthesis. A decrease in adrenal ascorbic acid levels also occurs after ACTH in some species but the physiological significance of this change is still obscure. In 1932, Cushing described a case of basophilic tumour of the pituitary gland and hypertrophy of the adrenal cortex. The symptoms of the disease (which now bears his name) are those produced by an excess of adrenal steroids. There may be virilizing effects in women since over-production of ACTH may stimulate androgen production by the adrenal cortex.

Potent factors capable of bringing about release of ACTH have been isolated from the hypothalamus. These corticotrophin-releasing factors (termed CRF) are probably polypeptides of low molecular weight.

The assay of ACTH is complicated by the fact that many stimuli produce the rapid release of this hormone from the adenohypophysis. Satisfactory assay procedures are therefore restricted to hypophysectomized animals. Three important methods are: (a) the adrenal ascorbic acid depletion test of Sayers, (b) the release of corticosteroid into the adrenal vein of dog or rat, and (c) the release of steroid into the plasma of mice. The release of corticosteroids from adrenal segments incubated *in vitro* has also been used as an assay procedure.

FOLLICLE-STIMULATING HORMONE (PROLAN A, FSH). This is a glyco-protein, with molecular weight about 29,000, secreted by basophilic staining cells of the adenohypophysis. As a result of the action of FSH, follicles develop in the ovary of the female, and spermatogenesis and testicular growth occur in the male. The sex glands are discussed in detail in Chapter 15. The final maturation of the ovarian follicle (and the production of the ovarian hormone or oestrogen) requires the presence of the luteinizing hormone. The follicle-stimulating hormone is excreted by the kidney and small amounts may always be detected in the urine. There is a dramatic increase in urinary FSH after, for example, surgical removal of the ovaries or the natural reduction of ovarian function at the menopause. These observations suggest that the secretion of FSH is influenced by ovarian hormones.

LUTEINIZING HORMONE (INTERSTITIAL CELL-STIMULATIN GHOR-MONE, PROLAN B, LH OR ICSH). An ovarian follicle which has matured under the influence of FSH ruptures and releases the ovum, and its remains then develop into a corpus luteum in the presence of the luteinizing hormone. During the ripening stage the follicle also produces and secretes oestrogens under the stimulus of both gonadotrophins. Corpora lutea are maintained by the continued secretion of LH, which is also a protein. The secretion of progesterone by the corpora lutea is controlled by LH alone or in combination with the lactogenic hormone. Administration of purified luteinizing hormone to hypophysectomized animals has little effect upon the ovaries. If, however, both FSH and LH are given together, the observed increase in ovarian weight is greater than the sum of the effects of the two hormones given separately. In the male, LH stimulates the production of the male sex hormone, testosterone, from the interstitial cells of the testis (the cells of Leydig).

During pregnancy, the placenta (the uterine structure through which the foetus receives its food and oxygen from the mother) also produces gonad-stimulating hormones. In the pregnant human being, the gonadotrophin has activity similar to that of LH. It is called *human chorionic gonadotrophin* (HCG) and large quantities are excreted in the urine during pregnancy. It causes folli-cular development in immature intact rodents, and then ovulation and luteini-zation of the corpora lutea. The serum of pregnant mares has been found to contain a gonadotrophin which is predominantly FSH-like in action. This hormone is termed *pregnant mare's serum gonadotrophin* (PMSG) and appears during the first third of gestation.

LACTOGENIC HORMONE (PROLACTIN, LUTEOTROPHIC HORMONE, LTH). The lactogenic hormone is secreted by acidophilic staining cells of the adenohypophysis. The activation of the corpus luteum to a functional state is generally accepted as one of the principal effects of LTH. In most species (the cow is an exception), it stimulates the production of milk by the mammary gland. This effect occurs in pregnancy and in experimental animals in which mammary gland development has been stimulated by pre-treatment with oestrogen and progesterone. Lactation ceases when hypophysectomy is performed in a lactating animal but re-commences when treatment with lactogenic hormone is started. The luteotrophic action of lactogenic hormone has only been adequately studied in the rat, where follicular development and corpora lutea formation follow FSH and LH treatment but progesterone secretion only occurs in response to LTH release from the adenohypophysis. The importance of the luteotrophic action in man is not clear.

Biological methods of assay of gonadotrophins include the following: *FSH*—In the hypophysectomized immature rat, FSH activity may be estimated by determining the amount of material necessary to re-initiate follicular growth. Alternatively, LH may be added to the unknown preparation to ensure maximum augmentation and then the amount of material required to double the ovarian weight in the intact immature animal is determined. *LH*—Advantage is taken of the fact that LH causes testosterone production in the male, so that the increase in the weight of the ventral prostate gland of the immature hypophysectomized male rat affords a sensitive and specific method. Two newer methods depend on the fact that highly purified preparations of LH induce a decrease in both ovarian ascorbic acid and cholesterol. *LTH*—The most commonly employed technique is that based upon the increase in weight of the crop gland in pigeons produced by LTH. *HCG*—The pharmaco-poeal assay depends upon the production of changes in the vaginal smears of immature female rats. HCG stimulates the immature ovary to secrete oestrogens which, in turn, induce the appearance of cornified cells in the vaginal smear. This assay is not specific since oestrogens themselves induce similar vaginal changes in ovariectomized rats. Other bio-assay methods include stimulation of ovarian growth in weanling rats and uterine hypertrophy in immature mice. HCG also increases the ventral prostrate weight in immature male rats. *PSMG*—The methods most frequently used depend upon PMSG-induced increases in ovarian and uterine weight in immature rats or mice.

The pars intermedia. The pars intermedia is, in fact, derived from the adenohypophysis and its secretion is chemically related to the hormones produced by the anterior lobe of the hypophysis. The hormone of the pars intermedia (the melanocyte stimulating hormone, MSH) stimulates dispersion of the melanin granules in melanocytes of the skin of fish, amphibia and reptiles, with a resulting darkening of the skin; this may explain the pigmentation found in patients with Cushing's disease.

The neurohypophysis. During the development of the neurohypophysis from the floor of the third ventricle, the central cavity disappears and three parts may be located in the gland. The lobular portion associated with the adenohypophysis is the infundibular process or neural lobe (*pars nervosa*); the connecting limb is called the *infundibular stem*; and the upper expanded portion is the *median eminence* of the tuber cinereum. Although the median eminence and infundibular stem comprise only 15% of the neurohypophysis they are functional parts. The histological appearance of the neurohypophysis is quite distinct from that of the adenohypophysis; there are many nerve cells and non-myelinated fibres which extend into the hypothalamus at the base of the third ventricle (see Fig. 14.2). There are also numerous spindle-shaped cells with a granular cytoplasm (pituicytes) and blood vessels.

The usual techniques of hypophysectomy only allow for the removal of the infundibular stem and neural lobe with the adenohypophysis. Functional neurohypophysial tissue is therefore left behind and the effects of hypophysectomy are mainly due to removal of the adenohypophysis. Extracts of the pars nervosa (posterior pituitary extracts) have been shown to possess three separate physiological properties. (1) They cause an increase in the reabsorption of water by the kidney tubules—the anti-diuretic action. (2) They produce powerful contractions of the uterus (see page 408)—the oxytocic action. (3) In larger doses they cause constriction of all arterioles, including coronary vessels, with a consequent increase in blood pressure—the vasopressor action. In most vertebrates, two hormones are found in the neurohypophysis, one exerting primarily oxytocic activity (named oxytocin) and the other primarily vasopressor and anti-diuretic (ADH) activity (named vasopressin). Both hormones appear to be formed in certain nuclei of the hypothalamus, the part of the brain to which the neurohypophysis remains attached throughout life by means of the infundibular stalk. The hormones are thought to travel down the hypothalamico-hypophysial tract to the pars nervosa, where they are stored and thence released.

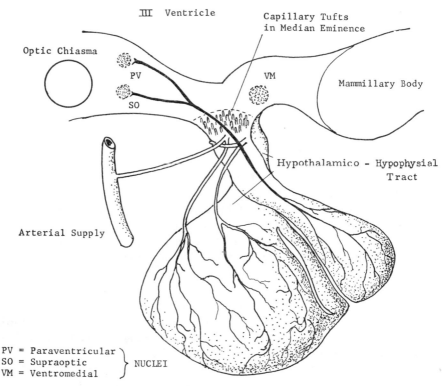

FIG. 14.2. General diagram of the blood supply to the adenohypophysis and of the nerve supply to the neurohypophysis.

Oxytocin and vasopressin are nonapeptides of molecular weight about 1000. They are similar to each other in structure. The amino-acid sequences were determined by du Vigneaud and his colleagues in 1953 and the hormones have since been synthesized. Each contains nine amino acids including two cystine residues linked by a sulphur bridge, and six of the amino acids are common to both (aspartic amide, cystine, glutamic amide, glycine, proline and tyrosine). There are some species differences; in the pig, for example, arginine in vasopressin is replaced by lysine, whereas in fish, amphibia and birds, a hybrid hormone named arginine-vasotocin has been found, in which the leucine of mammalian oxytocin is replaced by arginine.

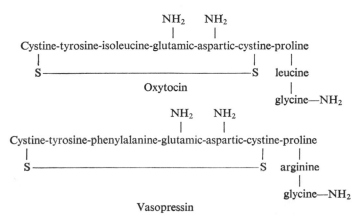

OXYTOCIN. The motility of the uterus of all species is increased by oxytocin. The sensitivity of the uterine muscle to oxytocin is greatly increased at the termination of pregnancy and during the immediate post-partum period. The hormone assists, therefore, in the expulsion of the foetus at the appropriate time. There is some evidence that oxytocin-induced uterine movements also assist sperm transport after mating, particularly in cattle. After parturition, oxytocin has a most important action on the mammary gland. Under the influence of oestrogen, progesterone and lactogenic hormone, the mammary gland develops and secretes milk which is stored in the alveoli. However, ejection of the milk only occurs under the influence of oxytocin. This 'milk let-down' effect is induced by suckling, thereby implicating the central nervous system in the regulation of oxytocin release. Oxytocin has an effect on the cardiovascular system, being pressor in large doses in the rat and dog but depressor in the chicken. Oxytocin is broken down by the enzyme oxytocinase which is produced in large quantities by the placenta during pregnancy.

VASOPRESSIN. Vasopressin increases the arterial blood pressure of mammals but the doses needed are greater than those required to produce an anti-diuretic effect. As both haemorrhage and fainting lead to secretion of vaso-pressin, this hormone may exert a physiological role in the maintenance of blood pressure. The pressor effect is due to constriction of arterioles. Constriction of coronary vessels is so marked that rapid injection of large doses of vasopressin intravenously may produce cardiac ischaemia and arrest. Anaesthetized animals usually exhibit tachyphylaxis (or tolerance) to the pressor action of vasopressin. In the chicken, this hormone, like oxytocin, exerts a depressor action.

The anti-diuretic effect of vasopressin is of great importance. The volume of urine in healthy adults is about $1\frac{1}{2}$ litres per day but when the neurohypophysis is damaged and vasopressin secretion fails, the volume may rise to 12 litres per day. This condition is known as *diabetes insipidus* and should not be confused with *diabetes mellitus* when glucose is present in the urine. Vasopressin is usually effective for the treatment of diabetes insipidus. It has little or no effect on the amount of glomerular filtrate formed, but increases the reabsorption of water in the tubules, principally in the distal convoluted tubule. Changes in blood osmotic pressure are thought to initiate the secretion of vasopressin. Osmo-receptors are present in the hypothalamus, and an intra-carotid injection of hypertonic saline solution produces a rapid release of anti-diuretic hormone, which causes water retention. About 85% of the amount of water reabsorbed in the tubules is transported passively but the effects of vasopressin on the small portion that is actively transported is sufficient for the regulation of osmotic pressure of the body fluids.

The isolated intestine is contracted by vasopressin, but it has not been established that the hormone plays a physiological role in peristalsis. Vasopressin also stimulates uterine contractions, especially in the non-pregnant state; this oxytocic activity is possessed by synthetic vasopressin and there is also a positive effect on milk ejection but only at relatively high dose levels. Oxytocin possesses slight vasopressin-like activity. Thus each of the two peptides has an oxytocic effect, a depressor action in birds, a milk-ejecting effect, a pressor action in mammals, and an anti-diuretic effect. These effects are shown by pure synthetic hormones, and thus the overlap of activity represents inherent properties of both molecules.

Anti-diuretic activity may be measured quantitatively after water-loading either dogs or rats. Oxytocic activity may be estimated on the isolated rat uterus although the fall in blood pressure in the hen is also used. Vasopressor activity is usually determined in the anaesthetized rat.

The thyroid gland

The thyroid gland is composed of two lobes, situated below the larynx on either side of the trachea. In most species, the lobes are linked by a narrow isthmus across the ventral aspect of the trachea (see Fig. 14.3). The blood supply arises from the superior and inferior thyroid arteries and provides a rich vascular network within the gland The thyroid is innervated by both vagal and sympathetic fibres but these are possibly of importance only in the control of the calibre of the blood vessels. Sheets of connective tissue divide the gland into lobules in which there are numerous spherical *acini*. Each acinus, or vesicle, is lined with a single layer of cubical epithelial cells and contains a variable amount of a homogeneous colloid material.

Removal of the thyroid gland leads to a reduction in the basal metabolic rate, which is a measure of the oxygen uptake of an animal under standard conditions of fasting, rest and temperature. As a consequence, all bodily functions are depressed and in young animals growth and sexual development are retarded. These effects are reversed by the administration of thyroid extracts or purified thyroid hormone. An active principle was isolated in

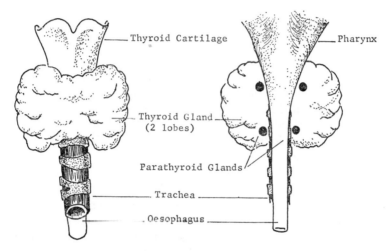

FIG. 14.3. Diagrams to show the position of the thyroid and parathyroid glands.

crystalline form in 1919 and the chemical structure was elucidated in 1927; for many years this substance, known as thyroxine, was believed to be the only thyroid hormone. However, in 1952 another substance, tri-iodothyronine, was found to be present in both thyroid tissue and the blood-stream. In certain circumstances, tri-iodothyronine has considerably greater physiological activity than thyroxine and it is now accepted as a second thyroid hormone. The thryroid hormones are synthesized by the acinar cells and then stored in the colloid material within the acinus.

The striking characteristic of the thyroid hormones is their high concentration of iodine. Both may be considered as derivatives of tyrosine, substitution in the meta positions being vital requirements for activity. Replacement of the iodine by other halogens decreases the physiological activity.

Iodine is an essential dietary trace element, the normal daily requirement

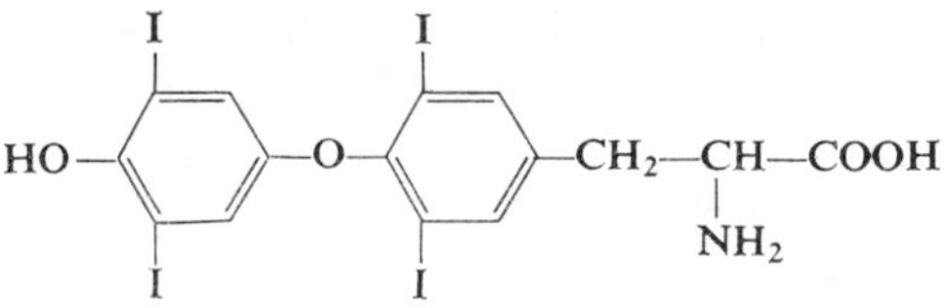

Thyroxine (tetra-iodothyronine)

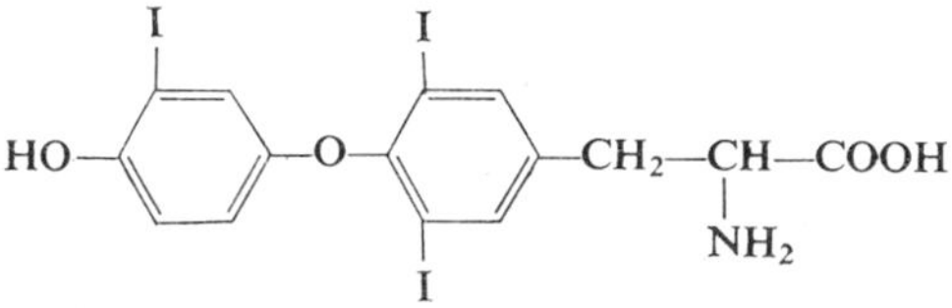

Tri-iodothyronine (3,5,3'-tri-iodothyronine)

being about 0·15 mg. The element is rapidly absorbed as iodide ion and is chiefly found in the extracellular fluid. The thyroid gland has a particular affinity for iodide but the mechanism of this 'trapping' process is unknown. The concentration of iodide in the thyroid is considerable and the usual ratio of thyroidal to serum iodine is 25 to 1. Intracellular iodide is oxidized to elemental iodine by an unidentified oxidase enzyme, and under the influence of peroxidase-enzymes, iodination of tyrosine in the *meta*-positions takes place. It is unlikely that tyrosine exists as the free amino acid within the thyroid cell, and more likely that it is held as part of a globulin molecule. Iodination proceeds to the di-iodotyrosine stage before condensation between two di-iodotyrosyl groups takes place to yield tetra-iodothyronine. The iodo-thyronine–globulin complex is called *thyroglobulin* and when synthesis has been completed the molecule is extruded into the lumen of the acinus where it is stored (see Fig. 14.4). When the thyroid hormone is required, thyroxine is split off from thyroglobulin by a proteolytic enzyme. The products of proteo-lysis, which include tri-iodothyronine and di- and mono-iodotyrosine, pass back into the thyroid cell, thyroxine and tri-iodothyronine being liberated into the blood-stream. Very little di- or mono-iodotyrosine is found in the blood and it is thought that de-iodination of these compounds occurs in the thyroid cell. The liberated iodide is subsequently used in the synthesis of new thyro-globulin. Once in the blood stream, both thyroid hormones become bound to a circulating plasma protein (probably an α-globulin). Precipitation of all plasma proteins therefore includes the circulating thyroid hormones and the con-centration of 'protein-bound iodine' (PBI) is used as an index of thyroid activity.

Most of the circulating thyroid hormone is thyroxine, and the percentage of tri-iodothyronine is quite small. However, there is a long latent period of action of thyroxine and this has led some workers to suggest that tri-iodo-thyronine, which acts faster, is the active hormone at the cellular level and that thyroxine is converted into the tri-iodo compound before exerting its physiological actions.

FUNCTIONS OF THE THYROID HORMONES. The thyroid hormones act as general stimulants to all metabolic processes. This action is reflected by an increase in oxygen consumption and in heat production. In physiological doses, thyroid hormones stimulate intermediary metabolism resulting in anabolism, although excess amounts induce catabolic changes. Thyroid hormones are necessary for other hormones such as the growth hormone and most of the 'trophic' adenohypophysial hormones to exert their full activity. The cardiovascular actions of the catecholamines are potentiated by thyroid hormones and diminished in their absence.

The role of thyroid hormones in development and sexual maturation is particularly important. In the lower orders, the effects of lack and excess of thyroid activity are most striking. Thyroidectomized tadpoles continue to grow without metamorphosing into frogs whereas addition of thyroxine to water containing immature tadpoles hastens their metamorphosis into miniature frogs. In man, lack of thyroid hormone leads to the failure of the development of bone from cartilage and to retarded gonadal function; blood levels of lipid and cholesterol increase but the conversion of carotene to vitamin A is reduced.

CONTROL OF THYROID SECRETION. The proper functioning of the thyroid gland is controlled by the thyrotrophic hormone of the adenohypophysis (TSH). Hypophysectomy results in a decrease in thyroxine output and a reduction in the iodine-trapping capacity of the thyroid. Histologically, there is a decrease in acinar cell height, and the acini are distended with a mass of inactive colloid. Ultimately, there is thyroid atrophy. On the other hand, the administration of thyrotrophic hormone to a normal animal is followed by an increase in acinar cell height and a decrease in the amount of colloid. There is an increase in mitotic rate within the thyroid, with hyperplasia and hyperaemia, and hence thyroid hypertrophy. The primary action of TSH appears to be stimulation of the activity of the proteolytic enzyme responsible for breakdown of thyroglobulin, with the resultant increase in thyroid hormone secretion. TSH also accelerates thyroidal-iodide trapping, and increases the rate of organic combination of iodine by affecting the enzymes involved in the synthesis of thyroid hormones.

The production of thyroid hormone is also governed by the availability of inorganic iodine, an essential raw material. Reduction of iodine intake leads to a decrease in thyroxine production and in the circulating level of the hormone.

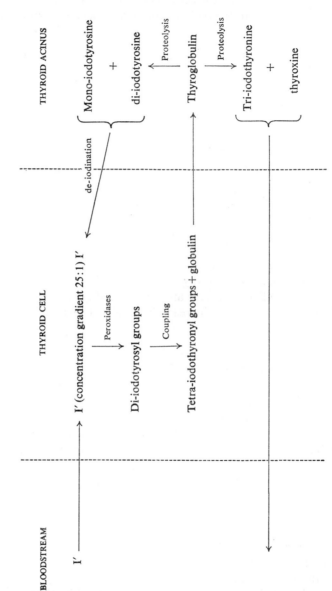

Fig. 14.4. Diagrammatic representation of synthesis and release of thyroid hormones.

In turn, the reduced blood thyroxine level stimulates the adenohypophysis to release more TSH. As a consequence there is a 'stepping-up' of all thyroid activities, hypertrophy of the gland and an attempt to make better use of the low iodine levels available. Hypertrophy of the gland leading to swelling in the neck is commonly seen in people living in areas where there is a chronic deficiency of the iodide in the diet, the condition being termed *endemic goitre*. Inclusion of adequate amounts of iodide in the diet restores this to normal but excess iodide may produce thyroid inhibition. The normal level of plasma iodide is 0·3 to 0·5 μg/100 ml, but when this is raised ten-fold or more there is an increased level of inorganic iodine in the thyroid. In some way, this reduces the rate of synthesis and release of the thyroid hormone.

The thyroid hormones have an effect on the output of TSH from the adenohypophysis. Release of this pituitary hormone is inhibited by excesss amounts of both thyroxine and tri-iodothyronine in the blood. This type of auto-regulation is termed *negative feedback*, for, as previously mentioned, decreased levels of thyroid hormones lead to increased TSH secretion. In addition, there is also involvement of the central nervous system in the control of thyroid secretions, probably at the hypothalamic level.

Thyroid disease may be associated with low iodide intake, hypersecretion or hyposecretion of thyrotrophin and primary hyperfunction or hypofunction of the thyroid. Endemic or simple goitre results from iodide deficiency and in most civilized countries it is prevented by addition of iodide to table salt. If underactivity of the thyroid occurs before sexual development, it leads to the condition of *cretinism*. In addition to the failure of proper physical development, there is usually an associated mental retardation. In the adult, hypothyroidism produces the condition called *myxoedema*. Hyperthyroidism in mild forms may show up in increased appetite, activity and restlessness. In severe forms, usually associated with excess thyrotrophin production, there is marked thyroid hypertrophy and protrusion of the eyes due to deposits of fat behind the orbits. This condition is known as thyrotoxicosis, Graves' disease or *exophthalmic goitre*. Development of benign functional thyroid tumours (toxic adenoma) may also give rise to hyperthyroidism, but malignant thyroid tumours rarely occur.

Although the pure thyroid hormones may be determined chemically, biological assessment of activity is sometimes required. The development of thyroid hypertrophy or goitre which follows treatment with some uracil derivatives is due to blockade of thyroxine synthesis and excess TSH production. Thyroid hormones suppress TSH secretion and so it is possible to compare potential thyroid analogues on their ability to prevent goitre formation. Alternatively, thyroid hormone suppression of TSH release may be judged by reduction of radioactive iodine uptake by thyroid tissue.

Thyrocalcitonin is another hormone secreted by the thyroid. It reduces the serum calcium levels, probably by increasing the uptake of calcium by bone.

The parathyroid glands

The parathyroid glands occur as small oval structures lying on the dorsal surface of the thyroid gland (see Fig. 14.3) although they are of independent embryological origin. Usually there are two pairs of glands. The blood supply is derived from the thyroid arteries and there is accompanying vasomotor innervation. Two types of cell are apparent in microscopic section: (1) the *chief cells* which possess a clear cytoplasm and which are believed to be responsible for the production of the parathyroid hormone. (2) Larger *oxyphil cells* which contain acidophilic granules but which do not appear until the approach of puberty; their function is unknown.

When the parathyroid glands are removed, death from asphyxia, through spasm of the laryngeal and thoracic muscles, occurs in a few days. Initially, there is a fall in plasma calcium and a rise in plasma inorganic phosphate. The urinary excretion of both calcium and phosphorus is reduced. Muscular twitching is observed due to an increase in excitability (pages 198–199) and finally convulsions occur. The symptoms are alleviated by intravenous administration of a soluble calcium salt. The condition, known as *tetany*, may be prevented by injection of parathyroid extracts after removal of the glands. Recently, a relatively small polypeptide of molecular weight about 8500 has been isolated from parathyroid extracts, and this is the active principle (parathormone). To understand its role, it may be helpful to consider the importance of calcium and phosphorus in more detail.

The level of calcium in the plasma is usually 10 mg per 100 ml, whereas that of phosphorus is about half this value. The solubility of most calcium salts is low and when the concentration of calcium and phosphate ions exceeds a certain value termed the solubility product, precipitation of calcium phosphate occurs. The pH of plasma also affects the solubility of calcium ions, increased alkalinity leading to decreased solubility. Approximately half of the plasma calcium is non-diffusible and is associated with protein. Calcium ions are essential for the efficient functioning of blood clotting mechanisms and for the formation of bones and teeth. They also play important parts in maintaining the excitability of nerve and muscle cell membranes, in the release of neuro-humoral transmitters and exocrine gland secretions, and in the contractile mechanism of muscles. Phosphate is of great importance in the buffering of body fluids and formation of the high energy phosphate compounds, e.g. ATP. Both vitamin D and bile salts are necessary for the efficient absorption of calcium from the intestine.

FUNCTIONS OF THE PARATHYROID HORMONE. The parathyroid hormone acts to maintain the level of plasma calcium, chiefly by mobilizing the calcium present in bone. Parathyroid hormone administration to normal animals causes *osteitis fibrosa*. In this condition, there is decalcification of bone which loses its strength and assumes a fibrous appearance. In addition, parathyroid hormone increases both the reabsorption of calcium by the renal tubule and the rate of calcium absorption by the gut, has a phosphaturic effect on the kidney, affects the distribution of phosphate between fluid compartments, and increases the uptake of phosphorus by the liver.

CONTROL OF SECRETION. Injections of parathyroid hormone result in an increase in serum calcium which persists for several hours, whereas parathyroidectomy is followed by a prompt decrease in the serum calcium. It was thought for many years that the level of serum calcium governed the output of parathyroid hormone by a negative feedback mechanism, a fall in serum calcium leading to an increase in parathyroid hormone release and vice versa.

Artificial manipulation of the serum calcium level in animals without parathyroid glands has revealed the inadequacy of this hypothesis. Not only does the level rise more slowly after reduction, but it also falls more slowly after elevation. The intravenous infusion of a chelating agent effectively reduces the serum calcium in intact dogs, and when the infusion is stopped, plasma calcium rebounds to normal values and abruptly levels off. If the parathyroid glands are removed at the end of the infusion, plasma calcium continues to rise to abnormally high concentrations. Recent studies have shown that a blood calcium-reducing factor (thyrocalcitonin) is present in the thyroid. Other endocrine secretions such as those of the adrenal cortex and sex glands also affect the levels of calcium and phosphorus in the blood.

The symptoms of hypoparathyroidism are less severe than those seen in experimental animals. Occasionally, spasms of facial muscles may occur and these may be exacerbated at times of high calcium requirement, e.g. pregnancy. Hyperparathyroidism leads to decalcification and resorption of bone which becomes fragile. Calcium deposits may occur in the renal tubules. In cases of lead poisoning, some deposition of lead in bone may occur, and parathyroid hormone may then be used to reverse this effect. Parathyroid hormone may be estimated by its ability to increase serum calcium in dogs or in parathyroidectomized calcium-depleted rats.

The adrenal gland

The adrenal glands, one lying above each kidney, consist of two separate parts. Although they are closely associated anatomically, they have a different structure and origin (see Fig. 14.5). The central *medulla* develops from the neural crest which also gives rise to the ganglion cells of the sympathetic nervous system. The outer *cortex* is of mesodermal origin. In microscopic section, the medulla appears as a mass of closely packed cells containing granules which stain with ferric chloride and salts of chromic acid. They are often called *chromaffin cells*. The adrenal cortex shows three distinct layers of cells. On the outside, beneath a capsule of connective tissue, is the *zona glomerulosa* with

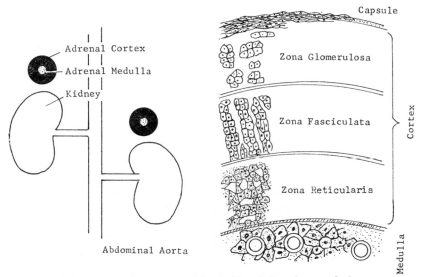

FIG. 14.5. Diagrams to show the position (left) and the microscopical appearance (right) of the adrenal gland.

cells arranged in circular or oval patterns. The middle layer, the *zona fasciculata*, is larger and is composed of columns of cells arranged radially. The inner *zona reticularis*, which surrounds the medulla, is a mass of irregularly arranged cells. Many of the cortical cells contain fine lipid droplets which take up lipid stains. All parts of the gland share a common blood supply and there is a generous distribution of sinusoids. The medulla receives pre-ganglionic sympathetic nerve fibres from the splanchnic nerve and the individual medullary cells may be regarded as analogous to post-ganglionic sympathetic neurones.

THE ADRENAL MEDULLA. The hormones produced by the cells of the adrenal medulla are noradrenaline and adrenaline. Their actions have already been discussed on pages 150–152. There is no condition known to be associated with hypofunction of the adrenal medulla, but hyperfunction, as when a medullary tumour secretes excess hormone, results in an abnormally high blood pressure. The condition is known as phaeochromocytoma (page 164).

THE ADRENAL CORTEX. Unlike the adrenal medulla, the adrenal cortex and its secretions are essential for life. After bilateral adrenalectomy, there is a loss of appetite, a rapid loss of weight and pronounced diuresis. The body temperature falls, hypotension follows, and the basal metabolic rate declines. The blood becomes more concentrated as plasma water is lost, and the blood concentrations of urea and potassium rise. There is a dramatic loss of sodium in the urine. Ultimately, there is renal failure and severe muscular weakness precedes death. The adrenalectomized animal is highly susceptible to changes in environmental temperature, traumatic injuries, burns, infections and toxic substances. These stimuli are often termed *stresses* and administration of adrenocortical extracts greatly improves the resistance of the adrenalectomized animal. Such extracts also prolong the survival time of adrenalectomized animals and reverse the symptoms which follow adrenalectomy. Chemical extraction and purification of the adrenal glands has yielded over thirty compounds all of which are related to cholesterol. It is likely that only seven of these occur in the adrenal secretion, the remainder being either artifacts of the purification procedures, precursors, or metabolites. Two types of hormone have been identified; one influencing carbohydrate metabolism, termed *glucocorticoids*, is secreted mainly from the zona fasciculata, whilst the other, influencing water and mineral metabolism, termed *mineralocorticoids*, is secreted from the zona glomerulosa.

CHEMISTRY OF THE ADRENAL CORTICOIDS. The biologically active hormones have three structural features in common: (1) There is an α-ketol group in the side-chain attached in the 17-position (i.e. $-CO-CH_2OH$). (2) There is a ketone group in the 3-position. (3) There is a double bond between carbon atoms 4 and 5, which gives the molecule the characteristic absorption spectra of an $\alpha:\beta$-unsaturated ketone. The presence of a hydroxyl group in

| Numbering in the nucleus | Structural features in biologically active hormones of the adrenal cortex | Hydrocortisone (cortisol) | Aldosterone |

the 17-position results in an increase in the activity of the steroid on carbo-hydrate metabolism. Usually the compounds lacking an oxygen at C-11 are active on salt metabolism, but the exception is aldosterone which has an oxygen atom at C-11 and yet is extremely active as a mineralocorticoid. The adrenal cortex is rich in both cholesterol and ascorbic acid, and their concentrations decrease as the tissue is stimulated to increase synthesis and release of its hormones under the influence of ACTH.

The principal steroids secreted by the adrenal cortex are *corticosterone*, *hydrocortisone* (17-hydroxycorticosterone) and *aldosterone*. Corticosterone and hydrocortisone are elaborated by the cells of the zona fasciculata and are under the control of ACTH. Aldosterone is secreted by the glomerulosa cells. The amounts of adrenal steroid stored in the gland are small but they are synthesized at a rapid rate when required. The human adrenal gland normally has a daily secretion of about 15 mg hydrocortisone, 3 mg corticosterone and 0·15 mg aldosterone. Hypophysectomy results in atrophy of the adrenal cortex but this is not immediately fatal; adrenalectomy, however, is always followed by death. Histological examination after hypophysectomy shows that most of the adrenocortical atrophy occurs in the zona fasciculata, with little or no change in the zona glomerulosa, and so hypophysectomy does not seriously disturb salt and water balance. Similarly, the adrenal hypertrophy after chronic dosage with ACTH is mainly confined to the zona fasciculata.

The glucocorticoids, hydrocortisone and corticosterone, exert profound effects on carbohydrate metabolism. They increase the blood sugar level and antagonize the effects of insulin, but they also promote the deposition of glycogen in the liver. This is due to an increased rate of gluconeogenesis and inhibition of the peripheral utilization of glucose. Consequently, there is a drain on protein reserves and an increased loss of nitrogen in the urine. Fasting is followed by hypoglycaemia and rapid depletion of liver glycogen stores. The glucocorticoids increase the resistance to stress and there is a rapid increase in their plasma concentration under stressful conditions. Gluco-corticoids also increase the efficiency of muscular contraction and reduce inflammatory reactions.

The most important mineralocorticoid is aldosterone, although most of its properties are shared by deoxycorticosterone. Despite its high potency on salt and water metabolism, aldosterone is as effective as hydrocortisone as a glucocorticoid. Since it is present in such small amounts, the physiological significance of this observation is in doubt. The most striking effects of aldo-sterone are in the kidney where it promotes the tubular re-absorption of sodium and excretion of potassium. After adrenalectomy, the loss of sodium and chloride ions, with accompanying water, leads to haemoconcentration, a fall in blood pressure, and bradycardia. An increase in sodium intake may offset the renal loss of sodium and, in the rat, prolongs survival of the adrenal-ectomized animal. Aldosterone also plays an important role in regulating sodium and potassium balance at the cellular level, particularly in the heart.

CONTROL OF ADRENOCORTICAL SECRETIONS. The secretion of cortico-sterone and hydrocortisone is dependent upon the release of ACTH from the pituitary. Three mechanisms are probably involved in this release (see Fig. 14.6). *Firstly*, adrenaline increases the circulating level of adrenocortical hormones in the intact animal but does not do so in the hypophysectomized animal; in fact, direct perfusion of the adrenal gland with adrenaline is not followed by an increase in steroid output. The adreno-medullary secretion is therefore a stimulator of the adrenocortical secretion acting via the adeno-hypophysis and ACTH release. However, this explanation does not fit all the facts since adreno-demedullated animals release ACTH as efficiently as intact ones. Similarly, sympathectomy and demedullation do not significantly shorten the survival time of animals placed in a cold environment whereas total adrenalectomy does. *Secondly*, a negative feedback mechanism produced by chronic treatment with adrenocortical hormones lead to adrenal atrophy because ACTH secretion is suppressed. However, atrophy of the adrenal cortex is prevented by concomitant administration of ACTH with cortical hormone. In addition, the acute release of ACTH in response to stress is blocked by glucocorticoids. Thus, ACTH secretion may be regulated by the level of adrenocortical hormones in the blood; in a stressful situation, the peripheral utilization of steroids may be increased and this, in turn, may reduce the circulating hormone levels and so may stimulate ACTH secretion. When the demand is satisfied, blood steroid levels increase and ACTH release is reduced. ACTH release occurs in the chronically adrenalectomized animal in response to stress. *Thirdly*, there are no nerve fibres passing directly to the adenohypophysis and yet the activity of the central nervous system modifies ACTH release. Electrical stimulation of certain areas of the hypo-thalamus results in ACTH secretion but this does not occur if the pituitary stalk is cut. Since there are no nerve fibres, the stimulus has to be conveyed by a neurohumor passing in the blood-stream from the hypothalamus to the adeno-hypophysis. This neurohumor (termed CRF) is a polypeptide similar to vasopressin in structure but not in molecular weight or activity. All three mechanisms probably contribute to the control of glucocorticoid secretion which is so important for the maintenance of homeostasis.

The rate of aldosterone secretion is independent of variations in ACTH blood levels, and, at present, the mechanism of its regulation is not clearly understood. A number of factors are known to play a part, including the ratio of sodium to potassium ions in the plasma. A lowered blood pressure increases aldosterone secretion by activating the baroreceptors in the vena cava and the carotid sinuses. Further, angiotensin, produced in response to renal ischaemia stimulates aldosterone secretion. Complex inter-relationships exist between ionic balance on the one hand and cardiovascular function on the other, and a co-ordinating role may be played by the central nervous system.

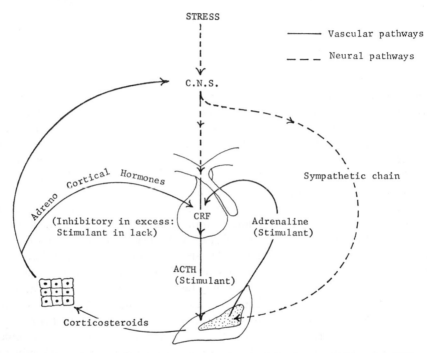

FIG. 14.6. Diagram illustrating pathways involved in the regulation of ACTH release.

Hypofunction of the adrenal cortex is usually known as Addison's disease and may result from an infection of the gland or failure of ACTH secretion. Hyperfunction leads to excess deposition of fat on the face and back, hyperglycaemia and hypertension. This condition is known as *Cushing's syndrome* when the primary fault is in the adrenal itself or as *Cushing's disease* when it occurs as a result of ACTH over-production. In some cases, there is functional hypertrophy of the zona glomerulosa, with excessive production of aldosterone. This condition is described as primary aldosteronism, and symptoms include severe muscular weakness and marked derangement of mineral metabolism, with accompanying polyuria.

Most of the adrenocortical hormones may be determined chemically. Earlier bio-assay techniques involved measurement of liver glycogen deposition, involution of the thymus gland, or prolongation of survival after adrenalectomy.

The pancreas

Scattered throughout the pancreas are irregular groups of cells which stain less darkly than the remainder of the tissue. These cells comprise the endocrine component of the pancreas and are known as the *islets of Langerhans*. They are not connected to the pancreatic duct system and, unlike the acinar cells, do not degenerate after ligation of the main pancreatic duct. Although all the islet cells contain granules, most contain granules which are alcohol-soluble (the beta cells) whereas the remaining alpha cells have water-soluble granules.

The surgical removal of the pancreas is followed by a series of changes in metabolism which are invariably fatal if untreated. Carbohydrate, protein and fat metabolism are all affected. The level of glucose in the blood rises and, when the renal threshold is exceeded, sugar appears in the urine. At the same time, there is a dramatic fall in the concentration of glycogen in both the liver and the muscles. Degradation of glucose to yield energy is depressed and there is a shortage of pyruvate (see Fig. 14.7). The inability of the pancreatectomized animal to utilize glucose effectively results in an increased conversion of protein to carbohydrate in an attempt to combat the deficiency. This leads to even higher blood sugar levels without providing any useful energy. More seriously, it results in muscle wasting because the rate of utilization of protein is increased and the incorporation of amino acids into new protein is decreased. As a result of increased de-amination in gluconeogenesis, the amount of nitrogen in the urine is increased. The only remaining source of energy is fat and the rate of oxidation of fatty acids is increased, thereby reducing the respiratory quotient. As there is a shortage of pyruvate, only a limited amount of acetyl-coenzyme A enters the tricarboxylic acid cycle and there is an accumulation of the two-carbon fragments. These condense to form ketone-bodies which appear in excessive concentrations in both blood and urine. The stores of adipose tissue become depleted and fat deposition is markedly reduced. Since the ability of the kidney to concentrate the urine is limited, the increased amount of solutes after pancreatectomy results in an increased urinary volume. This, and the fact that its sugar content gives urine a sweet taste, led to the condition being called *diabetes mellitus*. The increased water loss leads to dehydration of the tissues and thirst. The metabolic changes are followed by severe emaciation and finally the animal enters into a diabetic coma with high blood sugar and ketone levels and dies. All the changes and symptoms may be rapidly reversed by the parenteral administration of pancreatic extracts, as first shown by Banting and Best in 1922. The active principle is *insulin* and lack of it results in all the metabolic changes which occur after removal of the pancreas.

After the administration of the chemical, alloxan, metabolic changes very similar to those following pancreatectomy occur; alloxan destroys the beta cells of the islets of Langerhans. As extracts of pancreas from alloxan-treated animals do not ameliorate the symptoms of pancreatectomy, it has been

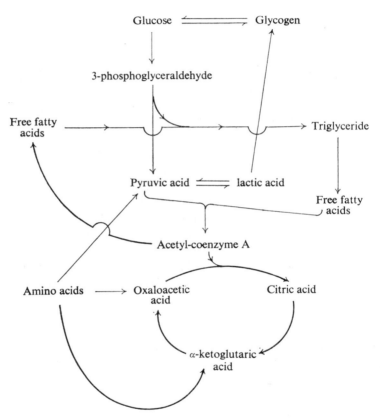

FIG. 14.7. Schematic drawing of metabolic inter-relationships.

concluded that insulin is synthesized and secreted by the beta cells. The pancreatic islet tissue also produces a second hormone called *glucagon*. In contrast to insulin which lowers blood sugar levels, glucagon is a hyperglycaemic factor. It is synthesized by the alpha cells which may be selectively destroyed by cobalt salts. Glucagon promotes the breakdown of glycogen in the liver but its physiological role is not yet well understood.

Both insulin and glucagon are complex polypeptides. Purified insulin was isolated in crystalline form as a zinc salt in 1926 but its structure was not elucidated until 1955. It consists of two straight chains of amino acids linked by two disulphide bridges. In all, there are fifty-one amino acid residues with a molecular weight of 4800. Glucagon has twenty-nine amino acid residues.

As indicated by the effects of pancreatectomy, insulin has profound effects upon intermediary metabolism. The injection of insulin is followed by a prompt lowering of the blood sugar level and by an increase in liver and muscle glycogen. There is an increase in the oxidation of glucose by the tissues and an increased incorporation of amino acids into new protein. The level of free fatty acids in the blood is decreased as a result of a lowered rate of lipolysis and a raised rate of lipogenesis. The conversion of glucose to fatty acids in the liver and adipose tissue is increased. Insulin also increases the permeability of cell membranes to glucose, effectively increasing its volume of distribution. It is not known what further actions insulin has inside the cell or what actions are due to increased cellular glucose content *per se*. The secretion of insulin appears to be completely regulated by the concentration of glucose in the blood passing through the pancreas. A rise in blood sugar stimulates the beta cells to secrete insulin which returns the sugar level to normal, whereas insulin secretion is inhibited by low blood sugar levels. There is little or no evidence of pituitary control of insulin secretion.

Inter-action of other hormones with insulin. The repeated injection of *growth hormone* into adult cats and dogs leads to diabetic symptoms associated with exhaustion of the pancreatic beta cells. Growth hormone increases the blood sugar level and depresses glycogen synthesis, probably by inhibiting hexokinase, whereas in its absence, the animal exhibits a greatly increased sensitivity to insulin. The antagonism between the effects of growth hormone and insulin on blood sugar levels may be shown in the dog where the symptoms of pancreatic diabetes are ameliorated by hypophysectomy. Unlike insulin, growth hormone promotes lipolysis and increases the level of plasma free fatty acids, but only when the insulin secretion is low. There is much evidence to support the hypothesis that metabolism is dominated alternately by the action of insulin or of growth hormone or of the combined effects of both in a three-phase cycle which is regulated by the intake of food. Immediately after a meal, alimentary hyperglycaemia ensures adequate supplies of insulin which encourage the storage of energy as carbohydrate and fat. Later, exposure to growth hormone and insulin encourages protein synthesis. Finally, in the 'post-absorptive period', exposure to growth hormone encourages mobilization of fatty acids from adipose tissue and the peripheral oxidation of fatty acids to yield energy, but antagonizes the deposition of glucose in muscle and fat. Some of these changes are diagrammatically represented in Fig. 14.8.

The *glucocorticoids* antagonize the effects of insulin and increase the conversion of protein to carbohydrate. In some way, they also facilitate the storage of glycogen, since adrenalectomized animals are unable to store adequate amounts. Adrenalectomy reduces the severity of pancreatic diabetes and increases the sensitivity to insulin. Excessive amounts of glucocorticoids or ACTH induce so-called 'steroid diabetes', with hyperglycaemia and glycosuria.

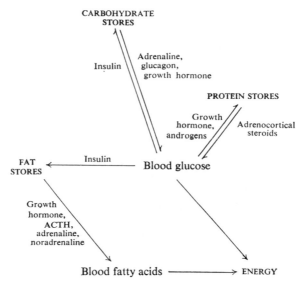

FIG. 14.8. Effect of hormones on intermediary metabolism.

Under stressful conditions, *adrenaline* released from the adrenal medulla stimulates the breakdown of glycogen in both liver and muscle. There is an increase in the blood levels of glucose and lactic acid as a result of glycogenolysis, but some of the lactic acid may then be re-converted into glycogen by the liver. The *thyroid hormones* also oppose the actions of insulin by promoting gluconeogenesis but there is no immediate change in blood sugar after their administration.

DIABETES MELLITUS. The condition of diabetes mellitus in man is most frequently diagnosed by the appearance of glucose in the urine, coupled with an elevated blood sugar level after an overnight fast. The normal fasting blood sugar level is 80–100 mg per 100 ml but in diabetic subjects it may exceed 300 mg %. The diabetic is unable to dispose of a large amount of glucose as efficiently as a normal person and this altered *glucose tolerance* is another diagnostic aid (see Fig. 14.9). It was formerly assumed that the varying degrees of clinical severity of diabetes mellitus were associated with different degrees of insulin deficiency. Plasma insulin assays show that most diabetics fall into one of two principal categories. The first group, having very low or zero blood insulin levels, develop symptoms during childhood or adolescence and, if untreated, become emaciated, dehydrated and die in diabetic coma. The second group, however, with normal or even elevated plasma insulin levels,

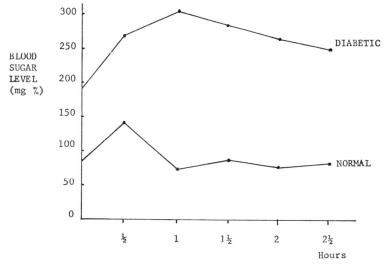

FIG. 14.9. Glucose tolerance curves in normal and diabetic individuals. Blood sugar levels are shown at different times after oral ingestion of 50 g glucose in the fasting state.

develop symptoms usually in middle age and instead of becoming emaciated they are frequently obese; they are often resistant to insulin treatment but may be kept alive for many years by careful attention to diet. The first group are said to be *insulin dependent* diabetics, whilst the second group are *non-insulin dependent* diabetics.

Insulin promotes the uptake of glucose by both muscle and adipose tissue, with subsequent conversion into glycogen and neutral fat. In the serum of diabetic patients, however, there is usually an anti-insulin factor which antagonizes the actions of insulin upon glucose uptake by muscle, without impairing its actions in adipose tissue. Whereas insulin-dependent diabetics show an absolute lack of insulin, non-insulin dependent patients suffer from a relative insulin deficiency, and conversion of glucose into neutral fat is not

13

prevented by the anti-insulin factor. It is not yet known whether the two categories represent the extremes of a range of diabetic conditions or are two diseases of separate aetiology.

The two well-established methods for the bio-assay of insulin depend upon the reduction of blood sugar in fasting rabbits and the induction of convulsions in fasting mice.

The central nervous system and endocrine function

Much evidence has been obtained which implicates participation of the central nervous system in the regulation of hormone secretion. In the case of the neurohypophysis and the adrenal medulla, the neural pathways involved are established. However, beyond a scanty vasomotor innervation of doubtful significance, there are probably no such neural pathways leading to the adeno-hypophysis, the thyroid, the adrenal cortex and the gonads.

The negative feedback mechanism which regulates the secretion of the adeno-hypophysial hormones and the output of the target glands does not explain all the observed facts. For example, from the relationship between ACTH and the corticosteroids, it may be predicted that minimal blood steroid levels after bilateral adrenalectomy should initiate maximal secretion of corticotrophin. In the adrenalectomized animal, ACTH titres are high, yet exposure to stress results in a still further release of ACTH. In the absence of circulating cortico-steroids, a neural mechanism is revealed which controls the release of ACTH, independently of feedback modifications.

As there are no simple neural links between the brain and the adeno-hypophysis, particular attention has been paid to the anatomy and physiology of this area. The adenohypophysis is derived from an upgrowth of the buccal ectoderm whereas the neurohypophysis develops from a downgrowth of neural tissue of the floor of the third ventricle. The area above the neuro-hypophysis is the *hypothalamus*. It is bounded at the front by the optic chiasma, at the back by the mamillary bodies and laterally by the optic tracts. It is divided medially by the third ventricle and contains a number of bilaterally placed nuclei and nerve tracts. The more important nuclei are the supra-optic, paraventricular and ventromedial nuclei. A clearly defined nerve tract passes from the hypothalamus, through the median eminence of the tuber cinereum, down the infundibular stalk and ends in the neural lobe. This tract is known as the hypothalamico-hypophysial; its fibres originate in the supra-optic and paraventricular nuclei (see Fig. 14.10).

The arterial blood supply to the adenohypophysis is of a complex type. Small arterial vessels arising in the Circle of Willis penetrate the pars tuberalis and then pass to the median eminence of the tuber cinereum where they form a mass of capillary loops. A series of vessels draining this highly vascular area run along the anterior surface of the pituitary stalk and finally penetrate the pars distalis forming numerous sinusoids (see Fig. 14.11). These *hypophysial portal vessels* provide the major source of arterial blood to the pars distalis in most species, although in the rabbit the pars distalis receives in addition a direct arterial twig from the internal carotid.

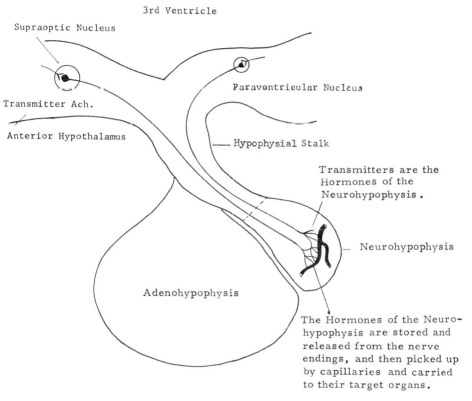

3rd Ventricle

Supraoptic Nucleus

Paraventricular Nucleus

Transmitter Ach.

Anterior Hypothalamus

Hypophysial Stalk

Transmitters are the Hormones of the Neurohypophysis .

Neurohypophysis

Adenohypophysis

The Hormones of the Neurohypophysis are stored and released from the nerve endings, and then picked up by capillaries and carried to their target organs.

FIG. 14.10. Diagram of the nerve supply to the neurohypophysis.

CNS and the neurohypophysis. Removal of the pituitary gland is followed by diabetes insipidus which only lasts for 2–3 days. However, when the hypothalamic-hypophysial tract is sectioned in the hypothalamus, permanent diabetes insipidus occurs and the neurohypophysis undergoes atrophy. These results indicate, first, that the median eminence of the tuber cinereum, together with the neural tract, produce adequate secretion of vasopressin in the absence of the neural lobe, and secondly, that the vital role of the hypothalamico-hypophysial tract is demonstrated in the maintenance of neurohypophysial function. Analysis of hypothalamic extracts shows that they possess considerable quantities of both oxytocin and vasopressin. Centrifugation of homogenates of hypothalamic tissue yields so-called 'neurosecretory granules' which possess anti-diuretic and oxytocic activity. Histochemical methods show the presence of neurosecretory granules within the nerve fibres of the hypothalamico-hypophysial tract. The amount of stainable material increases

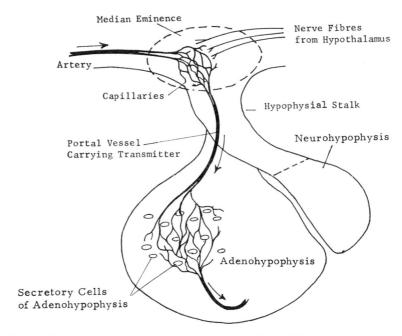

FIG. 14.11. Diagram of the humoral control of secretions of the adenohypophysis by transmitters carried in the hypophysial portal system.

under conditions of dehydration where release of anti-diuretic hormone is high, and decreases to zero after tract section.

Retention of water after emotional disturbance was noticed by various workers who subsequently found that the phenomenon was abolished by cutting the hypothalamico-hypophysial tract. Studies with hypertonic saline solutions led to the postulate of the existence of osmo-receptors, sensitive to minute changes in osmotic pressure. In some way, the osmo-receptors regulate vasopressin release by a mechanism involving the hypothalamico-hypophysial tract. There is evidence suggesting the participation of a cholinergic component.

The indirect stimulation studies have been extended by the direct stimulation experiments of Harris. Using rabbits, he inserted electrodes into the hypothalamus, taking leads to a coil which was sewn under the skin of the back. When the animal had regained consciousness, it was placed in a cage which acted as a primary coil to the indwelling secondary. By this means, Harris was able to show that stimulation of the hypothalamico-hypophysial tract was followed by anti-diuresis, a slight rise in blood pressure and increased intestinal activity. In oestrogen-treated rabbits, stimulation produced uterine contractions and, in the lactating animal, milk ejection. Such evidence affords proof of the neural control of neurohypophysial hormone secretion.

CNS and the adenohypophysis. Section of the hypothalamico-hypophysial tract does not result in atrophy of the adenohypophysis. However, proper functioning of the adenohypophysis is dependent upon close anatomical association with the hypothalamus and the median eminence. Transplantation of the pituitary gland to the anterior chamber of the eye or beneath the capsule of the spleen or kidney, is followed by reduced growth and size of the target organs. The atrophy is not as great as that after hypophysectomy, and although the neural lobe disintegrates, the pars distalis remains viable.

Interruption of the hypophysial portal vessels by cutting the pituitary stalk interferes with secretion of the adenohypophysial hormones. If regeneration of the portal vessels is prevented by the insertion of a wax plate between the median eminence and pituitary body, hormone secretion remains greatly reduced.

The direction of blood flow in the portal vessels is from the median eminence to the adenohypophysis. Much evidence has been marshalled in support of the hypothesis that neuro-transmitters are carried in the portal blood to regulate the secretion of the adenohypophysial hormones.

The Reproductive System

The sex of an individual is determined at the moment of conception by the complement of chromosomes in the fertilized ovum. The chromosomal pattern which determines the development of a human female is twenty-three pairs, one pair consisting of the so-called X or sex chromosomes. Development of a human male is determined by a chromosome pattern in which the pair of sex chromosomes are unmatched; one is an X and the other is the shorter so-called Y chromosome (see Fig. 2.12, page 53).

The particular set of sex chromosomes determines the development of the *primary* sex organs, or *gonads*. In the female these are the *ovaries*, and in the male they are the *testes*. The gonads have two functions: they provide the germ cells, the *ova* and *spermatozoa*, on which reproduction ultimately depends, and they also act as endocrine glands secreting various sex hormones. The genital organs include the gonads together with other organs which are essential for procreation. There are other differences between males and females, known as *secondary sexual characteristics*. They include the development of mammary glands, and sex differences in skeletal and muscular structure, in distribution of body fat and hair, and in the pitch and timbre of the voice. Sex differences in behaviour in humans are largely determined by the customs of society rather than by solely physiological factors, but in animals the sex hormones are important determinants of behaviour.

Male genital organs

The male genital organs are illustrated in Fig. 15.1. The external genitalia are the penis which contains the urethra and erectile tissue, and the scrotum which contains the testes. Each testis is surrounded by a tough connective tissue capsule and is divided by connective tissue septa into wedge-shaped compartments which are filled with masses of *seminiferous tubules* in which *spermatogenesis* takes place (see Fig. 15.2a). The tubules are lined by several layers of *spermatogenic cells*. Those close to the basement membrane are called *spermatogonia* or *germ cells*, and they divide mitotically to produce *primary spermatocytes*. These, in turn, divide meiotically into *secondary spermatocytes* containing only half the number of chromosomes, and divide again into *spermatids* which mature into *spermatozoa*. Half of the spermatozoa contain an X chromosome, and half contain a Y chromosome. The tubules also contain the elongated *cells of Sertoli,* which are believed to be concerned with the nutrition of the spermatogenic cells. Spermatogenesis in the adult testes is stimulated by follicle stimulating hormone (FSH) from the adeno-hypophysis.

The spermatozoa pass from the lumen of the seminiferous tubules into a series of irregular cavernous spaces known as the *rete testis,* and from there a

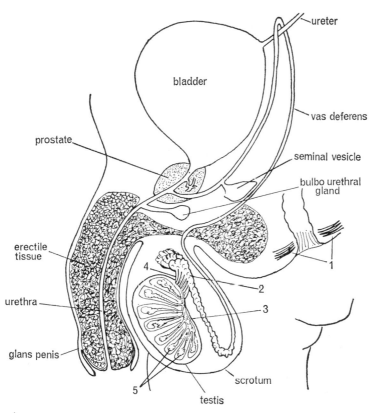

FIG. 15.1. Male genital organs. (1) External anal sphincter; (2) epididymis; (3) rete testis; (4) vasa efferentia; (5) convoluted seminiferous tubules.

number of ducts, the *vasa efferentia,* convey the spermatozoa into the *epididymis.* The distal portion of the epididymis is a single, long, highly convoluted tube which merges with a wider, thicker-walled tube, the *vas* (or *ductus*) *deferens.* The vas deferens runs from the scrotum into the pelvic cavity in the *spermatic cord,* which also contains arteries, veins, lymphatic vessels and nerve trunks. The terminal portion of the vas deferens, after uniting with the duct of the *seminal vesicle*, becomes the *ejaculatory duct*. The ducts from each side run through the *prostate gland* receiving secretions from it and finally empty into the urethra. The secretions of the seminal vesicles and prostate glands, which together with the spermatozoa constitute semen, are discharged immediately before ejaculation. The secretion of the *bulbo-urethral* (or Cowper's) glands joins the semen in the urethra. The spermatozoa are ciliated

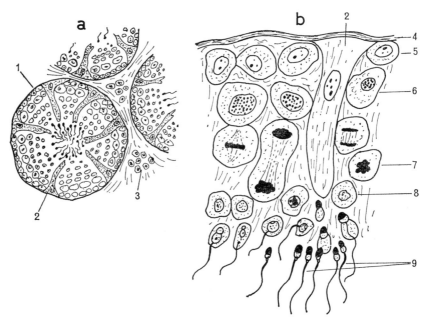

FIG. 15.2. Spermatogenesis in the testis. (*a*) Cross section through part of testis; (*b*) greater magnification of part of seminiferous tubules. (1) Seminiferous tubule; (2) Sertoli cell; (3) interstitial cells of Leydig; (4) basement membrane; (5) spermatogonia; (6) primary spermatocytes; (7) secondary spermatocytes; (8) spermatids; (9) spermatozoa.

in the seminiferous tubules but do not become fully motile until they are incorporated into semen. Their movement through the various passages is assisted by their rate of formation, by ciliated epithelium in the vasa efferentia, and by contraction of the muscular walls of the epididymis and vas deferens.

The spermatogenic function of the testes takes place only at a temperature from 1–3°C below that in the abdominal cavity. The scrotum is adapted to maintain this lower temperature, being well supplied with sweat glands and containing muscular structures which act to alter the rate of heat loss. The wall of the scrotum contains a sheet of smooth muscle, the *dartos*, which is relaxed at high temperatures and contracted at low temperatures, thus altering the surface area. In addition, filaments of striated muscle, the *cremasters*, running from the lower abdominal wall, are attached to the coat of each testis. These muscles are relaxed in a warm environment and the testes are low in the scrotum, but in the cold, they are contracted and the testes are drawn against the body surface; in some species (e.g. the rat) they may be withdrawn into the body cavity. In the human, the testes usually descend into the scrotum towards the end of the foetal period. There is a condition known as *cryptorchidism* in which the testes do not descend and the subject is infertile, since the temperature in the abdominal cavity is too high for spermatogenesis. It is alleged that the use of frequent hot baths impairs spermatogenesis and it is reported that the Romans used them with the intention of reducing fertility. However, the endocrine function of the testes is not impaired.

The endocrine activity of the testes is carried out by cells known as *interstitial cells* or *cells of Leydig*, which occur in groups in the connective tissue between the seminiferous tubules (Fig. 15.2). The hormones elaborated by these cells and released from them into the blood stream are known as *androgens* (Fig. 15.3). Testosterone, which has been isolated from the testes, is the principal androgen. It is metabolized, after release, into androsterone which is less active and is excreted in the urine. The production of testosterone is stimulated by a hormone from the adenohypophysis called *interstitial cell stimulating* hormone or ICSH (which is identical with *leutinizing hormone* (LH) in the female, page 363). The release of ICSH from the pituitary begins at puberty, and the subsequent release of testosterone is responsible for the maturation of the genital organs and the development of the secondary sexual characteristics which occur at this time.

If the testes are removed before the development of the secondary sexual characteristics in the operation known as castration or orchidectomy, further development follows a different path. A man so afflicted is a eunuch; he has little or no facial or body hair, a high pitched voice, and a 'feminine' distribution of sub-cutaneous fat. Animals are castrated to render them more tractable (geldings), or to yield more meat (bullocks and capons), or to ensure that only the best stock is allowed to breed. Dysfunction of the endocrine activity of the testes is usually the result of disturbances of the pituitary. In atrophic conditions of the pituitary, the onset of physical and sexual maturity is delayed whereas in hypertrophic conditions it may be accelerated, giving rise to precocious sexual development.

Biological assays of the potency of androgens depend on their ability to promote the growth of genital organs such as the seminal vesicle in the immature rat, or to stimulate development of secondary sexual characteristics such as the comb in the castrated cock.

13*

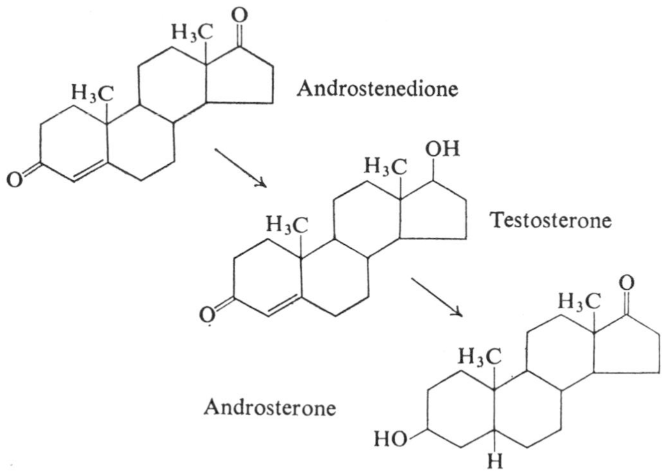

Androstenedione

Testosterone

Androsterone

FIG. 15.3. Structure of some androgenic steroids.

Female genital organs

The genitalia in the female consist of the *mons pubis*, the *labia*, erectile tissue and glands. The mons pubis is a pad of subcutaneous fat in front of the pubic symphysis, the anterior transverse bone of the pelvis. The labia are folds of skin which cover the orifices of the vagina and urethra. The erectile tissue includes the clitoris which is situated beneath the outer labia and anteriorly from the urethral orifice; it is analogous to the erectile tissue of the penis. The vestibular glands which secrete mucus at the orifice of the vagina are analogous to the male bulbo-urethral glands. The internal genital organs of the female are the *ovaries*, the *uterine* (or *Fallopian*) *tubes*, the *uterus* and the *vagina* (Fig. 15.4).

The Fallopian tubes are analogous to the oviducts of birds and reptiles. They convey the ova, after they have been released from the ovary, into the uterus. The wall contains three layers: an inner mucosa consisting of pseudo-stratified ciliated epithelium; a muscular layer consisting of spirally-arranged smooth muscle, the deep layers of which are predominantly circularly arranged, whereas the outer layers are nearly longitudinal; and an outer serous coat of connective tissue containing blood vessels, lymphatics and nerve bundles.

The uterus is that part of the genital system in which the foetus develops. The upper part of the uterus is the *fundus* (or body), the constricted middle part is known as the *isthmus,* and the lower part is the *cervix* through which runs the narrow *cervical canal* connecting the interior of the uterus with the vaginal passage. The human uterus contains only one cavity, but in many animals the uterus is bicornate, that is, divided into two horns which unite in a small fundus (in such animals the foetuses develop in the horns). The wall of the uterus contains three layers. The outer serous layer of connective tissue is in part continuous with peritoneum. A band of fibrous connective tissue known as the broad ligament attaches the uterus to the body wall, and the vascular and nerve supply of the uterus run with it. The thick middle coat contains

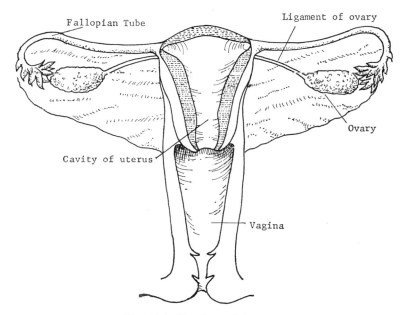

FIG. 15.4. Female genital organs.

smooth muscle and is termed the *myometrium*. The bundles of muscle fibres in the fundus run in various directions, but in the cervical region they are predominantly circular and form a sphincter. The structure of the inner layer, or *endometrium*, of the fundus changes during the menstrual cycle, as outlined below. The endometrium of the cervix contains many mucus-secreting glands.

The ovaries are situated low in the abdominal cavity, one at each side, and are attached by connective tissue to the ligaments of the uterus. The mass of the ovary consists of a fibrous tissue stroma containing *ovarian follicles* which arise from the germinal epithelium (Fig. 15.5). The follicles, which number about 400,000, are formed during foetal life. About 400 of them develop into *ova* during adult life. The remainder of them degenerate by a process known as *atresia*, in which the central cell is affected first. This usually occurs in undeveloped follicles, but it may occur at any stage during development. All the follicles are lost at the onset of the menopause. The course of follicular development is indicated in Fig. 15.5. At first, the follicle contains a central cell, the *primordial ovum* which is surrounded by a layer of *granulosa cells.* At puberty, under the influence of *follicle stimulating hormone* (FSH) from the adenohypophysis, the cells of the ovarian stroma surrounding one of the follicles

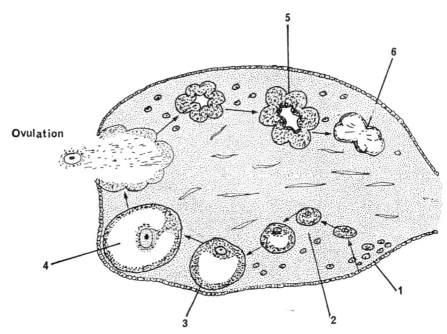

FIG. 15.5. Diagrammatic representation of a section through an ovary to show the development of an ovum and the subsequent production of the corpus luteum and corpus albicans. (1) Germinal epithelium; (2) developing Graafian follicle; (3) zona granulosa; (4) liquor folliculi; (5) corpus luteum; (6) corpus albicans.

start to proliferate and form a cavity. The primordial ovum divides meiotically into a *secondary oocyte* which retains most of the cytoplasm, and a polar body: each portion contains half the original number of chromosomes. The oocyte divides again after longitudinal splitting of the chromosomes to form an ovum and another polar body (the original polar body may also divide, so that three are produced in all). Meanwhile the follicle has been enlarging and protrudes through the wall of the ovary. Ovulation occurs when rupture of the follicle is stimulated by luteinizing hormone (LH) from the adenohypophysis. The ovum, with its surrounding granulosa cells, is released into the abdominal cavity and is swept into the Fallopian tube by the ciliary activity of cells at the mouth of the tube.

In women, an ovum is produced from one ovary or the other about every 28 days during the period from puberty (at 9 to 18 years of age) until the menopause (at 45 to 55 years of age), except when the process is interrupted by pregnancy. This rhythm is imposed by the cyclic activity of the adeno-hypophysis in releasing follicle stimulating hormone and luteinizing hormone. After discharging the ovum, the remainder of the follicle in the ovary forms the *corpus luteum*. At first, the follicular cavity contains a fluid, the *liquor folliculi*. Then, the granulosa cells lining the follicle proliferate and contain a yellowish lipoid material. If pregnancy does not occur, the corpus luteum degenerates, leaving a whitish scar, the *corpus albicans*, on the surface of the ovary. However, if pregnancy does occur, the corpus luteum develops further and in humans does not degenerate until the fifth or sixth month of pregnancy.

Two types of steroid hormone are elaborated in the ovary; *oestrogens* which are produced by the developing follicle, and *progestins* which are produced by the corpus luteum. The formulae of ovarian hormones are shown in Fig. 15.6. Oestradiol is the most active oestrogen to be isolated from ovaries. Progesterone, the most active progestin, has been isolated from the corpus luteum. It is rapidly metabolized to pregnanediol which is excreted in the urine. The increased production of oestrogens at puberty, under the influence of both the pituitary gonadotrophic hormones (FSH plus LH), is responsible for the maturation of the sex organs and the development of the secondary sexual characteristics. The ovary is not the only tissue in which these hormones are made; they are present in the adrenal cortex, and during pregnancy they are formed in the placenta.

Biological assay of the potency of oestrogens depends on their ability to produce cornification of the vaginal epithelium in immature rats or mice. The effect is detected by examination of vaginal smears. The potency of progestins is assayed by their effect on the uterus of immature rabbits previously treated for a week with oestrogens. Several days after injecting the progestin the uterus is removed and the degree of hypertrophy of the endometrium is examined histologically.

In adults, the ovary and the sex organs undergo rhythmic changes in activity. In women these take the form of the *menstrual* cycle (which also occurs in other primates) and in many lower animals there is an *oestrous cycle*. The menstrual cycle involves changes in the inner layer of the wall of the fundus of the uterus. This part of the endometrium consists of connective tissue and is richly supplied with blood vessels. It is lined by an epithelium containing simple tubular glands. After the first ovulation at puberty, the corpus luteum develops from the discharged follicle and produces progesterone. This hormone produces hypertrophy and an increase in the vascularity and secretory activity of the endometrium. Then the production of progesterone in the corpus luteum ceases. The superficial layers of the hypertrophied endometrium degenerate and slough off, and a fluid consisting of autolysing cells, blood and mucus passes out through the vagina: this is the menstrual fluid. The first menstruation is known as the *menarche*.

By convention, the menstrual period is reckoned to begin with the onset of bleeding. This usually lasts from 3 to 5 days. During the next 9 to 11 days the

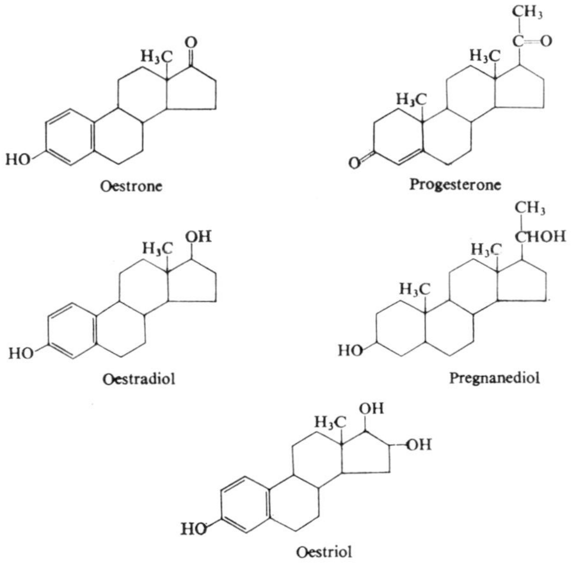

FIG. 15.6. Structure of some ovarian steroids.

endometrium slowly regenerates as another follicle ripens. At approximately the fourteenth day after the onset of bleeding, ovulation occurs and during the subsequent two weeks, proliferation of the endometrial mucosa takes place. Some 28 days after the previous endometrial breakdown, menstruation occurs again. The time up to ovulation is known as the *follicular phase* and the second part as the *luteal phase*. There is widespread variation in the length of the cycle in different women, and the time between onset of bleeding and ovulation is not constant. A convenient index of ovulation is the change in body temperature which occurs after ovulation and which is due to increased blood progesterone levels. It is best to take the temperature before rising in the morning when an increase of about $0\cdot8°$ F may be seen after ovulation. Careful temperature records over several menstrual periods are necessary in order to determine the ovulation time for any given individual.

Abnormalities of menstruation. There are many menstrual disorders and most of them are capable of correction using appropriate hormone therapy or other measures. Detailed discussion is beyond the scope of this book but a list of the more common abnormalities follows. (1) In *primary amenorrhoea*, menstruation fails to start at puberty as a result cither of congenital under-development of the reproductive organs or of disease or suppression of the pituitary. (2) In *secondary amenorrhoea*, cessation of established menstruation occurs as a result of disease or suppression of the pituitary. (3) In *metropathia haemorrhagia*, there is irregular or prolonged uterine bleeding in the absence of ovulation. It is often preceded by a period of amenorrhoea: the condition is due to an upset in the ovarian–pituitary feedback mechanism, as there is degeneration of Graafian follicles and absencc of active corpora lutea in the ovaries and the oestrogen, being secreted continuously, is unopposed by progesterone. (4) In *menorrhagia*, there is excessive menstrual loss after ovulation as a result of some pathological lesion in the pelvis. (5) In *polymenorrhoea*, there is frequent (every 14–21 days) but regular and normal menstruation. (6) In *hypomenorrhoea*, there is scanty menstrual bleeding but usually the ovarian and uterine cycles are normal and no treatment is needed. (7) In *oligomenorrhoea*, menstruation is delayed by up to 3 weeks, this condition often precedes amenorrhoea. (8) In *ovular bleeding*, bleeding occurs at the time of ovulation as a result of an endometrial defect or a temporary decrease in oestrogen levels just before ovulation: the condition may give rise to sterility. (9) In *pre-menstrual tension*, menstruation is preceded by anxiety, irritability, headache and a nausea as a result of an upset in the oestrogen–progesterone balance so that oestrogen predominates. (10) In *dysmenorrhoea*, menstruation is painful, possibly as a result of an oestrogen–progesterone imbalance in which progesterone predominates.

Oestrous cycle. This is best studied in rats and mice. *Pro-oestrus* is the phase during which maturation of the follicles takes place under the influence of FSH and oestrogen is released. In *oestrus*, ovulation is stimulated by LH, and several ova are released. During *post-oestrus*, the corpora lutea start to develop and produce progestins, and then regress. The period between oestrus and the next pro-oestrus is termed *dioestrus*. In rats the complete cycle takes about 4 days. There are changes in the blood supply and the epithelium of the uterus, but no degeneration (and hence no menstruation) during dioestrus. There are changes in the epithelial cells of the vagina which may be identified in vaginal smears and used to determine the phase of the cycle.

In some animals the sexual cycle is discontinuous. The bitch comes into heat twice in a year, that is, there are two mating seasons each year and during each of them there is a single oestrous cycle. Sheep and ferrets, however, have only one mating season each year (autumn and spring respectively) during which there are a series of oestrous cycles. The time of year at which breeding occurs in seasonally-breeding animals may be altered by artificially varying external environmental factors such as temperature or the amount of light to which the animal is exposed each day. In these animals, environmental factors influence the discharge of pituitary gonadotrophins. The period between discontinuous oestrous cycles is known as *anoestrus*.

There are relationships between sexual mating and the phase of the oestrous cycle in many animals (but not in humans). In rats and mice, the female is only receptive and the male only stimulated to copulation during the oestrus phase, and the same is true of animals which breed at certain seasons. In some animals, for example the rabbit and the cat, the oestrous cycle is initiated by copulation which occurs during anoestrus.

Sexual intercourse (copulation, coitus). As a result of sexual excitement, the penis becomes erect and enlarges due to engorgement with blood. This blood is contained in the erectile tissue which consists of a sponge-like network of vascular spaces supplied by thick muscular walled arteries and drained by thin-walled veins. The erectile tissue within the penis consists of three portions: the two *corpora cavernosa* which occupy each side of the shaft, and the *spongiosa* which surrounds the urethra and forms the glans at the free end of the penis. All three erectile bodies continue into the perineum (the region between the scrotum and the anus) to form the root of the penis (Fig. 15.1).

Sexual excitement leads to increased activity in the branches of the sacral parasympathetic nerves (the nervi erigentes) which innervate the arteries of the erectile tissue. These are dilated and the rate of blood flow into the cavities of the erectile tissue increases. The rise in pressure compresses the veins which drain the spaces. A similar change occurs in the erectile tissue of the vulva and mucus is secreted from the vestibular glands, thus facilitating penetration. During copulatory movements, the sensory stimulation of receptors in the skin of the glans penis by the vaginal walls elicits reflexes which culminate in ejaculation and orgasm. Sympathetic nerves supplying the epididymis, vas deferens, seminal vesicles and the prostate cause the discharge of sperm and of the secretions which together constitute semen. Ejaculation of the seminal fluid is produced by rhythmic contractions of striated muscles which compress the urethra in the root of the penis. Orgasm is the pleasurable sensations accompanying ejaculation; it also occurs in the female, although it is not essential for procreation. The sympathetic reflexes initiated during ejaculation also result in constriction of the arteries supplying the erectile tissue; the blood slowly drains away, and the erected tissues return to a flaccid state. Damage or drug blockage of the parasympathetic innervation of the penis results in failure of erection. Impairment of the sympathetic innervation causes failure of ejaculation (but the sensation of orgasm may persist). In animals, sexual intercourse is largely governed by endocrine activity and by instinctive responses to various stimuli; however, in humans, many psychological and sociological factors play a dominant role in reinforcing or inhibiting the basic reflexes.

Fertilization. The semen which is deposited within the vagina by ejaculation consists of about 3 ml of fluid containing up to 600 million spermatozoa. The activity of the ciliary tails of the spermatozoa renders them highly motile; they travel at about 1 mm per min. The sperm traverse the cervical canal, enter the uterine cavity and then pass into the Fallopian tubes by virtue of their motility. Fertilization of the ovum takes place only within the Fallopian tube, and since the ovum is only present in the tube for a few days after ovulation the time of mating is limited to these days if fertilization is to be achieved; coitus at other periods during the cycle is infertile. This is the basis of a technique of birth control but it is not always successful, partly because of irregularities in the cycle. Only one sperm fuses with the ovum, but fertilization does not occur unless millions of spermatozoa are present. The reason for this is not understood. The sperm of one species does not usually fertilize the ovum of another. It has been reported that the ovum contains a protein called *fertilizin* which reacts with an anti-fertilizin on the surface of the sperm of the same species but not with that on others. Once the two substances interact, the sperm becomes firmly attached and is then drawn into the interior of the ovum. Other sperms are prevented from entering the same ovum by changes which occur in the outer membrane of the ovum. The nuclei of the ovum and the spermatozoan fuse to form a zygote containing the full complement of forty-six chromosomes (23 pairs).

If two separate ova are released at ovulation and both are fertilized, fraternal (dizygotic) twins develop, which may be of the same or of opposite sex. Identical (monozygotic) twins develop from a single fertilized ovum which divides into two at some stage after fertilization. Occasionally there may be partial fusion of monozygotic twins with separation possible after birth, or there may be extensive fusion of bone and tissue resulting in inseparable 'Siamese twins'. About one in seventy human births results in twins and about one-third of these are identical twins. With identical twins, tissue from one, grafted on to the other, does not stimulate antibody formation. The graft is not rejected since the tissue is not recognized by the host as 'foreign'. It developed under the influence of genetic control identical with that of the host's own tissues.

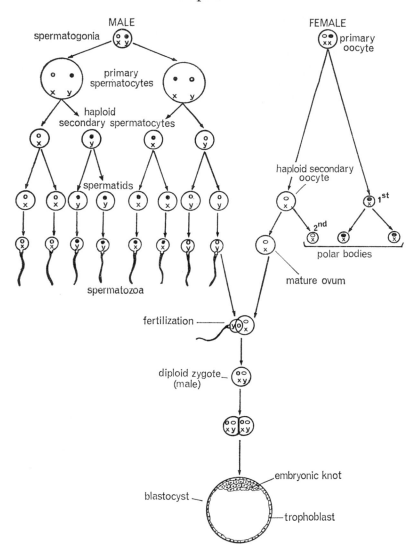

Fig. 15.7. Diagrammatic representation of the formation of male and female germ cells, fertilization and subsequent development to the blastocyst stage. The sex chromosomes are represented by X and Y; the remaining chromosomes are represented by the filled and open circles or ovals. Only four chromosomes are shown in each diploid cell; in man each diploid cell nucleus contains forty-six chromosomes. In the diagram, fertilization results in a male zygote (XY). A female zygote (XX) would result from fertilization with a sperm containing an X chromosome in its haploid nucleus.

Implantation and development. The fertilized ovum begins to divide mitotically almost immediately and is gradually passed down the Fallopian tube towards the uterus. This movement results from rhythmic contractions of the tube, assisted by activity of the ciliated epithelium. In women, the process takes about 3 days. During this time, the endometrium is hypertrophying under the influence of progesterone from the corpus luteum. The superficial layers of the endometrium become compact; it consists of enlarged cells known as *decidual cells* as they are shed after the birth of the offspring. Below the decidual cells, the glands are enlarged and the blood vessels widely dilated. Division of the zygote leads to a morulla of cells with a cavity in the centre. The cells at one pole accumulate to form the *embryonic knot*, which is the primordium of the foetus. The remainder of the cells, known as trophoblasts, become transformed into structures concerned with the nutrition of the foetus. The whole structure is termed a blastocyst. Figure 15.7 illustrates the development of male and female germ cells, fertilization and subsequent development to the blastocyst stage.

The trophoblast cells are responsible for attaching the embryo in the process known as *nidation*. The blastocyst lodges in an endometrial gland and the trophoblasts grow into projections, the *chorionic villi*, which penetrate the endometrium beneath the embryo. The villi burrow down to blood vessels, which enlarge into vascular spaces, the *lacunae*, in which the villi are immersed. In this way, the developing foetus is able to draw nourishment from the maternal blood. Trophoblast cells may invade tissues other than the endometrium. For example, the fertilized ovum occasionally remains in the Fallopian tubes or may even enter the abdominal cavity. The trophoblasts then invade whatever structure the blastocyst is attached to. In this event an *ectopic* pregnancy ensues: usually the embryo does not develop, but if it does the pregnancy must be terminated surgically. Experimentally it has been shown that trophoblasts invade the blood vessels of a number of organs in which they are implanted. Trophoblasts differ from other cells in that they do not elicit the usual responses to foreign cells and proteins (e.g. production of antibodies, invasion by lymphocytes). Thus they impose a barrier between the genetically different tissues of foetus and mother. In the rare instances in which foetal cells cross the barrier, the mother forms antibodies against them, for example, in Rh incompatibilities (page 242). The lack of antigenic activity on the part of trophoblast cells is so marked that they develop and invade tissues after experimental implantation into different species. The invasion of trophoblasts into the endometrium is limited by the appearance of resistant decidual cells. These form a layer surrounding the area of nidation.

Parts of the blastocyst that have invaded the endometrium produce progesterone, which maintains the integrity of the endometrium and thus prevents the degeneration which would otherwise culminate in menstruation. Furthermore, these cells produce a substance, known as *chorionic gonadotrophin*, which stimulates the growth of the corpus luteum and prevents its degeneration: its actions resemble those of pituitary gonadotrophins. Chorionic gonadotrophin appears in the urine in large amounts during pregnancy from about the fourteenth day after conception. This fact has been exploited in various tests for the diagnosis of pregnancy. In the Ascheim-Zondek test, the urine under test is injected into immature mice and a positive result is indicated by hypertrophy of the uterus and the appearance of blood spots on the ovary resulting from rupture of follicles. The Friedman test depends on the production of blood spots on the ovary of the rabbit. Another test depends on the production of ovulation in the *Xenopus* toad. A different type of test has recently become available since the introduction of the orally active progesterone analogues (which are used as oral contraceptives). The problem of pregnancy diagnosis is to decide whether or not a missed menstrual period is due to pregnancy or to some other cause. Administration of an oestrogen together with the progesterone analogue induces endometrial development and if there is no pregnancy, menstruation occurs when administration of these drugs is stopped. But if there is pregnancy the endometrium is maintained by endogenous progesterone. In a newer serological test, gonadotrophin in the urine is detected by the use of an anti-human gonadotrophin serum.

The embryonic knot at first differentiates into two layers, the *ectoderm* cells and the *endoderm* cells, and two cavities appear each surrounded by one of these cell layers. The ectoderm layer forms the amniotic membrane surrounding the *amniotic cavity*; the endoderm cells surround the *yolk sac*, or extra-embryonic gut. The cells in the region where the walls of these two cavities are in contact form a plaque-like mass called the *embryonic disc* from which the body of the embryo develops. A third layer of cells, the *mesoderm*, is formed in the embryonic disc between the endoderm and ectoderm, and all the organs of the foetus develop from these three primary cell layers as indicated in Fig. 2.17 (page 58). Mesoderm cells also develop adjacent to the trophoblast cells and these two layers together form another membrane, the *chorion*. The walls of the amnion gradually expand and come into contact with the inner surface of the chorion so that a double-layered sac filled with amniotic fluid is formed. The growth of the amnion squeezes the structure attaching the embryo to the chorionic villi into a narrow cord, the *umbilical cord*. The yolk sac persists as a narrow core to this structure. Blood vessels develop from mesoderm, and two umbilical arteries and a single umbilical vein are formed. Figure 15.8 is a diagrammatic representation of stages in the development of the early embryo, and the time course of further development of the human embryo is given in Table 15.1.

The chorionic attachment to the uterus increases in size until it occupies about half the endometrium at about the third month of pregnancy. The trophoblast cells decrease in size until they become only a thin membrane. At

TABLE 15.1. Stages in the development of the human embryo.

Time after fertilization	Development
4 weeks	Head and tail folds, neural groove and heart are present
5 weeks	Lens of eye, rudiments of face, gill-arches and stumps of limb buds appear. Embryo about 0·5 cm long
6 weeks	Body curved, head approximating to tail, umbilical cord attached to belly, liver enlarges and limb buds grow out and are demarcated into their segments
8 weeks	Body straightens, tail disappears, eyes, ears and nostrils formed, external genitalia differentiated and fingers and toes begin to form. The embryo is about 2·5 cm long and is now known as a *foetus*
18 weeks	Hair appears, foetus is about 20 cm long
25 weeks	Head becomes proportionately smaller, sex organs differentiate, sense organs well developed, foetus capable of movement, skin becomes covered with greasy secretion
30 weeks	Eye-lids open, testes descend into scrotum. Foetus capable of living if born prematurely
40 weeks	Full-term, weighs about 7 lb. At birth the foramen ovale closes and the ductus arteriosus begins to close. The umbilical vein becomes a round ligament of the liver

this stage the attachment (chorionic villi plus decidua) is known as the *placenta*. The blood on the foetal side of the placenta is then separated from maternal blood by two thin membranes: the trophoblastic membrane and the capillary endothelium. The nutrition of the embryo and the elimination of waste products of metabolism occur by diffusion across the placental membranes. The placenta is also an endocrine organ, secreting progesterone, and towards the end of pregnancy it secretes increasing amounts of oestrogens.

After about the fourteenth week of human pregnancy, the sex of the foetus may be determined by cytological examination of the cells in the amniotic fluid. Appropriate fixing and staining of the cells has shown that the sex chromatin within the nuclei is more conspicuous in female cells than in male cells and this difference forms the basis of the test. Until mid-pregnancy the sample of amniotic fluid is obtained by puncture from the vagina, but later on the puncture is made through the abdominal wall. These rather drastic procedures mean that, at present, the test is mainly of experimental interest only.

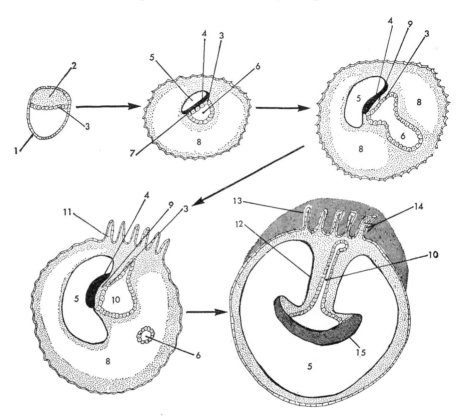

FIG. 15.8. Diagrammatic representation of development of the early embryo from the blastocyst stage to the age of about 4 weeks. (1) Trophoblast; (2) embryonic knot; (3) endoderm; (4) ectoderm; (5) amniotic cavity; (6) primary yolk sac; (7) embryonic disc; (8) extra-embryonic coelom; (9) mesoderm of embryo; (10) secondary yolk sac; (11) mesoderm of chorionic villus; (12) umbilical cord; (13) placenta; (14) chorion; (15) embryo.

Abnormalities of pregnancy

Abortion. About one in five human pregnancies end in abortion; that is, the foetus is expelled before the baby is able to live an independent existence (before 28 weeks). The causes are many and include chronic ill-health, disease of the uterus, high body temperature, syphilis, and lack of progesterone production. Habitual abortion is the term used when two or more pregnancies have ended in abortion.

Hydatidiform mole. In this relatively rare condition, the trophoblast proliferates excessively and the ovum dies. There is an excessive production of chorionic gonadotrophin by the trophoblast and the pregnancy tests are therefore positive. Eventually the uterine contents are wholly or partly aborted.

Antepartum Haemorrhage. In this condition, there is bleeding from the placental site after the twenty-eighth week of gestation. In some cases, the pregnancy is allowed to continue, whereas, in others, Caesarean section has to be performed.

Vomiting. Loss of appetite, nausea and vomiting, particularly in the mornings, are common during the first 3 months of pregnancy. Excessive and prolonged vomiting (*hyperemesis gravidarum*) may lead to dehydration and emaciation. The liver may become so depleted of glycogen that carbohydrate metabolism is disturbed and ketone bodies appear in the urine. The cause of excessive vomiting is unknown. Treatment includes dietary control and the use of anti-emetic drugs.

Pyelonephritis. This condition is not peculiar to pregnancy but is aggravated by it as a result of the effect of progesterone in relaxing smooth muscle. The ureters become dilated and kinked and may be compressed by the growing uterus so that urine flow is retarded. The bowel is also relaxed leading to constipation, and organisms from the bowel may pass via the blood vessels and lymphatics to the static urine and then to the kidneys which become infected. Treatment includes the use of sulphonamides and antibiotics.

Anaemia. The haemoglobin concentration usually falls during pregnancy as there is a greater increase in plasma volume than in the number of erythrocytes. However, true anaemias are also common during pregnancy, especially iron-deficiency (microcytic) and occasionally folic acid-deficiency (megaloblastic) anaemias, which are treated with iron or folic acid therapy respectively.

Varicose veins. Varicose veins are common in pregnancy due to the combined effects of the growing uterus and the relaxing action of progesterone on the smooth muscle of the vessel walls. The condition usually improves after delivery.

Hypertension and proteinuria. Raised blood pressure, sometimes associated with albuminuria, oedema and excessive weight gain, is fairly common in pregnancy after about the twenty-fourth week of gestation, and is one of the most common causes of maternal and foetal mortality. The cause of the generalized vasoconstriction which gives rise to the hypertension and the oedema is unknown. Various suggestions have been made and these include increased pressure on the renal veins and ureters and inside the uterus leading to excessive levels of angiotensin or noradrenaline, abnormalities in endocrine secretion, dietary (including vitamin) deficiencies, or the liberation of toxins by the placenta. When the condition is severe, it is called *pre-eclampsia*; it may lead to convulsive fits (*eclampsia*) during the later part of pregnancy or soon after delivery. Prophylaxis consists of careful dietary control. Treatment includes the use of sedative, diuretic and anti-hypertensive drugs. It may be necessary to terminate the pregnancy if there is no improvement.

Acute yellow atrophy. This disease is believed to be the final stage of infective hepatitis to which pregnancy is predisposing. The symptoms include jaundice, rapid pulse and respiration, epigastric pain, vomiting, dizziness, drowsiness, diminished urine output, weight loss and necrosis of the liver. Intravenous glucose is given to protect the liver from further damage. Foetal loss is high and pregnancy is usually terminated to protect the mother.

Parturition (Birth)

The period of intra-uterine life is termed *gestation*. In women it is about 270 days. Towards the end of gestation the placenta releases a protein hormone, *relaxin*, which causes softening of the pubic symphysis (this effect is pronounced in guinea-pigs and is used for bioassay of the hormone) and dilatation of the cervical canal. At term, contractions of the uterus in the first stage of labour force the amniotic sac into the cervix of the uterus which is expanded allowing the head of the foetus to enter the cervical canal. The amniotic fluid from the ruptured amnion lubricates the cervical canal. The amount of oxytocin released into the blood from the neurohypophysis increases until about mid-term, after which it remains at a constant elevated level. There is a similar increase in the circulating level of another 'oxytocic substance' which is possibly of placental origin. At the onset of labour, there is no further increase in pituitary oxytocin but there is an abrupt increase in the titre of the other oxytocic substance which is stimulated by the stretching of the cervix. These hormones stimulate the uterine contractions and the oxytocic substance, rather than oxytocin itself, may be the more important hormone in controlling the onset and duration of labour. In some cases where labour has lasted longer than usual, the amount of pituitary oxytocin was found to be normal, but the level of the other oxytocic substance was less than usual.

In the second stage of labour, uterine contractions become more rapid and the voluntary abdominal muscles aid the uterus in expelling the foetus from the vagina. Immediately after delivery the umbilical cord is severed leaving a scar which persists as the navel. The uterus is sensitized to the contracting action of the oxytocic principles by oestrogens (the secretion of which increases

TABLE 15.2. The main hormones concerned with sex and reproduction.

Hormone	Source	Function
Testosterone	Cells of Leydig in the testes. Some present in adrenal cortex	Maturation of male primary sex organs and development of secondary sex characteristics. Influences libido in males and females
Oestradiol	Developing follicle of ovary. The placenta in pregnancy. Some present in adrenal cortex	Maturation of primary female sex organs and development of secondary sex characteristics. *Menstrual cycle:* Maturation of ovum *Pregnancy:* Essential for maintenance of pregnancy; growth of mammary tissue; inhibits lactation until parturition; relaxes pelvic girdle and sensitizes uterus to the action of oxytocins during labour *Post-partum:* Maintains lactation; causes involution of uterus and prepares for fresh menstrual cycle
Progesterone	Corpus luteum of ovary. Placenta in pregnancy. Some present in adrenal cortex	*Menstrual cycle:* Hypertrophy and increase in vascularity and secretory activity of endometrium *Pregnancy:* Essential for maintenance of pregnancy; nidation; inhibits maturation of further follicles; relaxes uterine muscle; causes growth of mammary tissue *Post-partum:* Maintains lactation
Follicle stimulating hormone	Basophil cells of adenohypophysis	Stimulates ripening of follicles in females and spermatogenesis and growth of seminal tubules in males
Lutinizing or interstitial cell— stimulating hormone (L.H. or I.C.S.H.)	Eosinophil cells of adenohypophysis	*Female:* Stimulates rupture of follicles and development of corpus luteum. Together with FSH stimulates oestrogen formation. Together with prolactin stimulates progesterone formation *Male:* Stimulates production of testosterone by cells of Leydig
Lactogenic hormone Prolactin	Eosinophil cells of adenohypophysis	Concerned directly and indirectly in the development of mammary glands. Stimulates lactation. Has luteotropic action in animals but gonadotropic action in human beings is uncertain

Chapter 15

TABLE 15.2.—*continued*

Hormone	Source	Function
Chorionic gonadotrophin	Langerhans cells of the chorionic villi	Takes over the function of LH in pregnancy maintaining the functional corpus luteum. (Pituitary secretion of LH is blocked in pregnancy by oestrogens and progesterone)
Oxytocin	Neurohypophysis	Stimulates contraction of uterus in labour. Stimulates milk ejection post-partum
Oxytocic substance	Placenta	Stimulates contraction of uterus in labour
Relaxin	Placenta	Causes softening of the pubis symphysis, dilatation of the cervical canal and sensitizes the uterus to the action of oxytocic principles

greatly just before delivery) and by relaxin. In the third stage of labour, which may be several hours later, the placenta and membranes are expelled.

Lactation

The mammary glands, whose basic structure resembles that of sweat glands, are present in a rudimentary form in males where development is hindered by androgenic hormones. In the female, mammary growth is rapid after puberty under the influence of oestrogens. In the non-pregnant state, the mammary glands possess a fairly well developed duct system draining a series of lobes each of which is divided into lobules containing numerous elongated sacs—the alveolar ducts. In pregnancy, the raised blood levels of progesterone stimulate the release of a hormone, *prolactin* from the adenohypophysis. Prolactin and progesterone act together to increase the growth and activity of the lobules and alveoli, but the secretion of milk is inhibited by the high levels of circulating oestrogen released from the placenta. After expulsion of the placenta, this inhibiting influence is removed.

After delivery, milk (or rather at first a water fluid called colostrum) is ejected in response to the stimulus of suckling. Reflex secretion of pituitary oxytocin is necessary for this response. Maintenance of lactation is partly ensured by the continued suckling stimulus, in association with prolactin, growth hormone and ACTH. The source and functions of the main endocrine secretions concerned with sex and reproduction are summarized in Table 15.2.

Foetal abnormalities

Teratology is the science which investigates the nature and causes of foetal abnormalities, a great variety of which may occur. Structural abnormalities include missing fingers, arms, ears or other parts, excessive development or duplication of parts, persistence of structures which normally degenerate before birth (e.g. a tail), abnormal splitting of parts (e.g. cleft ureter), failure to split (e.g. double finger), failure to fuse (e.g. cleft palate), excessive fusion (e.g. horse-shoe kidney), failure of openings to close, and excessive narrowing of an opening and abnormal misplacement of parts.

Chemical, hormonal or vitamin deficiencies, radioactive substances, micro-organisms and some drugs may cause foetal abnormalities. German measles during early pregnancy, for example, may cause deaf-mutism and circulatory disorders in the offspring. Tests for teratogenic side-effects of drugs are very important (see pages 561–562).

CHAPTER 16

The Special Senses

The eye

The eyeball is situated in a bony cavity of the skull called the orbit. In man, it is approximately spherical having a mean diameter of about 24 mm and a weight of about 7 g. It possesses three distinct coats: The outermost protective coat is the *sclera* which continues anteriorly as the *cornea* where it is covered by the *conjunctiva*. The middle nutritive coat is the *choroid* with its specialized portions, the *ciliary body* and *iris*; these structures are concerned with the regulation of light entering the eye. The innermost light-sensitive coat is

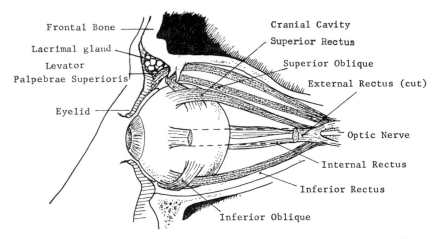

FIG. 16.1. Lateral aspect of the eye-ball in the orbit showing the attachments of the extra-ocular muscles.

the *retina* containing the nervous elements whose fibres ultimately transmit to the *optic nerve*. The interior of the eyeball contains the *lens*, the *aqueous humour*, and the *vitreous humour*. The aqueous humour is in two compartments—the anterior chamber contained between the cornea, the anterior surface of the iris and central portion of the lens, and the posterior chamber contained between the posterior surface of the iris, ciliary body, suspensory ligaments and the edges of the lens. These structures are illustrated in Figs. 16.1 and 16.2.

The movements of each eyeball within its socket are produced by six *extra-ocular muscles*. These are striated muscles attached between the orbit and tendons inserted into the sclera (Fig. 16.1). One pair on opposite sides of the eyeball produce horizontal movements, and the four remaining muscles produce rotation round oblique axes. Four of the muscles are innervated by motoneurones of the oculomotor nerve, one by fibres from the trochlear nerve and one by fibres from the abducens nerve. The extra-ocular muscles are the only mammalian muscles known to possess fibres with multiple-innervation

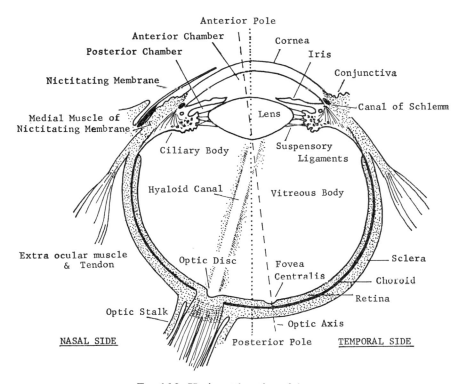

FIG. 16.2. Horizontal section of the eye.

(page 207). Movements of the eyeballs are co-ordinated so that the optical image of the object in view is directed to the portion of the retina possessing the greatest visual acuity. This process is called *fixation*. The optical axis of each eye converges on the object in view, and information about the degree of convergence is one of the clues used in the assessment of distance. Children with squint learn to ignore the information from one of their eyes. Since suppression of perception occurs in the visual cortex it may lead to deterioration of perception of the visual image in that eye. Failure of convergence in adults may occur acutely from damage to extra-ocular muscles, from extreme fatigue or from alcoholic intoxication, and visual perception is severely impaired. Binocular fixation of the object in view is maintained by reflexes below the level of consciousness.

THE SCLERA is a tough connective tissue containing bundles of collagen fibres providing a firm framework for the optical system of the eye. Its thickness varies from 0·4 to 1 mm. At the entrance of the optic stalk, the sclera is continuous with the connective tissue capsule of the optic nerve and blood vessels, thus protecting these structures when the eyeball is rotated in its orbit. The sclera withstands normal intra-ocular pressure without distending, but high intra-ocular pressure causes it to bulge outwards at its weakest point where it is penetrated by the optic stalk.

THE CORNEA is a protruding disc inserted into the anterior segment of the sclera. The special property of the cornea is its transparency. Opacity of the cornea results from injury to its surface and from inflammatory conditions, but small defects are repaired by rearrangement of the epithelial cells which cover each surface. The epithelium of the outer surface is the corneal conjunctiva which is composed of stratified squamous cells and has no blood vessels. It is continuous with the scleral conjunctiva, the blood vessels of which supply the tissue fluid containing nutrients and wandering lymphoid cells to the corneal conjunctiva. The sensory nerve endings in the corneal conjunctiva subserve only pain and touch.

THE SCLERAL CONJUNCTIVA over the anterior surface of the eyeball is reflected back to form the inner lining of the eyelid (the palpebral conjunctiva). Here it consists of a columnar epithelium containing mucus-secreting goblet cells. The reflection of the scleral conjunctiva with the palpebral conjunctiva of the upper eyelid is called the *superior fornix* whilst that with the lower is the *inferior fornix*. The conjunctival surfaces in apposition to each other form the conjunctival sac. The sac is loosely attached to the fat tissue which supports and cushions the eyeball within the orbit. The conjunctiva, except that over the cornea, is well supplied with blood vessels and lymphatic channels, and this accounts for the rapid absorption of drugs when placed in the conjunctival sac.

THE EYELIDS protect the anterior surface of the eye. The gap between the upper and lower eyelid is the *palpebral fissure*. The junctions between the eyelids are the *palpebral commissures*. The outer surface of the eyelids is composed of skin containing sweat glands and sebaceous glands. The eyelashes are inserted along the edges of the lids. The fine, striated *orbicular muscle* fibres, innervated by branches of the facial nerve, are situated beneath the subcutaneous layer of the eyelids. This muscle is responsible for gentle closing of the eyelids. The upper eyelid is held open by the *levator palpebrae* muscle, innervated by a branch of the oculomotor nerve. This muscle is attached to a sheet of connective tissue lying beneath the orbicular muscles. There are both striated and smooth muscle fibres in the levator palpebrae: their functional importance varies between species. In man the smooth muscle fibres are sympathetically innervated. Stimulation of the sympathetic nerves causes widening of the palpebral fissure. There is a reflex closing of the eyelids when

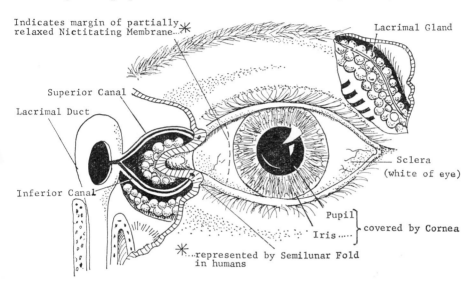

Indicates margin of partially relaxed Nictitating Membrane

Lacrimal Gland

Superior Canal

Lacrimal Duct

Inferior Canal

Sclera (white of eye)

Pupil
Iris } covered by Cornea

represented by Semilunar Fold in humans

FIG. 16.3. Anterior aspect of the eye showing the lacrimal apparatus.

the conjunctiva is touched or when there is a sudden movement towards the eye. The conjunctival touch reflex is one of the last reflexes to fail under general anaesthesia.

THE NICTITATING MEMBRANE. In man, the bulbar conjunctiva in the nasal commissure is thrown into a fold, the *semi-lunar fold* (Fig. 16.3). This is the vestigial remnant of the *nictitating membrane* which is present in most other vertebrates. The part of the nictitating membrane sliding over the anterior surface of the eye is composed of a sheet of cartilage covered with conjunctiva. The inner surface contains many mucus cells. The nictitating membrane in mammals is retracted by two bundles of smooth muscle lying within the intra-orbital space; they are attached to the nasal wall of the orbit. The smooth muscle of the nictitating membrane is innervated by post-ganglionic sympathetic nerve fibres arising from the superior cervical ganglion. In birds, reptiles and amphibia the nictitating membrane contains striated muscle which *closes* it rapidly; in some species (e.g. tortoise) the membrane is closed by striated muscle but retracted by smooth muscle, so that it is closed rapidly and then slowly retracted.

The eyeball is cushioned in the orbit by a deposit of fat. In the hyperthyroid state known as exophthalmic goitre, the eyeball protrudes from the orbit and the eye is widened, giving a startled, staring appearance to the face. It is now considered that this is due to excessive deposition of fat in the orbit. In experimental animals, administration of thyroxine does not cause exophthalmus, but thyroid-stimulating hormone from the pituitary gland causes deposition of orbital fat.

THE LACRIMAL GLANDS lie in the upper temporal part of the orbit (Fig. 16.3) and are innervated (and stimulated to secrete) by parasympathetic fibres from the facial nerve. The secretion of tear fluid is discharged on to the conjunctival surfaces. It is a dilute aqueous solution chiefly of sodium, potassium, chloride and bicarbonate ions. The fluid washes foreign bodies from the conjunctival surfaces and dilutes irritants. The enzyme lysozyme is found in tears: it hydrolyses the glycosidic link of bacterial mucopolysaccharides. Lysozyme, together with γ-globulins which are also present in tear fluid, protect the conjunctiva from bacterial invasion. Tear fluid accumulates in the *internal canthus* of the eye, beneath the nasal commissure, to form the *lacrimal lake*. It passes through *lacrimal ducts* (two in each eye) into the *lacrimal sac*, and then via the *nasolacrimal duct* into the nose. The normal daily rate of secretion of tear fluid is about 1 ml, but this may be increased by reflex stimulation of the lacrimal glands following irritation of the conjunctiva (watering of the eyes) or by reflexes associated with emotional displays (crying).

The internal structure of the eyeball

THE CANAL OF SCHLEMM is a series of channels running in a ring beneath the interior surface of the sclera, just posterior to the cornea. They communicate at intervals with the anterior chamber of the eye and contain aqueous humour. Their function is to regulate intra-ocular pressure by the resorption of aqueous humour.

THE CHOROID, or middle coat of the eyeball, is a thin sheet of tissue carrying a dense network of blood vessels and melanin-containing cells. The brown pigment, melanin, absorbs light and prevents stimulation of the retinal cells by reflected light. The absence of reflected light from the interior of the eye explains why the *pupil*, or aperture in the centre of the iris, appears black.

The pigment cells in the iris render it opaque to light and give the colour to the eye. Blue eye colour is due to the appearance of the pigment on the posterior surface of the iris when viewed through the iris. Albinos are congenitally unable to lay down melanin and the iris appears pink and the pupil red because of light reflected from the blood in their vascular structures. Albinos are photophobic and avoid bright light.

THE IRIS contains two sets of smooth muscle which control the diameter of the pupil and hence the amount of light entering the eye. The set arranged radially is called the *dilator pupillae* and these fibres are innervated by post-ganglionic sympathetic nerve fibres arising from cells in the superior cervical ganglion. Stimulation of these nerve fibres or the injection of noradrenaline results in *mydriasis,* that is, contraction of the radial smooth muscle and dilatation of the pupil. The set of smooth muscle fibres arranged concentrically is called the *constrictor pupillae* and these are innervated by post-ganglionic parasympathetic nerve fibres arising from cells in the ciliary ganglion. Stimulation of these nerve fibres, or the injection of acetylcholine, results in *miosis,* that is, contraction of the concentric smooth muscle and constriction of the pupil. The two most important stimuli which reflexly produce miosis are an increase in light intensity and convergence of the eyes to view near objects. The extent of the pupillary light reflex depends on the preceding conditions of illumination. For example, on changing from darkness to light the pupil contracts at first rapidly and then more slowly. As the retina adapts to the new light intensity the pupil may even dilate slightly. On changing from light to darkness the pupils dilate. The response to reduction in light intensity is much slower than that to an increase in intensity. This is because it is a passive dilatation resulting from relaxation of the circular muscle rather than contraction of the radial muscle. In the indirect light reflex, one eye is exposed to light but the other is covered: both eyes respond. Imagination or anticipation of a change of light intensity may produce the appropriate change in pupil diameter. The role of pupillary contraction in near vision is to diminish the spherical and chromatic aberration of the lens and to increase its depth of focus. During natural sleep and in surgical anaesthesia, there is miosis. Reflex dilatation of the pupil may be observed when sensory nerves from any part of the body are stimulated. Emotional states, loud noises, noxious odours or the sudden exposure to cold all result in pupillary dilatation as a result of sympathetic stimulation.

THE CILIARY BODY contains smooth muscle fibres which help to control the focal length of the lens and thus contribute to the mechanism of accommodation in the eye (Fig. 16.2). They are innervated by parasympathetic post-ganglionic fibres which arise from the ciliary ganglion, and stimulation of these

14

nerve fibres or the injection of acetylcholine produces contraction of the muscle and the eye is focused for near vision. The reflex control of the ciliary muscle is regulated centrally to retain on the retina the most distinct image of the object under fixation. Both eyes are focused simultaneously, even if the image is excluded from one. Drugs which block accommodation are called *cycloplegics*.

When the ciliary muscle fibres are relaxed the suspensory ligaments are taut and the lens is flattened by the tension placed on the capsule. In this condition the lens is focused for distant vision. Focusing of the lens for near vision, termed accommodation, is achieved by contraction of the ciliary smooth muscle fibres. This narrows the diameter of the ciliary ring and pulls the ciliary body forward, the tension on the suspensory ligaments is diminished and the elasticity of the lens causes it to bulge, thus diminishing its focal length. The range of accommodation can be found by determining the nearest point to the eye at which an object is clearly in focus. In children, the near point of vision is less than 10 cm, but with increasing age the lens loses its elasticity and does not become so convex when the suspensory ligaments are slackened, and the near point becomes further away. The gradual diminution in the power of accommodation with increasing age is termed presbyopia.

THE LENS is a transparent, round, elastic structure, about 9 mm in diameter and 4 mm thick. The body of the lens is composed of sheets of modified epithelial cells which are elongated, hexagonal prisms in close apposition to each other. The intercellular cement has the same refractive index as the cytoplasm. The nuclei of the cells are situated in the peripheral parts and receive nutrients from the aqueous humour by diffusion as there is no blood supply. The lens is enclosed in a capsule to which is attached the suspensory ligaments which also connect to the ciliary bodies. Opacity of the lens is termed *cataract* and it is caused by degenerative changes in the cells of the lens.

THE AQUEOUS HUMOUR is largely formed by ultra-filtration of the plasma across the membranes of blood vessels on the surfaces of the ciliary body and posterior surface of the iris, but active secretory processes also play a part in its formation. It carries nutrients to the bloodless structures within the eye. The mean intraocular pressure is determined principally by the rates of formation and absorption of the aqueous humour. The interior of the eye-ball is at a pressure of about 24 mmHg and this varies slightly with the systemic blood pressure. Tension on the eye-ball increases the intraocular pressure. The aqueous humour from the posterior chamber passes between the lens and the iris into the anterior chamber, and then into the angle between the iris and the corneal-scleral junction. This is known as the *filtration angle*. The passage of the humour is assisted by the movements of the ciliary body and the iris, by variations in intra-ocular pressure, and by thermal convection currents. Absorption of aqueous humour occurs across the membranes of the *canal of Schlemm*, the fluid being carried away by the veins associated with them. *Glaucoma*, that is, abnormally raised intra-ocular pressure, may arise from excessive production of aqueous humour or from diminished absorption. When the iris is retracted (that is, the pupil is dilated) and the muscle of the ciliary body is relaxed, the filtration angle is reduced and access of the aqueous humour to the canal of Schlemm is hindered. Conversely, widening of the filtration angle and relief of glaucoma may follow from contraction of the ciliary muscles and constriction of the pupil, as with parasympathomimetic drugs (Chapter 28 and pages 892–894).

The aqueous humour does not normally contain significant amounts of antibodies, and antigens implanted in the anterior chamber do not stimulate antibody production. These facts have been utilized in the study of drugs inhibiting the growth of certain pathogenic organisms, particularly the tubercle bacillus. When this is introduced into the chamber, it grows in a medium which is physiological and the responses to anti-tubercular drugs are uncomplicated by immunological effects. The behaviour of tissue implants in the anterior chamber has also been studied. Transplantation and survival of the cornea and lens is possible because of the insulation of these structures from the antibodies of the blood.

THE VITREOUS HUMOUR is similar in composition to that of the aqueous humour and exchanges solutes with it by diffusion. It has a firmer consistency and contains a gel of mucoprotein (a polymer of hyaluronic acid and albumin).

Optics of the eye. Rays of light passing obliquely from one transparent medium to another of different optical density are bent or refracted, the degree of refraction being greater, the greater the difference between the optical densities of the two media and the more oblique the incident rays. Rays which strike the second medium at right angles are not refracted. When the second medium is surrounded by the first, oblique rays are refracted at both surfaces. In passing from the medium of lower to the one of higher optical density, the rays are bent towards the perpendicular, while in passing from the higher to the lower optical density, refraction is away from the perpendicular. The formation of an image on the retina is illustrated in Fig. 16.4. Divergent rays emitted from all points on the object are brought to a focus on the retina where they form the image which is smaller than the objected and inverted. Re-inversion of the image is an automatic cerebral function probably developed through the integration of visual and other sensations. For simplicity, divergent rays from only the two ends of the object are shown in Fig. 16.4. Rays indicated by dotted lines are unrefracted, either because they strike the surfaces at right angles, or because the two surfaces of the media are parallel so that the refraction occurring at the first is cancelled by the refraction occurring at the second. The eye has three main refracting surfaces—the anterior surface of the cornea, the anterior surface of the lens and the posterior surface of the lens. The difference between the optical densities of adjacent media is greatest at the air/cornea interface (Fig. 16.4) and the greatest degree of refraction therefore occurs at

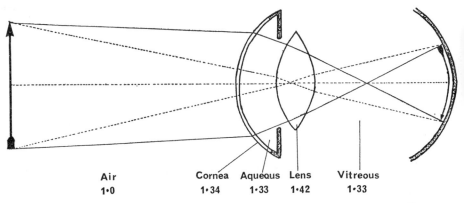

Air			Cornea	Aqueous	Lens	Vitreous
1·0			1·34	1·33	1·42	1·33

FIG. 16.4. Formation of the retinal image. The numbers denote the refractive indices of the different transparent media through which the light rays from the object (large arrow) pass before being focused on the retina. Note that the difference in refractive index is greatest between the air and the cornea, and refraction is therefore greatest at this interface.

this point. The fine control of focusing by the lens is due to its ability to undergo changes in curvature (accommodation); a fixed lens system provides clear images of objects situated at one distance only.

Parallel rays striking the peripheral parts of an ordinary convex lens are refracted more strongly and come to a focus nearer the lens than do rays transmitted through more central regions. A blurred image (spherical aberration) is therefore formed. In the eye, the optical density of the lens is not uniform, being greater at the centre, and this corrects spherical aberration. The iris, which shields the peripheral parts of the lens, also helps to prevent aberration.

Parallel rays entering the normal eye from an object at a distance greater than 6 m are brought to a focus on the retina without any effort of accommodation. The refractive state of the normal eye is called *emmetrophia*.

In *myopia* (short sight), the eye-ball is too long relative to its refractive power and parallel rays are brought to a focus in front of the retina so that the image of distant objects is blurred. Only divergent rays, as from a near object, can be focused on the retina. In *hypermetropia* (long sight) the eye is too short for its refractive power and parallel rays after refraction fall on the retina before they have come to a focus. Accommodation is necessary in order to focus the parallel rays on the retina. Myopia is corrected by means of concave (diverging) lenses, and hypermetropia is corrected by convex lenses. *Astigmatism* is present in all eyes to some extent and it is only when the defect is pronounced that it is considered abnormal. It is caused by inequalities in curvature in the meridians of the cornea or, occasionally, of the lens. Rays are refracted more strongly through meridians with a greater curvature and are brought to a focus in front of rays passing through meridians of lesser curvature. Astigmatism is corrected by means of lenses which are convex in the meridian corresponding to that of the cornea having the lesser curvature.

Sense of vision

THE RETINA is the actual receptive portion of the eye. It originates as an outgrowth from the embryonic brain. The detailed structure of the retina is shown diagrammatically in Fig. 16.5. The surface can be viewed through the pupil using an ophthalmoscope which enables the viewer to look along a beam of light projected into the chamber of the eye (Fig. 16.6). Ophthalmological examination of the retina may reveal lesions occurring primarily in the retina or changes resulting from systemic diseases or from increased intracranial pressure. The point of insertion of the optic nerve fibres and blood vessels supplying the retina is called the *optic disc* and it lies slightly to the nasal side of and above the posterior pole. The *maculata lutea* or yellow spot lies slightly to the temporal side of the posterior pole, its colour being due to a yellow pigment. The pigment called visual purple is present in other parts of the retina. The shallow depression in the middle of the yellow spot is known as the fovea.

Two types of sensory receptors in the retina, the rods and cones, respond to stimulation by light. The fovea centralis has only cones, each having a separate connection with a fibre of the optic nerve. The cones are densely packed, about 160,000 occupy an area of 1 sq. mm. The nervous elements overlying the cones in the fovea centralis are displaced laterally, allowing freer access of light, and there are no blood vessels in this region. These features explain the particular visual acuity of the fovea. Other parts of the retina have both rods and cones, and here there are many sensory elements converging on a single fibre of the optic nerve. The optic nerve fibres unite at the optic disc (Fig. 16.2) where there are no rods or cones and which is called the blind spot.

The cones function in bright light and are concerned with the detection of colour; they respond selectively to various wavelengths of visible light. The rods function in dim light and they do not detect differences in the wavelengths of the light which excite them. Dimly lit objects cannot be seen clearly when the gaze is directed at them (no rods in the fovea) but reappear if the gaze is shifted slightly to one side. Visual acuity is poor in dim light as many rods are

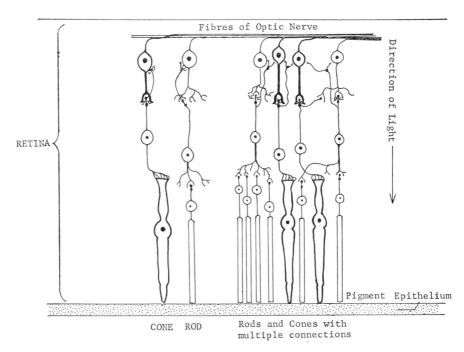

FIG. 16.5. Layers of the retina. The light-sensitive rods and cones are connected through bipolar neurones to the ganglion cells, the axons of which form the optic nerve. Note that the light has to pass through the nerve fibres and bipolar cells to reach the rods and cones except at the fovea where the bipolar cells and nerve fibres are displaced to the side.

connected to a single optic nerve fibre. Animals active at night have mostly rods whilst those who move by day have cones.

Variation in sensitivity of vision from different parts of the retina may be mapped out with an instrument called a *perimeter*. This is a large disc held in a framework so that its centre is transfixed by the visual axis and its plane is at right angles to the axis. The gaze is fixed at the centre of the disc which has concentric and radial lines marked on it to locate the position of test spots of various colours and intensities. Each test spot is moved away from the centre along the radii of the disc until the subject can no longer perceive it. The line joining the outermost points for each test spot is called an isopter.

COLOUR BLINDNESS is a condition in which the individual cannot match any given hue by mixing the three primary colours—red, green and blue—in suitable proportions. The common form is red blindness, in which red objects appear dark, though blue and green appear normal. Red–green colour blindness is rarer and more severe, both reds and greens are indistinguishable from yellowish-brown. Its inheritance is due to a sex-linked recessive gene occurring in about 4% of males and 0·4% of females.

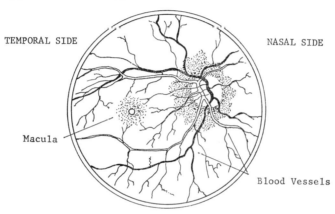

FIG. 16.6. The surface of the retina of the right eye as seen through the pupil using an ophthalmoscope. The optic disc is seen to the nasal side of the macula.

PHOTOCHEMISTRY OF VISION. The rods of the dark-adapted eye contain the pigment, visual purple or *rhodopsin*, which is formed by the cells of the retinal pigment layer. If the retina is strongly illuminated, the pigment disappears but is completely resynthesized in about 1 h after returning to darkness. The rate of destruction of rhodopsin depends upon the wavelength of the light, blue-green light being the most effective. Retinene, which is formed when rhodopsin is bleached by light, is a yellow pigment and an aldehyde of vitamin A (page 31).

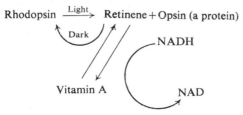

A supply of vitamin A is necessary for the synthesis of rhodopsin and deficiency of vitamin A leads to night blindness or *nyctalopia*, the failure of the eye to become dark adapted. The first sign of deficiency of vitamin A is night blindness, and this can be tested by bleaching the visual purple of the retina with a strong light and then measuring the rate at which dark adaptation occurs. A later stage of deficiency is degeneration of mucous membranes so that the access of bacteria is made easy and ulcers and infection result. These changes are particularly marked in the mucous membranes of the eye, giving rise to the state of *xerophthalmia* where the conjunctiva is keratinized and opaque and the lacrimal secretion fails. Vitamin B_2 (riboflavin) is also important for the normal functioning of the eye; deficiency leads to keratinization of the cornea and cataract.

THE ELECTRORETINOGRAM. Excitation of the retina by light leads to the appearance of a bioelectric potential. This phenomenon was discovered by a Swedish physiologist, Holmgren, in 1866. The electroretinogram can be detected by placing one electrode on the cornea and the other (indifferent) electrode on the skin of the temple or in the mouth. The electroretinogram can be elicited from an excised eye, in which case the second electrode is placed on the posterior pole of the eye-ball.

Action potentials in the optic nerve can be detected throughout the period of illumination. A rapid burst of action potentials occurs at the 'on effect' of the electroretinogram, and another at the 'off effect'. The frequency of the optic nerve action potentials depends on the intensity of the stimulus and the area of the retina illuminated.

VISUAL PATHWAYS. The optic nerve fibres (Fig. 16.5) arising from the nasal half of each retina cross over at the optic chiasma into the optic tract of the opposite side, while those arising from the temporal half of each retina continue uncrossed into the corresponding optic tract of the same side. The majority of the optic tract fibres end in the lateral geniculate bodies. A smaller number pass to the superior colliculi which are centres for light reflexes and for correlation of impulses from the retinae with movements of skeletal muscles. From the lateral geniculate bodies, visual fibres radiate to the visual area of the occipital cortex. Co-ordination of visual sense with other activities occurs in association areas adjacent to the visual cortex.

The sensation of smell (olfaction)

The receptors for smell are bipolar cells called olfactory rods, situated in the mucous membranes of the upper part of the nasal septum and lateral nasal walls. It has been estimated that the olfactory epithelium of the rabbit contains fifty million olfactory rods. A diagrammatic representation of the olfactory epithelium containing bipolar olfactory receptors is shown in Fig. 16.7. The long central processes of the receptors collect together to form the non-myelinated olfactory nerve (Ist cranial nerve) which passes through the roof of the nose and terminates in the olfactory bulb lying on the under surface of the frontal lobes of the cerebrum. The axons passing from the olfactory rods synapse in the olfactory bulb with the dendrites of other neurones, the axons of which form the olfactory tract. The olfactory tract terminates in the smell-receiving area of the cerebrum where integration results in the conscious

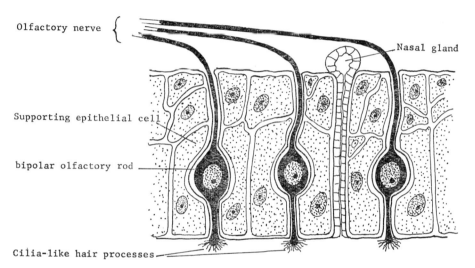

FIG. 16.7. The olfactory epithelium.

perception of smell. Fibres in the olfactory tract synapse in the cortex with neurones whose axons pass through various parts of the rhinencephalon and make connections with the hypothalamus, the mamillary bodies, the reticular formation and the limbic system. Nerve fibres also run from the brain back to the peripheral receptors and in this way the brain varies the sensitivity of the olfactory receptors.

The main stream of inspired air does not impinge directly on the olfactory epithelium. In order to possess a smell, a substance must be volatile so that the particles are transmitted to the upper part of the nose by diffusion and convection currents. However, the most volatile substances do not necessarily possess the strongest smell; the physico-chemical properties of odiferous substances which are involved in the excitation of olfactory receptors and which

14*

give rise to differences in odour are not known. It is thought that odiferous molecules enter into chemical combination with substances in the olfactory epithelium and in some way this causes depolarization of the receptor membrane. The generator potential so produced initiates propagating action potentials in the olfactory nerve fibres. Particular groups of olfactory rods may be specially sensitive to particular kinds of smell.

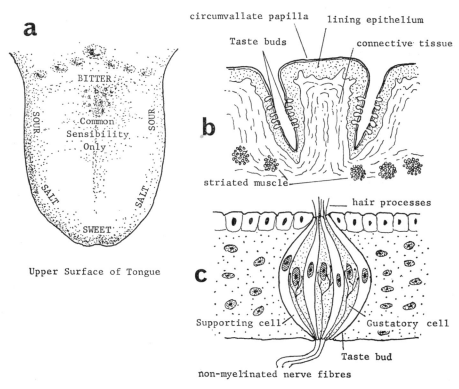

FIG. 16.8. Taste receptors. (*a*) The upper surface of the tongue showing the positions at which the basic qualities of taste are perceived. (*b*) Vertical section through the covering membrane of the tongue showing the position of the taste-buds in the walls of the papillae. (*c*) A taste-bud.

The sensation of taste (gustation)

The receptor organs for the sensation of taste are called taste-buds, and these are present in large numbers (about 9000 in adult man) at the tip, at the sides, and on the surface of the back of the tongue (Fig. 16.8a). The middle region of the upper surface of the tongue has no taste sensitivity. Taste-buds are also scattered over the surfaces of the palate and epiglottis. The covering membrane of the tongue is thrown up into papillary projections and the taste-buds lie in the epithelial walls of these papillae (Fig. 16.8b). A taste-bud is a cluster of from two to twelve spindle-shaped gustatory cells, with supporting cells arranged like the staves of a barrel. The gustatory cells terminate in hair processes projecting from the surface through a pore at the apex of the bud (Fig. 16.8c). Unlike the olfactory rods, the gustatory cells themselves do not conduct impulses but simply serve to generate the stimulus which, in some way, then excites the endings of non-myelinated nerve fibres lying in close contact with them. These fibres are chiefly carried in the chorda tympani branch of the facial (VIIth) and the lingual branch of the glosso-pharyngeal (IXth) nerves; those from taste-buds near the epiglottis are carried in the vagus (Xth) nerve. The cell bodies of these nerve fibres are located in the sensory ganglia of these cranial nerves. The central processes of the neurones are grouped together in the grey matter of the medulla oblongata as the *tractus solitarius*. They terminate in the *nucleus solitarius* where they synapse with second-order neurones ending in the thalamus. From the thalamus, third-order neurones relay the taste impulses to the taste centre in the lower end of the post-central gyrus of the cerebral cortex. Collaterals from the first-order neurones synapse directly or indirectly in the salivary nuclei, axons from which innervate the salivary glands. These pathways constitute the arcs involved in the reflex secretion of saliva in response to a taste stimulus. The taste pathways are illustrated in Fig. 16.9.

Taste has four basic qualities: sweet, salt, sour and bitter. Sweet tastes are most easily perceived at the tip of the tongue, bitter at the back, sour at the edge towards the back, and salt at the edge towards the tip (Fig. 16.8a). All the afferent nerve fibres from the tongue, both of taste and of common sensibility (touch, temperature and pain) follow a closely associated course to the thalamus and cerebral cortex, and what is commonly considered a taste is really a mixture of gustatory, common sensibility and olfactory sensations. To be tasted, substances must be soluble in water and saliva therefore assists in the sense of taste by acting as a solvent. As with smell, attempts to correlate chemical constitution with taste sensation have largely failed. Some examples of the difficulty of this problem may be mentioned. Thus, L-tryptophan is bitter, DL-tryptophan is sweet, and D-tryptophan is nearly tasteless. Epsom salts taste bitter when placed at the back of the tongue but salty at the sides. Phenylthiocarbamide tastes bitter to about 70% of persons but tasteless to the remaining 30%; the ability to taste this substance is inherited according to Mendelian laws. Sodium chloride produces the typical salt-taste sensation but the chlorides of potassium and calcium, as well as the bromide, iodide, sulphate and nitrate of sodium, also possess a salt taste. Sucrose, glycerol, saccharine, α-amino acids and the salts of lead and beryllium are examples of substances possessing a sweet taste. It is only in the case of sour-tasting substances that some relationship to chemical constitution is evident, since they are all acidic. The degree of sourness of an acid seems to be due to the

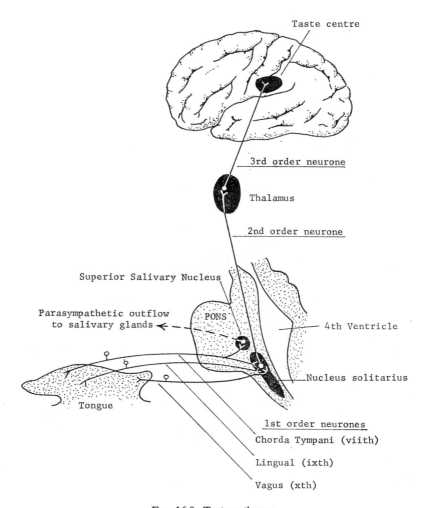

Fig. 16.9. Taste pathways.

anion and the undissociated molecule, as well as to the hydrogen ion. The taste stimulus is probably generated by inhibition of one or more of the enzymes present in the taste-buds, so that substances with the same taste, no matter how they differ chemically, may inhibit the activity of the same enzymes.

The sensation of hearing

The auditory apparatus is divided into three parts: the external ear, the middle ear or tympanic cavity, and the internal ear or labyrinth. The external ear, the only part outside the skull, consists of the pinna, a funnel-shaped organ composed of elastic fibrocartilage for the collection of sound waves, and the external auditory meatus, a channel about 2·5 cm long, lined by inturned skin possessing wax secreting glands and terminating in a fibrous membrane—the eardrum or tympanic membrane. The middle ear is a small cavity in the temporal bone, connected to the back of the nose by the narrow Eustachian tube which serves to keep the atmospheric pressure the same on both sides of the eardrum. The middle ear is bridged by three small bones or auditory ossicles, named the malleus (hammer), the incus (anvil) and the stapes (stirrup) on account of their shapes. The handle of the malleus is fixed to the eardrum and the head is joined to the incus which in turn connects with the stapes. The foot-plate of the stapes fits into an oval window in the wall of the bony internal ear or labyrinth, part of which is the essential organ of hearing. Situated a little below the oval window in the wall of the internal ear is the round window, which is closed by a thin membrane. Part of the internal ear—the vestibule and the semi-circular canals—is concerned with the sense of balance and has already been described on pages 107–108. The remaining part of the internal ear is known as the cochlea, on account of its resemblance to a snail's shell, and this is concerned with sound detection. The bony cochlea is a spiral canal making two and a half turns round a central pillar of bone known as the *modiolus*. A spiral shelf projects into the canal from the modiolus, and a membrane—the basilar membrane—joins the edge of the shelf to the outer wall so that the spiral canal is divided into upper and lower compartments which communicate at the apex of the cochlea. The upper compartment of the spiral canal is divided by a second membrane so that the original canal is divided into three spiral compartments named the membranous cochlea, the scala vestibuli and the scala tympani, as illustrated in Fig. 16.10. All three compartments are filled with fluid. The scala vestibuli is separated from the middle ear by the oval window and from the scala tympani by the round window. The basilar membrane forms the floor of the membranous cochlea and an elaborate structure sits on it known as the organ of Corti which, like the basilar membrane, spirals from base to apex of the cochlea. The organ of Corti contains rows of elongated hair cells, the specialized receptors for sound. Nerve endings lie in contact with the base of the hair cells and these collect together to form the cochlear nerve, which joins the vestibular nerve from the semi-circular canals to form the VIIIth cranial nerve (stato-acoustic) passing into the cranial cavity through the *internal auditory meatus*.

Sound waves cause the eardrum to vibrate at the same frequency as the stimulating tone. The ossicles of the middle ear then accurately transmit the vibrations of the eardrum to the footplate of the stapes which moves backwards and forwards in the oval window setting up waves in the fluid contained in the cochlea. The round window, by yielding to pressure, allows the fluid movements to occur. The arrangements of the auditory ossicles and the relative sizes of the eardrum and oval window are such that the force of the eardrum motion is amplified about ten times. Reflex contractions of two small muscles in the middle ear damp down over-vigorous movements of the

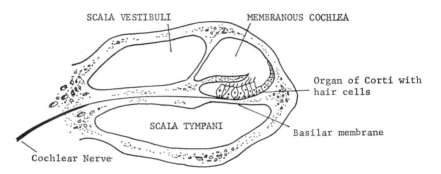

SCALA VESTIBULI
MEMBRANOUS COCHLEA
Organ of Corti with hair cells
SCALA TYMPANI
Basilar membrane
Cochlear Nerve

FIG. 16.10. Cross-section of the cochlea.

ossicles resulting from loud noise, and so protect against injury to the internal ear. The fluid waves in the cochlea are transmitted to the membranous cochlea and to the basilar membrane which, when displaced, cause a bending deformity of the hair processes in the organ of Corti. This mechanical deformation of the hair processes generates nerve impulses in the cochlear nerve. The frequency of nerve impulses in the cochlear nerve bears no relation to the frequency of the sound waves but is determined by the loudness. A weak tone sets up a low frequency of nerve impulses and a loud tone a high frequency. Appreciation of pitch appears to be related to the area of maximum disturbance of a particular part of the membranous cochlea. However, there are many aspects of the subjective interpretation of the complex physical properties of sound waves which are not yet understood.

Each cochlea is linked to the acoustic areas in both temporal lobes of the cerebral cortex by complex pathways involving at least four neurones. Synapses in the auditory pathways occur in the cochlear nuclei, the superior olives, the inferior colliculi and the medial geniculate nuclei.

CHAPTER 17

Body Temperature

Man is a *homothermic* animal, as are most mammals and birds; that is, the body temperature is held constant within narrow limits. Animals whose temperature varies with that of the environment are termed *poikilothermic*, examples being amphibia and reptiles. Some animals temporarily suspend their homothermic state and enter into a period of torpidity or hibernation during which they are poikilothermic. These animals are termed *heterothermic*.

In normal healthy man, the body temperature is maintained at 36–37·5° C (97–99·5° F). The temperature is usually measured in the mouth, the rectum, the axilla (armpit) or the groin. There are minor regional differences in temperature through the body. For example, the rectal temperature is about 0·3° C above mouth temperature, whereas that in the axilla is about 0·6° C lower. Blood leaving the lungs is slightly cooler than that entering the lungs as there is some heat exchange with the inspired air. Blood leaving the liver is about 0·2° C higher than that entering the liver as heat is released from metabolic processes. The testes lose heat and are about 1° C below the body temperature; spermatogenesis is more active at temperatures below 37° C.

There is a diurnal variation in temperature of about 1° C, the lowest temperatures being recorded in the early morning after some hours of sleep, and the highest being at night. A change in activities, as, for example, by a worker going on night shift, reverses the diurnal rhythm. In women the body temperature is at its lowest during menstruation. The temperature rises gradually until ovulation, and then it increases to about 0·5° C above the average and remains at this level until menstruation re-occurs.

The body temperature depends on the balance between heat gain and heat loss, and follows from purely physical and physico-chemical considerations:

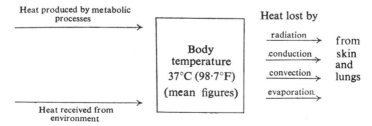

Heat production. The *basal metabolic rate* (B.M.R.) is the rate of heat production measured under standard conditions. For the test, the subject is completely

431

rested, both physically and mentally, in a comfortable environment, and about 12 h have elapsed after a meal. The rate of oxygen consumption is measured over a few minutes, using an apparatus known as a respirometer. The rate of energy production is calculated from a knowledge of the energy yielded in a calorimeter when oxygen is used up in the combustion of foodstuffs (see page 29). When 1 litre of oxygen (at N.T.P.) is used up in the combustion of carbohydrate, about 5 calories of energy appears as heat, whilst the combustion of pure fat liberates 4·8 Cal. Carbon dioxide is produced by the combustion, and the ratio of CO_2 produced to the O_2 consumed is called the respiratory quotient (R.Q.). For the combustion of carbohydrate this ratio is 1, whereas it is 0·7 for fat. The simultaneous determination of O_2 consumption and CO_2 production gives the value for the R.Q. and hence the amount of heat energy liberated can be estimated. For example, when the R.Q. is 0·75, the energy liberated when 1 litre of O_2 is consumed is 4·82 Cal. In practice, only the oxygen consumption is measured and the R.Q. is taken to be 0·75 as this is the ratio usually obtained after 12 h of fasting. For clinical purposes, a B.M.R. is sometimes expressed as the percentage deviation from an accepted average for persons of the same height, weight, age and sex. Thus, for a man aged 40 years, a B.M.R. of 38 Cal/sq. m/h is the norm (see Fig. 17.1); if the B.M.R. is measured at 76 Cal/sq. m/h, this value may be expressed as $+100\%$, or if it is 30 Cal/sq. m/h, it may be expressed as -21%, the calculation being $(30-38) \times 100/38$.

The resting metabolic rate in animals of different sizes varies considerably, and it is more closely related to the surface area than to its body weight (Table 17.1). The German physiologist, Rubner, first noticed that the metabolic rate was proportional to the surface area and suggested that the rate of heat production was governed by the rate of cooling from the surface. This is, however, an oversimplification of the balancing mechanisms involved.

The surface area of humans may be estimated using the following formula developed by Du Bois in 1916:

$$\log A = (0 \cdot 425 \times \log W) + (0 \cdot 725 \times \log H) + 1 \cdot 8563$$

where A is surface area in sq. cm, W is weight in kg, and H is height in cm.

FACTORS AFFECTING METABOLIC RATE. Age and sex are two factors influencing the B.M.R. (see Fig. 17.1). The metabolic rate also depends on *habitat*; for example, wild animals have a higher metabolic rate than animals of the same species kept in captivity or domesticated. Further, animals in polar regions have a higher metabolic rate (per sq. m of body surface) than those in tropical regions. This is an expression of adaptation to the environment. Human beings also alter their metabolic rate when the *external temperature* changes. In addition, the *body temperature* itself has an effect on metabolic rate; thus for every 1° F rise in body temperature, the B.M.R. increases by about 12%. When the body temperature is raised, as in fever, the increased metabolic rate

TABLE 17.1. Metabolic rates of different animal species

Species	Weight (kg)	Metabolic rate in Cal/h		
		Total	Per kg body wt	Per sq. m body surface
Rabbit	2·5	7·2	2·9	39
Dog	15	33	2·2	43
Man	70	72	1·0	40
Pig	130	102	0·8	45
Horse	440	208	0·45	39

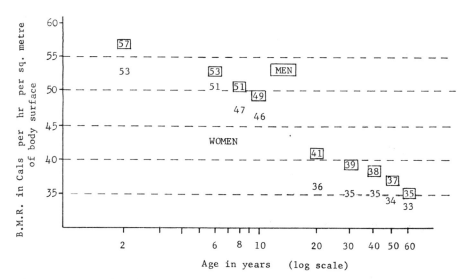

FIG. 17.1. The relationship between basal metabolic rate and age of men (figures in squares) and women.

is matched by an increase in pulmonary ventilation; this explains the rapid respiration rate seen in fevered patients. The food intake also influences the metabolic rate, as it is decreased in starvation and raised after feeding. After eating carbohydrate or fat, about 5 to 10% of the calorific value of the meal is released as heat, giving an increase in the metabolic rate over a period of 2 or 3 h.This metabolic increase is due to the energy expended in the synthesis of glycogen. However, after eating protein, as much as 40% of its calorific value appears as heat: this effect is known as the *specific dynamic action*. The heat production reaches a peak in about 3 h and continues until 7 or 8 h after the meal. The release of energy from the dynamic action of foodstuffs in a normal mixed diet amounts to 100 to 200 Cal a day. The diurnal variation of body temperature is due in part to this dynamic action of foodstuffs. The *thyroid hormone* also has a marked influence on metabolic rate; in thyrotoxicosis, the B.M.R. may be +100% above normal, whilst in myxoedema, it may fall as low as −40%. The secretion of the *anterior pituitary gland* influences the metabolic rate as it indirectly affects the thyroid. *Adrenaline* increases the metabolic rate.

In basal conditions, heat production occurs at the rate of about 1700 Cal/day in man and 1500 Cal/day in woman. The metabolic activity of the liver and brain together account for more than half of the B.M.R. of the body. The greatest output of metabolic energy results from muscular activity; thus, the rate of O_2 uptake may increase from 250 ml/min at rest to 3500 ml/min during violent muscular exertion. The muscular activity involved in shivering also liberates substantial amounts of heat. Shivering is more efficient than co-ordinated muscular activity as a means of increasing heat production to maintain body temperature in the cold, since in exercise the heat losses resulting from convection and vascular dilatation are greatly increased.

The daily energy output for various types of occupations has been computed, as follows:

Rest in bed	1700–1800 Cal
Sedentary work (clerical work, tailoring)	2200–2500 Cal
Light muscular work (housewife's duties, driving a car, light machining)	2600–2800 Cal
Muscular work (machining, building work)	3200–4000 Cal
Heavy muscular work (mining, sawing, harvesting)	4500–6000 Cal

HEAT RECEIVED FROM ENVIRONMENT. In high air temperatures heat is gained by the body, and the only way by which it may then be lost is by evaporation. On immersion in a bath of water at or above body temperature, this route of heat loss no longer operates and the temperature rises rapidly. Heat may also be gained from radiation, independently of air temperature. Skin absorbs (and radiates) infra-red wavelengths of between 5 and 20 μ, and it is interesting to note that skin colour, which is due to reflection of visible light, is immaterial.

Heat loss. The proportion of heat lost at an environmental temperature of 20° C in a subject at rest are:

(1) conduction and convection: 20–40%,

(2) radiation: 40–60%,

(3) evaporation: 20–25%.

Heat lost by conduction and convection depends largely on the extent to which the surrounding air is warmed, this route being only available when the air temperature is lower than the skin temperature. Similarly, heat loss from radiation only occurs if surrounding objects are at a lower radiation temperature. Evaporation results in a heat loss of 0·58 Cal per 1 g of water evaporated at 34° C (average skin temperature), and this takes place from the skin (as sweat) and in the lungs. The efficiency of evaporation as a route of heat loss varies with the saturation of the surrounding air with water vapour. Heat losses by conduction, convection and evaporation also depend considerably on the amount of body exposure, the nature of the clothing and the movement of the surrounding air.

Mechanisms for temperature regulation

Skin. Mechanisms for regulating heat exchange by radiation, conduction, convection and evaporation are present in the skin. In a comfortable environment, the temperature of the skin of the face is about 33° C, and that of the hands is about 30° C. The maximum temperature of the skin (37° C) is only a little above this so that the maximum loss by radiation is limited. In normally-clothed people in a temperate climate, about 900 cal/day are lost by radiation. Australian aboriginals, living a tribal life, sleep naked under a clear night sky, and thus are exposed to the greatest possible radiation temperature differential; they lose a considerable amount of heat, although they are reported to sleep curled up, so reducing the area of their radiating surface by about one half. Their skin temperatures drop to a point which would be extremely uncomfortable for people unaccustomed to their type of life. Heat loss by radiation is diminished by constriction of blood vessels of the exposed skin. The rate of heat loss by conduction to the surrounding air and by setting up convection currents in it also depends on the skin temperature.

Heat is transferred from the deeper structures of the body to the skin by the blood. The subcutaneous adipose tissue conducts heat but at a rate about one-quarter that of skin, and so it offers a barrier to heat loss by conduction. In aquatic mammals living in polar seas, the thick layer of blubber is very important for the conservation of heat. In man, the blood vessels of the skin of the face, the neck and the extremities are particularly adapted to regulate the body temperature. The skin of other regions may be involved in other animals; for example, the blood vessels in the skin of the ears of the rabbit, the wing of the bat, the tail of the rat, and the vessels in the mucosa of the tongue of the dog are all adapted for heat loss.

There are two mechanisms for regulating the blood flow through the skin. First, the arteries supplying the skin may be constricted so that the total blood arriving in the skin is diminished; and secondly, the way in which the blood is distributed through the skin may be altered by arterio-venous anastomoses (page 280). Constriction of the anastomotic channels shunts the blood through the capillary bed, thus exposing a greater surface area and allowing more time for heat exchange. When the blood flows rapidly through the anastomoses, less heat is lost.

The calibre of the blood vessels of the skin is controlled by the sympathetic nervous system. Noradrenaline and adrenaline cause blanching of the skin by constriction of the cutaneous blood vessels, whilst dilatation of these vessels is believed to result from cessation of sympathetic nerve impulses, less nor-adrenaline impinging on the vascular smooth muscle. However, there may be some sympathetic fibres which when stimulated cause dilatation by releasing acetylcholine, particularly those involved in the sudden dilatation of blushing and flushing of the skin.

In furred or feathered animals, the air entrapped in layers next to the skin provides a thermal barrier serving to conserve heat. Man adopts clothing and so achieves the same end. In many other animals, there is a cycle of hair growth which reaches a peak in early winter and is followed by a moult in spring. An immediate response to cold in these animals is fluffing up the hair (piloerection) or feathers, thereby increasing the thickness of the entrapped air layer. In man, the response of piloerection has persisted (although without any apparent functional value) as 'gooseflesh', pitting of the skin at the points of attachment of the contracted arrector pili muscles (see Fig. 17.2). These muscles are innervated by sympathetic adrenergic fibres.

Heat is lost by evaporation of water from the skin. The so-called 'insensible perspiration' is water which diffuses through the skin and then evaporates. About 600–850 ml pass through human skin in 24 h, and this results in a heat loss of 350–500 Cal. The heat lost by this route is fairly constant. The other source of water evaporated from the skin is the sweat, and sweating is par-ticularly important in the regulation of body temperature.

The two kinds of sweat glands in man are called the eccrine and the apocrine glands. The eccrine glands secrete a watery fluid which contains 2% or less of solute, chiefly urea, lactic acid and sodium chloride. The concentration of sodium chloride varies from 0·1 to 0·4%, depending upon the activity of the adrenal cortex. The eccrine sweat glands are innervated by sympathetic cholinergic nerve fibres, but sweating may also be elicited by local injections of noradrenaline and adrenaline. The sweat glands are reflexly stimulated to secrete by a rise in skin temperature of 0·2° to 0·5° C, but the maximum rate of sweating (about 1 to 1·5 litres/h) is not sustained for long periods. The maximal daily rate of sweat is about 5–10 litres each day, and as each litre loses 580 Cal on evaporation the daily heat loss may be nearly 6000 Cal. The drinking of cold liquids to replace the sweat lost is a comparatively ineffective means of cooling, as only 37 Cal are absorbed when the temperature of 1 litre of liquid at

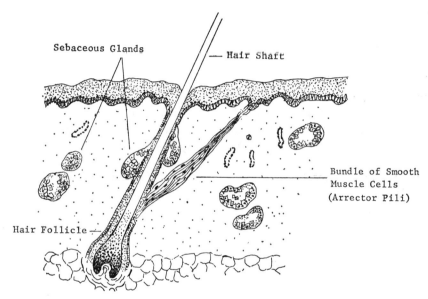

Fɪɢ. 17.2. Diagram of a hair follicle in the skin and its accompanying arrector pili muscles.

0° C is raised to body temperature. However, sweating only leads to heat loss if evaporation occurs. There is little or no loss of heat from sweating in a hot bath, or when the air surrounding the body is saturated with water vapour, or when the sweat falls off the skin in drops or is wiped off.

Apocrine sweat glands are related to the sebaceous glands of hair follicles. They occur in the axilla and also in the skin of the genital and anal region. Their secretion contains chiefly the products of disintegration of secretory cells; it does not contribute to heat loss in man. In the horse, however, there are only apocrine sweat glands, and these are concerned with heat loss. Apocrine glands are not innervated but are stimulated by adrenaline from the blood-stream. Noradrenaline is less effective than adrenaline in this respect.

Lungs. Expired air is saturated with water vapour in the lungs, besides being warmed to body temperature. However, the fraction of heat lost by this route depends on the temperature and humidity of the inspired air. In man it may average about 200 Cal/day. Some animals (for example, dogs) have no sweat glands, and heat losses by evaporation and convection are made by increasing the rate of respiration. Panting (also called *thermal* polypnoea) results in increasing air movements over the tongue and through the mouth, and heat is readily conducted from these surfaces as the mucosal blood vessels are dilated. In addition, there is evaporation of the thin copious saliva which is secreted during panting.

Metabolism. The rate of production of heat through metabolic processes is influenced by the temperature of the environment. Shivering generates heat since muscular activity is involved, and is an immediate response to a fall in temperature. However, on acclimatization to cold environments, there is a higher basal metabolic rate. Endocrinal influences also play some part in this adaptation. Both thyroxine and adrenaline, for example, increase heat production by increasing the rate of oxidative metabolism (see Fig. 17.3).

Temperature receptors. Exploration of the skin with fine heat-controlled probes reveals the presence of 'hot' or 'cold' sensitive spots, which may be associated with specific receptors. Stimulation of these spots with thermally indifferent stimuli gives rise to the sensations of warmth or cold. In between these spots, application of heat or cold does not give rise to temperature sensations. There are more cold-sensitive than heat-sensitive spots, but the total number varies greatly. The nerves conveying impulses from the temperature sensitive spots are fine myelinated fibres of the A group and non-myelinated C fibres (see pages 69–73).

Temperature receptors are extremely sensitive; a rise of $0.007°$ C in 3 sec is the threshold for warmth and a fall of $0.012°$ C in 3 sec is the threshold for cold. However, the intensity of temperature sensation depends on the area of skin stimulated. If, for example, a hand is immersed in water at $37°$ C and a finger is immersed in water at $40°$ C, the water on the hand feels hotter. The ability to discriminate different temperatures depends on the temperature in the skin ($28°$ C gives optimal sensitivity), on the density of temperature sensitive spots, and also on the thermal conductivity of the skin. Thickly keratinized skin is relatively insensitive for this reason. Intense thermal stimulation gives rise to the sensation of pain.

Thermal sensations from the temperature-sensitive receptors of the skin arise not only from heat or cold applied externally but also from temperature changes within the skin resulting from alterations in the blood flow. Hence there is a feeling of warmth from inflamed skin or in blushing where the blood supply is greatly increased.

There are temperature-sensitive receptors in the respiratory passages and in the gastro-intestinal tract. There are also regions in the hypothalamus,

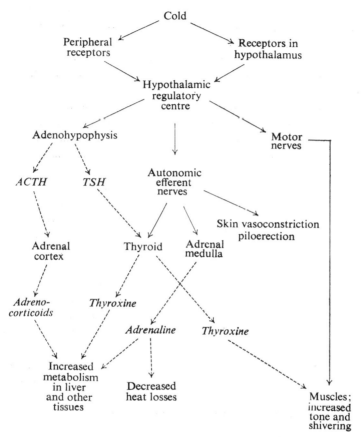

FIG. 17.3. Schematic diagram of nervous and hormonal responses to cold (adapted, in part, from Hardy, 1961). The dotted lines indicate hormonal mechanisms.

which are sensitive to changes in the temperature of the blood reaching this part of the brain.

Control of body temperature

The simplest response to raising the temperature of a patch of skin is dilatation of the blood vessels resulting from stimulation of an axon reflex. The local injection of acetylcholine or nicotine produces sweating and piloerection, both of which are believed to be mediated via axon reflexes. At the next level of complexity there are spinal reflexes invoking responses of the skin blood vessels, sweat glands, piloerection and allied phenomena (goose-flesh). Nerve fibres conveying temperature information ascend the spinal cord and relay in the thalamus. From the thalamus, other fibres pass to the cerebral cortex, thereby giving rise to perception of temperature, whilst others pass from the thalamus to the hypothalamus, which is under the control of the cerebral cortex. Impulses from the hypothalamus set in motion the various mechanisms concerned with the immediate control of temperature. These relationships are given diagrammatically in Fig. 17.4.

After removal of the cerebrum, or after sectioning between the cerebrum and the hypothalamus, the body temperature is held within normal limits, provided that the extremes of environmental temperatures are avoided. If the hypothalamus is removed, or if section of the spinal cord is made below it, the animal becomes poikilothermic.

There may be two centres in the hypothalamus which are concerned with temperature regulation. Stimulation of the anterior hypothalamus activates mechanisms leading to heat loss: these include vasodilatation of skin blood vessels, sweating and panting. Removal of the anterior hypothalamus does not impair the regulation of temperature when in a cold environment, but the responses to a hot environment are absent. On the other hand, stimulation of the posterior hypothalamus results in activation of mechanisms leading to increased heat production: these include vasoconstriction of skin blood vessels, pilo-erection, an increase in heart rate, shivering and liberation of adrenaline which causes a rise in blood sugar and in metabolic rate. After removal of the anterior hypothalamus, the responses to cooling are lost. Recent evidence indicates that the release of noradrenaline or 5-HT from the region of the hypothalamus may be responsible for initiating the responses which alter the body temperature. In the cat, noradrenaline applied to the hypothalamic region produces hypothermia whereas 5-HT produces hyperthermia.

Response to exercise. The blood flow through the skin increases during exercise, allowing an increased loss of heat by radiation and convection. There is also an increase in sweating. These thermoregulatory mechanisms are brought into play before there is an appreciable increase in temperature. If the muscular activity produces heat more rapidly than it is lost, the temperature rises, and the thermoregulatory mechanisms continue after exercise.

Responses to high environmental temperature. Sweating provides the main route of heat dissipation in hot climates. The body temperature rises when heat

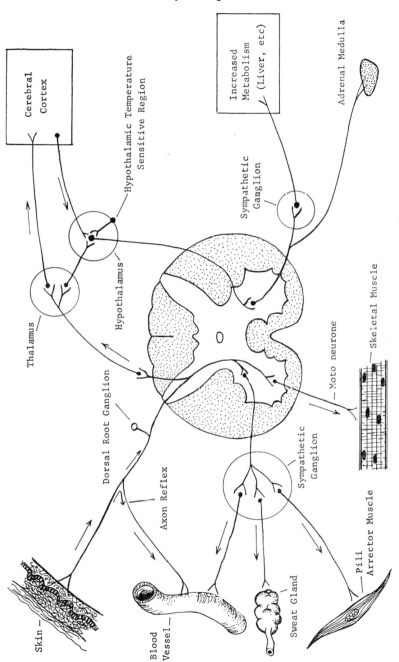

Fig. 17.4. Nervous regulation of body temperature.

loss is impaired when the humidity is high, or when heat production increases as a result of exercise. The loss of water by sweating leads to a decrease in blood volume (haemoconcentration) and in the rate of urine formation. The increased blood flow through the skin requires a higher cardiac output to hold the blood pressure constant, and when the increase in cardiac output is not forthcoming fainting occurs. The salt loss incurred by sweating may result in muscular cramps and headache, since as much as 20 g of salt per day may be lost in the sweat of unacclimatized persons. Other symptoms caused by high temperatures (before adaptation occurs) are the loss of appetite (anorexia), diarrhoea, fatigue (heat exhaustion), a listless attitude, dizziness and signs of inco-ordination. The replacement of water and salt lost in sweating *and* the reduction of the body temperature are necessary to produce full recovery. Adaptative responses to continued high temperatures are brought into play through the activity of the pituitary. Thus, thyroid function is depressed, which results in a lower rate of metabolism, and ACTH is secreted to produce a discharge of adrenal corticoids, with a retardation of Na^+ during sweat secretion, resulting in less salt depletion.

Hyperthermia. An increase in body temperature occurs whenever heat production exceeds heat loss. It may result from excessive production, from failure of thermoregulatory mechanisms, or from 'resetting' the temperature control at too high a level. Death occurs at body temperatures of 43–45° C. Neurogenic hyperthermia results from lesions of the hypothalamus, and is largely due to an increase in the rate of metabolism in the liver. In hyperthyroid states, there is often an elevated temperature, resulting from the increased metabolism.

Drugs producing hyperthermia. Dinitrophenol (DNP) increases the rate of oxidative processes, so a larger amount of heat is liberated. It acts by 'uncoupling' phosphorylation from oxidation (page 42). It was at one time used to reduce obesity, as it increases the utilization of the body's fat stores to produce heat which is wasted. Amphetamine and other sympathomimetic amines also produce hyperthermia by increasing oxidative metabolism. Cocaine is hyperthermic, possibly by potentiating the action of catecholamines (see page 774). Drugs which block the nervous impulses to the sweat glands (e.g. atropine or hexamethonium) also produce hyperthermia. Caffeine may raise the body temperature through an action on the hypothalamus. Pyrogens are substances which cause fever (pyrexia). The injection of protein or protein hydrolysates often raises the body temperature. In conditions in which there is extensive breakdown of tissue, as, for example, extensive bruising or crushing, neoplastic diseases, thrombotic occlusion of blood vessels (page 232) and haemolytic diseases (page 240), the temperature is also above normal. In some infectious diseases, the fever is caused by bacterial pyrogens which are usually lipopoly-saccharides. These pyrogens act by setting the hypothalamic controlata higher level. Antipyretics (page 646) act by resetting the hypothalamic control at a lower level, although they do not lower the temperature of a normal person.

Responses to low environmental temperature. The immediate response to cooling is the diversion of blood from the skin by constriction of the cutaneous blood vessels. In some regions of the skin there is a cold vasodilatation, particularly in the fingers, over the knee and elbow and parts of the face. If integrated body movements are not taking place, or if they are insufficient to replace the heat loss, there is shivering and 'goose-flesh'. Heat production is increased as the metabolic rate is increased by adrenaline, which is released from the adrenals through reflex stimulation (see Fig. 17.4). Adaptation to a cold environment involves an increased activity of the thyroid and adrenal glands.

The minimum environmental temperature at which an animal is capable of maintaining its body temperature for 1 h is termed the *lower critical temperature*. For the dog, the lower critical temperature is − 100° C. The lower critical temperature for man depends on his microclimate, that is the closely surrounding environment he creates with clothing and housing. Polar explorers and others exposed to extreme cold are overcome by lassitude as their body temperature falls and thay fall asleep when their temperature falls to about 25° C. Death follows cooling to about 20° C.

Hypothermia is induced in patients as a prelude to some forms of surgery for two reasons: (1) hypothermia itself produces an anaesthetic state, and (2) in anaesthetized patients it lowers the metabolic rate of tissues and the blood supply may then be temporarily interrupted without causing damage. Local hypothermia of limbs is sometimes used for amputations. Whole body hypothermia is used for cardiovascular surgery and some brain surgery. Cooling to 25° C reduces the metabolic rate to about one-third of normal, and consequently the circulation may be interrupted for three times as long as usual. The cerebral circulation may be cut off for 8 min at 30° C and for 45 min at 15° C, both with normal recovery from the operation. The EEG waves (page 132) disappear at about 18–20° C on cooling and reappear at 20–22° C on rewarming. Hypothermia for surgery is produced by cooling the body surface or by passing the blood through a heat-exchanging coil. Various drugs may be used to facilitate the production of hypothermia. Chlorpromazine works by dilating blood vessels, blocking the action of adrenaline and centrally inhibiting shivering. Anaesthetics cause hypothermia by blocking hypothalamic control of body temperature. Neuro-muscular blocking drugs work by paralysing muscular movements which include shivering.

During hypothermia, the heart slows due to cooling of the sino-atrial node (page 211), and cardiac activity usually ceases at about 15°C. There is a pronounced risk of ventricular fibrillation, particularly at temperatures below 30°C. During cooling, this is not such a problem as the object of cooling is to allow circulatory arrest.

PART 2

General and Systematic Pharmacology

CHAPTER 18

Principles of Drug Action

Sources of drugs. The first drugs known to man were obtained from natural sources; they were either from plants like the poppy (opium) and foxglove (digitalis), or they were simple inorganic substances like Epsom salts and arsenic. Later, the development of organic chemistry led to the introduction of synthetic drugs, and at present some 100,000 compounds have been tested for pharmacological activity. The growth of knowledge of biochemistry and physiology, which led to the concept of the chemical control of biological processes, has been of particular importance for pharmacology. The vitamins and endocrine hormones have long been used as medicines (that is, drugs) to cure diseases resulting from their deficiency.

Classification of drugs. There is no single comprehensive system of classifying drugs, but there are various approaches which are of some use in gathering together certain aspects of the subject matter.

(a) DRUGS FROM PLANTS. It is still common to refer to these drugs in terms of the species of plant from which they are obtained e.g., *cinchona* alkaloids, *solanaceous* alkaloids. This classification is often convenient for drugs with closely related chemical structures and pharmacological properties that occur together in plants of related species (e.g., *ergot alkaloids*), or when a plant extract containing a mixture of drugs is used therapeutically, e.g., *digitalis glycosides*. A limitation of this botanical classification is that drugs of completely unrelated pharmacological properties may occur together in a single plant extract; for example, *opium* contains the analgesic, morphine, and the smooth muscle relaxant, papaverine.

(b) CHEMICAL STRUCTURE OF DRUGS. Within a few series of chemicals, pharmacological activity is fairly closely related to chemical structure, and sometimes drugs may be grouped on the basis of a characteristic feature in their structure. Some examples are the *barbiturates*, the *organic nitrites*, the *phenothiazines*, the *sulphonamides* and the *quaternary ammonium bases*. However, pharmacological activity may change qualitatively as well as quantitatively in members of a homologous series. Hence the chemical classification of

447

drugs is inadequate as a means of presenting a systematic account of pharmacology, although the presence of certain types of pharmacological activity can sometimes be predicted from the chemical structure.

(c) USES OF DRUGS. From the practical point of view, this classification has much to recommend it, therapeutics being the most important branch of applied pharmacology. The physician wants to know what drugs bring about a particular result, such as the lowering of blood pressure, or the relief of pain. Drugs may therefore be grouped together according to their therapeutically useful actions, e.g., *antihypertensives*, and *analgesics*. From the scientific point of view, this method of classification is less useful. There are many drugs that have no place in therapeutics; nevertheless, the study of such substances may give an insight into the basic mechanisms of drug action, and this can result in a new approach to the treatment of disease.

(d) SITES OF ACTION OF DRUGS. It is a common practice to group drugs according to the part of the body on which they exert their effects. Thus, we speak of *central nervous system stimulants* ranging from psychomotor stimulants through analeptics to convulsants; these names indicate grades of 'stimulant' action on the central nervous system. Further examples of classification of drugs on the basis of their sites of action are: *cardiac* and *oxytocic* drugs (acting on organs, namely the heart and uterus respectively); *antiinflammatory* and *haematopoietic* drugs (acting on tissues, namely, connective tissues and bone marrow); and ganglion-stimulant drugs (acting on one type of cell, namely, ganglion cells).

TABLE 18.1. 'Overlap' of pharmacological activity, to illustrate the problem of classification of drugs.

Drug	Relative activity, quinidine (=100%)*	'Classification'
Quinine	110	Anti-fibrillatory (cinchona alkaloid)
Procaine	80	Local anaesthetic (synthetic)
Cocaine	620	Local anaesthetic, mydriatic, psychomotor stimulant (alkaloid)
Pethidine	83	Analgesic, spasmolytic (synthetic)
Papaverine	50	Spasmolytic (opium alkaloid)
Syntropan	130	Spasmolytic, antimuscarinic (synthetic)
Ephedrine	30	Sympathomimetic, psychomotor stimulant, bronchial dilator, vasoconstrictor (alkaloid)

[From Dawes, 1946, *Brit. J. Pharmacol.*, **1**, 90].

* The drugs were compared for their ability to reduce the maximum rate at which isolated rabbit atria could be driven by electrical pulses.

(e) PROTOTYPE DRUGS. A well-known drug is often taken as a prototype of compounds possessing a particular type of pharmacological activity. For example, drugs producing effects like those of atropine might be described as atropine-like. The limitation of this classification is that every drug has a variety of actions. This can be seen by inspection of Table 18.1, which shows the relative activity of a number of drugs in a 'screening test' (i.e. a means of identification) for drugs possessing quinidine-like activity.

(f) MECHANISM OF ACTION. In principle, this is the best method of classification, but there are relatively few drugs for which the mechanism underlying their pharmacological action is known. The following section considers this more fully.

Drug action in relation to the level of biological organization

To understand the mechanism of action of a drug it is necessary to consider the effects produced on biological systems at various levels of complexity of organization: these are the actions on enzyme systems; then on subcellular structures; on cells; on isolated organs or organ systems; and finally, on the intact animal or on man, both in health and disease.

ACTIONS ON ENZYMES. Many drugs act specifically on an enzyme or a group of enzymes. The first stage in an enzymatic reaction is the combination of the substrate with the enzyme. A drug which combines with the active centre of the enzyme, but does not then undergo the reaction, inhibits the catalytic activity of the enzyme. The activity of some enzymes may also be altered by modifying co-factors such as Ca^{++} or Mg^{++}, coenzymes, or prosthetic groups. Although a drug may influence a particular enzyme reaction *in vitro*, it does not follow that all, or indeed *any*, of its pharmacological effects in the intact animal are a result of its effects on this enzyme. In the intact animal, the concentration of the drug in the vicinity of the enzyme may be too low to produce its effect; further, modification of the activity of an enzyme that is not concerned with a rate-limiting step in a series of reactions usually has no effect on the functioning of a system; and finally, the demonstration that a drug acts on an isolated enzyme does not preclude it from having other effects which may be of greater importance.

ACTIONS ON BIOCHEMICAL SYSTEMS. The over-all effect of a drug on a biochemical system may be known, although the particular enzyme which is affected may not have been identified. An example of this is provided by di-nitrophenol (DNP) which decreases the rate of formation of high energy compounds (energy-storing phosphorylated compounds) from oxidation reactions (see page 42). This is summed up by saying that DNP *uncouples*

15

oxidative phosphorylation. The inefficient utilization of foodstuff results in an increased metabolic rate and this (and other factors) leads to a loss of weight. (Dinitrophenol is extremely toxic and its use in the treatment of obesity has been abandoned.)

ACTIONS ON SUBCELLULAR STRUCTURES. Drugs may act on the cell nucleus to alter the processes of cell division. Thus colchicine interferes with the last stage of mitosis and prevents cell division *in vitro*: however, it is not effective *in vivo* in treating cancer—one of the lines of research directed towards drug treatment of cancer is the search for agents which selectively impair the division of the tumour cells. On the other hand, many chemical agents produce changes in the nucleus which result in the appearance of tumours; these are the so-called *carcinogens*. Another intracellular site of drug action is on the granular elements of the cytoplasm. The granules of tissue mast cells and basophils contain histamine and heparin, and those of chromaffin cells contain catecholamines. These substances, when released, exert their pharmacological effects, and drugs causing their release are said to act indirectly. A third sub-cellular structure on which drugs act is the microsome (see page 39), which may be disrupted or activated, or may have its enzymatic activity altered; the functional activity of the cell, and of the whole organism, is thereby modified (see pages 517–521).

ACTIONS OF DRUGS ON CELLS. A major impetus for the establishment of pharmacology as a scientific subject existing in its own right (as distinct from therapeutics or medicinal chemistry) began with the study of the actions of drugs on cells—particularly on nerve cells and on effector cells of muscular or secretory tissues. One of the tenets of the early pharmacologists was that pharmacological effects involved only quantitative changes in the functions of a cell; that is, the change in activity produced by a drug was only an extension (or an attenuation) of an inherent capacity of the cell. If the change in cellular activity cannot be ascribed to an action of a drug on a definite constituent of a cell, it is attributed to an action on a part of the cell called the 'receptor'.

ACTIONS ON TISSUES, ORGANS AND ORGAN SYSTEMS. Although many drugs are known to act on particular types of cell, there are still many examples of drug action where the knowledge is less precise, and the action is recognized as a response involving an organ or a system. There are two reasons why this is so. Firstly, techniques of investigation are limited; thus, the identification of the cellular site of action of drugs in the central nervous system depends largely on the application of the techniques only recently introduced into electrophysiology. Secondly, the action of the drug may be on many cells rather than on a particular type of cell. Thus, a drug which, say, relaxes the smooth muscle in the walls of blood vessels and so causes vasodilatation may also produce a reflex acceleration of the heart rate. The action on the blood vessels is exerted at the cellular level, but the effect on the heart is exerted at the physiological level of organization. The direct action of acetylcholine on the heart is to decrease the rate of beating, yet the intravenous injection of small amounts produces the opposite effect providing the homeostatic mechanisms are operating.

ACTIONS IN THE INTACT ORGANISM. The effects of a drug may alter with variation in the prevailing physiological state. Thus, drugs which abolish the sympathetic nerve control of blood vessels produce a marked lowering of blood pressure in subjects standing upright, but have considerably less effect if the subject is lying down. Alterations in behaviour produced by drugs depend on the function of the whole organism. The effects of drugs on mood, in man, depend partly on the structure of the personality. Sociological factors play a part as determinants of the response to certain drugs, notably alcohol, as well as to some illegally-used drugs such as marihuana, cocaine, and amphetamine and its derivatives. Psychological factors often modify drug effects and result in erroneous conclusions in evaluating the effects of drugs in man. An apparent improvement in the clinical condition of a patient may be due to the attention he is receiving during the trial of a new drug rather than to a genuine pharmacological effect (or it may be due to a spontaneous remission, unconnected with the treatment). To obviate these factors, a control group of patients is treated with a dummy inert medicament which is prepared in a form resembling the drug under trial. As an additional safeguard against complications arising from psychological factors in clinical trials, the identity of the medicament is concealed from the patient and from the person administering it, but is known by a third person who interprets the results. An inert medicament, such as is used for comparison with the drug in these trials, is known as a *placebo*. There is a relationship between certain types of personality (as defined by psychological tests) and the intensity of reaction to a placebo.

HEALTH AND DISEASE. The effect of a drug may depend on the presence of concurrent disease. For example, anticholinesterase drugs relieve muscular weakness in patients with myasthenia gravis, but do not increase muscular power in normal subjects. Again, cardiac glycosides increase the force of contraction of the failing heart, but have less effect on the contraction of the healthy heart.

*　　*　　*

The ultimate mechanism by which a drug exerts its action involves the interaction of the drug with the biological system at the molecular level, and the consequences of this interaction then appear as the response at a more complex level of organization. Although there are many known examples of the molecular effects of drugs, with most drugs only the consequences of the interaction are known. For example, the drug lysergic acid diethylamide produces hallucinations (pages. 629–630), but the chemical reactions responsible for this are unknown.

It is important to realize that the effects on a biological system cannot necessarily be predicted from a knowledge of the actions of a drug on one of the components of the system. For example, many of the effects of the anticholinesterase, physostigmine, on isolated tissues may readily be explained by the accumulation of acetylcholine in the tissue: the isolated heart beats more slowly and the isolated intestine goes into a spasm. But in the intact animal, physostigmine has more complex effects; for example, it produces, in the rat, a rise in blood pressure, which is probably due to the accumulation of acetylcholine at certain synapses in the central nervous system; this particular effect could not have been predicted from knowledge previously available.

The study of the effects of drugs and the analysis of their modes of action often provide essential clues for the elucidation of physiological and biochemical mechanisms. There are many illustrations of this aspect of pharmacology, particularly in connection with the physiology of the nervous system and the biochemical processes of neurones and nerve endings.

Drug receptors

The receptor. Many drugs are effective in extremely low concentrations. The drug does not supply the motive energy for the effect, but rather, it triggers off the response by an action on a specific part of the cell, termed the *receptor*. The concept of the receptor was introduced by Langley and by Ehrlich. Langley observed that nicotine caused a twitch only when it was applied to certain small areas on the muscle surface, and he postulated that there was a *receptive substance* at those points. The persistence of the effects of drugs after denervation also led to the idea that they acted on a receptive region of the muscle cell (hitherto it had been thought that they acted on the nerve endings). Ehrlich was responsible for the more general concept of the drug receptor. He observed that certain dyestuffs acted selectively, staining some cells more deeply or in a different way from other cells, and he suggested that drugs with selective actions on particular cells could be developed. After the discovery of drugs which acted on the cells of a parasite but not on those of the host, this selectivity was explained by a difference in the receptors of the cells. The pharmacological activity was thought to reside in the *pharmacophore* portion of the molecule, as an analogy to the chromophore which is the portion of the molecule responsible for conferring the property of colour.

Another line of work which engaged Ehrlich's attention was the problem of immunity. He proposed that the immunizing protein (i.e. the antibody) was a highly selective receptor of the protoplasm which united chemically with the toxin (i.e. the antigen).

The receptor then is a small region of the cell which combines chemically with a drug, and this chemical reaction leads to the biological response. The concept is similar to that of the active centre of an enzyme which combines chemically with the substrate molecule, and this leads to the enzymatically catalysed reaction. The similarity is strengthened by the following considerations. (*a*) In the case of optical isomers, one enantiomorph is usually more effective than the other in producing a pharmacological response or in being utilized as a substrate in an enzyme reaction. (*b*) In an homologous series of chemical compounds, one member exhibits the most marked pharmacological effect or is most effectively used as a substrate. (*c*) The pharmacological effect, or the enzyme activity, can be inhibited by substances which compete with the drug for the receptors or with the substrate for the active centre, respectively. In both cases, the kinetics of the competition can be studied by the application of the Law of Mass Action.

Combination of drug with receptor. An analogy for the action of a drug on a receptor is that of a lock (the receptor) and key (the drug): the image has been borrowed from enzymology, where the lock is the active centre of the enzyme and the key in the substrate. The analogy is crude, in that it is a mechanistic view of a chemical combination; nevertheless it does convey some valid implications. Firstly, the drug 'unlocks' the response. Secondly, the specificity of the 'locks' (receptors) as far as 'keys' are concerned is only relative; the lock may be turned by a number of different keys, and so a series of chemically related drugs may have the same pharmacological action. Thirdly, the 'lock' may be 'jammed', that is to say the pharmacological response may be blocked by an appropriate substance. Fourthly, the lock and key model of drug action often gives a useful guide to possible pharmacological activity in a new chemical compound. When there is a chemical similarity with a compound of known pharmacological action, then a similar action may be expected, since the same receptor combination may occur. A more realistic view of drug-receptor combination comes from a consideration of the forces of interaction which exist between small molecules (drugs) and protein surfaces. They are as follows:

(1) IONIC BONDS. These arise from the electrostatic attractive force which exists between two groups of opposite charge. The charged groups on protein surfaces may be *protein*-NH_3^+ or *protein*-COO^-, where these are the free

groups of diamino or dicarboxylic amino acids; the charge depends on the pH and the isoelectric point of the protein (pages 17–18).

(2) DIPOLE–DIPOLE BONDS. The unequal distribution of electron density within a molecule results in regions of relative electropositivity ($\delta+$) and negativity ($\delta-$). Intramolecular bonding is due to a weak electrostatic force between dipoles of opposite charge. The water molecule contains a dipole:

$$\overset{\delta-}{\underset{\delta+}{H{\nearrow}O{\nwarrow}H}}$$

The water of hydration around ions or charged groups is caused by the attraction of these dipoles.

(3) HYDROGEN BONDS. One type of hydrogen bond can be considered as a special case of dipole–dipole bonding between the hydrogen atom of one group and another electronegative group. The hydrogen atom, being shared between the two reacting groups, strengthens the bond. In drug-receptor interactions, the hydrogen-donating group is usually hydroxyl or amino and the electronegative group is a carbonyl oxygen. These are illustrated below with the hydrogen bond indicated by a dotted line.

$$\overset{\delta+ \qquad \delta-}{RO{-}H \cdots O{=}CR_2}$$
$$\overset{\delta+ \qquad \delta-}{RN{-}H \cdots O{=}CR_2}$$

The hydrogen is bound to the carbonyl group by sharing the lone pair of electrons on this oxygen atom with the hydrogen atom. The lone pair of electrons in nitrogen can also be partly shared to form a hydrogen bond.

$$RO{-}H \cdots NR_3$$

(4) COVALENT BONDS. In these, electrons are shared between atoms and this bond is much more powerful than the other types discussed above. Drugs which combine covalently are very peristent in their action. Examples are the combination of mercury or arsenic with thiol groups on proteins, phosphorylation of the active centre of cholinesterase by organophosphates, and alkylation of the catecholamine receptor by some antiadrenaline drugs.

(5) VAN DER WAALS' BONDS. These are weak bonds which occur between any two atoms or groups of atoms. The attractive force is inversely proportional

to the seventh power of the distance, and therefore it is effective only over a very short distance. The bond strength increases with atomic weight and is significant for carbon, nitrogen and oxygen. These bonds probably serve to reinforce stronger bonds which form between drugs and receptors. Antigen–antibody complexes are considered to be held together by both van der Waals' forces and hydrogen bonds.

Kinetics of drug-receptor combination

The administration of a drug can be represented by the following equation:

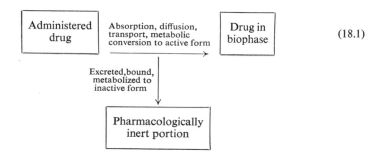

(18.1)

The drug in the *biophase* is physically in a position to react with the receptor. The amount may not be equal to that administered because of the factors listed in the above diagram. (These factors are considered in further detail in Chapter 19.) It is generally thought that the concentration administered and the concentration in the biophase are nearly equal in the case of the simplest type of pharmacological experiment on an isolated tissue when using a drug that is neither bound nor metabolized.

The combination of the drug with its receptor (to produce the pharmacological response) can then be expressed as:

$$\text{Drug (in biophase)} + \text{Receptor} \rightleftharpoons \text{Drug-receptor complex} \qquad (18.2)$$

This may be expressed in the following way:

$$D + \text{unoccupied receptors} \underset{k_2}{\overset{k_1}{\rightleftharpoons}} r \qquad (18.3)$$

where D = drug concentration, r = proportion of receptors combined with drug, and k_1 and k_2 are the rate constants for association and dissociation of the complex. The total number (or concentration) of receptors cannot be determined, but may be taken as unity; then, the proportion unoccupied during the action of a drug is $1 - r$. The concentration of drug is assumed to be in considerable excess, so that the amount taken up in the complex does not appreciably alter D.

The rate of formation of the complex depends on the drug concentration and the numbers of free receptors. Hence, rate of association $= k_1 D(1-r)$. Similarly, rate of dissociation $= k_2 r$. At equilibrium, the rates of association and dissociation are equal. Thus,

$$\frac{k_1}{k_2} = K_{\text{aff.}} = \frac{r}{D(1-r)} \tag{18.4}$$

where $K_{\text{aff.}}$ stands for the affinity constant, and represents a measure of the extent of formation of the drug receptor complex.

This treatment of the kinetics of drug-receptor combination is the same as that applied by Langmuir to the phenomenon of adsorption of a monomolecular layer of gas onto a solid surface, and equation (18.4) is analogous to the Langmuir adsorption equation. The reaction of an enzyme with its substrate may be similarly treated:

$$\text{Enzyme } (e) + \text{Substrate } (s) \underset{k_2}{\overset{k_1}{\rightleftharpoons}} \text{Complex } (p) \tag{18.5}$$

where $e =$ enzyme concentration, $s =$ substrate concentration and $p =$ concentration of enzyme–substrate complex. At equilibrium,

$$K_m = \frac{k_2}{k_1} = \frac{s(e-p)}{p}, \quad \text{and} \quad p = \frac{se}{(K_m+s)} \tag{18.6}$$

where K_m is called the Michaelis constant*. The affinity of the substrate for the enzyme is given by $1/K_m$.

It should be noted that the dissociation constant as applied to electrolytes has the form: $K_{\text{diss.}} = k_2/k_1$, as in the example:

$$\text{HCO}_3^- + \text{H}^+ \underset{k_2}{\overset{k_1}{\rightleftharpoons}} \text{H}_2\text{CO}_3$$

In this case, $K_{\text{diss.}}$ is a measure of the tendency of the acid to yield H^+, and the higher the value of $K_{\text{diss.}}$, the stronger the acid. The Michaelis constant, K_m, is a dissociation constant, but the drug affinity constant, $K_{\text{aff.}}$, is the reciprocal of a dissociation constant.

The formation of the drug-receptor complex is only the first step towards producing a pharmacological effect. The next step can be represented as:

Drug-receptor complex $\longrightarrow$ Pharmacological response (R)

* On a confusing point of terminology, some texts use the symbol K_s instead of K_m, and the constant is sometimes called the Michaelis–Menten constant.

Similarly, the enzyme–substrate complex is only the first step towards the over-all reaction:

$$\text{Enzyme-substrate complex} \longrightarrow \text{Enzyme} + \text{End product}$$

The reaction velocity (v) for the decomposition of the enzyme complex to yield the end-product of the reaction is proportional to the concentration of the complex (p). Hence, $p \xrightarrow{k'} e + \text{end-product}$, and

$$v = pk' \tag{18.7}$$

When there is a large excess of substrate the enzyme will be fully saturated; that is, $e = p$. The reaction velocity then attains its maximum value (V). This can be written as

$$V = ek' \tag{18.8}$$

Dividing equation (7) by (8),

$$\frac{v}{V} = \frac{p}{e} \tag{18.9}$$

Rearranging equation (6) and substituting,

$$\frac{s}{K_m + s} = \frac{v}{V} \tag{18.10}$$

Hence,

$$v = \frac{sV}{s + K_m} \tag{18.11}$$

This equation predicts that the rate of formation of the end-product is a rectangular hyperbola (Fig. 18.1) and the value of K_m can be read off from the point corresponding to 50% of the maximum velocity. This can be understood if $V/2$ is substituted for v in equation (11).

Equation (11) can be rearranged, thus:

$$\frac{1}{v} = \frac{1}{V} + \frac{K_m}{V} \times \frac{1}{s} \tag{18.12}$$

The graph of $1/v$ against $1/s$ gives a straight line (Fig. 18.2). The intercept of the line on the $1/s$ axis (when $1/v = 0$) gives the value of $-1/K_m$ (hence K_m) and is independent of the enzyme concentration. The intercept on the $1/v$ axis (when $1/s = 0$) gives the value of $1/V$; this varies with enzyme concentration. This useful procedure was first used by Lineweaver and Burk in 1934, and graphs such as that of Fig. 18.2 are often called Lineweaver–Burk plots. Graphs obtained experimentally agree with the predictions expressed in Figs. 18.1 and 18.2. Furthermore, the maximal velocity which can be obtained is directly proportional to the concentration of the enzyme (which follows

15*

from equation (8)). This experimental verification is strong evidence for the truth of the initial assumptions. The consequences which arise from the dissolution of the enzyme–substrate complex are the liberation of the enzyme and the formation of the end-products of the catalysed reaction. The concentration of an end-product can usually be measured without undue difficulty.

The situation is not so straightforward in the case of drug-receptor combinations. The consequence of the formation of the complex is a response, and this

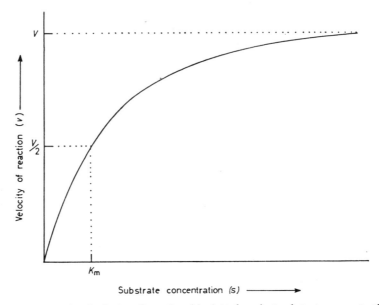

Fig. 18.1. Graph of velocity of reaction (v) plotted against substrate concentration (s) gives a hyperbolic curve which approaches the maximal velocity (V) asymptotically. The value of the Michaelis constant, K_m, can be read off the abscissa at the point corresponding to half the maximal velocity, $V/2$.

can be measured. However, the exact sequence of events between the formation of the drug-receptor complex and the observed effect are not known. Consider, for example, the contraction of smooth muscle produced by acetylcholine in an isolated segment of intestine. The first detectable effect is depolarization of the membrane, which can be recorded in a single cell (see page 223), but has not been used so far for quantitative work on drug kinetics. Next, the contractile protein of the cell is activated. The mechanisms which couple excitation of the membrane with contraction are not completely understood; indeed there is some doubt whether these are necessarily related as cause is to effect. The system by which a mechanical change in a smooth muscle cell is transmitted through the tissue introduces another element of uncertainty. Finally, the response of the tissue can be determined either as a shortening (if recorded *isotonically*), an increase in force (if recorded *isometrically*), or by a method in which the restoring force increases in proportion to the extent of shortening (i.e. recorded *auxotonically*): the relationship between the concentration of drug and response depends, in part, on which method of recording is used. These methods are shown diagrammatically in Fig. 18.3.

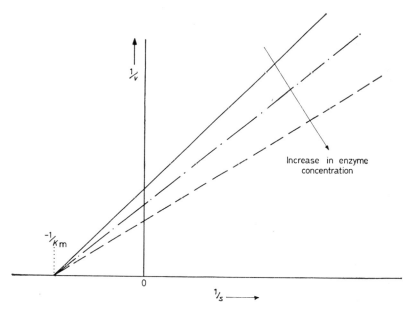

FIG. 18.2. Lineweaver–Burk plot of the reciprocal of the reaction velocity $(1/v)$ against the reciprocal of the substrate concentrations $(1/s)$. The intercept with the abscissa gives the value of $-1/K_m$, and is independent of the enzyme concentration. The intercept with the ordinate gives the reciprocal of the maximal velocity $(1/V)$ of the reaction.

A drug which produces a response of a tissue is termed an *agonist*: in smooth muscle, the response may be a contraction or a relaxation.

The difficulties in relating precisely the measured effect of an agonistic drug to its concentration introduce an element of uncertainty in using experimental results as a check on the assumptions made in the theoretical treatment. There are two main theories of drug action, but so far there have been insufficient experimental observations to enable one (or both) to be discarded, or substantiated. The older theory holds that the response depends on the proportion of receptors occupied, and is generally known as the *occupation theory*. It was first proposed by A. J. Clark about 30 years ago and has been modified more recently by Stephenson and by Ariens. The other theory, introduced by Paton, starts with the assumption that the response depends on the rate of combination of the drug with its receptors, and is known as the *rate theory*.

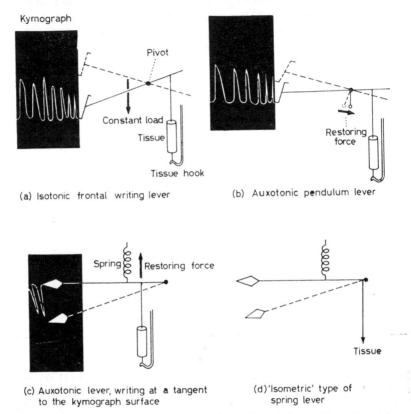

(a) Isotonic frontal writing lever

(b) Auxotonic pendulum lever

(c) Auxotonic lever, writing at a tangent to the kymograph surface

(d) 'Isometric' type of spring lever

FIG. 18.3. Methods of recording effects of drugs. Dotted lines indicate the position of the lever when the tissue is contracted. In the 'isometric' method illustrated in (d), a powerful spring is used and the small contraction is amplified by the lever: more commonly, a strain gauge is used and the increased tension produces an electrical change which can be amplified.

Response dependent on occupation of receptor

The relationship between agonist concentration (D) and the proportion of receptors occupied (r) in equation (4) was:

$$DK_{aff.} = r/(1-r)$$

If the response is proportional to r, then the graph of response against drug concentration will be a hyperbola (Fig. 18.4a). The graph of response against the logarithm of the dose is a sigmoid curve as shown in Fig. 18.4b. If it is assumed that the response is equal to the proportion of the receptors occupied (r), then half the maximal response will be produced when half the receptors are occupied; that is, $r/(1-r)=1$, and $K_{aff.}=1/D_{50\%}$ ($D_{50\%}$ is a convenient symbol for the dose producing 50% of the maximal response). This would provide a simple means of evaluating the affinity constants of drugs, since the value of $1/K_{aff.}$ can be read off from the dose-response curve as shown in Fig. 18.4. However, there is some reserve about accepting the assumption that the response is simply equal to the percentage of receptors occupied.

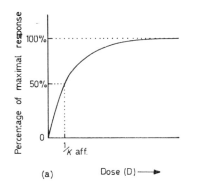 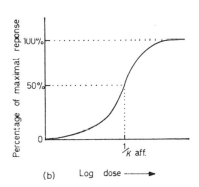

FIG. 18.4. Dose-response curves predicted by the occupation theory of drug action, assuming that the response is equal to the proportion of receptors occupied by the agonist.

Theoretical log dose-response curves have been drawn in Fig. 18.5 assuming three different values for the affinity constants so that the curves are displaced, but have the same form. It can be seen that the central portion of the sigmoid curve, corresponding to responses ranging from 20 to 80% of maximal, is approximately a straight line. Experimentally, it is found that a graph of response against log dose yields a straight line, within the limits of error of observation. Furthermore, it is observed that the log dose-response lines for different agonists are parallel provided that the agonists do not differ too much in potency.

Two drugs which act on the same receptor and are each capable of causing the same maximal response, but which differ in their affinity for the receptor, would have additive effects. Experimentally, this has been found for some pairs of agonists, for example, acetylcholine and tetramethylammonium. However, some weak agonists do not produce the same maximal response as a powerful agonist, and when given together with a powerful agonist the effects are less than additive, even though both agonists act on the same receptor. In order to explain this finding, another concept has been introduced: the response does not depend solely on the proportion of receptors occupied, but also on another property of the agonist which determines the effectiveness of the receptor complex in causing a response. This property is termed *intrinsic activity* (by Ariens) or *efficacy* (by Stephenson).

The assumption made about intrinsic activity (α) is that response $= r\alpha$. The maximal response is obtained for a drug-receptor complex when $\alpha = 1$ and $r = 1$; that is, all the receptors are occupied by an active agonist. Another agonist which acts on the same receptor, but which does not produce the same

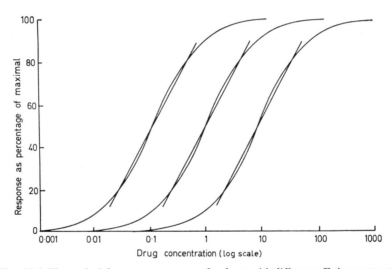

FIG. 18.5. Theoretical dose-response curves for drugs with different affinity constants.

maximal response is known as a 'dualist', and α for it is less than unity. A 'dualist' produces a response, but reduces the response to a more active agonist, i.e. it may behave as an agonist or as an antagonist. The value of α can be obtained by comparing the maximal response produced by a dualist with the maximal response caused by a highly active agonist acting on the same receptor; thus,

$$\alpha \text{ of dualist} = \frac{\text{maximal response to dualist}}{\text{maximal response to agonist with } \alpha = 1}$$

This fraction can be determined experimentally and α evaluated, as shown in Fig. 18.6.

The assumption made about efficacy (**e**) is that the product of affinity and efficacy gives the biological stimulus, S. Thus, $S=er$, and S can have any positive value. The relationship between S and the response is arbitrarily defined such that $S=1$ when the response is 50% of the maximal response with a highly active agonist. It follows from this that, if e is a high number, then the maximal response will be obtained when r is less than unity. That is, not all of the receptors are occupied. The receptors remaining unoccupied are termed *spare receptors*. Drugs that produce less than the maximal response which can be evoked from complete occupation of a given set of receptors by an active agonist are termed *partial agonists*. When a partial agonist is used in a concentration giving its maximal effect, all the receptors are occupied ($r=1$). If

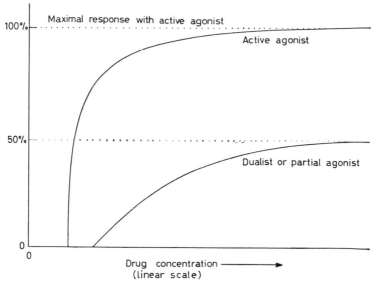

FIG. 18.6. Dose-response curves for active agonist and dualist or partial agonist. In this example, the maximal response to the weak agonist is 50% of that to the active agonist. The value of intrinsic activity, α, is 0·5. The value of efficacy, e, is 1 (see text).

the maximum is 50% of the absolute maximum obtainable with an active agonist (i.e., when by definition $S=1$), then $e=1$. From equation (4) and $S=er$

$$S = \frac{eDK_{aff.}}{1+DK_{aff.}}$$

For an active agonist, D is a small number, and $1+DK_{aff.} \rightarrow 1$, hence $S \rightarrow eDK_{aff.}$. It follows from this that the affinity constant cannot be determined from the concentration of agonist producing 50% of the maximal response. However, there is a way out of this difficulty for a partial agonist.

Assume that an active agonist with efficacy e and affinity K produces a response R in a concentration D, and that this response is matched by concentration P of a partial agonist having an efficacy of e' (Fig. 18.7). Further, assume that concentration D' of the active agonist produces response R', and that this is matched by a combination of concentration P of the partial agonist plus concentration D'' of the active agonist. Responses R are produced by the biological stimulus S; in the case of the partial agonists, $S=e'\,r'$, where r' is the fraction of the receptors occupied by the concentration of partial agonist, and for the active agonist, $S=eKD$. Responses R' are produced by the

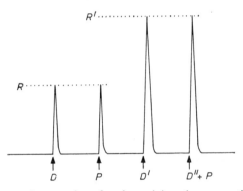

FIG. 18.7. Stephenson's procedure for determining the proportion of receptors occupied by a partial agonist in a concentration, P. R and R' are responses (contraction of a tissue). D, D' and D'' are concentrations of an active agonist (see text). [After Barlow.]

biological stimulus S'; for the active agonist, $S'=eKD'$, and for the partial agonist plus the active agonist, $S'=e'r'-eKD''(1-r')$. Combining these equations, $r'=1-(D+D')/D''$. If this procedure is repeated using different concentrations of the partial agonist, the concentration which produces 50% occupation of the receptors $(r'=0\cdot5)$ can be determined. The affinity constant of a partial agonist determined by this method is lower than that obtained by the relationship $K_{\text{aff.}}=1/D_{50\%}$. This finding constitutes an experimental verification of the concept of spare receptors.

Response dependent on rate of combination with receptors

According to Paton's rate theory of drug action, an active agonist combines with the receptor, but the complex rapidly breaks down to free the receptor, thereby allowing new combinations to form. The pharmacological response is proportional to the rate of formation of such combinations.

Taking the reaction considered previously:

$$\text{Drug} + \text{Receptor} \underset{k_2}{\overset{k_1}{\rightleftharpoons}} \text{Complex} \longrightarrow \text{Response}$$

In rate theory, the response is assumed to be directly proportional to the rate of association (Z) of the complex. At equilibrium, the rates of association and dissociation are equal, therefore,

$$Z = k_1(1-r)\,D \qquad (18.13)$$

and,

$$Z = k_2 r \qquad (18.14)$$

The proportion of receptors occupied is given by rearranging equation (4):

$$r = \frac{D}{D + k_2/k_1} \qquad (18.15)$$

Substituting for r between equations (14) and (15):

$$Z = \frac{Dk_2}{D + k_2/k_1} \qquad (18.16)$$

This equation predicts that the maximal response which is obtained when a high concentration of a drug is used is directly proportional to k_2, the dissociation rate constant. In other words, drugs which dissociate slowly are less effective in producing a response. The relationship between dose and response determined experimentally has the form predicted by equation (16), provided an auxotonic lever (Fig. 18.3) is used for recording the responses. Paton developed further equations from which theoretical predictions were made as to the relationship between response and time. The response predicted from rate theory is quite different in form from that predicted by occupation theory, as shown in Fig. 18.8. If one or the other response were observed in actual experiments, this would be strong evidence for the validity of the theory which predicted the response. In fact, responses resembling both types have been observed. The particular form of the response depends, in practice, on the tissue used and the way in which the response is recorded. One difficulty in the way of experimental verification of rate theory is that the drug concentration refers to drug in the biophase, and the time lag due to diffusion of the drug in or out of the biophase is a limiting factor. The initial assumption of rate theory, that the response is proportional to the rate of formation of drug-receptor combinations, can be modified to include a concept analogous to spare receptors: this is, 'that a maximum response can be obtained by a submaximal rate of combination with the receptors'. Paton also suggested an alternative view, which covers the situation for both rate and occupation theories, when the maximal response is obtained with less than the maximum possible receptor stimulation: 'that the tissue is incapable of responding to more than a limited degree of chemical excitation, and that signs of this incapacity are already present with quite low doses of agonist'.

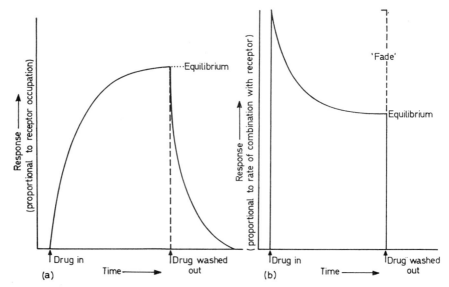

FIG. 18.8. Predicted forms of response based on (*a*) occupation theory, and (*b*) rate theory. According to occupation theory, the response rises exponentially with time to an equilibrium, and on washing out the drug the response decays exponentially. According to rate theory, the peak response is obtained instantaneously then fades to an equilibrium level, and on removing the drug the excitation ceases immediately. Records like those in (*b*) have been obtained experimentally with weak agonists acting on the guinea-pig isolated ileum with the responses recorded with an auxotonic lever. (It should be pointed out that a rather similar effect may be produced by strong agonists, but the explanation in this case is that the tissue is desensitized.)

Antagonism of drug action

An antagonist drug is one which prevents the action of an agonist. The agonist may be a substance which is playing a physiological role, like acetylcholine, or it may be an administered drug. The term antidote is often used in the latter connection, with the implication that the agonist is a poisonous substance or a drug given in an overdose.

There are three main categories of drug antagonism; chemical, physiological and pharmacological: in addition, there are a number of effects, which may be considered as drug antagonisms, but which do not fall within these categories.

Pharmacological antagonism. A pharmacological antagonist is one which abolishes or reduces the effect of an agonist by impairing the formation of the agonist-receptor complex. There are several ways in which antagonists may exert this action. If they combine with the receptor in much the same way as does the agonist, but the formation of the antagonist-receptor complex is weak or ineffective in promoting a response, they are termed *competitive antagonists*. One test for a competitive antagonism is that an increased concentration of agonist can break through the blockade. The blockade produced by a competitive antagonist is reversible, although usually slowly, as the antagonist-receptor complex dissociates slowly. Similarly, there are competitive inhibitors of enzymes which combine with the active centre but do not then proceed to a further reaction, or do so only slowly. Some antagonists act competitively at first, and then they undergo a chemical change which results in the receptor being altered irreversibly (e.g. dibenamine, see page 762). There are enzyme inhibitors which act similarly (e.g. organophosphates, see page 717). There are many instances of *non-competitive antagonism*, the most familiar example being the antagonism of the action of acetylcholine at the neuromuscular junction by depolarizing drugs such as decamethonium and suxamethonium (see pages 669–673).

Physiological antagonism. The response to a drug can be diminished or abolished by using another drug which has the reverse effect. For example, the contraction of isolated intestine or uterus produced by acetylcholine or histamine can be counteracted by adrenaline; in fact, this phenomenon is the basis of a very sensitive bioassay for adrenaline (de Jalon's method). Similarly, a fall in blood pressure to a dangerous level produced by a drug, as a result of overdosage, idiosyncracy, or poisoning, can be counteracted by giving another drug which elevates the blood pressure. Again, a severe depression of the respiratory centre caused by a drug (e.g. barbiturates, morphine-like drugs) can be treated with a respiratory stimulant drug (e.g. nikethamide).

Chemical antagonism. The biological activity of drugs can be considerably reduced or abolished by induction of a chemical change in the drug molecule. A simple illustration is provided by the emergency treatment of injury produced by corrosive chemicals, the action of the antidotes being to render the injurious agent less corrosive. Thus, a weak acid like acetic acid may be used for counteracting the action of corrosive alkalis (vinegar is used domestically), and sodium bicarbonate may be used to counteract acids. Phosphorus burns of the skin are treated by washing with weak copper sulphate solution, which forms copper phosphide with any remaining phosphorus. Weak solutions of potassium permanganate may be used in the treatment of poisoning with morphine, strychnine, aconitine and picrotoxin, any of these alkaloids remaining in the stomach being oxidized. Permanganate is ineffective against atropine or cocaine. Strong solutions of potassium permanganate solution taken by mouth cause severe damage and may be lethal. Crystals of potassium permanganate are applied topically as a remedy against snake bite; the wound is first deeply scarified to expose the venom.

Poisoning with heavy metals is treated by forming relatively non-toxic complexes of the metal with *dimercaprol* (BAL) or with *calcium ethylene-diaminetetra-acetate.*

Dimercaprol was developed by British scientists as a protection against the arsenical war gas, lewisite (Cl—CH:CH—AsCl$_2$), hence the abbreviation

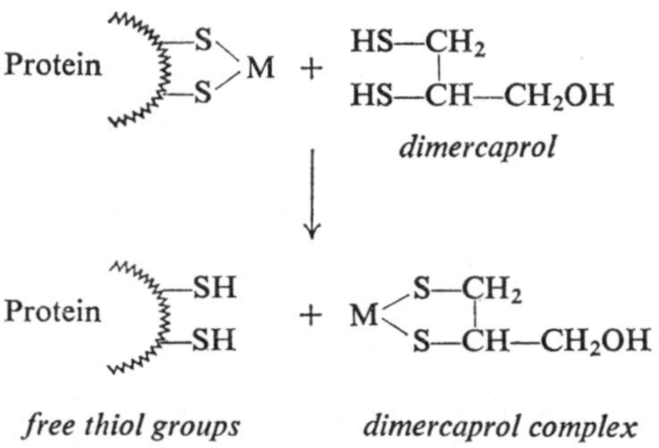

free thiol groups   *dimercaprol complex*

FIG. 18.9. The effect of dimercaprol (BAL) in removing a metal (=M) from its attachment to the sulphydryl groups of a protein. Dimercaprol is used in treating poisoning with arsenic, mercury, gold, tellurium, thallium or bismuth (it is *ineffective* in lead poisoning).

BAL from the initial letters of British Anti-Lewisite. Arsenic itself, and arsenic released in the body from organic compounds, combines with the free thiol (—SH) groups of proteins and this results in inactivation of certain enzymes (including some of the enzymes involved in the essential tricarboxylic acid cycle). The two thiol groups of dimercaprol, having a stronger affinity for the arsenic, capture it from the enzyme and the complex is excreted. The reactions are given in Fig. 18.9.

Ethylenediaminetetra-acetate, otherwise known as EDTA, edetate or versenate, is a chelating agent; that is, it incorporates a heavy metal ion into a ring structure with bonds, which, being partly covalent, are stronger than ionic bonds (Fig. 18.10). Sodium edetate forms a chelate complex with calcium. In order to avoid the loss of calcium from the tissues, sodium calcium-edetate is used. Metals that are more avidly bound into the complex replace the calcium. The strength of the complex formed with various metals is, in increasing order: calcium, magnesium; manganese; iron (Fe^{++}), cadmium;

cobalt, zinc; nickel; lead; copper (Cu++); mercury. Calcium edetate is particularly effective in treating lead poisoning, since lead is bound less firmly in the tissues than is iron, copper, cobalt or mercury. Some radioactive metals can be eliminated by exchange with calcium in the complex, including the radio-isotopes of calcium itself, strontium, radium, cobalt and yttrium, and the very toxic trans-uranic element, plutonium. A further example of a chemical

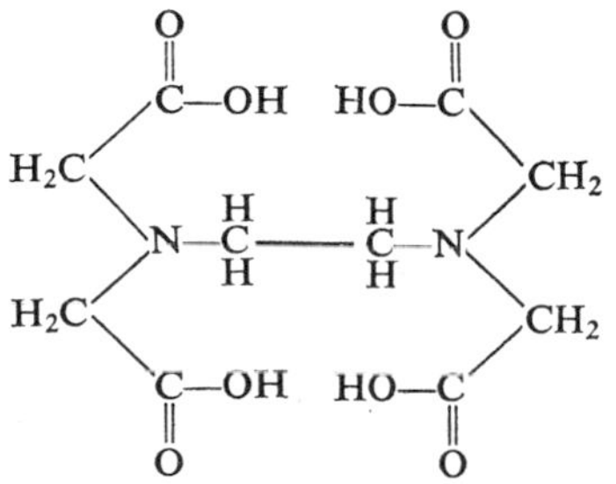

Ethylenediamine tetra-acetic acid

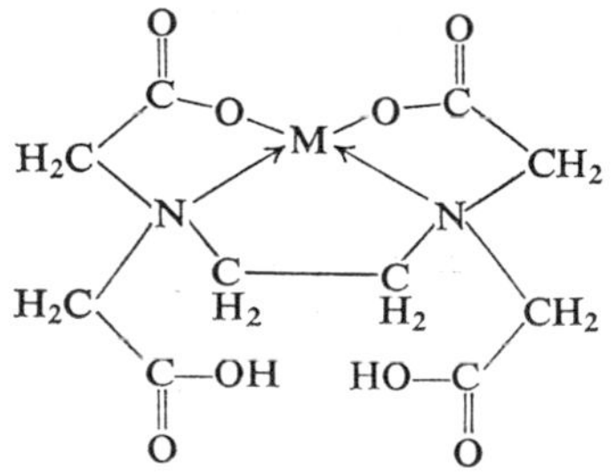

chelate complex

FIG. 18.10. (a) The sodium salt of the acid is known as sodium edetate, versenate or sequestrene. (b) The chelate complex formed with a metal (M). The disodium salt of calciumedetate is usually used in treating metal poisoning, the calcium in the complex being replaced by the heavier metal.

antagonism of a drug effect is provided by pyridine-2-aldoxime methiodide. This substance removes the phosphoryl group which has been attached to the active centre of cholinesterase by the irreversible organo-phosphorus inhibitors, and thereby re-activates the enzyme (details are given on page 717).

Other types of antagonism. Treatment of poisoning includes the use of emetic, cathartic or emollient drugs (each in appropriate circumstances depending on the poison ingested): these measures are intended to prevent any further absorption and are only effective against that portion of the poison not already absorbed. Diuretics help to eliminate bromide from the body in cases of brominism. There is a miscellaneous group of drugs, including local anaesthetics and quinine-like drugs, which depress the responsiveness of tissues to many agonists. They probably act on the cell membrane, making it less permeable, and hence less excitable. Drugs which have a specific action in blocking a particular receptor in low concentrations may act unspecifically in large concentrations to antagonize the actions of a variety of agonists.

The kinetics of competitive antagonism

It is convenient to deal firstly with the kinetics of competitive inhibition of enzyme activity before considering drug antagonism.

Enzyme inhibition. The formation of the inhibitor-enzyme complex may be represented as

$$\text{Inhibitor} + \text{Enzyme} \underset{k_4}{\overset{k_3}{\rightleftharpoons}} \text{Complex}$$

At equilibrium,

$$K_i = \frac{k_4}{k_3} = \frac{i(e-q)}{q}$$

where K_i is the dissociation constant for the inhibitor-enzyme complex, $i =$ concentration of inhibitor, and $q =$ concentration of enzyme combined with inhibitor (cf. equation (6)). Considering the case when substrate and inhibitor are both present:

$$\text{Substrate} + \text{Inhibitor} + \text{Enzyme} \rightleftharpoons \text{Substrate-complex} + \text{Inhibitor-complex}$$
$$\downarrow$$
$$\text{End-product}$$

The amount of free enzyme is $e-p-q$, since some is incorporated into each of the complexes. At equilibrium,

$$K_m = \frac{s(e-p-q)}{p} \tag{18.18}$$

and

$$K_i = \frac{i(e-p-q)}{q} \tag{18.19}$$

The unknown quantity, q, can be eliminated by the following steps. Rearranging equations (18) and (19):

$$p = s(e-p-q).\frac{1}{K_m}$$

$$q = i(e-p-q).\frac{1}{K_i}$$

Eliminating $(e-p-q)$ and rearranging:

$$q = ipK_m/sK_i \qquad (18.20)$$

But, from equation (19)

$$q = i(e-p)/(i+K_i)$$

Eliminating q and rearranging

$$es = pK_m(1+i/K_i)+sp \qquad (18.21)$$

Since the ratio of the reaction velocity to the maximal reaction velocity (v/V) is equal to p/e (see derivation of equation (18.9));

$$\frac{V}{v} = \frac{e}{p} = \frac{K_m(1+i/K_i)}{s}+1$$

Hence,

$$\frac{1}{v} = \frac{1}{s}\frac{K_m(1+i/K_i)}{V}+\frac{1}{V} \qquad (18.22)$$

When $i=0$, equation (22) becomes identical with equation (12). The graph of $1/v$ against $1/s$ is a straight line for the reaction in the presence of the inhibitor (Fig. 18.11a), just as it was in the absence of inhibitor. The maximum velocity of reaction obtainable in the presence of the inhibitor is the same as in its absence, which follows from the nature of a competitive inhibition given a sufficiently high concentration of substrate. The slope of the line of the inhibited reaction is steeper, the difference in slope being proportional to the inhibitor concentration. The intercept on the abscissa $(1/v=0)$ is $-1/K_m$ in the absence of inhibitor and $-1/[K_m+(1+i/K_i)]$ in its presence.

More useful information can be obtained by plotting $1/v$ against i (Fig. 18.11b), which is also a straight line with the following equation (rearranging equation (22)):

$$\frac{1}{v} = \frac{1}{V}\left(1+\frac{K_m}{s}\right)+i\left(\frac{K_m}{sK_i}\right) \qquad (18.23)$$

If the substrate concentration is changed, the slope changes and the intercept on the $1/v$ axis $(i=0)$ changes, but if the lines are extrapolated they intersect at a point corresponding with the value of $-K_i$ on the abscissa (i axis) and $1/V$ on the ordinate ($1/v$ axis).

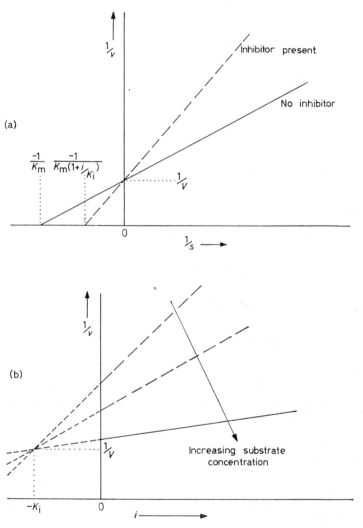

FIG. 18.11. Competitive enzyme inhibition. (a) Lineweaver–Burk plot (compare Fig. 18.2). The maximum obtainable velocity, $1/V$, is the same whether the inhibitor is present or not. (b) Plots of $1/v$ against inhibitor concentration, using 3 different concentrations of substrates. In the case of competitive inhibition, the extrapolated portions of the lines intersect at the same point, corresponding to $-K_i$ on the abscissa and $1/V$ on the ordinate.

In the case of *non-competitive inhibition,* it is assumed that the inhibitor combines equally well with the free enzyme or the substrate-enzyme complex, and in either case it inhibits the reaction. An equation corresponding to equation (22) may be derived:

$$\frac{1}{v} = \frac{1}{V}(1 = K_m/s)(1 = i/K_i) \qquad (18.24)$$

Graphs of the relationship between $1/v$ and $1/s$, and $1/v$ and i, are shown in

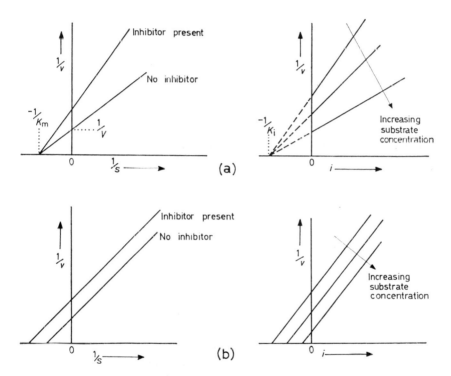

Fig. 18.12. (a) Non-competitive enzyme inhibition. (b) Uncompetitive enzyme inhibition. Compare with Fig. 18.11.

Fig. 18.12a. In non-competitive inhibition the value of K_m is not affected by changing the inhibitor concentration (since this is independent of the enzyme concentration), but the value of $1/V$ is changed (since this is proportional to the enzyme concentration).

A third type of inhibition, termed *uncompetitive,* arises when the inhibitor combines only with the substrate-enzyme complex. The following equation can be derived:

$$\frac{1}{v} = \frac{K_m}{sV} + \frac{1}{V}(1+i/K_i) \tag{18.25}$$

The graphs of the usual relationships are shown in Fig. 18.12b.

Examples are known of all three types of enzyme inhibition, the last being the least common.

Pharmacological antagonism. The reactions to be considered may be written

Agonist + Antagonist + Receptor $\rightleftharpoons$ Agonist–receptor + Antagonist–receptor
                                                   complex   complex

$\downarrow$

Response

The kinetic treatment of this for a competitive antagonist is carried out in a similar way as for a competitive enzyme inhibitor. The affinity constant of the agonist is

$$K_D = \frac{r}{D(1-r-u)} \tag{18.26}$$

and of the antagonist

$$K_G = \frac{u}{G(1-r-u)} \tag{18.27}$$

where u is the proportion of receptors occupied by the antagonist, and G = antagonist concentration. Eliminating u and rearranging gives

$$DK_D = \frac{r}{1-r}(1+GK_G) \tag{18.28}$$

Compare equation (28) with equation (4); the two equations are identical when the concentration of antagonist, G, is zero. A family of curves expressing the relationship between agonist concentration (D) and proportion of receptor occupied by agonist (r) in the presence of increasing concentrations of antagonist (G) is shown in Fig. 18.13. The linear portions of the theoretical dose-response curves are parallel, and this is in good agreement with the experimental finding that the log dose-response lines are displaced to the right by competitive antagonists, but remain parallel to the original line over a considerable range of concentrations of antagonists. However, it should be pointed out that such a parallel displacement of the line is not in itself sufficient to prove that the antagonism is competitive.

The theoretical prediction of log dose-response curves for non-competitive antagonists is a family of curves that are shallower (not parallel) with increasing concentrations of antagonist and that do not reach the maximal response

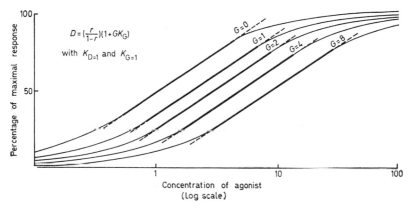

FIG. 18.13. Theoretical curves of response (assuming response = proportion of receptor occupied, r) against dose of agonist (D) in the presence of increasing concentration of antagonist, G.

produced by the agonist in the absence of inhibitor. Experimentally, it has been observed that low concentrations of a non-competitive antagonist may cause a parallel displacement of the log dose-response line, and the shallower

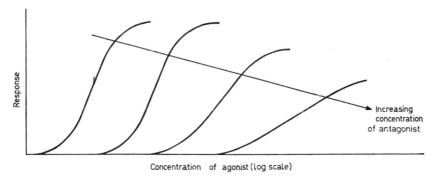

FIG. 18.14. Log dose-response curves in the presence of a non-competitive antagonist.

curves are obtained only with higher concentrations of the antagonist (Fig. 18.14). This result can be explained by the presence of spare receptors. The antagonism behaves as though it were competitive until all the spare receptors have been blocked by the non-competitive antagonist.

The value of K_G, the affinity constant of a competitive antagonist, can be determined in the following way. If the response produced by concentration D of an agonist is equal to that produced by concentration D' in the presence of an antagonist (concentration G), then, from equations (4) and (28),

$$DK_D = \frac{D'K_D}{1+GK_G}$$

which can be rearranged to

$$D'/D = 1+GK_G \tag{18.29}$$

When the concentration of antagonist is such that D' is twice D,

$$K_G = 1/G$$

This procedure for evaluating the affinity constant of an antagonist involves no assumption about the relationship of the response to the proportion of receptors occupied, since the responses are equal, and it is independent of the particular agonist used, provided only that the antagonist competes with it for the receptor.

Schild devised a scale for comparing the potency of antagonists in which the negative logarithm of the concentration of antagonist was taken, i.e. $1/[\log \text{antagonist}_x]$, where x refers to the ratio of equi-effective doses of agonists before, and in the presence of, the antagonist; he expressed this as pA_x. If the concentration of antagonist is such that twice the dose of agonist is required to reproduce the original response, then the negative logarithm of this concentration is the pA_2 value. It has become a common practice to determine the pA_2 or the pA_{10} value for antagonists. Table 18.2 gives some examples of pA values. A high specificity of antagonism is indicated by a high value (i.e. a small concentration of antagonist is effective). The pA_{10} value is less than the pA_2 value, as a higher concentration is necessary to produce the greater degree of antagonistic effect. Rather similar values are obtained for the same agonist–antagonist combination in a variety of tissues, suggesting that the receptors are similar. Low pA_2 values are obtained when the antagonism is unspecific, as for example, when antihistamine drugs are tested against acetylcholine, when atropine is tested against histamine, for the antagonism by atropine of the action of acetylcholine on frog rectus, and with the antagonisms of either histamine or acetylcholine by cinchonidine, cinchocaine or pethidine.

As pointed out before, when $x=2$, that is when $D'/D=2$, $K_G=1/G$; hence, $pA_2=\log K_G$, or, the affinity constant of the antagonist is antilog pA_2. Determinations of both pA_2 and pA_{10} have been used to provide a method for testing

TABLE 18.2. Comparison of pA_x values.

Isolated tissue	Antagonist	Agonist			
		Acetylcholine		Histamine	
		pA_2	pA_{10}	pA_2	pA_{10}
Guinea-pig ileum	Atropine	8·8	8·1	5·6	4·6
	Mepyramine	4·9		9·4	8·4
	Promethazine	7·7		9·2	
	Diphenhydramine	6·6		8·0	7·0
	Antazoline	5·5		7·7	
	Pethidine	5·9		6·1	5·0
	Cinchonidine	4·9			
	Cinchocaine			5·6	
Rat intestine	Atropine		8·1		
Guinea-pig trachea	Mepyramine			9·1	
	Diphenhydramine			7·8	
Guinea-pig perfused lung	Atropine	8·8	7·6	5·9	5·0
	Mepyramine			9·4	8·4
	Diphenhydramine			7·8	6·9
	Pethidine			6·2	5·1
Human bronchi	Mepyramine			9·3	
Chick amnion	Atropine	8·8			
Frog auricle	Atropine		8·3		
Frog rectus	Atropine		4·2		

[From Arunlakshana and Schild (1959), *Brit. J. Pharmacol*, **14**, 48, and Reuse (1948) *Ibid*, 3, 174].

whether an antagonism is competitive or not. The theoretical reasoning is as follows. In determining pA_{10},

$$D'/D = 10 \quad \text{and} \quad D'/D = 1 + G_{10} K_G \quad \text{(from equation (29))}$$

Hence, $\quad\quad\quad\quad G_{10} K_G = 9 \quad \text{and} \quad 1/G_{10} = K_G/9$

Taking logarithms, $pA_{10} = \log K_G - \log 9$, but $\log K_G = pA_2$

Therefore $\quad\quad\quad\quad pA_2 - pA_{10} = \log 9 = 0\cdot95.$

If the value of 0·95 is found, this is compatible with the antagonism in question being competitive, and figures in good agreement with this have been found experimentally (see Table 18.2).

A further procedure for examining the mode of action of an antagonist is given by rearranging equation (29) to

$$D'/D - 1 = K_G G$$

The graph of $\log(D'/D-1)$ against $\log G$ is a straight line if the antagonism is competitive, and when $D'/D=2$, $\log(D'/D-1)=0$, so the intercept on the $\log G$ axis gives the pA_2 value.

In the rate theory of drug action, an antagonist is a drug which dissociates slowly from its combination with the receptor. There are two consequences of this: firstly, it may be expected that an antagonist would have a vestige of a stimulant action, since it must at first combine with receptors; and secondly, an agonist must have some antagonistic activity, at least while it is acting (this is the cause of the 'fade' phenomenon, Fig. 18.7). It is well known that antagonistic drugs are rather persistent in their action, certainly more persistent than agonistic drugs, and the rate theory of drug action explains this fact quite nicely.

Tachyphylaxis and tolerance

Successive applications of the same dose of a powerful agonistic drug, like acetylcholine or histamine, usually produce constant responses (within the limits of biological variation), provided the drug is thoroughly washed out each time and a sufficiently long interval is allowed between doses to enable the tissue to recover from the response. However, with some drugs, the responses get smaller: this phenomenon is known as *tachyphylaxis*. The derivation of the word (from the Greek: *takhus* = quick, and *phulakterion* = a protection) suggests that the drug protects against, i.e., it blocks or antagonizes, its own action. Tachyphylaxis implies a fairly rapid diminution in responses, whereas the word *tolerance* is usually used to describe the more gradual decrease in the effectiveness of a drug given repeatedly over a longer period of time. Although the distinction is arbitrary, these terms are commonly used in different ways, which may be illustrated by reference to nicotine. The action of nicotine on ganglion cells is to stimulate them, and then to block them; there is tachyphylaxis to the stimulant action of nicotine. On the other hand, when a person first starts to smoke he may suffer some ill-effects from the nicotine but after some time he becomes accustomed to smoking; that is, he develops tolerance to nicotine.

The rate theory of drug action provides a simple explanation for the occurrence of tachyphylaxis; in fact it predicts the phenomenon for any agonist when the dissociation from the receptor is at a sufficiently slow rate that some receptors are still occupied and not free to engage in new combinations when the dose of the agonist is repeated. Thus, on rate theory, there is a continuum of types of drugs: agonist, partial agonist, tachyphylactic drug (or 'self-blocking' drug) and antagonist; these differ only in the relative rates at which they dissociate from the receptors.

Tachyphylaxis which is specific to one type of receptor of smooth muscle cells can be obtained with 5-hydroxytryptamine without appreciably affecting the responses to other agonists. It is more difficult to obtain a specific tachyphylaxis with histamine and almost impossible with acetylcholine. When excessively large doses of acetylcholine are used, the tissue certainly becomes less sensitive, but to all agonists: that is, there is a non-specific *desensitization*. This may be due to loss of intracellular potassium through the excited cell membrane, which has an increased permeability to K^+ (see page 78).

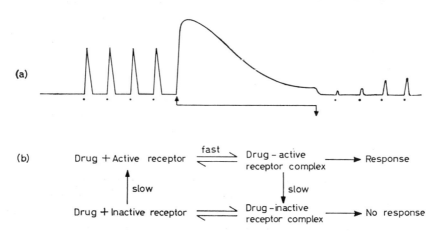

Fig. 18.15. (a) Microelectrode recording from motor endplate. At each dot, a brief test pulse of acetylcholine was applied with a micropipette. At the horizontal line, a continuous application of acetylcholine was given. The endplate depolarization was not maintained despite the continued presence of acetylcholine, and subsequently, the responses to the test pulses of acetylcholine were depressed. (b) Interpretation: the drug-receptor complex induces a response when it is first formed, then it is slowly transformed into an ineffective complex. The active complex formed by doses of acetylcholine applied for brief intervals yield only a small amount of ineffective complex. Large doses and prolonged contact favour the formation of the ineffective complex. The inactive receptor slowly reverts to the active form.

An explanation for desensitization which invokes and elaborates some elements of receptor occupation theory was proposed by Katz and Thesleff. A diagram of their experimental approach and their interpretation of the phenomenon observed is given in Fig. 18.15. They investigated the action of acetylcholine in causing depolarization of the motor endplate of striated muscle, but since this tissue cannot be stimulated by such a variety of agonists as smooth muscle, it is not clear whether their results and interpretations are applicable to tachyphylaxis with drugs acting at other receptors.

A completely different kind of tachyphylaxis is exhibited by some drugs that act indirectly, that is, drugs that owe their pharmacological activity to the release of an active agent within the tissues, rather than to a direct action on the receptors of the effector cells. Notable amongst such drugs are those that liberate histamine or noradrenaline. In fact, the phenomenon of tachyphylaxis was first recorded in connection with a protein-containing sea anemone extract which caused histamine-like effects, including a profound fall of blood pressure after intravenous injection in dogs. If the animals survived the first dose, they were completely unaffected by the second dose. The term, 'quick protection' (tachyphylaxis) distinguished between this effect and the more slowly developing protection (immunity), which involves the formation of antibodies following non-lethal doses of other toxins (e.g. typhoid toxin).* It is now known that the response to sea-anemone extract is largely due to the release of histamine. Tachyphylaxis occurs because the amount of histamine available for release is exhausted, and also because the receptors become desensitized after exposure to a considerable concentration of histamine. Noradrenaline-releasing drugs which exhibit tachyphylaxis to the most marked degree are arylethylamine derivatives with an α-methyl group on the ethyl side-chain (e.g. amphetamine, α-methyltyramine). These α-methyl substituted amines are not substrates for mono-amine oxidase. The corresponding non-methylated compounds (i.e. phenylethylamine, tyramine) exhibit only slight tachyphylaxis, but if mono-amine oxidase is inhibited, they become markedly tachyphylactic. This implies that the degree of tachyphylaxis depends on their persistence in the tissues, and probably their persistence at the storage site of noradrenaline.

Tolerance is the term usually applied to clinically used drugs when larger and larger doses have to be given to produce the desired effect. Important examples of drugs towards which tolerance develops are morphine and its congeners, and many of the ganglion blocking drugs and adrenergic neurone blocking drugs that are used in the treatment of hypertension. There is no satisfactory explanation of tolerance to these drugs, but one possibility is that there is a gradual physiological or biochemical adaptation which counteracts the effect of the drug.

The term *species tolerance* is sometimes used to describe the relative insensitivity of a particular species to a drug. The rabbit is particularly insensitive to atropine, because it has an enzyme, atropinase, which rapidly metabolizes the drug. A rat can survive a dose of a cardiac glycoside which would kill a man; but in this case it is unlikely that the more rapid metabolism in the rat can entirely explain the insensitivity.

Individual tolerance, or the relative insensitivity of some members of one

* On an historical point, the term anaphylaxis ('anti-protection') was introduced at about the same time: this describes sensitization to a substance after giving the first injection.

species to a drug may be simply a reflection of biological variability, the individual in question forming one extreme of the normal population (page 535), or it may be that the population is not homogenous with respect to the trait in question. Some rabbits are decidedly more resistant to atropine than others, and it seems that an inherited genetic factor determines the amount of atropinase. Similarly in man, the activity of blood cholinesterase, hence sensitivity to choline esters and to anti-cholinesterase drugs, is genetically determined. Recently it has been reported that rats are developing tolerance to the rat poison warfarin; this appears to be due to a mutation which obviously has high survival value and may be expected to spread through the rat population if the use of that poison is continued.

Acquired tolerance, or adaptation, to chemotherapeutic drugs has occurred in some pathogenic organisms. The resistance to the bactericidal effect of penicillin is due to secretion of an enzyme which destroys this antibiotic. Some staphylococci secrete a peroxidase which can destroy certain aminoacridines. Another mechanism by which bacteria become resistant is by secreting an antagonist to the chemotherapeutic drug, without actually destroying it. For instance, some staphylococci, pneumococci and gonococci resist the effects of sulphonamide drugs by secreting large quantities of PABA (see page 922). A further example of drug resistance is seen with the microorganism *B. lactis aerogenes*. This organism so alters its metabolism that it can grow in whatever concentration of proflavine it is placed. Hinshelwood suggested that proflavine upsets the metabolism responsible for division. Consequently the organism grows in size until it contains sufficient of the enzymes needed for division.

The development of adaptation to antibacterial agents is important in therapeutics since the resistant strains maintain their resistance in successive generations. The misuse of antibiotics has been responsible for the appearance of many strains which cannot be controlled with chemotherapeutic drugs.

Interaction between drugs

Antagonism of a drug's action is one example of interaction. When the resultant of the interaction is something other than a marked reduction or abolition of the action of one drug, the interaction is sometimes described as *synergism*; however, the term lacks precision. There is a convenient graphical method for expressing the resultant effect produced by the simultaneous action of two drugs. For this, a definite quantitative criterion of the pharmacological effect is chosen; it may, for example, be the contraction of muscle to 50% of the maximum obtainable contraction, or, the production of anaesthesia for a 10 min period in a rat. The doses of each of the two drugs are placed on the

16

axes of a graph, and a particular mixture of the two that produce the defined effect can be plotted as a point on the graph. The line joining a number of such points is called an *isobole*. If a quantitative change is made in the criterion (using the previous examples, contraction to 25% of the maximal, or anaesthesia lasting 5 min), then another isobole can be drawn on the same graph. A family of isoboles can be drawn to express the interactions between a pair of drugs. This procedure was introduced by S. Lowe in 1926; it has not been used extensively, largely because many experiments have to be carried out to construct an isobole, but it is a useful concept. There are three main types of isobole: (i) If the two substances each produce the effect being studied, the

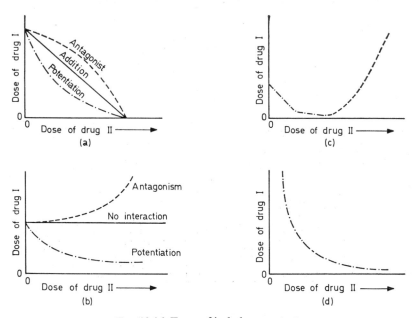

FIG. 18.16. Types of isoboles—see text.

isobole will touch both axes of the graph. Then a simple additive effect is a straight line joining the two points. The form of the isobole varies, depending on the nature of the interaction, as shown in Fig. 18.16a. A mutual enhancement of effects will be shown as an isobole which curves towards the origin; such an enhancement of the effects of one drug by another is termed a *potentiation*. A mutual suppression of the effect results in a curvature in the opposite sense; this is an antagonism, and such an effect is observed in the interaction between an agonist and a partial agonist. (ii) If one of the interacting drugs does not exhibit the effect in question when used alone, but moderates the action of the other drug, then the isobole will touch only one axis. The action of the one drug may be antagonized, potentiated or unaffected by a second drug (Fig. 18.16b). The nature of the interaction may change as the dose of interacting drug is increased. This happens, for example, with some anticholinesterases which potentiate the action of acetylcholine on the heart in low doses, but antagonize it in high doses. Fig. 18.16c illustrates an isobole representing such a phenomenon. (iii) Some pharmacological effects are known in which neither drug, when used alone, produces the particular effect that is seen with a combination of the drugs. An isobole representing this eventuality is illustrated in Fig. 18.16d.

Potentiation of drug action

The effect of one drug in enhancing the response to another may be brought about in a number of ways. Equation (1) (page 455) summarizes some of the factors which operate to divert an administered drug from the receptors. If any of these factors are eliminated, more of the drug reaches the receptors. Drugs which are rapidly metabolized have an enhanced action after inhibition of enzymatic destruction. The inhibition of cholinesterase by physostigmine results in a marked potentiation of acetylcholine and some other choline esters —this is dealt with in detail in Chapter 28. The actions of *some* sympathomimetic amines are potentiated by inhibition of mono amine oxidase or of catechol O-methyl transferase (see page 775). Drugs which are removed from the site where they exert their pharmacologically activity by being bound or taken up in the tissues have an enhanced action if the binding or uptake is prevented. For example, noradrenaline is taken up and bound in adrenergic neurones, and this constitutes the most important mechanism for terminating its action. There is a marked potentiation of the actions of noradrenaline if the uptake or binding mechanisms are impaired (page 774).

The sensitivity to drugs may be greatly altered after denervation of tissues. In the case of adrenergically innervated tissues, the increase in sensitivity after denervation is greatest to noradrenaline, because then uptake and binding is no longer possible and the noradrenaline persists in the vicinity of the receptors for a longer time and in a higher concentration. However, additional mechanisms are involved, since there is an increased sensitivity to acetylcholine and even to potassium. One possibility is that the receptors become more sensitive after prolonged rest. This is suggested by the findings of Emmelin and others that when an antagonist drug is given over a long period of time and is then stopped there is hyperactivity to an appropriate agonist. After denervation of focally innervated striated muscle, the receptors for acetyl-choline are distributed all over the muscle membrane instead of being confined at the site of the original neuromuscular junction. It is not known whether a similar change in the distribution of receptors occurs in autonomically innervated tissues.

The enhancement of drug action by reducing the rate of diffusion away from the site of action or by decreasing the rate of excretion from the body is dealt with in Chapter 19.

CHAPTER 19

Absorption, Distribution, Metabolism and Excretion of Drugs

When a drug is used in therapeutics, it is desirable to know about its rate and extent of absorption, its distribution in the body, and its metabolism and excretion. The physician treating a disease wishes to maintain an effective concentration of the drug at the site where its action is required, and the pharmacist has the task of formulating the drug into the most appropriate preparation for achieving this end. Chemists engaged on the synthesis of new drugs may be able to introduce modifications into the molecular structure of existing drugs that result in favourable changes in absorbability or duration of action.

Absorption of drugs

The principal factors which determine the absorption of a drug into the blood stream are its physico-chemical and pharmacological properties, the way it is formulated, and the site to which it is applied. Table 19.1 summarizes the routes of administration of drugs, together with the membranes which provide the barriers to absorption, and the types of preparations that are used. Drugs may be given with the intention of producing a local action, in which case absorption is a disadvantage. But when they are given to produce a systemic action or an action at a distant site, absorption is an essential first step.

A drug given by subcutaneous or intramuscular injection passes only through the endothelium of the capillaries or lymphatic vessels before entering the blood; these endothelial barriers are the most readily penetrated of all the boundary surfaces concerned in drug absorption. Injection of a drug directly into the blood stream circumvents this barrier. Drugs administered other than by injection must pass first through another barrier consisting of a mucous membrane or epithelium (Table 19.1) and then through the endothelium of the capillaries. There are four ways in which drugs can be absorbed through these membranes.

(1) *Lipid diffusion.* The barriers to the passage of drugs consist largely of lipid material. Drugs dissolve in the lipid phase and diffuse down their concentration gradient to the aqueous phase on the other side of the barrier. Most drugs are absorbed in this way.

485

TABLE 19.1. Site and methods of application of drugs.

Route of administration	Absorbing membrane	Types of preparation
By mouth	Mucous membranes of gastro-intestinal tract	Mixtures (solutions and suspensions), pills, tablets, cachets, capsules, pastilles
Sublingual	Mucous membrane	Lozenges, tablets
Rectal	Mucous membrane	Suppositories, ointments
Colonic	Mucous membrane	Enemas
Urethral	Mucous membrane	Bougies
Vaginal	Mucous membrane	Pessaries
Nasal	Mucous membrane	Drops, snuffs
By inhalation	Mucous membrane of respiratory tract	Aerosols, inhalers
	Epithelium of alveoli	Vapours, gases, smokes
Conjunctival	Mucous membrane of conjunctiva and epithelium of cornea	Drops, lotions, lamellae, ointments
Epidermis	Keratinized epithelium	Ointments, lotions, creams, liniments, pastes, powders
By parenteral injection*		
Subcutaneous Intramuscular	Endothelium of vascular and lymphatic capillaries	Solutions and suspensions, solid implants
Intravenous Intra-arterial Intrathecal	None	Solutions

* The term 'parenteral' means literally 'other than by the gut'; however, the term is often restricted to mean 'by injection'; this usage probably arose as an abbreviation of 'parenteral injection'.

(2) *Aqueous diffusion.* Lipid-insoluble drugs diffuse through the barriers at rates which depend on their molecular weight and their concentration gradient. Aqueous diffusion also contributes to the passage of lipid-soluble drugs of low molecular weight (e.g., ethanol). It is supposed that there are pores or interstices in the lipid material of the membrane that allow aqueous diffusion.

(3) *Active transport.* A few drugs that are chemically related to actively transported nutrients are absorbed by the same mechanism; for example, α-methyldopa is taken up from the gut by an amino acid-transporting mechanism.

(4) *Pinocytosis.* Drugs with large molecular weights, or which exist in solution in molecular aggregates, are probably taken up by pinocytosis.

Properties of drugs concerned in their absorption. The first requirement for absorption is solution in the aqueous phase in contact with the membrane, and the rate of absorption of a drug is proportional to its concentration in the aqueous phase. Insoluble substances are pharmacologically inert. Thus barium sulphate is taken by mouth as a 'meal' to provide an outline of the lumen of the gastro-intestinal tract in X-ray examination; soluble barium salts are absorbed and are extremely toxic. The rate of solution in the aqueous phase is an important factor in governing the rate of absorption, and this can be widely varied by appropriate formulation of the drug

The ability of drugs to be absorbed by lipid diffusion depends on their partition coefficient between the aqueous phase and the lipid phase of the membrane. Experimentally, a lipid material such as olive oil is used to investigate lipid/water partitioning and the aqueous phase is adjusted to a physiological pH (usually 7·4). Oil/water partition coefficients for a number of drugs

TABLE 19.2. Partitioning of drugs in lipid/water and chloroform/water systems (aqueous phase at pH 7·4).

Olive oil/water		Chloroform/water			
Drug	Partition coefficient	Drug	Partition coefficient	Drug	% extraction in chloroform
Sucrose	0·00003	Hexamethonium	0	Adrenaline	< 3
Urea	0·00015	Salicyclic acid	0·2	Dimethyl 5-HT	8
5-HT	0·06	Barbitone	1	Theobromine	11
Ethanol	0·1	Acetanilide	3	Theophylline	12
Phenazone	0·3	Amiphenazole	15	Caffeine	95
Morphine	0·4	Aniline	17	Physostigmine	95
Codeine	0·8	Quinalbarbitone	23	Mepacrine	95
Tryptamine	0·9	Phenazone	28	Caramiphen	95
Amidopyrine	1·3	Amidopyrine	73	SKF 525-A	95
Barbitone	1·4	Thiopentone	102	Pethidine	95
Allobarbitone	2·4			Noramidopyrine	95
Salicylamide	5·9			Ephedrine	95
Phenobarbitone	5·9				

are given in Table 19.2. A reasonable estimate of lipid/water partition coefficients can be obtained from partitioning between lipid solvents (e.g. chloroform or benzene) and water, or even from comparison of relative solubility in these solvents and in water. In general, the higher the partition coefficient, the higher is the affinity for lipid membranes and the more rapid is absorption.

The molecular structure of many drugs contains acidic or basic groups (or both) which may be ionized in aqueous solutions: only the non-ionized molecules are lipid soluble. The ability of such drugs to be absorbed through lipid membranes depends on the proportion of nonionized molecules, and this in turn depends on the pH of the aqueous solution (which is the reason for adjusting the pH in experimental studies on partition coefficients). The degree of ionization of a compound is expressed as its ionization constant. The pK_a is a more convenient expression than the ionization constant itself. For acidic drugs, the equation for ionization is $AH \rightleftharpoons A^- + H^+$: the ionization constant, K_a is $[A^-][H^+]/[AH]$; and $pK_a = -\log K_a$. For basic drugs, the equation is $B + H_2O \rightleftharpoons BH^+ + HO^-$; and the constant K_b equals $[BH^+][HO^-]/[B]$; the pK_a for a basic drug is $14 - pK_b$. The pK_a values of some drugs are given in Fig. 19.1.

The proportion of nonionized molecules of a drug present in the aqueous phase at a given pH can be calculated from the Henderson–Hasselbach equation: for an acid, $\log([\text{nonionized}]/[\text{ionized}]) = pK_a - pH$; and for a base, $\log([\text{nonionized}]/[\text{ionized}]) = pH - pK_a$.

When the pK_a of a drug equals the pH of the aqueous phase at the surface of the lipid membrane, the numbers of ionized and nonionized molecules are equal. The higher the pH, the higher is the ionization of acidic drugs and the lower is the ionization of basic drugs. Figure 19.2 expresses the relationship graphically. When the pK_a of the drug and the pH of the aqueous phase are known, the proportion of nonionized (i.e. lipid soluble) molecules can be read off from the graph. Table 19.3 gives the usual pH ranges encountered in

TABLE 19.3. Usual range of pH of aqueous
phases of absorbing membranes.

Mucous membranes of gastrointestinal tract:

Gastric contents	1·0–3·0
Duodenal contents	4·8–8·2
Jejunal and ileal contents	7·5–8·0
Colonic contents	7·0–7·5

Other mucosal surfaces:

Buccal cavity	6·2–7·2
Urethral mucosa	5·0–7·0
Vaginal contents	3·5–4·2
Conjunctival secretions	7·3–8·0

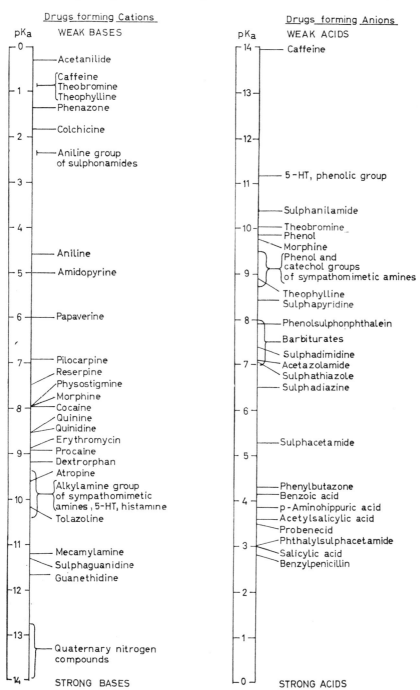

FIG. 19.1. pK$_a$ values of some drugs.

16*

the aqueous phases bathing various absorbing membranes. In the gastro-intestinal tract the pH is determined by three factors; the secretions, the diet, and the bacterial flora. Drugs are sometimes formulated in acidic, basic or buffered preparations in order to increase or retard their absorption.

To recapitulate, the factors determining the rate and degree of absorption of most drugs are (i) the solubility in aqueous media, (ii) the lipid/water

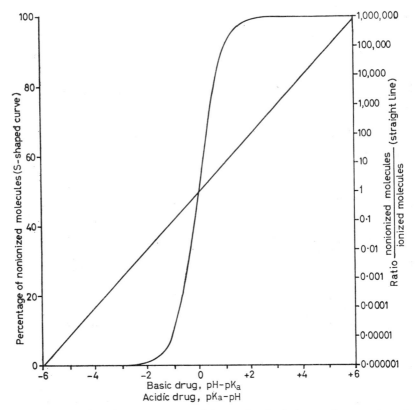

FIG. 19.2. Relationship between pK_a of drug, pH of solution, and proportion of nonionized (lipid soluble) molecules—on the left hand ordinate as the percentage not ionized, and on the right hand ordinate as the ratio of nonionized to ionized molecules.

partition coefficient, and (iii) the degree of ionization. The relative importance of these factors depends on the particular drug, as illustrated by the following examples: (a) Atropine is appreciably basic—the pH of a 1 mM solution is about 10. The pK_a is 9·5, and in the range of physiological pH values, only a small proportion of molecules are nonionized, as can be seen from Fig. 19.2. Nevertheless, it is well absorbed because of the very high lipid solubility of the nonionized molecules (It is 500 times more soluble in chloroform than in water.) (*b*) Quaternary ammonium compounds are very highly ionized. They are sometines referred to as 'permanent cations', but their ionization may be suppressed by raising the pH, as follows:

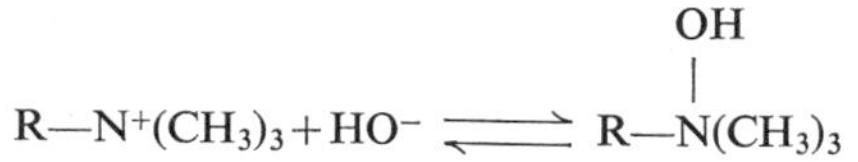

$$R—N^+(CH_3)_3 + HO^- \rightleftharpoons R—\overset{\overset{\displaystyle OH}{|}}{N}(CH_3)_3$$

However, at the pH of plasma, the ratio of nonionized to ionized molecules is only of the order of $1:10^6$. As a result of their high ionization they are very poorly absorbed (to the extent of 5 to 10%), and quaternary ammonium drugs which arc used for their systemic effects are usually given by injection. (*c*) The guanidine group is fairly basic, ionizing into the guanidinium ion:

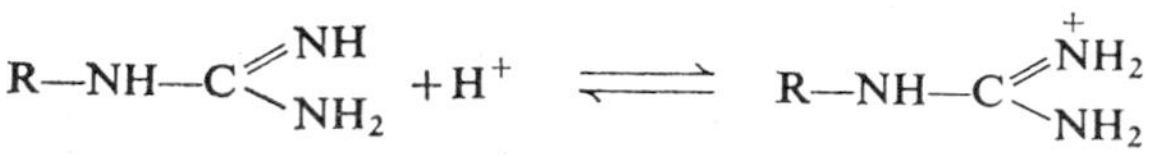

$$R—NH—C\underset{NH_2}{\overset{NH}{\diagup}} + H^+ \rightleftharpoons R—NH—C\underset{NH_2}{\overset{\overset{+}{NH_2}}{\diagup}}$$

Guanethidine, an antihypertensive drug, contains this group and is poorly absorbed. Nevertheless, the advantages of oral administration are such that guanethidine is usually given in this way. A guanidine derivative of the sulphonamides (sulphaguanidine) has been used for its local action within the gut, precisely because it is poorly absorbed. (*d*) The barbiturates have similar pK_a values and molecular weights, yet their rates of absorption differ widely. This is due to differences in their lipid solubility. For example, barbitone ($pK_a = 7.8$) with a chloroform/water partition coefficient of 0.75 is absorbed at about one-eighth of the rate of quinalbarbitone ($pK_a = 7.9$) which has a partition coefficient of 50. (*e*) Sulphonamides may ionize into anions or cations.

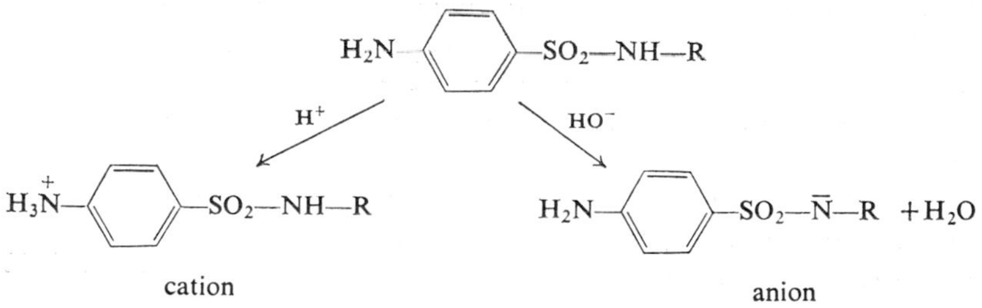

The weakly basic free anilinamino group of the unconjugated sulphonamides ($pK_a \simeq 2.4$) is almost completely nonionized in the pH range of the body, but the extent of anion formation varies considerably from one sulphonamide to another. In general, the higher is the pK_a of the acidic group, the less is the ionization, and the more rapid is the absorption. Thus:

	pK_a of acidic group	Blood level (mg%) 1 h after 4 g orally
Sulphadimidine	7·37	4·2
Sulphamerazine	7·06	3·0
Sulphadiazine	6·48	1·8

However, some other sulphonamides are rapidly absorbed even though their acidic pK_a values are relatively low. For example, sulphacetamide, sulphamethizole and sulphathiazole, have pK_a values of 5·4, 4·8, and 4·8 respectively; their rapid absorption is probably due to their very high aqueous solubility. The conjugated sulphonamides which are used for treating intestinal infection are poorly absorbed, partly because of their low acidic pK_a values and partly because of their low solubilities in both lipid and aqueous solvents.

Administration of drugs by mouth

Stomach. Nonionized drugs are readily absorbed from the stomach by lipid diffusion or by aqueous diffusion if the molecular weight is low. The low pH of the stomach contents is an important factor in the absorption of ionizing drugs. This was first demonstrated by placing strychnine (basic $pK_a = 8$) in the cat's stomach and confining it there by ligating the pylorus. As long as the stomach contents were acid, the strychnine was without action, but when they were made alkaline the strychnine was absorbed and killed the cat. Observations on absorption of drugs from the stomach of the dog and rat have shown how absorption is dependent on the pK_a: basic substances with pK_a values of more than 5, or acids with pK_a values of less than 2, are scarcely absorbed. This suggests that the *effective* pH at the lipid barrier is about 3·5 (i.e. less acid than the gastric contents, Table 19.3); absorption is not appreciable when less than 5% of the molecules are nonionized (Fig. 19.2). The absorption of many acidic drugs from the stomach may be hindered because of their lower aqueous solubility in an acid medium.

Drugs that are subject to acid hydrolysis in the stomach, or that cause vomiting, or that damage the gastric mucosa, may be given in gelatin capsules which disintegrate and liberate their contents only after passing into the intestine.

Small intestine. The mucous membrane of the small intestine is adapted for absorption (pages 315–316), and this is the principal site at which drugs are absorbed from the gastro-intestinal tract. The higher pH of the intestinal contents facilitates the absorption of basic drugs which are too highly ionized to be absorbed from the stomach. The lowest acidic pK_a value at which there is *rapid* absorption from the small intestine is about 3, and the highest basic pK_a value is about 8. This suggests that the *effective* pH at the absorbing surface is about 5, which is lower than the pH of the intestinal contents (Table 19.3) and may be representative of a lipid surface deep within the mucosa; absorption is rapid even when as few as 1 in 400 molecules is nonionized. Drugs which are more highly ionized than this are only slowly absorbed, and it is with these that absorption is erratic.

Colon. Absorption from the colon is less rapid than from the small intestine, but otherwise takes place by the same mechanisms.

FACTORS AFFECTING ABSORPTION FROM THE GASTRO-INTESTINAL TRACT. Blood flow may become the limiting factor in determining the maximum rate of absorption of drugs that are absorbed so rapidly that they attain equal concentrations in the lumen of the gut and in the plasma.

Drugs absorbed from the stomach and intestine into the blood stream are carried in the portal vein to the liver (Fig. 19.3). Here they are exposed to two factors which are of considerable importance in influencing pharmacological activity; the enzymatic detoxifying mechanisms of the liver and sequestration into the bile. The completeness with which the liver reduces the activity of certain drugs can be demonstrated by comparing the effect produced by a drug injected into the portal vein with the effect produced by injection into a systemic vein. Drugs which are taken into the bile are presented again to the intestine and reabsorbed; this cycle of events is termed an *entero–hepatic shunt*. The effect of the shunt is to prolong the duration of action; the drug is gradually lost by metabolism and by excretion. Examples of drugs which are cycled in this way are phenolphthalein, chloramphenicol and digitoxin.

The duration of action of an orally administered drug may be prolonged by giving it in a pill containing concentric layers of drug between soluble coats. Another method is to give a capsule containing many small pills whose coats are dissolved off at different rates. With either method, absorption is more erratic than with simpler preparations.

The convenience of oral administration is partly offset by a number of disadvantages, not the least of which is that patients are often unreliable in taking medicine. The amount of drug absorbed after oral administration may vary because of the following factors: (i) variations in the rate of passage through the stomach and intestine; (ii) variations in the pH of the contents of the gastro-intestinal tract; (iii) the presence of foodstuffs which may interfere with absorption by reducing the concentration of the drug, by obstructing access of drug to the absorbing surface, or by binding the drug.

Drugs given for their local action on the gastro-intestinal tract are dealt with in Chapter 31.

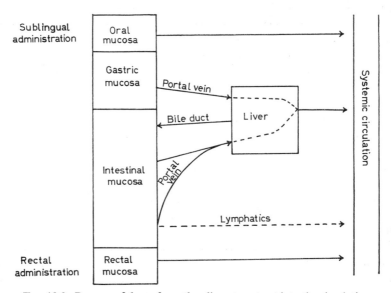

Fig. 19.3. Passage of drugs from the alimentary tract into the circulation.

Sublingual administration. A drug may be absorbed through the oral mucosa when it is given in lozenges or tablets which are placed under the tongue and allowed to dissolve; the subject is advised to refrain for as long as possible from swallowing the saliva containing the drug. The drug enters the systemic circulation without passing through the portal circulation (Fig. 19.3), thus avoiding the possibility of inactivation in the liver. The androgenic steroids are given sublingually for this reason. Absorption of lipid-soluble molecules through the oral mucosa is rapid and the effects of drugs given in this way may become apparent within 2 min. Consequently, this route is used for the administration of glyceryl trinitrate (a coronary vasodilator drug) at the first premonition of an impending attack of angina, and for the administration of isoprenaline which gives relief of bronchospasm in asthma. Drugs given for their local action in the buccal cavity include secretagogues (such as bitters) and expectorants (Chapter 31), disinfectants and antibiotics.

Rectal administration. Blood from the rectum reaches the vena cava without entering the hepatic portal circulation (Fig. 19.3); therefore drugs absorbed from suppositories through the rectal mucous membrane are not immediately exposed to detoxication in the liver. However, drugs given in an enema pass into the colon and may even reach the ileum. Some local anaesthetics are applied to the rectum in ointments or in suppositories to alleviate the pain and itching of haemorrhoids or other anal disorders.

Other mucous membranes. In most instances, drugs applied to the vagina, the urethra, the conjunctiva (Chapter 35) or the nose are given with the intention of obtaining their effects locally, but sufficient may be absorbed through the mucous membranes to produce systemic effects.

Absorption through the skin. The keratinized epidermal layer of the skin allows the passage of lipid soluble drugs. The skin is filmed over with the water-repellant secretion of the sebaceous glands which further hinders the penetration of hydrophilic drugs. The dermis is freely permeable and the penetration of drugs to the dermis can be assisted by incorporating them into vehicles which penetrate the epidermis. Ionized drugs can be driven through the skin by electrophoresis. Methacholine (page 704) has been used in this way to produce vasodilatation locally in cases of peripheral vascular spasm (page 830). Drugs applied to damaged skin surfaces may be rapidly absorbed. Drugs used for a local action on the skin include counter-irritants, antihistamines, local anaesthetics, steroid hormones, and drugs used in skin infections. Accidental contact with some industrial chemicals (c.g. aniline) or organophosphate anticholinesterases, may result in poisoning since these substances are highly lipid soluble and are rapidly absorbed. The poisonous gas, lewisite, also penetrates the skin rapidly.

Parenteral injection of drugs. Drugs which are not absorbed through mucous membranes or epithelium must be given by parenteral injection. Some drugs are destroyed in the gastro-intestinal tract, and these too are usually given by injection. It may also be necessary to inject a drug for the following reasons: (i) in order to produce a rapid response; (ii) the patient may be unconscious and unable to swallow; (iii) the drug may not be retained because of vomiting or purging. In experimental pharmacology, drugs are usually injected to avoid uncertainty about the amount absorbed. The main difficulty of parenteral injections is that, usually, they must be given by trained personnel; however, some people (e.g. diabetics), who depend on repeated injections, become skilful and self-sufficient. Parenteral injections may be given to achieve either a systemic action of the drug (intravenous, subcutaneous or intramuscular injection) or a local action (infiltration; intra-arterial or intrathecal injections).

Subcutaneous or intramuscular injections. The fluid injected spreads out through the loose connective tissue of the subcutaneous layer, or between the sheaths of muscle bundles (see page 191). Subcutaneous injections are more painful because of the rich sensory innervation of the skin. Larger volumes may be given intramuscularly than subcutaneously, and the greater spreading results in a more rapid absorption. Spreading of the injected mass may be facilitated by including hyaluronidase in the injection; this enzyme breaks down the intracellular matrix which is a polymer of hyaluronic acid. The drug is disseminated into the system after passage through capillary or lymphatic endothelium. Substances with molecular weights above about 20,000 are taken up principally into the lymphatics and those with molecular weights below about 3,000 are taken up by the capillaries. Increasing the blood supply to the site of injection by heating or by massage hastens the rate of dissemination.

PROLONGATION OF ACTION OF INJECTED DRUGS. The local action of an injected drug can be prolonged by decreasing the rate of removal of the drug from the site of injection, and this can be achieved by adding a vasoconstrictor drug to the injection; thus adrenaline may be mixed with local anaesthetic drugs to prolong the duration of action at the site of injection. Decreasing the rate of dissemination of a systemically acting drug gives the advantage of reduction in the number of injections required and a smoother control of blood levels. Drugs are formulated for this purpose into what are known as 'depot' preparations. Water-soluble drugs may be converted to a less soluble salt (e.g. procaine penicillin) or complex (e.g. protamine zinc insulin) which is injected as a suspension; the active drug is slowly released and passes into the circulation. Drugs injected as solutions in oil diffuse out slowly into the tissue fluid. Steroid hormones are often given in the form of pellets which are implanted under the skin, the drug being slowly dissolved before diffusing into the capillaries. The pellet becomes surrounded by fibrous connective tissue which slows its rate of dissolution still further. Implants of deoxycortone acetate may remain effective for up to 6 months. The effectiveness of testosterone pellets can be prolonged by using esters of this steroid: the higher the molecular weight of the esterifying acid, the more slowly it is hydrolysed and the longer the persistence: the following are used: acetate, propionate, isobutyrate, cyclopentylpropionate, heptanoate and phenylpropionate.

Intravenous injection. These give a rapid onset of action since the drug reaches the tissues in one circulation time (ca. 15 sec). Some drugs with an irritant action when injected into the tissues can be tolerated by intravenous injection, in which case, care is taken to ensure that none of the injection leaks out from the vein. A sustained level of drug in the blood stream can be maintained by giving an *intravenous infusion*. Injections into the bone marrow are sometimes given in infants where the veins are small or in adults when the superficial veins are collapsed or deeply buried in fat—the drug passes immediately into the blood stream.

Other methods of injection

Intradermal injections are used mainly for the administration of test sera for the identification of antigens causing allergic reactions, and in testing for the presence or absence of antibodies to various bacteria.

Intraperitoneal injections are rarely given in man as the danger of creating adhesions is considerable, but they are commonly used in animal experiments. Diffusion into the blood stream is rapid, owing to the large area of the absorbing surfaces.

Intrathecal injections are given into the subarachnoid space to produce a local action of a drug on the meninges or spinal nerve roots; antibiotics may be injected in this way for treatment of inction feand local anaesthetic drugs are sometimes used to produce regional anaesthesia.

Intra-arterial injections are often used in animal experiments when it is desired to localize the action of a drug to a particular organ (as for cxamplc, the close-arterial injection of acetylcholine into striated muscle). In man, substances that are opaque to X-rays may be injected intra-arterially as an aid in diagnosis. In the treatment of cancer, cytotoxic drugs are sometimes perfused for short pcriods through thc artcrics supplying the affected organ and the perfusate is collected from the veins leaving the organ so that the drug does not enter the general circulation. Injections intended to be intravenous are sometimes given by accident into an artery. If this occurs with thiopentone there is a risk of producing vasoconstriction and necrosis. *Intracardiac injections* are sometimes given for emergency resuscitation and during cardiac surgery.

Inhalation. Absorption is rapid for drugs given by inhalation since the surface area of alveoli is large and the alveolar epithelium is readily penetrated. The volatile and gaseous anaesthetics are the most important group of drugs given in this way. Inhalation of the vapour of amyl nitrite gives rapid relief of anginal attacks. Drugs given by inhalation to produce a local action in relieving bronchospasm include the vapours of some sympathomimetic drugs (amphetamine, ephedrine) and aerosols of isoprenaline, atropine or antihistamines. Drugs which are taken in by inhalation of smoke include nicotine (from tobacco), morphine (from opium) and tetrahydrocannabinol (from hashish, hemp or marihuana); atropine and ephedrine have been incorporated into cigarettes.

Distribution of drugs in the body

After absorption, drugs are disseminated through the body in the blood stream. Substances that permeate freely through cell membranes become distributed throughout the body water. Substances that pass through the capillary endothelium but do not permeate cell membranes become distributed throughout the extracellular fluid. Most drugs are not distributed equally throughout the body, but tend to be sequestered at particular sites.

Factors determining the sequestration of drugs

(a) DIFFERENCE IN pH ON EITHER SIDE OF A LIPID BOUNDARY. Consider a hypothetical system of two compartments, one with a pH of 5, the other of 7, separated by a membrane which is permeable only to nonionized (lipid soluble) molecules. A basic drug with pK_a 6 will be unequally distributed when the system is in equilibrium owing to the difference in the ratio between nonionized molecules and cations in each compartment. The concentration of the non-ionized molecules is the same in each compartment, but the ratio of nonionized to ionized molecules is 0·1 in compartment I, and 10 in compartment II.

Distribution of drug with basic $pK_a = 6$

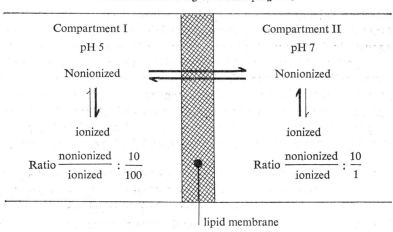

About 91% of the total amount of drug is in compartment I.

In general, basic drugs tend to accumulate in regions of low pH; conversely, acid drugs tend to accumulate in regions of high pH, providing always that the drug *can* penetrate the barrier between the regions. Even a small difference in pH across a boundary membrane, such as exists between cerebrospinal fluid (pH 7·3) and plasma (pH 7·4) may lead to unequal distribution.

(b) DIFFERENCES IN BINDING. Take a hypothetical case of a two compartment system with different degrees of drug binding in each; only the unbound drug molecules are able to pass from one compartment to the other.

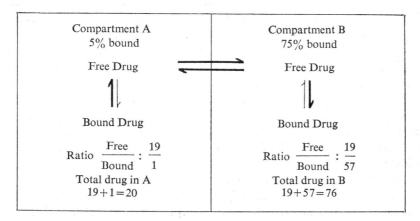

At equilibrium in this system, about 21% of the drug will be in compartment A and 79% in compartment B.

In general, the nature of the binding is immaterial it may be, for example, an attachment to protein, solution in lipid, the formation of a non-diffusible chemical compound, or attachment to a specific binding site in tissues.

(c) ACTIVE TRANSPORT. A drug that is moved across a membrane by active transport will be unequally distributed across that membrane. Two drugs which are actively transported by the same carrier mechanism are in competition for it, and the rate of transport of either one will be decreased in the presence of the other. A slowly transported drug inhibits the carrier mechanism.

Sequestration of drugs in various tissues. Interaction between these factors, which may act in the same or in opposite directions, determines the distribution of drugs in the body and accounts for the fact that drugs may become more concentrated in some tissues than in others. Some drugs are largely bound to blood constituents, and others form complexes with components of other tissues or are dissolved in the fat depots. Some drugs traverse the blood-brain barrier or the placental barrier whereas others do not. The sequestration of drugs in particular tissues is illustrated by the following examples.

BINDING TO BLOOD CONSTITUENTS. The binding of a drug to plasma protein or blood cells facilitates absorption by lowering the concentration of free drug in the aqueous phase of the plasma.

Drugs may be reversibly bound to *plasma proteins* (chiefly albumin) by ionic, hydrogen or van der Waals' bonds. Suramin, a trypanocidal drug, is so firmly bound to albumin that it persists in the blood for a considerable time, but enough is released from the bound form to exert a trypanocidal action. This confers an advantage in the treatment of sleeping sickness, since after a single dose the trypanosomes are suppressed for 3 months or more. Papaverine, a spasmolytic drug, also becomes bound to albumin, and this results in the termination of its relaxing action on smooth muscle. Other drugs that are largely bound to albumin in the blood include phenylbutazone (1 to 5% in the free form) and dicoumarol (less than 1% in the free form): the therapeutic doses of these drugs are such that there are sufficient amounts of the *free* drugs for them to act. The diagnostic agent azovan blue is also firmly bound to albumin and remains in the blood stream for some days: it is injected intravenously for the determination of cardiac output (page 262) and plasma volume.

Drugs permeate through the *erythrocyte* membrane at rates depending on their concentration, molecular weight and lipid solubility. Their distribution between the plasma and the erythrocytes depends on the extent of binding on each side of the membrane. Haemoglobin has an excess cationic charge and anions are bound preferentially. Carbon monoxide is firmly bound to haemoglobin, and so is sequestered in erythrocytes. *Phagocytic leucocytes* assist in the distribution of drugs that are injected subcutaneously or intramuscularly, in particular those given as suspensions or as emulsions in oil. *Platelets* bind 5-hydroxytryptamine and some other amines.

BINDING TO COMPONENTS OF OTHER TISSUES. *Basophilic components* of tissues, including *nucleoproteins*, bind acridine drugs which are therefore accumulated in cell nuclei and in some cytoplasmic particles. The antimalarial drug mepacrine (an acridine) rapidly disappears from the blood stream and a few hours after a single dose in the dog the concentration in various tissues (muscle, lung, spleen, and liver) was from 200 to 4000 times that in plasma. Daily administration for two weeks resulted in still further binding, the tissue concentrations being from 1100 to 21,000 times the plasma concentration. Mepacrine imparts a yellow tint to the skin as it is bound to the basophilic collagen bundles beneath the dermis.

Some drugs are taken up by *keratinous tissues* (skin, nails and hair). The accumulation of arsenic in hair and nails is of significance for forensic medicine in the detection of poisoning. Many other metals are accumulated in keratin. The formation of thiol compounds (page 468) is probably involved, since keratin is rich in cysteine (page 60). Drugs bound to keratin are not released back into the rest of the body.

Calcium in the *bones* can be exchanged against certain other metallic ions.

Lead and radioactive strontium (^{90}Sr) are accumulated in this way and give rise to toxicological hazards.

The *granules* of mast cells, chromaffin cells, enterochromaffin cells and sympathetic neurones normally contain pharmacologically active amines (see Chapters 5 and 6) and are capable of taking up and binding these amines; they also take up related substances. Various dyestuffs are taken up selectively by cytoplasmic inclusions and this is the basis of their histological identification. Certain dyestuffs, the so-called 'vital stains', are taken up by such components of the living cell as the mitochondria, lysosomes, the Golgi apparatus and the endoplasmic reticulum.

Pigmented tissues take up chloroquine, an antimalarial drug, and sufficient may be accumulated in the retina to produce disturbances of vision.

Many drugs are accumulated in the *viscera*, particularly in the liver and kidney in the course of drug detoxication or excretion. Iron accumulates in ferritin deposits in the walls of the intestine and in the spleen and liver (page 238). The entrapment of some drugs in reticulo-endothelial tissues may lead to the sequestration of large amounts of them in the spleen and liver.

The fat of *adipose tissue* may amount to as much as 20% of the body weight and can take up considerable amounts of lipid soluble drugs. These include the anaesthetic gases and thiopentone. The brief duration of anaesthesia produced by a single administration of ether or thiopentone is due to their rapid sequestration into fat; when they are administered continuously, the capacity of the fat to dissolve them becomes saturated, and then the rate of administration must be decreased. Dibenamine and phenoxybenzamine (α-adrenoreceptor blocking drugs) are also taken up in fat owing to their high lipid/water partition coefficient. The chlorinated hydrocarbon insecticides, dicophane (DDT), aldrin and dieldrin, are stored in the fat; in small amounts they are apparently harmless to man provided that they remain in the fat. However, if the fat is utilized, as during slimming, they are released into the body and may then produce toxic symptoms.

CEREBROSPINAL FLUID AND BRAIN. The blood-brain barrier was discussed on page 104. The barrier acts like a lipid membrane and is preferentially permeable to nonionized lipid-soluble molecules. The distribution of drugs depends largely on the extent of drug binding on either side of the barrier, and, for ionizing drugs, on their pK_a value and the pH difference across the barrier. Plasma protein binding retards passage into the CSF; the CSF protein content, being about 1/500 that of plasma, is negligible. Solution in brain lipids favours the accumulation of lipid-soluble drugs in the brain. Thus, thiopentone, the most lipid soluble of the barbiturates, is the one most readily taken up by the brain.

The ability to penetrate the blood-brain barrier is a requisite for drugs used in the treatment of infections of the brain. Of the antibiotics, chloramphenicol attains a concentration in the CSF of 27% that in plasma; penicillin permeates slightly through the normal barrier but passes through more readily when the membranes of the brain are inflamed, so that in meningitis sufficient is taken up for it to be effective; tetracycline does not pass into the CSF. Of the drugs used to combat tuberculosis, streptomycin and isoniazid are effective in treating infections of the CNS, but aminosalicylate is not. Of the sulphonamides, the concentration of sulphadiazine in the CSF reaches 75% of the plasma level; the other sulphonamides are less well absorbed owing partly to binding with plasma protein and partly to unfavourable pK_a values.

Some drugs are selectively taken up in the brain, and this is the reason for their acting predominantly on the CNS. Chlorpromazine reaches a brain : blood ratio of 80:1 and it is 99·8% bound in the brain. Imipramine is 97% bound in the brain and 82% bound in the plasma and it achieves a distribution ratio of 20:1 (this ratio is *higher* than the theoretical equilibrium distribution of 8:1 based on the degree of binding on each side of the barrier).

Quaternary ammonium drugs, being highly ionized, do not penetrate to any appreciable extent through the blood-brain barrier, and are generally without action on the central nervous system (unless injected locally). Related, non-quaternary drugs are effective, as in the following examples (the second of each pair crosses the blood-brain barrier):

Methylatropine—Atropine; Neostigmine—Physostigmine;
Hexamethonium—Mecamylamine; Tubocurarine—β-Erythroidine.

Drugs pass more readily from the CSF into the plasma than in the reverse direction. The pathway is via the villi in the sub-arachnoid space. There is a pressure gradient from the CSF to the blood capillaries which facilitates the outward movement of fluid and solutes, and in addition there is active transport of cations, including the ionized molecules of basic drugs. (It was pointed out on page 104 that the blood-brain barrier was not simply a physical barrier, and it is likely that the lack of effect of quaternary compounds on the CNS is due to their active removal as well as to their poor penetration.)

PLACENTA AND FOETUS. Nutrients, such as glucose and amino acids, are actively transported from the maternal blood stream. The passage of drugs across the placental membranes is largely by lipid diffusion. The two respects in which the penetration of drugs to the foetus is important are (i) the toxicity of drugs to the embryo including teratogenic effects (this is discussed on page 561) and (ii) the effects on the foetus of drugs used in parturition.

The volatile anaesthetics used during childbirth have less of a depressant effect on the foetus than on the mother. But barbiturates and drugs used to produce analgesia in the mother are less well tolerated by the foetus because of the absence of enzymes that detoxify them, and these drugs may depress the respiratory effort of the new-born baby. Morphine taken frequently during pregnancy may result in withdrawal symptoms appearing in the baby after parturition.

Practical applications of drug sequestration. The accumulation of drugs at the site of their desired action is often of great importance in therapeutics. Chloroquine, which was first introduced as an antimalarial drug, accumulates in the liver. This suggested its use for treating hepatic amoebiasis, in which it is highly effective. The antibiotic griseofulvin is deposited in developing keratin, and is particularly useful in the treatment of fungal infections of the nails which were formerly almost incurable. The accumulation of arsenic in the skin has been utilized in the treatment of eczema. Inflamed lung tissue takes up the diethylaminoethyl ester of penicillin (penethamate): the ester is hydrolysed and penicillin is released in a relatively high concentration at the site of infection. The treatment of hypertrophy of the prostrate gland with stilboestrol is facilitated by the selective accumulation of the steroid in the prostrate gland after administration in the form of the diphosphate ester: the alkaline phosphatase activity of the gland is high and the ester is rapidly hydrolysed resulting in the local deposition of stilboestrol. Brain tumours take up azobenzeneboronic acid: this is a radio-opaque substance and is useful in the location of the tumour in X-ray examination. The accumulation of radio-opaque iodine-containing substances in the biliary and urinary systems is utilized in diagnostic X-ray examination (Table 19.8). Iodine has an affinity for the thyroid (pages 369 to 370); a radio-isotope (^{131}I or ^{132}I) has been used in small doses in the diagnosis of thyroid disorders and in large doses to destroy part of the gland in patients with hyperthyroidism. Chromium is firmly bound in erythrocytes, and the radio-isotope (^{51}Cr) has been used in the diagnosis of anaemia. Phosphate is incorporated into bone, and neoplastic conditions of the haematopoeitic tissue in the bone marrow have been treated with phosphates containing a radio-isotope of phosphorus (^{32}P).

Drug metabolism

The enzymatic changes undergone by a drug in the body usually results in the attenuation or loss of pharmacological activity—the term *detoxication* describes the result of such metabolic changes. However, this is not the only possibility: a pharmacologically active metabolite may be formed from an inactive precursor, or *pro-drug*; or, the metabolites of a drug may have a different type of pharmacological action from that displayed by the administered drug.

Enzymes involved in drug metabolism are present in many tissues. In the gut they may be contained in the digestive secretions, the bacterial flora, or the intestinal wall. The enzymes of blood may be in the plasma or associated with the cells. The main organ concerned in drug metabolism is the liver and many drugs are attacked by enzymes contained in the microsomes of the hepatic cells. The kidney, lung and nervous tissue also contain drug-metabolizing enzymes.

When a substance which is a natural constituent of the body is administered as a drug, it is metabolized in the same way as the endogenous substance. Most drugs are 'foreign' to the body; nevertheless, if they are metabolized it is by enzymes that are normally concerned with the metabolism of the constituents of the body. For example, fluoroacetate, a rat poison, is converted to fluoroacetyl coenzyme A—just as acetate is converted to acetyl CoA (page 25). This metabolite enters the tricarboxylic acid cycle (Fig. 2.5, page 43) where the fluoroacetyl radicle condenses with oxaloacetate to form fluorocitrate. But fluorocitrate is not a substrate for aconitase, the next enzyme in the tricarboxylic acid cycle; in fact, it is an inhibitor. In this example fluorocitrate is a pharmacologically active metabolite, and fluoroacetate may be considered as a pro-drug. It is also an example of a *metabolic analogue* which is incorporated into a so-called *lethal synthesis*. This is also the case with the anticancer drugs 5-bromouracil and 8-azaguanine which are incorporated into nucleoproteins, but these do not have the functions of normal nucleoproteins and cell division is inhibited.

There are enzyme systems that appear to be concerned entirely with the detoxication of toxic by-products of normal metabolism. For instance, the urea synthesizing system (page 329) detoxifies the ammonia liberated during deamination of amino acids. Hydrogen peroxide which is formed in oxidative metabolism is rapidly detoxified by catalase and peroxidase. Cyanide is liberated in small amounts in normal metabolism and is detoxified by being converted to thiocyanate, which has less than 1% of the toxicity of cyanide. Cyanide, whether administered as such or split off aliphatic nitriles, is detoxified in the same way:

$$R.CH_2.CN \longrightarrow HCN + RCOOH$$

rhodanese
+S (from thiosulphate)

$$HSCN$$

The toxicity of nitriles is proportional to the rate at which they are metabolized to yield cyanide.

The enzymatic reactions to which drugs are subject can, in general, be classified according to the type of chemical change produced: these are *oxidation, reduction, cleavage* (including hydrolysis) and *conjugation.*

Oxidation

Alcohols are oxidized to aldehydes, and aldehydes to acids. Ethanol is completely catabolized to water and carbon diozide:

$$CH_3—CH_2OH \xrightarrow[\text{dehydrogenase}]{\text{alcohol}} CH_3—CHO \xrightarrow[\text{dehydrogenase}]{\text{aldehyde}} CH_3COOH \longrightarrow$$

$$\text{acetylcoenzyme A} \longrightarrow H_2O + CO_2$$

Inhibition of aldehyde dehydrogenase by disulfiram (page 586) results in the accumulation of a toxic metabolite, acetaldehyde, in the body. Methanol is oxidized to formaldehyde and then formic acid: these metabolites are toxic.

The enzymatic oxidations that are involved in the biosynthesis of catecholamines (page 160) occur with other drugs; thus, both *p*-hydroxyamphetamine and phenylpropanolamine are metabolites of amphetamine:

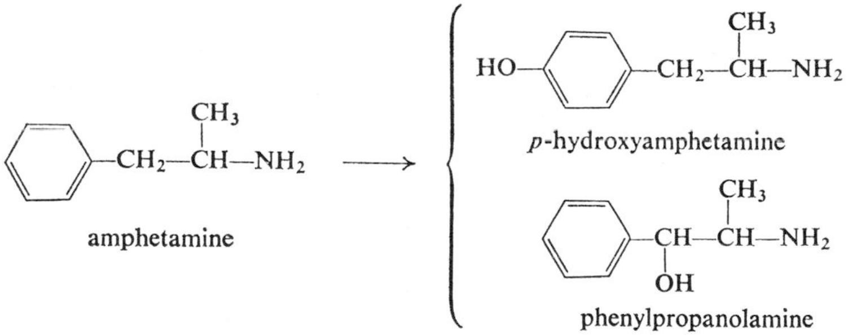

Similarly, the biosynthetic enzyme oxidizing tryptamine to 5-HT (page 179) oxidizes dimethyltryptamine. In these instances the metabolites have increased activity, and sometimes the type of action is altered.

Monoamine oxidase is mentioned in connection with the metabolism of catecholamines (page 165) and 5-HT (page 179); this enzyme acts on aryl-, alkyl- or long chain alkyl-amines and secondary amines, provided that the α-carbon atom is not substituted. *Histaminase* (page 175) catalyses the oxidation of a terminal amine in a number of di-amines. *Xanthine oxidase* which is concerned in the formation of uric acid, also oxidizes certain foreign purines that are used as cytotoxic agents (e.g. 6-mercaptopurine). Oxidative deamination usually results in the loss of pharmacological activity.

Examples of oxidations of metals which are of particular importance in pharmacology include the conversion of arsenic (in arsenicals) from the tri- to the penta-valent form and of iron from the ferrous to the ferric form.

Sulphides are oxidized to sulphates and sulphydryl compounds to sulphuric acid esters or sulphonic acids; the oxidized compounds are less toxic and are excreted rapidly. One metabolic route of thiopentone is oxidation to pentobarbitone, thus:

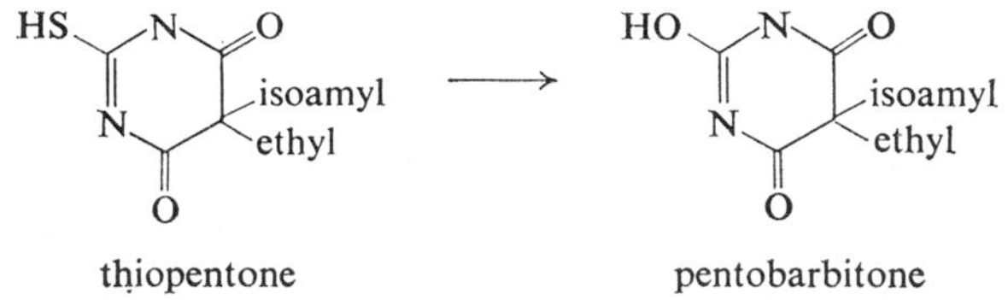

thiopentone   pentobarbitone

OXIDATIONS CATALYZED BY LIVER MICROSOMAL ENZYMES. These reactions include hydroxylation of aromatic rings and of alkyl side-chains, oxidative deamination, N-dealkylation and O-dealkylation, and sulphoxide formation. The microsomal enzymes involved utilize $TPNH_2$ and molecular oxygen (in this respect they differ from the mitochondrial $TPNH_2$-enzymes in which oxidation is through FAD and the cytochrome system, as shown in Fig. 11.7, page 300).

Hydroxylation. The aromatic substances undergoing this reaction are benzene, benzene derivatives (e.g., reaction A in Fig. 19.7) and polycyclic compounds including steroid hormones. There may be more than one site of hydroxylation, and more than one hydroxyl group added, thus:

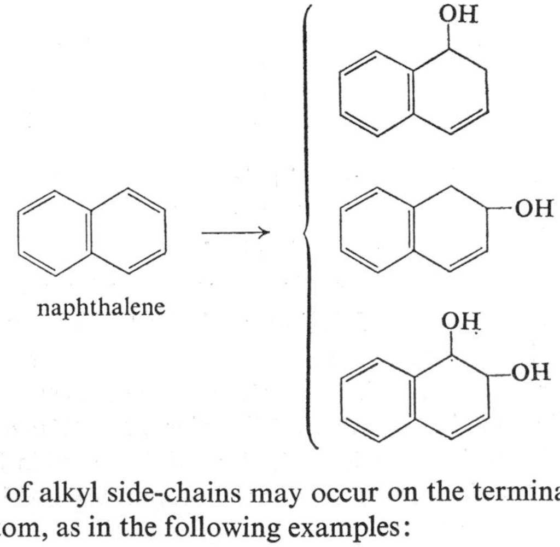

naphthalene

Hydroxylation of alkyl side-chains may occur on the terminal or the penultimate carbon atom, as in the following examples:

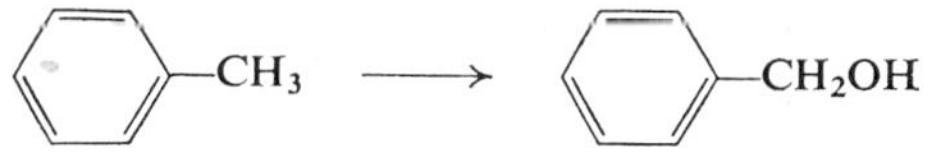

toluene   benzyl alchohol

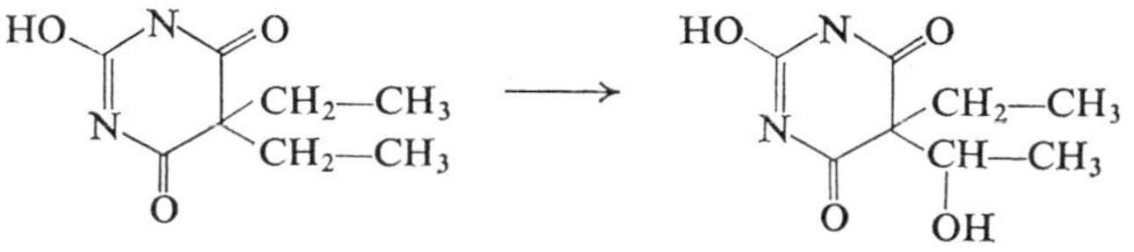

barbitone   hydroxybarbitone

The oxidation of the side chain of barbiturates results in the loss of sedative activity. However, hydroxylation often results in increased pharmacological activity. The hydroxyl group is subject to further alteration by conjugation: the conjugates are usually inactive; moreover they are rapidly excreted.

N-dealkylation and *O-dealkylation* is the result of decomposition of unstable intermediary oxidized compounds; the general reactions are as follows:

$$R{-}NH{-}CH_3 \xrightarrow{(\frac{1}{2}O_2)} [R{-}NH{-}CH_2OH] \longrightarrow R{-}NH_2 + HCHO$$
unstable

$$R{-}O{-}CH_3 \xrightarrow{(\frac{1}{2}O_2)} [R{-}O{-}CH_2OH] \longrightarrow R{-}OH + HCHO$$
unstable

The net result of these reactions amounts to a *cleavage* of the drug molecule and examples are given below under that heading.

Oxidative *deamination* of α-methylated amines takes place in a similar way; thus:

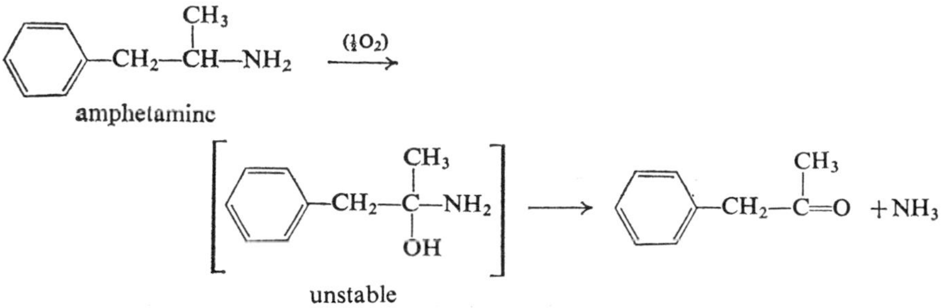

amphetamine

unstable

(Note that the microsomal enzyme differs from monoamine oxidase in that the latter does not attack α-methylated amines.) The aniline —NH_2 group is converted to hydroxylamine, and this leads to increased toxicity of the product (see reaction C, Fig. 19.7).

Sulphoxidation occurs in compounds containing a thio-ether group [R—S—R′], an example being the oxidation of phenothiazines, as shown below:

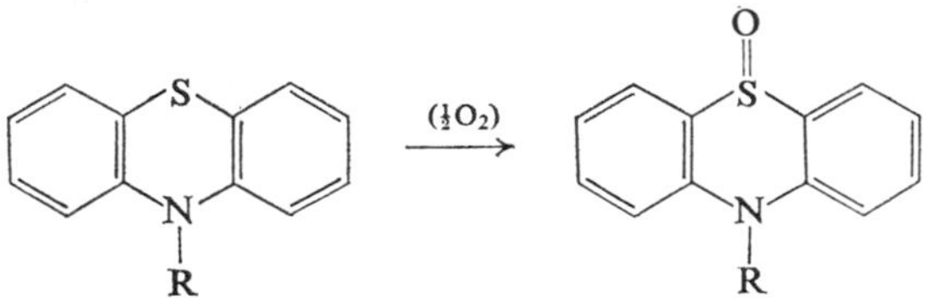

| phenothiazine | sulphoxide form. |

Hydrogenation (reduction)

This occurs less commonly than oxidation in drug metabolism. The reaction uses $TPNH_2$ or $DPNH_2$ plus FAD (Fig. 1.9, page 24) in a mechanism involving electron transfer (Fig. 11.7, page 300). Examples of reduction are conversion of aldehydes and ketones to primary and secondary alcohols, nitro groups to hydroxylamines and amines, azo groups to hydrazines and amines, hydroxamic acids to amines, pentavalent to trivalent arsenic, disulphides to sulphydryls, and saturation of double bonds. Three examples follow:

(i)

$$Cl_3C\text{—}CHO.H_2O \xrightarrow{(2H)} Cl_3\text{—}CH_2OH + H_2O$$
$$\text{chloral hydrate} \qquad\qquad \text{trichloroethanol}$$

Chloral hydrate is a pro-drug and must first be converted to trichlorethanol.

(ii)

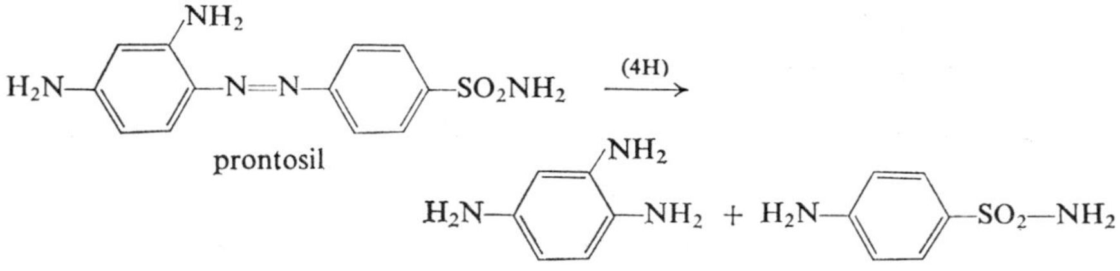

Prontosil has antibacterial activity, but is rather toxic; the metabolite, sulphanilamide, has greater activity and is less toxic.

(iii) Chloramphenicol is a substituted nitrobenzene compound (see Fig. 19.5 for formula); its metabolites include substituted phenylhydroxylamine and aniline—these have no antibiotic activity.

Cleavage

Hydrolysis. In general, esters are subject to hydrolysis by enzymes in the blood, liver, kidney and other tissues. Cholinesterases have been dealt with elsewhere (pages 156 to 158). Other examples of reactions catalysed by esterases which result in loss of pharmacological activity are as follows.

Atropine $\longrightarrow$ tropine + tropic acid

Cocaine $\longrightarrow$ ecgonine + methanol + benzoic acid

Pethidine $\longrightarrow$ methylphenylisonipecotic acid + CH_3CH_2OH

Procaine $\longrightarrow$ *p*-aminobenzoic acid + $HO-CH_2.CH_2.N(C_2H_5)_2$

Procaine amide $\longrightarrow$ *p*-aminobenzoic acid + $H_2N.CH_2.CH_2.N(C_2H_5)_2$

Procaine is hydrolysed by a plasma cholinesterase and by a liver microsomal esterase. Pethidine is hydrolysed only by liver microsomal enzymes. In rabbits, atropine is hydrolysed by a plasma enzyme.

Amide esters are hydrolysed more slowly than alcohol esters—procaine and procaine amide have similar cardiac actions, but the greater persistence of the amide in the body makes it more suitable for the treatment of atrial fibrillation (page 819); another advantage is that it lacks the central stimulant action of procaine. Examples of amide hydrolysis that result in greater pharmacological activity are as follows: (*a*) Fluoracetamide is hydrolysed to yield fluoroacetic acid. (*b*) Amide ester hydrolysis of phthalyl- and succinylsulphathiazole by bacterial enzymes in the colon liberates the antibacterial sulphathiazole:

Glucosidases. The sugar residues of cardiac glycosides (page 799) are removed one at a time by glucosidases. Some purgatives are glycosides and attain their pharmacological activity after hydrolysis (page 796).

Decarboxylation. This has been dicussed in connection with the biosynthesis of catecholamines, (page 159), histamine (page 174) and 5-HT (page 178). The antihypertensive drug, α-methyldopa, must be decarboxylated before it becomes effective in lowering the blood pressure (page 841).

Dealkylation. An example of removal of O-methyl groups (after decomposition of an unstable oxidized compound, page 507) is given below:

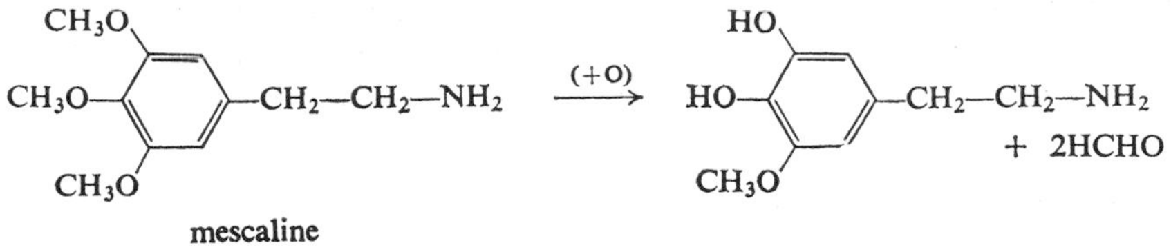

mescaline

This results in a loss of hallucinogenic activity but an increase in sympathomimetic activity.

Further examples of drugs undergoing O-demethylation are codeine (to morphine) and metanephrine (to adrenaline). An example of removal of an O-ethyl group is given in reaction B, Fig. 19.7. In general, O-dealkylation increases pharmacological activity.

N-demethylation is undergone by ephedrine, methyl-amphetamine and related drugs: the products have greater activity than the original compounds. Methylphenobarbitone (a short-acting barbiturate) is converted to phenobarbitone (long-acting). N-demethylation of pethidine, codeine and morphine reduces pharmacological activity, largely because the products are more rapidly excreted, being more water-soluble. N-methyl groups can be removed one at a time from tertiary amines (e.g., imipramine).

Conjugation

N-Methylation. Activated methionine (page 50) is the methyl donor. The transferases, which occur in various tissues, are relatively specific. The N-methylation of nicotinamide is shown below:

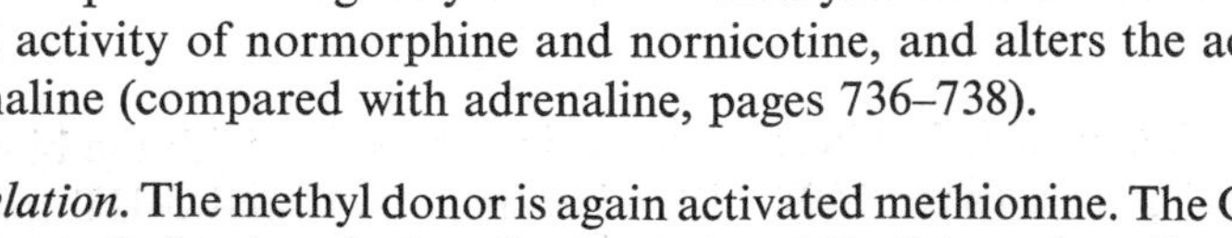

Another example is the N-methylation of histamine (Fig. 6.1, page 175); the metabolite is pharmacologically inactive. N-methylation increases the pharmacological activity of normorphine and nornicotine, and alters the activity of noradrenaline (compared with adrenaline, pages 736–738).

O-Methylation. The methyl donor is again activated methionine. The O-methylation of catecholamines is described on page 165. Other phenolic and polycyclic alcohols, including the steroid hormones, are subject to O-methylation.

N-Acetylation. Acetylcoenzyme A is the source of the acetyl radicle; it is transferred by various *acetyl transferases*. The compounds that are conjugated are alkyl- and aryl-amines, including *l*-amino acids, *p*-aminobenzoic acid, and sulphonamides, as in the example:

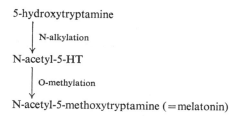

sulphonamide   acetylated
             sulphonamide

In the case of sulphanilamide, acetylation of the amide N also occurs.

Both N- and O-alkylations may occur in the same molecule. For example, noradrenaline is converted to adrenaline (page 160) and is also converted to normetanephrine (page 165). An example of alkylation producing a change in pharmacological activity has recently been worked out (Axelrod), as follows:

5-hydroxytryptamine
  | N-alkylation
  ↓
N-acetyl-5-HT
  | O-methylation
  ↓
N-acetyl-5-methoxytryptamine (= melatonin)

Melatonin inhibits the oestrous cycle; it has been suggested that melatonin is a pineal gland hormone.

Sulphate conjugation. A phenolic hydroxy group may be converted to a sulphanilic acid: $ROH \rightarrow ROSO_3H$. The 'active' sulphate is transferred from adenosine-3-phosphate-5-phosphosulphate. This conjugation frequently follows ring hydroxylation.

AMINO ACID CONJUGATIONS. (i) *Glycine* conjugates with acids. The reaction is activated in the following way:

$$\text{Acid} + \text{ATP} + \text{CoA} \longrightarrow \boxed{\text{Acyl}}\text{—CoA} + \text{AMP} + 2 \,\, \circled{P}$$

$$\Big\downarrow \text{glycine}$$

$$\boxed{\text{Acyl}}\text{—glycine}$$

$$+ \text{CoA}$$

The conjugation of benzoic acid to form hippuric acid (benzoyl glycine, $C_6H_5.CO.NH.CH_2.COOH$) was the first example discovered of a conjugation reaction, and indeed, the first example of detoxication. Other acids that undergo glycine conjugation are nicotinic acid and cinnamic acid. Long chain fatty acid side chains are first broken down by β-oxidation (Fig. 2.7, page 45), before being conjugated, thus:

phenylbutyric acid $\longrightarrow$ phenylacetic acid $\longrightarrow$ phenylacetylglycine
(phenaceturic acid)

(ii) *Glutamine* conjugation is confined to man and the anthropoid apes. The substances undergoing it are phenyl- and indole-acetic acids. These are the abnormal metabolites that accumulate in *phenylketonurics* (Fig. 6.5, page 186): in this disease the urine contains increased amounts of the glutamine conjugates as well as the free acids. The acids are converted into active complexes with coenzyme A before reacting with glutamine:

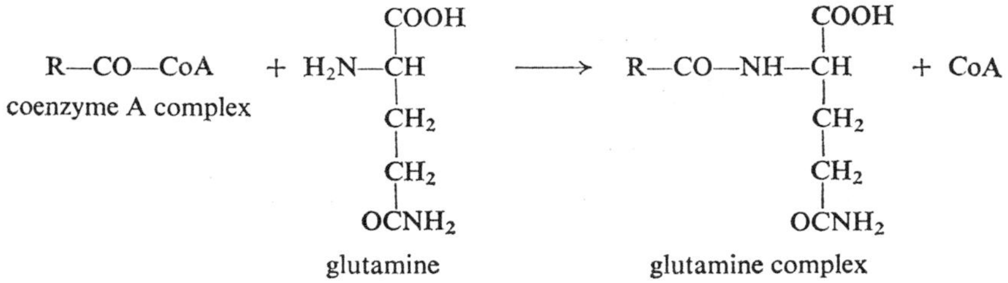

$$
\begin{array}{ccccc}
 & & \text{COOH} & & \text{COOH} \\
 & & | & & | \\
\text{R—CO—CoA} & + \text{H}_2\text{N—CH} & \longrightarrow & \text{R—CO—NH—CH} & + \text{CoA} \\
\text{coenzyme A complex} & | & & | \\
 & \text{CH}_2 & & \text{CH}_2 \\
 & | & & | \\
 & \text{CH}_2 & & \text{CH}_2 \\
 & | & & | \\
 & \text{OCNH}_2 & & \text{OCNH}_2 \\
 & \text{glutamine} & & \text{glutamine complex}
\end{array}
$$

(R = phenylacetyl- or indoleacetyl-)

(iii) *Mercapturic acid* conjugation takes place in two steps. First, there is conjugation through the sulphydryl of cysteine. The source of the cysteine has not been decided upon: it may be from glutathione (page 25), or it may be from a protein chain. In any event, the amino group of the S-cysteine conjugate is then acetylated to form the mercapturic acid conjugate. An example is shown below:

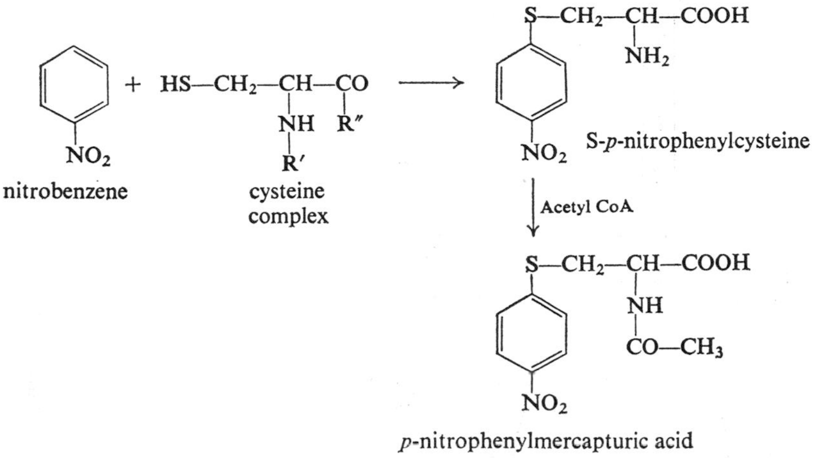

p-nitrophenylmercapturic acid

This conjugation is also undergone by alkyl and aryl halogenated or nitrated compounds, benzene and polycyclic hydrocarbons.

(iv) *Other amino acid* conjugations are known; a few compounds are conjugated with serine and lysine, and ornithine conjugation occurs in birds and reptiles, often with compounds that form glycine conjugates in mammals.

GLUCURONIC ACID CONJUGATION. The formation of 'active' glucuronic acid and the transfer of this group is summarized in Fig. 19.4. In many animals, (e.g. rat, dog) UDP-glucuronic acid is further metabolized to yield ascorbic acid, but this does not happen in man, the monkey or the guinea pig (hence the dependence of these animals on exogenous vitamin C). The *UDP-glucuronic acid transferase* which catalyses the conjugation is located in the microsomes

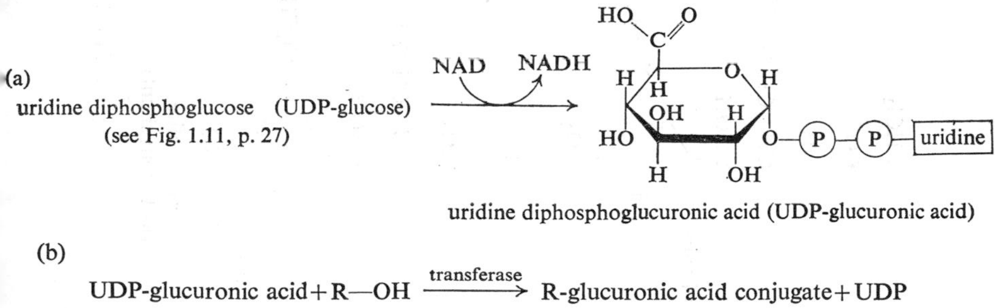

(a)
uridine diphosphoglucose (UDP-glucose)
(see Fig. 1.11, p. 27)

uridine diphosphoglucuronic acid (UDP-glucuronic acid)

(b)

UDP-glucuronic acid $+$ R—OH $\xrightarrow{\text{transferase}}$ R-glucuronic acid conjugate $+$ UDP

FIG. 19.4. (a) Formation of UDP-glucuronic acid. The role of UDP-glucose in glycogen-glucose exchange is shown in Fig. 2.8 (page 46). (b) Glucuronic acid conjugation reaction. [R—OH = alcoholic, phenolic or aromatic carboxylic compound.]

17

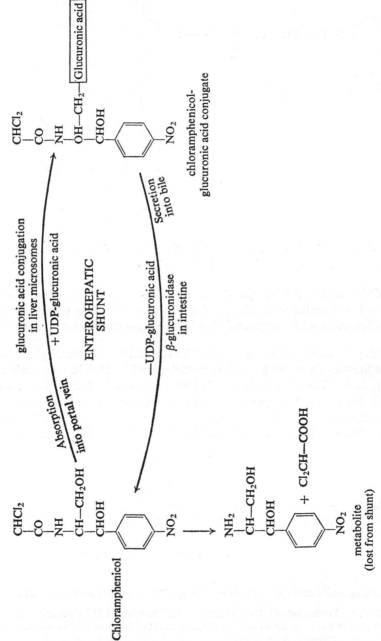

FIG. 19.5. Metabolic cycle of chloramphenicol in entero-hepatic shunt.

of hepatic cells. Normal constituents of the body that are conjugated with glucuronic acid include bilirubin and the steroid hormones. Both the carboxylic groups of bilirubin (Fig. 8.4, page 236) are conjugated to yield the diglucuronic acid derivative, which is excreted in the urine much more rapidly than bilirubin itself. A deficiency of UDP-glucuronyl transferase results in the accumulation of bilirubin in the body (jaundice). Steroid-glucuronic acid conjugates are also rapidly excreted.

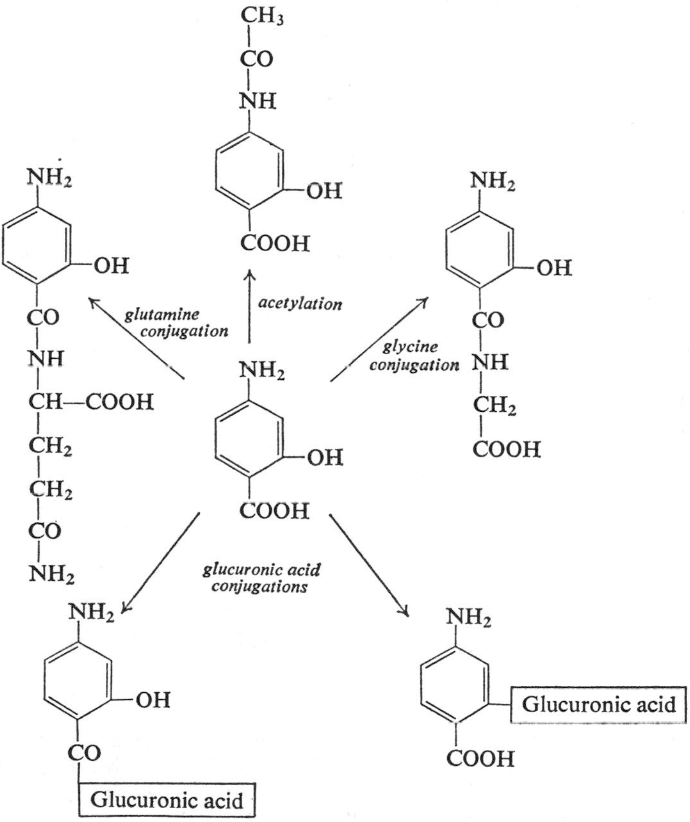

FIG. 19.6. Metabolic conversions of *p*-aminosalicylic acid.

Glucuronic acid conjugates are secreted into the bile then enter the intestine. An enzyme, β-glucuronidase, may then hydrolyse the conjugate. The drug which is released may then be reabsorbed, carried into the portal vein to the liver and again conjugated. This metabolic cycle occurs with phenolphthalein and chloramphenicol (Fig. 19.5).

Multiplicity of routes of metabolism. Some drugs are conjugated almost exclusively in one way. Phenylacetic acid, for example, appears in the urine as phenylacetylglycine corresponding to about 90% of the amount administered.

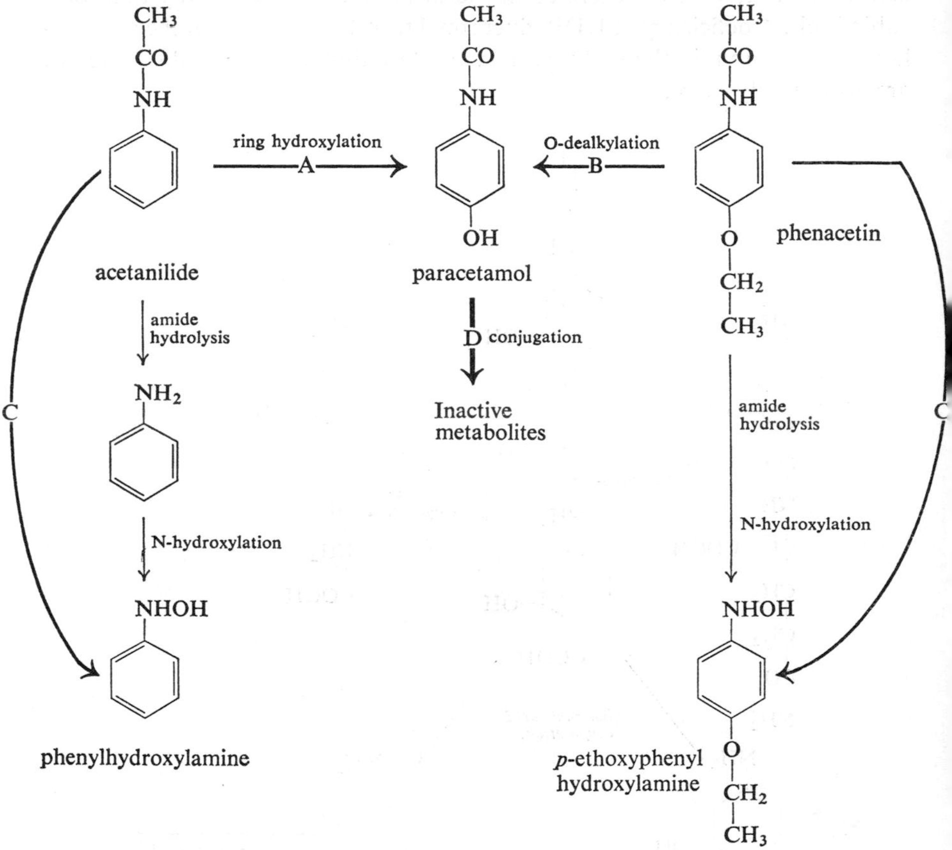

FIG. 19.7. Types of metabolic conversion. A and B—increased pharmacological activity (analgesia) of metabolites; C—altered pharmacological activity (the hydroxyl-amines convert haemoglobin to methaemoglobin); D—detoxication. (Adapted from Axelrod, see Brodie and Gillette in 'Further Reading'.)

However, many drugs are subject to several alternative conjugations, as shown for *p*-aminosalicylic acid in Fig. 19.6. Metabolism may proceed not only by different pathways but also to various degrees of completeness before the metabolites are excreted. Thalidomide gives rise to at least 17 metabolites that have been identified in the urine, and this posed quite a problem in attempts to determine which of these substances was responsible for the teratogenic effects observed after thalidomide administration. The possibilities that are inherent in drug metabolism for changing the intensity or the nature of the pharmacological effects can be seen in the simpler case of the acetanilide analgesics (Fig. 19.7). The pathways of metabolism of a drug may vary from one species to another (page 559).

The role of liver microsomes in drug metabolism. The most important group of enzymes involved in drug metabolism is in the liver. Within the liver cells, drug metabolizing enzymes are present in the cytoplasm and in mitochondria, but the microsomes of the liver cells contain the most versatile range of enzymes.

Certain of the metabolic changes described above are entirely or predominately brought about by liver microsomal enzymes. To summarize briefly these are the following:

Oxidations	hydroxylation of aromatic ring and alkyl side chains; oxidative deamination and dealkylation; formation of sulphoxides.
Reductions	conversion of nitro and azo groups to amines.
Cleavages	hydrolysis of esters and amides.
Conjugations	formation and transfer of glucuronic acid.

In general, the effect of these metabolic changes is to increase the water solubility, hence the rate of excretion, of the metabolites. The microsomal enzymes act only on substances that have a high lipid solubility. This suggests that diffusion through the lipid membrane of the microsome is the deciding factor in determining which drugs are metabolized by them. The striking aspect of drug metabolism by the microsomal enzymes is that the rate of metabolism can be changed considerably, being either increased or decreased.

ACTIVATION OF LIVER MICROSOMAL ENZYMES. Activation of liver microsomal enzyme activity was first observed with the cyclic hydrocarbons, 3-methylcholanthrene and 3,4-benzpyrene. Later it was observed with barbiturates, analgesics and a wide range of other drugs (Table 19.4). These activators have nothing in common as far as their pharmacological activity or their chemical structures are concerned, but they *are* all subject to metabolism by microsomal enzymes systems. However, it should be pointed out that activation of the microsomal enzymes does not necessarily follow from the presentation of substrate to these enzymes.

The increase in activity of the microsomal enzymes can be measured *in vitro* as the rate of utilization of a substrate. *In vivo*, the increased enzyme activity

TABLE 19.4. Effects of drugs on activity of liver microsomal enzymes.

Type of drug	Stimulate activity	No effect	Depress activity*
Anaesthetics	Ether, Chloroform Nitrous oxide	Divinyl ether, Halothane	Ether (sl.)
Hypnotics and sedatives	Barbiturates, Glutethimide Urethane, Chlorobutanol, Carbromal, Pyridione, Methylprylone	Ethinamate, Hydroxydione, Thalidomide, Paraldehyde	Ethanol (sl.) Chloralhydrate (sl.) Chloralose (sl.)
Tranquillizers	Phenaglycodol, Meprobamate, Chlorpromazine, Triflupromazine	Promazine, Chlordiazepoxide	Meprobamate (sl.)
Anticonvulsants	Primidone, Phenytoin, Methoin, Paramethadione	Troxidone	Phenytoin (sl.)
Muscle relaxants	Orphenadrine, Carisoprodol, Mephenesin	Zoxazolamine	
Analeptics and psychomotor stimulants	Nikethamide, Bemegride, Imipramine, Iproniazid	Leptazol, Amphetamine	Pheniprazine, Iproniazid
Analgesics	Phenylbutazone, Amidopyrine, Pethidine		Morphine (and congeners)
Antihistamine	Diphenhydramine, Chlorcyclizine		
Sulphonamides	Tolbutamide, Carbutamide	Sulphanilamide	
Antibiotics			Chloramphenicol
Steroids	Androgens, Adrenocorticoids, Dihydrocholesterol, -ergosterol		Oestrogens, Progesterones
Polycyclic hydrocarbons	3,4-Benzpyrene, 3-Methylcholanthrene, 1,2,5,6-Dibenzanthracene		
Insecticides	Chlorinated hydrocarbons (DDT, dieldrin, aldrin, etc.)	Pyrethrum Piperonyl butoxide	

* sl. = slight effect. Note some drugs entered in more than one column, for explanation, see text.

results in a decrease in the effectiveness or the duration of action of drugs that are inactivated by these enzymes. Two examples are given in Fig. 19.8; strychnine is less effective in rats that metabolize it more rapidly because of pretreatment with microsomal enzyme activators; and zoxazolamine produces a shorter lasting effect when microsomal metabolism has been activated.

Drugs which increase microsomal enzyme activity enhance their own rates of metabolism. For instance, the duration of the anaesthesia produced by phenobarbitone becomes shorter with repeated trials and the increase in the rate of metabolism explains the appearance of this tolerance.

The hypothesis that the production of new enzymes is induced by the administration of substances foreign to the body was proposed by Abderhalden in 1910; he termed these new enzymes *protective ferments*. The intravenous injection of sucrose in dogs gives rise to the appearance of sucrase (invertase) in the plasma, and the oral administration of lactose induces the presence of

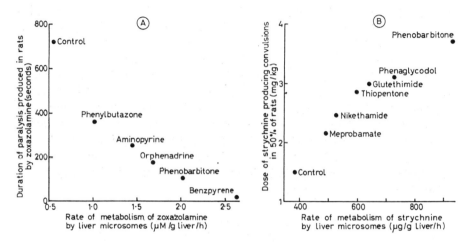

FIG. 19.8. Effects of pretreatment with drugs that activate liver microsomal enzymes. A. On duration of action and rate of metabolism of zoxazolamine. Results determined on the day after the following pretreatments: phenylbutazone, 125 mg/kg/day for 4 days; aminopyrine 125 mg/kg/day for 4 days; orphenadrine, 50 mg/kg/day for 4 days; phenobarbitone, 75 mg/kg day for 4 days; benzpyrene, 25 mg/kg on 1 day. (Adapted from Conney, see Brodie and Gillette in 'Futher Reading'.) B. On convulsive dose and rate of metabolism of strychnine. Results determined 48 hours after the following pretreatments: meprobamate, 200 mg/kg; nikethamide, 150 mg/kg; thiopentone, 30 mg/kg; glutethimide, 80 mg/kg; phenaglycodol, 130 mg/kg; phenobarbitone, 90 mg/kg. (Adapted from Kato, R., Chiesara, E. and Vassanelli, P. (1962). *Biochem. Pharmacol.*, **11**, 913.)

lactase in the pancreatic juice. These special instances of enzyme induction are overshadowed by the capacity for induction of the microsomal enzymes.

In the new born, the activity of microsomal enzymes is low, and generally increases gradually after birth, but administration of an activating drug rapidly accelerates their rate of appearance. Similarly in adult animals and man, when microsomal enzymatic activity is low, it can be considerably boosted by giving activating drugs. Microsomal enzyme activity is low during starvation, and in patients with cancer, liver disorder (e.g. obstructive jaundice), or severe burns, and in animals with alloxan-induced diabetes. Under these circumstances there is also a deficiency of other enzymes that are produced in the liver (e.g. plasma cholinesterase).

Polycyclic hydrocarbons activate principally the microsomal hydroxylating enzymes and produce this effect rapidly whereas the other activators induce a wider range of enzymes but their effect is slower in onset and less intense. The stimulation of the glucuronic acid conjugating mechanisms is reflected in an increase in the excretion of glucuronic acid in the urine (there is also an increased excretion of ascorbic acid in the dog and the rat). After being activated the enzyme activity gradually reverts back to its original level. The increased enzyme activity is due to the production of new enzyme and can be prevented by the following substances that impair protein synthesis in various ways: (i) Ethionine, an antimetabolite of methionine, combines with ATP to form S-adenosyl-ethionine. This blocks transmethylations which require S-adenosyl-methionine; these are necessary to produce some of the amino acids required in protein synthesis (see Fig. 2.11). (ii) Puromycin, an antibiotic, blocks the transfer of RNA-bound amino acids to the new protein chain. (iii) Actinomycin D, an antibiotic, is bound to DNA and blocks the synthesis of nuclear (messenger) RNA.

INHIBITION OF MICROSOMAL ENZYME ACTIVITY. Table 19.4 lists some drugs that decrease the activity of the liver microsomal enzymes. The compound known as SKF 525-A is a powerful inhibitor of these enzymes. It is believed to act by preventing the penetration of drugs into the microsomes. The structures of SKF 525-A and a number of other inhibitors of microsomal enzymes are shown in Fig. 19.9.

After repeated administration of some of the inhibitors, the activity of the microsomal enzymes recovers and then increases; this has been shown for iproniazid, tolbutamide, carbutamide, CFT 1201 and SKF 525-A.

Iproniazid is an inhibitor of monoamine oxidase and of other extra-microsomal enzymes, and SKF 525-A also inhibits a number of other enzymes. They have been termed 'multi-potent' enzyme inhibitors.

Sex differences in response to drugs are largely due to the influence of sex hormones on microsomal enzyme activity; androgens stimulate activity, whereas oestrogens and progesterone inhibit. It has been shown that male rats metabolize hexobarbitone more rapidly than do females, and that the duration of hexobarbitone anaesthesia is shorter in males than in females. Strychnine is more toxic to female than to male rats, but after depressing microsomal enzyme activity with SKF 525-A, strychnine is more toxic to both sexes, and there is no difference between them in their sensitivity.

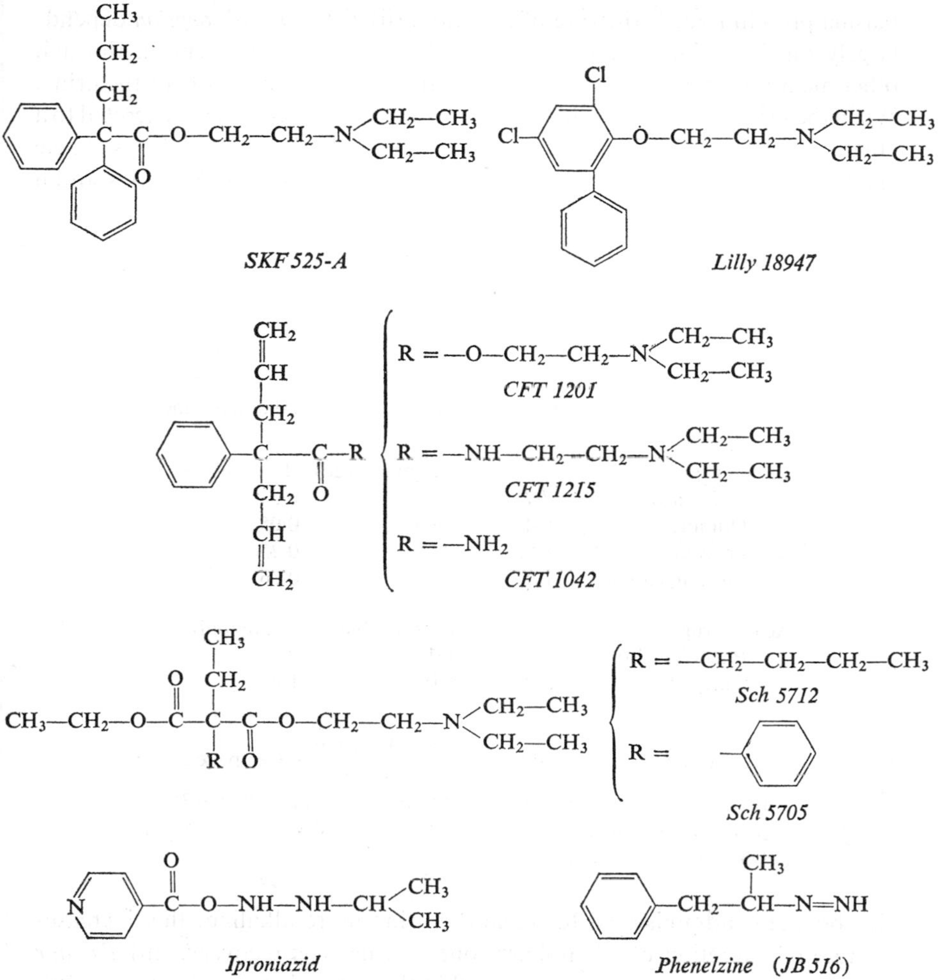

CH₃—CH₂—CH₂— ... (chemical structures)

SKF 525-A

Lilly 18947

R = —O—CH₂—CH₂—N(CH₂—CH₃)(CH₂—CH₃)

CFT 1201

R = —NH—CH₂—CH₂—N(CH₂—CH₃)(CH₂—CH₃)

CFT 1215

R = —NH₂

CFT 1042

R = —CH₂—CH₂—CH₂—CH₃

Sch 5712

R =

Sch 5705

Iproniazid

Phenelzine (JB 516)

Fɪɢ. 19.9. Some inhibitors of liver microsomal enzyme activity. Many of these compounds have not been assigned familiar names or approved names and are designated by laboratory serial numbers.

Drug excretion

The principal route of excretion of drugs and drug metabolites is in the urine, the rate and extent of urinary excretion being governed by three factors: glomerular filtration, tubular reabsorption and tubular excretion. (i) *Glomerular filtration* of any substance proceeds at a rate which depends on its molecular weight and on its concentration in free solution in the plasma. Binding to

17*

plasma protein retards the rate of filtration. (ii) *Tubular reabsorption* depends largely on the lipid/water partition coefficient (as does absorption through other membranes) and for ionizing drugs this depends on the pH of the urine. When the urine is acid, basic drugs are more highly ionized and are excreted to a greater extent than in alkaline urine; the converse holds for acid drugs (Table 19.5). In the treatment of overdosage with phenobarbitone (pK_a 7·2), sodium

TABLE 19.5. Dependence of rate of urinary excretion of drugs on degree of ionization.

Drug	pK_a	Rates of urinary clearance*	
		Acid urine	Alkaline urine
Basic drugs		(more ionized)	(less ionized)
Quinacrine	7·7	3·0	0·5
Quinine	8·4	0·65	0·05
Procaine	8·95	2·25	0·25
Mecamylamine	11·2	4·6	0·06
Acidic drugs		(less ionized)	(more ionized)
Phenobarbitone	7·2	0·1	0·7
Salicylate	3·0	0·02	1·6

* Clearance ratios, equal to $\dfrac{\text{clearance of substance}}{\text{clearance of inulin}}$ (see page 349).

Ratios higher than 1 imply tubular secretion (see pages 349 to 351). [Data from Milne, M.D., Scribner, B. H. and Crawford, M.A. (1958) *Am. J. Med.*, **24**, 709.]

bicarbonate is administered to make the urine more alkaline: this increases the rate of excretion of phenobarbitone and hastens recovery. (iii) *Tubular secretion* is one of the factors concerned in the formation of urine (page 350).

The cells of the proximal convoluted tubule actively transport certain substances from the plasma into the tubular urine; there are at least two transport mechanisms—one for acidic, the other for basic substances (Table 19.6). It is the *ionized* molecules that are transported. Substances that are transported by the same mechanism compete with each other; the more slowly a substance is transported the more effectively this substance inhibits the transport of another. The effect of a number of acidic dyes in inhibiting the transport of phenolsulphonphthalein is shown in Table 19.7.

Drugs which are insoluble in lipid are usually excreted in the urine in an unchanged form, whereas lipid soluble drugs usually undergo metabolism

TABLE 19.6. Examples of drugs and drug metabolites that are actively excreted into the renal tubules.

Acids	Bases
Penicillin	Quaternary ammonium compounds
Chlorothiazide	(e.g. choline, tetraethylammonium,
Salicylic acid	N-methylnicotine, N-methylnico-
Phenolsulphonphthalein	tinamide)
Diodone	Guanidine derivatives
Carinamide	Tolazoline
Probenecid	Quinine
Cinchophen	Mepiperphenidol
p-Aminohippuric acid and other	
glycine conjugates	
Glucuronic acid conjugates	
Sulphuric acid conjugates	

before being excreted. The metabolic changes that facilitate excretion are those in which the products are more polar and less lipid soluble. The formation of conjugates with sulphate, amino acids and glucuronic acid is particularly effective in increasing the polarity of drug molecules.

TABLE 19.7. Relationship between rate of tubular secretion of some acidic substances and their ability to inhibit the tubular secretion of phenol-sulphonphthalein (PSP; phenol red). (Observations in the chicken.)

Substances	Rate of secretion		Inhibition of PSP secretion	
	T_m* μM/min	Relative rate of secretion (PSP = 100%)	μM/min producing 50% inhibition	Relative inhibitory potency (BCB = 100%)
Phenolsulphonphthalein	3·	100	—	—
Carinamide	2	67	1	1
Xylenol blue	1	33	0·7	1·4
Chlorophenol red / Bromophenol red	0·5	17	0·2	5
Bromochlorophenol red / Thymol blue	0·1	3·3	0·04	25
Bromothymol blue	0·06	2	0·03	33
Bromophenol blue	0·04	1·3	0·01	100
Bromocresol purple / Bromocresol blue (BCB)	0·03	1	0·01	100

* The determination of the maximal rate of tubular secretion (T_m) is dealt with on page 351.
[Adapted from Sperber, I (1954). *Arch. Int. Pharmacodyn.* **27**, 221.]

POTENTIATION OF DRUG ACTION BY INHIBITION OF TUBULAR SECRE-
TION. At the time when penicillin was scarce and expensive, the inhibition of
its tubular secretion by drugs was a practical procedure for prolonging the
action of a small dose. With improved methods of penicillin production this is
no longer necessary and prolongation of action is obtained with depot preparations. The drugs that were used to inhibit tubular secretion are probenecid
and carinamide (Fig. 19.10). These two substances are acids, and being actively

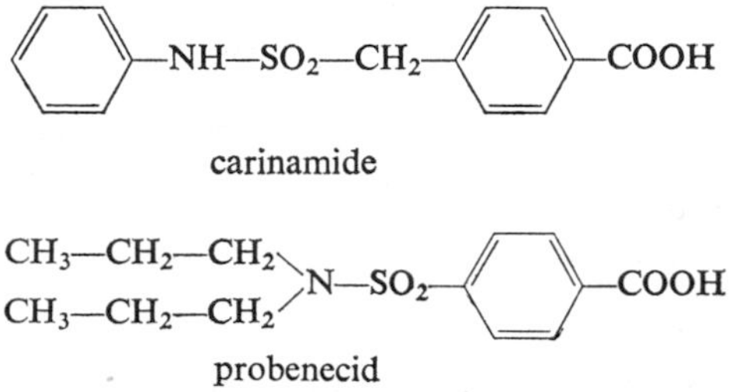

carinamide

probenecid

FIG. 19.10. Competitive inhibitors of active transport of anions across epithelium
of renal tubules into urine.

transported into the urine by the same mechanisms that transport other acids,
they competitively inhibit acid transport. Thus they potentiate and prolong the
action of a variety of acidic drugs.

Active transport through the tubular epithelium is also concerned in the
reabsorption of some constituents of the glomerular filtrate (page 350) and is
inhibited by the same agents that inhibit secretion. Probenecid and salicylates
are used to promote the urinary excretion of uric acid and are termed *uricosuric*
agents.

EXCRETION OF DRUGS INTO THE INTESTINAL TRACT. The factors which
determine the absorption and the distribution of drugs in the body are also
concerned in the elimination of drugs and metabolites in the faeces. The important considerations are (i) the relative proportion of lipid diffusing molecules in the plasma and the gut, and (ii) active transport into the gut. Metals
that combine with fatty acids to form insoluble soaps are eliminated with the
faeces. Active transport into the gut takes place mainly by way of the bile.
There are two transport mechanisms; one for lipid-insoluble carbohydrates
(e.g. dextran, mannitol, sucrose, inulin), and another for acids. The mechanism
for transporting acidic drugs into the bile resembles that of the kidney in that
ionized molecules are transported. Normal constituents of the body that are
transported into the bile include bilirubin and bile acids; diagnostic agents
that are transported include the dyes, phenolsulphonphthalein and fluorescein,
and iodine-containing radio-opaque substances; drugs that are transported

include penicillin; drug-conjugates with glucuronic acid that are transported into the bile and subsequently hydrolysed and reabsorbed were mentioned in connection with the enterohepatic shunt (page 515). Radio-opaque substances that undergo active transport into the bile or into the urine are put to practical use in outlining the biliary or the urinary tract in X-ray examination: their formulae are shown in Table 19.8.

TABLE 19.8. Radiocontrast media secreted into the urine or bile.

Compounds given by intravenous injection for outlining the urinary tract (urography) or renal pelvis (pyelography).

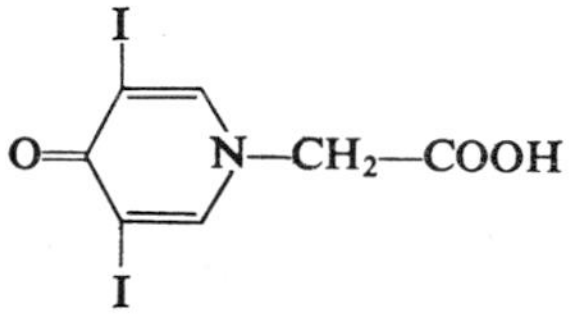

diodone

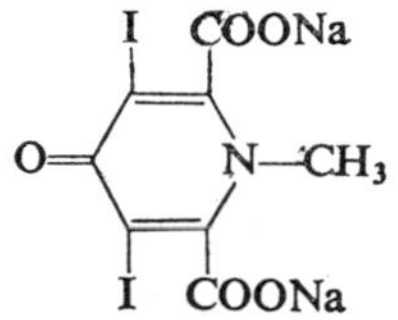

iodoxyl

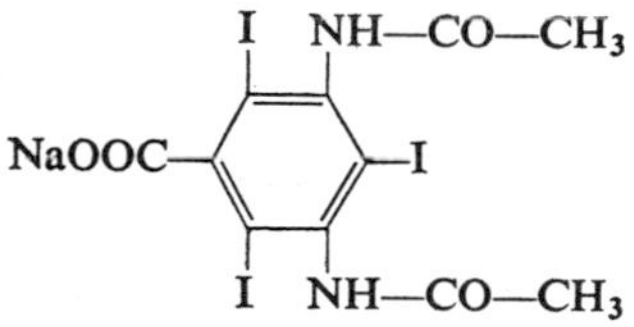

sodium diatrizoate

methiodal sodium

Compounds given by intravenous injection for outlining the gall bladder (cholecystography) or bile duct (cholangiography).

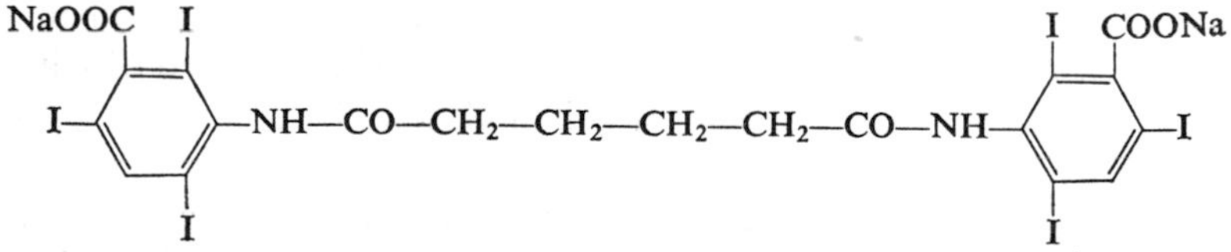

iodipamide (di-sodium salt; also used as di-methylglucamine salt).

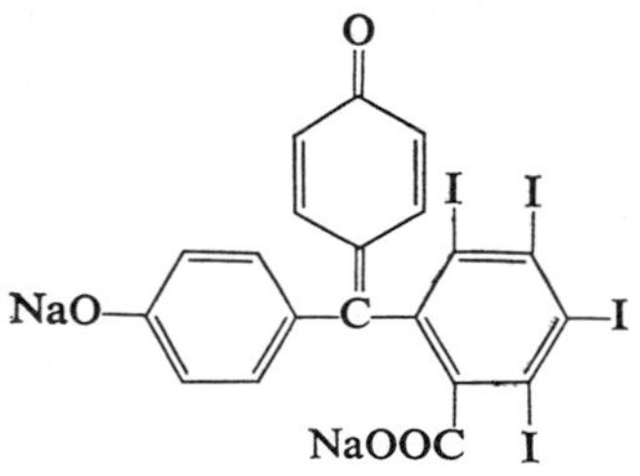

tetraiodophthalein

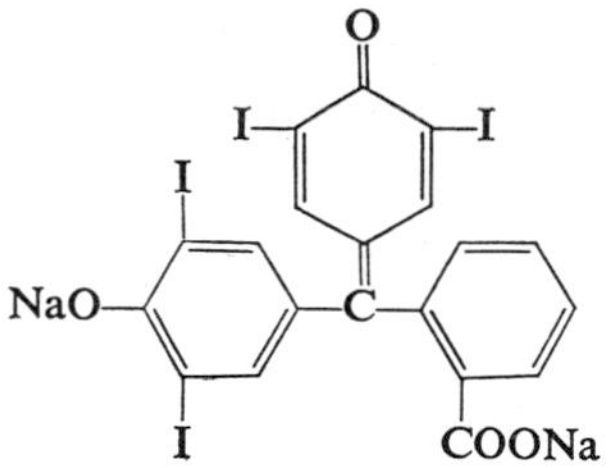

iodophthalein

TABLE 19.8—*continued*

Compounds given by mouth for outlining the gall bladder. (The phenolphthalein derivatives above may also be given by mouth.)

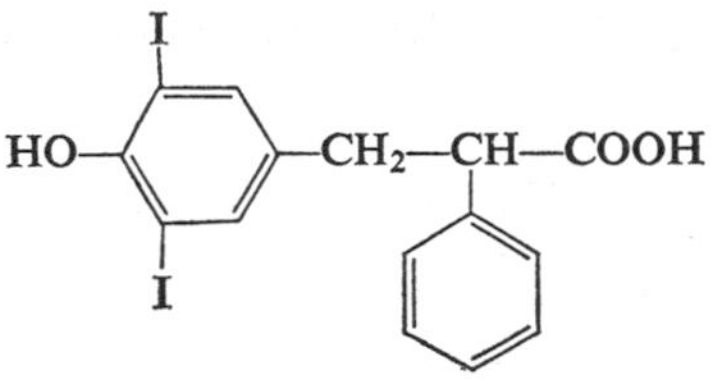

pheniodol

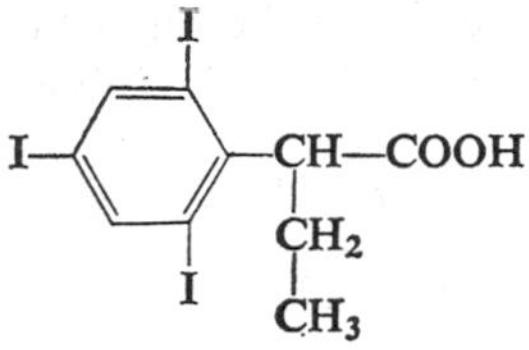

phenobutiodil

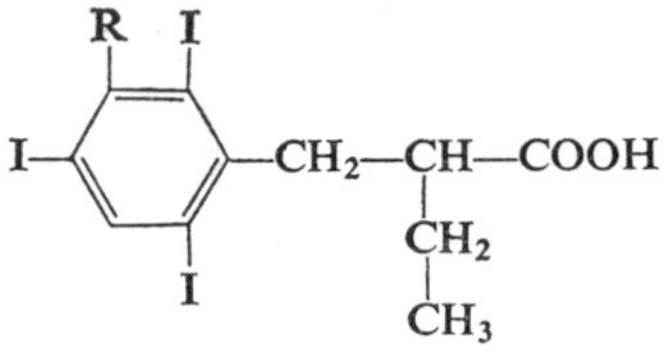

R = —NH$_2$ iopanoic acid

R = —OH   iophenoxic acid

MINOR ROUTES OF DRUG EXCRETION include the lungs, and the fluid of saliva, tears, sweat and milk. Few drugs or metabolites are actively transported into these fluids; one exception appears to be the secretion of thiocyanate into saliva. Most drugs pass into the fluids from the plasma by lipid diffusion and are distributed in accord (i) with the proportion of ionized molecules and (ii) with the degree of binding on either side of the membranes of the gland; since the volumes of the secretions are small, only small amounts of drugs are lost. The presence of drugs in the milk may affect a breast-fed child. Small amounts of penicillin are present in the milk of cows that have been treated with it and it has been suggested that ingestion of this milk may be a cause of penicillin hypersensitivity.

The gaseous and volatile anaesthetics are eliminated from the body in the same way as they are absorbed—by diffusion through the alveolar epithelium in accord with their concentration gradient. For other drugs, elimination through the lungs is insignificant, although pronounced odours may be imparted to the breath.

General considerations in drug administration

The concentration of a drug in the blood depends on the balance between the rate at which it is absorbed and the rate at which it is lost. The loss is due to a combination of binding in the tissues, metabolism and excretion. The rate of loss of many drugs is proportional to their concentration in the blood, and the graph of concentration against time is an exponential 'decay' curve. Such a decay can be characterized by its 'half-life'; in this case, the time for the concentration in the blood to decrease by one-half. When the concentration of drug is high, its rate of loss is fast, but as the concentration falls, the rate of loss becomes slower. When a drug is given intravenously, the concentration in the blood reaches its peak value almost immediately and so the rate of loss is high. In Fig. 19.11a, curve A illustrates the blood concentration after intravenous administration of a drug which has a half-life of 45 min. When the same drug is given by routes in which the time taken for absorption introduces a delay, the peak concentration is lower; furthermore, the rate of loss from the blood is less rapid, partly because of the lower peak concentration, and partly because absorption and loss are going on simultaneously. The slower the rate of absorption, the lower the peak concentration and the longer the persistence in the blood (compare curves B, C and D in Fig. 19.11a). If the

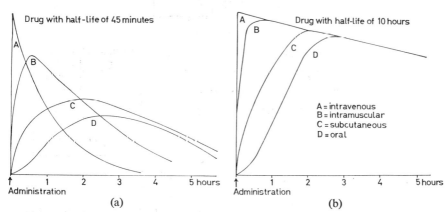

Fig. 19.11. Blood concentrations of drugs with different half-lives after administration by various routes.

route of administration imposes a delay due to absorption and, if the rate of loss of a drug from the blood is rapid, a larger dose is needed to reach a given blood level than when the drug is injected intravenously; moreover, if the doses given by two different routes are adjusted so that they give rise to the same peak concentration, then the persistence in the blood is longer for the route from which there is slower absorption.

Some drugs which are rapidly lost from the blood produce only a transient effect when a single dose is injected intravenously; this is observed, for example, with choline esters, catecholamines, and many other pharmacologically active substances which occur in tissues; synthetic drugs that rapidly disappear from the blood include thiopentone, suxamethonium and trimetaphan, and with these the *rate* of intravenous injection is adjusted to produce the desired level of *effect*. Drugs that are lost slowly are only given intravenously if a rapid onset of action is required, since the blood level reached after administration by other routes is nearly as high (assuming complete absorption): this situation is illustrated in Fig. 19.11b.

What has been said above about the concentration of a drug in the blood also applies to the concentration of the drug in any other tissue, where the amount present at any time depends on the rate of arrival and the rate of loss. The calculation of the amount of a drug at its site of action, or in another tissue, may be difficult when there are many interacting factors to be taken into account; as for example, in the hypothetical, but by no means far fetched, situation pictured below:

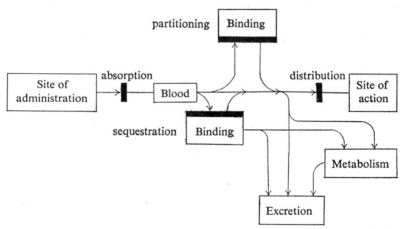

Recently, computers have been used to analyse such situations, both in hypothetical models, and in studies where actual measurements have been made. Using this approach, it has been possible to assign quantitative values to the rates of exchange of drug between blood and other tissues.

The rate of elimination of a drug determines the regime of dosage. Fig. 19.12 shows the blood concentrations of a drug with a half-life of 16 h when it is given once daily, and when one-third of the daily dose is given at 8-hourly intervals. The large dose given once daily produces a high peak concentration straight away but there is a pronounced downwards swing until the next dose is given. The smaller dose given 3 times a day results in a slow build up of the blood concentration but this is then maintained at a much steadier level than with daily dosage. The practice of giving a large initial dose and then a series of small doses is employed with many drugs. The first dose, or priming dose, rapidly raises the concentration of drug to the effective level, and it is then maintained there by giving repeated small doses. Sulphonamides are usually given in this way, the first dose being twice the maintenance dose. Another example is digoxin, where the 'digitalizing dose' (as the priming dose of digitalis and the cardiac glycosides is called) is 1 to 1·5 mg, and the maintenance dose is 0·25 mg daily or twice daily.

When the rate of administration of a drug exceeds the rate of elimination, the amount in the tissues steadily accumulates. This is a more likely occurrence

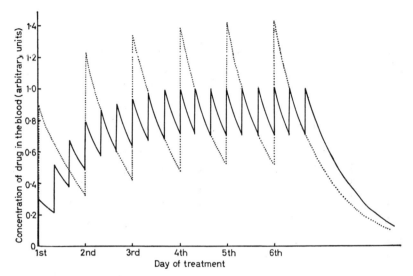

FIG. 19.12. Blood concentrations of a drug with a half-life of 16 h, administered in daily doses (----) and in divided doses given 8-hourly (——). If it is assumed that the effective concentration is 0·7 unit per ml. of blood, then: daily dosage produces this for 7 h in the 1st day, 12 h in the 2nd, and 16 h in the 3rd and every subsequent day; 8-hourly dosage does not produce this level in the 1st day, produces it for 13 hours in the 2nd day, 22 h in the 3rd day, and thereafter, 24 h a day.

with drugs that are slowly eliminated, and such drugs are said to be *cumulative*. Figure 19.13 illustrates the difference in accumulation of two drugs, each given daily in the same dose: one has a half-life of 80 h in the body and the other of 16 h. Cumulation is pronounced for the drug with the longer half-life. Some substances are retained in the body for considerable periods, and have half-lives measured in weeks, months, or even years. Prolonged retention constitutes a hazard with certain poisonous substances encountered by workers in various industries, lead poisoning being a well-recognized example. The longer the period of retention, the greater the risk that repeated exposure will lead to cumulation of an amount that produces toxic effects. With very prolonged retention, the *total* of previous exposures throughout the life of the individual may be a better indication of the risk of toxic cumulation than the interval between exposures.

The term cumulation is applied not only to the retention of a drug or poison in the body, but also to the persistence of the *effect*. The effect may outlast the presence of the drug, as in the case of some organo-phosphorus cholinesterase inhibitors; for example, dyflos (page 719) does not persist as such in the body,

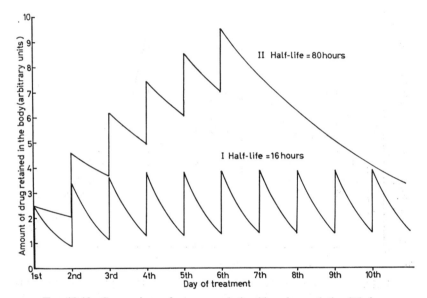

FIG. 19.13. Comparison of a noncumulative (I) and cumulative (II) drug.

but its effect persists since the recovery of cholinesterase activity depends on the formation of new enzyme—a slow process. The possibility of cumulation is particularly insidious when the action of the poisonous substance is to destroy or damage permanently a portion of the tissues, especially if the action is so slight as to be undetectable after a single exposure. The liver damage produced by carbon tetrachloride is such an effect, and irreparable damage to tissues produced by substances that give off ionizing radiations is another.

The therapeutic concentrations of drugs may also be built up slowly; although it is not customary to refer to this as cumulation, it may amount to the same thing. The slow build up in concentration of the drug given at 8-hourly intervals in Fig. 19.12 portrays this eventuality. The therapeutic effect may be cumulative even though the drug is eliminated; an example of this is encountered in the treatment of mental illness or hypertension with reserpine, when each of the twice or thrice daily doses goes a little further in producing the effect (probably, depletion of catecholamines, see page 839); small doses are usually given and the therapeutic effect may take as long as 5 days to come on; large doses act more rapidly but cause a number of unpleasant side effects. A latent period between the administration of a drug and the appearance of the response may also occur when a pro-drug has to be metabolized into an active form. Imipramine, a drug used to relieve mental depression, may have to be given for longer than a week before useful results are obtained, but one of its metabolites, desmethylimipramine, is effective in a day or two.

CHAPTER 20

Evaluation of Drug Action

The quantitative aspects of drug action are concerned with the potency of drugs in producing effects, and the qualitative aspects are concerned with the nature of the various actions produced by drugs. Most of the following chapters are concerned with the qualitative aspects of drug action, but it should be borne in mind that in pharmacology, as in other sciences, measurement and the quantitative expression of data is a central problem.

This chapter deals firstly with the statistical concepts and procedures that are used in the quantitative evaluation of drug action. These were developed largely in connection with *bioassay* and with comparisons between drugs.

The object of bioassay is the measurement of the amount of a drug in terms of its biological activity. Comparisons of the potency of different drugs in producing the same action are also of value for a number of reasons, as, for example, in determining the relationship between chemical structure and pharmacological activity, and in 'screening' compounds that are being assessed for their ability to produce a certain action. The quantitative evaluation of drug action is of considerable importance in comparing the relative efficacy of treatment of patients with different drugs. Frequently it is necessary to consider qualitative differences in drug action in addition to quantitative differences. This is particularly so in the screening of potential therapeutic agents when it is necessary to reject compounds having untoward or dangerous actions in addition to the desired action.

Variability in pharmacological responses

Repeated measurements of the same amount do not yield identical results. This holds just as much for the so-called exact sciences as in the biological sciences. This variability arises from errors in measurement, and its extent largely depends on the method used. There are two classes of error in measurement. In the first place, there are systematic errors which yield results that are consistently too high or too low: such errors are said to be *lacking in accuracy* and are not amenable to statistical treatment. Then there are results which differ at random from the true value, some being larger and some smaller: errors of this type are *lacking in precision* and can be treated statistically.

In biology, there is another source of variability in that the thing being measured may vary in magnitude from one individual to another or from time to time in a single individual. It is a matter of common observation that biological material is by its nature variable, so much so that, amongst human beings, differences are taken for granted (for example, in height, weight, colouring, or in shape of features), whereas similarities provoke comment. Almost any biological phenomenon which can be measured is found to vary from one individual to another.

In pharmacology, the main concern is with variability in responses to drugs. When the lethal dose of a drug is determined in a number of animals, the dose is found to vary from one animal to another. Again, when responses to a fixed dose of a drug are elicited from time to time in the same animal (or in a preparation of isolated tissue), they are found to vary. In addition to graded differences, there is another type of variation between otherwise closely related individuals and this consists of the presence or absence of a particular characteristic. In pharmacology, this shows itself in the presence or absence of a response to the same dose of a drug given to a number of animals. The experimental material used by pharmacologists is a group of animals, an animal or a preparation consisting of animal tissue. Considerable time and trouble has been spent in many pharmacological laboratories in establishing stocks of animals that are as homogeneous as possible with the object of reducing the variability in response to drugs. Although this improves the precision of quantitative data, there is the limitation that the findings may be of less general applicability.

Quantitative observations in pharmacology are frequently subject to rather large experimental errors (error, in this context, implies variability in experimental results due to the random operation of chance factors). There are two ways of reducing the error. One is to refine the techniques of observation and measurement, although, in pharmacological experiments, the biological variability of the experimental matter provides a limitation on this type of refinement. The other is to repeat the experiments and to take the average (mean) result. The error of a mean is inversely proportional to the square root of the number of observations; thus, the average of four observations has one-half the error of a single observation, with sixteen observations it is one quarter, and with a hundred observations it is one-tenth. However, there may be limitations on the number of times an experiment can be repeated; these are largely imposed by consideration of time and money, and a compromise must be made between these factors and the degree of precision required in the results.

The variability in responses of a piece of tissue to repeated applications of the same dose of a drug is illustrated in Fig. 20.1. The measured heights of the responses are given in Table 20.1. These results can be summarized by calculating the average (or *mean*) response. The response is usually designated as Y, the sum of responses as SY, the number of observations as N, and the mean as $\bar{Y}$. Then $\bar{Y} = SY/N$, and using the data in Table 20.1, $\bar{Y} = 132 \cdot 9/19 = 6 \cdot 995$ or 7 as a reasonable approximation.

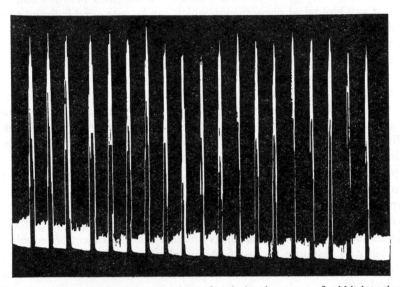

FIG. 20.1. Variability in the contractions of an isolated segment of rabbit intestine produced by acetylcholine (0·1 μg/ml). The preparation was in a bath of Tyrode's solution maintained at 35°C and bubbled with air. The contractions were recorded with an isotonic lever, magnification 4-fold, exerting a tension of 1·5 g on the tissue. The acetylcholine was left in contact for 30 sec before washing it out, and applications were repeated at intervals of 3 min.

TABLE 20.1. Results from the experiment illustrated in Fig. 20.1.
Responses (in cm to nearest 0·5 mm), Y

6·80	6·85	7·00	7·10
6·95	7·30	7·30	7·15
6·90	6·80	7·00	7·25
7·00	6·40	6·95	6·95
7·15	6·65	7·40	

Sum of responses $= SY = 132 \cdot 90$
Number of observations $= N = 19$
Mean response $= \bar{Y} = 6 \cdot 995$
Sum of squares of responses $= SY^2 = 930 \cdot 66$
Sum of squares of deviation from mean $= Sy^2 = SY^2 - (SY)^2/N$
$$= 930 \cdot 66 - (132 \cdot 9)^2/19$$
$$= 1 \cdot 0595$$

It is clearly desirable to indicate, in addition to the mean, the degree of variability of the responses, and one way of doing this is to give the *range*. For the data in Table 20.1, the mean is 7 cm with a range of 6·4 to 7·4 cm. The disadvantage of the range is that it is determined by only two observations— the most extreme ones—and takes no account of the way in which other results are distributed about the mean. In the example given, it can be seen that the response at the lower limit of the range (6·4 cm) is due to a single aberrant response. A better way to describe the variability of the responses is to relate them to the normal distribution curve.

The normal distribution. When variability is due to a number of random factors, the pattern of distribution of the values obtained from a large number of measurements is known as a *normal* or *Gaussian distribution* or a *normal error curve* (Fig. 20.2). It is immaterial whether the variability arises from lack of

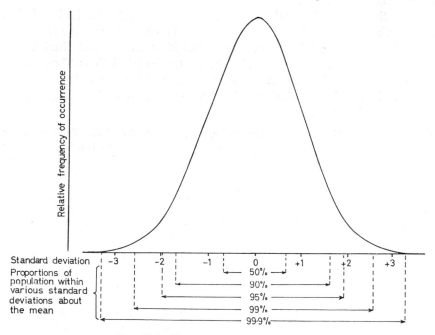

Fig. 20.2. The normal distribution curve.

precision in measurement or from biological variability; the errors from these two sources are usually indistinguishable and can be treated together. In a normal distribution, the values are distributed equally on either side of the mean and tend to cluster about the mean: values that are widely divergent from the mean occur less commonly. This distribution can be described mathematically; in fact, the curve was first produced as a result of the theoretical consideration of chance occurrences. The height on the ordinate of a point on the curve represents the frequency of an occurrence and the corresponding co-ordinate on the abscissa is in a unit known as a *standard deviation*. The area beneath a segment of the normal distribution curve is proportional to the fraction of the population of measurements that comprises the distribution, and this fraction represents the probability with which a single observation will fall within the particular area. There are published tables giving the number of standard deviations on each side of the mean which will enclose an area corresponding to any particular fraction of the population, (i.e. the probability that any single measurement will yield a value falling within this area, or lying within these standard deviations from the mean). Some values are given in Table 20.2 (first and second columns). These values have also been transferred to the curve in Fig. 20.2.

In the theoretical distribution curve discussed above, the standard deviation has been assigned a value of 1 (standard deviation unit), and the mean has been placed at the origin (zero). Figure 20.3 illustrates normal distributions that have different mean values and different standard deviations. These curves can be 'normalized', that is, converted to a scale with a mean of zero and the 'spread' in standard deviation units, and when that is done they can be exactly superimposed.

TABLE 20.2. Proportion of observations falling within standard deviation limits about the mean for an infinitely large sample and for smaller samples. This table is taken from Table III of Fisher, R. A. & Yates, F. (1963) *Statistical Tables for Biological, Agricultural and Medical Research*, 6 ed. Oliver & Boyd, Edinburgh and by permission of the authors and publishers.

Fraction of population between standard deviations each side of mean (or probability of occurrence)	Standard deviation units (values of t at $N=\infty$)	Values of t for small samples (column 1 refers to probability of occurrence of values)		
		$N=2$	$N=5$	$N=25$
1/2 = 50%	0·67	1·00	0·74	0·68
9/10 = 90%	1·65	6·31	2·13	1·71
19/20 = 95%	1·96	12·71	2·78	2·06
99/100 = 99%	2·58	63·66	4·60	2·80
999/1000 = 99·9%	3·29	636·62	8·61	3·75

Although the normal distribution curve is the distribution that is found for an infinitely large number of observations (that is what is meant by a population), it can be applied to measurements made on a small sample. In this case, there is a reduced probability of the measurements falling within any pair of standard deviation limits. This can be stated in another way; namely, the smaller the sample size, the broader are the standard deviation units (values of t, see p. 539) on either side of the mean which will contain a given fraction of the sample. The statistic 't' has been calculated for sample sizes ranging from 2 to 200, and a few values are given in Table 20.2 (last 3 columns).

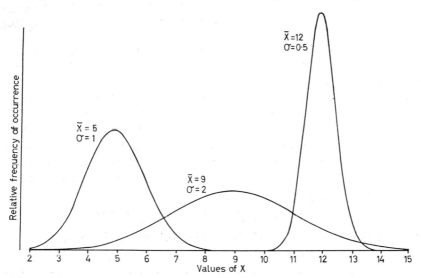

FIG. 20.3. Distributions having different mean values ($\bar{X}$) and standard deviations (σ).

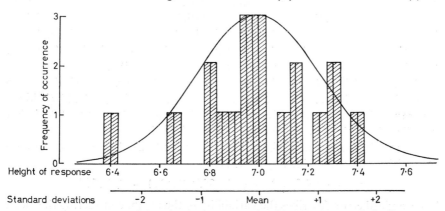

FIG. 20.4. Histogram of data from Fig. 20.1 and Table 20.1. A normal distribution curve with the same standard deviation as the experimental results has been superimposed on the histogram.

The experimental results from a small sample may be plotted in the form used for the normal distribution curve, that is, with the value of the variant on the abscissa and the frequency of occurrence of each value on the ordinate. A graph prepared in this way is known as a histogram. The data provided in Fig. 20.1 have been plotted as a histogram in Fig. 20.4. The resemblance between the form of this graph and that of the theoretical normal distribution is sketchy. Fortunately, however, any distribution with a peak near the mid-point can usually be assumed to be normally distributed, especially when the sample is small, and in any case normality may be checked by the χ^2 test (see p. 539).

Calculation of variance, standard deviation and standard error. The first step in calculating the variability of experimental data is to determine the sum of the squares of the differences of each response from the mean. There are two methods of computation. *First method:* The difference is determined for each observation $[(\bar{Y}-Y)]$, each of these differences is squared $[(\bar{Y}-Y)^2]$, and the squares are summed $[S(\bar{Y}-Y)^2$, which may be written as Sy^2 where y indicates a difference]. This method is tedious when there are many observations. *Second Method:* Each response is squared $[Y^2]$, the squares are summed $[SY^2]$, and then the sum of the squares of differences from the mean is given by the following equation:

$$Sy^2 \quad \text{or} \quad S(\bar{Y}-Y)^2 = SY^2-(SY)^2/N$$

Returning to the example used above (Fig. 20.1 and Table 20.1),

$$Sy^2 = 930{\cdot}66-132{\cdot}9^2/19 = 1{\cdot}0595.$$

The two methods are in fact algebraically identical, but the second method is much simpler in computation, especially when a calculating machine is used.

The variance (v) is the sum of squares of differences from the mean divided by the number of *degrees of freedom* (n) in the set of observations. In the example, one degree of freedom has been used up in assigning the mean, therefore $n=(N-1)$, Hence, $v=Sy^2/n=1{\cdot}0595/18=0{\cdot}0589$.

The *standard deviation* (symbolized as σ, the Greek letter, *sigma*) is the square root of the variance. Hence, $\sigma=\sqrt{(Sy^2/n)}=\sqrt{0{\cdot}0589}=\pm0{\cdot}2425$ (being a square root it has both a positive and a negative value). The standard deviation describes the variability of the observations *about* the mean.

The *standard error* (abbreviated to S.E., or symbolized as σ_m) is the square root of the variance divided by $\sqrt{N}$. Hence

$$\sigma_m = \sqrt{(Sy^2/Nn)} = \sqrt{(1{\cdot}0595/19 \times 18)} = \pm0{\cdot}0557$$

The standard error describes the variability *of* the mean, considering the mean of the particular set of observations as one of a number of possible values which might have been obtained from other similar sets of observations drawn from the same population.

Fiducial limits of a mean. The published tables of values of t corresponding to various probabilities (at the appropriate number of degrees of freedom) provide a way of calculating the limits within which the true mean of a set of observations will lie at a given level of probability. The assumption that underlies this calculation is that the experimental results are a sample from a population of results which are normally distributed about the mean of the population, and the means of a number of such samples would also be normally distributed about the population mean. The mean of the experimental data and the standard error of the mean are calculated. In the example, these figures are 7 ± 0.0557. When it is desired to know what are the limits within which 95% of the mean values determined in separate but similar experiments will fall, the value of t corresponding to a probability of 0.05 (at 18 degrees of freedom) is read from tables: it is 2.10. Then, the 95% fiducial limits for the mean are given by the following calculation: $\bar{Y} \pm \sigma_m \times t$. That is,

$$7 \pm 0.0557 \times 2.10 = 7 \pm 0.12 = 6.88 \text{ and } 7.12$$

Probability. This is a statistical term which expresses on a numerical scale the degree of certainty (or uncertainty) with which an assertion can be made. The scale runs from 0 to 1, or from 0 to 100%. Zero probability means that the assertion is completely unjustified, and a probability of 1 or 100% means that it is definitely true. The assertion that is generally made in a statistical analysis is that any difference between the experimental result and some theoretical result (or the result from another experiment) arose from chance alone and that in fact the difference in results is merely what would be expected from different samples drawn from the same population: this type of assertion is described as a *null hypothesis*.

The statistical tests commonly used in the analysis of pharmacological experiments are the following:

STUDENT'S 't'-TEST. This compares the difference between the mean values of two sets of observations, or the difference between a mean value from an experiment and some other theoretical value. It yields the value known as 't' (see p. 540).

FISHER'S ANALYSIS OF VARIANCE. The variance is a measure of the variability of experimental data and this analysis consists of determining the ratio of two variances. It yields a value known as 'F'.

THE χ^2 TEST. This compares the observed distribution of sets of experimental observations with some other distribution which might be expected on theoretical grounds. It yields a value known as 'χ^2'. (χ^2 is sometimes written as 'chi-squared'; χ is a Greek letter, pronounced kye.)

Each of the values, t, F and χ^2 is described as a *statistic*, and the values of these statistics corresponding to various levels of probability have been computed and are published in statistical tables. The statistic obtained from the analysis of the experimental data is compared with the published values in order to estimate the probability of the assertion made in the analysis. If the probability is low then the assertion may be rejected, whereas if the probability is high then the assertion is confirmed. Where the assertion has been a null hypothesis and the probability obtained from the analysis is low, then it follows that the difference that was tested was unlikely to have been due to chance factors and was probably due to the difference in the experimental conditions.

Level of significance. The decision about what particular level of probability will be accepted as significant is decided by the experimenter. A probability of 0·05 (5%) is usually sufficient to allow the experimenter to reject the null hypothesis and the difference is described as being *statistically significant*. This indicates that the experimenter believes that there is a true difference in the effects produced by two different experimental treatments, since if there were no real difference it would occur by chance only once in 20 similar experiments. Probabilities of 0·01 (1%) and 0·001 (1 in 1000) are sometimes called statistically highly significant and statistically very highly significant respectively. A higher probability than 0·05 does not indicate that the null hypothesis is correct but suggests that the results *could* be explained by chance factors alone. The following examples illustrate the reasoning involved in interpreting statistical analyses.

(1) THE USE OF THE t-TEST. The effects of equal doses of hexobarbitone and pentobarbitone, administered intraperitoneally, were compared. Two rats were injected with each drug and the duration of anaesthesia produced was hexobarbitone, 10 min and 12 min, and pentobarbitone, 14 min and 16 min. The null hypothesis was set up that the difference between the mean values (11 min and 15 min) could have arisen by chance and was not due to any real difference in duration of action between the two barbiturates. The value of t can be calculated from the formula

$$t = (\bar{Y}_A - \bar{Y}_B) \bigg/ \sqrt{\left\{ \frac{(N_A + N_B - 2) N_A N_B}{(Sy_A^2 + Sy_B^2)(N_A + N_B)} \right\}}$$

where suffixes A and B refer to the two samples. The calculated value of t for the data is 2·84 and the values of t from the published tables (at 2 degrees of freedom) are 1·89 and 2·92 corresponding to probabilities of 0·2 and 0·1 respectively. This means that by chance alone, without there being any difference between the two drugs, such a difference would be expected to occur between 1 and 2 times in every ten similar experiments. It would obviously be rash to consider that there was a difference in duration of action between the drugs, and even though there may be other reasons for thinking that there is a difference, it has not been demonstrated in the experiment. It is worth considering the effect of increasing the size of the experiment. Suppose that two additional rats were injected, and the results were hexobarbitone, 10, 11 and 12 min; and pentobarbitone, 14, 15 and 16 min. The mean values have remained the same, but the errors of each set of results has been decreased by repetition of the experiment. The calculated value of t is now 4·9 and the values of t (at 4 degrees of freedom) are 4·60 for a probability of 0·01 and 8·61 for a probability of 0·001. The experimental results would have occurred by chance between 1 in 100 and 1 in 1000 times in similar experiments if there was no difference between the drugs. It is unlikely therefore that the difference was due to chance, the null hypothesis is rejected, and the difference is described as statistically (highly) significant.

In the context of a statistical analysis, 'significant' has a technical (but arbitrary) meaning in describing the probability of an event in terms of a hypothesis of its occurrence. Accordingly, the particular statistical test used and the level of probability which corresponds to the derived statistic should be quoted. Thus, in the last example used above, the difference between the means would be described as 'statistically significant (t-test, $0·01 > P > 0·001$)'. In this usage as a technical term, 'significant' should not be confused with 'large' or 'important'. Nor should the experimenter fall into the trap of much repetition of experiments merely to produce a (statistically) significant difference if the difference, though real, is trivial. This last consideration is important in the clinical trial of a new drug which is intended for the treatment of a minor ailment, because the unknown risks which might accompany its use militate against its widespread employment unless it promises worthwhile improvement in therapy.

(2) THE USE OF ANALYSIS OF VARIANCE. Patients were being selected for use in a trial of an antihypertensive drug; of the 10 patients available, 5 were in one ward (ward A) and 5 in another ward (ward B). Their systolic blood pressures (mmHg) are given below:

| Patients in ward A | 200 | 210 | 180 | 190 | 200 |
| Patients in ward B | 150 | 190 | 240 | 200 | 200 |

The mean systolic pressure was the same in each ward, but it can be seen that the range of pressures in one group (A) was from 180 to 210, whereas in the other group (B) it was from 150 to 240. It is necessary to determine whether the variability within each group is the same, i.e., whether the two samples can be considered as coming from the same 'population.' (They could be from different populations if, for instance, there were differences either in the way the pressures were measured or in the criteria for admission to the wards.)

The null hypothesis is that there is no real difference between the samples, the differing degrees of variabilities being what might be expected by chance in samples of this size.

The variances of each group are calculated:

$$\text{For A, } Sy_A^2 = 520 \quad \text{and} \quad n = 4, \text{ hence, } v_A = 130$$

$$\text{For B, } Sy_B^2 = 4120 \quad \text{and} \quad n = 4, \text{ hence, } v_B = 1030$$

Then the ratio of the larger to the smaller variance is calculated. This ratio is termed F:

$$F = v_B/v_A = 1030/130 = 7\cdot92$$

The tables of variance ratio give the values of F corresponding to the number of degrees of freedom of each sample. There is a separate table for each probability level. The tables are entered with n_1 corresponding to the higher variance (here, $n_1 = n_2 = 4$). The values of F for probabilities of 0·05 and 0·01 are 6·4 and 16. The F ratio calculated in the example lies between these, so the probability is between 0·05 and 0·01. That is, such a difference in variability would occur between 1 in 20 times and 1 in 100 times by chance if the two samples were drawn from a single population. Accordingly, the null hypothesis has little chance of being correct and must be rejected. The result can be stated in the following way: there is a significant difference in variability of systolic pressure between the two groups of patients (analysis of variance, $0\cdot05 > P > 0\cdot001$).

(3) THE USE OF THE χ^2 TEST. The mydriatic action of ephedrine was tested on sixty subjects by instilling a 2% solution into the conjunctiva. Half of the subjects were European and the other half were non-European. The extent of the dilatation of the pupil produced in these two groups of subjects is shown below.

	Dilatation of pupil 1 mm or more	Dilatation of pupil less than 1 mm	Row totals
Europeans	23	7	30
Non-Europeans	3	27	30
Column totals	26	34	60

The results observed suggest that in European subjects the iris is more sensitive to the effect of ephedrine than in non-European subjects. However, there is the possibility that such a distribution of results may have been due to chance alone and this probability was estimated by calculating χ^2. The calculation is as follows:

$$\chi^2 = \text{Sum} \left\{ \frac{(\text{observed value} - \text{expected value})^2}{\text{expected value}} \right\}$$

The expected values in this instance (assuming a null hypothesis; i.e. no difference in the effect of ephedrine on European and non-European irides) are given in the following table.

Expected mydriatic responses:

	Dilatation 1 mm or more	Dilatation less than 1 mm	Row totals
European	$\dfrac{30 \times 26}{60} = 13$	$\dfrac{30 \times 34}{60} = 17$	30
non-European	$\dfrac{30 \times 26}{60} = 13$	$\dfrac{30 \times 34}{60} = 17$	30
Column totals	26	34	60

Then

$$\chi^2 = \frac{(23-13)^2}{13} + \frac{(7-17)^2}{17} + \frac{(3-13)^2}{13} + \frac{(27-17)^2}{17}$$

$$= \frac{100}{13} + \frac{100}{17} + \frac{100}{13} + \frac{100}{17}$$

$$= 7 \cdot 69 + 5 \cdot 88 + 7 \cdot 69 + 5 \cdot 88$$

$$= 27 \cdot 14$$

There are published tables giving the values of χ^2 corresponding to various levels of probability. The tables also take into account the number of degrees of freedom. In the example used, there is one degree of freedom since only one value can be fitted into the block of four by choice, the remaining three being then fixed in order that the row and column totals remain constant. The value of χ^2 found by calculation in the example exceeds the value corresponding to a probability of $0 \cdot 005$. Therefore it can be stated that the observed distribution of values would occur by chance less often than once in 5000 similar experiments. In other words it is extremely unlikely that the results are due to chance and there is a correspondingly strong probability that there is a difference in sensitivity of the iris to ephedrine in European and non-European subjects. [The reader is cautioned against accepting this conclusion as the last word on the matter and is referred to the paper by Obianwu and Rand (*Brit. J. Ophthalmology*, **49**, 264, 1965) for a fuller account.]

The χ^2 test is simple to apply and is often useful in making a preliminary analysis of experimental data. However it should not be used when the number of items which would be expected to occur in any group, on the null hypothesis, is less than 5.

The relationships between dose and response

These may be divided into two types: in the first, the response is *graded* between zero and the maximal value, the magnitude of the response being dependent on the dose; in the second, the response is *quantal*, being either present or absent, and the proportion of positive responses to the total number of trials depends on the dose.

Dose-response lines with graded responses. A typical example of this category is the relationship between the dose of an agonist, such as acetylcholine or histamine, and the response of an isolated tissue preparation, such as the contraction of guinea-pig isolated ileum. The theoretical aspects of dose-response relationships of this type were discussed on page 461 where it was pointed out that there was close agreement between the form of the experimentally obtained dose-response curve and the curve predicted by theory. The important practical consideration is that the response is directly proportional to the logarithm of the dose providing that the response is within the limits of 20 to 80% of the maximal. In other words, the graph of response versus log dose is a straight line.

The experimentally obtained points on a graph which gives a linear relationship between response and dose are scattered about the line, owing to the variability which is to be expected in the determination of the response at each dose. However, there is a statistical procedure for determining the line which gives the best fit to the experimental points; this line is termed the *regression* for response on dose (or log dose). The regression line passes through the point on the graph which corresponds to the mean point of all the observations (i.e., the point corresponding to $\bar{X}$, $\bar{Y}$) and its inclination to the x-axis of the graph, where dose or log dose is plotted on the abscissa according to the usual practice, is described by the regression coefficient which is symbolized as b.

THE CALCULATION OF REGRESSION OF RESPONSE ON DOSE. The data which will be used to illustrate the procedure are contained in Table 20.3, and the outline of the calculations is given below the Table.

The calculated regression line is drawn on the graph in the following way. The mean point of all the observations is plotted ($\bar{X}$, $\bar{Y}$), then a second point on the line is determined by moving parallel with the x-axis for 1 unit and parallel with the y-axis for b units, as illustrated in Fig. 20.5. The regression line runs through these two points.

The variance of the regression line is given by $(Sxy)^2/Sx^2$, which equals 2260 in the example, and there is one degree of freedom associated with it. The variance *about* the regression line is obtained by the following calculation:

$$\frac{Sy^2 - (Sxy)^2/Sx^2}{n} = 18 \cdot 3$$

TABLE 20.3. Duration of anaesthesia produced by various doses of pentobarbitone in rats.

Dose of pentobarbitone mg/kg X	Duration of anaesthesia minutes Y	Squares and products		
		X^2	Y^2	XY
30	11	900	121	330
30	12	900	144	360
30	13	900	169	390
30	15	900	225	450
40	28	1600	784	1120
40	30	1600	900	1200
40	31	1600	961	1240
40	35	1600	1225	1400
40	35	1600	1225	1400
40	37	1600	1369	1480
50	46	2500	2116	2300
50	50	2500	2500	2500
50	53	2500	2809	2650
$SX=470$	$SY=361$	$SX^2=19100$	$SY^2=13303$	$SXY=15420$

$N=12$ (12 pairs of observations) $Sx^2=SX^2-(SX)^2/N=692$
$\bar{X}=SX/N=39.2$ $Sy^2=SY^2-(SY)^2/N=2443$
$\bar{Y}=SY/N=30$ $Sxy=SXY-(SXSY)/N=1251$

The term Sxy is the sum of the products of the deviations of the X's and the Y's from their respective means. The regression coefficient, b, is given by $Sxy/Sx^2=1.81$.

where n, the number of degrees of freedom, is equal to the numbers of pairs of observations (N) minus 2, since one degree of freedom has been used up in the calculation of the regression coefficient and another in the calculation of the mean. The variance *about* the regression line is also known as the *residual variance* and is analogous to the variance about a mean. It can be used to calculate the fiducial limits of regression lines at any desired level of probability by taking the square root and multiplying it by the appropriate value of t. In the example, the value of t corresponding to 10 degrees of freedom and a probability of 0.05 is 2·23 and the square root of the residual variance is 4·24, giving a product of 9·46, which is the displacement above and below the regression line in units of the y-axis which include 95% of the observations; these lines are plotted in Fig. 20.5. The significance of the regression can be assessed by comparing the variance of the regression with the residual variance. In the example, the variance ratio, $F=2260/18.3=123$ with $n_1=1$ and $n_2=10$. The value of F from tables for a probability of 0·001 is 21. The calculated value is

18

considerably in excess of this figure, indicating that the regression is very highly significant.

The statistical estimation of a regression line gives not only the line of best fit, but also an estimate of the precision of the fit. The procedure is relatively simple when there is a linear relationship, and advantage is taken of this fact by transforming the measurements of dose and response in such a way that a

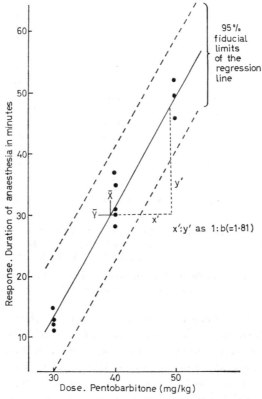

Fig. 20.5. Regression of response (duration of anaesthesia in rats) on dose of pentobarbitone (injected intraperitoneally). The data is taken from Table 20.3. The individual observations are indicated by black dots.

linear relationship is obtained. In the example used to illustrate the calculation, no transformation was necessary. However, as was pointed out previously, log dose is frequently employed.

Dose-response relationship with a quantal response. This category of dose-response relationship is encountered in experiments of the type in which a drug is given at various doses to groups of experimental animals and observations are made of the proportion of animals in each group which react in some characteristic way. The reaction may be the death of the animal, or it may be any other effect which allows a definite classification of each animal into one of two classes—reacting or not reacting. When the results of such an experiment are plotted on a graph, with the proportion reacting on the *y*-axis and the log dose on the *x*-axis, an *S*-shaped curve is produced. The curve can be

TABLE 20.4. Toxicity text (hypothetical data) showing relation between dosage and mortality. (The probit values corresponding to percentage mortalities are obtained from published tables.)

Dose (mg/kg)	Log Dose	Proportion killed	% Mortality	Probit
1·6	0·20	0/15	0	—
2·0	0·30	1/15	7	3·52
2·5	0·40	2/15	13	3·87
3·2	0·51	7/15	46	4·90
4·0	0·60	10/15	67	5·44
5·0	0·70	12/15	80	5·84
6·3	0·80	14/15	93	6·48
8·0	0·90	15/15	100	—

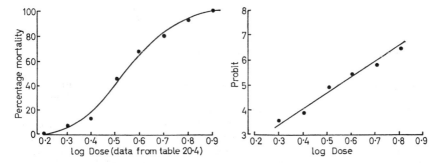

FIG. 20.6. Effect of probit transformation in converting sigmoid curve of percentage mortality versus log dose (left hand graph) to straight line (right hand graph). The graph lines are fitted to the points by eye; however, the regression line could be readily calculated for the probit versus log dose relationship.

converted into a straight line by re-scaling the *y*-axis. The proportion (or percentage) of animals responding is transformed into another unit known as a *probit* (see p. 547). The regression line is then calculated from the probits corresponding to the percentage responding and the log dose administered to the animals in each group. This is illustrated by the data given in Table 20.4 and the graphs in Fig. 20.6. The regression line which fits the linear relationship between log dose and probit can then be calculated and subjected to statistical analysis by the methods described above.

A value which has been obtained by transformation of the original datum (or *parameter*) is known as a *metameter*. In the use of log-dose probit relationships, both dose and response metameters are employed. The selection of the metameter is determined by the effect of the transformation: if it results in a

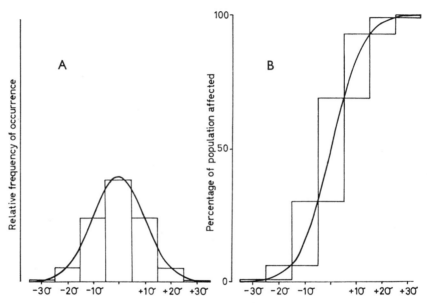

FIG. 20.7. A. Normal distribution curves. The proportion of the population lying between various limits (at one standard deviation intervals; $-3\cdot5$ to $-2\cdot5$, $-2\cdot5$ to $-1\cdot5$, $-1\cdot5$ to $-0\cdot5$, $-0\cdot5$ to $+0\cdot5$ and so on) are represented by the histogram of rectangles. B. Cumulative frequency distribution. The rectangles from A, each representing a fraction of the population lying between certain defined limits, are added together along the ordinate; they then form the sigmoid curve which characterizes relationships such as that between percentage mortality and dose. This curve would be converted to a straight line by transforming the ordinate into probits.

straight line relationship and does not unduly distort the scatter of responses at the different dose levels, then the transformation is justified. It may be that there is also justification for the transformation on theoretical grounds, as in the adoption of log-dose rather than dose, but the more important consideration is the empirical one that it results in a linear relationship.

The rationale of the probit transformation depends on the considerations illustrated in Fig. 20.7. The lowest dose level affects only the most susceptible members of the population, represented by the block at the extreme left of the normal distribution curve which lies between -3.5 and -2.5 standard deviations from the mean in Fig. 20.7A. The next higher dose level affects not only these, but also an additional group of members; in the normal distribution curve shown, this additional group is the proportion of the population lying between -2.5 and -1.5 standard deviations from the mean. In order to represent the sum of the two groups, the blocks must be added. Similarly, a still higher dose level affects all those members previously affected, plus a further additional group. If this process is continued, the addition of blocks of positive responses results in an S-shaped curve (Fig. 20.7B). This curve is a cumulative normal distribution, and represents the probability of occurrence of a response (e.g. mortality) in terms of standard deviation units on each side of the dose which is effective (or lethal) for 50% of the population (the ED_{50}, or LD_{50}). Mathematically, the cumulative probability curve can be converted to a straight line and the published tables give the probit values corresponding to percentages. The term probit is derived from 'probability unit'.

The use of dose-response lines in comparing potency

The relative potency of two samples of a drug can be determined from the amounts of each required to produce a given response. However, more information can be gained from a comparison based on dose-response regression lines; this applies both to graded and to quantal responses.

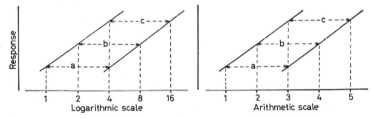

FIG. 20.8. The value of log dose in comparisons of potency. The graph on the left represents two parallel response-log dose lines and the graph on the right represents another pair of lines which are straight and parallel when plotted as response against dose (*not* log dose). The horizontal distance between the pairs of lines expresses the relative potency. The findings may be summarized in tabular form:

Relative potency

	a	b	c
Response vs. log dose	1:4	2:8 (=1:4)	4:16 (=1:4)
Response vs. dose	1:3	2:4 (=1:2)	3:5 (=1:1.7)

It is clear that the comparison is independent of the level of response or the particular dose level in the case of the response-log dose lines.

Where the response is linearly related to the log dose, the comparison is facilitated since the relative potency is independent of the magnitude of the response (provided the two regression lines are parallel). This is illustrated in Fig 20.8. The horizontal distance between the regression lines for response on log dose is the logarithm of the relative potency; this distance is usually termed *M*. Statistical procedures are available for determining the fiducial limits of *M*. These depend on the variability of responses about each regression line. The precision of comparisons based on regression lines is greater the steeper the line; the ratio of the variance to the regression coefficient is known as the *index of precision* (this ratio is sometimes called λ).

Biological Assay

Biological assay (or bioassay) is used to measure the concentrations of pharmacologically-active substances in pharmaceutical preparations or in tissue extracts when there are no suitable chemical or physical methods. Bioassay may be the only method of measurement, as in the assay of insulin. An advantage of bioassay methods is their sensitivity and they may be employed when the concentration of active substance is below the limit detectable by chemical or physical methods; for example, acetylcholine released from cholinergic nerves may be assayed by this means. Bioassay is convenient when the pharmacological action of the drug is the result of two or more active principles which, though chemically similar, may differ in potency (as, for example, in the assay of digitalis leaf). Although often more sensitive, bioassays are generally less accurate and more laborious to perform than are chemical or physical assays.

The disadvantage of bioassay is its relative lack of precision, which stems from the fact of biological variation. The assay method must therefore be designed to minimize and to compensate for biological variations as far as is possible, and to allow the results obtained to be treated statistically so that the experimenter may estimate the precision of his assay by calculating the probability that the true potency is within certain 'limits of error'. Statistical calculations based on the fact that drug responses are usually normally or log-normally distributed enable the bioassayist to estimate the internal error of his assay. The essence of bioassay is that the test and standard are compared under as near as possible identical conditions.

Most drugs and pharmaceutical preparations are intended for use in man but their assay is usually carried out in another species; however, there have been exceptions. For example, batches of digitalis have been standardized in human volunteers using as the response the change in the T-wave of the ECG (see page 255), and patients with pernicious anaemia have been used for the standardization of antianaemia preparations; in both these cases, the need for biological assay of the drug preparations has been greatly reduced as pure substances (which can be assayed by more exact methods) have been introduced.

The response which is used in bioassay may be the same as the response which will be elicited in the human patient by the drug. Thus insulin preparations may be assayed by measuring the decrease in blood glucose they produce in rabbits. However, often the bioassay response differs considerably from the required response in patients. For instance, oxytocin preparations may be assayed by making use of the fall in blood pressure produced in the anaesthetized fowl.

Bioassay methods may be used for standardizing drug preparations regardless of the species used or of the nature of the effect observed. The only necessity is that the biological response is dependent on the dose of active principle of the preparation. The validity of bioassay depends on whether the preparation responds selectively to the active principle being measured and is unaffected by the presence of other materials which may be present. This is an advantage which some bioassays possess over some chemical assays. A chemical method may be unable to distinguish between closely related chemical substances, but their biological activity may differ widely: pharmacologically-active polypeptides are a good example of this. In the bioassay of pharmacologically-active substances in tissue extracts, evidence that the substance being assayed is the same as the standard is obtained by using several different assay preparations.

The results of a bioassay are usually determined as the strength of a preparation, relative to the strength of a standard preparation of the same substance; they are only rarely expressed in terms of the response.

BIOLOGICAL STANDARDS. Drugs cannot be assayed reliably in terms of their action because of the variability between batches of animals and the other varying factors in biological experimentation. However, they can be assayed in suitably designed experiments in such a way that the strength of one sample can be compared with that of another. If one particular sample of the drug is designated as 'standard', then the relative strength of other samples can be determined in terms of this standard.

The first biological standard was set up by Ehrlich in 1897. It consisted of a certain weight of a dried preparation of diphtheria antitoxin. Other preparations of diphtheria antitoxin were compared with the designated standard in their ability to protect guinea-pigs from the effects of diphtheria toxin. Ehrlich's standard, or rather a preparation standardized from it, was adopted by the League of Nations as the International Standard in 1921. International standards were originally declared under the auspices of the League of Nations Health Organization but are now under the World Health Organization. The first reference laboratories having the responsibility for custody and issue of the standards were the Danish State Serum Institute, which was responsible for immunological standards (sera and vaccines), and the British National Institute for Medical Research, which in 1925 held the standards for digitalis, pituitary (posterior lobe) extract, insulin, neoarsphenamine and sulpharsphenamine. The division of biological standards into immunological preparations (under Danish custody) and all other preparations (under British custody) has continued to the present day. In Britain, the Therapeutic Substances Act and Regulations laid down standards for all therapeutic substances which could not be reliably assayed by chemical or physical methods and these national standards are also maintained by the National Institute. The Department of Biological Standards in the Institute is responsible for research into improved methods of biological assay and the establishment of methods for the assay of new substances. The Department collaborates with other laboratories in making recommendations about amendments to the Regulations governing national standards and also collaborates with corresponding bodies in other countries for the purpose of advising the Committee on Biological Standardization of the World Health Organization.

Official Bioassays. Table 20.5 gives brief details of biological assays included in the 1963 British Pharmacopoeia (other than those for antibiotics and for serological and bacteriological products, which are outside the scope of this book).

These bioassays may be divided into two main classes—those performed entirely upon one animal or upon one piece of isolated tissue (direct comparisons) and those performed on numbers of animals. This latter class may be further subdivided into those in which the response in each animal is measured, those in which the percentage of positive effects is measured (a quantal assay), and those in which the threshold or minimal effective dose in each animal is measured.

Experimental design in bioassay. The repetition of part of an experiment to obtain additional measurements is known as replication. This is necessary to provide an estimate of the error by statistical analysis. It is often necessary that several pieces of information must be obtained in the same experiment. For example, in a bioassay depending on direct comparison, the responses of a tissue or an animal to various amounts of a standard solution of a drug and of a solution of unknown strength are determined. In order to avoid any bias being imparted to the results, it is usual to apply the solutions in a random order, and the replicates are also given in random order. Then, any changes in responsiveness of the preparation, either a progressive increase or decrease

TABLE 20.5. Bioassays of the British Pharmacopoeia 1963

Active principle	International standard	Response observed or measured	Type of assay
Chorionic gonadotrophin	An extract of the urine of pregnant women	Production of a majority of cornified cells in vaginal smears from 4 groups of immature female rats	Quantal
Corticotrophin	Dry corticotrophin	Ascorbic acid depletion in adrenal glands from 6 groups of hypophysectomized rats. A test for prolongation of effect is also included	Response in each animal measured
Insulin injection	Pure dry crystalline insulin	Death, convulsions or loss of righting reflex in 4 groups of mice	Quantal
Protamine zinc insulin injection	As above	(*a*) In mice as above	Quantal
		(*b*) Level of blood sugar determined in 4 groups of rabbits—cross-over assay. A test for prolongation of effect is also included	Response in each animal measured
Oxytocin injection	An extract of acetone dried powder obtained from posterior lobes of ox pituitary glands	(*a*) Fall in arterial blood pressure of anaesthetized chicken	Direct comparison in same animal or tissue
		(*b*) Contraction of isolated uterus of a rat in dioestrus	
Vasopressin injection	As for oxytocin	Rise in arterial blood pressure of anaesthetized male rat	Direct comparison in same animal
Prepared Digitalis	A sample of dried powdered leaves of *Digitalis purpurea*	Cessation of heart beat in anaesthetized guinea-pigs	Measurement of threshold dose
Heparin	Dried sodium salt of heparin prepared from the crystallized barium salt of ox heparin	Time to clot of sulphated fresh blood to which a standard amount of thrombokinase extract has been added. The relationship between log coagulation time and log concentration is linear	Direct comparison on the same tissue
Vitamin D	Crystalline Vitamin D$_3$	By reference to a standard scale, the extent to which rickets is cured is measured by histological staining of bones or X-ray examination in 4 groups of young rats fed on a rachitogenic diet	Measurement of response in each animal

18*

in sensitivity, or spontaneous fluctuations, produce random variation in the responses. Providing the experimental design is appropriate, there are statistical procedures for reducing the error which is contributed by the random variations. In the case of the comparison of two solutions, a standard (S) and an unknown (U), in which observations are made at two dose levels, high (H) and low (L), there are 4 treatments which may be designated SH, SL, UH, and UL. If each treatment is repeated 4 times, there are 16 observations. The order in which each set of treatments is given may be varied in such a way that each one occupies a different position in the set in each replication. This may be represented in the following way:

SH UL SL UH
UL SL UH SH
SL UH SH UL
UH SH UL SL

This arrangement is known as a 4×4 Latin square, of which the example is one of a number of possible designs. It should be noted that each treatment occurs once in each column. If there were no variability on replication, the sums of the results in each row and in each column would be equal. However, in practice there are differences in these figures. By appropriate statistical analysis, it is possible to determine the variability attributable to the arrangement of the sets of treatment in rows and in columns. The variation from this source can be subtracted from the total variation of the determination and the degree of uncertainty in the comparison of the two solutions can be thereby decreased.

When the assays are performed on numbers of animals, all possible steps are taken to minimize errors due to differences between animals, and the environment is closely controlled. The most important of these steps are: (1) the use of as many animals as possible for both standard and test group (the minimal number necessary to give the required accuracy may be calculated statistically); (2) the determination of the responses to the standard and test preparations of the drug are made as nearly as possible at the same time; (3) the use of littermate animals of the same sex, maintained under the same conditions of diet, housing and hygiene; and (4) the use, when the effect of the drug is not lethal, of a 'cross-over assay', in which the assay is performed twice on the same animals, those initially receiving the standard subsequently receiving the test, and those initially receiving the high doses subsequently receiving the low doses. The statistical calculation of the result from the combined responses yields a lower error of estimate than if the cross-over method is not used.

In assays which depend on the measurement of the response in each animal, the animals are randomly divided into four equal groups. The groups are given high and low doses of the standard and high and low doses of the solution of unknown strength. The ratio of the large dose to the small dose should be the same for the standard and the test solutions for convenience in calculation. The doses of standard and unknown are adjusted from preliminary experiments to be such that the effects are approximately equal. An example of this type of bioassay is that for protamine zinc insulin using rabbits. The response measured in each rabbit is the fall in blood sugar. A 'cross-over' design is usual in this assay.

In bioassays where the response is quantal, the criterion of the response must be distinct and may be, for example, death, occurrence of oestrus, or hypoglycaemic convulsions. Animals are randomly distributed, usually into four equally sized groups. High and low doses of standard and unknown solutions are used. The percentage of animals responding in each group is converted to the corresponding probit value and the relative potency is determined from the regression of probit on log dose. An example of a quantal assay is the assay of insulin using mice in which the percentage incidence of convulsions is determined.

Introduction of new drugs

There are two phases in the pre-clinical evaluation of new drugs. Firstly, potentially useful chemicals must be selected by using suitable pharmacological tests. Secondly, those that are dangerous must be recognized and rejected.

Ways of finding new drugs. Many of the drugs first used in medicine were obtained from plants (e.g. morphine, digitalis), and there are probably still useful drugs to be found from further surveys of plants. These may be selected on the basis of folk lore, or because related plants are known to contain active principles of pharmacological interest. Reserpine, which was only recently introduced into Western medicine as a tranquillizer and antihypertensive drug, was obtained from an Indian plant which had been used for centuries in folk remedies.

Some useful drugs have been discovered by synthesizing compounds chemically related to existing drugs obtained from plant or animal sources. The stimulus behind this approach may be a desire to produce drugs which are more selective and possess fewer side-effects, or are more readily absorbed or more slowly metabolized (as in the development of synthetic hormones), or to replace a naturally occurring drug when the demand for it exceeds the supply (as in the development of gallamine because of the difficulty of obtaining adequate quantities of tubocurarine from natural sources), or to produce a drug which can be patented. Many drugs have been produced by making slight alterations in the chemical structure of a drug which had already been successfully marketed by another pharmaceutical company. This practice, which had been described as 'molecular manipulation', has been criticized on the grounds that it is motivated largely by profit rather than by the lack of useful drugs for particular purposes. Drugs developed in this way include many of the ganglion blocking drugs which followed the clinical use of hexamethonium (pp. 690-694), some of the diuretics resembling chlorothiazide (pp. 881-882), and the host of barbiturates (pp. 588-591), local anaesthetics (Chapter 25) and antihistamine drugs (pp 780-782) that are available.

The greatest effort put into the search for new drugs is spent in making extensive surveys of large series of chemicals. The sorts of compounds to be tested can be selected in various ways, but usually there is an attempt to produce compounds for which there are reasons to believe a particular type of pharmacological activity is likely. The reasons may be based on available knowledge about relationship between chemical structure and activity, but one must expect agonists, partial agonists or blocking drugs to be found.

Sometimes compounds that have pharmacological activity of a completely different kind from that predicted are found. Examples of drugs with interesting pharmacological properties unrelated to those that first led to their development are chlorpromazine, a tranquillizer which was found in a trial designed to produce antihistamines, and xylocholine, an adrenergic neurone blocking drug and the prototype of the antihypertensive drugs, bretylium and guanethidine, and which was one of a series of compounds being investigated for their local anaesthetic action.

Another technique in the search for new drugs is to use a more random approach in which new series of compounds are submitted to a battery of screening tests designed to show up a variety of types of biological activity. Often, the first test is to observe the effects in mice; in this case compounds of high toxicity are usually subjected to further investigation since this is often a reflection of potent pharmacological activity.

Screening tests. The role of the pharmacologist is to devise screening tests that discriminate all the compounds that have the particular action which is being sought. The screening test is selected in the first instance by its ability to detect the action of all of the drugs that are already known to be effective in a particular condition. Tests which are simple to operate and are as cheap as possible are preferred as large numbers of compounds may be tested. The tests are designed, as far as possible, to have relevance to the pathological condition in which it is hoped to employ the drugs clinically, although it is often not necessary to mimic the condition precisely. For example, in screening for antihypertensive drugs, it is not desirable to run preliminary screens on animals who have been made hypertensive in the laboratory; if the compounds are likely to reduce blood pressure by interfering with sympathetic transmission, it is simpler to use an isolated, sympathetically innervated organ as a test, such as innervated rabbit intestine. When less information is available about the precise mechanism of action of a drug, reliable screening tests are more difficult to devise. Traditionally, antianginal drugs have been screened for their ability to produce dilatation of the coronary vessels in an isolated, perfused heart; however, more recent evidence suggests that this may be an unsuitable model, because in patients susceptible to anginal attacks, atherosclerotic lesions of the coronary vessels may render them unresponsive to dilator drugs. It may prove better to screen antianginal drugs on the basis of their ability to reduce either the work done by the heart or the energy requirements of the heart. It is not possible in this chapter to consider more than the principles involved in the selection of suitable screening tests for the evaluation of the activity of new drugs. Many books have been written about screening tests, and some of these are indicated in the list of further reading for this chapter.

Many uses for drugs introduced for some other property may be found from observation of the patients receiving them. The carbonic anhydrase inhibiting action of some sulphonamides (page 879) and the hypoglycaemic action of others (page 854) are examples of new and useful actions of drugs discovered by careful observations of the side-effects of the sulphonamides. Similarly, the development of the monoamine oxidase inhibitors (page 623) stems from the observation that iproniazid, originally used as an antitubercular drug, possesses antidepressive properties.

Toxicity testing. Toxicity tests in animals are carried out before a new drug is offered for clinical trial, and responsible physicians require evidence that this has been done before using a drug in man. The rationale of these tests depends on the assumption that man reacts in the same way as the species used for the toxicity studies in the laboratory. The assumption is often supported by the results obtained in clinical trials, but there is no logical justification for it, since different species frequently exhibit different manifestations of toxicity. In fact, many drugs have been withdrawn from clinical use owing to the occurrence of serious toxic effects in man, although when they were introduced into medicine they were thought to be free from undue toxicity on the basis of animal tests. Examples of such drugs include thalidomide (page 593), triparanol (p. 918), dithiazanine, zoxazolamine (p. 613) and etryptamine (p. 622).

All drugs are potentially dangerous and may produce unwanted effects. The object of toxicity testing is to determine the nature of these effects in animal experimentation. With many drugs, the main toxic effect is an extension of the therapeutically desired effect and the hazard is in overdosage. However, toxic effects of drugs may also be due to actions that are unrelated to the desired effect, in which case they may be termed *side-effects*. Both types of toxicity may be present. For example, tubocurarine paralyses respiratory movements, this being an extension of its muscle relaxant action, and it may also cause bronchospasm, this being due to a histamine-liberating action.

Unexpected toxic effects may result from interaction between two or more drugs taken concurrently, or even between a drug and a constituent of diet. Drugs deserving special mention in this respect are barbiturates taken in conjunction with ethyl alcohol (page 591), and the antidepressive monoamine oxidase inhibitors which may potentiate the action of a variety of other drugs, and even interact with amines derived from the diet (pages 625–626). Formulated mixtures of two or more drugs require toxicity testing even though the individual toxicities of the constituents are known, since the toxicity of the combination may differ from that of the ingredients given alone.

CHOICE OF ANIMALS USED IN TOXICITY TESTING. The use of as many species as possible is recommended, but practical considerations limit the species used. Tests employing rats and mice are favoured owing to their cheapness and the ease with which they can be housed and fed. Additional tests are generally also carried out in at least one species other than rodents. Of the commonly available laboratory animals, the dog is usually employed.

Much work is being carried out to devise suitable animal tests for detecting some of the serious toxic effects which may be produced by drugs in man. In the past, there has been difficulty in predicting certain types of toxicity, including hypersensitivity and allergic reactions, photosensitivity, aplastic anaemia, agranulocytosis, some types of liver damage and peripheral neuritis. Recently it has proved possible to produce contact sensitization with hydrallazine and with benzylpenicillin, by using guinea-pigs, and to produce anaemia with chloramphenicol by using ducks; these drugs occasionally produce such toxic reactions in man. The manifestation of a toxic effect in one species may be due to an anomolous sensitivity, as with penicillin which has high toxicity in guinea-pigs. Undue reliance on such a result could lead to a useful drug being unnecessarily discarded.

There may be qualitative differences between species in their reaction to a drug. Thus, morphine sedates man, rats and dogs, but excites cats. Again, in the toxicity tests of a new antibacterial drug, it was found that irreversible structural changes were produced in the lens and cornea of guinea-pigs, there were less severe effects in rabbits and monkeys, whereas there were no such effects in rats, mice or dogs.

Quantitative differences in drug action between species are commonly encountered. These are largely, but not entirely, due to species differences in rates of metabolism.

SPECIES DIFFERENCES IN DRUG METABOLISM. This question is of importance in the choice of animals for the evaluation of potentially useful drug action as well as for drug toxicity. Phenylbutazone is metabolized very rapidly in most laboratory animals, consequently it is practically inactive; in fact, its anti-inflammatory activity was first discovered in man. Pethidine is metabolized in man at the rate of 17% of the amount present per hour, and a single dose is effective for 3 to 4 h, but in dogs, which metabolize 70 to 90% of the dose per hour, the effects of a single dose are correspondingly short-lasting. Mice metabolize hexobarbitone twenty times as rapidly, and phenazone sixty times as rapidly, as man. In rats, many drugs are metabolized more rapidly in males than in females, thus the duration of anaesthesia produced by the same dose of hexobarbitone is four times longer in female than in male rats. This sex difference in rates of metabolism is not seen in mice, guinea-pigs, rabbits and dogs.

As well as differences in rate of drug metabolism, there are also different pathways of metabolism. Thus, the major metabolic alterations reported for amphetamine are deamination in rabbits, demethylation in dogs, and hydroxylation in rats. In certain species, enzyme systems may be absent, as shown in the following examples: (a) in dogs, acetylation of primary amines does not occur; (b) in guinea pigs, mercapturic acid conjugates are not formed; (c) in cats, UDP-glucuronic acid transferase is absent and glucuronic acid conjugates do not occur; this enzyme is also deficient in the newborn guinea-pig and the human baby.

These considerations indicate the difficulty of extending observations made with animals to man. Tests with human subjects are necessary to determine the rate and route of metabolism of a new drug in man. Some toxic effects of drugs in man are due to inherited differences in drug-metabolizing enzymes. This occurs, for example, with suxamethonium and isoniazid which are known to produce unusually prolonged effects in a few patients.

NUMBERS OF ANIMALS USED IN TESTING FOR TOXICITY. If a toxic side-effect occurred frequently in a new drug investigation, the drug would probably never reach clinical trial, or if it did, its use would soon be discontinued. However, most clinically established drugs exhibit some incidence of toxicity; for example, chloramphenicol produces aplastic anaemia in about 1 in 100,000 patients. It is of interest that this toxic effect of chloramphenicol can be readily demonstrated on cultured human marrow cells in which it inhibits the incorporation of iron into haem. Pre-clinical toxicity testing should, as far as possible, give some clue about the nature of even these rare toxic effects. Unfortunately, it is usually not feasible to carry out animal tests which detect a toxic effect which has a low incidence since the probability of observing a toxic effect depends on the number of animals used in the test. If the effect has an incidence of one in

100 animals, about 300 animals would be needed in order to detect the effect at the 5% level of probability. Furthermore, from this group of animals, information would be obtained about the toxic effects at only one dose level. Even if it were practicable to administer a drug to some hundreds of animals, it would be impossible to give each animal more than a superficial examination. It is generally acknowledged that thorough examination of smaller numbers of animals provides more valuable data. Consequently, toxic effects of low incidence usually escape detection in animal tests and preliminary clinical trials, and for this reason it is necessary to keep watch for toxic effects of drugs after their introduction into clinical practice.

DURATION OF TOXICITY TESTS. It is relatively easy to establish the nature of acute toxic effects of drugs in animal experiments, and these are rarely a problem in clinical trials because the usual practice is to begin with a low dose and gradually increase it. The determination of chronic toxicity presents a more serious problem. The duration of toxicity tests is usually related to the intended use of the drug in question in man. Many drugs are given only once, or on only a few occasions to any one patient (e.g. an anaesthetic). Other drugs are given over long periods (e.g. oral contraceptives, hypoglycaemic drugs, antihypertensive drugs). Clearly, toxicity testing of long duration is necessary in the latter case. However, toxicity tests of more than 2 years duration are approaching the length of the normal life span of rats and mice. Many authorities in toxicity testing consider that most information about the toxicity of a drug is obtained in the first 3 months of tests in animals, although the production of cancerous changes by drugs may only become manifest after longer periods of testing.

Prolonged toxicity tests impose a delay in the introduction of drugs into medicine, and this delay may not be justified in the case of a drug which provides a major advance in therapeutics. In such cases, a drug may be used clinically after preliminary toxicity tests, while the long term toxicity tests are still in progress.

DOSES AND ROUTES OF ADMINISTRATION USED IN TOXICITY TESTS. The usual practice in pharmacological laboratories is to determine the acute LD_{50} of a drug by a number of routes (intravenously, subcutaneously and orally). In tests for chronic toxicity, the dose levels are chosen to be as high as possible, but to allow a high proportion of the animals to survive for the required duration of the test. The route of administration used in chronic testing is the same as that used for the drug in man. The influence of the route of administration on the appearance of toxicity can be illustrated by reference to griseofulvin, which produced no deleterious effects after oral administration in animals, but with parenteral injection it was a powerful mitotic inhibitor. Since griseofulvin was intended for oral use in man, these results did not preclude its clinical trial, although they indicated need for caution, and it was found to be safe when given orally to patients.

TESTS FOR TERATOGENICITY. The birth of malformed children to mothers who took thalidomide during the early weeks of pregnancy has focused attention on the need to test for the effects of drugs on the development of the embryo. Teratology, the study of antenatal malformations and monstrosities, has now become a recognized branch of pharmacology.

Thalidomide had not been tested for teratogenic activity before its introduction into medicine; however, this manifestation of toxicity had never been encountered to any significant extent with other drugs. Thalidomide was singularly free from toxicity in other respects and it was largely for this reason that it was widely prescribed. The tragedy arose from the fact that it was given to alleviate the symptoms of morning sickness. This disorder is more likely to occur and is most troublesome during the first 3 months of pregnancy which corresponds to the period when the foetus is most prone to teratogenic effects.

Screening for teratogenic activity is of vital importance to those responsible for the introduction of new drugs. Now that a wide range of compounds have been tested and shown to have teratogenic effects in animals it is known that there are at least three important factors which must be considered.

Firstly, the foetus is sensitive to teratogenic effects only during a limited critical period of its development in early pregnancy, corresponding to the period of greatest organization and greatest mitotic activity. The compound being tested for teratogenicity may however be cumulative in its effects and may therefore be effective when given some time before the critical period. Secondly, the dose of a teratogenic drug may be critical. There is a relatively narrow band of dosage which is capable of producing deformed young. If too much of the drug is given, the foetuses die *in utero* and are aborted or resorbed, and if too little is given the young are not deformed. Probably, most drugs which can kill a foetus will exhibit teratogenicity when given at a lower dosage. Thirdly, the species in which teratogenic tests are carried out may determine to some extent the abnormality, as there is considerable variation in the effects seen when the same drug is given by the same route to several species. With thalidomide, for example, it is relatively easy to obtain hindlimb malformations in rabbits but difficult to achieve this in rats.

Not all mothers who took thalidomide early in pregnancy gave birth to malformed babies. In experimental teratology, it is also known that not all animals in an experiment produce malformed young, even though they are of the same genetic stock and all are given the same treatment. Furthermore, not all the young in any one litter are malformed. It has been suggested that teratogencity may be linked with the nutritional requirements and the hormonal activity of the foetus and the mother; but other factors may be important.

Fresh light has been thrown on the action of thalidomide by the finding that this drug delayed the rejection of skin heterografts in rats. It was suggested therefore that the deformed young were born because they were not rejected, rather than that the drug produced the deformities. Additional work is required before this explanation can be fully accepted.

TESTS FOR CARCINOGENICITY. The tendency of some chemicals to produce cancer in animals has been known for about 50 years, but tests for carcinogenic effects of drugs have assumed importance only with the relatively recent development of a larger number of drugs intended for prolonged use.

As yet, no simple procedure for detecting carcinogenicity is available. When a substance under test is chemically related to a known carcinogen, then procedures similar to those which detect the effect of the known carcinogen should be used for the new substance. For example, hydrocarbons painted onto the skin of mice or rabbits, and aromatic amines administered orally or parenterally to dogs are often carcinogenic. Some chemicals may produce cancer after a single dose, while others are carcinogenic only when administered in small doses over prolonged periods. Many otherwise harmless substances (even glucose) may produce tumours in rats when repeatedly injected subcutaneously. Carcinogenic activity may be due to a metabolic product, and cancer occurs only in those species which form the metabolite. For example, it has been shown that 2-naphthylamine is converted to a carcinogenic metabolite, 1-hydroxy-2-naphthylamine, in man and the dog, but not in the rabbit or rat.

The numbers of animals used in tests for carcinogenicity should be sufficient to ensure that a considerable number survive for their accepted life-span. Carcinogenicity is indicated when the number of tumours in the treated groups is statistically significantly higher than that in the untreated control groups. The predictive power of animal tests for carcinogenicity is low and it is never possible to say that a compound will not be carcinogenic in man.

Therapeutic index: the ratio of toxic to therapeutic doses. The concept of the therapeutic index was introduced to express the relative safety of drugs: the higher the index, the safer the drug. In the preliminary pharmacological evaluation of a new drug, the lethal dose determined in an acute toxicity test and the effective dose used in the screening test may be used, then, the ratio of LD_{50} to ED_{50} is used to give a guide to the therapeutic index.

The therapeutic index is more valid when applied to toxic effects which are extensions of the therapeutic effect than to side effects. Where the therapeutic and toxic effects are related to each other, the doses tend to have normal distributions of the same form (i.e. with equal standard deviations). This is the case with cardiac glycosides, which have a therapeutic index of about 3 (dose to produce cardiac arrhythmias/dose to improve cardiac performance) and with barbiturates, with an index of about 10 (dose to produce fatal level of central depression/dose to produce sedative level of central depression).

Where the therapeutic and toxic effects are quite unrelated, it is most likely that the doses have different forms of distribution. There is then little justification for comparing the ratio of means. In recent years, the great concern about drug toxicity has led to more conservative ratios being adopted. Some authorities maintain that the ratio should be calculated on the minimum toxic dose (TD) and the maximum therapeutically effective dose (ED), the values used being, say, TD_1 and ED_{99}.

Extrapolation of data from animal experiments. Dosages of drugs are usually computed on the basis of body weight. However, there is no justification for using relative body weights in experimental animals and in man as a basis for selecting suitable doses of drugs for trial in man. Reasonable results have usually been obtained by using relative surface areas for predicting dosage. Ideally, information would be needed about the concentrations of drugs at their sites of actions, in respect of both therapeutic and toxic actions. However, differences between absorption, distribution and metabolism of drugs between man and laboratory animals does not allow accurate prediction of effective concentrations in man. The dose in man may be adjusted to give a concentration of a drug in the blood which is equal to that producing the desired effect in animals. In practice, the first time a new drug is given to man, a very small dose is used. However, before a full clinical trial is started, it is necessary to ensure that the dose is adequate. From the above considerations, it is clear that animal experiments give no more than an indication of the dose of a drug that will be suitable in man; this raises practical problems, but there is no particularly serious risk. A more important question is the value of toxicity tests in animals for predicting the nature of the toxic effects that are likely to occur in patients treated with a new drug. The magnitude of this problem was demonstrated by Litchfield in 1962. He compared the unwanted effects in man reported for a series of six drugs in established clinical use with the toxic effects that could be observed in toxicity experiments with dogs and rats. Of the 53 unwanted effects that occurred in man, 29 of these were detected in experiments with dogs and 18 in experiments with rats. There appeared to be only a marginal advantage in using both the dog and the rat for chronic toxicity studies in this particular study, because only 1 of the 18 toxic reactions seen in rats was different from those found in dogs. Many of the toxic effects that occur in animals are not encountered in patients who are treated with the drug. Litchfield found that the dog, while giving an indication of about half of the unwanted effects that did occur, also provided indications of 24 unwanted effects that have so far not been encountered with these drugs in man.

Apart from predicting the nature of the toxic effects that occur in man on the basis of animal experiments, there is the far more difficult question of predicting their frequency. It has been mentioned above that it is possible in toxicity tests to use only a very small number of animals relative to the large numbers of patients who are likely to receive the drug when it becomes established in clinical use. There is a margin of safety provided by toxicity testing in animals since patients will be exposed to a lower dose of the drug than that which has been used in animals during chronic toxicity tests. Nevertheless, there always remains an element of risk, since toxic effects have occurred in man without there being any counterpart in animal experiments. The most serious of these are allergic reactions, skin lesions, neurological disorders, and some blood dyscrasias. Toxicity tests in animals also fail to reveal such minor unwanted effects as headache, nausea or mild depression, which constitute no great hazard to the patient, but which often preclude the use of a drug in any but the more serious diseases.

It is not possible to propose a standard of 'maximal permissible toxicity' for a drug before it is administered to man. Moral decisions are involved. Where the prognosis of the disease for which the drug is intended is poor and the existing drugs are unsatisfactory, a lower standard may be acceptable than if satisfactory drugs are already available. There may be in fact greater risk to the patient if a potentially useful drug is not used. The responsibility of administering the drug rests with the clinician in charge of the patient. In order to accept this responsibility, it is essential that he should understand and appreciate the meaning and limitations of toxicity tests in animals.

Control over the introduction of drugs into medicine. The evaluation of drug toxicity is not always at the discretion of individuals. In the United States, there has been for some years government control over the introduction of new drugs into medicine; this is exercised by a body known as the Food and Drug Administration (FDA) which was first established under regulations passed in 1906 and subsequently brought up to date. Officials of the FDA must evaluate the data on the potential usefulness and the toxicity of all new drugs before they are released for sale; they may also review existing drugs and cause them to be withdrawn if they are considered to be worthless or have undue toxicity. There is no equivalent British organization, but public concern about the increased incidence of toxicity, which has accompanied the recent expansion in drug development, led to the establishment in 1963 of a committee on safety of drugs known as the Dunlop committee, named after its first (and present) chairman. This committee assesses the evidence on the efficacy and the toxicity of newly developed drugs and decides on whether clinical trials are justified and then on whether the drug should be marketed. It also reviews reports on toxicity of drugs already in use. The decisions of the committee are adhered to by voluntary agreement on the part of those concerned with the development and promotion of drugs.

Clinical trial of new drugs. After laboratory investigations have indicated that a drug may be worthy of trial in patients, the first use of the drug in man may be confined to a few selected subjects who have volunteered to act as 'guinea-pigs'. Often they are people who have been engaged on the development of the drug. Close attention is paid to these subjects in order to determine the pharmacology of the drug in man and in case of deleterious unforeseen actions.

The clinical trial itself has as its object the assessment of the efficacy of the new drug in treating disease. Thus, the trial is in the nature of an experiment which should be conducted with due regard to appropriate design and statistical analysis. This has not always been done. Bradford Hill has pointed out some of the pitfalls that are encountered when the trial is not planned properly. (1) The patients given the new drug may be chosen by applying special criteria: they may be, for example, the most severely ill, or refractory to previous methods of treatment. (2) The new drug may be given only to patients who volunteer. It cannot be assumed, without proof, that volunteers are comparable to those who do not volunteer. (3) The results from the exclusive use of a new drug by one doctor, or in one hospital, are compared with the results obtained by another doctor, or in another hospital. Again, the two groups of patients are not necessarily comparable. A further difficulty that arises is that the response of patients to many drugs depends in part on the particular doctor or hospital. (4) The results obtained with a new drug may be compared with results obtained previously; that is, there is a 'historical' control group. The problems in this case are that the severity of the disease may have changed (the marked changes in the virulence of influenza virus are well-known), the method of diagnosis may differ, and the criteria for assessing the results of treatment are unlikely to remain constant.

The experimental design of clinical trials cannot be discussed without consideration of medical ethics. The efficacy of a drug in treatment of diseased patients could be most readily assessed if some patients received no treatment and acted as controls. When the consequences of withholding drug treatment from a control group may be the risk of death (or severe or permanent damage to health), then it would be unethical to assign patients to such a fate and there can be no control group. However, there are many disorders in which the effectiveness of medical treatment is not definitely established, and then there is no reason to believe that there is any risk in withholding treatment (the common cold, headache and acne are three examples). Where the object of the trial is to compare a new drug with an established drug, then the ethics of the situation require that the experimenter should have grounds for believing that the trial is worthwhile. Frequently, the evidence for this belief is provided by laboratory findings of lower toxicity or greater effectiveness in the new drug.

In selecting patients for clinical trial, due consideration is needed of unwanted side-effects that may result from disease. For example, tuberculosis and other infections may be activated and exacerbated by anti-inflammatory drugs related to the adrenal steroids.

The division of patients into groups is carried out in accordance with the same principles that guide the division of stocks of experimental animals into comparable groups. The sex and age of the patients are obvious factors to be considered, but additional factors include the severity of the disease, the previous response to treatment, and the presence of complications and concurrent disease. The allocation into the groups of patients who are matched in all obvious respects is ideally made by a random procedure, such as tossing a coin. In the simplest case, the patients are divided into two groups: one is treated with the new drug, the other is given either an existing drug or a dummy preparation (placebo) depending on the nature of the disease and other factors.

It is usual to carry out clinical trials in such a way that neither the attendant physician nor the patients knows which treatment is being given; the treatments are coded by someone not directly involved in the trial (e.g. the hospital pharmacist). This procedure is known as a *double-blind trial*. It eliminates bias in the physician's asssessment of the degree of improvement of the patient. Furthermore, any changes in the patient's condition are unlikely to be affected by his attitude to the treatment; patients make judgements about the treatment they are receiving, and often respond in the way they think is expected of them. For example, in a trial where special enquiries were made about the incidence of stuffy noses, there was as much complaint among patients who received placebo as among those who took the active drug (reserpine).

In clinical trials, as in bioassay, the dose of drug and the measurement of the response must be considered, as well as the experimental design. As far as possible, information about dosage is gauged from preliminary trials. While it would be desirable to investigate the effects of more than one dose level, this introduces difficulties and often insufficient patients are available. It is often worthwhile to choose the maximum dose that can be tolerated by each individual rather than select an arbitrary dose which can be tolerated by all, but which may be less than optimal for many. In addition to the dose administered, the formulation and presentation of the drug should be optimal to ensure that absorption and persistence of effect are adequate. The response of a patient to drug treatment may not always be amenable to quantitative measurement. In some cases, the response can be expressed numerically, for example, with a diuretic, there is the volume of urine voided, or with an antihypertensive, there is the fall in blood pressure. However, the relief of pain by an analgesic, or the decrease in arthritic symptoms with an anti-inflammatory drug, is more difficult to express in quantitative terms. In such cases, the response may be graded in terms of an arbitrary rating scale.

Sequential analysis. There is a recently developed statistical method that is of particular use in the analysis of clinical trials in which one drug (treatment A) is compared with another or with a placebo (treatment B). Matched pairs of

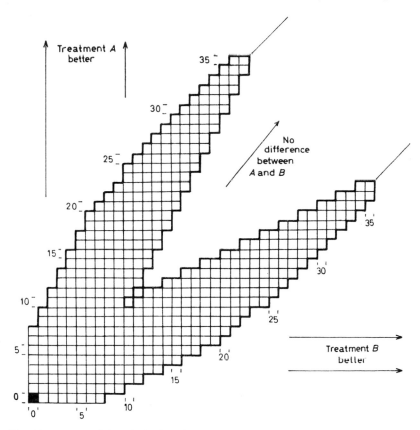

FIG. 20.9. Sequential analysis chart for pair difference (between treatment A and B) at 95% significance level. The result from each pair of patients is entered in the chart by filling in the square above the black corner square if A is better than B, or the square to the right if B is better than A. No entry is made if there is no difference. This process is continued up or across the chart with successive pairs of patients until a barrier is crossed, when the statement indicated can be made. Charts with other significance levels can be constructed.

suitable patients are selected and the decision about which of each of a pair is to receive which treatment is made at random (say, by tossing a coin). The two treatments are given to the pair of patients and one of three possible judgements is made about the result: treatment A is better, or treatment B is better, or there is no difference between the treatments. This result is entered into the appropriate place in a specially prepared chart such as that shown in Fig. 20.9; its use is described in the figure legend. The trial is continued in this way until a statistically meaningful statement can be made about the comparison between the treatments. This method of analysis has the advantage that no decision has to be made before beginning the trial about the number of patients to be used.

CHAPTER 21

General Anaesthetics

Drugs producing depression of the activity of the central nervous system (CNS) may be classified according to the part of the nervous system affected and the degree of depression produced. General anaesthetics are one class of CNS depressant drugs; other classes are described in Chapters 22 and 24. The word anaesthesia means *without sensation*, and implies a state of unconsciousness. Some CNS depressant drugs are termed *narcotics* as they produce narcosis (derived from the Greek word meaning stupor). In the United States of America, the word narcotic has come to have a rather different meaning, and is applied only to drugs capable of causing addiction.

General anaesthetics produce a reversible loss of consciousness which allows surgical operations to be carried out. Most of them are gases or volatile liquids and are given by inhalation (inhalation anaesthetics). Non-volatile general anaesthetics are administered by intravenous injection; they may also be used in lower doses as basal anaesthetics before an operation. The patient then arrives in the theatre asleep or drowsy so that his anxiety is allayed and full anaesthesia is easier and safer to accomplish.

Inhalation anaesthetics

Structure–action relationships. These are mostly simple aliphatic compounds. Within an homologous series of compounds, anaesthetic potency generally increases with increase in the length of the carbon chain up to a maximum, beyond which potency decreases. Solubility in water also varies with chain length. The abrupt decrease in potency in many series is probably linked with the lower solubility of the compounds in plasma. The saturated straight-chain *paraffins* have anaesthetic activity although they are not used in medicine for this purpose; anaesthetic potency increases up to hexane, beyond which a stimulant action becomes evident. Each member of the *olefine* series is a more potent depressant than the corresponding paraffin and in fact ethylene is employed as an anaesthetic. Members higher than ethylene are increasingly more potent in inducing cardiac arrhythmias. In the *acetylene* series, there is also an increase in potency with increase in chain length; however, members higher than acetylene are too unstable to allow their use as anaesthetics. Halogen substitution of the paraffins, olefines, and acetylenes increases

569

anaesthetic potency, chlorine substitution being most often used as these compounds are more stable. The potency of chlorine-substituted compounds increases with increase in chain length, with progressive unsaturation, and with an increase in the number of substituent chlorine atoms although with complete chlorination there is a slight fall-off in potency. Thus, chloroform is more potent than carbon tetrachloride, and trichloroethylene is more potent than tetrachloroethylene. The introduction of chlorine atoms, while increasing depressant activity, also leads to unwanted effects such as the production of degenerative changes in liver and kidney and depression of the heart. The incidence of these side-effects increases with increase in the number of chlorine atoms. The addition of a hydroxyl group reduces but does not abolish anaesthetic potency; the greater the number of hydroxyl groups, the less is the activity. Thus ethane is more potent than ethyl alcohol, which in turn is more potent than glycol; glycerol has practically no activity. Tertiary alcohols have more activity than primary alcohols. In fact, tertiary amyl alcohol (amylene hydrate) was once used in medicine. The introduction of hydroxyl groups results in an unwanted irritant action as the tissues are dehydrated and protein is precipitated. Halogen substitution in the alcohols again leads to increase in depressant potency, and tribromethanol is a useful basal anaesthetic. Substitution of an alkyl group for the hydrogen in the hydroxyl group gives an *alkyl oxide* or *ether*, and these compounds form an important group of anaesthetic agents although the higher members in a homologous series of ethers possess unwanted side-effects. Substitution of an amine group in a hydrocarbon nucleus to form an alkylamine usually abolishes anaesthetic activity.

In the choice of anaesthetic agents for clinical use, it is necessary to take into account anaesthetic potency, intensity of unwanted effects, and chemical stability.

Anaesthesia. With increasing concentration, general anaesthetics produce an irregular descending depression of the central nervous system; the functions depressed first are, in general, those which were formed last in phylogenetic and embryological development. The order of depression is cerebral cortex (probably indirectly through the brain stem reticular formation), basal ganglia, cerebellum and spinal cord. Sensory functions of the cord are depressed before motor functions. With toxic doses, the respiratory and vasomotor centres of the medulla oblongata are depressed.

The progress of anaesthesia produced by an inhalation anaesthetic may be divided into three merging stages.

STAGE 1. The effects seen in this stage are due to depression of higher cortical functions. Consciousness is not lost but thoughts are blurred and there may be hallucinations. All reflexes are present. Smell and pain sensations are lost towards the end of this stage which is sometimes called the *stage of analgesia*. Anaesthesia limited to stage 1 is sometimes used in the first stage of labour.

STAGE 2. This begins with the onset of unconsciousness. The cortical inhibitory centres are depressed before the motor centres and this gives rise to exaggerated reflexes, increased and irregular breathing, increased muscle tone, and increased autonomic activity. The patient may laugh or sing and make uncontrolled movements; reflex vomiting may occur. Hence this stage is sometimes called the *stage* of *excitement* or *delirium*. Most deaths resulting from anaesthesia have occurred during this stage. After a period of apnoea, the patient may take a few deep breaths and these rapidly produce a toxic concentration of anaesthetic in the blood. Cardiac arrhythmias may occur as a result of vagal inhibition of the heart or of sensitization of the heart by the anaesthetic to circulating adrenaline and noradrenaline released from cardiac sympathetic nerves. There is further depression of sensory areas and the senses of hearing and sight are lost. The pupils are dilated and the eye-balls roll. There is flushing of the skin, temperature control is lost, and the patient becomes poikilothermic. No surgical operations are performed during this stage. Stages 1 and 2 together form the *induction* phase of anaesthesia.

STAGE 3. This is the *stage of surgical anaesthesia*, the *first plane* of which is recognized by the return of regular, slightly slowed breathing and constriction of the pupil. The cough and vomiting centres are depressed, although passive regurgitation of stomach contents may occur at any time in stage 3. It is therefore necessary to fast the patient before the operation so as to avoid the risk of aspiration of stomach contents into the trachea. The pharyngeal and cutaneous reflexes disappear towards the end of the first plane. In the *second plane*, the eye-balls become fixed and the pupils begin to dilate again. Respiration becomes shallower and the pharyngeal and laryngeal reflexes completely disappear. The larger skeletal muscles relax and only the peritoneal and deeper reflexes remain active. The corneal reflex disappears towards the end of the second plane. Before the introduction of muscle relaxants (page 678), only relatively minor operations were performed in the first and second planes. In the *third plane*, breathing becomes further depressed and thoracic respiratory movements lag behind abdominal respiration. The pupil becomes further dilated and muscular relaxation becomes marked. The peritoneal reflex disappears, permitting abdominal surgery even in the absence of specific muscle relaxant drugs. The blood pressure decreases towards the end of the third plane. In the *fourth plane*, depression of medullary centres becomes more marked; the blood pressure falls, the pulse is rapid and feeble, and respiration becomes shallow, weak and irregular. All reflexes are completely abolished and the pupils are widely dilated. Surgical anaesthesia is never intentionally allowed to pass beyond this point as the medullary centres become completely paralysed, respiration ceases, and the heart and circulation fail. This stage of overdosage is sometimes designated *stage* 4.

With various inhalation anaesthetics, the *relative* duration of the stages is about the same but the time to reach plane 4 varies widely. For example, the time is short with vinyl ether but relatively long with ether. During recovery from anaesthesia, function returns essentially in the reverse order to that in which it disappeared, although the stage of excitement is usually milder than during induction.

Uptake and elimination of anaesthetics. The depth of anaesthesia produced by a particular drug depends on its concentration in the central nervous system. The uptake of an inhalation anaesthetic depends on the concentration of the drug in the inspired air, the rate and depth of breathing, the permeability of the alveolar-capillary membrane to the drug, the blood flow to the lungs, the solubility of the drug in the blood, the blood flow to the brain relative to that to other tissues, and the partition coefficient of the drug between the blood and brain tissue.

When anaesthesia is first induced, the concentration gradient from alveolar air to blood is steep and absorption into the blood is therefore rapid. With time, blood and tissue levels approach equilibrium with alveolar air and absorption slows until finally diffusion is equal in both directions. When administration of the anaesthetic is stopped, the reverse process occurs, elimination being rapid at first and then slower. With a relatively water-soluble anaesthetic such as ether, the approach to saturation of the blood is slow and is chiefly limited by the respiratory minute volume. Premedication with morphine may cause respiratory depression and so reduce the amount of anaesthetic inhaled and absorbed. On the other hand, stimulation of respiration (as, for example, with CO_2) results in an increased amount of anaesthetic being absorbed. The alveolar-capillary membrane is usually highly permeable to the anaesthetic and there is free diffusion across it, although excessive secretion of mucus may impede diffusion. The cardiac output and rate of blood flow to the lungs is only important in determining the speed of induction with anaesthetics which are sparingly soluble in water.

The fact that the rich blood supply to the brain receives a large percentage of the total cardiac output (page 104) may explain the selective action of anaesthetics on the central nervous system. The membranes of the closely-packed neurones and glial cells of the brain are composed partly of lipids, and anaesthetics must be capable of passing from the aqueous blood phase and of penetrating lipid barriers to exert their depressant action. It was shown by Overton and Meyer and others at the turn of the twentieth century that the potency of anaesthetics (measured in tadpoles) increases with their solubility in lipid compared with that in water. However, many classes of drugs are soluble in lipids but have no anaesthetic activity. Although anaesthetics are lipid-soluble, the concentration in fat depots of the body is slow to reach equilibrium with that in the plasma as the blood supply to these depots is usually poor. When anaesthetic administration is discontinued after short-lasting operations, the brain contains a high concentration of the anaesthetic and diffusion from the brain to other tissues, including the lungs, occurs rapidly down the steep concentration gradient. After long operations, however the body tissues are saturated and diffusion from the brain is slower. Most inhalation anaesthetics are eliminated from the body by the lungs although a proportion of some is metabolized in the liver.

Site and mechanism of action. The drugs capable of producing general anaes-thesia vary widely in chemical structure. They are relatively unspecific in their action in the sense that with high concentrations all excitable tissues of the body are affected by them. Their type of action therefore differs from that of more specific drugs; for example, atropine-like drugs (Chapter 28), neuro-muscular blocking drugs (Chapter 26), or antihistamines (Chapter 30) which have a high affinity for particular receptor sites, with relatively little effect on other structures. The apparently selective action of anaesthetics on certain areas of the brain is probably the result of these areas having high lipid con-tents, relatively large blood supplies, and delicately balanced metabolic mechanisms which are highly susceptible to disturbances. There is evidence that several anaesthetics preferentially depress the ascending reticular activa-ting system (page 133) which is known to be concerned in maintaining wakefulness. As a result, there is a decrease in the electrical activity of the cortex as recorded with the EEG, and sensory stimulation no longer produces the characteristic arousal reaction.

The structural non-specificity of anaesthetics suggests that their mechanism of action depends upon their physico-chemical properties. In fact, Ferguson in 1939 stated that the same *relative* saturation of the brain with different anaesthetics should produce the same degree of depression. Thermodynamic activity (which is a measure of the proportion of molecules free to react with the target site) should therefore be a suitable index of anaesthetic activity. The thermodynamic activity at the site of action (i.e. the nervous tissue) cannot be measured directly. When a steady level of anaesthesia is produced during long-continued administration, however, the concentrations of anaesthetic administered and those present in the various tissues are in equilibrium. Then, the thermodynamic activity at the site of administration is proportional to that in the nervous tissue. The thermodynamic activity (μ) is given by the formula: $\mu = RT \log_e(P/P_s)$, where R is the gas constant, T the absolute temperature, P the partial pressure of the anaesthetic in the inspired gas mixture and P_s, the saturated vapour pressure of the pure anaesthetic. Since R and T are constants, Ferguson used the factor P/P_s as an index of thermodynamic activity. Even though the concentrations of different anaesthetics necessary to produce a given degree of anaesthesia vary widely, the value of the ratio P/P_s was found to be fairly constant. Although this gives no information about the actual mechanism of action, Ferguson's result supported the idea that anaesthetic agents act through some physical mechanism rather than by chemical combination with a specific receptor site.

At the neuronal level, possible mechanisms of action of anaesthetic drugs include (i) depression of conduction along axons, (ii) depression of the release of excitatory transmitters from presynaptic nerve endings, and (iii) depression of the sensitivity of post-synaptic neuronal membranes to the released transmitters. There are technical difficulties involved in testing these possibilities in the brain itself, as well as a lack of knowledge concerning the nature of central transmitters (see pages 167–171). There is little direct evidence for one or other of these actions as yet. However, the rather unspecific nature of the mode of action of anaesthetics may permit analogies to be drawn from their known actions on the spinal cord and on simpler peripheral organizations such as isolated nerves, autonomic ganglia, the neuromuscular junction, and the nerve plexuses of the gut.

The volatile anaesthetics depress conduction along isolated nerve fibres and decrease excitability without markedly affecting the resting membrane potential (i.e. they act as membrane stabilizers, page 88), but high concentrations are required to produce these effects. They are more active in impairing transmission at synapses. Concentrations which impair transmission through the stellate ganglion of the cat and through the superior cervical ganglia of cats and rabbits are much lower than those which affect conduction in the pre-ganglionic nerve trunks; the concentrations which impair ganglionic transmission are comparable with those which produce surgical anaesthesia. Ether depresses the monosynaptic reflex pathway of the spinal cord (page 114) by acting at the synapse. In the guinea-pig ileum, volatile anaesthetics produce a marked reduction of acetylcholine release in response to electrical stimulation of the intra-mural nerve network; they also reduce the response of the smooth muscle to stimulant drugs. In striated muscle, ether and halothane decrease the sensitivity of the motor end-plates to acetylcholine. It seems probable, therefore, that volatile anaesthetics interrupt synaptic transmission in the brain by depressing the release of transmitters and by depressing the excitability of post-synaptic membranes. The concentration of acetylcholine in the brain is increased during anaesthesia suggesting that its release and consequent destruction by cholinesterase, may have been depressed.

Several mechanisms have been postulated to explain the depressant effects of anaesthetics on central synaptic transmission. (1) Anaesthetics may act by depressing respiratory enzymes systems. Reduced cerebral oxygen uptake has been demonstrated during anaesthesia produced by barbiturates, and the oxygen uptake of isolated stimulated brain slices is also depressed. However, the concentrations of drug required are high and the effect is accompanied by a rise, rather than by a fall, in the concentration of energy-rich phosphate compounds suggesting that the reduced oxygen uptake may be the result, and not the cause, of anaesthesia. (2) Mullins suggested that molecules of anaesthetic agents enter some non-aqueous polar lattice in the cell membrane decreasing its permeability to ions. He considered the size of the molecule as well as the concentration to be important and showed that the product of the thermodynamic activity and the molecular volume is constant for many anaesthetics. (3) Some compounds in solution form complexes in which aggregates of solute molecules are completely enclosed within cavities formed by the union of molecules of solvent around them. Miller noted that many anaesthetics formed such complexes (known as *gas hydrates* or *clathrates*) in water and suggested that this effect, occurring at a neuronal surface, affects its electrical and permeability properties. Pauling independently put forward a similar suggestion but considered that the simple gas hydrates are stabilized by interaction with the charged side-chains of proteins and other tissue constituents.

Inhalation anaesthetics used in surgery

The chief inhalation anaesthetics in clinical use are listed in Tables 21.1, 21.2 and 21.3. None of them is free from unwanted effects and, where possible, attempts are made to correct their imperfections by the simultaneous use of adjuvant drugs. The ideal anaesthetic should (i) be free from unpleasant smell, (ii) be non-irritant, (iii) produce rapid pleasant induction and recovery, (iv) be non-explosive, (v) not increase capillary bleeding, (vi) produce complete muscular relaxation, (vii) possess a wide margin of safety, (viii) be highly potent so that adequate amounts of oxygen may be mixed with it, (ix) be free from side-effects, (x) be absorbed and excreted rapidly thereby allowing accurate control of depth of anaesthesia and (xi) be cheap to manufacture and purify, and be stable during storage.

The main volatile liquids used as general anaesthetics are *ether* (diethylether), *chloroform*, *halothane*, *divinylether*, *ethylchloride* and *trichloroethylene* (Fig. 21.1). The first three of these, when mixed only with adequate amounts of air or oxygen, may be considered as major anaesthetics in that the vapours are capable of producing anaesthesia to planes 3 or 4 and adequate muscle relaxation for most operations. In practice, neuromuscular blocking drugs are often used as adjuvants. As halothane produces insufficient muscle relaxation for

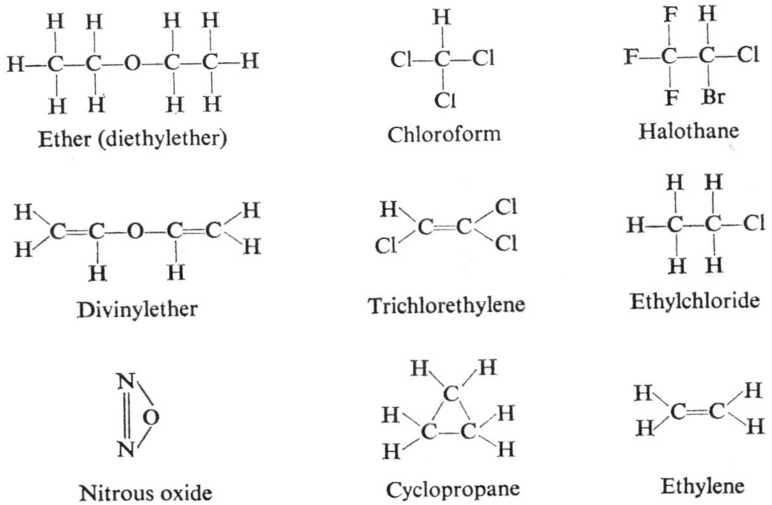

FIG. 21.1. Chemical formulae of some inhalation anaesthetics.

major abdominal surgery, a neuromuscular blocking drug is essential in this case. Some of the properties of ether, chloroform and halothane are compared in Table 21.1.

Divinylether, ethylchloride, and trichloroethylene are not used as the sole agents for major surgery. The depth of anaesthesia produced by divinylether is too difficult to control, and the depth of anaesthesia and degree of muscle relaxation that is produced with sub-toxic concentrations of ethylene chloride and trichloroethylene are inadequate. Some of the properties of these three agents are compared in Table 21.2.

The principal gases used as general anaesthetics are *nitrous oxide, cyclopropane* and *ethylene* (Fig. 21.1). Induction with these three agents is rapid and pleasant, and none of them is irritant to mucous membranes. They are often used for induction, and then anaesthesia is continued with one of the more potent anaesthetics, or they may be used as the sole anaesthetic for short-lasting minor operations. Toxic effects produced by the gaseous anaesthetics are chiefly due to anoxia and they should therefore be administered mixed with oxygen. When concentrations high enough to produce adequate muscle relaxation for major surgery are administered, it is impossible to include

TABLE 21.1. Some properties of the major volatile liquid anaesthetics.

Anaesthetic	Ether	Chloroform	Halothane
Boiling point	35°C	61°C	50°C
Inflammable and explosive	Yes	No	No
Induction	Slow and unpleasant	Rapid and pleasant	More rapid than ether and pleasant
Irritant to mucous membranes	Yes. Causes coughing, laryngeal spasm and profuse mucus secretion	Less irritant than ether because more potent and less is required	Non-irritant
Sensitizes myocardium to adrenaline	No	Yes, and may lead to cardiac arrhythmias	Yes, but less so than chloroform
Stimulates sympathetic system	Yes	No	No
Causes increased capillary bleeding	Yes	No	No
Heart and circulation	Heart rate and blood pressure not depressed until plane 3 is reached	Fall in blood pressure and in cardiac output due to depression of myocardium and vasomotor centre and direct dilator action on vessels	Causes hypotension and bradycardia due to depression of vasomotor centre and ganglionic blockade
Potentiates curare-like drugs	Yes	Very weakly	Yes, but less than ether
Post-operative complications	Nausea and vomiting after prolonged operation. No permanent liver damage	Nausea and vomiting May cause permanent damage to liver and kidneys	Minor and rare

sufficient oxygen to avoid anoxia. Consequently, the gaseous anaesthetics are not used as the sole agents for major operations. Some of the properties of these three gaseous anaesthetics are compared in Table 21.3.

The chief disadvantages of inhalation anaesthetics are as follows: (1) *Toxic decomposition products.* The volatile liquid anaesthetics are readily oxidized on exposure to air, light or moisture with the production of toxic and sometimes explosive impurities, such as peroxides from ethers and phosgene from the halogen-containing agents. Consequently special conditions of storage and the addition of preservatives (such as ethanol or thymol) are often necessary to prevent decomposition. (2) *Inflammable and explosive properties.* These are

19

TABLE 21.2. Some properties of minor volatile liquid anaesthetics.

Anaesthetic	Divinyl ether	Trichloroethylene	Ethyl chloride
Boiling point	28°C	87°C	12°C, therefore kept under pressure
Inflammable	Yes, and explosive in air or oxygen	Not inflammable in air but may be when mixed with oxygen	Yes
Induction	Very rapid and difficult to control	Rapid	Fairly rapid
Irritant to mucous membranes	Slightly	No	Slightly
Cardiovascular system	No serious effect	Cardiac arrhythmias are common but not serious	Sensitizes heart to adrenaline and depresses heart and blood vessels, as does chloroform
Other complications during anaesthesia	High potency and rapid action makes anaesthesia difficult to control. Convulsions occasionally occur	May cause rapid shallow respiration due to sensitization of pulmonary stretch receptors	May cause laryngospasm
Post-operative complications	Nausea and vomiting rare. May cause liver damage after prolonged use	Nausea and vomiting common. Liver and kidney damage rare	Nausea and vomiting and damage to liver and kidneys if inhalation prolonged
Use	Minor surgery and in obstetrics and dentistry. Induction prior to ether anaesthesia, sometimes mixed with nitrous oxide or ethylene	Short operations and in obstetrics and dentistry. Combined with oxygen and nitrous oxide for operations lasting up to 1 h	Minor surgery and in obstetrics and dentistry Induction prior to ether anaesthesia. Occasionally sprayed on skin to produce local loss of sensation—rapid evaporation cools the tissue

Table 21.3. Some properties of gaseous anaesthetics.

Anaesthetics	Nitrous oxide	Cyclopropane	Ethylene
Inflammable and explosive	No but supports combustion	Yes	Yes
Causes increased capillary bleeding	No	Yes	No
Sensitizes myocardium to adrenaline	No	Yes; may lead to cardiac arrhythmias	No
Other actions during anaesthesia	Exhilaration, euphoria and hallucinations during induction. Called 'laughing gas'	May cause laryngospasm during induction. Causes reflex bradycardia via the vagus	Usually none, provided sufficient oxygen present
Post-operative effects	Anoxia may occur if mixed with less than 20% v/v oxygen. Otherwise no serious post-operative effects	Excitement, nausea, vomiting and laryngospasm may occur. Anoxia occurs if insufficient oxygen is present	Nausea and vomiting. Anoxia occurs if insufficient oxygen is present
Use	Mixed with oxygen for dental surgery and obstetrics and to induce anaesthesia before giving a more potent anaesthetic. Surgery may be performed under nitrous oxide plus oxygen provided a neuromuscular blocking drug is used	Mixed with oxygen to induce anaesthesia or to supplement anaesthesia produced by a basal anaesthetic. May be used as sole anaesthetic agent, with oxygen, when a neuromuscular blocking drug is used	Mixed with oxygen for minor surgery, dental surgery and obstetrics. May be used in major abdominal surgery when combined with oxygen, a basal anaesthetic and a neuromuscular blocking drug

a serious disadvantage as any spark occurring in the electrical equipment present in an operating theatre may be sufficient to cause ignition. Further-more, electro-cautery cannot be used to stop small bleeding points; this is especially troublesome when, in addition, the drug increases capillary bleeding (as, for example, with ether and cyclopropane). (3) *Prolonged induction.* Induc-tion is particularly slow with ether as it has a relatively high water solubility (1 in 15 at 37°C). Saturation of the blood is slow and a considerable amount is taken up in the body water. When ether is to be used, anaesthesia is usually induced with a rapidly acting inhalation or intravenous anaesthetic. (4) *Irritant action.* Ether is particularly troublesome in this respect, producing broncho-constriction and increased secretion of mucus and saliva, both of which may obstruct the airways and cause laryngospasm. These effects are due to excita-tion of parasympathetic nerves and may be prevented by the previous admini-stration of atropine or hyoscine (page 728). (5) *Sympathetic stimulation.* Anxiety and fear in a patient before the operation increases the level of circu-lating adrenaline and this is raised further when induction is slow and strugg-ling occurs. This effect may be minimized by suitable pre-medication with a tranquillizer or basal anaesthetic and by the use of a rapidly acting anaesthetic for induction. Ether itself however stimulates the sympatho-adrenal mech-anism during induction, thereby temporarily raising the blood pressure and heart rate. Ether does not sensitize the myocardium to the action of circulating catecholamines, whereas this occurs with other anaesthetics, such as chloro-form, cyclopropane, halothane and ethyl chloride; it is then particularly important to prevent increased sympathetic activity in order to prevent the precipitation of ventricular fibrillation. Cardiac arrhythmias are more liable to occur in thyrotoxic patients (thyroid hormone sensitizes many tissues to the action of adrenaline), when there is hypoxia and CO_2 retention, and during operations carried out under hypothermia. The cardiac arrhythmias may sometimes be prevented by antifibrillatory agents (pages 817–820). The neuro-muscular blocking drugs, *tubocurarine* and *gallamine*, have also been reported to reduce the production of cardiac arrhythmias by anaesthetics in the presence of adrenaline. (6) *Other cardiovascular effects.* Ether depresses the myocardium but this effect is relatively unimportant as it occurs only with high concen-trations. Chloroform, on the other hand, depresses the heart and blood vessels from the start of induction and this effect, coupled with the sensitization to adrenaline, makes chloroform particularly liable to precipitate ventricular fibrillation during induction. For similar reasons sudden deaths have occa-sionally occurred with cyclopropane. When cyclopropane is withdrawn, there is occasionally a sudden drop in blood pressure. Halothane may cause a fall in blood pressure and bradycardia and these effects are enhanced by adjuvants possessing a hypotensive action (for example, other anaesthetic agents, ganglion blocking drugs or anticholinesterase drugs). The fall in blood pressure may be antagonized by pressor agents such as *methoxamine* (page 749) or by using a mixture of one part ether and two parts halothane (halothane-ether-azeotrope), when the sympathetic stimulation induced by ether tends to antagonize the vascular depression produced by halothane. (7) *Inadequate muscular relaxation.* None of the anaesthetics in Tables 21.2 and 21.3 by themselves in sub-toxic doses produce adequate muscle relaxation for major surgery. Those in Table 21.1 are capable of doing so but in practice the depth of anaesthesis is rarely allowed to reach planes 3 or 4 and muscle relaxation is achieved either by the use of neuromuscular blocking drugs or by nerve block produced by local anaesthetic drugs (e.g. lignocaine). Some general anaesthetics potentiate the action of the competitive neuromuscular blocking drugs, tubocurarine and gallamine. Ether is particularly effective in this respect but halothane, cyclopropane and to a lesser extent chloroform share this property. (8) *Post operative complications.* Several inhalation anaesthetics give rise to post-operative nausea and vomiting but this is rarely serious. Damage to the liver and kidney is a more serious complication and the production of hepatic necrosis by chloroform, together with its toxic effects on the heart and circulation, have resulted in its use as an anaesthetic being largely discontinued.

Adjuvants to anaesthesia. The drugs used in conjunction with general anaesthetics depend partly on the type of operation and partly on the anaesthetic used. As premedication for surgery, basal anaesthetics or sedative drugs (e.g. barbiturates) or tranquillizing drugs (e.g. chlorpromazine) are given to reduce the patient's anxiety. Analgesic drugs (e.g. morphine or pethidine) may be administered when the patient is in pain or when only a weak general anaesthetic agent is to be used. Atropine or hyoscine may be used to reduce bronchial and salivary secretions; these two drugs are also reputed to protect the heart from vagal inhibition but the dose usually used is unlikely to block the action of the vagus on the heart. Many of the drugs used in premedication potentiate the action of the main anaesthetic and the correct use and dosage of combinations of drugs requires knowledge and experience on the part of the anaesthetist.

Post-operatively, an analgesic drug (e.g. pethidine) may be used to relieve pain. Complications such as post-operative paralytic ileus and urinary retention may be treated by using carbachol to restore tone to the smooth muscle or an anticholinesterase drug to increase the effectiveness of the parasympathetic nerve impulses. Antagonists of competitive neuromuscular blocking drugs (e.g. neostigmine) or of hypnotic drugs (i.e. analeptics) may be necessary when spontaneous breathing shows no sign of recommencing at the end of the operation.

Intravenous anaesthetics. The intravenous anaesthetics produce a rapid and pleasant induction; the stages of anaesthesia described for the inhalation anaesthetics are not always seen unless the drug is injected very slowly. By themselves, they do not produce a sufficient depth of anaesthesia for major surgery but they are used as basal or induction anaesthetics in major operations and as the sole anaesthetic agent in short-lasting minor operations. The intravenous anaesthetics are mainly the sodium salts of the very short-acting barbiturates, principally *thiopentone* (pentothal), but also *buthalitone, thialbarbitone, hexobarbitone* and *methohexitone*. These drugs are described more fully with other barbiturates in Chapter 22.

Anaesthesia with thiopentone is induced by injecting about 2 ml of a 2·5% w/v solution and repeating this at about half minute intervals until the required depth of anaesthesia is reached. Great care is necessary to avoid overdosage which results in depression of respiratory activity. Laryngospasm and increased bronchial secretion are common, but these may be prevented by atropine. Solutions of thiopentone sodium are very alkaline and irritant to the tissues; when injected subcutaneously, the skin may slough; when injected into an artery, thrombosis may occur—heparin must be injected immediately and sometimes it is necessary to sympathectomize the limb; when injected near a nerve, permanent damage to the nerve may be produced; however it is safe by clean intravenous injection. Thiopentone is slowly metabolized in the liver. Its duration of action is very short since it is quickly taken up from the plasma into the fat depots of the body. After many injections have been given, the fat depots become saturated and a further dose then produces a prolonged effect. The other very short-acting barbiturates mentioned above are occasionally used to produce anaesthesia but they do not appear to possess any real advantages over thiopentone sodium.

Certain steroid substances have anaesthetic activity (but no hormonal activity) and one of them, *hydroxydione*, has a limited use as an intravenous anaesthetic. Induction is slow but pleasant, and respiratory and circulatory depression are said to be minimal.

Hydroxydione sodium succinate
(21-hydroxypregnane-3,20-dione sodium hemisuccinate)

During recovery there are no unpleasant after-effects such as nausea and vomiting. In cats, it inhibits adrenaline-induced cardiac arrythmias and this is an advantage when it also occurs in man. Its major disadvantage is that it produces pain and venous thrombosis unless injected in very dilute solutions. It is metabolized to 21-dihydroxy 5β-pregnane-20-one which is excreted in the urine.

Basal anaesthetics

These are drugs used to produce a state of unconsciousness which is not deep enough to allow surgery.

Thiopentone is often given by rectum as a 5% solution up to a maximum of 1·5 g, or rarely 3 g. Other drugs used as basal anaesthetics include the following: *Tribromoethanol, an unstable* white powder which is administered rectally as a solution in amylene hydrate; *Bromethol*, a drug which has largely been replaced by the barbiturates for basal anaesthesia although it is still used to prevent convulsions in eclampsia of pregnancy (page 408); and *Paraldehyde*, an irritant inflammable liquid with a very unpleasant smell, is a relatively safe hypnotic. As 10 to 30% of the dose is excreted unchanged in the breath, its offensive smell constitutes its major disadvantage. For basal anaesthesia it is given by rectum (up to 25 ml of a 10% solution); it is also used as an anticonvulsant in status epilepticus, tetanus and eclampsia of pregnancy.

Anaesthetics for animal experiments. Many general anaesthetics are used for animal experiments but when recordings are to be made during anaesthesia (e.g. blood pressure or muscle contraction), the use of adjuvant drugs must be restricted as they may influence the results obtained. When the animal is to be allowed to recover from the anaesthesia, ether or a barbiturate (such as thiopentone sodium or pentobarbitone sodium) provide a suitable short-lasting anaesthesia. These anaesthetics may also be used for acute experiments in which the animal is killed at the end of the recording before it regains consciousness. However, chloralose and urethane are particularly useful for this purpose. Chloralose is not used in man, and urethane has only a limited use.

Chloralose is prepared by heating a mixture of anhydrous glucose and anhydrous chloral. For injection, it is usually made up as a 1% solution by boiling in 0·9% w/v NaCl solution. The solution is injected (at a temperature of 30 to 40°C) before the chloralose comes out of solution on cooling.

Cats and dogs require about 80 to 100 mg/kg (8 to 10 ml/kg of 1% solution). The solution may be injected intravenously or intraperitoneally. During induction, convulsions may occur but these can be prevented by mixing a small dose of pentobarbitone sodium (about 6 mg/kg) with the chloralose solution. Alternatively, when the nature of the experiment permits, anaesthesia may be induced with ether or ethyl chloride and the chloralose solution may then be injected intravenously. However, increased capillary bleeding produced by ether, as well as its depressant action at the neuromuscular junction, make its use inadvisable in some experiments. Anaesthesia produced by chloralose lasts for over 10 h and vasomotor tone is usually well maintained throughout.

Urethane: This is usually made up as a 25% solution in water; it does not precipitate on cooling and is stable. The solution may be injected intravenously or intraperitoneally, the dose to produce anaesthesia usually being 1·5 g/kg (i.e. 6 ml/kg of a 25% w/v solution).

$$H_2N—C—O—CH_2–CH_3 \quad \text{Urethane (Ethyl carbamate)}$$
$$\underset{O}{\overset{\|}{}}$$

Urethane stimulates the adrenal medulla and cortex and this may be a disadvantage in some experiments. Mixtures of urethane and chloralose are sometimes used to produce anaesthesia in animal experiments.

Urethane has a limited use in mild cases of insomnia in man. It has also been used in certain forms of leukaemia as it has the property of depressing cell division in the bone marrow and lymphoid tissues.

Aliphatic alcohols

The aliphatic alcohols are included in this chapter as they exert a depressant action on the central nervous system which is qualitatively similar to that of the inhalation anaesthetics.

Ethyl alcohol (ethanol) is the main alcohol present in beers, wines and spirits, but small amounts of higher alcohols, esters and ethers are also present. The initial effects of ethanol are due to depression of the integrating activity of the reticular formation of the brain stem on the cortex; this results in impairment of judgement, observation and attention; behaviour at this stage depends on the personality of the individual and on his environmental conditions and company. In stimulating surroundings, the drinker may become expansive, over confident and excited, or noisy and aggresive. But in other surroundings, and especially when alone, the drinker may become morose, dull and sleepy. In general, mental and physical ability is reduced by ethanol. However, strongly inhibited introverted people, or those whose normal performance is impaired through anxiety and nervous tension, may show a distinct improvement in ability after small doses, because of a selective depression of cortical inhibitory centres.

With increased intake, further depression of higher centres occurs, and self-restraint and sense of responsibility is lost; there may be depressed motor co-ordination, reduced visual acuity, reduced sensitivity to sound, taste, smell and pain, nystagmus, vertigo, and slurred speech. Further intake causes sleep from which the drinker awakes, usually with the characteristic 'hangover'.

When a very large quantity of ethanol has been taken, loss of consciousness and anaesthesia result, as with the inhalation anaesthetics. All the stages of anaesthesia leading to medullary paralysis are passed through when the amount absorbed is large enough, but the margin of safety between loss of consciousness and medullary paralysis is smaller than with the general anaesthetics. However, deaths from acute ethanol poisoning are relatively rare as its emetic action usually prevents the absorption of lethal concentrations. Most deaths are due to the inhalation of vomit during unconsciousness.

The rate of absorption of ethanol depends on the amount imbibed and on its concentration; absorption is delayed by the presence of food. About 20% is absorbed from the stomach and the rest from the small intestine. In high concentrations, ethanol inhibits peristalsis in the stomach and so delays its entry into the small intestine. Absorption is also delayed by fat and carbohydrate, especially in the form of milk. Food intake hastens the metabolism of ethanol; the mechanism of this effect is not understood. Ethanol is metabolized at the rate of 10 to 15 ml per hour so that cumulative effects occur if the rate of consumption exceeds this. Regular drinkers show tolerance and may take up to about two and half times the amount needed to produce a similar effect in a non-drinker. The tolerance is not the result of increased metabolism and is probably explained by their having learned to compensate to some extent for the depressant action. More than 90% of absorbed ethanol is metabolized in the liver by oxidation through acetaldehyde, to acetate and then to carbon dioxide and water. These reactions are catalysed by the enzymes *alcohol dehydrogenase* and *aldehyde dehydrogenase* (page 505). The remainder is excreted unchanged in the breath, urine and sweat.

Other actions of ethanol include the following: (1) It lowers body temperature through peripheral vasodilatation resulting from depression of the vasomotor centre. It is therefore unwise to take ethanol when in a cold environment. (2) The emetic action of ethanol is exerted partly on the vomiting centre and partly reflexly through its local irritant effect on the stomach. In small amounts, the irritant action of ethanol reflexly stimulates the flow of saliva and gastric and pancreatic juices. Hence the value of alcoholic drinks as aperitifs. Larger quantities depress the secretion of digestive juices. As it has an irritant action, ethanol may cause gastritis and is contra-indicated in patients with peptic ulcer. (3) It possesses a diuretic action by inhibiting the secretion of antidiuretic hormone from the posterior lobe of the pituitary gland. (4) It depresses liver function and depletes liver stores of glycogen. Prolonged use may cause fatty liver and serious liver disease. It is contra-indicated in patients with liver disfunctions. (5) As a food, ethanol supplies 7 Calories per gram (cf. caloric values of foods on page 29), and may therefore be useful in debilitated patients. (6) The depressant effects of ethanol are additive with those of other CNS depressants, including tranquillizers and some antihistamines.

19*

Patients taking these drugs should therefore not drink ethanol as severe depression, coma, or even death, may result.

MEDICAL USES OF ETHANOL. In the past, ethanol was used as a general anaesthetic. It is still occasionally used as an analgesic and hypnotic in elderly patients and as a sedative in status asthmaticus. Its lack of depressant effect on respiration is a particular advantage in asthmatic patients. It is occasionally injected into the region of nerves to relieve intractable pain, and it is used externally as an antiseptic (70% w/v solution is optimal) and a rubifacient or astringent (e.g. to prevent bed sores).

Chronic alcoholism: Chronic alcoholics suffer from loss of appetite and gastritis and many of the symptoms observed, including hepatic cirrhosis, are as much due to malnutrition, especially vitamin B deficiency, as to ethanol itself. In severe cases, there is loss of memory, optic neuritis, delirium tremens and epileptic-like blackouts; resistance to disease is low. Sudden withdrawal of ethanol may produce an acute psychotic state and severe collapse.

DISULFIRAM. This compound inhibits the enzyme *aldehyde dehydrogenase*

$$CH_3CH_2 \diagdown \qquad \diagup CH_2CH_3$$
$$NC-S-S-CN$$
$$CH_3CH_2 \diagup \underset{S}{\overset{\|}{}} \qquad \underset{S}{\overset{\|}{}} \diagdown CH_2CH_3$$

Disulfiram (tetraethylthiuram disulphide)

(page 505) in the liver and so the metabolism of ethanol stops with the formation of acetaldehyde; this accumulates and produces extremely unpleasant symptoms. Aldehyde dehydrogenase is a copper-containing enzyme and disulfiram inhibits it by combining with the copper. Dilsulfiram is occasionally used to reinforce an alcoholic's own desire to be cured. Convulsions, leading to circulatory collapse and death may follow a large ethanol intake in its presence, and it must therefore be used with caution and only under supervision. The effects of a single dose of disulfiram persist for several days. *Citrated calcium carbimide* produces a similar effect to that of disulfiram but its duration of action is shorter (about 12 hours).

Methyl alcohol (methanol) has similar actions to ethanol but it is metabolized more slowly and less completely so that cumulation is greater and its actions are more prolonged. When ethanol and methanol are mixed (as in industrial methylated spirits) and taken together, ethanol is preferentially metabolized and methanol persists even longer than when given alone. The toxic effects of methanol are mainly due to its oxidation products, formaldehyde and formate. These give rise to a severe acidosis and may cause damage to the retina, atrophy of the optic nerve, and permanent blindness.

Hypnotics, Sedatives, Tranquillizers, Anticonvulsants and Centrally Acting Muscle Relaxants

Hypnotics and sedatives

Hypnotics are drugs used to produce sleep whilst *sedatives* quieten patients without producing sleep. Large doses of some hypnotics may be used to produce general or basal anaesthesia whereas small doses are often used for sedation. The choice of a hypnotic depends largely on the condition of the patient. For example, a quick but short-acting hypnotic may be useful when the patient has difficulty in getting to sleep whereas a longer-acting drug with slower onset of action may be required when the patient consistently wakes early. In some patients, hypnotics may be addictive, particularly when repeated large doses have to be used, but the liability to addiction is less serious than with morphine-like drugs.

Bromides. Bromide has been used as a hypnotic and sedative for over 100 years and is still occasionally used; it is usually given orally as the potassium or sodium salt. In therapeutic doses, bromides cause sedation and only slight drowsiness but larger doses produce sleep which may be followed by a hangover. The absorption, distribution and excretion of bromide resembles that of chloride. The ratio of chloride to bromide absorbed depends on the ratio of the two ions, and the ratio of the amounts passing into cells similarly depends on the ratio in the extracellular fluid; the ratio of chloride to bromide excreted in the urine, however, is higher as bromide is more readily reabsorbed in the tubules of the kidney. It is thought that depression of the neurones of the CNS results when a critical proportion of the chloride ion is replaced by bromide, whereas peripheral tissues are less sensitive and remain functional until a greater level of replacement is reached. This may explain why bromides exert a selective depressant action on the CNS. The amount of chloride which is replaced by bromide is slight when a single large dose of bromide is given but builds up gradually when repeated doses are given over several days. Chronic poisoning with bromides (termed *bromism*) produces rashes, dermatitis, vomiting, loss of appetite, constipation and disturbance of behaviour (bromide psychosis). The rate of elimination of bromide ion in such cases is increased by increasing the chloride intake, by giving large volumes of fluids, and by diuretic drugs. Bromides have a limited use in cases of epilepsy which prove to be resistant to other treatments.

Chloral hydrate. This is usually administered orally or rectally and may be used as a hypnotic or as a basal anaesthetic in larger doses. It is metabolized in the body to trichloroethanol (page 508) which probably is the active agent. It is

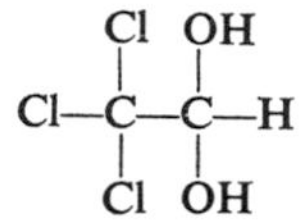

$$\begin{array}{c} \text{Cl} \quad \text{OH} \\ | \qquad | \\ \text{Cl}-\text{C}-\text{C}-\text{H} \\ | \qquad | \\ \text{Cl} \quad \text{OH} \end{array}$$

often used in patients in whom barbiturates have undesirable effects. However, it is irritant to the stomach and a number of its derivatives are now in use. These include *chloral glycerolate, trichloroethylphosphate, chloralformamide,* and *butylchloral.*

Paraldehyde. This drug is used both as a sedative and as a hypnotic. It has a

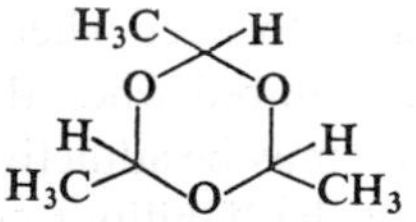

wide margin of safety. Paraldehyde is administered by mouth, by rectum or by injection. It imparts an unpleasant smell to the breath. Its use as a basal anaesthetic is described on page 583.

Barbiturates. The barbiturates were discovered during the search among compounds related to urea for drugs with hypnotic activity like that of urethane (ethyl carbamate). They are formed by condensing malonic acid or its derivatives with urea, as shown in the following equation:

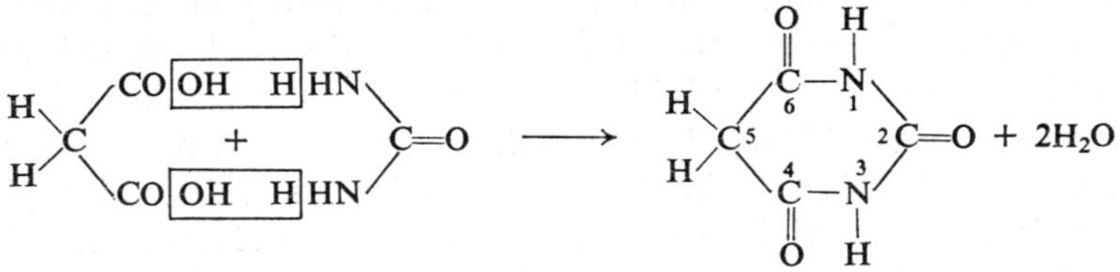

Malonic acid + urea   Barbituric acid + water.

Barbituric acid is without depressant activity but active derivatives are prepared by substitution of alkyl or aryl radicals on the C(5) and also by substitution on the N(1) or N(3) atoms. The thiobarbiturates are prepared from thiourea and possess a sulphur atom in place of the oxygen at C(2). Barbiturates are acidic in nature and form salts which are more water-soluble.

The following generalizations can be made with regard to structure-activity relationships: (i) Both hydrogen atoms on C(5) must be substituted to produce depressant compounds. (ii) Increases in the length of the alkyl side-chain on C(5) to 5 or 6 carbon atoms increases depressant activity but compounds with still longer chains may have stimulant activity; the depressant barbiturates are the only ones used clinically. (iii) Compounds with branched chains on C(5) have short duration of action; cyclohexenyl or cyclopentenyl rings in this position give compounds with a very short duration of action. (iv) Compounds in which the groups on C(5) are derived from secondary alcohols, and which have unsaturated bonds in the side chains on C(5) have increased depressant activity. (v) Compounds in which a phenyl group is substituted on C(5) possess anti-convulsant activity. (vi) Compounds derived from thiourea have a shorter duration of action than those derived from urea.

SITE AND MECHANISM OF ACTION. The barbiturates depress the activity of all parts of the CNS. However, different regions vary in their sensitivity, the order of depression resembling that produced by the volatile anaesthetic agents. Under barbiturate hypnosis, the EEG resembles that in natural sleep. Barbiturates depress the neurones and synapses of the ascending reticular formation of the brain stem in doses which have little action elsewhere and this effect is probably responsible for the reduction in electrical activity of the cortex. Unlike the powerful general anaesthetics (e.g. ether), the barbiturates in the usual dose range do not depress the direct afferent pathways to the thalamus and cortex, and therefore have less analgesic action. The basis of the anti-convulsant activity of certain barbiturates is believed to be an increase in the threshold to stimulation of some regions of the CNS resulting in depression of the intensity of reverberating after-discharge.

Studies on single neurones in the spinal cord have shown that the barbiturates depress the excitability of both pre- and post-synaptic membranes, the pre-synaptic membrane being more susceptible, and this suggests that the depressant effect may be due to decreased release of transmitter. Barbiturates, like chloralose, also increase and prolong pre-synaptic inhibition and the associated pre-synaptic depolarization (see page 91). These actions on synapses in the spinal cord may reflect the action of barbiturates at synapses in the brain stem and elsewhere.

THERAPEUTICALLY USEFUL BARBITURATES. The duration of action of barbiturates depends upon the speed with which they are removed from their site of action, metabolized to inactive compounds, and excreted. The most stable compounds have the longest duration of action and most of these have straight saturated chains or a phenyl ring on C(5). Barbitone (Table 22.1) is particularly stable and most of it is excreted unchanged. The other barbiturates

Table 22.1. Commonly-used barbiturates

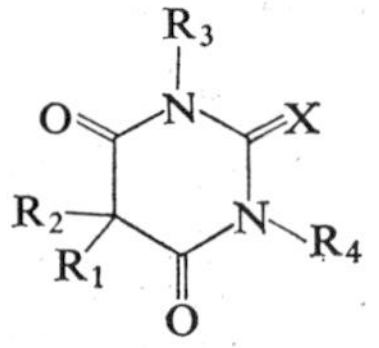

Group	Barbiturate	R₁	R₂	R₃	R₄	X	Fate in the body	Use
Longer-acting group (effect of hypnotic dose lasts more than 8 h)	Barbitone	Ethyl	Ethyl	H	Na	O	Excreted unchanged	Sedative (oral)
	Phenobarbitone	Ethyl	Phenyl	H	Na	O	About 80% metabolized in liver and 20% excreted unchanged	Anticonvulsant and sedative (oral) The sodium salts may be injected intramuscularly or subcutaneously but not intravenously
	Methylphenobarbitone	Ethyl	Phenyl	CH₃	Na	O		
Shorter-acting group (effects last less than 8 h)	Butobarbitone	Ethyl	n-Butyl	H	Na	O		Hypnotics (sedatives in smaller doses) (oral)
	Amylobarbitone	Ethyl	iso-Amyl	H	Na	O		
	Cyclobarbitone	Ethyl	Cyclohexenyl	H	H	O	Metabolized in the liver	The sodium salts may be injected intramuscularly, subcutaneously or intravenously
	Pentobarbitone	Ethyl	1-Methylbutyl	H	H	O		
	Quinalbarbitone	Allyl	1-Methylbutyl	H	Na	O		
Very short-acting group (effects last less than 2 h)	Hexobarbitone	Methyl	Cyclohexenyl	CH₃	Na	O	Stored in fat depots and then metabolized in the liver	Hypnotic and intravenous anaesthetic
	Thiopentone	Ethyl	1-Methylbutyl	H	Na	S		Intravenous anaesthetics
	Thialbarbitone	Allyl	Cyclohexenyl	H	Na	S		

are metabolized at differing rates in the liver, and undergo oxidation and conjugation reactions before being excreted by the kidneys. Derivatives of thiobarbituric acid (e.g. thiopentone) or of N-methylbarbituric acid (e.g. hexobarbitone) have a very short duration of action because the lipid-water partition coefficient of the undissociated form is exceptionally high and hence they are rapidly taken up into the fat depots of the body and so removed from the plasma. After several doses, each of which produces only a brief effect, the fat depots may become saturated so that a subsequent dose persists in the circulation and produces an unexpectedly prolonged depression. These barbiturates are finally metabolized in the liver.

The formulae and uses of the principal barbiturates used in medicine are given in Table 22.1. It has been customary, on the basis of animal experiments, to classify barbiturates into long-, intermediate-, short- and very short-acting types. Clinical experience indicates that the classification of some into a very short-acting group is valid but the remaining barbiturates may be conveniently divided into only two groups, as shown in Table 22.1. The Table does not include all the barbiturates used in therapeutics but the remaining ones have few, if any, advantages over those that are included. Additional hypnotic barbiturates which belong to the shorter-acting group are *allobarbitone, aprobarbital, butabarbital, probarbital, butallylonal, cyclopal, heptabarbitone, hexethal, propallylonal,* and *vinbarbitone.* Additional very short-acting barbiturates used occasionally as intravenous anaesthetics are the sodium salts of *buthalitone, methitural,* and *thioamylal.*

BARBITURATE POISONING. Barbiturates in high doses depress the medullary centres and the first effect of overdosage is usually respiratory depression due to decreased sensitivity of the respiratory centre to carbon dioxide, so that the stimulus to breathing then becomes oxygen-lack. Respiratory depression is followed by depression of the vasomotor centre and possibly by a direct depression of the myocardium leading to circulatory failure. There may be renal failure due to a decreased systemic blood pressure and to the action of barbiturates in stimulating the release of antidiuretic hormone. The course of acute poisoning is therefore coma with respiratory depression, followed by circulatory failure and death. Treatment consists of emptying the stomach, applying artificial respiration, producing an alkaline urine to suppress tubular reabsorption, dialysing the blood when poisoning is due to one of the long-acting barbiturates, and occasionally, in an emergency, administering an analeptic drug such as bemegride or picrotoxin (page 626).

The depressant action of barbiturates is additive with that of other CNS depressant drugs; for example, the usual hypnotic dose may be fatal when taken in conjugation with ethanol or antihistamines.

Allergic reactions to barbiturates are rare, but hypersensitivity reactions, especially rashes, occasionally occur with phenobarbitone.

BARBITURATE ADDICTION. Barbiturates are drugs of addiction, addicts showing symptoms similar to those of alcoholics (childishness, mental confusion, violent emotional outbursts, depression and suicidal tendencies) except that food intake is usually not reduced. Withdrawal symptoms are characterized by loss of appetite, weakness, delirium and convulsions.

Disulphonemethanes. In the past a number of sulphones were used as hypnotics. These included *sulphonal, methylsulphonal* and *diethylsulphone diethylmethane*. All of them had several disadvantages and toxic actions on the liver, kidney and blood were common. They are now obsolete, having been replaced by the barbiturates and newer drugs.

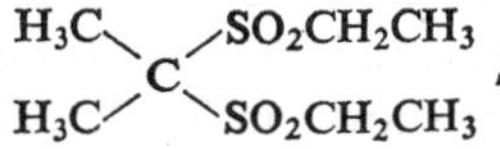

$$\begin{array}{c} H_3C \\ \diagdown \\ H_3C \diagup \end{array} C \begin{array}{c} SO_2CH_2CH_3 \\ \diagdown \\ SO_2CH_2CH_3 \end{array} \quad \textit{Sulphonal}$$

Carbamates. Urethane (ethylcarbamate) has already been mentioned (page 584). It finds a limited use in mild cases of insomnia. The secondary (*hedonal*) and tertiary (*apronal*) amyl esters of carbamic acid, as well as dichloroisopropyl carbamate (*aleudrin*) and trichlorethyl carbamate (*voluntal*) have also been used as hypnotics. They are more toxic than urethane and are now obsolete. However, a urethane derivative known as *ethinamate* (1-ethinyl-cyclohexyl carbamate) is useful when a rapid short-acting hypnotic effect is needed.

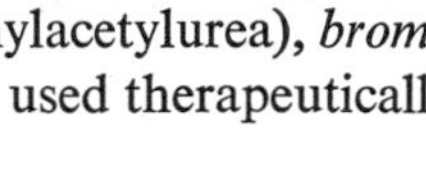

$$\begin{array}{c} \diagup OCONH_2 \\ \diagdown C \equiv CH \end{array} \quad \textit{Ethinamate}$$

Unlike urethane itself, ethinamate has no effect on dividing cells and does not reduce the production of blood cells.

Acylureas. A number of acylureas possess weak hypnotic activity. Of these *carbromal* (bromodiethylacetylurea), *bromvaletone* (bromoisovalerylurea) and *levanil* (acetylurea) are used therapeutically.

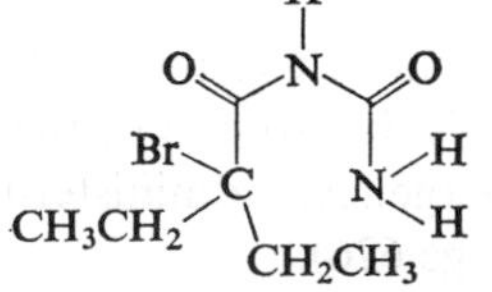

Carbromal and *Bromvaletone* structures

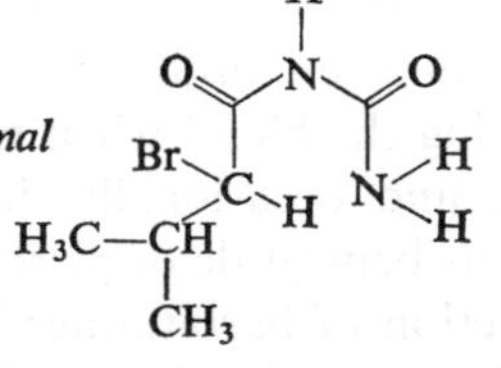

Sedormid (allylisopropylacetylcarbamide or 2-(isopropyl-4-pantanoyl) urea) frequently causes thrombocytopenic purpura and its use has been abandoned.

GLUTARIMIDE DERIVATIVES. In glutarimide, all the R-groups in the

$$
\begin{array}{c}
\text{H} \\
\text{O}\!\!=\!\!\overset{\text{N}}{\diagdown}\!\!=\!\!\text{O} \\
\overset{\text{R}_1}{\underset{\text{R}_2}{\diagdown}} \\
\overset{\diagup}{\text{R}_3}\ \overset{\diagdown}{\text{R}_4}
\end{array}
$$

formula above are hydrogen. Compounds formed by substituting various groups for these hydrogens may possess either stimulant or depressant actions on the CNS, and several are used therapeutically.

Glutethimide (α-phenyl-α-ethyl-glutarimide) is probably the most useful sedative of this series. Taken orally, its effect lasts for about 6 h. In glutethimide, R_1 is phenyl, R_2 is ethyl, and R_3 and R_4 are hydrogen.

Thalidomide in which R_1 is phthalimido- and R_2, R_3 and R_4 are hydrogen, is a more effective sedative than glutethimide. In males and non-pregnant females, thalidomide has a wide margin of safety and is relatively free from serious side-effects although the occurrence of rashes and irreversible peripheral neuritis may occur after taking the drug for several months. However, thalidomide has been withdrawn from use as it may give rise to congenital abnormalities, many involving the limbs, when taken during the first 3 months of pregnancy.

Other derivatives of glutarimide which are therapeutically useful include the stimulant drug *bemegride* (page 626) and the atropine-like drug, *phenglutarimide*, which is used in the treatment of Parkinsonism.

Acetylenic carbinols and derivatives. Examples of this class are *methylparafynol* (methylpentynol) and its carbamate, and *ethchlorvynol*.

$$
\begin{array}{cc}
\underset{\text{H}_3\text{C}}{\overset{\text{CH}_3\text{CH}_2}{\diagdown}}\!\!\overset{\diagup}{\underset{\diagdown}{\text{C}}}\!\!\overset{\text{OH}}{\underset{\text{C}\!\equiv\!\text{CH}}{\diagup}} & \text{\textit{Methylparafynol}}
\end{array}
\qquad
\begin{array}{cc}
\underset{\underset{|}{\text{HC}\!=\!\text{HC}}}{\overset{\text{CH}_3\text{CH}_2}{\diagdown}}\!\!\overset{\diagup}{\underset{\diagdown}{\text{C}}}\!\!\overset{\text{OH}}{\underset{\text{C}\!\equiv\!\text{CH}}{\diagup}} & \text{\textit{Ethchlorvynol}} \\
\text{Cl}
\end{array}
$$

These drugs are used to allay anxiety. They also have some anticonvulsant activity.

Methylprylone. This is comparable in potency and duration of action to quinalbarbitone. It has been reported to produce pruritus, rashes and diarrhoea.

$$
\textit{Methylprylone}\quad
\begin{array}{c}
\text{H} \\
\text{O}\!\!=\!\!\overset{\text{N}}{\diagdown} \\
\underset{\text{CH}_3\text{CH}_2}{\overset{\text{CH}_3\text{CH}_2}{\diagdown}}\!\!\!\!\overset{\diagup\text{CH}_3}{\underset{\diagdown\text{H}}{}} \\
\text{O}
\end{array}
$$

Tranquillizers

The tranquillizers comprise one of the groups of drugs used in the treatment of mental disease. Another important group is the *antidepressives* described in Chapter 23. These two groups of drugs, together with the *psychotomimetics*, (page 629) are known as *psychotropic drugs*. Tranquillizers restore hyperactive behaviour to normal, abolish mental confusion including delusions and hallucinations, and allay the patient's anxiety and nervous tension without impairing consciousness. The major tranquillizers are sometimes termed *ataractics* (from a Greek word meaning 'undisturbed'). When the patient sleeps under the influence of a tranquillizer, he is easily aroused without the residual clouding of consciousness characteristic of the hypnotics.

Tranquillizers differ from the hypnotics (which can also be used in small doses for their tranquillizing effect) in that they do not produce anaesthesia in large doses, although the use of all of them results in some degree of drowsiness or lethargy. In animals, very large doses of the major tranquillizers, and of some minor tranquillizers, have been shown to produce a state of *catalepsy* in which the animal remains motionless and relaxed in any position in which it is placed, although there is no anaesthesia. Some of the minor tranquillizers (for example, the derivatives of propanediol) in large doses produce relaxation of skeletal muscle by an action exerted mainly in the spinal cord, but again there is no anaesthesia. Before the development of the tranquillizers (which began with *chlorpromazine* in 1951), the hypnotic drugs were the only drugs used in Western medicine to quieten disturbed patients.

Mental illnesses in which tranquillizers may be used are divisible into two major categories, the *psychoses* and the *neuroses*. *Psychotic* patients, particularly schizophrenics are generally unaware that they are ill. Their behaviour differs qualitatively from that of normal people, and may be characterized by disorientation, hallucinations, aggressiveness, unco-operativeness, destructiveness and violence. The behaviour of *neurotic* patients differs only quantitatively from that of normal persons. They are usually aware of their illness and there are no marked changes in personality. Their behaviour may be characterized by acute anxiety, apprehension or excitement.

Drugs used as tranquillizers are obtained from a variety of chemical classes: they include phenothiazine derivatives, indole alkaloids from Rauwolfia species, diphenylmethane and propanediol derivatives. All of them are readily absorbed from the gastro-intestinal tract, although some may be administered rectally or by injection. The *major tranquillizers*, which include some phenothiazine derivatives and the Rauwolfia alkaloids, are effective in hyperactive psychotic states, particularly when of recent origin, but are of less value in neurotic conditions. They may not prevent delusions and hallucinations but by promoting emotional detachment, they reduce the extent to which these trouble the patient. The *minor tranquillizers* are used in neurotic conditions but are of little value in the psychoses. This group includes the less active phenothiazine derivatives and derivatives of diphenylmethane and propanediol. There is no doubt that tranquillizers are valuable in the treatment of mental disease but the extent of their value is difficult to assess. This is mainly because (1) the aetiology of mental disease and the precise site and mechanism of action of the drugs are largely unknown, (2) treatment of large numbers of patients suffering from the same mental disease is not often possible and statistical assessment of the results is rarely attempted, and (3) placebos often produce an unusually high proportion of improvements. By reducing the symptoms of mental disease, tranquillizers may break a cycle of events and thereby cause a temporary improvement which renders the patient more susceptible to psychotherapy. Most tranquillizers are capable of producing dangerous or unpleasant side-effects and should not be used indiscriminately. The popular supposition that they are able to allay ordinary everyday worries has been disputed.

Major tranquillizers

1. PHENOTHIAZINE DERIVATIVES. The first tranquillizer to be extensively used was *chlorpromazine*, and this is still used for this purpose; in addition, it is useful as an adjuvant in anaesthesia and as an anti-emetic. Its synthesis followed the discovery of the sedative properties of the anti-histaminic drug *promethazine*, which is also a derivative of phenothiazine (page 782).

The chemical formulae of the principal phenothiazine derivatives used as major tranquillizers are given in Table 22.2. Chemically they may be divided into three groups: those in the first group possess an aliphatic side chain which terminates in a dimethylamine group, those in the second group contain a piperidine ring in the side chain, and those in the third group contain a piperazine ring in the side chain. The third group contains the most potent compounds, *trifluoperazine* and *perphenazine* which are 5 to 10 times more potent and *fluphenazine* which is about 25 times more potent than chlorpromazine. The potencies of the remaining compounds in Table 22.2 are similar to or slightly greater than (2 to 3 times) that of chlorpromazine. All possess similar pharmacological properties but their relative abilities to produce the various effects differ.

CHLORPROMAZINE. In therapeutic doses, chlorpromazine reduces spontaneous motor activity and causes calmness and indifference to the external environment. It also causes some indifference to pain. It produces sedation and drowsiness from which the patient is easily awakened. It may cause

TABLE 22.2. Formulae of major tranquillizers derived from phenothiazine.

Approved Name	R	R′
Chlorpromazine	Cl	$(CH_2)_3N(CH_3)_2$
Methoxypromazine	OCH_3	$(CH_2)_3N(CH_3)_2$
Acepromazine	$COCH_3$	$(CH_2)_3N(CH_3)_2$
Triflupromazine	CF_3	$(CH_2)_3N(CH_3)_2$
Alimemazine	CH_3	$(CH_2)_3N(CH_3)_2$
Methotrimeprazine	OCH_3	CH_3 | $CH_2 \cdot CH . CH_2 N(CH_3)_2$
Mepazine	H	
Thioridazine	SCH_3	
Perazine	H	
Prochlorperazine	Cl	
Trifluoperazine	CF_3	
Perphenazine	Cl	
Fluphenazine	CF_3	
Thiopropazate	Cl	

severe mental depression and reduce the ability to perform complex rapid movements. In cats, it prevents the sham-rage which can be induced by suitable stimulation after severing the brain immediately above the hypothalamus (page 134). It pacifies savage monkeys and suppresses conditioned avoidance behaviour in rats. Electrophysiological studies in animals show that chlorpromazine synchronizes the cortical EEG giving the characteristic pattern of sleep, raises the threshold of the arousal response to sensory stimulation and to electrical stimulation of the reticular formation, and slightly enhances the thalamic recruiting response (page 133). It potentiates hypnotics, anaesthetics, analgesics, local anesthetics and, in large doses, neuromuscular blocking agents. In animals, it has been shown to protect against convulsions produced by nicotine or nikethamide but not those produced by leptazol, picrotoxin, strychnine or cocaine. Small doses antagonize the muscular spasm of tetanus (resulting from the toxin of *Cl. tetani*) but large doses may enhance the spasm. Small doses, of chlorpromazine exert an anti-Parkinson effect, but in large doses, it may produce rigidity and tremor resembling the symptoms of Parkinson's disease (page 120); this is called the 'extra-pyramidal syndrome'. It may precipitate epileptiform seizures in patients predisposed to the disease. It exerts an antiemetic action by depressing the chemo-sensitive trigger zone of the medulla. Thus, it protects against vomiting produced by apomorphine and ergot alkaloids but has little action against that produced by cardiac glycosides or copper sulphate. It is effective against vomiting in pregnancy and in disease of the labyrinths, but it is inactive against vomiting that occurs after X-irradiation and in motion sickness in man, although in dogs it prevents sickness produced by swinging.

Chlorpromazine has pronounced anti-adrenaline activity and may cause a fall in blood pressure and postural hypotension. It produces a fall in body temperature which is due to peripheral vasodilatation, to an effect on the heat regulating centre, and to diminution of muscular movement. It depresses the secretion of ACTH and of gonadotrophic hormones from the adenohypophysis, probably through an action exerted in the hypothalamus. It antagonizes the actions of histamine, of 5-hydroxytryptamine and of acetylcholine at both muscarinic receptor sites and at autonomic ganglia; consequently therapeutic doses of chlorpromazine may give rise to blurred vision and constipation.

Chlorpromazine has local anaesthetic, antipruritic and quinidine-like actions, and it inhibits some enzymes (e.g. cytochrome oxidase and adenosine triphosphatase). It prevents inflammation, oedema and shock due to various causes, and reduces the number of deaths produced by irradiation. It stimulates appetite and produces a gain in weight.

The uses of chlorpromazine are (i) as an antipsychotic, (ii) as an antiemetic,

(iii) as an antipruritic, (iv) in premedication before anaesthesia where it allays anxiety and potentiates the analgesic and anaesthetic action of other drugs, (v) in severe pain where it potentiates the action of analgesics and renders the patient more indifferent to pain, and (vi) to aid the production of hypothermia in operations performed at a low temperature. The principal side-effects which occasionally occur during treatment with chlorpromazine are excessive drowsiness, hypotension, extra-pyramidal syndrome, skin rashes, blood disorders and jaundice; these occur sufficiently frequently to necessitate great care and discretion in its use.

None of the newer phenothiazine derivatives listed in Table 22.2 has provided an improvement over chlorpromazine in every respect. Side-effects are said to be produced less frequently than with chlorpromazine by the compounds in the first group of Table 22.2 although *acepromazine* is more likely to produce hypotension. Side-effects produced by *thioridazine* are said to be rare and extra-pyramidal symptoms less severe. On the other hand, most of the compounds in the third group of Table 22.2 produce extra-pyramidal symptoms more frequently than does chlorpromazine, although jaundice is said to be less common with *trifluoperazine*. *Triflupromazine, prochlorperazine, trifluoperazine and perphenazine* have been used as antiemetics.

Prothipendyl is a newer compound which is a derivative of azaphenothiazine.

(CH₂)₃·N(CH₃)₂
Prothipendyl

It is said to differ from the other phenothiazine tranquillizers in that it combines tranquillizing properties resembling those of chlorpromazine with those of a sedative. Its peripheral actions resemble those of chlorpromazine, antiemetic and antihistamine actions being particularly pronounced. It is claimed to be relatively free from serious side-effects.

Phenothiazine derivatives in which the substituent group at R′ in Table 22.2 is a 2-substituted ethyl or 2-substituted propyl side-chain, lack tranquillizing properties. Among these, the presence of a terminal diethylamino group gives anti-Parkinsonian activity while antihistamine activity is given when a terminal dimethylamino group is present. Numerous phenothiazine derivatives, which are not used as tranquillizers but as antihistaminics, antipruritics, anti-Parkinsonian drugs or antiemetics, have been synthesized. Some of these are referred to in other chapters.

2. RAUWOLFIA ALKALOIDS. The root of *Rauwolfia serpentina* has long been used in the treatment of mental disorders in India but it was not introduced into Western medicine until 1953. The principal alkaloid is *reserpine*, but *deserpidine* and *rescinnamine* (Fig. 22.1), which are also present, have similar properties. The Rauwolfia alkaloids and related substances are used principally in the treatment of hypertension and their use in this respect is described on pp. 839-841.

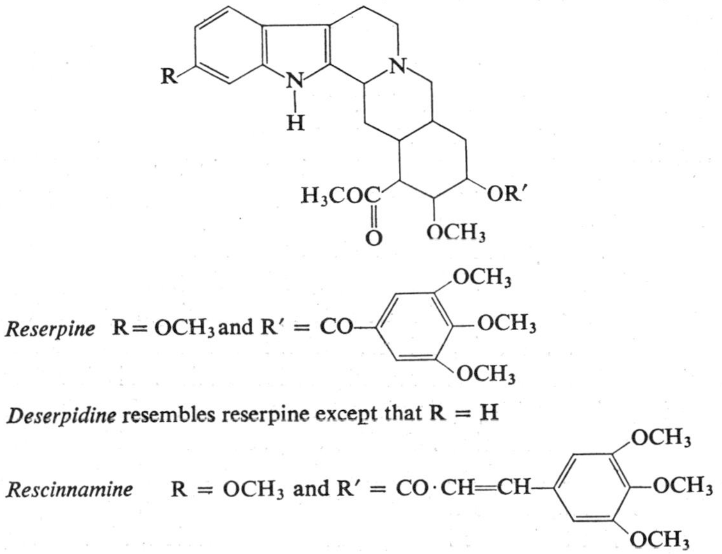

Reserpine R = OCH₃ and R′ = CO—

Deserpidine resembles reserpine except that R = H

Rescinnamine R = OCH₃ and R′ = CO·CH=CH—

FIG. 22.1. Chemical formulae of Rauwolfia alkaloids with tranquillizer actions.

As a tranquillizer, reserpine is used in similar conditions to those in which chlorpromazine is used. However, it has toxic side-effects in large single doses which make it necessary to administer it in small daily doses, and the onset of therapeutic effect is therefore slower than with chlorpromazine. It is unsuitable for psychiatric outpatients and its use in psychiatric medicine is generally restricted to hospitalized patients who have failed to respond to the phenothiazine derivatives. Reserpine produces many of the effects of chlorpromazine listed above, but it also produces the effects enumerated below, most of which are not shared by chlorpromazine.

(1) Reserpine does not synchronize the cortical EEG which shows a continuously alert pattern even when the animal is asleep, and it has no effect on the thalamic recruiting response. However, like chlorpromazine, it raises the threshold of the arousal response to sensory or reticular stimulation. Hypnotics and anaesthetics produce the EEG pattern of sleep, completely block the arousal reaction, and enhance thalamic recruitment. The effects of chlorproma-

zine therefore more closely resemble those of a hypnotic than do those of reserpine. Whereas hypnotics abolish the arousal reaction and produce unconsciousness, chlorpromazine and reserpine only raise the threshold for arousal and reduce alertness. (2) In animals, reserpine potentiates the convulsant action of drugs such as nikethamide, leptazol and caffeine, and of electro-shock treatment, but it does not potentiate convulsions produced by strychnine. In man, it reduces the anti-epileptic activity of barbiturates and phenytoin (page 608), and appears to facilitate the spread of activity associated with epileptiform seizures. (3) Although chemically related to yohimbine (page 766) which also occurs in *R. serpentina*, reserpine differs from yohimbine (and from chlorpromazine) in having no peripheral anti-adrenaline action. However, it releases catecholamines and 5-hydroxytryptamine from central and peripheral storage sites, thereby depleting the brain and peripheral tissues of these amines. It also lowers the concentration of γ-aminobutyric acid (page 187) in the CNS. Many of the actions of reserpine can be reversed by treatment with monoamine oxidase inhibitors (see pages 623–626). (4) Reserpine possesses a pronounced parasympathomimetic action, producing hypotension, bradycardia, flushing of the skin, miosis, salivation, nasal stuffiness, increased peristalsis and diarrhoea, and increased gastric secretion. It is therefore contraindicated in patients with peptic ulcer. These effects are largely the result of depletion of peripheral amines. Cardiac output and renal blood flow are not much affected. (5) Reserpine may cause dyspnoea sometimes associated with heart failure. It may cause fluid retention and oedema. It decreases libido and may give rise to intense lethargy, severe depression, nightmares, mental confusion and suicidal tendencies.

The phenothiazine derivatives and reserpine are the most potent tranquillizers used as antipsychotics but a few other drugs with slightly less activity are also useful and may be classed as major tranquillizers.

3. TETRABENAZINE. This compound is chemically related to reserpine although it lacks the indole nucleus. It has similar central actions, causing depletion of noradrenaline and 5-hydroxytryptamine from the brain, but it does not deplete peripheral tissues of these amines and is therefore weaker in its peripheral actions causing fewer side-effects.

Tetrabenazine

It acts more quickly and for a shorter time than does reserpine.

4. THE BUTYROPHENONES. Two compounds in this class, *haloperidol* and *triperidol*, are used clinically as major tranquillizers. Their properties resemble those of chlorpromazine and include antiemetic activity. Triperidol is the more potent antipsychotic of the two but it is more likely to cause extra-pyramidal side-effects.

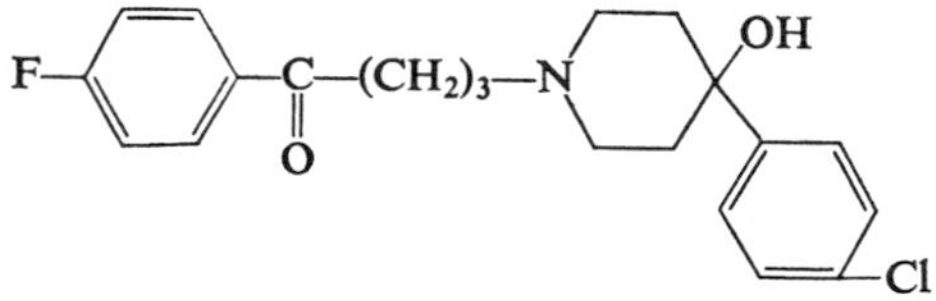

Haloperidol

(In triperidol,
Cl is replaced by CF$_3$)

5. CHLORPROTHIXENE. This compound, although not a phenothiazine derivative, is chemically related and its properties are similar to those of chlorpromazine except that its atropine-like action is stronger. In addition, it possesess antidepressive properties (page 623).

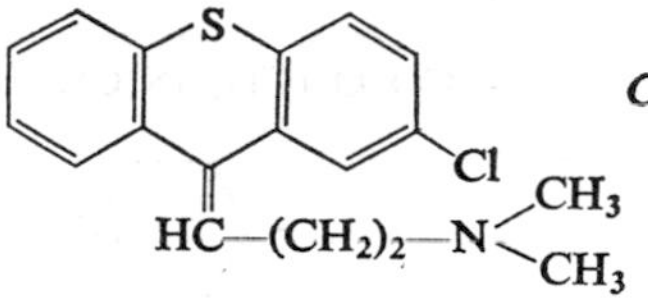

Chlorprothixene

Minor tranquillizers

The agents in this group have not been shown to exert a beneficial effect in psychotic patients. They may be of some value in the treatment of anxiety and tension in neurotic patients. The phenothiazine derivatives in this group and the derivatives of diphenylmethane, although much less potent, qualitatively resemble the major tranquillizers in some of their effects on behaviour in animals and man, and produce catatonia in large doses. The derivatives of propanediol, often classified as *tranquillo-sedatives*, depress polysynaptic spinal and brain stem reflexes leading to muscular relaxation in large doses. Their tranquillizing and sedative effects are independent of their muscle relaxant properties. With the exception of chlordiazepoxide, the minor tranquillizers, like the major tranquillizers, potentiate barbiturate sleeping time in mice.

1. PHENOTHIAZINE DERIVATIVES. Phenothiazine derivatives with minor tranquillizing properties include *promazine, promethazine* and *ethopropazine*. Promazine resembles chlorpromazine chemically except that the chlorine group is replaced by H. Promethazine differs from promazine in that the substituent group on the nitrogen (R' in Table 22.2) is CH$_2$.CH(CH$_3$).N(CH$_3$)$_2$ and ethopropazine differs from promethazine in that the terminal dimethylamine group is replaced by a diethylamine group. In addition to their mild tranquillizing action, promethazine possesses potent antihistaminic and antiemetic actions while ethopropazine possesses marked atropine-like action and is used in the treatment of Parkinson's disease (page 732).

2. DIPHENYLMETHANE DERIVATIVES. The names and formulae of the principal members of this class used as minor tranquillizers are given in Table 22.3. Chemically related compounds are used as spasmolytics, antidepressants, antihistaminics or antiemetics.

TABLE 22.3. Diphenylmethane derivatives used as minor tranquillizers.

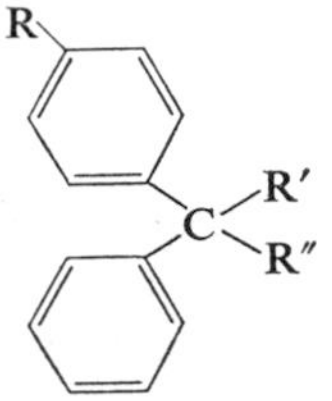

Name	R	R′	R″
Benactyzine	H	OH	$-CO.O.(CH_2)_2N(CH_2CH_3)_2$
Azacyclonol	H	OH	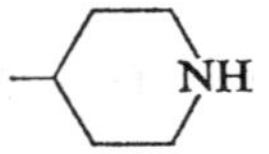 (image: piperidine ring) NH
Captodiamine	$-C_4H_9S$	H	$-S \cdot CH_2 \cdot CH_2 \cdot N(CH_3)_2$
Buclizine	Cl	H	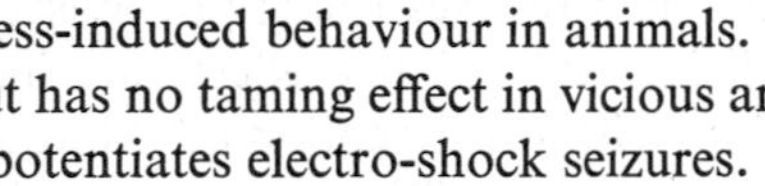 $-N$ (piperazine) $N \cdot CH_2-$ (phenyl) $-C(CH_3)_3$
Hydroxyzine	Cl	H	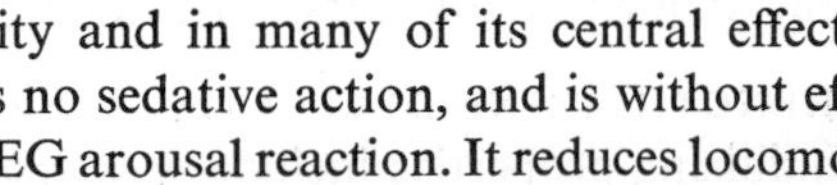 $-N$ (piperazine) $N \cdot CH_2 \cdot CH_2 \cdot O \cdot CH_2 \cdot CH_2 \cdot OH$

Benactyzine is said to normalize stress-induced behaviour in animals. It suppresses the EEG arousal reaction but has no taming effect in vicious animals; it increases locomotor activity and potentiates electro-shock seizures. Benactyzine possesses atropine-like activity and in many of its central effects it resembles hyoscine. *Azacyclonol* has no sedative action, and is without effect on conditioned reflexes and on the EEG arousal reaction. It reduces locomotor activity and protects against electro-shock convulsions. It restores the EEG to normal after desynchronization by psychotomimetic drugs (e.g., lysergide and mescaline, page 629). Its use in man stems from a report that it suppresses hallucinations produced by lysergide or mescaline. Azacyclonol is a structural isomer of the stimulant drug, pipradol (page 618). *Captodiamine* potentiates analgesics and protects against electro-shock convulsions but not those produced by leptazol or strychnine. *Buclizine* and *hydroxyzine* have sedative actions and share to a mild degree many of the effects of chlorpromazine including antiadrenaline, antiemetic, analgesic and local anaesthetic actions. They are also fairly potent antihistaminics.

3. DERIVATIVES OF PROPANEDIOL. The best known representative of this group is *meprobamate*. This compound has sedative properties and exerts a taming effect on aggressive animals. It synchronizes the cortical EEG and has some inhibitory effect on reticular arousal and thalamic recruitment. It does not affect the autonomic nervous system and does not produce extra-pyramidal symptoms.

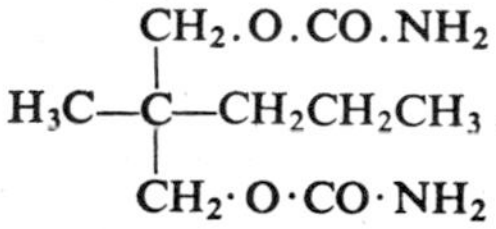

$$
\begin{array}{c}
CH_2.O.CO.NH_2 \\
| \\
H_3C-C-CH_2CH_2CH_3 \quad \textit{Meprobamate} \\
| \\
CH_2 \cdot O \cdot CO \cdot NH_2
\end{array}
$$

In large doses it produces muscle relaxation by blocking interneurones in the spinal cord and brain stem, and in animals it protects against convulsions which occur after strychnine, leptazol and electric-shock. A number of severe allergic reactions have been reported to follow its use, and the drug is habit forming in some patients.

Other propanediol derivatives and related compounds with mild tranquilizing activity include *promoxolane, phenaglycodol, oxanamide* and *emylcamate*. Some related compounds with central muscle relaxant activity are described on pages 610–614.

4. CHLORDIAZEPOXIDE. This drug is chemically unrelated to the other tranquillizers. It is reported to exert a more powerful taming effect on aggressive animals than chlorpromazine and reserpine, and has a pronounced ability to abolish fear in doses which do not decrease spontaneous activity. It possesses muscle relaxant properties resembling those of mephenesin (page 610), and anticonvulsant activity equivalent to that of phenobarbitone (page 608). It

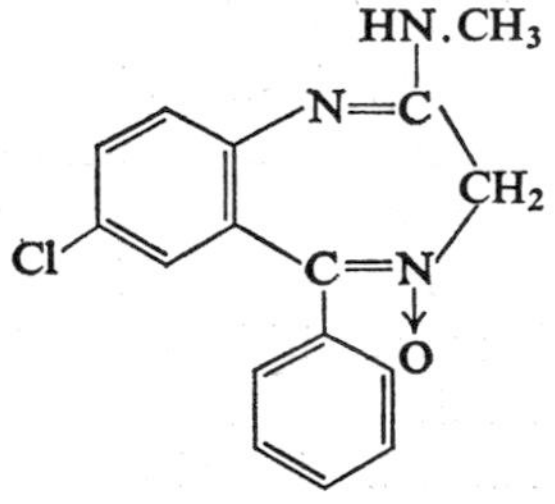

Chlordiazepoxide (Librium)

stimulates appetite, has little effect on the autonomic nervous system, and appears to be relatively free of serious side-effects. Unlike the other tranquillizers, chlordiazepoxide does not potentiate the action of barbiturates and other depressants.

Chlordiazepoxide has been used with success to relieve emotional tension and to allay anxiety and fear.

In the symptomatic treatment of the neuroses, sedatives are used widely in addition to the minor tranquillizers. Despite the large amount of work and expense involved in the development of the minor tranquillizers, there is no convincing evidence of their superiority to small doses of the barbiturates.

Site and mechanism of action of the tranquillizers. The precise sites and mechanisms of action of the drugs used as tranquillizers are unknown; it is unlikely that all of them act in the same way. The chief action of the major tranquillizers which distinguishes them from other drugs is their ability to alter the emotional state of psychotic patients, an action which may be analogous to their taming effect on aggressive animals.

The limbic system of the rhinencephalon (including the hippocampus and the amygdala—page 102) appears to be concerned with the conscious experience of emotion and may determine the level of sensory input at which the outward signs of emotion are brought into play; in other words, the limbic system may determine the attitude of the individual towards the environment.

It has been postulated that, at the hypothalamic level, the homeostatic control of the emotional reaction to the environment is determined by two opposing systems—an *ergotropic* system which produces arousal activity and increased sympathetic tone, and a *trophotropic* system which has the opposite effects, causing reduced activity and increased parasympathetic tone. Similarly, at the higher level of the limbic system, the hippocampus and the amygdala appear to exert opposing influences; stimulation of the hippocampus or inhibition of the amygdala produces docility, whereas the reverse procedures produce rage reactions. Abnormal EEG patterns have been recorded from the region of the limbic system in schizophrenic patients, especially during disturbed periods. The sensory input signalling external environmental conditions and visceral sensations is conveyed via the reticular formation to the thalamus, hypothalamus and limbic system. There are two-way neuronal connections between all of these regions, and the experience and expression of emotion follows integration of the sensory input by this complex system. There is good evidence that the tranquillizers act within this system, but the precise sites are difficult to determine, as an action at any one part of the system is reflected by altered activity at others. The behavioural non-reactivity and indifference to the environment produced by the major tranquillizers might be explained by blockade of the sensory inflow to the reticular formation so that the individual is less aware of his environment. Lesions in the amygdala or stimulation of the hippocampus in animals produce depressed behavioural effects which resemble those produced by the major tranquillizers, and these drugs alter the EEG recorded from the region of the limbic system. However, the fact that the drugs abolish sham rage produced in animals by separating the cerebral structures from the hypothalamus indicates a site of action below the limbic system. Possibly the drugs exert effects at three levels—reticular formation, hypothalamus and limbic system.

Attempts have been made to relate the effects of the tranquillizers to interaction with substances normally present within the brain, principally noradrenaline, 5-hydroxytryptamine and acetylcholine (see pages 184–189). Among the Rauwolfia alkaloids and related compounds, only those which cause release and depletion of amines in the CNS possess tranquillizing action, and there is suggestive evidence that amine depletion and tranquillizing action are related. Brodie has postulated that the transmitter in neurones of the ergotropic system is noradrenaline, and that of the trophotropic system is 5-hydroxytryptamine. Both amines are present in high concentration in the hypothalamus. Brodie suggested that reserpine, by releasing 5-hydroxytryptamine from its binding sites, causes the synapses of the trophotrophic system to be exposed to a continuous low concentration of this amine so that the parasympathetic nervous system is activated. Chlorpromazine, on the other hand, is suggested to act centrally as an antiadrenaline drug, blocking the adrenergic synapses of the ergotrophic system. Effects similar to those of reserpine are produced by chlorpromazine because, by inactivating the ergotrophic system, the trophotrophic system is allowed to predominate. This is an attractive hypothesis because it explains how similar effects of the major tranquillizers might be produced through different mechanisms. However, other findings appear to contradict it, especially as it now appears that the actions of 5-hydroxytryptamine in these regions of the brain are predominantly stimulant. It may be that the tranquillizing effects of reserpine and related drugs are the result of depletion of both types of amine, while the similar effects produced by chlorpromazine and related drugs are due to blockade of their action. Whatever the details of the mechanism, it is generally accepted that the tranquillizing action, at least of reserpine, is a consequence of its ability to modify brain amine levels. Some workers have suggested that alteration in 5-hydroxytryptamine levels may effect brain metabolism through an action on the neuroglial cells.

The evidence that acetylcholine is a chemical transmitter in some areas of the brain is summarized on pages 169–171. The anticholinesterase drug, physostigmine, may produce convulsions and EEG seizures and arousal patterns, whereas antagonists of acetylcholine, such as atropine, abolish these effects producing an EEG characteristic of sleep, although without impairing alertness. Benactyzine is the main tranquillizer possessing significant atropine-like activity, and it may be that it exerts its effects by blocking cholinergic synapses, possibly in the reticular formation. The atropine-like drug, hyoscine (page 723), possesses a minor tranquillizing action resembling that of benactyzine.

Tests for tranquillizing activity in animals. It is impossible to duplicate in animals the ill-defined psychiatric conditions for which tranquillizing drugs are used in man, and, as with all new drugs, but particularly with those which are potential tranquillizers, their value in therapeutics can only be accurately assessed by carefully controlled clinical trials in patients, together with long experience of their use. However, from a knowledge of the effects of established tranquillizers in animals, pharmacologists have devised a battery of animal tests to which new drugs may be submitted. From the results of these tests, and of toxicity tests, a decision is made as to whether the potential tranquillizer should be submitted to clinical trial in psychotic or neurotic patients. Results of some pharmacological tests which may indicate potential tranquillizing action are listed below: (1) Taming of naturally aggressive animals (e.g. Rhesus monkeys or Siamese fighting fish). (2) Abolition of sham rage in operated animals. (3) Suppression of behavioural arousal response to noise or to electrical stimulation of the reticular formation. (4) Prevention of abnormal behaviour produced by psychotomimetic drugs such as mescaline, lysergide or harmine (page 629). (5) Suppression of EEG arousal reaction to sensory stimulation or to stimulation of the reticular formation. (6) Suppression of conditioned reflex responses of various kinds (see Pavlovian conditioning, page 135), suggesting that the animal is less aware of incoming sensory information or less anxious or afraid. (7) Reduction of spontaneous locomotor activity and impairment of muscular co-ordination (care is necessary to exclude a peripheral paralysing action, or reduced activity which is simply due to the animal being made too ill to move). (8) Potentiation of depressant drugs (e.g. barbiturates), and antagonism of stimulant drugs (e.g. amphetamine). (9) Depletion of amines present in the CNS and antagonism of their action.

Anticonvulsant drugs

All anaesthetic and hypnotic drugs act as anticonvulsants but with most of them suppression of convulsions is produced only by anaesthetic or hypnotic doses. *Antiepileptic drugs* are a special class of anticonvulsants which are capable of suppressing epileptic seizures in doses smaller than those which produce hypnosis or loss of consciousness.

Epilepsy. Epilepsy is due to an abnormal paroxysmal discharge of neurones. The discharge may spread locally (possibly ephaptically, page 84) to neighbouring groups of neurones, or may travel via the axons to more distant groups of neurones, where the effect may be excitation or inhibition. The site of origin of the discharge is called the 'focus'. The record from an EEG electrode represents the activity from only a small proportion of the total surface of the brain, but during an epileptic episode abnormal activity from the focus spreads out and the EEG pattern is usually changed. The manifestations of the epileptic attack depend on the neurones involved. When the discharge remains confined to a small part of the cortex and is of short duration, it may not lead to any obvious symptoms but yet may be detected in the EEG. When the motor system is involved, there is loss of voluntary power and usually tonic (increased tone) and/or clonic (repetitive contraction and relaxation) spasms. When a large part of the cortex or specific parts of the reticular activating system are involved, the patient loses consciousness. When the discharge is confined to sensory areas of the cortex, the patient will experience hallucinations involving sight, hearing, smell, taste or sense of time.

There are several classifications of epilepsy based on the site of origin of the discharge, on the clinical manifestations, or on the EEG changes. In *focal epilepsy*, the discharge is confined to one portion of the cortex; when it is confined to the motor area, it is called *Jacksonian epilepsy*; and when it is in certain parts of the temporal lobe concerned with mood, it is called *psychomotor epilepsy*. Tumours, injuries or infections may produce a focus. A focal cortical seizure may spread to involve the whole cortex and cause a *grand mal* seizure (i.e., a fit) with unconsciousness, convulsions and incontinence. When the spread from the initial focus is slow, the initial focal symptoms give rise to a warning (or aura) of the impending fit. In *idiopathic epilepsy*, which is often due to an inherited predisposition, there may be multiple foci, or a varying focus, or such rapid spread over the cortex that an aura may be absent. *Status epilepticus*, in which the episodes of grand mal occur without intervening recovery of consciousness, is serious and may be fatal unless treated rapidly. It may require the use of intravenous thiopentone and muscle relaxants.

Three types of epilepsy arise from subcortical foci and are often called *centrencephalic* epilepsy. *Petit mal*, which is more common in children than in adults, involves a sudden loss of consciousness without accompanying motor symptoms and usually lasts less than 15 sec. In *akinetic seizures*, there is a sudden loss of postural control and the patient falls to the ground but does not lose consciousness. In *myoclonic epilepsy*, there are brief jerky movements without loss of consciousness. Myoclonic epilepsy is very resistant to drug treatment and large doses of spinal relaxant drugs (e.g. mephenesin) may have to be used.

A patient may have more than one type of epilepsy. In susceptible patients, certain stimuli such as a flickering light or a fever may precipitate an epileptic discharge.

There is no single drug which is effective in all types of epilepsy. Numerous antiepileptic drugs are available; most of them are believed to prevent the spread of activity to normal grey matter rather than to depress the neurones in the foci of origin. The choice of drug depends upon the form of epilepsy being treated and upon the response of the individual. An antiepileptic drug

TABLE 22.4. The principal antiepileptic drugs.

Class of compounds	Name	Type of epilepsy	Side-effects
Barbiturates	Phenobarbitone Methylphenobarbitone Metharbitone	Grand mal	Sleepiness which usually wears off with continued treatment. Occasional rashes
Hydantoins	Phenytoin sodium Methoin	Grand mal and focal	Ataxia, tremors, gastric upset, blurred vision, confusion, blood disorders and rashes
Pyrimidinediones	Primidone	Grand mal and focal	Sleepiness, nausea, ataxia which often wear off with continued treatment. Megaloblastic anaemia
Acylureas	Phenacemide Pheneturide	Grand mal, psychomotor and mixed forms	Personality changes, liver damage, blood disorders, rashes, gastric upset
Oxazolidinediones	Troxidone Aloxidone Paramethadione	Petit mal	Infrequently causes drowsiness, photophobia, gastric upset, severe blood disorders and rashes
Phenylsuccinimides	Phensuximide Methsuximide	Petit mal	Sleepiness, headaches, rashes, vomiting, kidney damage and leucopenia
Succinimides	Ethosuximide	Psychomotor and petit mal	Sleepiness, dizziness, vomiting and leucopenia but incidence less than with phenylsuccinimides
Propionamides	Beclamide	Grand mal and focal	Not yet assessed

is given in increasing doses until either the episodes are prevented or toxic effects occur, in which case the procedure is repeated with another drug. A combination of drugs is often more effective than a high dose of a single

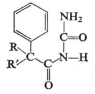

Barbiturates
Phenobarbitone: R = Et, R′ = Ph, R″ = H.
Methylphenobarbitone: R = Et, R′ = Ph,
                R″ = Me
Metharbitone : R = Et, R′ = Et, R″ = Me

Hydantoins
Phenytoin: R = R′ = Ph, R″ = H.
Metholn: R = Et, R′ = Ph, R″ = Me

Pyrimidinedione
(Primidóne)

Oxazolidinediones
Troxidone: R = Me, R′ = Me, R″ = Me
Aloxidone: R = Me, R′ = H, R″ = $CH_2CH:CH_2$
Paramethadione: R = Me, R′ = Et, R″ = Me

Succinimides
Phensuximide: R = H, R′ = Ph, R″ = Me
Methsuximide: R = Me, R′ = Ph, R″ = Me
Ethosuximide: R = Me, R′ = Et, R″ = H.

Acylureas
Phenacemide: R = H, R′ = H.
Pheneturide : R = Et, R′=H

FIG. 22.2. Chemical formulae of antiepileptic drugs. Me=methyl, Et=ethyl and Ph=phenyl.

drug. When a drug is of no benefit, it should be withdrawn; sudden withdrawal of an effective drug, however, often results in status epilepticus.

Many of the newer drugs have been discovered through experiments on animals. Drugs active in grand mal have been found to depress convulsions in

20

animals produced by electrical stimulation applied through electrodes attached to the cornea or to the ears. Experimental convulsions produced in this way do not mimic clinical epilepsy and the order of clinical potency is not the same as that obtained from animal experiments. Nevertheless, drugs active in the animal tests possess anticonvulsant activity in epilepsy and the tests therefore form a useful means of detecting this type of action.

Bromide was the first effective antiepileptic drug but it is now obsolete. *Phenobarbitone, methylphenobarbitone* and *metharbitone* are barbiturates possessing anticonvulsant activity in major epilepsy in doses below those causing heavy sedation. Useful drugs have been found among other classes of compounds and the uses and side-effects of the principal ones are given in Table 22.4. Their chemical formulae are given in Fig. 22.2. Phenobarbitone, methylphenobarbitone or phenytoin sodium are drugs of first choice in grand mal, phenytoin sodium in psychomotor epilepsy, and troxidone (trimethadione) or ethosuximide in petit mal.

Fig. 22.2 illustrates the parts of the molecules which are common to all of the antiepileptic drugs. For activity against grand mal, an aromatic substituent at R' in Fig. 22.2 seems to be important. The substituent at R is usually a small alkyl group except in phenytoin where both R and and R' are phenyl. When the substituent on the nitrogen at R" is a methyl group, potency is increased probably because N-methylation decreases ionization allowing easier penetration of lipid barriers *en route* to the site of action. One carbonyl group appears to be essential and two increase potency.

ACETAZOLAMIDE. This drug is an inhibitor of the enzyme *carbonic anhydrase*; it possesses a diuretic action and is described more fully on page 879. Favourable results have been reported following its use alone, and in combination with other drugs, in the treatment of both grand mal and petit mal. It is not known whether its anticonvulsant activity is due to inhibition of enzymes concerned with neuronal activity, or to the production of a metabolic acidosis. It appears to exert its depressant action on the neurones in the focus of origin, rather than by preventing the spread of activity to normal grey matter. Side-effects, including drowsiness, thirst, nausea, headache and dizziness, are fairly common. Occasionally serious allergic reactions and blood dyscrasias occur.

Centrally-acting muscle relaxants

Mephenesin. Berger and Bradley studied the pharmacological properties of a series of glycerol ethers and found that some of them produced a flaccid paralysis of skeletal muscles without loss of consciousness. Mephenesin (3-ortho-toloxyl-1,2-propanediol) was the most active of the series.

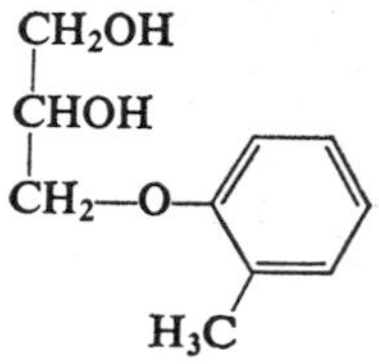

CH₂OH

$$\text{CH}_2\text{OH}$$
$$|$$
$$\text{CHOH}$$
$$|$$
$$\text{CH}_2\text{—O—}$$

H₃C

Analysis of the action of mephenesin showed that it was without *direct* effect on the lower motoneurones, on the neuromuscular junction, or on skeletal muscle. It was shown to act within the spinal cord and to be more selective in depressing polysynaptic than monosynaptic reflexes. Fig. 22.3 illustrates experiments on cats which point to spinal interneurones as the site of action of mephenesin. Reflex contractions of the same quadriceps femoris muscle were elicited alternately by tapping the patellar tendon (knee jerk: a stretch reflex) and by stimulating the central stump of the cut contralateral sciatic nerve (crossed-extensor reflex). Fig. 22.3b is a simplified diagram of the neuronal pathways involved in these reflexes (see also pages 111–115), and Fig. 22.3a illustrates the muscle contractions recorded on a kymograph. An intravenous injection of mephenesin abolished the crossed extensor reflex but did not depress the monosynaptic stretch reflex, which was slightly potentiated. Since the motoneurones innervating the quadriceps muscle are the final common path in both reflex arcs, mephenesin cannot be acting on the motoneurones, the neuromuscular junction or the muscle itself, but is most probably acting at some point on the chains of interneurones, only one of which is illustrated in the diagram. Although the knee jerk is a monosynaptic reflex, it is normally partially inhibited through polysynaptic pathways. The small potentiation of the knee jerk produced by mephenesin is therefore probably due to depression of these polysynaptic inhibitory pathways. Fig. 22.3c illustrates the complex action potentials recorded from a ventral root in response to stimulation of the corresponding ipsilateral dorsal root. The arrangement of the electrodes is shown in Fig. 22.3d. There is an initial large synchronous action potential which represents the monosynaptic pathways, and this is followed by an irregular series of asynchronous action potentials recorded after passage through interneurone chains. Mephenesin did not depress the initial large 'monosynpatic' action potential indicating its selective action on polysynaptic pathways. Mephenesin antagonises convulsions produced by strychnine but has little effect against convulsions in mice produced by leptazol, picrotoxin, amphetamine or electrical stimulation applied to the cornea or the ears.

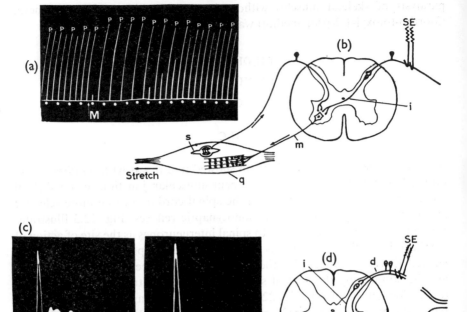

FIG. 22.3. Effects of mephenesin on spinal reflexes. (a) Kymograph recording of contractions of the quadriceps femoris muscle of an anaesthetized cat elicited every 30 sec, alternately by tapping the patellar tendon (monosynaptic stretch reflex— contractions labelled P) and by stimulating the central end of the cut contra-lateral sciatic nerve (polysynaptic crossed-extensor reflex—contractions unlabelled). At M, 15 mg/kg of mephenesin was injected intravenously. Mephenesin blocked the crossed-extensor reflex but slightly potentiated the patellar reflex. (b) shows the neuronal pathways involved in the experiment illustrated in (a). *SE*, stimulating electrodes; *i*, spinal interneurone; *m*, motoneurone innervating extrafusal fibres of *q*, the quadriceps muscle; *s*, muscle spindle. (c) Action potentials recorded from a ventral root of a spinal cat in response to stimulation of the ipsilateral dorsal root with a single shock. Between the two records, 15 mg/kg of mephenesin was injected intravenously. Mephenesin blocked the asynchronous action potentials which had travelled over chains of interneurones within the cord, but was without effect on the initial synchronous action potential. (d) shows the neuronal pathways involved in the experiment illustrated in (c). *SE*, stimulating electrodes; *d*, dorsal root; *i*, interneurone; *v*, ventral root; *RE*, recording electrodes leading to cathode ray oscilloscope (Cro).

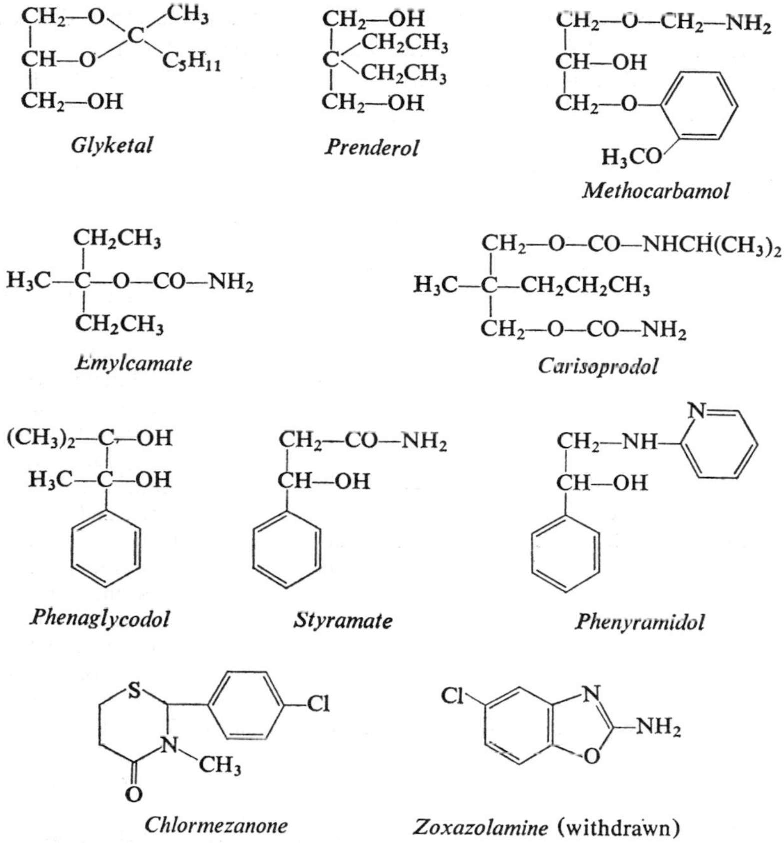

Glyketal

Prenderol

Methocarbamol

Emylcamate

Carisoprodol

Phenaglycodol

Styramate

Phenyramidol

Chlormezanone

Zoxazolamine (withdrawn)

FIG. 22.4. Chemical formulae of some centrally-acting muscle relaxants.

The action of mephenesin is not confined to spinal polysynaptic pathways. It also causes sedation through an action on the reticular formation of the brain stem. Its properties are very similar to those of *meprobamate* described on page 603. With meprobamate the tranquillizing properties are relatively more pronounced while with mephenesin the spinal interneurone blocking action is the more important.

Mephenesin possesses a local anaesthetic action equivalent to that of procaine (page 656) but this action does not contribute to its effects after systemic administration. It is not used as a local anaesthetic, as it also possesses a local irritant action.

Mephenesin is useful as a muscle relaxant in the treatment of tetanus in which it is administered continuously as an intravenous infusion. It may also be used in acute muscle spasm and to relax muscles during the manipulation of dislocated or fractured bones. Side-effects occasionally include nystagmus, weakness, muscular inco-ordination, loss of appetite, nausea and vomiting. Death from overdosage is the result of respiratory depression.

TABLE 22.5. Actions and uses of some centrally acting muscle relaxants.

Derivative of	Name	Additional pharmaco-logical properties	Use
Glycerol	Prenderol	Stimulates higher centres of CNS	As for mephenesin
	Glyketal	—	As for mephenesin
	Methocarbamol	Inhibits leptazol, electro-shock and strychnine convulsions	Mild tranquillizer and muscle relaxant in rheumatism, lumbago and sprains
Butanediol	Phenaglycodol	—	Anticonvulsant, sedative and tranquillizer
Benzoxazole	Zoxazolamine	Longer acting than mephenesin	Cerebral palsy and spasticity and as for mephenesin, but use abandoned because of occasional occurrence of serious hepatic toxicity
Aryl-metathiazanone	Chlormezanone	Similar to meprobamate but more active	Tension and anxiety states
Phenylalkyl carbamate	Styramate	Similar to mephenesin but longer acting	As for mephenesin
Propanediol	Carisoprodol	Depresses decerebrate rigidity in cats. Depresses facilitating activity of mid-brain reticular formation. Inhibits mono- as well as polysynaptic spinal reflexes. Analgesic	Relief of pain in muscles, joints and bones. Used in rheumatism, lumbago, sprains etc
Aminopyridine	Phenyramidol	Similar to carisoprodol	As above
Propylcarbamate	Emylcamate	More potent tranquillizer than meprobamate	Tension and anxiety states

Other compounds. A number of other compounds combine mephenesin-like properties with other actions and have a limited use in therapeutics. Their chemical formulae are given in Fig. 22.4 and their actions and uses are summarized in Table 22.5.

Nicotine. Nicotine paralyses skeletal muscles by an action exerted in the spinal cord and this effect occurs in doses much smaller than those necessary to block neuromuscular transmission. Nicotine is not used in medicine but it seems probable that sufficient nicotine is absorbed by smokers to exert a weak muscle relaxant action, and relief of muscular tension may be one of the beneficial effects felt by smokers. Nicotine paralyses both mono- and polysynaptic reflexes, the knee jerk and the crossed extensor reflex being about equally sensitive to its action while the flexor reflex is more resistant. Nicotine acts primarily by stimulating the inhibitory Renshaw interneurones (page 115) which are cholinoceptive, and which are activated in the body by acetylcholine released from axon collaterals of the lower motoneurones.

CHAPTER 23

Central Nervous System Stimulant Drugs

The mechanism of action of drugs which stimulate the CNS is largely unknown. Some appear to exert a direct stimulant action on particular areas of the CNS, whereas others may act indirectly by blocking central inhibitory mechanisms or by stimulating peripheral sensory receptors. CNS stimulants may be divided into three main classes according to the region of the CNS affected by the smallest effective doses and to the type of stimulation produced. The classes are (1) *psychomotor stimulants*, which affect the higher levels of the cerebral cortex, (2) *analeptics*, which act primarily on the midbrain and medulla, and (3) *spinal cord stimulants*. A drug in one class may stimulate other areas of the CNS when given in large doses and with most of them the stimulant action is followed by a depressant action.

Psychomotor stimulants. These are often referred to as *psycho-activators* or *psycho-analeptics*. They elevate the mood (euphoria) and stimulate mental activity. They also increase wakefulness and produce increased motor activity. Some of the newer drugs in this class are termed *antidepressant drugs, psychic energisers*, or *thymoleptics*; they are used to counteract the depression characteristic of some mental diseases. Antidepressant drugs in general are effective only in depressive states whereas the remainder of the psychomotor stimulants increase mental and physical activity in all individuals.

Some psychomotor stimulants possess appetite-suppressant activity (that is, they are anorexigenic) and are used in the treatment of obesity.

Analeptics. These drugs stimulate the nerve cells in the mid-brain and medulla, but with larger doses motor areas of the brain are stimulated so that finally co-ordinated convulsions occur and these are accompanied by unconsciousness. The chief use of analeptics is to stimulate the vasomotor and respiratory centres in the brain stem and so to antagonize the respiratory depressant action of other drugs.

Spinal cord stimulants. The main drug in this class is strychnine which blocks inhibition in the spinal cord and so enhances the reflex responses to sensory stimulation giving rise to tonic convulsions without loss of consciousness. Strychnine has no great value in medicine although it is still used as an ingredient of tonics and bitters.

Psychotomimetics. These drugs produce mental derangements resembling those occurring in some psychotic states and are sometimes called *hallucino-*

616

genic drugs. Their mechanism of action is unknown and it may be incorrect to describe them as stimulants of the central nervous system. Some clinicians believe that these drugs facilitate psychotherapy and they use them in the treatment of mental illness. Many hallucinogenic drugs derived from plant sources have been used since ancient times in religious and tribal festivals in Africa, Asia, and South America. Psychotomimetics, antidepressant drugs and tranquillizers (page 594) are collectively known as *psychotropic drugs.*

Psychomotor stimulants

The Chinese have used the herb 'ma-huang' from the genus *Ephedra* for thousands of years and during the late nineteenth century its active principle, *ephedrine,* was isolated. Ephedrine is a sympathomimetic amine and this action is described on pages 750–752. In addition to its peripheral sympathomimetic actions, ephedrine has a stimulant action on the cerebral hemispheres and mid-brain, and this led to the synthesis of similar compounds which possess this action. *Amphetamine* is a synthetic sympathomimetic amine possessing a more pronounced central stimulant action than ephedrine. *Dexamphetamine,* the (+) isomer, is about twice as potent as amphetamine (which is the racemic compound) and (+) *methamphetamine* is still more potent. The amphetamines are not substrates of monoamine oxidase (MAO) and are weak inhibitors of this enzyme. Their CNS stimulant action is probably not due to inhibition of MAO.

Amphetamine

Methamphetamine

Their primary site of action appears to be the reticular-activating system. They produce feelings of wakefulness, alertness and elation in most subjects. There is a greater ability to concentrate and an increased amount of mechanical work is possible, especially with methamphetamine, although the rate of recovery from exhaustive work done under the influence of these drugs is not increased. The action of these drugs is short-lasting and the period of stimulation may be followed by deep depression. This is especially apparent after repeated doses have been used over a long period, and may be the basis of amphetamine addiction. The amphetamines increase locomotor activity in animals. This effect is more marked in animals that are in a new environment than in animals that are in their usual surroundings. The emotional dependence of amphetamine addicts on this drug is pronounced, but there is no physical dependence and therefore no definite abstinence syndrome. Prolonged use leads to tolerance.

20*

The amphetamines are of some use in mental exhaustion and in non-psychotic mental depression, but because of their short duration of effect they are of most value when the depressive state is confined to a particular part of the day; otherwise repeated doses are necessary. They are of little or no value in endogenous psychotic depressive states. They possess an analeptic action and have been used to antagonize the anaesthesia and the respiratory depression produced by barbiturates and other CNS depressants. They are of use in *narcolepsy*, a disease characterized by periodic attacks of an overwhelming desire to sleep, and they may be used by normal individuals to give a feeling of freedom from fatigue when faced with an unusually boring or strenuous mental or physical task. They have some use in the treatment of Parkinson's disease (page 733) and their anorexigenic (anti-appetite) effect is of some use in the treatment of obesity.

Undesirable effects resulting from the central action of amphetamines include irritability, tension, agitation, tremor, increased reflex activity, dizziness, a feeling of panic, and with large repeated doses, hallucinations, mental confusion, and delirium. Peripheral side-effects are mainly those resulting from their sympathomimetic action.

Mixtures of amphetamines and barbiturates are sometimes used (e.g. Drinamyl tablets—dexamphetamine 5 mg plus amylobarbitone 30 mg). The barbiturate is believed to depress the excessive irritability and tension characteristically produced by the amphetamines. Animal experiments have shown that such mixtures are more potent in increasing motor activity than is dexamphetamine alone, possibly because the dose of barbiturate is sufficient to depress cortical inhibitory mechanisms preferentially, or because a decrease in anxiety and fear produced by the barbiturate augments performance. The relative proportions of the two drugs in Drinamyl tablets is optimal for this effect. Addiction to mixtures of this type is more common than with the stimulant drugs alone.

Other drugs with similar central actions to the amphetamines but with little peripheral sympathomimetic action have been developed in attempts to reduce side-effects. These include *methylphenidate, pipradol*, and *deanol*. None of these drugs possesses appetite-suppressant activity.

Methylphenidate and pipradol have similar mild stimulant actions and are

Methylphenidate

Pipradol

relatively free from toxic effects although habituation to them may occur. They are of doubtful value in the treatment of mild depression and apathy. Pipradol is a structural isomer of the minor tranquillizer, azacyclonol (page 602).

Deanol is the tertiary analogue and precursor of choline. Unlike quaternary ammonium compounds such as choline, it readily penetrates the blood-brain barrier, after which it is believed to be converted to choline which in turn is acetylated, thus increasing the level of acetylcholine in the brain. It is not certain however that its central stimulant action is the result of the increased acetylcholine levels. Its action is slow in onset (up to 3 weeks) and slow to disappear when the drug is discontinued. Side-effects are said to be mild and it is claimed not to produce habituation. It was once claimed that deanol increased intelligence.

$$HO-CH_2-CH_2-N\begin{array}{c}CH_3\\CH_3\end{array}\quad Deanol$$

Appetite-suppressant drugs. Dexamphetamine has a pronounced anorexigenic action and was formerly used extensively in the treatment of obesity. The central control of appetite and the site of the anorexigenic effect of amphetamine are discussed on pp. 134 and 332. The pronounced side-effects of amphetamine and its tendency to produce habituation led to attempts to synthesize powerful anorexigenic agents which were free from the central stimulant effects of the amphetamines.

Phenmetrazine (Preludin) is chemically related to amphetamine and possesses a powerful suppressant effect on appetite. Although less pronounced, the sympathomimetic effects and central stimulant and habit-forming actions of phenmetrazine are similar to those of the amphetamines.

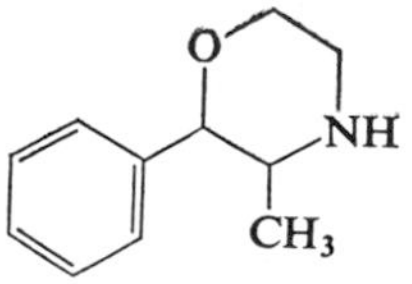

Phenmetrazine

Newer drugs developed as appetite-suppressants include *chlorphentermine* and *diethylpropion* (Tenuate). These drugs are claimed to be free from amphetamine-like side effects, although there have been reports of their use by amphetamine addicts.

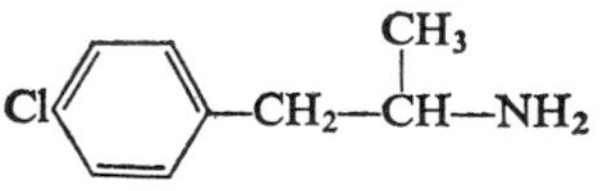

Chlorphentermine

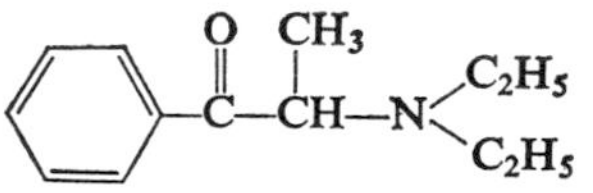

Diethylpropion

The Xanthines. Caffeine, theophylline and theobromine are purine derivatives related to xanthine. They stimulate all parts of the CNS but in the usual doses their effect is confined chiefly to higher cortical centres and results in increased mental activity and reduced or delayed fatigue; they also hasten recovery after exhaustive exercise. In addition to their action on the CNS, they affect the heart and smooth muscle and possess a diuretic action (pages 873–874).

Tea contains caffeine and theophylline, coffee contains caffeine, and cocoa contains caffeine and theobromine. The cola nut and drinks prepared from it contain caffeine.

Caffeine—R = CH_3, R′ = CH_3
Theophylline—R = CH_3, R′ = H
Theobromine—R = H, R′ = H

All three xanthine alkaloids have qualitatively similar actions but they are quantitatively different. Theobromine is weakest in all types of activity and has no clinical value. Caffeine has the most powerful action on the CNS. Regular tea and coffee drinkers have what amounts to an habituation. Excessive chronic consumption causes headache, restlessness, anxiety, insomnia and confusion. The medicinal uses of caffeine are few. It is occasionally used as a respiratory stimulant and has been combined with mild analgesics where it is believed to potentiate their action. Theophylline has wider uses, especially as a mixture with ethylenediamine (then called aminophylline), but these do not depend on its central stimulant effects and are described elsewhere. The mechanism of the central action of the xanthines is unknown.

Cocaine. Cocaine is an alkaloid obtained from *Erythroxylon* species. It is a local anaesthetic used chiefly for the production of surface anaesthesia (page 655) and this is its only medical use. Taken internally, it stimulates the cerebral cortex, facilitates mental activity, and reduces fatigue. Overdosage results in delirium and convulsions. It is a drug of addiction or at least strong habituation. Cocaine potentiates the peripheral actions of adrenaline and noradrenaline. It is an inhibitor of monoamine oxidase and prevents the uptake of adrenaline and noradrenaline into storage sites in the body (page 774). Such effects on catecholamine metabolism or uptake in the brain may be the basis of its actions on the CNS.

Antidepressant drugs

The depressive states of some forms of mental illness may be broadly divided into *endogenous psychotic depressions* in which there is no external cause and the apparent grief and depression are of pathological origin, and the *reactive depressions* in which there is an abnormal depressive reaction to environmental factors which is accompanied by emotional tension and instability. The dividing line between the two types is not always distinct. About thirty years ago, depressed patients were subjected to convulsive therapy and this was found to improve the condition of many patients. Convulsions were originally produced by administering analeptic drugs such as leptazol (page 626); later insulin was used for this purpose, the convulsions resulting from hypoglycaemia. Subsequently, the method of electro-convulsive therapy (ECT) was developed and found to be safer. The convulsions, which resemble major epileptic fits, are induced by passing an AC current for a fraction of a second through electrodes fixed to the scalp. Before ECT, the patient is anaesthetized with intravenous thiopentone and then a short-acting neuromuscular blocking drug is injected to prevent damage to the limbs during the violent convulsions. The treatment is repeated about twice a week for several weeks, and sometimes produces a complete cure; the mechanism is unknown. Possibly, the cycle of events leading to the depressive symptoms is broken by flooding the brain with electrical activity, thus allowing the neuronal activity to return to normal. However, ECT has been shown to increase the level of free amines in the brain, and another possibility is that its beneficial effect in depressed patients is due to this.

Imipramine. During a search among the phenothiazine derivatives for new tranquillizers, it was observed that the compound *methotrimeprazine,* in contrast to chlorpromazine, produced a beneficial effect in depressed patients. More active antidepressant drugs of this type were developed and finally imipramine came into use. Imipramine (Fig. 23.1) is chemically related to the phenothiazines and shares some of their peripheral pharmacological properties, but in contrast to most of the phenothiazines it possesses an antidepressant rather than a sedative action. Imipramine is still the most widely used antidepressant drug in endogenous psychotic depression and has replaced ECT to a large extent, especially when the depression is moderate. Combined ECT and antidepressant therapy is reserved for more seriously affected patients, or those in whom an effect is required quickly, perhaps because of suicidal tendencies. However, several cases have been reported in which patients unresponsive to ECT were benefited by imipramine. Imipramine does not antagonize the symptoms of agitation and tension which sometimes accompany mental depression and may even augment them. In these cases imipramine is often administered in combination with a phenothiazine tranquillizer or a sedative.

The side-effects of imipramine are not serious. Like chlorpromazine, it possesses atropine-like, antihistamine, antiadrenaline and anti-5-hydroxy-tryptamine actions. Autonomic side-effects associated with these actions are common initially but tend to disappear with continued treatment. Other side-effects which occasionally occur include insomnia, tremor, skin reactions and blood changes such as eosinophilia. It does not produce liver damage or jaundice. The therapeutic effect of imipramine is achieved slowly, up to 1 or 2 weeks of continued treatment being necessary before an anti-depressant

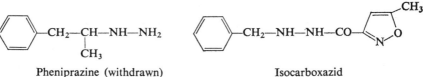

FIG. 23.1. Chemical formulae of some antidepressant drugs.

effect is observed. The slow onset is partly due to the fact that imipramine owes its action to a metabolite, desmethylimipramine; this has the approved name, *desipramine*, and is available for clinical use. The action of desipramine is similar to that of imipramine except that it is more rapid in onset. *Amitriptyline* is chemically related to imipramine (Fig. 23.1) and its peripheral actions and side-effects are similar although they are claimed to be less severe. It is said to differ from imipramine in that it is effective against agitation and anxiety. Its action, therefore, appears to resemble that of a combination of imipramine and chlorpromazine although its antidepressant effect is weaker. *Chlorprothixene*, described under tranquillizers (page 601), is also said to combine anti-depressant and tranquillizing properties.

The mechanism of action of imipramine and amitriptyline is unknown. Unlike the antidepressant drugs described below they are not inhibitors of monoamine oxidase: the basis of their action may be to affect brain amine levels by interfering with their uptake into binding sites.

Monoamine oxidase inhibitors. The development of the antidepressive mono-amine oxidase (MAO) inhibitors followed from the observation that the anti-tubercular drug *iproniazid* (for formula see Fig. 23.1) possesses marked antidepressant activity and inhibits MAO. The effect with small daily doses develops gradually over about 2 weeks and takes a similar period to disappear when the drug is discontinued. Iproniazid may cause a number of side-effects, the most serious being acute hepatic necrosis which is occasionally fatal. Because of this, the use of iproniazid as an antidepressant has been discontinued. The MAO-inhibiting action of iproniazid in the brain may be responsible for its antidepressant properties. Inhibition of MAO is not confined to that in the brain, and the MAO of the blood platelets, liver, spleen and kidneys is also inhibited. It has been suggested that inhibition of MAO of the liver renders this organ susceptible to a virus infection which occasionally causes fatal hepatitis. Other compounds have been studied in an attempt to find MAO inhibitors with a more selective action on the brain enzyme. Most of those now available for therapeutic use as antidepressants are claimed to be active mainly against the brain enzyme, and the incidence of serious liver damage is less than with iproniazid. Nevertheless, because they are MAO inhibitors, the possibility of liver damage remains, and these drugs should therefore be used only under supervision, and never in patients with a history of liver disease. *Pheniprazine*, one of the compounds related to iproniazid, proved to be more liable than others to cause liver damage and has been withdrawn from use.

Iproniazid is a derivative of hydrazine. Other hydrazine derivatives available for use as antidepressives are *nialamide, phenelzine, isocarboxazid* and *phenoxy-propazine* (Fig. 23.1). These are all slowly reversible noncompetitive inhibitors of MAO. Their side-effects are similar although they are said to be less severe than those of iproniazid; these include, in addition to the serious one of occasional liver damage, headache, vertigo, dry mouth, constipation, urinary retention, insomnia, postural hypotension, tremor, skin reactions, oedema, impotence and bone decalcification. Most of these side-effects subside with continued treatment or when the drug is withdrawn. Side-effects with nialamide are probably the least serious but this drug is also the least effective in its antidepressant action. These drugs antagonize depression and produce a feeling of well-being and elation. They also produce greater motor activity which usually occurs much earlier than the improvement in the patient's depressed condition. When first introduced, the MAO inhibitors were thought to be useful in all types of depression. However, the value of antidepressant drugs in clinical practice is difficult to assess accurately because depressive illnesses tend to improve spontaneously and, in clinical trials, placebo-reactions are common. It is difficult to determine the type of depressed patient likely to respond and in many cases it is a matter of trial and error. When no improvement occurs after a month, some other form of treatment is indicated. Recently, prolonged clinical trials on psychotic patients with endogenous depression have demonstrated no significant difference between the beneficial effects of MAO inhibitors and those of a placebo, although imipramine and ECT produced striking improvements. As a result, many psychiatrists are coming to the conclusion that the MAO inhibitors are chiefly of value in reactive depression, where they are also reputed to relieve emotional tension and instability. It is doubtful whether in these conditions they are any more effective than a combination of imipramine with a phenothiazine tranquillizer. Whatever the drug treatment, any improvement is only symptomatic; the most that can be hoped for is that natural remission will occur.

Two reversible competitive inhibitors of MAO which are not derivatives of hydrazine have been developed as antidepressants. These are known as *tranylcypromine* and *etryptamine* (Fig. 23.1). Their action is quicker in onset and, on cessation of treatment, disappears more rapidly than that of the hydrazine inhibitors. Side-effects associated with the hydrazine inhibitors are less pronounced but states of collapse associated with hypertension have been reported in a clinical trial with tranylcypromine. Etryptamine has recently been withdrawn from use because of its liability to produce blood dyscrasias.

MECHANISM OF ACTION. There is much evidence to suggest that the degree of psychomotor activity of the cortex is in some way dependent on the balance between 5-HT, dopamine and noradrenaline in the hypothalamus. Recently, increased levels of the 5-HT metabolite, 5-HIAA (page 178), have been detected in the CSF of depressed patients during periods of depression. These amines are substrates of MAO, the function of which appears to be to inactivate them when they are in the unbound form. The MAO inhibitors may produce their antidepressant effect by inactivating the enzyme and restoring the balance of these amines towards normal. There is a rough correlation between *in vitro* MAO-inhibiting power and clinical effectiveness of these compounds, and the onset and termination of the clinical effect corresponds with the onset and termination of the enzyme inhibition. In animal experiments, these drugs potentiate the central stimulant effects of injections of dopa and 5-hydroxytryptophan. These amino acids (pages 160 and 178) are the precursors of dopamine and 5-hydroxytryptamine, and they penetrate the blood-brain barrier after systemic injection; the amines themselves do not. The reduction in brain noradrenaline and 5-hydroxytryptamine produced by reserpine or tetrabenazine in animals (page 600) is reversed in the presence of MAO inhibitors, and the sedation which these tranquillizers normally produce is converted to excitement. However, in a clinical trial on depressed patients, the administration of dopa or 5-hydroxytryptophan was found to be without beneficial effect although the patients responded well to iproniazid, but the balance of amines produced by injection of the amino acids may not have been optimal to produce an antidepressant effect. One difficulty in relating brain amine levels to changes in behaviour is that some drugs which are MAO inhibitors, and which penetrate the blood-brain barrier, do not possess antidepressant activity.

OTHER ACTIONS OF MAO INHIBITORS. Besides producing psychomotor stimulation, the MAO inhibitors possess other actions, the most important of which are enumerated below. MAO inhibitors are also referred to on pages 775, 825 and 843. (1) Those compounds, which are derivatives of hydrazine, stimulate appetite; this is in contrast to the anorexigenic effect of amphetamine which is also a MAO inhibitor. (2) Most have an analgesic effect which is especially useful in the treatment of angina pectoris. (3) They potentiate the cardiovascular actions of amines which are substrates of MAO (e.g. 5-HT, dopamine, and tyramine), and cause accumulation of endogenous 5-HT and dopamine in peripheral tissues. (MAO is not an important pathway in the destruction of exogenous adrenaline and noradrenaline in peripheral tissues.) (4) Some have been shown to prevent the release of noradrenaline from storage sites in adrenergic neurones and to inhibit the uptake of this amine into these sites. (5) The hydrazine inhibitors protect mice and rats against electro-shock and leptazol convulsions. (6) Many inhibit a number of other enzymes including *diphosphopyridine nucleotidase, spermine oxidase, succinic dehydrogenase, guanidine deaminase, histaminase* and the *liver microsomal enzymes.* (7) Most potentiate the actions of other drugs, and numerous toxic and occasionally fatal reactions have occurred during combined therapy. These drugs include barbiturates, pethidine and other CNS depressants, atropine-like drugs. imipramine-like drugs, and steroids such as cortisone. Hypertensive crises have resulted when drugs such as ephedrine, amphetamine, tryptophan and methyldopa have been administered to patients undergoing therapy with MAO inhibitors, and similar effects have been reported even after eating certain cheeses which are rich in amines such as tyramine, or in amino-acids such as tyrosine which may be decarboxylated in the body to form pressor amines normally inactivated by MAO. (8) Many MAO inhibitors produce a slowly developing, reversible block of transmission through the superior cervical ganglion of the cat by a mechanism which is not yet understood although it appears to be a consequence of MAO inhibition. (9) Several MAO inhibitors cause abortion but only when given during early pregnancy in animals. Abortion is also produced by 5-HT but this is not limited to a particular stage of pregnancy.

Analeptics

The principal drugs in this class are those listed in Table 23.1; in addition, amphetamine and caffeine may occasionally be used as analeptics. The chemi-

TABLE 23.1. Some analeptic drugs

Drug	Use
Picrotoxin	Used in barbiturate poisoning when it is given in divided doses until corneal and pupillary reflexes return. Onset of effect occurs about 15 min after injection
	Unsatisfactory in poisoning by monoureides or alcohol. Dangerous if given in morphine poisoning as the two drugs synergize to produce convulsions
Leptazol	Rapid onset and brief duration of effect when given parenterally
	Useful in poisoning by monoureides as well as by barbiturates. Relatively more active on the cerebral cortex than is picrotoxin. Usually given as a single dose
Nikethamide	Similar to leptazol in its actions but less potent and has longer duration of action than leptazol. Useful in morphine poisoning as well as barbiturate poisoning. Usually given in divided doses until the desired effect obtained
Bemegride	Similar in its actions to the other analeptics but longer duration of effect than nikethamide. Mainly used in mild barbiturate poisoning in which it is given in divided doses until the desired effect is obtained
Amiphenazole	Less pronounced but longer-lasting analeptic action than the other drugs. Has been used together with bemegride in barbiturate poisoning. Is sometimes combined with large doses of morphine in patients with intractable pain. It is said to reduce the toxicity of morphine without antagonizing the analgesic action

cal formulae of the chief analeptics are given in Fig. 23.2. The main use of analeptics in therapeutics is to antagonize excessive depressant effects of drugs such as morphine and the barbiturates on the respiratory and vasomotor centres. Table 23.1 gives brief details of their use. The antagonistic action of analeptics to depressant drugs is due to their producing the opposite pharmacological effect. In large doses they produce convulsions and they are often used to produce this effect in animal experiments designed to test anticonvulsant drugs. When dosage is continued, the CNS is depressed and this

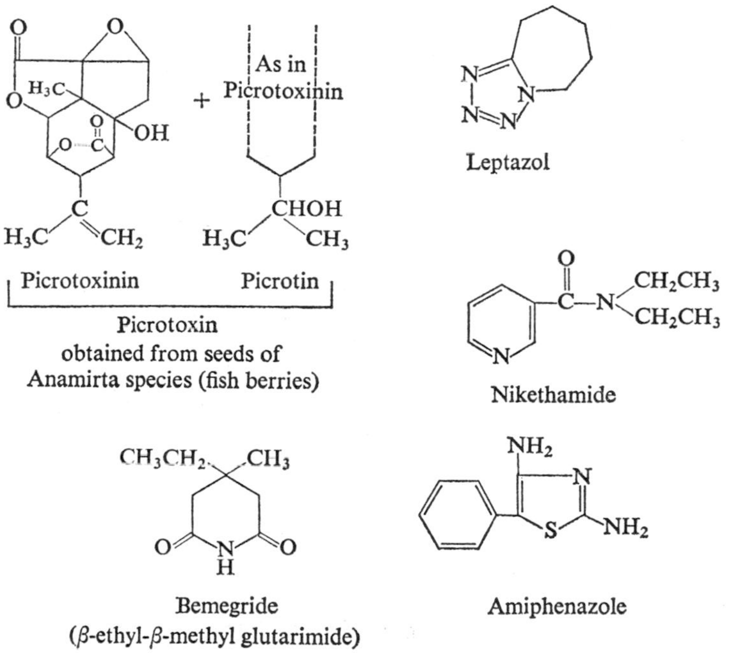

Picrotoxinin Picrotin

Picrotoxin
obtained from seeds of
Anamirta species (fish berries)

Leptazol

Nikethamide

Bemegride
(β-ethyl-β-methyl glutarimide)

Amiphenazole

FIG. 23.2. Chemical formulae of some analeptic drugs.

results in medullary paralysis and death. The mechanism of the medullary stimulant effect of leptazol, amiphenazole and bemegride is unknown. Picrotoxin appears to owe part of its stimulant effect to blockade of pre-synaptic inhibition (page 91). Nikethamide stimulates respiration through a direct action on the respiratory centres and through a stimulant action on chemoreceptors in the cartoid body.

Camphor, menthol and thujone possess analeptic activity which is exerted at least partly through reflex stimulation of the respiratory centre. They are not used clinically for this effect. Alkaloids of lobelia (lobeline), hemlock (coniine) and tobacco (nicotine) stimulate carotid body chemoreceptors and reflexly increase respiration. These alkaloids are only occasionally used therapeutically: nicotine is sometimes used to stimulate respiratory activity in new-born babies when the usual measures have proved unsuccessful.

Spinal cord stimulants

The most important member of this group is strychnine, an alkaloid obtained from the seeds of *Nux vomica*. Its chief action is on the spinal cord; large doses also stimulate the medulla and mid-brain. Very large doses may cause death through depression of the respiratory centre without first producing convulsions. Strychnine renders the senses of touch, smell and hearing more acute but the dose necessary to produce this effect is too close to the convulsive dose for any use to be made of it. It also increases visual acuity and field of vision by a local action on the retina when applied topically to the conjunctiva (page 904).

Strychnine

The action of strychnine on the spinal cord results in enhanced reflex responses. Larger doses produce tonic convulsions interspersed with periods of fatigue. The convulsions are reflex in origin, being initiated by even the slightest sensory stimulus of any type. All muscles take part in the convulsions but since extensor muscles are stronger than flexor muscles the trunk and limbs are rigidly extended, the back being arched (opisthotonus) and the facial muscles contorted. Each convulsion lasts 1 to 2 min and then all muscles relax. Mammals, including man, die from asphyxia after a few convulsions. Frogs, which absorb oxygen through the skin, survive much longer.

Strychnine has no medicinal value but it is still an ingredient of tonics and of pesticides, and cases of poisoning occasionally occur. Treatment consists of administering an inhalation anaesthetic to control the convulsions quickly. This is followed by a short-acting barbiturate and, as far as possible, the patient is isolated from sources of external stimuli. Mephenesin and similar drugs are effective antidotes to strychnine but are less convenient than the volatile anaesthetics and barbiturates.

Strychnine produces its stimulant effect on the spinal cord by blocking the action of the inhibitory transmitter (see pages 90–91), and it has been called 'the curare of spinal inhibitory mechanisms'. It has no direct stimulant effect. As a result of its action, any incoming sensory stimulus spreads to all motoneurones so that an unco-ordinated tonic (or tetanic) contraction results. The effects of strychnine poisoning resemble those of *tetanus toxin*, and there is evidence which suggests that tetanus toxin acts on inhibitory neurones in the spinal cord preventing the release of inhibitory transmitter from them, so that the end result is similar (cf. the action of botulinum toxin on cholinergic nerves, pages 156 and 664). Convulsions due to tetanus toxin, like those produced by strychnine, may be controlled by mephenesin or barbiturates. However, chlorpromazine also controls tetanus convulsions but is without effect in strychnine poisoning suggesting that the two conditions are not similar in all respects.

Brucine is another alkaloid from *Nux vomica* with strychnine-like activity; it is less potent than strychnine itself. In addition, a number of unrelated synthetic substances have been shown to possess strychnine-like activity. These include diphenyldiazadamantanol, 4-formyl-4-phenyl-*N*-methyl piperidine and hexahydromethylspirocyclohexane oxazine pyrazine.

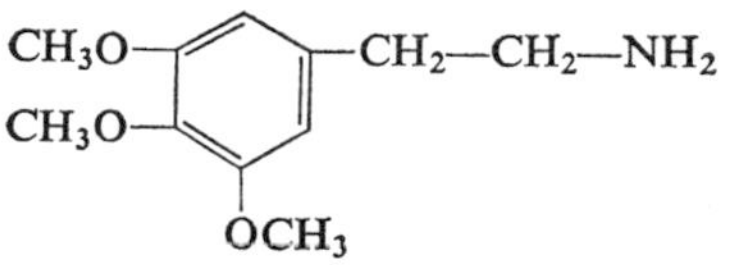

Mescaline
from the cactus,
Lophophora williamsi.

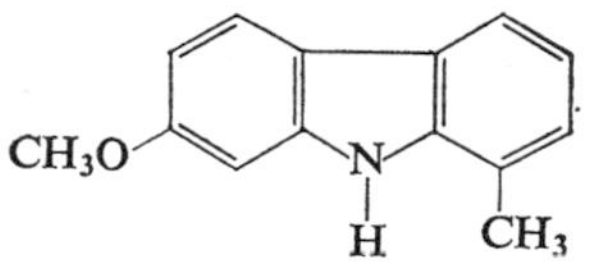

Harmine
from *Bannisteria caapi* and
Pegana harmala

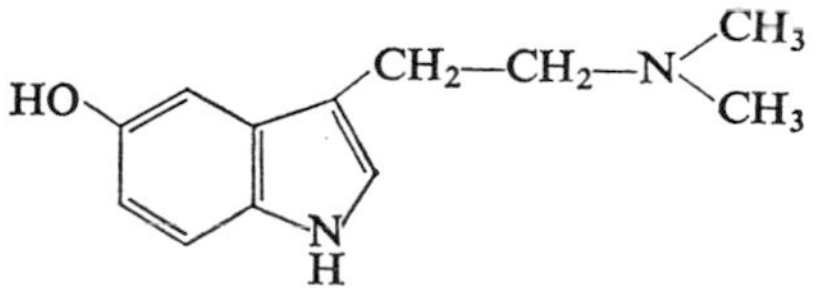

Bufotenine
from *Piptadena peregrina*

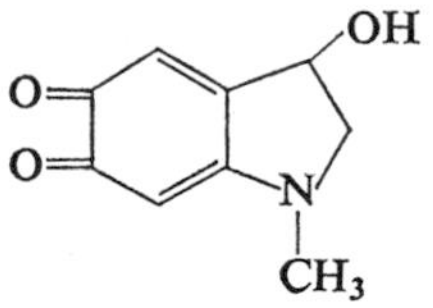

Adrenochrome
an oxidation product
of adrenaline

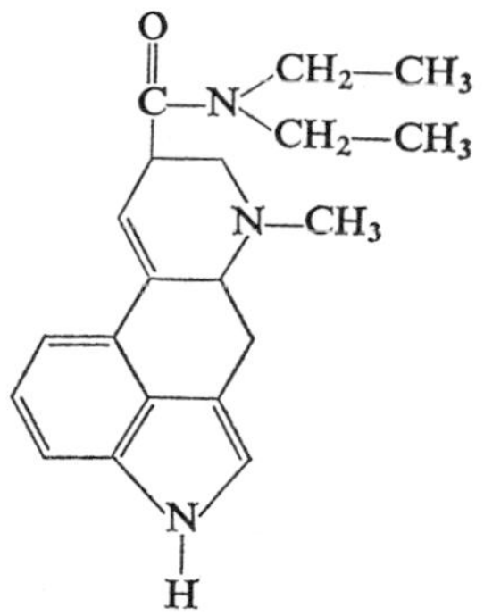

Lysergide
(+)-lysergic acid diethylamide
(partially synthetic)

FIG. 23.3. Some psychotomimetic drugs.

Psychotomimetic (hallucinogenic) drugs

The names, sources and chemical formulae of the chief drugs capable of causing symptoms in man which resemble to some extent those seen in some psychotic patients are given in Fig. 23.3. These drugs usually cause initial autonomic disturbances (tachycardia, dilatation of the pupil, tightness in the chest and abdomen, and nausea) followed by vivid visual hallucinations, anxiety and delusions. Lysergic acid diethylamide is active in oral doses as small as 50 μg in man. Many of these drugs bear some chemical relationship either to 5-hydroxytryptamine or to noradrenaline, and it is possible that their central effects are due to antagonizing, potentiating or mimicking these endogenous amines. Harmine is a MAO inhibitor. However, others possess atropine-like activity and atropine itself may produce psychotomimetic effects in toxic doses. This has led to the suggestion that some of these drugs may exert their effects by blocking the action of acetylcholine at some central sites.

CHAPTER 24

Analgesics

The drugs discussed in this chapter relieve pain without producing general anaesthesia. They are of two types—*narcotic analgesics* such as morphine and allied drugs which produce analgesia with depression of the central nervous system, and *non-narcotic analgesics* such as the salicylates and pyrazolone derivatives which possess both analgesic and antipyretic activity.

Narcotic analgesics

Opium. This is the dried milky exudate of the incised unripe seed capsules of the poppy plant, *Papaver somniferum*. Preparations of the opium poppy have been used in medicine for a long time to relieve pain, and in 1803 a crystalline sample of the chief alkaloid, morphine, was isolated. Later it was shown that the analgesic activity of crude opium is almost entirely due to the morphine it contains, although several other alkaloids are present in small amounts. The alkaloids in opium are benzylisoquinoline and benzylisoquino-line-derived compounds; the chief ones are listed in Table 24.1. Morphine, codeine and thebaine have analgesic activity. Papaverine depresses the activity of smooth muscle and is discussed elsewhere (page 827); narcotine is a cough suppressant, and narceine is a very insoluble alkaloid with little pharmacological activity.

TABLE 24.1. The most important alkaloids of opium.

	Alkaloid	Percentage of total solids
Analgesic	Morphine	10·0
	Codeine	0·5
	Thebaine	0·2
Non-analgesic	Papaverine	1·0
	Narcotine	6·0
	Narceine	0·3

Morphine. Morphine is the most important alkaloid present in opium and is the most commonly used narcotic analgesic. Most of the properties of the potent analgesics differ from those of morphine only in detail and hence morphine is discussed at length. It is optically active; the (−)-isomer is responsible for the pharmacological activity, the (+)-isomer being inactive.

The structure of morphine (Fig. 24.1) has a partially reduced phenanthrene ring system as an obvious structural unit, although it may also be considered as a dibenzofuran, or better as a benzylisoquinoline. Its hydroxyl groups are phenolic (3 position) and a secondary alcohol (6 position) respectively. These oxygen functions are important since their esterification or etherification modifies analgesic potency considerably.

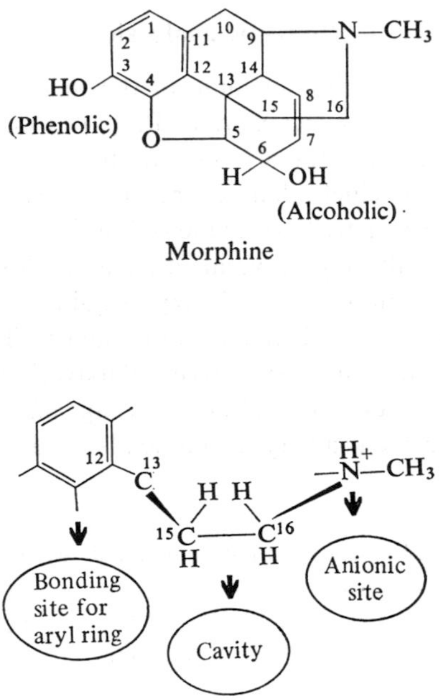

Morphine

FIG. 24.1. The structure of morphine and the Beckett and Casy concept of its fit with the receptor.

STRUCTURE-ACTION RELATIONSHIPS IN MORPHINE-LIKE ANALGESICS. It has been proposed that morphine and morphine-like compounds possess three characteristic chemical features of importance to their activity: (1) a methyl group attached to the tertiary nitrogen atom, (2) several oxygen-containing groups situated at a distance of 7 to 9 angstrom units from the tertiary nitrogen, and (3) at least one aryl nucleus attached to an asymmetric carbon which is joined by a short hydrocarbon chain to the tertiary nitrogen. Beckett and Casy attempted to deduce the nature of the morphine receptor from the chemical structures of compounds with analgesic activity and arrived at the following conclusions: (1) The protonated tertiary nitrogen is attracted to an anionic site in the receptor surface. (2) The flat aryl nucleus is attached to a flat surface on the receptor by van der Waals' forces. (3) The alkyl chain between carbon 13 and the tertiary nitrogen has a semi rigid steric configuration and is accommodated in a cavity. The geometry of this structure explains the large difference in potency between the (+)- and the (−)-isomers. All the morphine-like analgesics possess these three features but so do several other compounds which are not analgesics. Furthermore, several potent analgesics do not possess these features.

PHARMACOLOGICAL PROPERTIES OF MORPHINE. Morphine depresses activity throughout the central nervous system. The depression, however, differs from that produced by the general anaesthetics, which (with the exception of nitrous oxide) produce analgesia only after unconsciousness. It is usually possible to rouse a person from the sleep produced by morphine.

Analgesia. Morphine produces analgesia chiefly by acting on the cerebral cortex although it also has some action on the diencephalon. It depresses pain-induced reverberation in cortical neurone circuits. Its action in reducing pain appears to be specific as the sensitivity of the central nervous system to other stimuli such as touch, smell and hearing is little altered, although it may depress visual perception since acuity is often raised during the cure of addiction. Morphine raises the threshold to pain, so that a pain-producing stimulus must be stronger to be detected. This effect is best seen when morphine is administered before applying a painful stimulus. When morphine is given for the treatment of long-standing pain, pain may still be felt but the emotional response of the patient is altered in such a way that the pain becomes tolerable. Alleviation of fear and anxiety associated with pain and with the anticipation of pain is an important component in the analgesic action of morphine. Morphine has no significant local anaesthetic action and there is little pharmacological basis for its use in lotions and ointments. However, when given systemically, its central action adds to the peripheral pain-relieving action of local anaesthetics.

Respiration. Morphine has a depressant effect on respiration, even in doses which do not dull consciousness. Overdosage produces death through respiratory failure. The sensitivity of the medullary respiratory centre to the CO_2 content of the blood is reduced, and after morphine treatment, the response to inhalation of a mixture of 95% O_2 and 5% CO_2 is reduced. The decreased sensitivity to CO_2 results in a change in the electrolyte balance of the blood. Morphine readily passes the placental barrier, and in obstetric use it depresses the baby's respiration; it is therefore unwise to use morphine as an analgesic in childbirth.

The electroencephalogram. Morphine addicts usually have an abnormally large amount of slow α activity. This suggests that activity in the corticothalamic region is depressed (page 132) but the effect is not always reversed when the subject ceases to be addicted. However, in some addicts in which marked delta rhythm occurs, recovery is common when morphine is withdrawn. In non-addicts, morphine produces only slight effects on the EEG, even in amounts that produce pronounced effects on mood and behaviour.

The hypothalamus. Morphine causes a rise in the body temperature, hyper-glycaemia and antidiuresis. There is depletion of the catecholamine stores in the hypothalamus and these effects indirectly result in depletion of both adrenal medullary and cortical hormones. Antidiuresis is probably the result of the release of ADH from the neurohypophysis (page 366) although morphine may also affect renal haemodynamics. Depletion of the adrenocorticoids and hyper-plasia of the zona reticularis result from the release of ACTH by morphine.

The cough centre. Morphine is a powerful depressant of the cough centre and it also reduces awareness of coughing. It is therefore valuable in the treat-ment of severe cough, as for example that caused by neoplasms of the respira-tory passages.

Vomiting. Morphine produces vomiting by stimulating the chemoreceptor trigger zone in the medulla oblongata, and not by a direct effect on the vomiting centre. The emetic action is most frequently seen in ambulatory patients and is much less common in patients lying down. When the dose of morphine is increased, it tends to exert an anti-emetic action, preventing the effects of other emetics. *Apomorphine*, obtained by treating morphine with mineral acids, is more potent than morphine in stimulating the chemosensitive trigger zone; it is injected subcutaneously to produce this effect.

The spinal cord. Morphine stimulates most monosynaptic reflexes and in the dog and cat it first stimulates and then depresses the knee-jerk. It depresses polysynaptic reflexes; flexor and crossed extensor reflexes are markedly depressed by small doses, but the responses to stretch are either unaffected or enhanced. The tail of a rat or a mouse is held rigid and erected across the back of the animal in a S-shaped curve when morphine is administered (the Straub reaction); this reaction is due to contraction of the sacro-coccygeus dorsalis muscle but the lumbo-sacral cord with its peripheral nervous outflow must also be intact.

The eye. Morphine produces miosis in man and dog but not in cat and mouse.

The 'pin-point' pupil in man is a characteristic sign of morphine administration provided that the dose is not so large as to produce anoxia which dilates the pupil. The mechanism of the miosis is not fully understood: it is not a peripheral effect since morphine has no miotic action when applied locally or to excised eyes. A further account is given on page 899.

Action on the gastro-intestinal tract. Morphine prevents the release of acetylcholine from cholinergic nerves innervating smooth muscle, and many of its effects on the gut may result from this action. It causes constipation and has been used in the treatment of diarrhoea since ancient times. It reduces the motility of the stomach and initially reduces the secretion of hydrochloric acid. The pyloric sphincter is constricted. Denervation of the stomach does not affect these action, which indicates that they are exerted peripherally. Morphine slows the movements of the small intestine although tone is increased. The secretion of bile and pancreatic juice is reduced. Reduction in the propulsive movements of the large intestine also occurs. The anal sphincter is contracted. These effects, together with a decreased responsiveness to the stimulus for defaecation, are responsible for the constipating action of morphine.

Action on ureter and bladder. Morphine increases the tone and amplitude of contraction of the ureter in man. The detrusor and trigone muscles of the bladder are also contracted. These effects, together with the fact that morphine depresses the responsiveness of the subject to the stimulus for micturition, lead to retention of urine.

Release of tissue histamine. Morphine releases tissue-bound histamine, and this is probably responsible for the itching, urticaria and reddening of the skin which often occur with morphine treatment. Morphine occasionally produces allergic and anaphylactic reactions in susceptible patients, and may produce sufficient bronchoconstriction in asthmatic or bronchitic patients to hamper respiration.

Tolerance and addiction. Tolerance develops to the actions of morphine on the CNS (such as analgesia, respiratory depression and sedation) but not to the action on the gastro-intestinal tract. Thus the patient on prolonged therapy, or the addict, suffers from severe constipation. Furthermore, tolerance developed to one morphine analogue applies to another, so it is usually impossible to overcome tolerance by changing from one drug to another. The euphoria produced by morphine may be the cause of addiction; tolerance to the euphoric effect may result in the addict taking more and more of the drug to produce the desired effect. The sensations that occur when the addict is deprived of his drug are so appalling that he takes higher doses to keep them at bay. At this stage, the addict is both mentally and physically dependent on the drug. This liability to cause addiction is the most serious drawback in the clinical use of morphine, as addiction is likely to occur after only a few doses.

Thus, in the long-term suppression of pain, the use of morphine has to be carefully controlled.

When the addict no longer obtains supplies of morphine, he experiences withdrawal symptoms. They vary in severity from lachrimation and perspiration to tremor, insomnia, vomiting, diarrhoea, loss of weight and cramp. The body temperature and systolic blood pressure both increase and respiration becomes rapid. Withdrawal symptoms usually appear about 24 h after the last dose of morphine. Addiction to morphine is treated by the gradual withdrawal of the drug or by its replacement with methadone and then the gradual withdrawal of methadone. Sudden and complete withdrawal of morphine is dangerous and may cause death. Addicts are also given sedatives and psychotherapy.

DISTRIBUTION, METABOLISM AND EXCRETION OF MORPHINE. Morphine is readily absorbed from the gastro-intestinal tract. The liver is the principal site of metabolism; a small amount undergoes N-demethylation but most is conjugated with glucuronic acid. The main excretory route for both free and conjugated morphine is through the kidneys, although some free drug is often found in the sweat and faeces. There is some evidence that the proportion of conjugated morphine excreted decreases as tolerance develops.

NATURALLY-OCCURRING MORPHINE-LIKE ANALGESICS (see Fig. 24.2). *Codeine (methylmorphine)*. The analgesic activity of codeine is less than that of morphine, and although it may be used in large doses as an analgesic its main use is as a cough suppressant. In therapeutic doses, only slight respiratory depression is observed but toxic doses produce marked respiratory stimulation, with excitement and convulsions. Codeine has little effect on the pupil. It produces the Straub effect in mice. Its actions on the gastro-intestinal tract are similar to, but slightly weaker than those of morphine, constipation often being a prominent side-effect. Codeine is a much safer drug than morphine and although tolerance and addiction may occur, cases of primary addiction (i.e. addiction produced by taking codeine alone) are rare. It does not produce the same degree of euphoria as does morphine, and addicts regard it as inferior, resorting to codeine only when supplies of morphine are unobtainable.

Thebaine (dimethylmorphine). Thebaine possesses only slight respiratory depressant and analgesic actions and its main effect is central stimulation resulting in convulsions. The convulsions in the frog are said to be produced by a decrease in the central inhibition of spinal reflexes.

Papaveretum (omnopon, pantopon, pantopium). Papaveretum is a mixture of the opium alkaloids in about the same proportions as they occur in the crude drug. There is about 50% of morphine in the mixture, which does not appear to

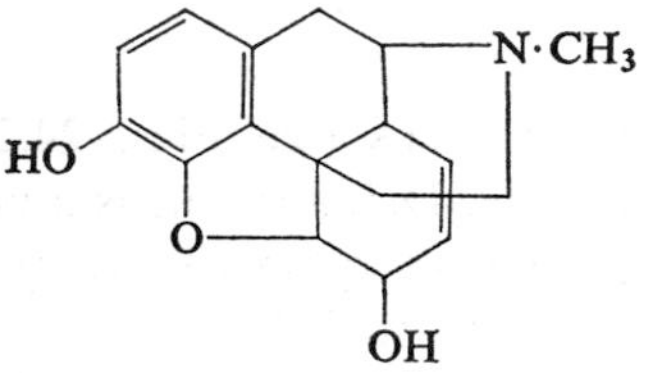

Morphine

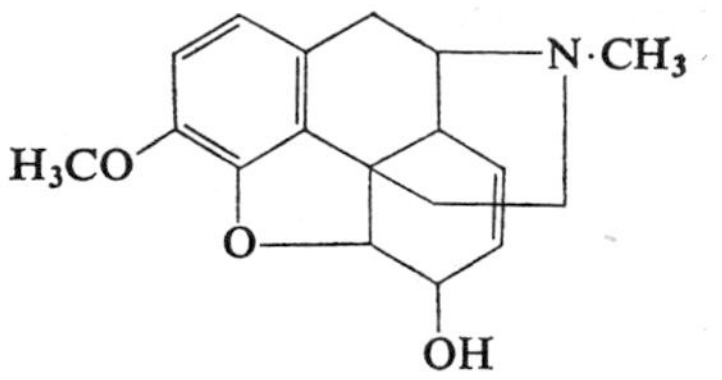

Codeine

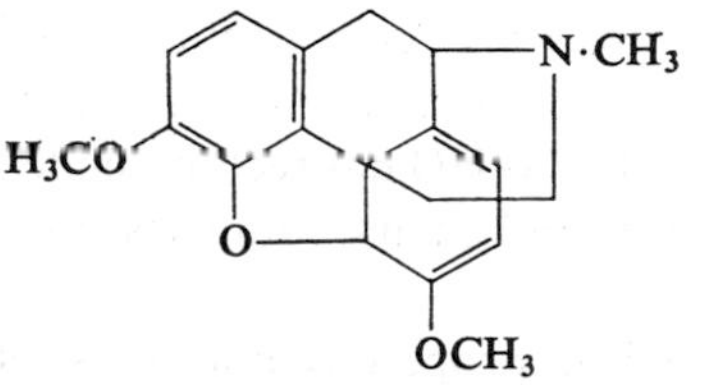

Thebaine

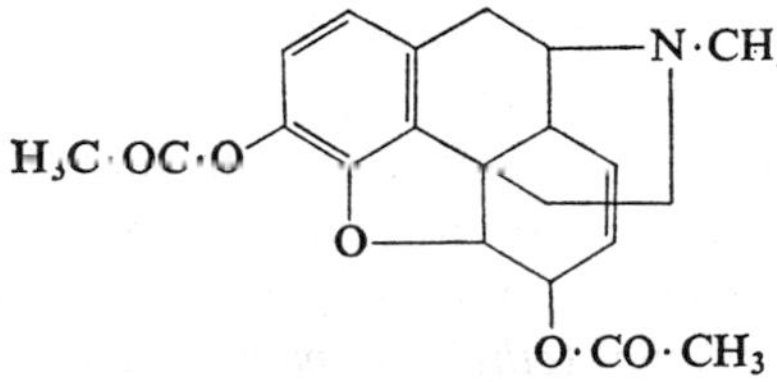

Diamorphine

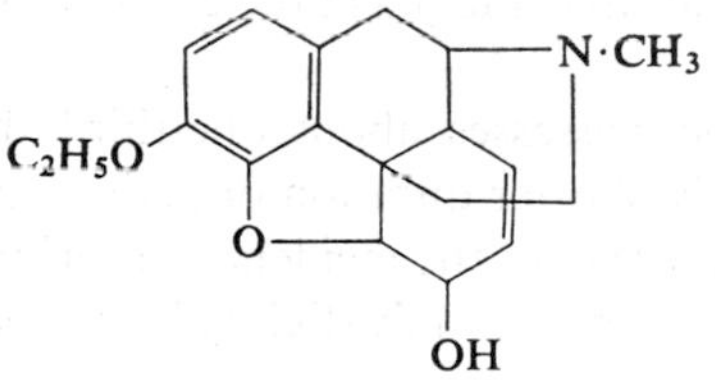

Dionin

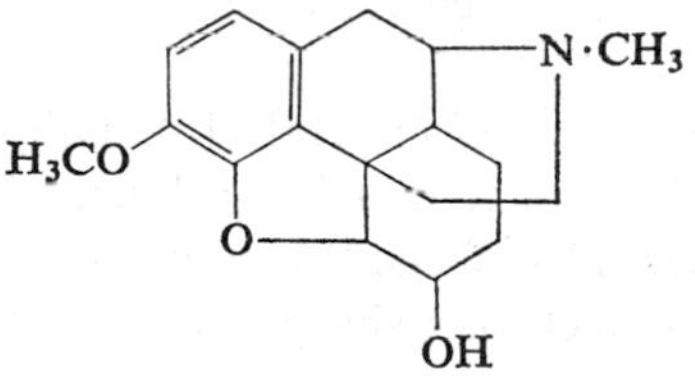

Dihydrocodeine

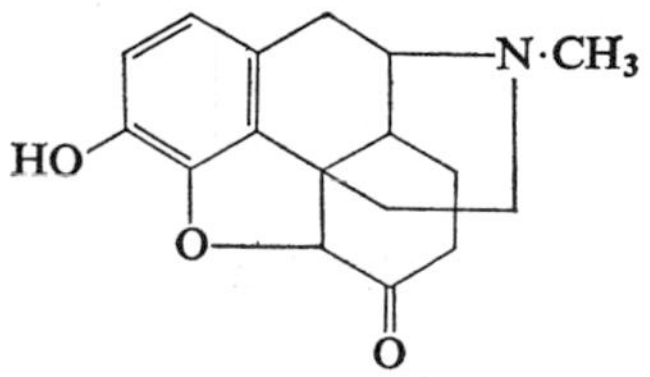

Dihydromorphinone

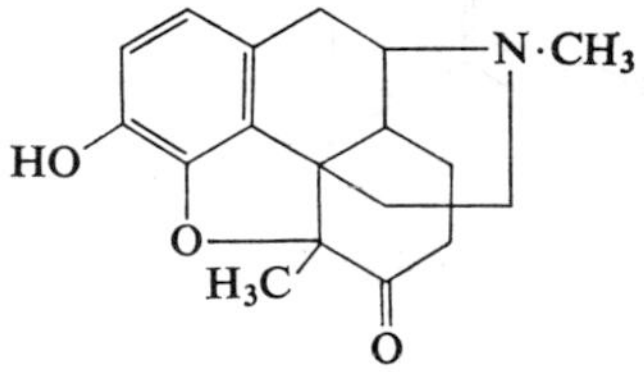

5-Methyldihydromorphinone

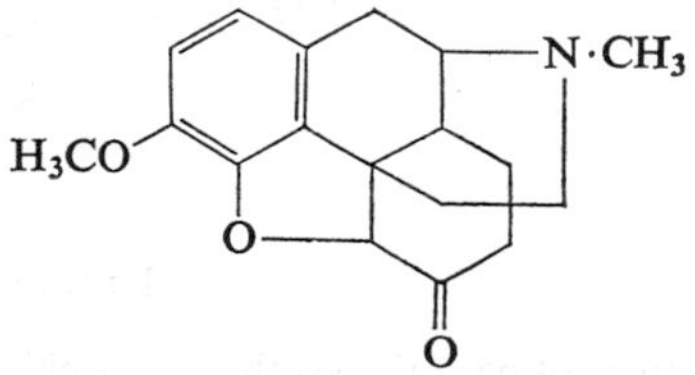

Dihydrocodeinone

FIG. 24.2. Formulae of some of the more important morphine-like analgesics.

have an advantage over either pure morphine or prepared opium, except that it can be injected.

PARTIALLY SYNTHETIC MORPHINE DERIVATIVES (see Figs. 24.2 and Fig. 24.3). *Diamorphine (diacetylmorphine, heroin).* Diamorphine is a powerful analgesic being about 4 to 5 times as active as morphine. Its respiratory depressant action is also correspondingly greater and it is more potent in suppressing the cough centre but less active as an emetic. Diamorphine is more rapid in action but shorter lasting than morphine. It is metabolized in the body by hydrolysis to morphine. Diamorphine produces euphoria and excitement and it is particularly prone to cause addiction. The diamorphine addict is very difficult to cure and often relapses. The WHO has recommended a total ban on its manufacture and medical use, and many countries have complied with this request.

Dionin (ethyl morphine). The pharmacological properties and uses of dionin closely resemble those of codeine. The drug is also occasionally used in ophthalmology as a counter-irritant to produce hyperaemia in the conjunctiva and eyelids.

Dihydrocodeine (DF118). Dihydrocodeine possesses about one-third the analgesic activity of morphine, with a slightly shorter duration of action and fewer side-effects. When the dose is greatly increased, the incidence of serious side-effects rises sharply although the analgesic action is only slightly increased.

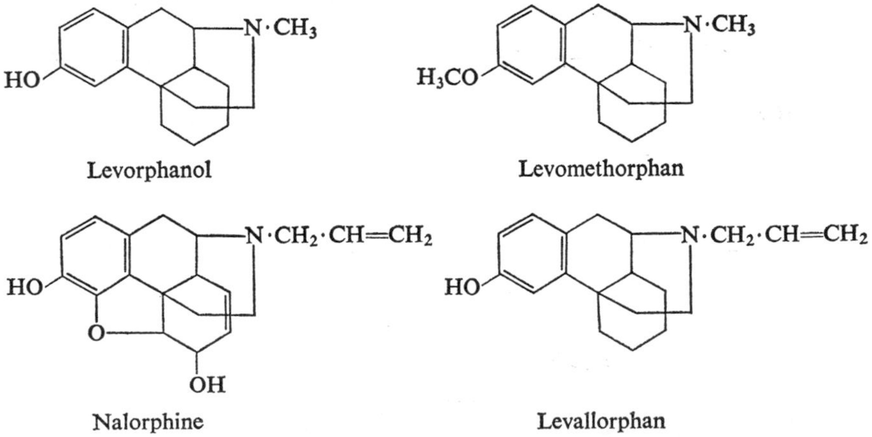

FIG. 24.3. Formulae of partially synthetic morphine derivatives.

Dihydromorphinone (Dilaudid). This compound has actions similar to those of morphine, but is about 6 times more potent. It is considerably shorter in duration of action. It has a greater depressant effect upon the respiratory and cough centres but is less constipating and emetic than is morphine. The drug may give rise to tolerance and addiction.

Methyldihydromorphinone (*metopon*). The drug is about 10 times more potent than morphine as an analgesic, particularly when given orally. Tolerance develops more slowly. It does not substitute completely for morphine in subjects addicted to the latter drug. It is very expensive to prepare as the synthesis is difficult.

Dihydrocodeinone (*Dicodid, Hycodan*). Dihydrocodeinone is slightly more potent than codeine. It is used in the treatment of cough and is preferred to codeine by addicts to tide them over a morphine shortage.

Levorphanol (*levorphan, Dromoran*). Levorphanol lacks the oxygen bridge, the alcoholic hydroxyl group and the 7:8 double bond of morphine; it is the *laevo* isomer of 3-hydroxy-N-methyl-morphinan. It is far more toxic than the *dextro* isomer, which is devoid of analgesic activity. Its actions closely resemble those of morphine but it is about 5 times more active. Its effects are longer lasting and it produces less sedation than does morphine, although tolerance and addiction occur to about the same extent.

Levomethorphan. This drug is closely related to levorphanol and possesses potent analgesic activity. The dextro-isomer (dextromethorphan, Romilar), which is devoid of analgesic activity, is used as a cough suppressant.

SYNTHETIC MORPHINE-LIKE ANALGESICS (see Fig. 24.4). *Pethidine* (*meperidine, dolantin*). Pethidine was discovered during a search for drugs with atropine-like properties. Its actions on the central nervous system are said to be less pronounced than are those of morphine; 100 mg of pethidine produces an analgesic effect similar to, but of shorter duration than, 10 mg of morphine. Pethidine is more effective against pain arising from the viscera than against pain of skeletal origin. When administered to man, it usually produces dysphoria (restlessness), and euphoria occurs in some patients.

In therapeutic doses, pethidine does not seriously depress the respiratory centre or the cough centre, and the size of the pupil is unchanged. The EEG usually shows the presence of slow waves which become progressively slower and increase in amplitude as treatment proceeds. Toxic doses of pethidine produce central excitement.

Pethidine exerts a mild spasmolytic action on the gut. Constipation does not occur as readily with pethidine as with morphine. Gastric secretion is also only slightly affected. Side-effects are usually not serious and consist mainly of sweating, nausea, vomiting, dry mouth and dizziness. Tolerance and addiction, although slower in onset than with morphine, constitute a serious hazard in the use of pethidine. The drug is rapidly metabolized and inactivated in the liver, and this necessitates doses at frequent intervals to maintain a suitable blood level.

Many compounds based upon the relatively simple pethidine structure have been prepared. One of them, *ketobemidone* (in which the —$CO.O.C_2H_5$ group

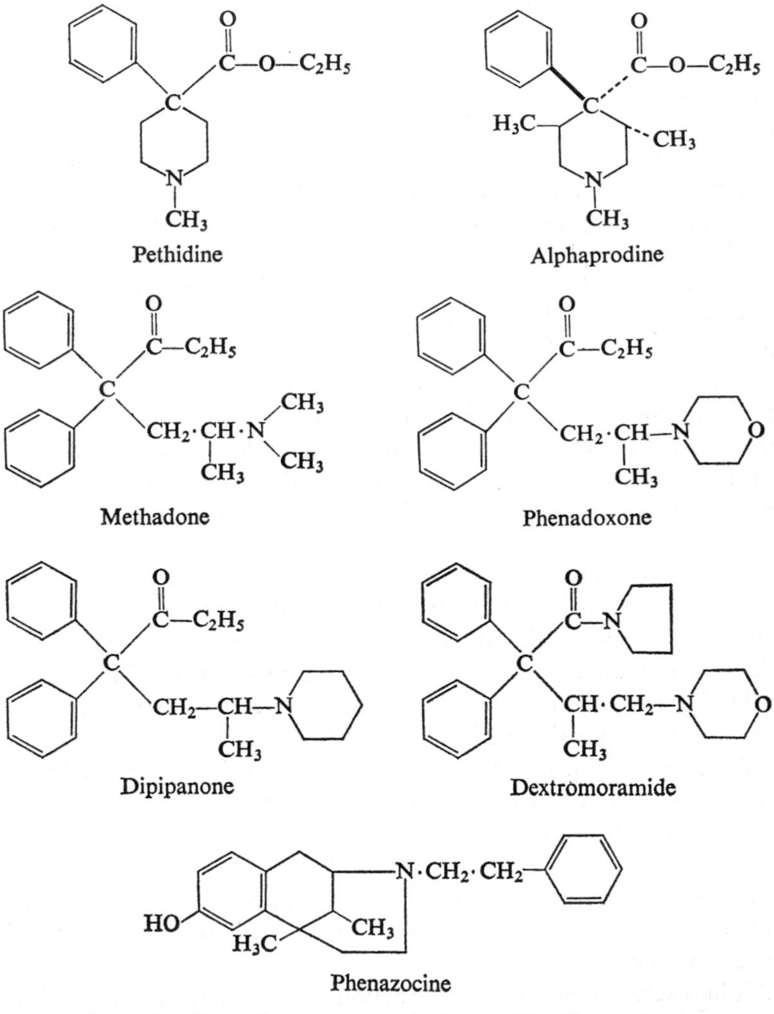

FIG. 24.4. Formulae of some synthetic morphine-like analgesics

of pethidine is replaced by —$CO.C_2H_5$ and a meta —OH is inserted in the phenyl ring), has been reported to be 30 times more potent than pethidine as an analgesic in animals. However, addiction occurs so rapidly that it is impossible to use the drug clinically.

Alphaprodine (Nisentil). This drug, which is closely related to pethidine, is slightly more potent and has a shorter duration of action; it has been tried in obstetrics but does not possess any advantage over pethidine.

Methadone (Amidone, physeptone). The chemical structure of this drug is little related to that of morphine. It is prepared as the racemic mixture in which the $(-)$-isomer is up to 50 times more potent than the $(+)$-isomer. Its pharmacological effects are similar to those of morphine, with an approximately equipotent analgesic action. It is only slightly less depressant on the respiratory centre and this precludes its use in obstetrics. It is less sedative and constipating, and produces less miosis. Methadone is a powerful inhibitor of the cough centre and is used in the treatment of the chronic cough of malignant disease of the respiratory tract. The risk of addiction is serious. Minor side-effects including dizziness, nausea and vomiting may occur.

Phenadoxone (Heptalgin). Phenadoxone is a closely related compound to methadone with similar activity.

Dipipanone (Pipadone). This drug is the piperidine analogue of methadone: it has similar properties but also possesses some atropine-like activity.

Dextromoramide (MCP875). Dextromoramide has only recently been synthesized (1965). It is about 10 times more potent as an analgesic than morphine in animals but equipotent in man. It is not a sedative in therapeutic doses and the development of tolerance and addiction is slow. It is useful in alleviating the symptoms of morphine withdrawal. The incidence of euphoria is low and it is not an attractive drug to the potential addict. Cases of severe respiratory depression produced by dextromoramide have been reported.

Phenazocine (Narphen, Prinadol, NIH75190). This is about 5 times as potent as morphine. The effect also lasts longer than does an equiactive dose of morphine. It does not produce nausea, vomiting or constipation. There is little sedative or respiratory depressant action, and tolerance and addiction are less of a problem. This drug represents an improvement on the other morphine-like analgesics.

ANTAGONISTS OF THE MORPHINE-LIKE ANALGESICS (see Fig. 24.3).
Nalorphine (N-allylnormorphine). It has been known for many years that N-allylnorcodeine antagonizes respiratory depression produced by morphine. In 1953, nalorphine was introduced as an antagonist of morphine. When given alone, nalorphine has analgesic activity but it is not used to produce this effect. It antagonizes the analgesic, respiratory depressant and sedative actions of morphine-like analgesics, whether administered before or after them. It can be a life-saving drug in the treatment of the severe respiratory depression which occurs with an overdose of morphine and related analgesics. It does

21

not antagonize the depressant action on the cough centre and the effects of the two drugs at this site may be additive.

The precise mode of action of nalorphine is not well understood. It has been suggested that there is competitive antagonism on the receptor surface for which nalorphine has a greater affinity than has morphine. However, nalorphine is able to antagonize several times its molecular concentration of morphine. Nalorphine antagonizes all the morphine-like analgesics and produces withdrawal symptoms in addicted subjects, regardless of the addicting drug. In addicts, nalorphine precipitates withdrawal symptoms which may be so serious as to cause death.

Levallorphan (*Lorfan*). Levallorphan is the compound in the morphinan series analogous to nalorphine in the morphine series. It has properties similar to those of nalorphine.

Some analeptic drugs (page 626) may also be used to antagonize the effects of morphine overdosage.

NEWER ANALGESICS. During the course of studies on the structure-activity relationships in analgesics, rigid analogues of morphine were prepared from thebaine by the inclusion of an extra alicyclic ring joining carbons 6 and 14. These were then substituted in the 16 position to produce a series of primary and secondary alcohols with analgesic potencies of up to about 8000 times that of morphine. The series is shown in Fig. 24.5.

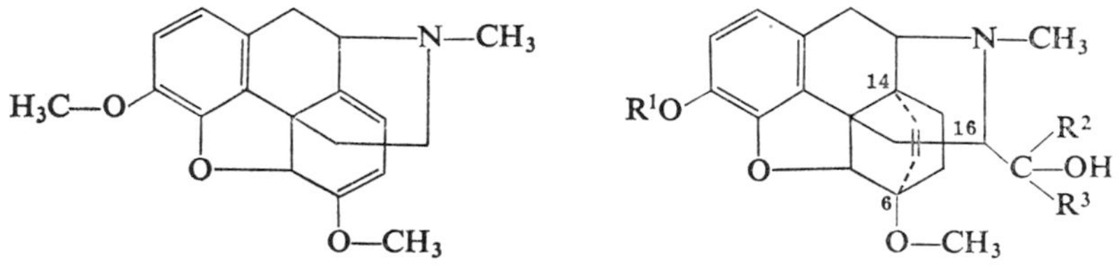

Thebaine

FIG. 24.5. Formulae of thebaine and its potent derivatives. Maximum activity is when $R^1 = H$, $R^2 = CH_3$, and $R^3 = CH_2.CH_2.CH(CH_3)_2$.

Although these derivatives (for example M99 or *etorphine*) have such high analgesic activities when compared with morphine, their toxicities are not increased to the same degree. When injected they produce analgesia, depression of the respiratory and the cough centres, inhibition of gastrointestinal motility, lowering of body temperature and other characteristic signs of morphine-like drugs. All the depressant effects are antagonized by nalorphine or levallorphan. The introduction of the second bridged system into the molecule and the addition of further substituents opens up a fresh approach to elucidation of the nature of the morphine receptor site. These new compounds have a more rigid molecular structure than morphine and thus may fit the receptor surface more closely. Another highly selective binding site for the additional group has been postulated.

Tests for analgesic activity. Two procedures are in general use; one is based on a graded response and the other on a quantal response. In both, groups of animals are given various doses of the drugs under test, and after a suitable time interval the response of each animal to a stimulus is determined. Graded responses are measured in terms of threshold stimulus intensity to produce pain, or of reaction times. Quantal responses depend on the presence or absence of a response to a stimulus of fixed intensity: these are quicker to obtain.

ANIMAL TESTS

Radiant heat. Heat is focused on to the tip of a rat's tail, and when a sufficiently high intensity is reached, there is a typical twitch of the tail. This is taken as a sign that the animal feels pain. Pain thresholds are measured in terms of the reaction time or the stimulus intensity required for a response.

Pressure. The tip of the rat's tail is subjected to pressure, and that pressure which produces a squeak is taken as a measure of pain threshold. This procedure allows either for a graded response in which activity is assessed in terms of increased threshold pressure, or for a quantal response in which analgesia is indicated when the threshold is raised to at least twice the control value.

Hot plate. Mice are placed on to a heated metal plate and the times taken for a reaction (such as hind limb movement) are noted. This may also be adapted to a quantal response, the animals showing analgesia when they fail to respond within a given time, for instance, 15 seconds.

Electric shock methods. Electrodes are inserted in holes drilled in the incisor teeth of guinea-pigs, and the strength of the stimulus necessary to produce a rapid upward thrust of the head is determined. In another method using mice, electric shocks are given to the tail and the response is a squeak.

In some laboratories, the so-called *analgesic triple test* is used. Each mouse is subjected to three tests in which its reaction to thermal, mechanical and electrical pain stimuli are observed. This arrangement differentiates analgesics from other depressants of the central nervous system. Morphine and pethidine are slightly more potent against thermal pain than against mechanical and electrical pain; acetylsalicyclic acid is also active against all three types of pain stimulus, but only at doses approaching lethal levels.

TESTS IN MAN. Tests for analgesia in man involve either experimentally induced pain or pathological pain. Commonly, heat is focused on to a blackened spot upon the forehead of the subject for exactly 3 sec. If no pain is experienced, the procedure is repeated at 60-sec intervals with increasing heat intensity until pain is felt. The heat intensity at this point is measured by a radiometer and is considered to be the minimum stimulus for pain. This value represents a measure of the pain threshold and its elevation after drug administration gives an assessment of analgesic potency. Although similar methods in animals give reliable results, those obtained in man are often inconsistent.

Methods using electro-dental stimulation have been used and contraction of muscle deprived of its blood supply (ischaemic muscle) has been applied to the study of deep pain.

Clinical trials using pathological pain have also been adapted to give quantitative data.

TESTS FOR ADDICTIVE LIABILITY. Addicts are stabilized by the regular administration of morphine and then the drug under test is substituted for morphine. The intensity of the abstinence syndrome is compared with that after total withdrawal of morphine. Another method is to give nalorphine after administration of the drug under test. A withdrawal syndrome may be produced if the drug produces physical dependence.

Non-narcotic analgesics

Salicylates. The salicylates are analgesic drugs with antipyretic properties. Salicylic acid as such is far too irritant to administer internally. It possesses a keratolytic action and may be applied topically to the skin in the treatment of corns and warts. Methyl salicylate (oil of wintergreen) is also too irritant to be used internally. It is often incorporated in liniments as a counter-irritant. Sodium salicylate and acetylsalicylic acid (aspirin) are less irritant and are used internally. Weight for weight, aspirin is a more potent analgesic than sodium salicylate.

The salicylates are readily absorbed from the upper intestinal tract and then distributed to all organs of the body. About 80% of the dose given is eliminated in the urine, over half of this in the first 24 h. The urine contains unchanged salicylate, salicyluric acid, gentisic acid and conjugates of glucuronic and salicylic acids (see Fig. 24.6).

ANALGESIC ACTION OF SALICYLATES. The salicylates reduce the sensation of pain by an action on the central nervous system. The site of action is probably cortical in origin as analgesic doses of salicylates have no effect on sensations other than those of pain, produce no mental disturbances, and have no anaesthetic effect. They may act on the conduction of pain-induced impulses

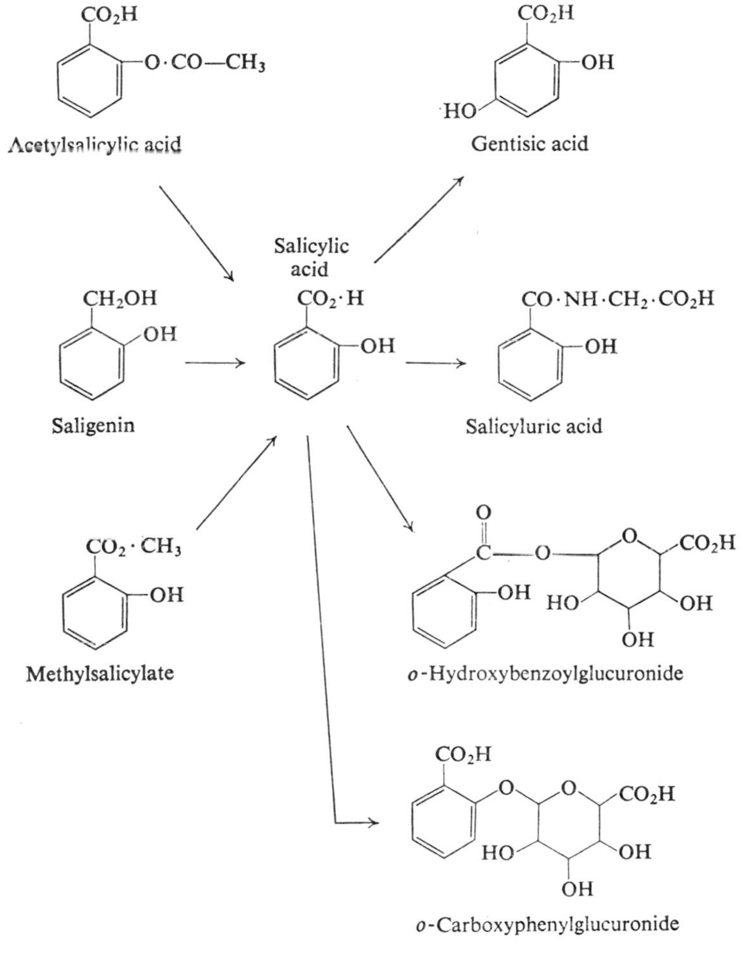

FIG. 24.6. Metabolism of salicylates.

through the thalamus. There is also evidence that part of the action of salicylates is peripheral, and pain caused by locally produced or injected bradykinin is selectively blocked by acetylsalicylic acid and related drugs. Salicylates do not affect the receptors of sensory nerves subserving sensations other than pain (such as touch or pressure). Salicylates are effective in the treatment of headache, muscle pain and rheumatic pain but are not effective against pain arising from viscera or against severe traumatic pain. The writhing response produced in rats or mice by the intraperitoneal injection of dilute acetic acid is inhibited by the antipyretic-analgesic drugs, but this test is non-specific as many compounds without analgesic action in man also prevent the response. The inflammatory response produced in a rat's paw by an injection of formalin or brewer's yeast is reduced by salicylates, and some of the effects in rheumatoid conditions may be due to local effects on capillary permeability.

ANTIPYRETIC ACTION OF SALICYLATES. The effect for which the salicylates were first used was to lower the body temperature in fever; they have no effect unless the body temperature is raised. In fever, the hypothalamic temperature-controlling mechanism is set at at higher level than that at which the body temperature is usually maintained, and the antipyretic-analgesics in general reset the central mechanism at a lower level. Sweating is the most obvious feature of the heat loss produced by salicylates, but a fall in temperature still occurs even when the sweat glands are inhibited by atropine. The loss of heat under these conditions is produced by peripheral vasodilatation.

SIDE-EFFECTS OF SALICYLATE TREATMENT. Oral administration of salicylates especially over long periods of time (e.g. in the treatment of arthritis) may lead to gastric irritation. Patients receiving long-term salicylate therapy may lose a few millilitres of blood from the gastro-intestinal tract each day. Usually the amount lost is small and the patient suffers no ill-effects. However, haematemesis (blood vomiting) sometimes occurs. The use of soluble and buffered preparations of aspirin reduces the incidence of gastric irritation. Allergic reactions to salicylates are rare and disappear when the drug is withdrawn.

The salicylates are antagonists of vitamin K, and large doses may lead to prolongation of the prothrombin time; the salicylates therefore should not be given to patients receiving anticoagulant therapy. In toxic doses, salicylates produce hyperpnoea through a central stimulant action and sodium salicylate in the dose range used in rheumatic fever may cause hyperventilation. Overdoses produce central stimulation and convulsions, and finally death.

Salicylamide (2-hydroxybenzamide)

$$\text{CO·NH}_2$$

OH

This drug is equipotent with aspirin as a mild analgesic. It causes slightly less gastric disturbance and does not affect the prothrombin time. Toxic doses cause central nervous and respiratory depression.

Cinchophen (2-phenylquinoline-4-carboxylic acid).

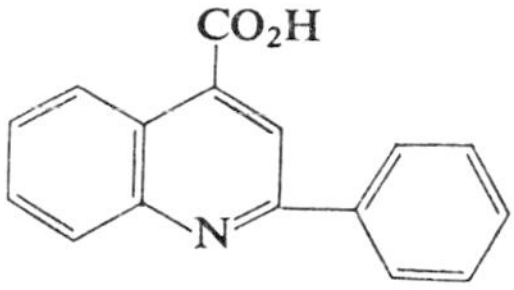

$$CO_2H$$

Cinchophen is similar in its analgesic and antipyretic effects to the salicylates, but it is too toxic for long term administration as it produces severe and often fatal liver damage. Other less toxic derivatives have been used (e.g. neocinchophen and hydroxyphenyl cinchoninic acid) but they have no advantage over the salicylates.

PARA-AMINOPHENOL DERIVATIVES. Para-aminophenol and its more important derivatives differ from the salicylates in being effective analgesics

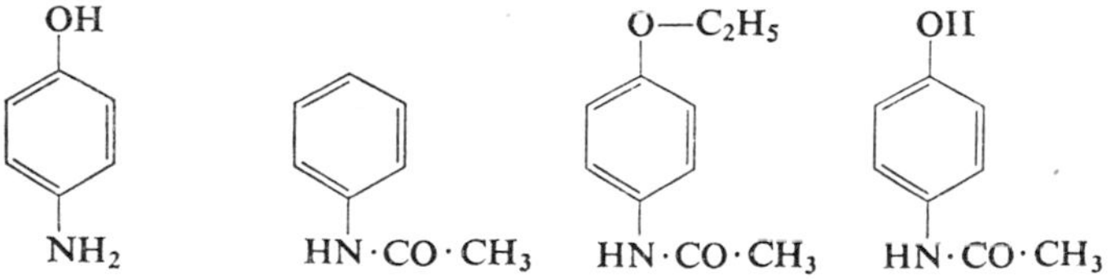

OH		$O-C_2H_5$	OH
NH_2	$HN \cdot CO \cdot CH_3$	$HN \cdot CO \cdot CH_3$	$HN \cdot CO \cdot CH_3$
p-Aminophenol	Acetanilide	Phenacetin	Paracetamol

and antipyretics with little or no effect on the 'collagen diseases', e.g. rheumatism, arthritis and rheumatic fever. Acetanilide (antifebrin), introduced in 1886, was found to be effective but toxic and this provoked a search for less toxic compounds. Para-aminophenol itself was also tried but this was also too toxic for use. Phenacetin (acetophenetidine) later became the drug of choice in this group, but toxic effects on the liver and kidney have been reported recently, especially arising when mixtures of phenacetin and aspirin are used.

Toxicity. Both acetanilide and phenacetin produce cyanosis, due to the formation of methaemoglobinaemia. This is brought about by metabolites of the drugs (Fig. 19.7, page 516). Very severe anaemia and kidney damage may ensue. The latter effect is caused by blockage of the renal tubules by cell fragments and is particularly common with acetanilide.

Absorption and metabolism. Both phenacetin and acetanilide are rapidly absorbed from the gastro-intestinal tract. Acetanilide is rapidly metabolized, particularly in the liver, to form a small amount of aniline, and this in turn is converted to phenylhydroxylamine which is responsible for the production of methaemoglobin. The bulk of the acetanilide, however, is metabolized to N-acetyl-*p*-aminophenol (paracetamol), which is analgesic in man and does not cause methaemoglobinaemia as it is not metabolized to phenylhydroxylamine. A small proportion of phenacetin is converted to *p*-phenetidin which in turn is converted to a hydroxylamine derivative which promotes methaemoglobin formation, but the bulk of the phenacetin is metabolized into paracetamol. The analgesic action of both acetanilide and phenacetin has been attributed to their conversion to paracetamol, and as this is far less toxic it is sometimes used to replace phenacetin. However, there is some contention over the correctness of this hypothesis.

Pyrazolone derivatives. Phenazone (antipyrine) and its close relative aminopyrine (amidopyrine, pyramidon) were introduced into medicine in the last century as antipyretics.

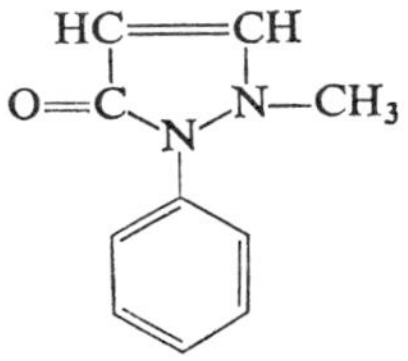

Phenazone 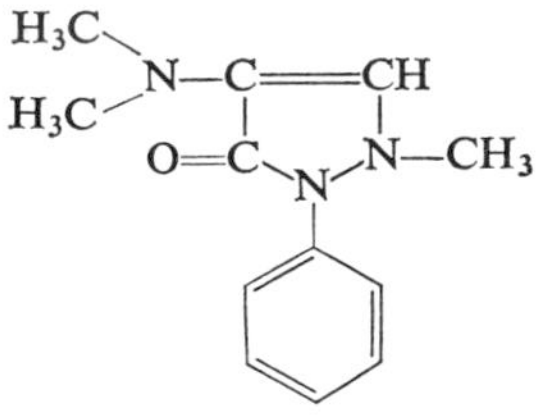   Amidopyrine

They are also analgesics with modes of action similar to those of salicylates. Although they do not cause methaemoglobinaemia, they are too toxic to justify their use. Their toxicity mainly lies in their ability to produce agranulocytosis. Skin rashes which persist for months after withdrawal of the drugs may also occur.

Phenylbutazone (Butazolidin).

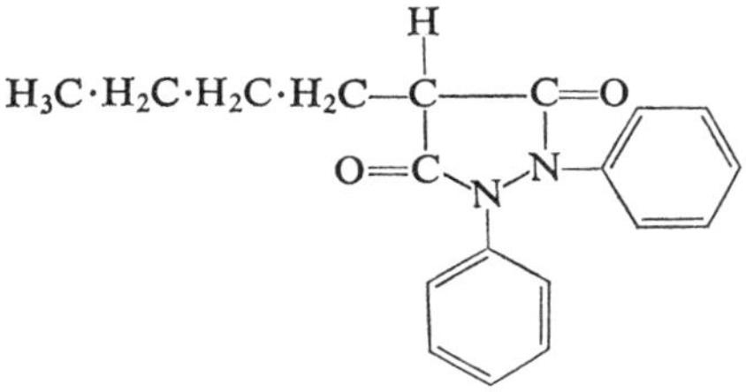

Phenylbutazone was first synthesized in 1946 and introduced into medicine in a mixture called 'Irgapyrin'. This contained 15% of amidopyrine and 15% of phenylbutazone in water. It was later shown that the clinical potency of the

mixture was due at least in part to the phenylbutazone although this had been included only as a solvent for the amidopyrine. This mixture is no longer used.

Phenylbutazone is an antipyretic-analgesic of particular value in chronic painful conditions, e.g. arthritis. It has been used in rheumatic fever, gout, osteoarthritis, ankylosing spondylitis and superficial thrombophlebitis. It was at one time thought that the drug exerted its action in a similar manner to that of ACTH or cortisone. However, it has no effect on ketosteroid excretion, eosinophil count, and erythrocyte sedimentation rate, and it does not deplete the adrenal ascorbic acid content in the rat. Its analgesic action resembles that of the salicylates. It is slow in onset and so is unsuitable for the treatment of pain of relatively short duration, e.g. headaches. Its antipyretic activity is also similar to that of the salicylates.

Phenylbutazone possesses some anti-inflammatory action which is shown by its effects in delaying the erythema produced by ultra-violet light and in reducing the oedema in rats' paws after injections of egg-white or formalin. It prolongs the actions of many drugs in the body, probably by retarding their elimination. This effect, for example, is present when phenylbutazone is given with morphine or pethidine. After a single dose of phenylbutazone, the majority is bound to the plasma protein. The rate of metabolism in man is slow, only about 10 to 20% disappearing in 24 h. Several metabolites are excreted in the urine and some are active analgesics.

Phenylbutazone has many toxic side-effects which make it a difficult drug to use clinically. It causes fluid retention which may be controlled by reduction of sodium intake in the diet and by administering a diuretic. It often causes skin rashes which usually disappear when the drug is withdrawn, but occasionally a severe generalized skin reaction occurs that may persist after discontinuing the drug. It may cause gastrointestinal irritation of sufficient severity to cause ulceration. All the above effects may become serious but perhaps the most serious is the production of blood dyscrasias. These take the form of depression of the white cells. Although usually reversible when the drug has been withdrawn, there have been several fatalities.

Chlormethoxezin (valtorin).

This drug is equipotent with aspirin as an analgesic in man but is slightly more effective than aspirin and has a longer duration of action in animals. It has some anti-inflammatory action, reducing the inflammation produced in the rats' paw by formalin, dextran or egg-white. It is metabolized in the body to

21*

gentisates and to other as yet unidentified metabolites. It is possible that the gentisates are responsible for the analgesic actions. It is effective in the treatment of pain of short duration and of pain associated with muscle spasm.

Colchicine.

This drug has been used in the treatment of gout. It does not relieve the pain of any other condition so it is not really an analgesic. It stops mitosis in metaphase but this does not seem to be responsible for its potent action in the acute phase of gout. Its mode of action is unknown.

CHAPTER 25

Local Anaesthetics

Local anaesthetics are drugs which produce a *reversible* blockade of conduction in nerves. They are applied locally to produce a loss of sensation or of motor power in a particular area of the body. Conduction in all types of axons is blocked by local anaesthetics, but in general small diameter fibres are more susceptible to their action, and are slower to recover, than are large diameter fibres. However, fibre size is not the only factor determining the sensitivity of neurones to local anaesthetics, since conduction in small diameter myelinated fibres (for example, fibres of the A delta group, page 71) is blocked before conduction in some non-myelinated C fibres, even though the C fibres have the smaller diameter.

If a local anaesthetic is applied to a nerve trunk, the sensory functions of the nerve are blocked in a definite order. The sensation of pain is the first to disappear and this is followed in turn by disappearance of the sensations of cold, warmth, touch and deep pressure. This order of susceptibility of the various sense modalities may be because pain sensation is conveyed by the smallest diameter fibres, deep pressure by the largest, and temperature and touch by fibres of intermediate size. Conduction in nerve trunks may also be blocked by the application of pressure and here the largest diameter fibres are the first affected, so that the order in which the different sensations are lost is the reverse of that produced by local anaesthetics. When a local anaesthetic is applied to the trunk of a nerve supplying a skeletal muscle, reflex contractions of the muscle elicited by stretching its tendon (the stretch reflex, page 114) are blocked by concentrations of the drug smaller than those necessary to block contractions elicited by electrical stimulation of its motor nerve fibres. Sensory afferent fibres originating in the muscle are no more sensitive to local anaesthetics than are motor efferent fibres, both being large myelinated fibres of the A group, but the small motor fibres (the γ-efferents) which innervate the muscle spindles and upon which the stretch reflex depends (page 107) are more sensitive, and this fact accounts for the selective abolition of the reflex contractions.

The action of local anaesthetics is not exerted specifically on sensory terminals and afferent and efferent axons of the peripheral nervous system; conduction in all types of excitable membrane is depressed by them. Thus, transmission at synapses and neuro-effector junctions is blocked as a result of actions both on the nerve endings and on the post-junctional membranes, and excitation of all types of muscle fibre is depressed. However, different tissues exhibit different sensitivities and again the size of the cells concerned is one of the factors determining this. For example, conduction in small nerve endings is blocked more readily than conduction in the membranes of large muscle fibres.

The chief methods by which local anaesthesia may be produced are shown in Table 25.1. In *surface* anaesthesia, the local anaesthetic is applied directly to the mucous membrane which is to be anaesthetized. Local anaesthetics which penetrate such surfaces are applied to relieve pain or to allow observation of an injured or damaged surface. In *infiltration* anaesthesia, the local anaesthetic is injected in and around the area in which the effect is desired; this method of local anaesthesia is used for minor operations on the skin and in dentistry. In *block* anaesthesia, the local anaesthetic is injected near to the peripheral nerve trunk. Transmission of impulses in the sensory nerve fibres originating in the operative area is then interrupted, and, as transmission in motor fibres is also blocked, muscle relaxation results. Operations on limbs are made possible by using block anaesthesia. In *spinal* anaesthesia, the local anaesthetic is injected into the subarachnoid space so that it reaches the roots of the spinal nerves

TABLE 25.1. Methods of producing local anaesthesia.

Method of local anaesthesia	Tissue affected	Type of preparation used	Examples of drugs used	Therapeutic use
1. Topical or surface	Sensory nerve endings of mucous membranes such as in the nose or the eyes, and of dermis	Solution, ointment, cream, powder	Cocaine, Benzocaine, Amethocaine, Cinchocaine	Relief of pain or itching. Examination of conjunctiva
2. Infiltration	Sensory nerve endings in sub-cutaneous tissues or in the dermis	Injection	Procaine, Lignocaine	Minor operations such as the removal of cysts or teeth
3. Block	Nerve trunk	Injection	Procaine, Amethocaine, Cocaine, Lignocaine	Dental operations and operations on limbs. Muscle relaxation
4. Spinal	Spinal roots (via cerebrospinal fluid)	Injection	Cinchocaine, Amylocaine, Lignocaine	Abdominal operations. Muscle relaxation

supplying the site of the operation. The patient remains conscious although anaesthesia may be extended as high as the chin. This method of local anaesthesia is often used for operations upon the pelvic viscera.

When absorbed systemically in sufficient concentration, local anaesthetics first stimulate and then depress the CNS. The stimulant action, which probably arises from conduction block in inhibitory neurones, is evidenced by restlessness, tremor and sometimes clonic convulsions; these may be prevented and treated by hypnotic drugs such as the barbiturates. The secondary depressant action results in deep hypnosis, coma and respiratory arrest. Analeptic drugs (pp. 626–628) are ineffective in antagonizing the respiratory depression and artificial respiration must be applied.

Determination of local anaesthetic potency. The evaluation of local anaesthetics requires not only determination of their local anaesthetic potency but also elucidation of their systemic and local toxicity. The simpler animal tests for local anaesthetic potency include inhibition of the corneal reflex in rabbits, production of local anaesthesia in guinea-pig skin, and production of plexus anaesthesia or nerve block in frogs.

In rabbits, the drug under test is applied to one conjunctival sac and the corneal reflex is tested at intervals until it is first abolished and then recovered; it is a common practice to compare potency with that of cocaine which is applied to the other conjunctival sac, and calculations are made after carrying out cross-over tests. In guinea-pigs, the comparison is made after intradermal injection of the compound being tested, local anaesthesia being determined when the animal no longer squeaks on application of a mechanical stimulus to the injected area. In frogs, the hindquarters of pithed animals are dipped into an acid solution which stimulates the sensory nerves and so produces a flexor or withdrawal reflex. The drug under test is then applied to the ventral lymph sac, local anaesthesia being judged from the abolition of the flexor reflex.

A number of new methods or variants of these earlier methods have been reported during the last few years. For example, local anaesthetics have been shown to prevent the passage of impulses in afferent fibres of the vagus nerve from the lungs of anaesthetized guinea-pigs when these nerves have been stimulated by veratrine. Blockade of conduction in sensory nerves may be directly studied by recording action potentials. Tests in man have included abolition by local anaesthetics of the pain produced when a mechanical stimulus is applied to the skin and the production by local anaesthetics of bilateral ulnar block. Some workers prefer to use abolition of the pain produced by electrical stimulation of dental pulp. This method is probably the most useful one available for experimental evaluation of local anaesthetics in man.

The evolution of local anaesthetics began with the isolation of cocaine from coca leaves in 1865. The alkaloid was soon accepted as a potent and valuable drug although its toxic effects and addictive properties prompted an intensive search for substitutes. Forty years later, the first potent and safer synthetic agent—procaine—was introduced into medicine. This drug, with its relatively low toxicity and its blandness for the tissues, soon dominated most fields of local anaesthesia and, although a large number of active synthetic agents were prepared and tested in the next 40 years, none of them seriously threatened the supremacy of procaine. The introduction of lignocaine in 1948, a compound with a higher therapeutic index than that of procaine, has resulted in its widespread use in recent years.

CHEMICAL CONSIDERATIONS. The structure of a local anaesthetic may be briefly summarized as consisting of a lipophilic centre, an intermediate chain, and a hydrophilic centre. The lipophilic centre generally consists of an aromatic or heterocyclic nucleus, although it may be an aralkyl or an alkyl group. The hydrophilic centre in nearly all local anaesthetics in clinical use is a secondary or tertiary amino group; an alkoxy or a hydroxy group replaces the amino group only in a few compounds with local anaesthetic action. The intermediate chain between the lipophilic and hydrophilic centres consists of a hydrocarbon bridge or a group of atoms such as —CO.O—, —CO.NH—, or —CO— (see Fig. 25.1). Compounds which have a centre with too great a

Type 1. Aminoalkylesters, e.g. cocaine, procaine.

R—CO.O—alk—N<

Type 2. Esters of aminobenzoic acid, e.g. benzocaine.

>N—R—CO.O—alk

Type 3. Aminoalkylketones, e.g. falicaine.

R—CO—alk—N<

Type 4. Aminoacylamides, e.g. lignocaine.

R—NH—CO—alk—N<

Type 5. Aminoalkylamides, e.g. cinchocaine.

R—CO—NH—alk—N<

FIG. 25.1. Five types of local anaesthetics.

hydrophilic activity are not effective as local anaesthetics, and those with a centre having too great a lipophilic activity are not readily soluble in water. The balance within the molecule of these two portions is probably the key factor in determining the behaviour of the molecule on cell membranes. Many of the local anaesthetics used clinically differ from cocaine only in so far as the ester linkage (—CO.O—) in the intermediate chain between the lipophilic aromatic nucleus and the hydrophilic amino group has been exchanged for other linkages.

Mechanism of action of local anaesthetics. Local anaesthetics are believed to block conduction by inhibiting the transient increase in the permeability of excitable membranes to sodium ions, a process which is necessary for the generation and propagation of an action potential. Conduction block produced by cocaine in isolated nerve is abolished by raising the extracellular sodium concentration. Local anaesthetics also reduce the permeability of the resting membrane to potassium and other ions. Since all ions are affected, there is little change produced in the resting membrane potential, and abrupt changes in potential are prevented (i.e. local anaesthetics act as membrane stabilizers, page 88).

The relative local anaesthetic potency of a series of compounds has been found to match their relative potency in increasing the surface pressure of monomolecular films of lipids, and it has been suggested that the drugs reduce membrane permeability by increasing the surface pressure of the lipid layer of the membrane (see page 40).

Another theory concerning the mode of action of local anaesthetics depends on Nachmansohn's hypothesis that acetylcholine is involved in axonal conduction (see page 173). The molecules of many local anaesthetics bear some structural resemblance to that of acetylcholine and are capable of antagonizing its stimulant action on various peripheral tissues. This led Nachmansohn to suggest that local anaesthetic drugs block conduction by antagonizing the action of acetylcholine within the membrane. However, there is a lack of correlation between the local anaesthetic potency and the antiacetylcholine activity of numerous compounds of different types, and the hypothesis lacks rigorous proof.

Local anaesthetics are usually available in the form of their stable water-soluble salts, but the free undissociated base must be liberated in the body for the drug to penetrate to its site of action and produce a local anaesthetic effect. Most local anaesthetics are secondary or tertiary amines and therefore the non-ionized amine and the positively charged cation coexist, the ratio depending on the pK_a of the compound and the pH of the body fluid. Most evidence indicates that the cation is the active form.

COCAINE. Cocaine is an alkaloid derived from leaves of the coca plant, *Erythroxylon coca*, which grows in Peru, Chile and Bolivia. The natives in these countries chew the leaves to lessen their hunger (possibly by a central anorexigenic action) and increase their endurance (through its stimulant action on the central nervous system). Chemically, it is benzoyl methylecgonine a near relative of atropine. Like most other alkaloids, it is soluble in acids but not in alkalis. It is readily absorbed from mucous membranes but not through undamaged skin.

Cocaine blocks conduction along nerves but it is no longer extensively used as a local anaesthetic for general purposes as it is too toxic and patients often show an idiosyncrasy to it. Its chief use is to anaesthetize mucous membranes. For example, anaesthesia of the cornea of the eye is achieved with a 0·25% (w/v) solution. Cocaine applied to the conjunctiva causes dilatation of the pupil and constriction of the conjunctival blood vessels (page 896). The formation of conjunctival fluid is impaired and, in some cases, this may lead to ulceration of the cornea. The heart rate is first slowed by cocaine and then increased, and the body temperature rises. Cocaine sensitizes tissues to the actions of noradrenaline and adrenaline and to the effects of stimulation of adrenergic nerves and this accounts for its sympathomimetic effects (see page 774).

On the central nervous system, cocaine produces stimulation of the highest centres which spreads after large doses to the spinal cord. Thus, there is at first restlessness and excitement, with an increased capacity for work, and later convulsions. The stimulation is followed by depression.

Cocaine is a drug of addiction. The cocaine addict differs from the morphine addict in being more extroverted. However, after prolonged use, those addicted to cocaine become moody, experience hallucinations, and often imagine they are being pursued. Treatment of cocaine addiction depends largely on psychotherapy; recently barbiturates have been used to produce sedation which helps to break the addiction.

PROCAINE (Novocaine). Procaine has been in use for about 60 years and is still widely used. It is preferred to cocaine for injections as it is more stable and less toxic. It is poorly absorbed from mucous surfaces and therefore is not used for surface anaesthesia. Infiltration anaesthesia (using a 0·2 per cent solution) and nerve block anaesthesia (using a 2 per cent solution) are prolonged by including adrenaline in the solution of procaine. The vasoconstrictor action of adrenaline (in a strength of about 1 in 100,000) keeps the procaine localized longer and so prolongs the local anaesthetic action.

Procaine (for formula, see Fig. 25.2) is rapidly metabolized in the liver and plasma to para-aminobenzoic acid and diethylamino-ethanol. The toxic side-effects of procaine are rarely seen; they include cardiovascular collapse and stimulation of the central nervous system. The effects on the CNS can usually be controlled by the injection of a barbiturate such as sodium thiopentone. Sensitization of the heart by cyclopropane to the arrhythmic action of adrenaline is antagonized by procaine, but this effect is brief and stimulation of the central nervous system may also result; it is safer to use procainamide (page 819) for suppressing cardiac arrythmias. Procainamide has a longer duration of action and does not stimulate the CNS.

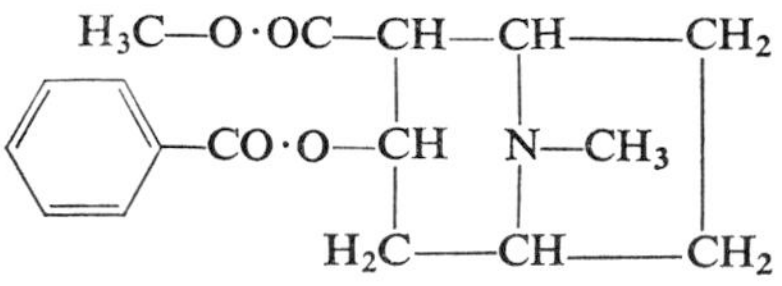

H_3C—O·OC—CH—CH——CH_2
| | | |
〈benzene〉—CO·O—CH   N—CH_3 |
| | |
H_2C——CH——CH_2

Cocaine

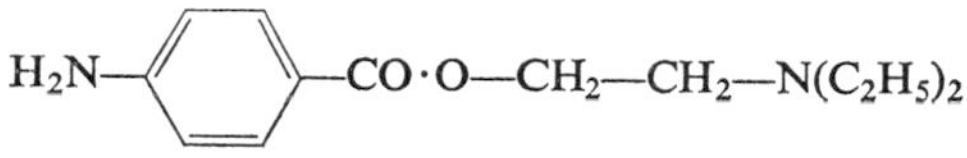

H_2N—〈benzene〉—CO·O—CH_2—CH_2—N(C_2H_5)_2

Procaine

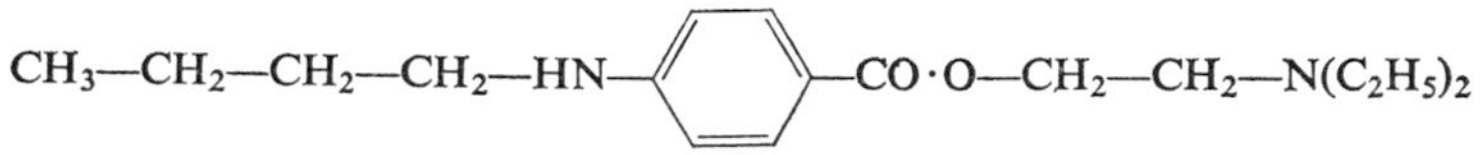

CH_3—CH_2—CH_2—CH_2—HN—〈benzene〉—CO·O—CH_2—CH_2—N(C_2H_5)_2

Amethocaine

H_2N—〈benzene〉—CO·O—CH_2—CH_2—CH_2—N(CH_2—CH_2—CH_2—CH_3)_2

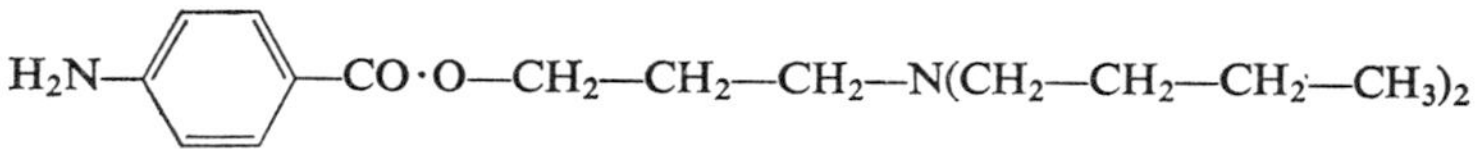

Butacaine

FIG. 25.2. Formulae of local anaesthetics containing an ester group.

AMETHOCAINE (Pontocaine, Tetracaine). This compound (see Fig. 25.2) is closely related chemically to procaine and is about 10 times more potent. It is well absorbed from mucous surfaces and has been particularly valuable as a spray for nose and throat anaesthesia. It may cause skin reactions.

BUTACAINE (Butyn). This compound (see Fig. 25.2) penetrates mucous membranes and is commonly used as a topical anaesthetic, especially for the eye. Its action is rapid in onset and of long duration. It has largely replaced cocaine for use in ophthalmic surgery, as it lacks the undesirable mydriatic and vaso-constrictor actions of cocaine.

BENZOCAINE. This compound is very insoluble in water and is only slowly absorbed by the tissues. It is used as a dusting powder for a painful mucous

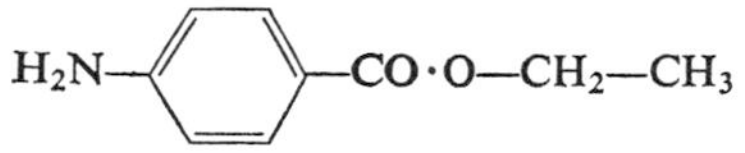

H_2N—〈benzene〉—CO·O—CH_2—CH_3

surface or open wound or it may be incorporated into suppositories, ointments or lozenges. Benzocaine is non-irritant and relatively free from toxicity.

FALICAINE. This compound has been used in Eastern Germany for anaesthesia and is an example of a ketone anaesthetic. It is about 10 times as active as procaine but also about 10 times as toxic. In surface anaesthesia, it is roughly equal to amethocaine in potency.

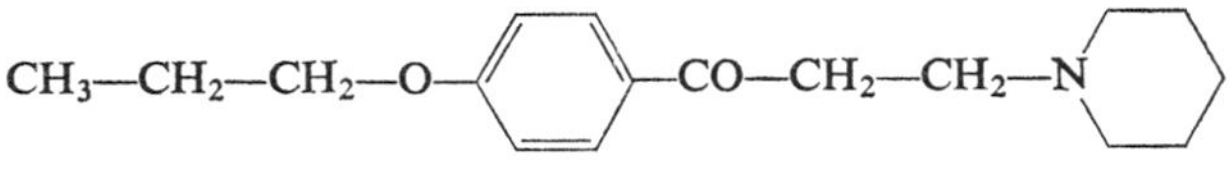

$$CH_3—CH_2—CH_2—O—\langle\text{ring}\rangle—CO—CH_2—CH_2—N\langle\text{ring}\rangle$$

LIGNOCAINE (Xylocaine). This is probably the most commonly used of the local anaesthetics; it has largely replaced procaine for infiltration anaesthesia and nerve block or spinal anaesthesia, as it is slightly more potent and less toxic. Its onset of action is more rapid and it has a longer duration. It is widely used in dental surgery. Its formula is shown in Fig. 25.3.

MESOCAINE. This is the para-methyl derivative of lignocaine (see Fig. 25.3) which was originally discovered, like lignocaine, in Sweden.

PRILOCAINE. This is a recently introduced local anaesthetic (see Fig. 25.3). It is intended for all types of local anaesthesia. It is relatively non-toxic.

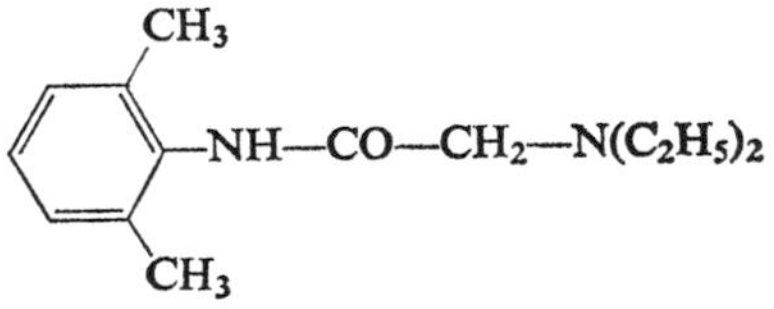

$$\text{(ring with }CH_3\text{, }CH_3)—NH—CO—CH_2—N(C_2H_5)_2$$

Lignocaine

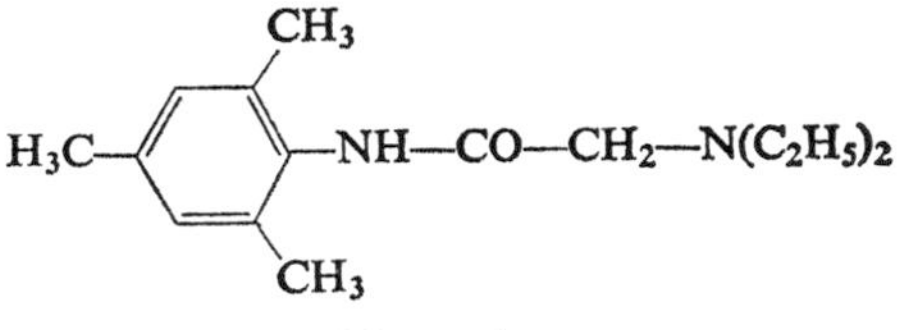

$$H_3C—\text{(ring with }CH_3\text{, }CH_3)—NH—CO—CH_2—N(C_2H_5)_2$$

Mesocaine

$$\text{(ring with }CH_3)—NH—CO—CH—N\langle\begin{array}{l}H\\CH_2—CH_2—CH_3\end{array}\qquad(\text{with }CH_3\text{ on }CH)$$

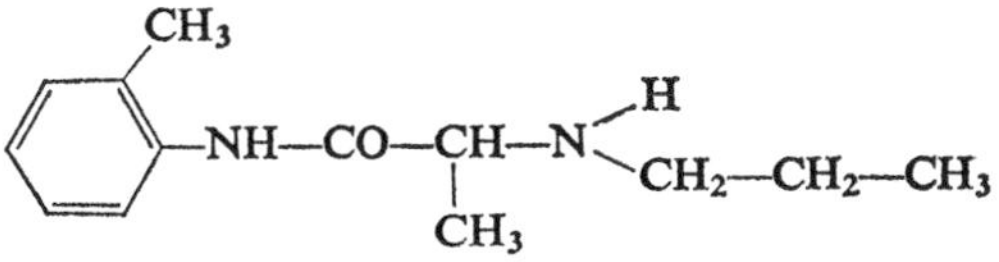

Prilocaine

FIG. 25.3. Formulae of local anaesthetics containing an amide group.

CINCHOCAINE (Nupercaine). Cinchocaine is the most potent of the local anaesthetics in general use, being 8 to 10 times as potent as cocaine; it is however about 10 times as toxic. It can be used for all types of local anaesthetic procedures but onset of action is slow. Toxic side-reactions are uncommon. Cinchocaine is especially useful as a topical anaesthetic for the ear, nose and throat.

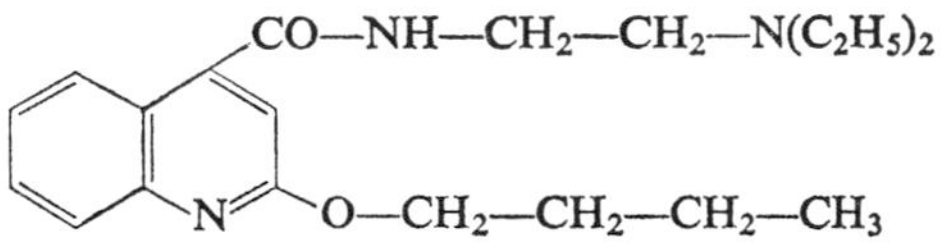

$$CO\text{---}NH\text{---}CH_2\text{---}CH_2\text{---}N(C_2H_5)_2$$

$$O\text{---}CH_2\text{---}CH_2\text{---}CH_2\text{---}CH_3$$

CHAPTER 26

Drugs Modifying Neuromuscular Transmission

The processes of neuromuscular transmission, described in Chapter 7, may be interrupted or facilitated by drugs. The term 'neuromuscular', although logically applicable to all nerve-muscle junctions, is generally restricted to that junction between a somatic motor nerve and striated muscle; it is in this sense that it is used here.

Neuromuscular Block

Compounds described as neuromuscular-blocking agents interrupt neuro-muscular transmission but do not affect conduction of the nerve impulse along the motor axons, nor modify the contractile power of the muscle itself as judged by its response to direct electrical stimulation. Tubocurarine is a typical neuromuscular-blocking drug as shown by the experiments illustrated in Fig. 26.1 which demonstrate that its site of action is located at the neuromuscular junction.

Neuromuscular-blocking drugs may be broadly classified into those which act prejunctionally on the fine non-myelinated nerve endings and those which act postjunctionally on the motor endplates.

Pre-junctional block. Drugs may act on the motor nerve endings to block transmission by reducing the amount of acetylcholine released by nerve impulses. As soon as the quantity of acetylcholine released falls below that required to produce the critical degree of endplate potential necessary to initiate the muscle fibre action potential, the muscle fibre fails to contract. If a drug acts entirely prejunctionally, the response of the muscle to injected acetylcholine is unaltered and in this way such drugs may be distinguished from those which act on the motor endplates.

There are two general mechanisms whereby drugs acting prejunctionally may reduce acetylcholine output from the nerve endings: these are (1) depression of synthesis of acetylcholine and (2) prevention of its release.

(1) DEPRESSED SYNTHESIS. The important factors necessary for the synthesis of acetylcholine were briefly described on pages 152–153 and a lack of any of these components decreases the ability of the nerve to manufacture its trans-mitter. During nerve activity, the loss of acetylcholine by release from the nerve

endings is balanced by a corresponding increase in its synthesis. There is good evidence that sodium ions within the nerve endings are necessary for

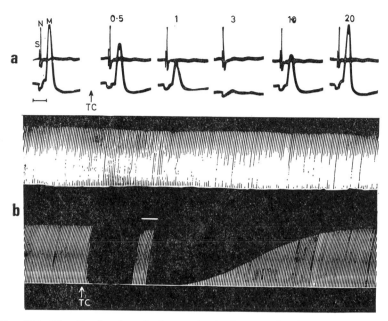

FIG. 26.1. The site of action of tubocurarine in the cat under chloralose anaesthesia.

a. Action potentials recorded from the motor nerve (N) and from the tibialis anterior muscle (M) in response to nerve stimulation every 10 sec; S denotes the stimulus artifact. At TC, 0·5mg/kg of tubocurarine was injected intravenously. The numbers denote the time in minutes after injection of tubocurarine. Time calibration, 10 msec. Tubocurarine abolished the muscle action potentials but was without effect on the nerve action potentials showing that it does not affect nerve conduction. **b.** Twitches of a chronically denervated tibialis anterior muscle in response to direct electrical stimulation every 10 sec (upper record) and of the contralateral innervated muscle in response to motor nerve stimulation at the same frequency (lower record). At TC, 0·5 mg/kg of tubocurarine was injected intravenously. The twitches evoked by nerve stimulation were blocked but those elicited by direct stimulation were unaffected. During the period marked by the horizontal bar, the muscle was stimulated directly. The results in **a** and **b** show that tubocurarine does not affect conduction in the nerve or the response of the muscle to direct stimulation, and its action must therefore be located at the junction between the two. (From W. C. Bowman; Chapter 16 in 'Evaluation of Drug Activities: Pharmacometrics'. Ed. by D. R. Laurence and A. L. Bacharach, Vol. 1 Academic Press 1964.)

the synthesis of acetylcholine and they may provide the link which gears synthesis to release by the following mechanism. Sodium enters the axoplasm during the rising phase of the action potential (page 77); therefore, the greater the frequency of nerve impulses, the higher is the intracellular concentration of sodium ions. Deficiency of sodium ions causes transmission failure as soon as the preformed transmitter is exhausted. Action potentials cannot be conducted in the absence of sodium ions, and in experiments in which the effects of sodium deficiency are studied, acetylcholine release from the nerve endings cannot be induced by electrical stimulation; some other procedure, such as the addition of excess potassium chloride, must therefore be used. The action of sodium ions on synthesis may be to control the membrane transport of metabolic substrates such as glucose and choline.

Excess sodium ions accumulate within the nerve endings when the sodium pump (pages 74 and 811) is inhibited. This may be achieved by reducing the extracellular potassium concentration or by adding high concentrations of the cardiac glycosides, *digoxin* or *ouabain* (page 811), to the perfusion fluid. The increased intracellular sodium level stimulates acetylcholine synthesis and there is an increase in the spontaneous release of transmitter giving rise to irregular muscular twitchings. At the same time, the transmission of nerve impulses across the junction is blocked, probably because the reduced concentration gradient of sodium ions across the membrane of the nerve endings extinguishes the nerve action potential.

Prevention of acetylcholine synthesis by inhibition of *choline acetyltransferase* is a theoretically possible way of producing pre-junctional block. No compound is yet known which, after systemic administration, specifically and directly inhibits this enzyme. However, a series of compounds synthesized by Long and Schueler in 1954 have been shown to inhibit choline acetyltransferase by an indirect mechanism. The molecules of these compounds contain two choline-like moieties and spectroscopic evidence shows that they undergo hemi-acetal formation in solution. Schueler coined the name *hemicholiniums* to denote them; the formula of the most active member of the series, known as *hemicholinium No. 3* or *HC-3*, is given on page 153. Experiments on perfused sympathetic ganglia, skeletal muscles and homogenates of brain tissue have shown that HC-3 depresses acetylcholine synthesis, not by inhibiting choline acetyltransferase directly, but by preventing the access of choline to the enzyme. HC-3 is believed to compete with choline for a transport mechanism in the membranes of the nerve endings and of the subcellular particles enclosing the enzyme. It therefore blocks the transport of choline to the sites of its acetylation and the nerve endings become deficient in acetylcholine. The neuromuscular transmission failure produced by HC-3 is slow in onset and occurs only when the frequency of nerve impulses is high, since the preformed acetylcholine stored in the nerve endings must first be used up. The effects of HC-3 on cholinergic transmission are reversed by choline.

Some simple analogues of choline (particularly the triethyl analogue, $(CH_3CH_2)_3N^+CH_2CH_2OH$) produce a failure of neuromuscular transmission which is similar to that produced by HC-3, and recent experiments indicate that many other quaternary ammonium compounds may also exert this effect. With large doses of HC-3 and of triethylcholine neuromuscular block is also partly due to a post-junctional action on the motor endplates.

Drugs of the HC-3 type provide useful tools in animal experiments for investigating cholinergic mechanisms and may in the future find a use in the symptomatic treatment of some forms of muscle spasticity in man in which a high rate of nerve discharge is responsible for maintaining the spasms (e.g. tetanus); such a drug may produce transmission failure and a selective relaxation of the affected muscles.

(2) PREVENTION OF RELEASE. The dependence of acetylcholine release on the extracellular *calcium* and *magnesium* ion concentrations was referred to on page 155. Lack of calcium or excess of magnesium produces neuromuscular transmission failure by preventing the release of acetylcholine from the nerve endings in response to nerve impulses; the frequency of the spontaneously occurring miniature endplate potentials is also depressed. Excess phosphate inhibits acetylcholine release by reducing the amount of ionized calcium. When endplate potentials are recorded with fine intracellular electrodes from single muscle cells, the ionic composition of the bathing solution is often deliberately adjusted so that the amount of acetylcholine released on stimulating the nerve produces endplate potentials which are too small to initiate propagating action potentials in the muscle fibre membrane. Muscle contraction, which might break or dislodge the microelectrode, therefore does not occur and the endplate potentials may be studied without the complications of action potentials. Sodium ions, in addition to their role in the generation of the action potential and in acetylcholine synthesis, are also important in the mechanism of acetylcholine release. Possibly the increased concentration of sodium ions along the inside of the membrane during the rising phase of the action potential acts, together with the altered membrane potential itself, to displace calcium ions from the membrane. The freed calcium ions then trigger the release mechanism.

High dosage of the antibiotics, neomycin, streptomycin and kanamycin produce a neuromuscular block which is similar to that produced by calcium-lack and which may be the result of depression of acetylcholine release. This effect of the antibiotics may be an important unwanted action in patients in whom neuromuscular transmission is already depressed, either by other drugs or by disease.

Harvey first showed in 1939 that the intra-arterial injection of the local anaesthetic, *procaine*, decreases the amount of acetylcholine released from the motor nerve, and other local anaesthetics have a similar action. These drugs prevent conduction along the axons although their action after systemic administration is probably first exerted on the non-myelinated nerve endings. There, they may act by stabilizing the membrane of the nerve endings so that the nerve impulse is abolished before it produces transmitter release. The action of procaine, however, is not only on the nerve endings; it also acts on the motor endplates, depressing their sensitivity to acetylcholine. This motor endplate blocking action of procaine is due partly to stabilization of the post-junctional membrane and partly to block of acetylcholine receptors; the structure of the procaine molecule (page 657) bears some similarity to that of acetyl-choline. The neuromuscular-blocking action of procaine has little clinical importance except in three circumstances where it should be administered with caution: firstly, in patients with myasthenia gravis who are extra-sensitive to any procedure which reduces acetylcholine release or which antagonizes the action of acetylcholine; secondly, in patients with low plasma esterase activity, as procaine is destroyed by an enzyme which is probably the pseudocholinesterase of plasma; and thirdly, in patients receiving suxamethonium during a surgical operation (see page 672) because suxamethonium is also destroyed by the pseudocholinesterase of plasma and the combination of procaine with this enzyme reduces its ability to hydrolyse other substrates.

The effects of the toxin of the organism *Clostridium botulinum* are due to a selective blocking action on the mechanism of release of acetylcholine from cholinergic nerves. Electron microscope studies with ferritin-tagged toxin suggest that the toxin molecules may mechanically obstruct the site of release of acetylcholine from the nerve endings. Unlike the majority of bacterial toxins, botulinum toxin is active when administered by mouth. It is extremely potent; as little as one microgram of toxin from some strains of *C. botulinum* is lethal in man. Most research with the toxin is carried out in chemical warfare laboratories.

Motor endplate (post-junctional) block. The main use of neuromuscular-blocking agents is to produce adequate muscle relaxation during surgical anaesthesia (see page 576). Those in current use produce motor endplate block and are believed to act by combining reversibly with the receptors to which acetylcholine becomes attached. Some of these drugs are *agonists* and, like acetylcholine itself, depolarize the motor endplates; some are *antagonists*, in which case their combination with the receptors does not result in depolarization but simply prevents the reaction of acetylcholine with them, and some are *partial agonists*, producing an initial depolarization followed by receptor block. These three terms are defined in Chapter 18, and the different types of action may be explained by the theories of drug action outlined in that chapter.

In focally-innervated mammalian muscles (page 207), all three types of drug block neuromuscular transmission and produce a *flaccid* (limp) paralysis, although if a depolarizing action is present, the paralysis is preceded by a stimulant effect.

COMPETITIVE BLOCK. This type of block is produced by antagonists of acetylcholine. Drugs which appear to act in this way do not always fulfil *in vivo* the strict criteria of 'block by competition' and for this reason the less precise term 'non-depolarization block of the motor endplates' may be preferred. The blocking actions of drugs which act in this way are additive. Antagonism to competitive block may be brought about by an increase in the local concentration of agonist (acetylcholine) in the region of the motor endplates. Experimentally, an increased acetylcholine concentration may be achieved in a number of ways but, when rapid antagonism of a competitive neuromuscular blocking drug is required in a patient, it is usually achieved by the use of an anticholinesterase drug. Anticholinesterase drugs prevent the hydrolysis of the acetylcholine, and as a result the concentration builds up and it competes with the blocking drug. The most effective anticholinesterase drug used for this purpose is neostigmine (page 715) and it is an important characteristic of block by competition that it is rapidly reversed on injection of neostigmine. Transmission from the γ-efferents to the muscle spindles is cholinergic and competitive blocking drugs also block at this site.

Curare and the purified alkaloid (+)-tubocurarine chloride (Fig. 26.3) are the most widely studied substances which produce neuromuscular block by competition with acetylcholine and their action will be described here in detail. The study of the action of these substances resulted in major advances of knowledge concerning the physiological processes underlying neuromuscular transmission (see page 146).

The first examples of this are the classical experiments of Claude Bernard, published in 1851, on the site of action of curare in the frog (see page 138). Curare is a generic term for various crude extracts obtained from different plants of the species, *Strychnos* and *Chondodendron*. It was and still is used by some South American Indians to make the poison tip for blow-pipe darts. Since curare is poorly absorbed by mouth, animals poisoned by it may be eaten without ill-effect.

The most important curare alkaloid possessing neuromuscular blocking activity is (+)-tubocurarine, isolated from tube-curare by King in 1935. It is still widely used as a muscle relaxant during surgical anaesthesia. Tubocurarine prevents the response of skeletal muscle to motor nerve impulses and to applied acetylcholine (Fig. 5.4, page 146). During the paralysis, conduction in the nerve continues and the muscle fibres themselves retain their responsiveness to direct electrical stimulation (Fig. 26.1). The depolarizing action of excess potassium ions on the muscle membrane, including the endplate region, is not affected. Under the influence of tubocurarine, the endplate potentials produced by successive shocks applied to the nerve (cf. Fig. 7.3, page 196) rapidly diminish in size and the muscle fails to contract when the endplate depolarizations are insufficient to initiate propagating action potentials. At

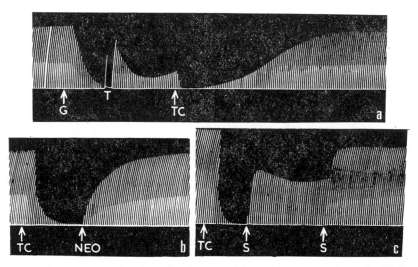

FIG. 26.2. Characteristics of non-depolarization block of the motor endplates in tibialis anterior muscles of cats under chloralose anaesthesia. Maximal twitches were elicited every 10 sec by stimulation of the motor nerves. Intravenous injections: at G, 1·5 mg/kg gallamine triethiodide; at TC in (a) 0·1 mg/kg tubocurarine; at TC in (b) and (c) 0·4 mg/kg tubocurarine; at NEO, 75 μg/kg neostigmine. At S, 2 μg suxamethonium were injected close-arterially. At T, a tetanus was elicited by stimulation of the nerve at 50/sec for 10 sec. (Source as for Fig. 26.1.)

this stage, there are insufficient receptors remaining free to combine with the acetylcholine released from the nerve. Further addition of tubocurarine completely abolishes the endplate potentials. A similar effect on endplate potentials may be produced by substances which decrease the amount of transmitter released from the motor nerve. However, Dale, Feldberg and Vogt in 1936 perfused muscles with a physiological salt solution and found that the amount of acetylcholine released into the perfusion fluid on stimulating the motor nerve was not diminished when the muscle was completely paralysed by the addition of tubocurarine.

When tubocurarine, or a similarly acting drug, is injected in an amount sufficient to cause an incomplete paralysis of maximal twitches elicited by motor nerve stimulation, the picture illustrated in Fig. 26.2 is obtained. (1) The block is not preceded by a stimulant action. (2) The blocking action summates with that of drugs with a similar type of action (e.g. gallamine, Fig. 26.2a). (3) During the block, high-frequency stimulation of the motor nerve produces a tetanus, the tension of which rapidly wanes while the stimulation continues. The tetanus is therefore not only depressed but is unsustained to the extent that its time course appears little longer than that of a twitch (Fig. 26.2a). The waning tetanus is probably due to the raised threshold of the endplates to the depolarizing action of acetylcholine, together with the fall-off in transmitter release which occurs during high frequency stimulation (page 154). (4) After the tetanus, the partially-blocked twitches are temporarily increased in tension. This post-tetanic decurarization is mainly due to an increase in the number of muscle fibres contracting; it is brought about by the increased transmitter release which occurs in response to single nerve impulses after a tetanus (pages 118 to 119, 199 to 203). (5) The block may be antagonized by any drug which depolarizes the motor endplates (such as acetylcholine, suxamethonium, or decamethonium). This effect of suxamethonium is illustrated in Fig. 26.2c. The endplate potentials produced by the acetylcholine released from the nerve then summate with the background depolarization produced by suxamethonium and in some fibres reach the threshold necessary to trigger action potentials. The dose of depolarizing drug is critical since such drugs themselves produce neuromuscular block. (6) The block may be antagonized by potassium chloride. Excess extracellular potassium ions produce depolarization by lowering the potassium ion concentration gradient across the cell membrane (pages 87 to 88); the action of potassium differs from that of the depolarizing drugs in that it is exerted on the nerve terminals and on the whole muscle fibre membrane as well as on the motor endplates. (7) The block may be antagonized by adrenaline, tetraethylammonium or guanidine. The mechanism of action of these three drugs is not fully understood but they are believed to act mainly on the nerve endings and in some way increase the amount of acetylcholine released by nerve impulses. (8) Finally, and most important from a clinical point of view, the block is antagonized by anticholinesterase drugs such as neostigmine (Fig. 26.2b). The effects of anticholinesterase drugs on skeletal muscle are described later in this chapter.

The *dimethyl ether of tubocurarine* (dimethyltubocurarine chloride or iodide), in which the two hydroxyl groups are replaced by methoxy groups, is 2 to 3 times more potent than tubocurarine but the duration of its effect is slightly less. It is also used as a muscle relaxant during surgical anaesthesia.

Of the numerous alkaloids isolated from the curares, *toxiferine I* is perhaps the next important to tubocurarine itself. This substance was isolated from the bark of *Strychnos toxifera* by King in 1949. Its mechanism of action is similar to that of tubocurarine but it is more potent and has a longer duration of action. Toxiferine I was at first believed to be monoquaternary but is now known to be bisquaternary like most other blocking agents (Fig. 26.3). It is unstable in solution, splitting up into two symmetrical monoquaternary compounds. The substance has recently undergone clinical trials and shows promise as a useful long-acting muscle relaxant. *Alcuronium chloride* (diallyl-nortoxiferine dichloride) is a derivative of toxiferine I. It has been used successfully as a medium-duration neuromuscular blocking agent, and is said not to lower blood pressure or to produce histamine release in the doses employed during surgical operations. Its blocking action is antagonized by neostigmine.

Another naturally-occurring alkaloid with neuromuscular blocking action is *β-erythroidine*, isolated from *Erythrina americana* by Folkers and Major in 1937. This substance and its more potent dihydro derivative (Fig. 26.3) have not been used much clinically. In animal experiments, they produce a neuro-muscular block which is similar in its characteristics to that produced by tubo-curarine, but their mechanisms of action may not be identical. The erythroidines are tertiary amines and are well absorbed after oral administration; they pene-trate the blood-brain barrier to exert a depressant action on the brain, and in the spinal cord they block the response of the Renshaw interneurones (pages 115, 170 and Fig. 5.3, page 145) to acetylcholine released from the axon collaterals of the lower motoneurones.

The expense and difficulty of obtaining pure alkaloids from natural sources stimulated efforts at synthesis and many hundreds of compounds have been screened for neuromuscular-blocking activity. *Gallamine triethiodide* (Fig. 26.3) introduced by Bovet and his colleagues in 1947 was the first to be widely used and it is still used extensively. It is about one-fifth as potent as tubocurarine and has a slightly shorter duration of action. Gallamine possesses an atropine-like action on the heart but not on other tissues, and it also reduces cardiac arrhythmias induced by adrenaline in the presence of cyclopropane anaesthesia.

Two other synthetic blocking agents which found a limited use as adjuvants to surgical anaesthesia are *benzoquinonium chloride*, introduced by Cavallito in 1948, and *laudexium methylsulphate*, introduced by Taylor and Collier in 1950. Benzoquinonium possesses a fairly pronounced anticholinesterase action and consequently produces unwanted muscarinic side-effects. Although its blocking action resembles that of tubocurarine, it is only weakly antagonized by anticholinesterase drugs and these disadvantages led to its being abandoned as an adjunct to surgical anaesthesia. The use of laudexium has also been abandoned; this drug is antagonized by neostigmine but its duration of action is long and cases have been reported of neuromuscular block returning after the effect of neostigmine has terminated. Gallamine is the only entirely synthetic drug of the curare-like type which is at present extensively used in surgical anaesthesia.

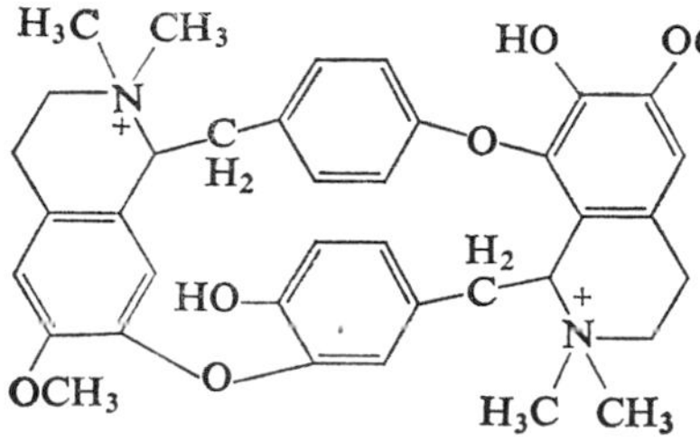

2Cl⁻ 5H₂O
Tubocurarine

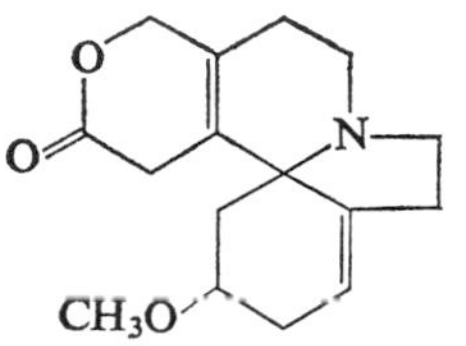

Dihydro-β-
erythroidine

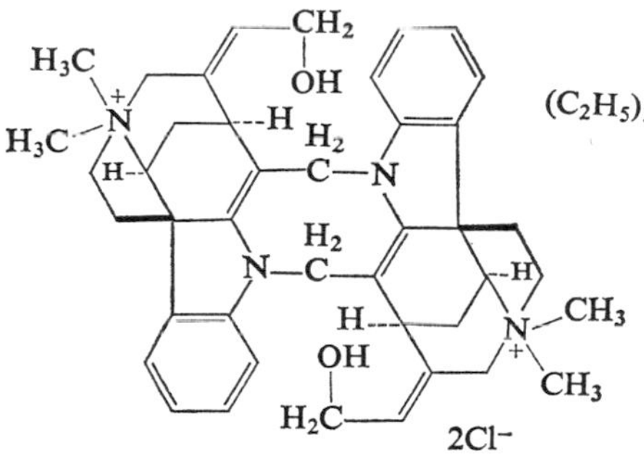

Toxiferine I

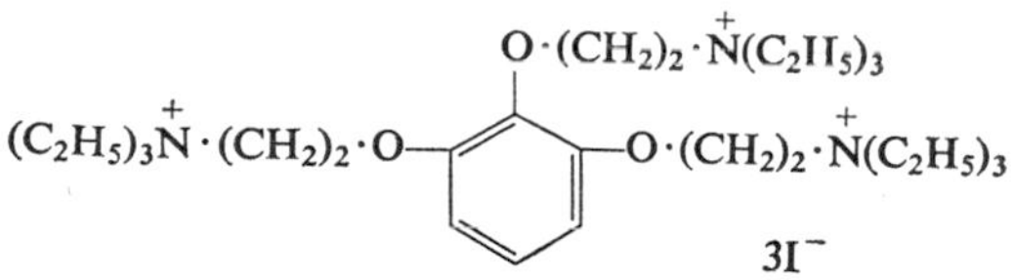

Gallamine
triethiodide

$$(CH_3)_3\overset{+}{N}\cdot(CH_2)_2\cdot O\cdot CO\cdot(CH_2)_2\cdot CO\cdot O\cdot(CH_2)_2\cdot\overset{+}{N}(CH_3)_3$$
2Cl⁻·2H₂O
Suxamethonium

$$(CH_3)_3\overset{+}{N}\cdot(CH_2)_2\cdot O\cdot CO\cdot NH\cdot(CH_2)_6\cdot NH\cdot CO\cdot O\cdot(CH_2)_2\cdot\overset{+}{N}(CH_3)_3$$
2Br⁻
Carbolonium

FIG. 26.3. Chemical formulae of some neuromuscular-blocking agents.

BLOCK BY DEPOLARIZATION. This type of block is produced by agonists including acetylcholine itself. When acetylcholine is injected into the artery supplying a focally innervated mammalian muscle, it produces a brief contraction (Fig. 7.4b, page 200) but its destruction by cholinesterase is so rapid that it has little effect on maximal twitches of the muscle elicited by motor nerve stimulation (Fig. 5.4a, page 146). After inhibition of cholinesterase by a large dose of an anticholinesterase drug, the contraction produced by a similar injection of acetylcholine is still short-lasting but the maximal twitches after the injection are now depressed (Fig. 5.4b). The depression of the twitches has been shown to be due to neuromuscular block, and acetylcholine therefore stimulates or blocks depending upon its concentration and upon the length of time it is allowed to persist in the region of the motor endplates. In 1951, Burns and Paton, using skeletal muscles of the cat, showed that the depolarization produced by large amounts of acetylcholine occurred, not only at the motor endplates, but also in a small area of muscle fibre membrane immediately surrounding them. The mechanism whereby nerve conduction is blocked by a sustained depolarization produced by a negative electrode is explained on pages 85 to 86, and the similar effect produced by acetylcholine at the neuromuscular junction is also referred to on page 198. The depolarized area of membrane surrounding the motor endplate therefore constitutes an inexcitable barrier between the endplate and the rest of the muscle fibre membrane. Endplate potentials produced by motor nerve stimulation cannot initiate propagating action potentials in this inexcitable region and, as a result of this conduction block, the fibre membrane is not excited and contraction does not occur. Depolarization of the muscle fibre membrane in the region of the motor endplates by a cathodal electrode produces a block which is similar to that produced by acetylcholine, and both types of block are reversed by applying an (hyperpolarizing) anodal electrode to the endplate region. In addition to acting on the motor endplates, acetylcholine and related drugs are now known to depolarize nerve endings in striated muscle, an action resembling that on non-myelinated sensory terminals (pp. 148 and 698). It is not known to what extent this pre-junctional action contributes to their effects on neuromuscular transmission.

Acetylcholine is not used clinically to produce neuromuscular block as huge doses are required by intravenous injection, its actions are too widespread, and full inhibition of cholinesterase is necessary. Most drugs which possess the nicotinic action of acetylcholine (e.g. carbachol, page 705) produce block by depolarization providing the dose is large enough. However, the potent actions of most of these drugs at other sites makes them useless as neuromuscular blocking drugs.

In 1948, Barlow and Ing, and Paton and Zaimis, independently studied a series of bisquaternary compounds (the methonium compounds) of the structure, $(CH_3)_3N^+$—$(CH_2)_n$—$N^+(CH_3)_3$, and found that *decamethonium* (C—10), the compound in which $n = 10$, possess a powerful neuromuscular-blocking action. The mechanism of action of decamethonium was subsequently elucidated, particularly by Zaimis, and for the next 10 years or so, it was used extensively as an adjuvant to surgical anaesthesia. A comparison

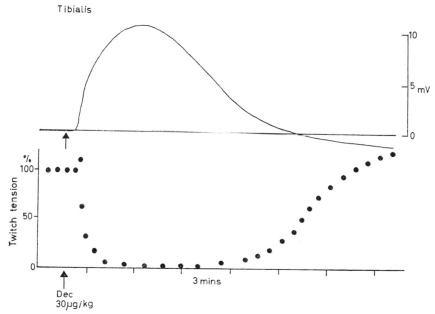

FIG. 26.4. Graphical representation of the effects of decamethonium (30 μg/kg intravenously) on the endplate potential (upper curve) and maximal twitches (lower curve) of the tibialis anterior muscle of an anaesthetized cat. The motor nerve was stimulated once every 10 sec. The twitches were recorded isometrically and simultaneously the gross endplate potential was recorded between a wick electrode placed on the muscle surface in the region of greatest endplate density and a second electrode in contact with the muscle surface near its tendon of insertion. Note that the time course of the endplate depolarization corresponds to that of the effect on the twitches. (Figure supplied by Dr. J. Maclagan.)

between Fig. 5.4b and Fig. 26.5a illustrates the similarity between the effects of a close-arterial injection of acetylcholine after inhibition of cholinesterase and those of an injection of decamethonium with cholinesterase functioning normally. Decamethonium differs from acetylcholine in that it is unaffected by cholinesterase, and it is effective in small doses after intravenous injection. Furthermore, unlike acetylcholine, it has little action elsewhere than in striated muscle. It is devoid of muscarinic action and has little effect on autonomic ganglia. In most of the muscles of the cat and of man, the block produced by decamethonium, like that produced by acetylcholine, is a consequence of persistent depolarization of the motor endplates. Fig. 26.4 is a graphical representation of the effects of decamethonium during a simultaneous recording of endplate depolarization and maximal twitch tension in the tibialis anterior muscle of the cat. Although the receptors with which depolarizing drugs react are situated on the external surface of the membrane, recent work indicates that during the depolarizing process the drugs penetrate to the inside of the muscle fibre. Penetration, which may be an essential part of the depolarization process, is prevented by a previous injection of tubocurarine.

Succinyldicholine (Fig. 26.3) is a neuromuscular-blocking agent of the depolarizing type, first examined for this action by Bovet and his colleagues in 1949. This drug has received the official name, *Suxamethonium*. Since 1951, it has been widely used as a muscle relaxant in operations. Suxamethonium is rapidly hydrolysed by the pseudocholinesterase of plasma, first to succinylmonocholine and then, 6 to 7 times more slowly, to succinic acid and choline. The primary break-down product, succinylmonocholine, has a much weaker blocking action than suxamethonium itself so that the duration of action of suxamethonium is very short. A single dose is given to relax the muscles of the larynx and so to facilitate endotracheal intubation at the start of an operation. For prolonged operations, suxamethonium may be administered in the form of a continuous intravenous infusion. The degree of muscle relaxation is then controllable throughout and spontaneous respiration usually returns rapidly on stopping the infusion. Unfortunately this does not always occur, and numerous cases of unduly prolonged apnoea have been reported after the use of suxamethonium. One cause is a low plasma cholinesterase activity but this does not account for all cases. Anticholinesterase drugs prevent the destruction of suxamethonium and greatly prolong its action.

Suxethonium was also examined in 1949 by Bovet and his colleagues; it differs from suxamethonium only by the substitution of an ethyl group for one methyl group on each quaternary nitrogen. Its action closely resembles that of suxamethonium but it is slightly less potent and its duration of action is even shorter. It is hydrolysed by plasma cholinesterase about one and a half times faster than suxamethonium.

Carbolonium (Fig. 26.3) is one of a series of compounds first synthesized and studied pharmacologically in 1953–54 by Cheymol and by Klupp and their associates. Its neuromuscular-blocking activity and potency are similar to those of decamethonium but its duration of action is longer. It is still used as an adjunct to anaesthesia in continental Europe.

The characteristics of depolarization block of the maximal twitches of the tibialis anterior muscle of the cat produced by intravenously injected decamethonium are illustrated in Fig. 26.5, and should be compared with those of non-depolarization block (Fig. 26.2). (1) The block is preceded by muscle fasciculations and potentiation of the maximal twitch (Fig. 26.5b and c). These

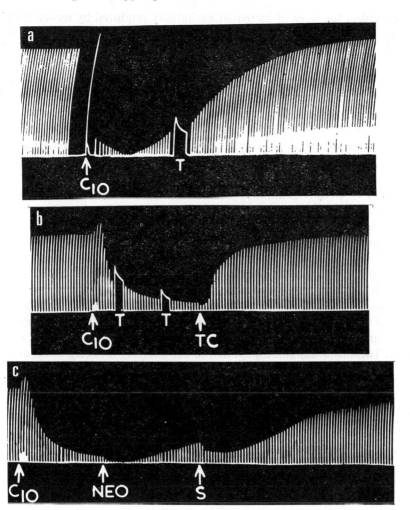

FIG. 26.5. Characteristics of block by depolarization in the tibialis anterior muscle of cats under chloralose anaesthesia. Maximal twitches were elicited by stimulation of the motor nerves once every 10 sec. In **a**, electrical stimulation was temporarily stopped and 5 μg of decamethonium (C_{10}) were injected close-arterially. Decamethonium caused a large contraction (cf. the effects of acetylcholine in Fig. 5.4b.). On recommencing electrical stimulation the twitches were blocked. In **b** and **c**, at C_{10}, 40 μg/kg decamethonium; at TC, 75 μg/kg tubocurarine; at NEO, 75 μg/kg neostigmine and at S, 15 μg/kg suxamethonium were injected intravenously. At T in **a** and **b**, a tetanus was elicited by stimulation of the motor nerve at 50/sec for 10 sec. (Source as for Fig. 26.1.)

effects reflect the stage of increased excitability produced by motor endplate depolarization. Depolarizing drugs also stimulate the intrafusal fibres of the muscle spindles (page 107), and when the nerve is left connected to the spinal cord the fasciculations may be more pronounced as reflex contractions are initiated by the contracted muscle spindles. (2) During the block, the tension of a tetanus, though depressed, is sustained throughout the period of stimulation (Fig. 26.5b). With a depolarizing drug, the *effect* of acetylcholine is depressed but the sensitivity of the endplates to it is not, and so the reduction in transmitter release occurring during the tetanus is not immediately reflected in the tension. (3) After a tetanus, the twitches are neither restored nor further depressed (Fig. 26.5b). In the absence of an anticholinesterase, the excess acetylcholine released by each impulse after a tetanus does not persist long enough to summate with the blocking drug. (4) Since the blocking drug has the same mechanism of action as acetylcholine, the injection of an anticholinesterase (e.g. neostigmine) does not antagonize, but slightly increases, the depth of paralysis (Fig. 26.5c). (5) The blocking action of other depolarizing drugs (e.g. suxamethonium) summates with that of decamethonium (Fig. 26.5b). (6) Any drug with a weak curare-like action (e.g. pentamethonium) antagonizes the excessive endplate depolarization and restores transmission. Sub-blocking doses of tubocurarine are effective in this respect (Fig. 26.5b). This antagonism is of experimental interest only since the dose is too critical to be of clinical value. There is no suitable antagonist to depolarizing blocking drugs and this constitutes one of their main disadvantages.

Depolarizing drugs may also be distinguished from other types of blocking drug by studying their effects on the multiply-innervated muscles of frogs or birds. Thus the rectus abdominis muscle of the frog and the gastrocnemius and neck muscles of the fowl respond to depolarizing drugs with a sustained contracture (see page 207 and Fig. 26.6a and b). In contrast, other types of blocking drug produce a flaccid block in all species and drugs acting like tubocurarine antagonize the contractural response to depolarizing drugs in frog (Fig. 26.6a) and avian muscles. A quick method for detecting a depolarizing action is to inject the drug intravenously into young chicks. The sustained contracture produced in some muscles by depolarizing drugs results in a spastic paralysis of the chick in which the legs are rigidly extended and the head thrust back (Fig. 26.6c). Non-depolarizing blocking drugs on the other hand produce a limp flaccid paralysis (Fig. 26.6d). Chronically denervated muscles of all species also respond to depolarizing drugs with a sustained contracture (see page 206). Occasionally, however, competitive blocking drugs such as tubocurarine and gallamine produce a similar, though weaker effect in chronically denervated muscles, which demonstrates that their initial combination with the receptors may result in a weak and transient depolarization.

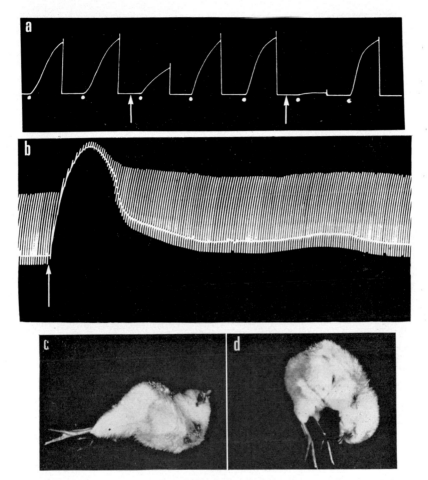

FIG. 26.6. Effects of neuromuscular-blocking drugs in muscles with multiple inner-vation. **a**. Isolated rectus abdominis muscle of frog. At the white dots, 3 μg/ml of suxamethonium was added to the bath. At the arrows, 0·5 μg/ml and 1 μg/ml of tubocurarine was added and left in contact with the tissue during the next response to suxamethonium. Note that tubocurarine depressed the response to suxamethonium. **b**. Maximal twitches of the gastrocnemius muscle of an anaesthetized chicken elicited by stimulation of the motor nerve once every 10 sec. At the arrow, 2 μg/kg of carbolonium was injected intravenously. Contrast this response with that in the cat to the similarly acting drug, decamethonium (Fig. 26.5). The effect of drugs like tubocurarine in the chicken is similar to that in the cat. **c**. Spastic paralysis of a chick produced by the intravenous injection of 3 μg decamethonium. **d**. Flaccid paralysis of a chick produced by the intravenous injection of 12 μg tubocurarine.

The extra-ocular muscles in man and other mammals have a multiple innervation and respond to depolarizing drugs with a sustained contracture like that produced in some avian and frog muscles. This effect of suxamethonium may contribute to the increase in intra-ocular pressure produced by this drug.

DUAL BLOCK. Dual block is produced by drugs which behave as partial agonists. The block of the maximal twitches is preceded by potentiation of the twitch and muscle fasciculations, indicating an initial depolarizing action.

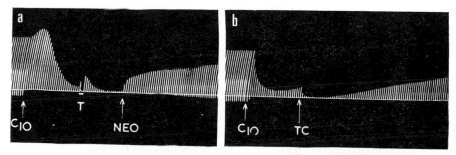

FIG. 26.7. Dual block produced by decamethonium in the tibialis anterior muscle of the ferret under chloralose anaesthesia. The motor nerve was stimulated once every 10 sec. At C_{10} in (a) 50 μg/kg and at C_{10} in (b) 150 μg/kg decamethonium; at NEO, 75 μg/kg neostigmine and at TC, 100 μg/kg tubocurarine, all injected intravenously. At T, a tetanus was elicited by stimulation of the motor nerve at 50/sec for 5 sec. (From W. C. Bowman, Chapter 3, in 'Progress in Medicinal Chemistry'. Vol. 2. Ed. by G. P. Ellis and G. B. West. Butterworth, 1962.)

However, the depolarization wanes although the receptors remain occupied by the drug molecules so that the block itself exhibits characteristics similar to those of non-depolarization block, being antagonized by a tetanus and by anticholinesterase drugs and intensified by tubocurarine. Decamethonium behaves as a partial agonist in the muscles of the ferret, and Fig. 26.7 illustrates dual block produced by decamethonium in the tibialis anterior muscle of this species. Figure 26.7 should be compared with Figs. 26.2 and 26.4. The two phases of dual block are mutually antagonistic and as a result large doses of the drug are required to produce it, and a marked tachyphylaxis is evident when successive doses are injected.

Drugs which produce block by depolarization in some species may produce dual block in others, and even in the same species different muscles may respond differently. Thus, decamethonium and suxamethonium produce block by depolarization in most of the muscles of man and of the cat, but in the soleus muscle of the cat and in the muscles of all other laboratory animals tested, these two drugs produce dual block. In contrast to their effect in normal man, these drugs also produce dual block in patients with *myasthenia gravis* (page 208). Myasthenic patients are therefore very resistant to decamethonium and this fact has been made the basis of a diagnostic test for the disease.

Tridecamethonium (C_{13}), in which a chain of 13 methylene groups separates the two quaternary nitrogens produces dual block in all species tested, including the cat.

The term *mixed block* was sometimes used to denote the uncertain type of block produced when both competitive and long-lasting depolarizing blocking drugs were unwisely administered during the same operation in man. It should not be confused with dual block which is produced by only one drug.

OTHER TYPES OF MOTOR ENDPLATE BLOCK. Thesleff and his co-workers have shown that, in isolated skeletal muscles bathed in an artificial solution, depolarizing drugs may produce a block which differs from block by depolarization and from dual block in the following ways. The period of depolarization produced by the drugs is fleeting and the motor endplates are rapidly repolarized; block starts during the period of depolarization but persists after the endplates have repolarized. Tubocurarine and gallamine, which antagonize block by depolarization (Fig. 26.5), augment the block in isolated muscle, and neostigmine, which antagonizes dual block (Fig. 26.7), also augments the block in isolated muscle. These results suggest that depolarizing drugs cause receptor desensitization in isolated skeletal muscle and the type of block produced is called *desensitization block*. It may arise because excessive depolarization causes an ionic imbalance across the muscle membrane which cannot be compensated for in the absence of the circulation and the kidneys. The extent, if any, to which desensitization occurs during depolarization block *in vivo* is difficult to determine.

Drugs may depress the sensitivity of the motor endplates in less specific ways than by combining with acetylcholine receptors. For example, some general anaesthetics, particularly *ether*, have this property. This effect of ether is particularly important in anaesthesia because it potentiates non-depolarizing neuromuscular-blocking drugs; the dose of tubocurarine necessary to produce adequate muscle relaxation may sometimes have to be reduced by as much as 60%. Ether has less effect on depolarizing blocking drugs but does tend to reduce their effectiveness.

Block by depolarizing drugs in man. In non-myasthenic patients, decamethonium, suxamethonium and carbolonium produce a depolarization block. However, after prolonged administration, the characteristics of the block often change and many anaesthetists have reported that neostigmine may then have some antagonistic action. There is no convincing evidence as to the cause of this change. The block does not appear to be the same as dual block, which, when it occurs in animals, is always produced by the first injection of the drug; nor does it resemble desensitization block. The change may be a consequence of inter-action with other drugs used as adjuvants to surgical anaesthesia (page 581); it may be the result of a weak hemicholinium-like action of the depolarizing drugs; or it may arise from depressed acetylcholine release due to depolari-zation block of the nerve endings (see page 670).

USES AND DISADVANTAGES OF NEUROMUSCULAR-BLOCKING DRUGS. *Surgical anaesthesia.* The most important use of neuromuscular-blocking drugs is to produce muscle relaxation during surgical anaesthesia. Tubo-curarine was the first drug to be used for this purpose, in 1942; since that time it has been used in conjunction with most anaesthetic agents. Neuromuscular blocking drugs increase the safety of operations, for without them the amount of anaesthetic necessary to abolish reflex activity and produce muscle relax-ation is large. Generally, the respiratory muscles are paralysed and artificial respiration must therefore be applied.

The depolarizing blocking drugs have a number of disadvantages. (1) There is no suitable antagonist to their action, should the need arise. (2) When a change in the characteristics of the block occurs as described above, the anaes-thetist is in a difficult position since he is uncertain whether to risk trying neo-stigmine when faced with a case of prolonged apnoea. Several cases of pro-longed apnoea have been reported particularly after long-lasting operations in which suxamethonium was used. As mentioned earlier, this is not always associated with a low plasma cholinesterase. (3) The powerful muscle fascicul-ations which precede the block produced by suxamethonium may cause damage to the muscle fibres which results in severe deep muscle ache after the operation. (4) Suxamethonium may raise the intra-ocular pressure, partly through its ganglion stimulating action causing local vascular changes and contraction of smooth muscle in the orbit, and partly through producing contracture of the extra-ocular muscles.

These disadvantages have largely restricted the use of depolarizing blocking agents, at least in Britain, to short-lasting operations. Decamethonium is no longer used, but suxamethonium and suxethonium are still widely employed, and carbolonium is used in some countries. If it existed, many anaes-thetists would prefer a blocking drug with a very short duration of action but of the non-depolarizing type. For long operations, adequate muscle relaxation could be produced by continuous intravenous infusion, thereby giving the anaesthetist full control of the degree of relaxation and allowing the rapid return of spontaneous respiration when the infusion is stopped.

The names, doses and some of the side-effects of the blocking agents used as adjuvants to surgical anaesthesia are given in Table 26.1. In the usual doses, the

Table 26.1. Neuromuscular Blocking Drugs used in Surgical Anaesthesia.

Name	Intravenous dose (mg)	Type of block	Duration (min)	Effect of Ether	Effect of Hypothermia	Histamine Release	Action on autonomic ganglia	Excretion	Contra indication
1. (+)-Tubocurarine (chloride)	15–20	Non-depolarization block of motor endplates	About 30	Potentiates	Reduces magnitude of block but does not affect duration	Marked	Blocks in same dose	30% excreted unchanged in urine	In bronchial asthma and other allergic conditions. In myasthenia gravis and renal insufficiency
2. Dimethyltubocurarine (chloride)	2–4		Slightly shorter than 30			Less marked	Less blockade	55% excreted unchanged in urine	Myasthenia gravis and renal insufficiency
3. Toxiferine I	2–4		Longer than 30			?	?	?	Myasthenia gravis and renal insufficiency
4. Gallamine triethiodide	80–100		Shorter than 30			Very little	Very little	100% excreted in urine	Cardiovascular disorders, hyperthyroidism, myasthenia gravis and renal insufficiency
5. Suxamethonium (chloride or bromide)	10–50	Depolarization block	Very short	No effect or slight antagonism	Increases magnitude and duration of block	Occasionally after prolonged infusion	Slight stimulation	Hydrolysed by pseudocholinesterase. Less than 3% excreted unchanged	Patients with low plasma cholinesterase
6. Suxethonium (bromide or iodide)	20–100		Very short			Slight	Very slight stimulation	As for suxamethonium	As for suxamethonium
7. Carbolonium (bromide)	2–5		About 30			Slight	No effect	100% excreted unchanged	Renal insufficiency

drugs used clinically do not penetrate the blood-brain barrier and do not therefore exert central actions.

Convulsions. Neuromuscular-blocking drugs may be used to control convulsions in tetanus and in electro-convulsive therapy.

Orthopaedics. These drugs have been used to produce relaxation while manipulating fractured or dislocated bones.

Myasthenia gravis. Myasthenic patients are very sensitive to competitive blocking agents and insensitive to depolarizing blocking agents. Tubocurarine and decamethonium are sometimes used as indicators in cases of uncertain diagnosis. In a few cases, myasthenic patients have shown a temporary improvement after a prolonged period of full curarization. This seems to be due to 'resting' the motor endplates. The symptoms of myasthenia gravis are described on pages 208 to 209.

STRUCTURE-ACTION RELATIONSHIP. In 1869, Crum Brown and Fraser demonstrated that the quaternary derivatives of various alkaloids, including strychnine and atropine, had neuromuscular-blocking activity. Since that time it has been realized that a strongly basic centre, giving rise to a positively charged ion, is necessary. Sulphonium, phosphonium, arsenium and stibonium radicals, which also carry a strong positive charge, similarly impart some degree of neuromuscular blocking activity to molecules containing them. However, most attempts to synthesize neuromuscular blocking drugs, especially since the elucidation of the structure of tubocurarine, have been confined to series of bisquaternary compounds. Consequently, little is known about the structural requirements for neuromuscular block apart from the fact that amongst the bisquaternaries with an inter-nitrogen distance of the order of 9–14 Å there are some active drugs.

In general, bulky molecules with large hydrocarbon skeletons tend to be competitive blocking agents, possibly because they present a large surface which may be bound to the receptor by van der Waals' forces. Bovet classified compounds of this type as 'pachycurares'. On the other hand, less bulky, more polar compounds with at least 2 methyl groups attached to the quaternary nitrogens tend to be depolarizing drugs; these were called 'leptocurares' by Bovet. In a series of related compounds, it is possible to pass from a structure optimal for competitive block, through a large number of structures of lesser potency and showing the characteristics of dual block, to a structure optimal for depolarization block.

β-Erythroidine, and its more potent dihydro derivative, produce neuromuscular block despite the fact that their molecules contain only one tertiary nitrogen atom (Fig. 26.3). Dihydroerythroidine is about 20 times less potent than tubocurarine in the cat, although its effect is much more rapid in onset. The rapid onset of effect may reflect the ability of tertiary amines to penetrate lipid barriers (e.g. the terminal Schwann cells enclosing the neuromuscular junction) more quickly than quaternary ammonium ions. Surprisingly, tests on frogs have shown that quaternization of the erythroidines reduces their potency. This is possibly because the reduced ability to penetrate lipid barriers may outweigh any increased affinity for motor endplate receptors.

Recently, a number of mono- and bis-quaternary compounds with a steroid nucleus have been tested for neuromuscular blocking activity. The duration of action of some of these drugs is brief and it may be that a useful very short-acting blocking drug of the non-depolarizing type will be found among compounds of this type.

Facilitation of Neuromuscular Transmission

Drugs may facilitate neuromuscular transmission in the following three ways:

INCREASED TRANSMITTER RELEASE. A few drugs are believed to facilitate neuromuscular transmission by an action on the nerve endings through which the amount of acetylcholine released by nerve impulses is increased. *Adrenaline, tetraethylammonium* and *guanidine* are examples of compounds said to possess this action, although the mechanism by which they produce this effect is probably different in each case. All possess an anticurare action and all have been shown to increase the size of endplate potentials elicited by motor nerve stimulation, but to be without effect on endplate potentials produced by applying acetylcholine from a micropipette. If their facilitating action depended upon sensitization of the motor endplates or upon an anticholinesterase action, there would be augmentation of endplate potentials produced by either method. Experiments in which acetylcholine released from the nerve endings was collected and assayed have supplied direct evidence that tetraethylammonium increases transmitter release in response to nerve impulses.

The prejunctional action of adrenaline is produced to a lesser extent by noradrenaline and probably contributes to the *Orbeli effect* described on page 151. It has no clinical value and it is doubtful whether it plays any part in physiological processes. However, it is possible that a similar effect of the related drug *ephedrine* accounts for its beneficial effect in some myasthenic patients. Adrenaline may augment transmitter release by hyperpolarizing the membrane of the nerve endings. Hyperpolarization of the nerve endings by anodal currents also augments transmitter release. In addition to its action on transmission, adrenaline exerts a direct effect on the muscle fibres themselves (page 152).

The main action of tetraethylammonium is a brief ganglion-blocking action of the competitive type (page 690). In its action in increasing transmitter release, it appears to act by increasing the duration of the spike potential in the nerve endings. Other actions of tetraethylammonium include the following: (*a*) it possesses a weak curare-like action on the motor endplates which probably accounts for its ability to antagonize block produced by depolarizing drugs; (*b*) it possesses a weak hemicholinium-like action which is evident when the motor nerve is stimulated at a high frequency; (*c*) it excites sensory nerve endings and produces a tingling sensation in the extremities in man; and (*d*) in frogs, it exerts a veratrine-like action (page 83), causes isolated nerves to discharge impulses in the absence of electrical stimulation, and is able to substitute for sodium ions in nerve conduction (page 87). Because of its widespread effects, tetraethylammonium is rarely used clinically.

The action of guanidine on neuromuscular transmission is of little clinical value but a few myasthenic patients find it of beneficial effect. However, in most patients it produces unpleasant side-effects.

INCREASED EXCITABILITY OF THE MOTOR ENDPLATES. Drugs may increase the excitability of the motor endplates by causing a sustained but sub-effective depolarization. This effect results in antagonism to curare-like drugs but, as already described, in non-curarized muscle the stage of facilitated transmission is fleeting and depolarization block soon develops.

INHIBITION OF CHOLINESTERASE. The anticholinesterase drugs provide the most important means of facilitating neuromuscular transmission. They are discussed in more detail on pp. 712–713. Their mechanisms of action at the neuromuscular junction are all fundamentally the same. Any apparent differences in their effects arise mainly from differences in the rapidity with which they combine with acetylcholinesterase and differences in the stability of the enzyme-inhibitor complex.

In the presence of an anticholinesterase, the endplate potential produced by the acetylcholine released by a single nerve impulse is greatly increased and prolonged. The endplate potential therefore outlasts the refractory period of the surrounding muscle fibre membrane so that more than one muscle action potential is initiated by a single nerve impulse (see pages 197–198), and the contraction is augmented (Fig. 26.7). In other words, anticholinesterases convert single twitches into brief, high frequency tetani, as illustrated in Fig. 26.8a. The repetitive action potential record of Fig. 26.8a shows a series of waning deflections. This is because it was recorded from the whole muscle, and not all of the muscle fibres respond more than once. When repetitive firing is recorded from a single muscle fibre, each spike obeys the all or nothing law and is equal in size to all the others. When the nerve action potential is recorded, as well as the

22*

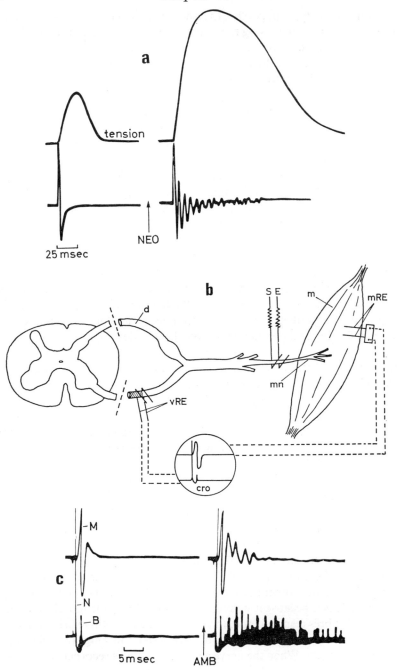

a

tension

NEO

25 msec

b

S E   m   mRE

d

mn

vRE

cro

c

M

N

B

5 msec   AMB

muscle action potential, by the method illustrated in Fig. 26.8b, both are seen to become repetitive in the presence of an anticholinesterase (Fig. 26.8c). This effect on the nerve action potential is not fully understood. There are at least three possible causes: (a) Anticholinesterases may have a direct action on nerve endings converting the single nerve impulse into a repetitive discharge. (2) When the nerve endings are no longer protected by cholinesterase, accumulated-acetylcholine may be capable of exciting them to fire repetitively, especially during the enhanced period of excitability corresponding to the negative after-potential (page 81). (3) The repetitive firing in the nerve may be due to ephaptic re-excitation of the nerve endings by the repetitive muscle action currents (see page 84). Whatever the cause of the repetitive firing in the nerve, it probably contributes to the occurrence of muscle fasciculations which are a characteristic sign of excessive anticholinesterase treatment. The fasciculations are not con-tractions of single muscle fibres but are synchronous contractions of the fibres in whole muscle units. This may be explained if repetitive firing initiated at one nerve ending is propagated by axon reflex into all the fibres of the motor unit so that all the muscle fibres of the unit respond almost simultaneously. Trans-mission from the γ-efferents to the muscle spindles is cholinergic (page 147) and anticholinesterase treatment therefore probably increases their sensitivity to stretch. Reflex muscle contractions initiated in this way may thus add to the fasciculations.

Repetitive firing of the muscle action potential does not occur when the frequency of nerve stimulation is greater than 2/sec. Repetitive firing is not therefore produced by anticholinesterase drugs during powerful voluntary movements (see page 208). In normal muscles, anticholinesterase drugs depress

---

Fig. 26.8 (opposite). Effects of anticholinesterase drugs on responses to single motor nerve shocks in cats under chloralose anaesthesia. **a.** Maximal isometric twitches (upper trace) and gross muscle action potentials (lower trace) of the tibialis anterior muscle were elicited by stimulation of the motor nerve once every 10 sec and recorded simultaneously on a cathode ray oscilloscope. The first record is a control response; the second record shows the increase in tension and the repetitive muscle action potential 2 min after the intravenous injection of 0·25 mg/kg of neostigmine (NEO). **b.** This illustrates the experimental arrangement for recording the results illustrated in **c**. The motor nerve was stimulated once every 10 sec through the stimulating electrodes SE, and the muscle action potential (upper trace in **c**) and the antidromic nerve action potential in the ventral root (lower trace in **c**) were recorded simultaneously on an oscilloscope (cro). mRE and vRE are the muscle and ventral root recording electrodes respectively. In **c**, M is the muscle action potential, N, the nerve action potential, and B, the back-response in the nerve produced by ephaptic re-excitation of the nerve by the large muscle action currents. Between the two records in **c**, 5 μg of ambenonium (AMB, a powerful anti-cholinesterase drug) were injected close-arterially into the gastrocnemius muscle. The record on the right shows the repetitive firing produced in both muscle and nerve 2 min after injection of ambenonium.

powerful voluntary contractions in the same way as they depress experimentally produced tetanic contractions (Fig. 26.9). This is because the acetylcholine,
released by the high frequency of nerve impulses, accumulates and produces
depolarization block of the motor endplates.

In muscles paralysed by competitive blocking agents and in patients with
myasthenia gravis, neuromuscular transmission is subnormal. In these cases,
excess acetylcholine improves transmission and restores muscular power by
increasing the number of muscle fibres contributing to the contraction. Repetit-

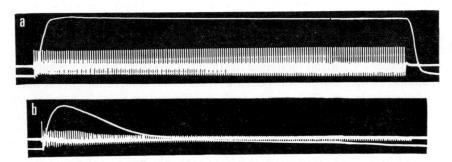

FIG. 26.9. Effect of anticholinesterase drugs on tetanic contractions of the gastrocnemius muscle of a cat under chloralose anaesthesia. Isometric tension and gross muscle
action potentials were recorded simultaneously in response to stimulation of the motor
nerve at 100 shocks/sec for about 1·5 sec every 30 sec, **a**, before and **b**, 5 min after
intra-arterial injection of 10 μg of neostigmine. The effect of anticholinesterase drugs
on tetanic responses of normal muscles is depressant. (From L. C. Blaber and W. C.
Bowman. *Brit. J. Pharmacol.* 1963, **20**, 326.)

ive firing of nerve and muscle fibres is not produced by anticholinesterase drugs
in the presence of tubocurarine. The anticholinesterase drugs used particularly
for their effects on skeletal muscle are *neostigmine, pyridostigmine* and *edrophonium* (page 715). Neostigmine and edrophonium possess a direct
acetylcholine-like action on the motor endplates in addition to their anticholinesterase action. This direct action is weak but may contribute to their effects.
When these drugs are used for their effects on skeletal muscles, atropine is usually injected to prevent muscarinic side-effects. Neostigmine methylsulphate
is the main *anticurare agent* and is usually given in a dose of 1 to 2·5 mg intravenously. The main anticholinesterase drugs used in myasthenia gravis are
neostigmine bromide (a total of 15 to 75 mg/day in 3 or 4 oral doses) and pyridostigmine bromide (a total of 60 to 300 mg/day in 3 or 4 oral doses).

Edrophonium has a very rapid onset of action but its effect is too short-
lasting to be of much therapeutic value. It is mainly used as a diagnostic for
myasthenia gravis and sometimes to enable an anaesthetist, faced with a case of

prolonged apnoea after a neuromuscular-blocking drug, to decide whether neostigmine would be of benefit.

Localization of site of action of neuromuscular blocking drugs

Waser carried out experiments in which he injected radioactively-labelled calabash curarine or decamethonium into mice. At the time of maximal neuro-muscular block or death, the thin diaphragms of the mice were removed and the endplates were located by staining for cholinesterase (page 158). The dia-phragms were then placed in contact with film to detect radioactivity. The endplates in the diaphragm are arranged in a circular band around the central tendon and, on developing the autoradiographs, the curarine molecules could be seen under the microscope to have been combined discretely within the endplate regions. The number of curarine molecules in combination with the receptor surface of one endplate was estimated from the radioactivity of one endplate. The picture obtained with labelled decamethonium differed slightly from that with curarine. With decamethonium the endplate band always had a diffuse blurred appearance suggesting that this drug combines with receptors, not only in the endplate region, but also further out on the muscle membrane around the endplate. Iontophoretic microapplication of acetylcholine (page 147) has shown that some acetylcholine receptors are scattered around the end-plate region beyond the area in apposition to the nerve ending. These extra-endplate receptors are considered not to play a part in the normal transmission process but decamethonium apparently combines with them, and this may explain the finding that depolarization produced by decamethonium extends a little beyond the endplate region. Presumably the more bulky curarine molecule is prevented from reaching these receptors because of diffusion bar-riers around the junctional gap. Acetylcholine released from the nerve endings is thought not to react with these receptors under normal conditions, because it is rapidly hydrolysed by the acetylcholinesterase in the endplates. Waser also carried out experiments in which mice were given a lethal dose of labelled curarine mixed with various doses of neostigmine. Although neuromuscular transmission was quickly restored even by small doses of neostigmine, the amount of curarine combined with the receptors was no less than usual, unless a 10 times normal dose of neostigmine was given. This result indicates that, in contrast to the once-held view, acetylcholine, accumulating in the presence of neostigmine, does not reverse curarine block by displacing it from the receptors. Rather, it may be that inhibition of the junctional cholinesterase allows the released acetylcholine to spread to the extra-endplate receptors (which are not occupied by curarine) and transmission is restored as a result of this.

CHAPTER 27

Drugs Acting at Autonomic Ganglia

The process of chemical transmission in autonomic ganglia is described on pp. 142–144. In many respects it is similar to transmission at the neuromuscular junction, although there are important differences. At both sites, acetylcholine exerts a 'nicotinic' action (page 139) and most drugs which are active at the one site are to some extent also active at the other. However, the differences between the two sites are such that many drugs are relatively specific in their action. For example, among the neuromuscular-blocking drugs only tubocurarine possesses significant ganglion-blocking activity (page 678); conversely, the neuromuscular-blocking action of the ganglion-blocking drugs developed for clinical use is too weak to be produced by the doses employed therapeutically.

Methods used for studying drugs acting at ganglia

The superior cervical ganglion of the cat. Because of its relative simplicity, this preparation has been used in most physiological and pharmacological studies on ganglionic transmission. Preganglionic fibres in the cervical sympathetic trunk form synapses in the superior cervical ganglion, and many of the postganglionic fibres leaving the ganglion innervate the nictitating membrane, a structure which is vestigial in man but which is well developed in the cat. Stimulating electrodes may be placed on both pre- and postganglionic trunks, the preganglionic trunk being sectioned centrally to the electrodes, and contractions of the nictitating membrane may be recorded (Fig. 27.1). Alternatively, electrical activity of the postganglionic neurones may be recorded on an oscilloscope. Drugs may be injected intravenously or directly into the arterial supply to the ganglion.

When it is desired to study the effect of a drug on the release of acetylcholine from the presynaptic nerve endings, the ganglion may be perfused through its arterial supply and the outflow collected from a cannula in the vein leaving the ganglion. The acetylcholine released into the fluid leaving the ganglion on stimulating the preganglionic fibres may be assayed both before and after adding the drug to the perfusion fluid. The superior cervical ganglion was first perfused by Kibjakow in 1933 and the method has since been improved and used extensively by Feldberg, Perry and MacIntosh and their colleagues. When acetylcholine is to be assayed, its hydrolysis is usually prevented by the inclusion of an anticholinesterase (e.g. physostigmine) in the perfusion fluid. However, MacIntosh has developed a method in which an anticholinesterase is not used. In this method the choline in the perfusate, which is formed by the hydrolysis of the acetylcholine, is reacetylated before assay.

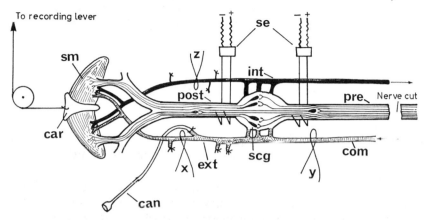

FIG. 27.1. Diagram of the blood and nerve supply to the nictitating membrane of the cat (not to scale), and the arrangement for pre- and postganglionic stimulation and for giving intra-arterial injections into the ganglion. *sm* and *car*, smooth muscle and cartilage of nictitating membrane; *can*, cannula tied into the lingual artery; *pre* and *post*, pre- and postganglionic nerve trunks; *se*, stimulating electrodes on both nerve trunks; *scg*, superior cervical ganglion in which most of the fibres form synapses; *int*, internal jugular vein; *com*, common carotid artery; *ext*, external carotid artery; *x, y, z*, loose ligatures. When intra-arterial injections are made, the ligatures, *x* and *y*, are pulled to occlude the artery so that the injection is forced into the ganglion. To perfuse the ganglion, ligatures *x* and *z* are tied tightly. An 'inflow' cannula is tied into the common carotid artery and an 'outflow' cannula into the internal jugular vein in the positions marked by the arrows.

ANALYSIS OF GANGLIONIC ACTION. Drugs which *stimulate* autonomic ganglia cause a discharge of action potentials in the postganglionic fibres and contraction of the nictitating membrane. The same effect is produced whether the drug is injected intravenously or into the arterial supply to the ganglion. Theoretically, drugs could produce ganglion stimulation by depolarizing the presynaptic nerve endings causing them to release acetylcholine. This effect could be detected by perfusing the ganglion and assaying the perfusion fluid. If this were the only action of the drug, its effect would be abolished when the preganglionic nerve had degenerated through denervation carried out a few days previously, or when substances (such as botulinum toxin) which prevent the release of acetylcholine had been previously injected. Injection of potassium chloride solution does actually depolarize the presynaptic nerve endings and so stimulates the ganglion, and there is evidence to suggest that drugs possessing a nicotinic action on ganglion cells (e.g. nicotine, carbachol and acetylcholine itself) may also act presynaptically. Koelle has incorporated this possibility into a modified theory of transmission. He suggests that when the nerve impulse arrives at the presynaptic nerve endings, it initially causes the release of only a small amount of acetylcholine. This small amount of acetylcholine then acts presynaptically to depolarize the nerve endings, thereby causing the release of a larger amount of acetylcholine which effects transmission by diffusing across the synaptic gap and exciting the postsynaptic membrane. This mechanism was postulated to explain the observation that most of the cholinesterase in autonomic ganglia (unlike that at the neuromuscular junction) is located presynaptically. However, most ganglion-stimulant drugs act mainly by directly depolarizing the postsynaptic cell membranes. Their action is not abolished by botulinum toxin or by degeneration of the preganglionic fibres, although it may be slightly reduced.

Drugs which *block* transmission through autonomic ganglia abolish the discharge of impulses in the postganglionic fibres and the contractions of the nictitating membrane produced by preganglionic stimulation. Contractions of the nictitating membrane produced by postganglionic stimulation are not affected (Fig. 27.3). Drugs which block transmission by an action on the presynaptic nerve endings reduce the amount of acetylcholine released into the fluid perfusing the ganglion but do not prevent the response of the ganglion cells to injected acetylcholine. Conversely, drugs which act only by blocking acetylcholine receptors on the postsynaptic membrane do not affect transmitter release but prevent the response to injected acetylcholine and to other drugs with a similar action. When the block is of the competitive type, it may be overcome either by injecting a large amount of acetylcholine into the arterial supply to the ganglion or by the administration of physostigmine (for some reason, neostigmine is ineffective in this respect).

Some drugs facilitate ganglionic transmission, not by directly causing the release of acetylcholine, but by increasing that released in response to nerve impulses. This type of action may also be detected by collecting and assaying the released transmitter.

The isolated superior cervical ganglion of the rat. Pascoe has developed a method for studying the action of ganglion-stimulant and ganglion-blocking drugs using this preparation. The ganglion, with short lengths of pre- and post-ganglionic trunks attached, is suspended vertically in Krebs' solution with the postganglionic trunk uppermost. One recording electrode is placed in contact with the postganglionic fibres and the other electrode is simply dipped into the Krebs' solution. By lowering the level of the Krebs' solution so that the post-ganglionic fibres and their electrode are in air, any potential difference between the postganglionic fibres and other parts of the preparation may be recorded, as the second electrode is effectively in contact with the part of the preparation at the air/liquid interface. Depolarizing drugs render the body of the ganglion negative with respect to the postganglionic fibres, and ganglion-blocking drugs prevent the effect of depolarizing drugs.

The ciliary ganglion of the cat. This ganglion contains the synapses of the parasympathetic supply to the constrictor pupillae (Fig. 4.11, page 125). Perry and his co-workers have used this preparation in the cat to study the action of drugs on parasympathetic ganglia. Pre- and postganglionic stimulation may be used and observations may be made either of constriction of the pupil or of the postganglionic action potentials. Drugs may be injected intravenously, or intra-arterially through a cannula in the lingual artery.

Dually-innervated cat heart. This preparation was used by Perry and Wilson to study the action of ganglion-blocking drugs simultaneously on sympathetic and parasympathetic ganglia. The experiment was carried out on artifically-respired anaesthetized cats with open chests. Stimulating electrodes were placed on the preganglionic vagus trunk, on the preganglionic sympathetic fibres between the second and third thoracic ganglia, and on the postganglionic sympathetic (accelerator) nerve. The vagal ganglia are inside the walls of the heart and electrodes could not therefore be placed upon the postganglionic vagal fibres. Arterial blood pressure, pulse rate and pulse pressure were recorded on a kymograph. Drugs were injected intravenously,

Numerous other preparations may be used to study drugs affecting autonomic ganglia. These include: (i) inhibition of salivary secretion, (ii) mydriatic activity in mice, (iii) pressure changes in the bladder, (iv) the isolated perfused rabbit heart with vagus nerves attached, (v) peristalsis in isolated ileum of guinea-pigs and (vi) a simple recording of arterial blood pressure in anaesthetized cats or dogs. None of these provides such clear-cut results as the preparations described above but much valuable information concerning the action of a new drug may be gained from them by using known ganglion blocking and stimulant drugs for comparison in the investigation.

Drugs interrupting transmission through autonomic ganglia

Drugs acting presynaptically. The output of acetylcholine in response to nerve impulses in the presynaptic nerve endings may be reduced by the same drugs and procedures as those which depress transmitter output at the neuromuscular junction (pages 660–664). In fact, much of the direct evidence for an effect on acetylcholine release was obtained first from the use of a perfused sympathetic ganglion. Thus, hemicholinium depresses acetylcholine synthesis and produces a delayed, choline-reversible, transmission failure during rapid preganglionic nerve stimulation. Sodium ions play the same role in acetylcholine synthesis in preganglionic neurones as in motor neurones; similarly botulinum toxin, procaine, lack of calcium or excess magnesium inhibit acetylcholine release in both types of neurone. Small doses of adrenaline facilitate ganglionic transmission while larger doses depress it. The effects of adrenaline are due, at least partly, to changes in acetylcholine release. None of these methods of interrupting ganglionic transmission is used clinically but they are sometimes employed in experimental pharmacology.

Some central nervous system depressants (e.g. general anaesthetics, paraldehyde and methylpentynol) have been shown to block transmission through the superior cervical ganglion by reducing transmitter release. This effect on peripheral ganglia is probably not produced by the doses used clinically, but a similar action at synapses in the CNS may account for the actions of these drugs on the brain.

Drugs acting postsynaptically. Ganglion block by depolarization may be produced by large doses of ganglion-stimulant drugs with a 'nicotinic' action. These drugs are described on pages 695–698. The term *ganglion-blocking drugs* is generally restricted to non-depolarizing drugs which act as antagonists to the nicotinic action of acetylcholine on the postsynaptic membrane. This class includes all those drugs which are or which have been used therapeutically to block ganglionic transmission.

The main clinical use of ganglion-blocking drugs is to lower the blood pressure in severe cases of *essential hypertension*. In essential hypertension, the cause of the high blood pressure is not known but block of transmission through the sympathetic ganglia abolishes vasoconstrictor tone, so that the blood vessels dilate, and the arterial pressure falls. The property of ganglion-blocking drugs to lower the blood pressure is occasionally made use of to reduce bleeding during surgery. Only the very short-acting drugs are used for this purpose. The names and chemical formulae of the principal ganglion-blocking drugs are given in Fig. 27.2.

In 1915, Burn and Dale demonstrated that *tetraethylammonium chloride* (TEA, $N^+(CH_2CH_3)_4Cl$) blocked the transmission of impulses through autonomic ganglia. Unlike *tetramethylammonium* (page 696), it does not depolarize the ganglion cells but simply blocks the action of acetylcholine upon them. Although for a short time TEA found a limited use in the treatment of hypertension, its duration of action is too brief for it to be of real value. It has also been used as a diagnostic to determine whether treatment with other ganglion-blocking drugs might be effective. Other actions of TEA are described on pages 680–681.

Symmetrical Bis-quaternary Compounds

$$H_3C—\overset{\overset{CH_3}{|}}{\underset{\underset{CH_3}{|}}{\overset{+}{N}}}—(CH_2)_n—\overset{\overset{CH_3}{|}}{\underset{\underset{CH_3}{|}}{\overset{+}{N}}}—CH_3$$

Pentamethonium, $n=5$ (C_5)
Hexamethonium, $n=6$ (C_6)

$$CH_3CH_2—\overset{\overset{CH_3}{|}}{\underset{\underset{CH_3}{|}}{\overset{+}{N}}}—CH_2—CH_2—\overset{\overset{CH_3}{|}}{\underset{}{N}}—CH_2—CH_2—\overset{\overset{CH_3}{|}}{\underset{\underset{CH_3}{|}}{\overset{+}{N}}}—CH_2CH_3$$

Azamethonium

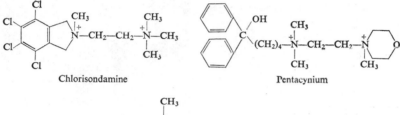

Pentolinium

Asymmetrical Bis-quaternary Compounds

Chlorisondamine

Pentacynium

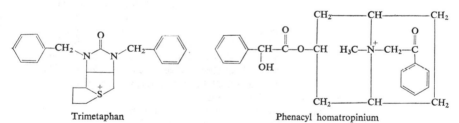

Trimethidinium

Short-Acting Compounds

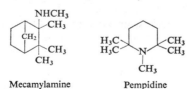

Trimetaphan

Phenacyl homatropinium

Orally-Active Secondary and Tertiary Amines

Mecamylamine

Pempidine

FIG. 27.2. Chemical formulae of some ganglion-blocking drugs.

Bis-quaternary ammonium compounds. The development and study of the *methonium compounds* by Paton and Zaimis in the years after 1948 has already been referred to on page 670. Two members of the series, pentamethonium (C5) and hexamethonium (C6), provided the first real advance in the drug

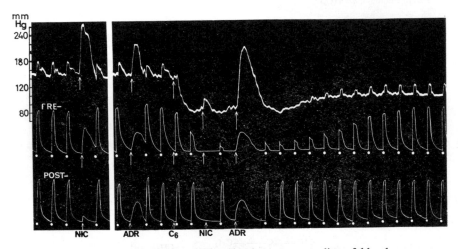

FIG. 27.3. Cat, chloralose anaesthesia. Simultaneous recording of blood pressure (upper record), contractions of the left nictitating membrane in response to preganglionic stimulation (middle record) and contractions of the right nictitating membrane in response to postganglionic stimulation (lowest record). The nerves were stimulated at the white dots at a frequency of 10/sec for 30 sec every 2·5 min except when nicotine or adrenaline were injected. At NIC, 200 μg/kg of nicotine and at ADR, 5 μg/kg of adrenaline were injected intravenously; electrical stimulation was stopped during the effects of these drugs. At C_6, 3 mg/kg of hexamethonium were injected intravenously. C_6 lowered the blood pressure, blocked the responses to nicotine and to preganglionic stimulation, but did not depress responses to adrenaline or to postganglionic stimulation. The preganglionically-stimulated nerve was sectioned centrally to the electrodes. The superior cervical ganglion was removed on the postganglionically stimulated side. The small contraction of the membrane produced by nicotine on the postganglionically-stimulated side was mainly due to release of catecholamines from the adrenal medullae. Note that the arrangement for this experiment differed from that illustrated in Fig. 27.1 in that contractions of both membranes were recorded simultaneously.

treatment of arterial hypertension. Hexamethonium was used successfully for some years before being replaced by other agents. It is still used extensively as a typical ganglion-blocking agent in pharmacological experiments.

In contrast to *decamethonium*, which is a *depolarizing* type of neuromuscular blocking agent, penta- and hexamethonium do not depolarize ganglion cells. Along with other bis-quaternary ammonium ganglion-blocking agents, C5 and C6 are believed to block the action of acetylcholine on the ganglion cells by combining with acetylcholine receptors in a competitive manner, although strict evidence for block by competition at this site is less complete than it is at other sites. The effects of hexamethonium on the blood pressure and nictitating membrane of a cat are illustrated in Fig. 27.3. Hexamethonium causes a fall in blood pressure and blocks the contractions of the nictitating membrane produced by preganglionic stimulation but not those elicited by postganglionic stimulation. The effects of the ganglion-stimulant drug *nicotine* are blocked, but the effects of adrenaline which acts directly on the smooth muscle are not. Note that during the effect of C6 the contractions of the membrane to preganglionic stimulation wane during the period of stimulation. This effect resembles the waning tetanic tension of skeletal muscle during block by competitive blocking agents (Fig. 26.2 and page 667). Similar effects are produced by other quaternary ganglion-blocking agents.

Following the successful use of hexamethonium, other *symmetrical* bisquaternary compounds were developed. These included *azamethonium* and *pentolinium*. Pentolinium showed some advantages over C6, being more potent, possessing a longer duration of action and being slightly better absorbed after oral administration. It is still occasionally used today. *Asymmetric* bisquaternary compounds were also developed and found to be yet more potent and to possess a still longer duration of action. Those that are used to some extent in man include *chlorisondamine, pentacynium* and *trimetaphan*. Although numerous other quaternary compounds with powerful ganglion-blocking activity have been studied in the laboratory, further development of them has slowed down, as more effective compounds with a different mechanism of action have been introduced for the treatment of hypertension (see pages 831–844).

In the doses used clinically, the methonium compounds have few effects other than those arising from ganglion block. They do not penetrate the blood-brain barrier and so do not exert central actions. They are excreted unchanged in the urine.

Disadvantages in the use of quaternary ganglion-blocking drugs. 1. Absorption after oral administration is irregular. Predictable blood concentrations are possible only after administration by subcutaneous, intramuscular or intravenous injections. This constitutes a serious disadvantage to hypertensive patients when several daily doses may be required. 2. All autonomic ganglia, both sympathetic and parasympathetic, are affected and this results in a wide range of unpleasant and occasionally fatal side-effects. Block of parasympathetic ganglia may cause dry mouth, reduced gastric secretion, paralytic ileus, constipation, urinary retention and blurred vision due to dilatation of the pupils and loss of accommodation. In addition to the desired effect of lowering the blood pressure, block of sympathetic ganglia causes postural hypotension because compensatory circulatory adjustments are prevented. Thus on standing, blood pools in the leg veins so that the venous return to the heart is reduced and cardiac output falls. Fainting may occur as the blood supply to the brain is then insufficient. Vasodilatation in the skin caused by sympathetic block leads to heat loss and lowering of body temperature, although this is counteracted to some extent by blockade of the sympathetic stimulation of the sweat glands. Impotence occurs due to a combination of parasympathetic and sympathetic block. Parasympathetic block prevents erection and sympathetic block prevents ejaculation (page 401). 3. Tolerance and cross-tolerance to the drugs occurs after repeated administration. The mechanism giving rise to tolerance is not understood although it may be connected with the fact that quaternary ammonium compounds in some way sensitize the blood vessels to the action of noradrenaline.

Short-acting ganglion-blocking drugs. *Trimetaphan camphorsulphonate* and *phenacyl homatropinium* are two short-acting drugs with a rapid onset of action which have been developed for use in *bloodless field surgery*. They are potent ganglion-blocking agents but in addition trimetaphan lowers blood pressure by a direct vasodilator action and by causing histamine release.

Secondary and tertiary amines. *Mecamylamine*, a secondary amine, was discovered in 1956 and was the first compound found to be fully effective in lowering the blood pressure after oral administration. Subsequently, in 1958, *pempidine*, an orally active tertiary amine was discovered. Both of these drugs cause ganglion block but it is not certain whether their mechanism of action is the same as that of the quaternary blocking agents. There is evidence which suggests that at least part of their ganglion-blocking activity is due to an *intra*-cellular action through which the sensitivity of the ganglion cells to acetylcholine is depressed. Although mecamylamine does not affect the synthesis of acetylcholine, there is some evidence that part of its action on autonomic ganglia is due to inhibition of the mechanism for transmitter release. In addition to its ganglion-blocking activity, mecamylamine may lower the blood pressure through actions on the heart and on the blood vessels themselves. Mecamylamine and pempidine are excreted in the urine. Excretion is hastened when the urine is acid but some tubular reabsorption occurs when the urine is alkaline.

Effectiveness on oral administration is a great advantage but mecamylamine and pempidine to some extent possess all the other disadvantages exhibited by the quaternary ganglion-blocking agents. The development of tolerance is rather less with these drugs but the occurrence of constipation is more pronounced. Both mecamylamine and pempidine penetrate the blood-brain barrier and may give rise to tremors of central origin. This effect is rare with pempidine, possibly because it is excreted more rapidly. Mecamylamine is no longer used clinically but a few hypertensive patients are still satisfactorily controlled with pempidine.

Reserpine and the diuretic *chlorothiazide* potentiate the hypotensive action of ganglion-blocking agents but do not potentiate their side-effects. Combinations of these drugs may be administered since they enable smaller doses of the ganglion-blocking agent to be used, thereby reducing the incidence of side-effects. Other types of drug used in the treatment of hypertension are described on pp. 831–845. The newer ones have largely replaced the ganglion-blocking drugs.

Drugs stimulating ganglion cells

The stimulant action of acetylcholine on autonomic ganglion cells is classically regarded as a 'nicotinic' action (see pages 147–148), and this type of action appears to be the principal one exerted by transmitter acetylcholine. However, more recent research work has demonstrated the presence of additional types of receptors on some ganglion cells, and it is therefore necessary to describe some ganglion stimulants under other headings (see pages 698–700).

Drugs with a nicotinic action. Drugs with this type of action depolarize the membranes of the postsynaptic dendrons and cell bodies of both sympathetic and parasympathetic ganglia causing them to discharge impulses along the postganglionic axons, which in turn release their transmitters on to the effector cells. Chromaffin cells in the adrenal medullae and elsewhere in the body are also stimulated and adrenaline and noradrenaline are released into the blood stream. The results of stimulation of ganglion and chromaffin cells are therefore due to the release of acetylcholine, adrenaline and noradrenaline, and may be prevented by antagonists of these substances (e.g. atropine and anti-adrenaline drugs). The depolarization of the ganglion and chromaffin cells may be antagonized by tubocurarine and the ganglion-blocking drugs described above. The effects of nicotinic stimulant drugs in the whole animal are complex and depend upon the species, upon the dose injected, and upon the balance between parasympathetic and sympathetic activity at the time of injection. The rate and force of the heart beat may be decreased through stimulation of vagal ganglia, or increased through sympathetic stimulation. The calibre of the blood vessels is almost entirely controlled by the sympathetic nervous system and ganglion stimulants invariably cause a rise in blood pressure by stimulating the ganglia of the vasoconstrictor nerves and by releasing catecholamines from the adrenal glands. The rise in pressure may be preceded by a fall due to slowing of the heart as a result of stimulation of vagal ganglia. Peristalsis and tone of the small intestine are usually enhanced due to stimulation of parasympathetic ganglia but movements of the rectum may be first inhibited due to stimulation of sympathetic ganglia. The bladder usually contracts due to parasympathetic stimulation. Secretions of saliva, mucus and sweat are usually increased.

Drugs possessing the nicotinic actions of acetylcholine on autonomic ganglion cells include those enumerated below.

(i) CHOLINE AND ESTERS OF CHOLINE. Choline and many of its esters depolarize ganglion cells. Some of these also possess the muscarinic actions of acetylcholine and the important drugs possessing both properties are listed in Table 28.1, page 704. Other choline esters possess a nicotinic action but little or no muscarinic action. Examples of the latter type are *benzoylcholine* and

$$\text{N} \diagdown \text{NH} \quad -\text{CH}=\text{CH}-\text{CO}-\text{O}-\text{CH}_2-\text{CH}_2-\overset{\overset{\displaystyle CH_3}{|+}}{\underset{\underset{\displaystyle CH_3}{|}}{N}}-\text{CH}_3$$

Urocanylcholine (murexine)

urocanylcholine (murexine), and many others have been synthesized. Urocanylcholine is of interest as it occurs naturally in large amounts in certain molluscs. Succinyldicholine (page 672) also stimulates ganglion cells to a small extent.

(ii) NICOTINE AND OTHER ALKALOIDS. Nicotine is the most important alkaloidal ingredient of tobacco. The free base is a liquid, but its neutral salts, such as the hydrogen tartrate or sulphate are crystalline solids. At the pH of the tissues, nicotine exists mostly as the univalent nicotinium ion and it appears to be this form, rather than the non-ionized base, which is active. Its actions at autonomic ganglia have been known since 1889 when Langley demonstrated them on the cat's superior cervical ganglion. However, Traube had previously shown in 1863 that its effect on the dog's heart was the result of an action at some point more central than the site of action of atropine but more peripheral than the vagus nerve trunk.

Other naturally-occurring alkaloids with a ganglion stimulant action resembling that of nicotine are *coniine*, obtained from hemlock (*Conium maculatum*), and *lobeline*, obtained from lobelia (*Lobelia inflata*).

(iii) TETRAMETHYLAMMONIUM SALTS. This simple quaternary ammonium ion ($N^+(CH_3)_4$) was shown by Burn and Dale to possess the nicotinic actions of acetylcholine, in contrast to tetraethylammonium which is an antagonist of these actions. Tetramethylammonium also possesses a weak muscarinic action.

(iv) 1,1-DIMETHYL-4-PHENYLPIPERAZINIUM SALTS (DMPP). This substance was first studied by Chen and his co-workers in 1951; it possesses the nicotinic actions of acetylcholine to a pronounced degree. In addition, DMPP has recently been shown to possess an action on adrenergic nerve endings resembling that of guanethidine (page 769).

DMPP

Ganglion block by nicotinic stimulants. Large doses of the ganglion-stimulant drugs mentioned above produce ganglion blockade. Acetylcholine injected intra-arterially also blocks ganglionic transmission when the dose is large enough, or when cholinesterase is inhibited. Acetylcholine, and the other drugs possessing a quaternary ammonium group, block the ganglia by producing a long-lasting depolarization. This mechanism is described on page 148 and is similar to block by depolarization at the neuromuscular junction (page 669). However, ganglion cells appear to be less susceptible to block by depolarization than is the neuromuscular junction. At the latter site, a dose of a stable depolarizing drug which is sufficient to cause muscle contraction, subsequently blocks transmission (see Fig. 26.5a, page 673). On the other hand, depolarizing drugs stimulate ganglion cells, causing them to discharge propagated action potentials in doses much smaller than those necessary to block transmission.

The ganglion blocking actions of nicotine, coniine and probably of lobeline are of the non-depolarizing type. These alkaloids, which are secondary and tertiary bases, therefore produce a type of ganglion block which in some respects is similar to dual block at the neuromuscular junction (page 675). The effects of ganglion-blocking doses of the drugs resemble those produced by the competitive ganglion-blocking agents. There is also evidence that part of the ganglion-blocking action of nicotine is presynaptic being due to impairment of transmitter output.

Other actions of nicotinic drugs. In addition to stimulating and blocking autonomic ganglia, nicotinic drugs exert actions at other sites in the body and these are listed below. (The list does not include the *muscarinic* actions of those parasympathomimetic drugs with a nicotinic action: these are dealt with in Chapter 28.) 1. All of the ganglion-stimulant drugs mentioned above first stimulate and then block at the neuromuscular junction. The intravenous doses required to affect the neuromuscular junction are larger than those required to raise the blood pressure. The neuromuscular blocking action of nicotine, coniine and lobeline is of a non-depolarization type. The stimulant action of the drugs at the neuromuscular junction is abolished by tubocurarine and similar drugs. 2. Many sensory receptors resemble autonomic ganglia in their reaction to nicotinic drugs. This has been demonstrated for stretch, pressure, temperature and pain receptors as well as for chemoreceptors such as those in the carotid body. Acetylcholine and other nicotinic drugs have been shown to cause a discharge of impulses in the afferent fibres from these sensory endings. Large doses block the effect of subsequent doses of the same or of a related chemical agent. The doses required to affect sensory receptors are little different from those required to affect autonomic ganglia, and reflex actions initiated by sensory stimulation must therefore contribute to the complex effects of nicotinic drugs in the whole animal. One of the reflex effects of nico-tinic drugs is respiratory stimulation arising through excitation of chemo-receptors in the carotid body. This action of lobeline accounts for its one time use as a respiratory stimulant. Ganglion-blocking drugs of the competitive type block the simulant action of the nicotinic drugs on sensory nerve endings. 3. Nicotinic drugs depolarize adrenergic nerve terminals causing them to dis-charge their transmitter. This effect, coupled with their ability to stimulate chromaffin cells, contributes to their sympathomimetic activity. These actions are also abolished by ganglion-blocking drugs. 4. The depressant action of nicotine on spinal reflexes is described on page 615. Large doses of the alkaloids also affect centres in the brain stem resulting in vomiting (stimu-lation of the chemo-sensitive trigger zone in the medulla), slowing and arrest of the heart (stimulation of vagal centre), respiratory stimulation followed by depression (stimulation and depression of the respiratory centre), a rise followed by a fall in blood pressure (stimulation and depression of the vasomotor centre), convulsions (action on subcortical nuclei of the extra-pyramidal system) and antidiuresis (stimulation of the supra-optic nucleus of the hypothalamus resulting in excessive release of antidiuretic hormone). This last effect of nicotine is fairly powerful and is detectable after smoking a single cigarette (equivalent to about 0·3 mg nicotine). The quaternary ganglion stimulants penetrate the blood-brain barrier poorly and do not exert central actions unless special methods of injection are used.

Muscarinic receptors on sympathetic ganglion cells

A number of drugs possessing the muscarinic actions of acetylcholine have been shown to stimulate sympathetic ganglion cells. The depolarization of the ganglion cells with the discharge of propagated spikes produced by these drugs, differs from that produced by the nicotinic drugs in that it is not blocked, and may even be potentiated, by ganglion-blocking drugs such as hexamethonium. However, the stimulant action of these drugs is readily blocked by small doses of atropine. Except in huge doses, atropine has no effect on the ganglion stimulation produced by nicotinic drugs.

Drugs which have been shown to produce a specific atropine-sensitive stimulation of sympathetic ganglion cells include muscarine, F2268, pilocarpine, acetyl-β-methylcholine (these drugs are described on pages 703–704) and 4-(*m*-chlorophenylcarbamoyloxy)-2-butynyltrimethylammonium chloride (McN-A-343). This last compound is of especial interest because its main action is on muscarinic receptors of sympathetic ganglion cells; it possesses only slight muscarinic action at other sites. Its injection, therefore, results in a rise in blood pressure, which is abolished by atropine. Injection of drugs such as

$$\text{—NH—CO—O—CH}_2\text{—C}\equiv\text{C—CH}_2\text{—}\overset{+}{\text{N}}(\text{CH}_3)_3 \quad \text{Cl}^-$$

Cl McN-A-343

acetylcholine, which possess both nicotinic and muscarinic actions, produce both types of ganglion stimulation—an initial depolarization which is selectively blocked by hexamethonium, and a delayed effect which is blocked by atropine.

The effects of preganglionic nerve stimulation may be completely abolished by drugs such as hexamethonium, and the physiological role of the muscarinic receptors, if any, in ganglionic transmission is not known. However, after inhibition of cholinesterase by dyflos (page 719), acetylcholine released by repetitive preganglionic stimulation has been shown to produce a secondary delayed discharge from the ganglion cells which is blocked by atropine.

In the isolated superior cervical ganglion of rabbits, R. M. Eccles has shown that the electrical response of the ganglion cells to a stimulus applied to the preganglionic fibres, is characterized by a complex wave form with three components: (i) an initial negative potential (N), (ii) a positive potential (P), and (iii) a late negative potential (LN). All of these potentials were absent after treatment with botulinum toxin, indicating that they are all due to acetylcholine. Tubocurarine abolished the N potential but enhanced the LN potential, whereas atropine abolished the P and LN potentials. (The P potential was also abolished by antiadrenaline drugs and this result is discussed below.) It therefore appears that transmitter acetylcholine combines with nicotinic receptors to produce the N potential, and with muscarinic receptors to produce the P and LN potentials.

It may be that the muscarinic receptors on the ganglion cells play a part in the development of tolerance to the antihypertensive action of ganglion blocking drugs in man. Although the nicotinic receptors continue to be blocked, sensitization of the muscarinic receptors by the ganglion-blocking drug may lead to them playing a more important part in the transmission process so that sympathetic nerve function is partly restored.

Other drugs stimulating ganglion cells

Histamine has been shown to stimulate ganglion cells and to cause the release of catecholamines from the adrenal medulla. In very large doses it exerts the opposite effect and depresses ganglionic transmission. Doses slightly smaller than those necessary to depress transmission potentiate the ganglion-blocking action of both competitive (e.g. hexamethonium) and depolarizing (e.g. tetramethylammonium) blocking drugs.

5-Hydroxytryptamine also stimulates some ganglion cells, including those in the superior cervical ganglion of the cat and the intestine of the guinea-pig. Part of the stimulant action of 5-hydroxytryptamine on some smooth muscle preparations (e.g. guinea-pig ileum) is an indirect one brought about through stimulation of parasympathetic ganglion cells and the consequent release of acetylcholine from the postganglionic fibres.

The actions of histamine and 5-hydroxytryptamine on the ganglion cells are not blocked by hexamethonium or by atropine showing that they do not act on either of the two cholinoceptive receptor sites.

Drugs facilitating ganglionic transmission

Small doses of most of the ganglion-stimulant drugs described above, including histamine and 5-hydroxytryptamine, have been shown to facilitate ganglionic transmission when preganglionic stimulation is submaximal. A number of other chemically unrelated drugs also produce this effect. These drugs include veratrine, guanidine, small doses of adrenaline (see page 680), and digoxin and ouabain. The cardiac glycosides exert their effects by causing accumulation of intracellular sodium ions, as at the neuromuscular junctions. No clinical use is made of the property of these drugs to facilitate ganglionic transmission.

Reserpine and the antiadrenaline drug *dibenamine* facilitate transmission through the superior cervical ganglion and this has been attributed to depletion (with reserpine) or blockade of the action (by dibenamine) of noradrenaline, present in adrenergic terminals impinging on the ganglion cells (page 144). The amounts of noradrenaline normally present are presumed to be sufficient to exert an inhibitory modulating influence on transmission. Both dibenamine and atropine abolish the hyperpolarization (P potential) which forms part of the triphasic response of the ganglion cells to a preganglionic stimulus, as described above. It has therefore been suggested that acetylcholine released from the presynaptic nerve endings acts on adrenergic axons (the atropine-sensitive site) to release catecholamines, which in turn act on the ganglion cells (the dibenamine sensitive site) to initiate the inhibitory P potential.

Accumulation of catecholamines in the ganglion after inhibition of mono-amine oxidase may explain the unusual type of ganglion blockade produced by inhibitors of this enzyme described on page 626.

Anticholinesterase drugs facilitate transmission through autonomic ganglia but their effects are less striking and more difficult to demonstrate than those produced at the neuromuscular junction.

The rise in blood pressure produced by lipid soluble anticholinesterase drugs such as physostigmine and dyflos may be blocked by atropine, and is partly of central origin and partly due to facilitation of cholinergic trans-mission at muscarinic sites in sympathetic ganglia.

Large doses of the quaternary anticholinesterase drugs, neostigmine and edrophonium, have been shown to depolarize ganglion cells by a direct nicotinic action, while large doses of physostigmine block transmission without initial depolarization.

CHAPTER 28

Parasympathomimetics and Drugs Modifying Their Actions: Anti-Parkinsonian Drugs

Parasympathomimetic drugs

Barger and Dale introduced the terms 'parasympathomimetic' and 'sympathomimetic' to describe those drugs whose actions mimicked the effects of parasympathetic and sympathetic nerve stimulation respectively. Sympathomimetic drugs are described in Chapter 29. Responses to parasympathetic nerve stimulation may be reproduced by drugs which excite parasympathetic centres in the brain stem, either directly or reflexly, and by drugs which stimulate parasympathetic ganglia. Drugs which inhibit cholinesterase thereby causing an accumulation of acetylcholine may also produce effects resembling the responses to parasympathetic nerve stimulation. However, the term *parasympathomimetic* drugs is usually taken to include only those drugs which combine with acetylcholine receptors on the effector cells. In other words, parasympathomimetic drugs are those drugs which exert direct *muscarinic* actions (page 147).

Acetylcholine and drugs with a similar action were at one time thought to act on parasympathetic nerve endings rather than directly upon receptor sites on the effector cells themselves. The direct action of these drugs was first demonstrated with pilocarpine (page 703). Thus, after section and degeneration of the postganglionic parasympathetic ciliary nerve to the cat's eye, pilocarpine still constricted the pupil showing that its action was independent of the nerves.

In addition to their important muscarinic actions, many parasympathomimetic drugs exert other actions at different sites. For example, acetylcholine itself, apart from having powerful muscarinic activity, stimulates ganglion cells and striated muscle.

The effects of parasympathetic stimulation are listed in Table 4.1, pp. 123–124 and many are referred to in more detail in the descriptions of the various organs affected. All of these actions are produced by injected acetylcholine and other parasympathomimetic drugs.

Acetylcholine (20 to 100 mg intravenously) has found occasional therapeutic use to terminate attacks of paroxysmal auricular tachycardia, but on the whole its actions are too widespread and, because of its rapid hydrolysis by both true and pseudocholinesterase, too fleeting to be of real therapeutic value.

Choline possesses all of the pharmacological actions of acetylcholine but its potency is very much less. Most of the choline in the body is combined as part of the lecithin molecule. Some is free in the plasma (about 1 μg/ml) and some is combined as acetylcholine. Choline is an essential constituent of diet and is considered to be part of the vitamin B complex (page 35).

Parasympathomimetic drugs from plant sources

MUSCARINE. Muscarine is an alkaloid obtained from a toadstool, *Amanita muscaria*. It produces all of the effects of parasympathetic nerve stimulation and muscarine provides the prototype for parasympathomimetic drugs (page 138); it has no nicotinic activity. Muscarine stimulates the CNS, possibly by combining with cholinoceptive receptors in the brain, and the fungus has been chewed to produce central stimulation by inhabitants of Eastern Siberia. Muscarine is not used in medicine because its actions are too widespread, but it is occasionally used to kill flies. Cases of poisoning with *A. muscaria* are rare. 'Mushroom poisoning' is more commonly produced by *A. phalloides* which possesses a different type of toxic principle.

Naturally-occurring (+)-Muscarine (2S-methyl-3R-hydroxy-tetrahydrofuryl-5S methyl trimethylammonium).

The naturally-occurring (+)-muscarine is 200 to 800 times more potent than the (−)-isomer. A synthetic compound known as F2268 is related to muscarine and is of interest because it is one of the most potent muscarinic substances known, being 10 to 50 times more potent than acetylcholine on some tissues. The (+) form of the cis isomer which has the 2S, 5S configuration is about a 100 times as active as the (−)-2R, 5R isomer.

F2268

PILOCARPINE. Pilocarpine is obtained from species of *Pilocarpus* and is available as the nitrate and hydrochloride. Its peripheral vasodilator actions were described by Langley as long ago as 1875. Its most prominent actions are to cause profuse salivation and sweating. It finds an occasional use in the treatment of glaucoma by virtue of its miotic action (see page 419), and to counteract mydriasis produced by atropine, but otherwise it is rarely used. Large doses of pilocarpine have a stimulant action followed by a depressant action on the CNS.

Table 28.1. Parasympathomimetic drugs used in medicine.

Names	Formula	Nicotinic activity	Usual dose in man	Main clinical use
Acetylcholine chloride or bromide	$(CH_3)_3\overset{+}{N}$—CH_2—CH_2—O—CO—CH_3	Yes	20 to 100 mg intravenously	Paroxysmal auricular tachycardia (obsolete)
Choline chloride, gluconate or dihydrogen citrate	$(CH_3)_3\overset{+}{N}$—CH_2—CH_2—OH	Yes	—	Not used for its parasympathomimetic action. Some use in treatment of liver disease
Pilocarpine nitrate	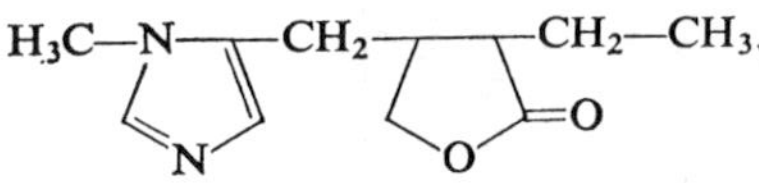	Very weak	1% solution in oil	Applied locally to the eye as a miotic
Arecoline	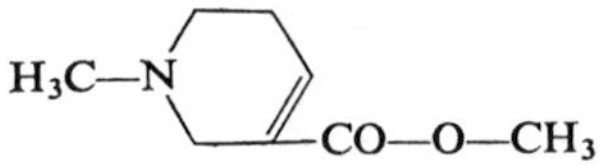	Yes	—	As a vermifuge in veterinary medicine. Not used in human medicine
Methacholine, acetyl-β-methyl choline chloride (Amechol, Mecholyl)	$(CH_3)_3\overset{+}{N}$—CH_2—CH—O—CO—CH_3 with CH_3	No	2.5 to 40 mg subcutaneously; 0.2 to 0.5% solution for iontophoresis	To slow the heart in cases of supra-ventricular tachycardias. To dilate the blood vessels in peripheral vascular diseases

Drug	Formula	Acts orally	Dose	Use
Carbachol, carba-minoyl choline chloride	$(CH_3)_3\overset{+}{N}-CH_2-CH_2-O-CO-NH_2$	Yes	0.2 to 0.5 mg subcutaneously or 1 to 4 mg orally	To produce motility of the gut in postoperative paralytic ileus and contraction of the bladder in non-obstructive urinary retention.
			Up to 3% solution	Sometimes applied locally in glaucoma
Bethanechol, carba-minoyl-β-methyl choline chloride (Urecholine, Mechothane),	$(CH_3)_3\overset{+}{N}-CH_2-\underset{\underset{CH_3}{\vert}}{CH}-O-CO-NH_2$	No	2 to 5 mg subcutaneously or 5 to 30 mg orally	As for carbachol
Meprochol bromide (Esmodil)	$(CH_3)_3\overset{+}{N}-CH_2-\underset{\underset{CH_2}{\Vert}}{C}-O-CH_3$	No	3 mg subcutaneously or intramuscularly	As for carbachol (withdrawn from use)
Furtrethonium iodide (Furmethide)	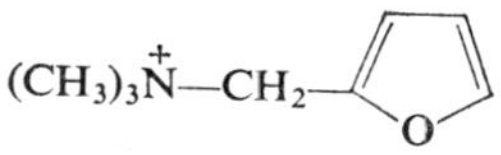 $(CH_3)_3\overset{+}{N}-CH_2-$ (furan ring)	No	5 mg subcutaneously	To contract the bladder in non-obstructive urinary retention

23

Although pilocarpine has been known the longest of all the parasympatho-mimetic drugs, its mechanism of action is difficult to understand from the point of view of structure–activity relationships, since chemically it differs from most other drugs in this class in that it does not possess a quaternary nitrogen group (Table 28.1).

ARECOLINE. Arecoline is present in the seeds known as 'betel nuts' which are habitually chewed by natives of many Oriental countries. Betel is probably used because of the central stimulant action of arecoline, although there is also increased salivary flow and digestion is said to be improved. It has no therapeutic use in man but is occasionally used as a vermifuge in veterinary medicine.

Synthetic parasympathomimetic drugs. Attempts have been made to synthesize more stable drugs than acetylcholine and with a more selective action on particular structures. The most important parasympathomimetic drugs and some of their uses and properties are listed in Table 28.1. In general they possess the same muscarinic actions as acetylcholine, but there is some select-ivity on particular structures. Thus, after systemic administration, *methacholine* is relatively more effective on the cardiovascular system, whereas *carbachol*, *bethanechol* and *furtrethonium* are relatively more active on the gastro-intestinal tract and on the bladder. Methacholine is the only medicinally-useful syn-thetic parasympathomimetic drug which is destroyed by cholinesterase to a significant extent (Table 28.1). However, unlike acetylcholine, which is a sub-strate both for acetylcholinesterase and for pseudocholinesterase, meta-choline is destroyed only by acetylcholinesterase. The Pharmacopoeal prep-aration of methacholine is the racemic compound. The (+)-S-isomer is about equal to acetylcholine in its muscarinic potency, but is destroyed by acetyl-cholinesterase at only about half the rate that acetylcholine is destroyed. The muscarinic activity of the (−)-R-isomer is only about 1/500 that of acetyl-choline. It is only very slowly destroyed by acetylcholinesterase and acts as a weak inhibitor of the enzyme.

Parasympathomimetic drugs are used (i) to stimulate the intestines and bladder in postoperative intestinal atony and urinary retention, (ii) to terminate attacks of paroxysmal auricular tachycardia, (iii) to lower intra-ocular pressure in glaucoma, (iv) to promote salivation and sweating, particularly to overcome the effects of atropine, and (v) to dilate peripheral blood vessels in conditions of vascular spasm, such as *Raynaud's disease* (page 281). Choice of the drug depends upon the condition being treated (Table 28.1).

Acetylcholine is injected intravenously since absorption by other routes is irregular and unpredictable owing to its rapid destruction. The other para-sympathomimetics are dangerous when injected intravenously and are usually administered by mouth or by subcutaneous injection. However, methacholine is particularly unreliable when given orally because it is largely destroyed in the intestine. When used for their effects on the eye, the drugs are instilled into the conjunctiva. In peripheral vascular disease, methacholine may be given by iontophoresis (page 830).

The therapeutic use of parasympathomimetic drugs depends upon their muscarinic actions but, like acetylcholine, some of them possess nicotinic actions in addition (Table 28.1). Nicotinic actions are not a serious disadvantage, however, as the doses required to produce them are much larger than those used therapeutically. Experimentally, a nicotinic action may be detected by the following tests. (1) After sufficient atropine has been administered to block muscarinic actions, large doses of parasympathomimetics which possess a nicotinic action cause a rise in blood pressure in the anaesthetized cat due to stimulation of the sympathetic ganglia of the vasoconstrictor and cardio-accelerator nerves, and to the release of catecholamines from the adrenal medullae. An experiment demonstrating the nicotinic action of acetylcholine in this way is illustrated in Fig. 5.1 (page 139). Hexamethonium abolishes these nicotinic actions, just as it abolishes the actions of nicotine itself (Fig. 27.3, page 692). (2) Drugs which possess a nicotinic action on skeletal muscle cause a contraction of the tibialis anterior muscle of the cat on close-arterial injection (Figs. 5.4, page 146 and 7.4b, page 200), and contracture both of the frog's rectus abdominis muscle and of certain avian muscles (Fig. 26.6, page 674), and of chronically denervated mammalian muscles (Fig. 7.4c, page 200). These effects on skeletal muscle are blocked by tubocurarine (Figs. 5.4a, page 146 and 26.6a, page 674).

Structure-action relationship among acetylcholine-like drugs. Extensive pharmacological studies of acetylcholine and closely related compounds have been made in an attempt to gain information about the drug-receptor. However, the nature of the receptor is still largely unknown and it is not yet possible to say which molecular features are essential for acetylcholine-like activity as there are exceptions to the various hypotheses advanced. Nevertheless much valuable information has been gained from these studies, and they serve to illustrate one method employed in the search for new drugs. The potency of acetylcholine-like drugs relative to that of acetylcholine itself varies widely according to the species and to the tissue being studied. Because of this, detailed figures for relative potency are not given in the discussion below. Widely differing potency ratios in different tests may mean that the configuration of the receptors differs in different species and tissues. One complication in attempting to reach conclusions concerning the nature of a receptor from studies of relative potencies of agonists is that agonistic potency is dependent on two properties—affinity for the receptor and efficacy (or intrinsic activity, see page 462). For example, the fact that a change in chemical structure may reduce the agonistic potency of a compound does not necessarily mean that it combines less efficiently with the receptor. There may be a decrease in efficacy but affinity for the receptors may remain the same or even be increased. Such a compound would then behave as a partial agonist. A further complication with esters of choline is that increased potency may be the result of decreased destruction by enzymic hydrolysis rather than increased efficacy or affinity.

The intramolecular portions of the acetylcholine molecule which play a part in combination with the receptor may be considered under the following headings.

THE CATIONIC HEAD. The quaternized nitrogen atom is positively charged and is referred to as the 'cationic head'. This part of the molecule gives acetylcholine its strongly basic character. A positively-charged centre with attached methyl groups appears to be very important for agonist activity (cf. the simple tetramethylammonium ion, page 696). Replacement of one or more of the methyl groups of the cationic head by hydrogen atoms results in loss of the positive charge and there is a decrease in both muscarinic and nicotinic activity. When two or all methyl groups are replaced, agonist activity is diminished as much as 500 to 40,000 times, depending upon the tissue. The importance of the positive charge suggests that the initial attraction between acetylcholine and its receptor is an electrostatic one and this implies a negatively charged *anionic* site on the receptor (Fig. 28.1).

An increase in the size of the cationic head also causes a loss of both muscarinic and nicotinic potency. This has been demonstrated with acetylcholine analogues in which the nitrogen atom was replaced by phosphorus, sulphur or arsenic, and also with analogues in which the methyl groups attached to the nitrogen atom were progressively replaced by larger alkyl radicals. It has been suggested that for agonistic activity the cationic head must fit into a hemispherical depression in the receptor surface (Fig. 28.1). Only two of the methyl groups are involved in this process. The compound in which one methyl group is replaced by an ethyl group has about a quarter of the potency of acetylcholine. The explanation of this relatively small loss of potency is that there is a reduced probability of the cationic head being in the correct position, with both methyl groups presented to the receptor surface. The replacement of two methyl groups by ethyl groups causes a very pronounced loss of activity (300 to 1500 times less potent than acetylcholine) because there is now much less possibility of the cationic head fitting into the hemispherical depression. These compounds behave as partial agonists. When all three methyl groups are replaced by ethyl groups, acetylcholine-like activity is lost and in some tissues the compound acts as a weak acetylcholine antagonist (cf. the tetraethylammonium ion, page 690).

THE ESTER-LINK. The ester-link is concerned in the combination with the receptor, and hence with agonist activity. When this is absent, as in *n*-amyltrimethylammonium ($(CH_3)_3.N^+$—CH_2—CH_2—CH_3—CH_2—CH_3), potency is many times less at both muscarinic and nicotinic sites. Both carbonyl and ether oxygens are involved in the combination with the receptor, the carbonyl oxygen being relatively more important for nicotinic activity and the ether oxygen for muscarinic activity. Thus, 4-keto-amyltrimethylammonium ($(CH_3)_3.N^+$—CH_2—CH_2—CH_2—CO—CH_3), is fairly potent in its nicotinic activity but weak in muscarinic activity; on the other hand, the ethyl ether of choline ($(CH_3)_3.N^+$—CH_2—CH_2—O—CH_2—CH_3) has high muscarinic but low nicotinic activity. Although less active than acetylcholine, both of these compounds are more potent than *n*-amyltrimethylammonium in both muscarinic and nicotinic activity.

THE ALKYLAMINE CHAIN. The distance between the nitrogen and the ester group is optimal in acetylcholine; the compound with one less —CH_2— group (acetylnorcholine) and that with one additional —CH_2— group (acetylhomocholine) are much weaker than acetylcholine; there is more loss of muscarinic than of nicotinic activity.

These results show that both the presence and position of the ester link are important for agonist activity and this suggests the presence of additional active sites on the receptor protein at approximately the same distances from the anionic site as the ether and carbonyl oxygens in acetylcholine are from the cationic head. However, it is interesting to note that the so-called 'reversed carboxy ester' of acetylcholine (CH_3—O—CO—CH_2—CH_2—$N^+(CH_3)_3$) is about equipotent with acetylcholine. The ester-link constitutes a dipole which presumably interacts with a dipole or so-called *esteratic site* on the receptor.

The total length of the chain attached to the onium group is also important, being optimal in acetylcholine. This is illustrated, for example, by the increase in activity of 5-methylfurtrethonium over that of furtrethonium itself. The formula of furtrethonium is given in Table 28.1. The additional methyl group is probably bound to the receptor protein by van der Waals' forces.

Branching of the alkylamine chain alters the activity of acetylcholine-like compounds. The addition of a methyl group to the β-carbon atom to produce acetyl-β-methylcholine (methacholine, Table 28.1) results in almost complete loss of nicotinic activity, but muscarinic activity of the (+)-S-isomer is retained. In contrast, acetyl-α-methylcholine retains nicotinic activity to about the same extent as acetylcholine. However the racemic compound has about 40 times less, the (−)-S-isomer about 90 times less, and the (+)-R-isomer about 25 times less muscarinic activity than acetylcholine. Similar variations in potency are produced when methyl groups are substituted in the molecule of carbachol; for example, bethanechol (Table 28.1) has very little nicotinic activity.

THE ACETYL GROUP. Choline (Table 28.1) possesses all of the pharmacological properties of acetylcholine but is 100 to 100,000 times less potent depending upon the tissue and the species in which they are compared. Even ethyltrimethylammonium $((CH_3)_3N^+CH_2CH_3)$ is more potent than choline, which suggests that the hydroxyl group of choline in some way impairs its reaction with the receptor. Possibly hydrogen bonding between the hydroxyl group of choline and water molecules of the extracellular fluid prevent its close approach to the receptor. Masking of the OH group of choline, by esterification with any of the lower fatty acids or by ether formation, enhances activity.

Esterification with acetic acid to give acetylcholine produces optimal muscarinic activity but nicotinic activity is greater with some of the higher molecular weight fatty acids. The relative potency varies in different tissues but formyl-, carbamoyl-, propionyl-, butyryl-, valeryl-, trimethylacetyl-, benzoyl-, phenylacetyl- and β-phenylpropionyl-cholines are all weaker than acetylcholine in their muscarine-like actions. Of these, the choline esters of aromatic acids are almost devoid of muscarinic action and esters with fatty acids higher than butyric possess atropine-like activity. However, many of these compounds are more potent than acetylcholine in nicotinic activity.

Cholinoceptive receptors. The foregoing discussion indicates that differences exist, at least in the spatial arrangement of the active sites, between muscarinic and nicotinic receptors. This is also borne out by a consideration of acetylcholine antagonists. Antimuscarinic drugs, such as atropine, bear little chemical relationship to antinicotinic drugs such as hexamethonium and tubocurarine. Furthermore, differences also appear to exist between the nicotinic receptors in different tissues, since ganglion blocking drugs are chemically distinct from neuromuscular blocking drugs. Tubocurarine has antinicotinic activity at both sites, but the remaining neuromuscular-blocking drugs are devoid of ganglion blocking activity and the ganglion blocking drug, hexamethonium, has little neuromuscular blocking activity. One additional cholinoceptive site, presumably differing to some extent from all of the others, is that on the enzyme cholinesterase. Antagonists of acetylcholine on receptors are usually not inhibitors of the enzyme, at least *in vivo*, and anticholinesterase drugs have, at the most, only weak antagonistic activity to acetylcholine at sites other than the enzyme.

Acetylcholine, being a flexible molecule, may combine with all of these cholinoceptive sites. A consideration of the position of important groups in

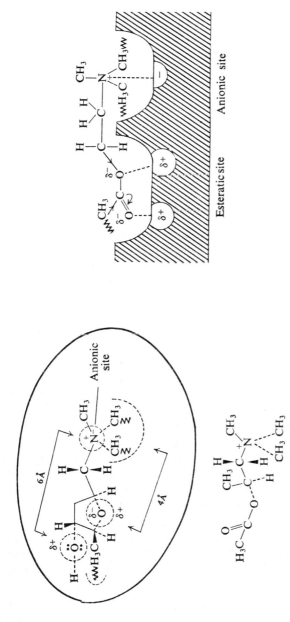

Fig. 28.1. Hypothetical structure of the muscarinic receptor. The diagram on the left shows a plan view of a molecule of (+)-2S:3R:5S-muscarine superimposed on the receptor. The dotted circles represent active sites on the receptor. The zig-zag lines (∿∿) indicate areas of van der Waals' binding. A molecule of (+)-S-acetyl-β-methyl choline with a configuration similar to that of (+)-muscarine is shown below. The diagram on the right shows a 'side-view' of a molecule of acetylcholine in combination with a muscarinic receptor. Ionic binding occurs at the anionic site and attraction between partial charges at the esteratic site. Van der Waals' binding occurs where methyl groups approach the receptor protein.

more rigid molecules provides information on the position of active sites on the receptor. The molecule of naturally occurring (+)-muscarine is rigid and it has high potency, therefore it lends itself to the analysis of the structure of muscarinic receptors. In (+)-2S, 3R, 5S-muscarine, the methyl group and the onium group are on the same side of the ring, being *trans* to the hydroxyl group. Any variation in the arrangement or orientation of these three groups, or omission of one or more of them from the tetrahydrofuran ring, markedly reduces muscarinic activity. These considerations have led to the hypothetical depictions of the muscarinic receptor illustrated in Fig. 28.1. It therefore appears that when acetylcholine, or a similar flexible molecule such as methacholine, reacts with muscarinic receptors they must exist in a form (Fig. 28.1) analogous to that of naturally occurring muscarine.

Anticholinesterase drugs

The cholinesterase enzymes and the methods of estimating the rates at which they hydrolyse acetylcholine and other choline esters are described on pages 156–158. Many drugs inhibit the *in vitro* enzymatic hydrolysis of acetylcholine when added to the enzyme-substrate mixture. However, this does not necessarily mean that the pharmacological effects of these drugs is a consequence of an anticholinesterase action. For example, the anticholinesterase activity of decamethonium may be readily demonstrated *in vitro* but it is unlikely that this effect contributes much to its *in vivo* pharmacological action. On the other hand, some drugs, which are inactive in *in vitro* experiments, may exert a powerful *in vivo* anticholinesterase action as a result of the enzyme-inhibiting properties of a metabolite. The organo-phosphorus compounds, schradan and parathion (Table 28.3), are examples; they are oxidized in the liver to highly active metabolites. The oxidation product of parathion, which is known as paraoxan, is commercially available.

The drugs classified as anticholinesterases are those whose primary action is to inhibit cholinesterase. In experiments on whole animals or on isolated tissues, they can be readily shown to potentiate the effects of cholinergic nerve stimulation and of injected acetylcholine. Most of them cause 50% enzyme inhibition *in vitro* in concentrations of the order of 10^{-6}M or less. When attempting to correlate the pharmacological effect of a drug on a particular tissue with its *in vitro* anticholinesterase activity, it is important that the enzyme preparation used in the *in vitro* work should be obtained from the same species and preferably from the same tissue; this is because enzymes from different species and tissues may vary in the type of substrates and inhibitors with which they combine. An extreme example of these differences is found in the cholinesterases from the domestic fowl which, unlike their mammalian counterparts, are incapable of combining with bisquaternary substrates or inhibitors. Thus, the cholinesterase in hen plasma cannot destroy suxamethonium, and the bisquaternary compound *ambenonium*, which is a very powerful inhibitor of mammalian acetylcholinesterase, is almost inactive against hen cholinesterases. Much of the work with acetylcholinesterases has been carried out on the enzyme present in the electric organ of certain fishes (particularly *Electrophorus electricus*) because it can be obtained in an almost pure form. However, relative enzyme-inhibiting potencies of anticholinesterase drugs calculated from *in vitro* studies using an enzyme preparation from a particular species are strictly applicable only to that species and serve as no more than a guide when applied to others.

Some anticholinesterases have a selective action in inhibiting only acetyl- or only butyrylcholinesterase. For example, bis(3-dimethylamino-5-hydroxyphenoxy)1,3-propane dimethiodide (3116CT) is 250,000 times more potent against the acetylcholinesterase of human red cells than against the butyrylcholinesterase of human plasma, whereas 10-(1-diethylaminopropionyl) phenothiazine hydrochloride (Astra 1397) is 10,000 times more potent against the plasma enzyme. These selective inhibitors are valuable tools for helping to classify the cholinesterases present in different tissues. The anticholinesterases used in medicine are less selective; in general they are slightly more potent against pseudocholinesterases than against true cholinesterases, but they inhibit both types. Inhibition of butyrylcholinesterases is probably of importance for stimulant action on the gut but on the whole the therapeutic use of anticholinesterases stems from their ability to inhibit acetylcholinesterase.

Anticholinesterase drugs act by combining with cholinesterase and so preventing the enzyme from hydrolysing acetylcholine. Acetylcholine liberated at the various sites in the body therefore accumulates and exerts its effects to a greater degree. The actions of anticholinesterase drugs at the neuromuscular junction and at autonomic ganglia are described on pages 681 and 701. Their effects on autonomically innervated structures are similar to those of acetylcholine itself; they differ only in their relative slowness of onset and more prolonged duration of action.

Anticholinesterase drugs can be divided into two main classes according to their chemical composition and to the stability of the enzyme-inhibitor complex. Those which dissociate from the enzyme when their concentration in the extracellular fluid falls (reversible anticholinesterases) bear some structural resemblance to acetylcholine itself (Table 28.2); those which form an irreversible complex with the enzyme are unrelated to acetylcholine and may be classed together as the organo-phosphorus anticholinesterases (Table 28.3). Most of the anticholinesterases used in medicine are of the reversible type. The organophosphorus compounds are mainly used as insecticides. Some of the latter (e.g.

23*

sarin and tabun) were developed as war gases; they are the so-called 'nerve gases'.

Reversible anticholinesterases. *Physostigmine* (eserine) is a naturally-occurring anticholinesterase drug obtained from the Calabar bean. It was first isolated in 1864 by Jobst and Hesse and synthesized in 1935 by Julian and Pike. Physostigmine contains a urethane group (Table 28.2) and synthetic compounds possessing this grouping include some of the most potent reversible anticholinesterase drugs. Urethane (ethylcarbamate) possesses some anticholinesterase activity and for this reason the effects of anticholinesterase drugs are sometimes difficult to demonstrate in animals anaesthetized with urethane.

After the elucidation of the structure of physostigmine, many compounds with a substituted carbamic acid grouping were synthesized and tested for anticholinesterase activity. Of these, *neostigmine* (Prostigmin), first studied by Aeschliman and Reinert in 1931, has proved to be the most successful, and remains the most widely-used synthetic anticholinesterase. Unlike physostigmine, neostigmine contains a quaternary ammonium grouping (Table 28.2). The strong onium charge increases its rate of association with the enzyme and the onset of action of neostigmine is therefore more rapid, although its potency *in vitro* is similar to that of the tertiary amine, physostigmine.

A hypothetical depiction of the reaction of neostigmine with cholinesterase is illustrated in Fig. 28.2. At the pH of the body physostigmine is positively charged and combines with the anionic site in a similar way to neostigmine, whilst the ester grouping interacts with the esteratic site. Kinetic studies have shown that these anticholinesterase drugs inhibit the enzyme in a competitive manner. The esteratic site is the part of the enzyme receptor which hydrolyses acetylcholine (see page 157). However, substituted carbamic esters like physostigmine and neostigmine are much more stable to hydrolysis and consequently they remain bound to the enzyme for a longer time. The enzyme-inhibitor complex dissociates as the drug concentration in the extracellular fluid is lowered through excretion and inactivation, and it is also probable that physostigmine and neostigmine are themselves slowly hydrolysed by the enzyme.

Wilson and Bergmann studied the effect of alterations of pH on the *in vitro* inhibitory activity of physostigmine and neostigmine, and their results form part of the evidence for the presence of an anionic site in the active centre of acetylcholinesterase. At a pH of 8 or less, physostigmine is largely in the cationic form and was highly active, but above 8, where the ionization is suppressed, the inhibitory potency of physostigmine declined. Neostigmine, being a quaternary compound, retains its positive charge over a wide range

TABLE 28.2. Reversible anticholinesterase drugs used in medicine.

Names	Formula	Route of administration and usual dose	Main clinical use
Physostigmine salicylate or sulphate (Eserine)	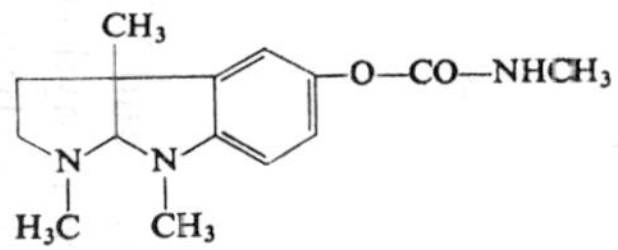	Applied to conjunctiva: 0·1 to 1% solutions or lamellae each containing 0·065 mg	Main use now restricted to its miotic action, especially in glaucoma
Neostigmine methylsulphate or bromide (Prostigmin)	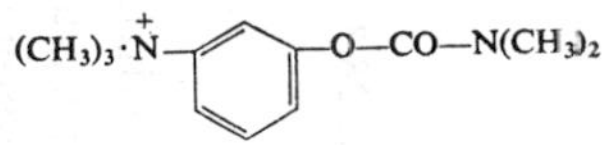	Orally: 15 to 30 mg of bromide. Intravenously: 0·25 to 1 mg of methylsulphate	To stimulate bowel and bladder movement and in myasthenia gravis. As an antagonist of tubocurarine and related drugs
Pyridostigmine bromide (Mestinon)	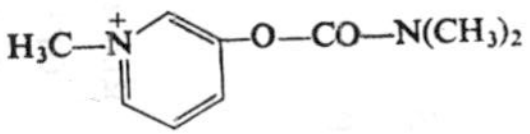	Orally: 60 to 300 mg/day	In myasthenia gravis (longer duration of action and fewer visceral side-effects than neostigmine.)
Benzpyrinium bromide (Stigmonene)	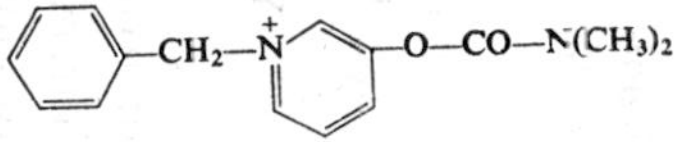	Intramuscularly: 0.5 mg.	To stimulate bowel and bladder movement (no advantage over neostigmine)
Edrophonium chloride (Tensilon)	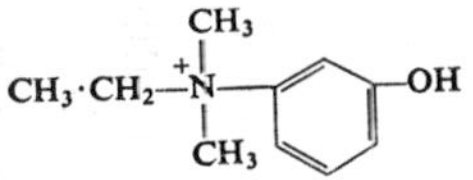	Intravenously: 10 mg.	As an aid to the diagnosis of myasthenia gravis. (Too short-acting for other uses.)
Distigmine bromide (Ubretid)	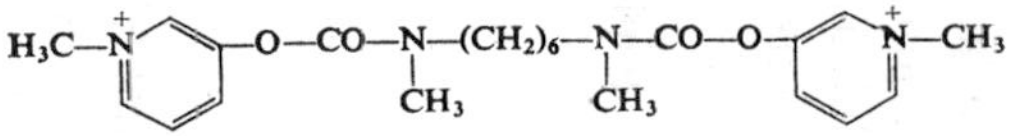	Orally: 5 to 15 mg every 3rd day. Intramuscularly: 0·75 to 1·5 mg every 3rd day	Functional insufficiency of the bladder. Urinary incontinence. Post-operative intestinal atony.

of pH values and its enzyme inhibitory potency was found to be independent of the pH of the medium.

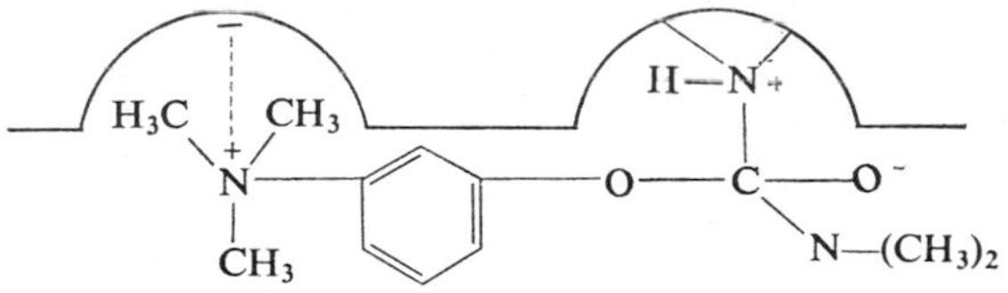

FIG. 28.2. Hypothetical depiction of the reaction of neostigmine with acetylcholinesterase. (Cf. reaction of acetylcholine with this enzyme, Fig. 5.7, page 157.)

Other medicinally useful anticholinesterase drugs related to neostigmine are *benzpyrinium, pyridostigmine* and *distigmine* (Table 28.2).

It is now known that the urethane grouping is not essential for anticholinesterase activity. An important compound without this grouping is *edrophonium*, which combines very rapidly with cholinesterase and has a very rapid dissociation rate on dilution. Consequently, its onset of effect is abrupt and its duration of action very short. Edrophonium produces only very weak muscarinic actions but is a potent anti-curare although its short duration of action limits its usefulness (page 684).

Organophosphorus anticholinesterases. These are mainly pentavalent phosphorus compounds with the general structure:

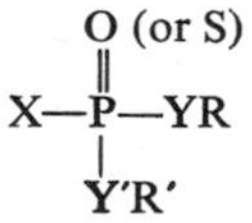

$$\begin{array}{c} O \text{ (or S)} \\ \| \\ X-P-YR \quad \text{(see Table 28.3)} \\ | \\ Y'R' \end{array}$$

R and R' denote alkyl or aromatic groups, or hydrogen; Y and Y' are usually oxygen but may be sulphur, nitrogen or carbon; X is an easily hydrolysed group which may be organic or inorganic. Some compounds have been synthesized in which the labile group, denoted as X, contains a quaternary nitrogen atom. These compounds are collectively known as the 'phosphostigmines' and are highly active inhibitors. The quaternary group presumably reacts initially with the anionic site of the enzyme by electrostatic attraction. The formulae of some of the more important organophosphorus anticholinesterases are given in Table 28.3.

The organophosphorus cholinesterase inhibitors which do not possess a quaternary nitrogen, react only with the esteratic site of cholinesterase. The reaction takes place in two stages. The first stage of this reaction is reversible, the enzyme-inhibitor complex dissociating when the concentration of inhibitor is reduced by dilution. The second stage involves the removal by hydrolysis of group X, with the result that the esteratic site becomes phosphorylated. Unlike the acetyl-enzyme which is produced during the break-down of acetylcholine (page 157), the phosphoryl-enzyme is stable and at this stage the cholinesterase is irreversibly inhibited. Dissociation of the phosphoryl group from the cholinesterase by hydrolysis, with the production of re-activated enzyme, is a

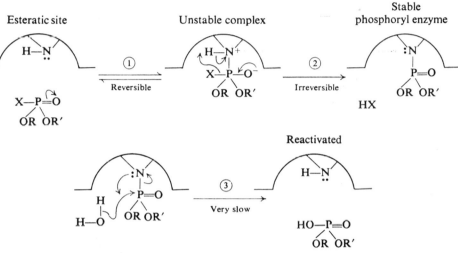

FIG. 28.3. Reaction of an organophosphorus compound with the esteratic site of cholinesterase.

slow process, and with some inhibitors (such as dyflos) it may take several months. The reaction of the organophosphorus agents with the esteratic site of cholinesterase is illustrated in Fig. 28.3 (cf. reaction with acetylcholine Fig. 5.7 on page 158). Hydrolysis of the phosphoryl-enzyme complex is very slow but more rapid reactivation of the enzyme can be brought about by nucleophilic agents such as choline or hydroxylamine (NH_2OH) which catalyse hydrolysis. The mechanism is probably as illustrated in Fig. 28.4.

A more potent compound than hydroxylamine in reactivating phosphorylated cholinesterase is *pralidoxime iodide* (2-pyridine aldoxime iodide, P-2-AM). This compound possesses a quarternary ammonium group (compound (*a*) below) which is attracted to the anionic site of acetylcholinesterase and holds the molecule in position so that the nucleophilic group is directed towards the phosphoryl group.

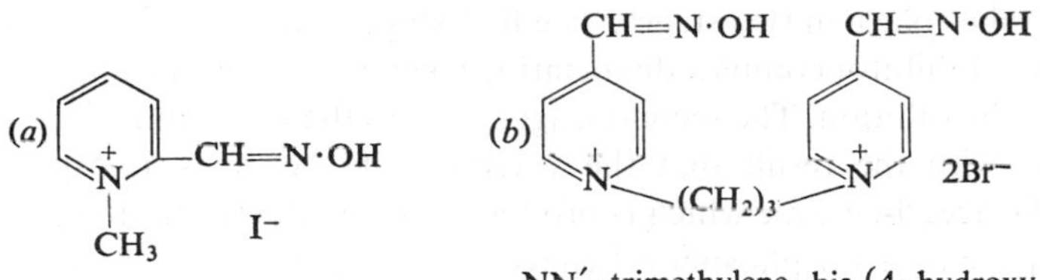

(a) Pralidoxime iodide

(b) NN′-trimethylene-bis(4-hydroxy iminomethyl-pyridinium)dibromide

Since the discovery of this action of pralidoxime, several more potent re-activators of phosphorylated cholinesterase have been synthesized. These compounds contain the —CH=NOH group and the most active are bis-quaternary derivatives of P4-AM. Of these NN′-trimethylene-bis(4-hydroxy-iminomethyl-pyridinium) dibromide (compound (b) above) is one of the most potent.

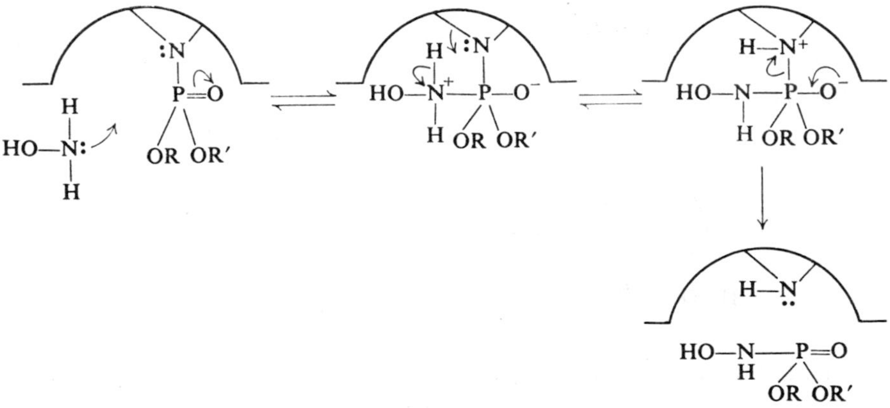

FIG. 28.4. Reactivation of phosphoryl enzyme by hydroxylamine.

In experiments in which phosphorylated cholinesterase has been stored for a long time, it has been found that less and less enzyme becomes capable of subsequent reactivation by nucleophilic agents. This seems to be due to the removal by hydrolysis of one alkoxy group; the resultant hydrogen phosphate form of the inhibited enzyme (Fig. 28.5) is resistant to nucleophilic agents.

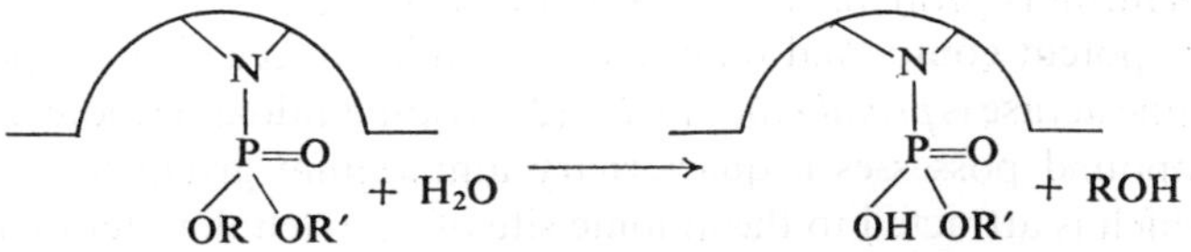

FIG. 28.5. Production of the hydrogen phosphate form of the inhibited enzyme after prolonged combination with an organophosphate inhibitor.

It is possible to protect animals from the lethal effects of an organophosphorus cholinesterase inhibitor by first administering a reversible inhibitor, such as physostigmine or neostigmine. The reversible inhibitor combines with some of the enzyme and prevents the combination of the organophosphorus compound. The organophosphorus compound is unstable in solution and its potency is lost before the effects of the reversible inhibitor have worn off. Thus, providing the dose of reversible inhibitor is big enough, sufficient enzyme to maintain life will be reactivated before the lethal effects of the organophosphorus compound occur.

Two important organophosphorus compounds which are used in medicine are *dyflos* (di-isopropylfluorophosphonate, DFP) and *ethylpyrophosphate* (tetraethylpyrophosphate, TEPP). On the whole, the cumulative, widespread and long-lasting effects of this type of compound make them unsuitable for systemic administration, and their use has been largely abandoned; an exception is the use of dyflos as a miotic in glaucoma. In this condition, the dyflos is dissolved in oil and applied locally to the eye. The fall in intraocular tension produced by a single application may last as long as 2 to 3 weeks.

Analogues of dyflos were prepared in 1932 and were studied in great detail during the Second World War as substances that could be employed as war gases; they are volatile and are absorbed through the lungs.

Dyflos inhibits both pseudo- and true cholinesterase but it is much more active (about 250 times) against pseudocholinesterases. Ethylpyrophosphate is more water-soluble although it is more unstable in solution than dyflos. It is relatively more effective against true cholinesterase than is dyflos and its onset of action is more rapid. The phosphorylated enzyme complex produced by ethylpyrophosphate dissociates more rapidly and the duration of action of ethylpyrophosphate is therefore shorter than that of dyflos.

Table 28.3 gives the names, formulae and LD_{50} values in mice or rats of a few of the hundreds of organophosphorus compounds that have been studied. Owing to their widespread use as insecticides, cases of poisoning are not uncommon; most are volatile and may be absorbed through the lungs, and some, such as parathion, may be absorbed through intact skin. A few (such as malathion and dipterex) are more toxic to insects than to mammals (Table 28.3) because of differences in metabolism.

Some research workers believe that, in addition to inhibiting cholinesterase, many anticholinesterase drugs stimulate the release of acetylcholine from nerve endings. When anticholinesterase drugs are added to isolated segments of gut, the usual effect is a gradually developing spasm of the smooth muscle. However, the organophosphorus anticholinesterase *mipafox* is said not to

TABLE 28.3. Organophosphorus anticholinesterases.

Names	Formula	Intraperitoneal LD$_{50}$ values (mg/kg)
Isopropylmethylphosphoro-fluoridate (Sarin)	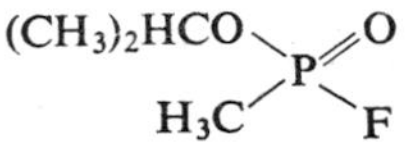 (CH$_3$)$_2$HCO, H$_3$C — P=O, F	0·42 (mice)
Diisopropylfluorophospho-nate (Dyflos, DFP)	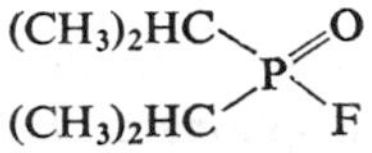 (CH$_3$)$_2$HC, (CH$_3$)$_2$HC — P=O, F	4 (mice)
Ethyl-N,N-dimethylphos-phoramidocyanidate (Tabun)	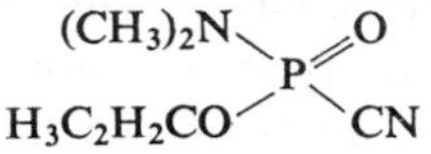 (CH$_3$)$_2$N, H$_3$C$_2$H$_2$CO — P=O, CN	0·6 (mice)
N,N′-Diisopropylphosphoro-diamidic fluoride (Mipafox)	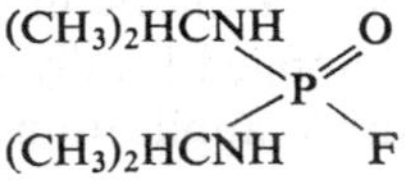 (CH$_3$)$_2$HCNH, (CH$_3$)$_2$HCNH — P, O, F	90 (rats)
Dimethyl 2,2,2-trichloro-1-hydroxyethyl phosphonate (Dipterex)	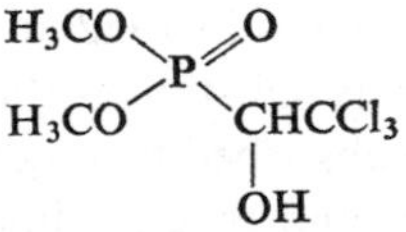 H$_3$CO, H$_3$CO — P=O, CHCCl$_3$, OH	500 (mice)
O,O′-diethyl S-(2-ethylthio-ethyl) phosphorothioate (Systox)	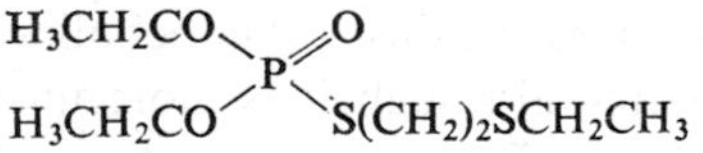 H$_3$CH$_2$CO, H$_3$CH$_2$CO — P=O, S(CH$_2$)$_2$SCH$_2$CH$_3$	5·8 (mice)
O-Ethyl O-(4-nitrophenyl) phenylphosphonothioate (EPN)	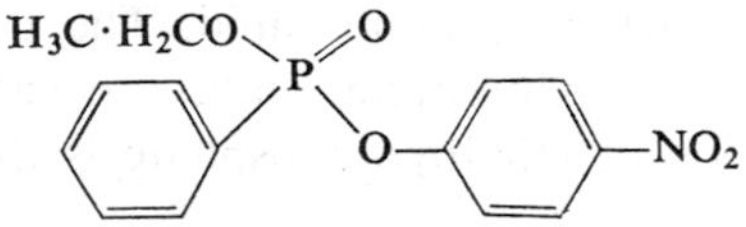 H$_3$C·H$_2$CO, C$_6$H$_5$ — P=O, O—C$_6$H$_4$—NO$_2$	48 (mice)
O,O′-Diethyl O-(4-nitrophenyl) phosphorothioate (Parathion)	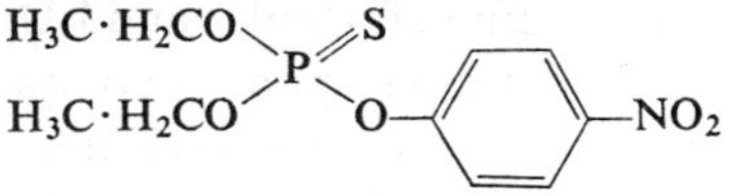 H$_3$C·H$_2$CO, H$_3$C·H$_2$CO — P=S, O—C$_6$H$_4$—NO$_2$	10 to 12 (mice) (subcutan-eously)
O,O′-Dimethyl S-(1,2-dicarb-ethoxy ethyl) phosphoro-dithioate (Malathion)	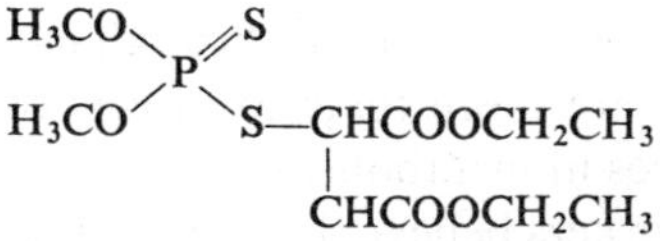 H$_3$CO, H$_3$CO — P=S, S—CHCOOCH$_2$CH$_3$, CHCOOCH$_2$CH$_3$	750 (rats)
Tetraethylpyrophosphate (Ethyl pyrophosphate, TEPP)	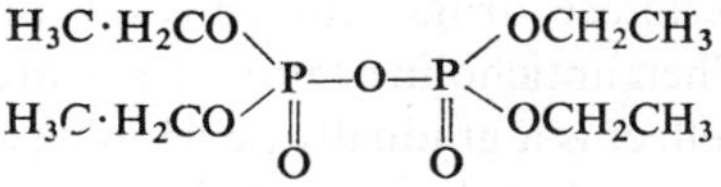 H$_3$C·H$_2$CO, H$_3$C·H$_2$CO — P—O—P, OCH$_2$CH$_3$, OCH$_2$CH$_3$ (both P=O)	0·7 (mice)

TABLE 28.3—*continued*

Names	Formula	Intraperitoneal LD$_{50}$ values (mg/kg)
Octamethylpyrophosphor-tetramide (Schradan, OMPA)	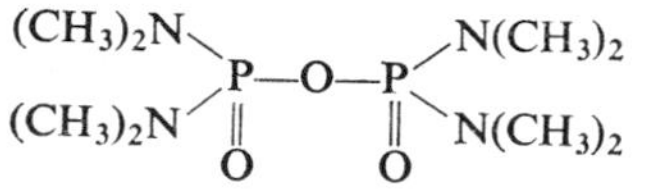 $(CH_3)_2N$ $\sim$ P—O—P $\sim$ N$(CH_3)_2$ / $(CH_3)_2N$ $\parallel$ $\parallel$ N$(CH_3)_2$ / O O	17 (mice)
2-Trimethylammonium-1-methyl-ethyl methyl phosphono-fluoridate (a phosphostigmine)	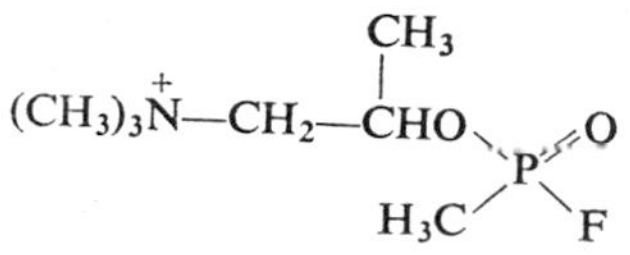 $(CH_3)_3\overset{+}{N}$—CH_2—CHO $\sim$ ... CH$_3$ / P $\rightleftharpoons$ O / H$_3$C F	0·07 (mice)

cause spasm of the gut. This is possibly because it does not stimulate acetylcholine release, but whatever the reason, mipafox is useful in producing a sensitive preparation of isolated intestine for the assay of acetylcholine.

Actions of anticholinesterase drugs on the CNS. In general, lipid-insoluble anticholinesterase drugs such as neostigmine exert a mainly depressant action on the CNS whereas lipid-soluble drugs such as physostigmine and DFP are predominantly excitatory, although very large doses cause depression. The site of action of the drugs therefore appears to depend upon their lipid solubility. Central actions are not produced by the doses employed clinically. Most central actions of anticholinesterases are blocked by atropine.

In animal experiments, chiefly using rats, physostigmine causes a rise in blood pressure. The site of action of this effect is in the midbrain and it is blocked by atropine. Surprisingly, the discharges in the vasoconstrictor fibres responsible for effecting the pressor response are not blocked by hexamethonium, and it appears that transmission at the synapses between the presynaptic fibres and the sympathetic ganglion cells involve the ganglionic *muscarinic* receptors described on pages 147 and 698.

Poisoning with anticholinesterase drugs. The toxic symptoms consist of effects associated with overactivity of the parasympathetic nervous system, coupled with powerful fasciculations of skeletal muscle. Death is caused through pulmonary oedema or by depression of the respiratory centre; powerful fasciculations or even neuromuscular block of the respiratory muscles may contribute to the respiratory failure.

Treatment consists of administering atropine to prevent both the powerful muscarinic actions and the depressant effect on the respiratory centre. In the case of the organophosphorus compounds, it may be necessary to administer for several weeks large doses of atropine which may be many times the usual lethal dose and this may be coupled with the use of a nucleophilic agent to reactivate the enzyme. Atropine does not prevent the distressing muscle fasciculations and the use of tubocurarine is impractical, so endotracheal intubation and artificial respiration may be necessary.

NEUROTOXICITY PRODUCED BY ORGANOPHOSPHORUS COMPOUNDS. Many organophosphorus compounds, including certain triaryl phosphates and alkylorganophosphorus compounds, give rise to delayed but long-lasting neurotoxic effects. These consist of polyneuritis, with flaccid paralysis of the distal muscles of the extremities and degeneration of the myelin sheaths and axons of the medulla, the spinal cord and the sciatic nerve. Many of the cases of poisoning have been caused by triorthocresyl phosphate; this substance, which has anticholinesterase activity, is present in certain mineral oils used as a substitute for cooking fats in Germany during the Second World War. All of the potent compounds which cause neurotoxicity are inhibitors of butyryl cholinesterase and this enzyme is present in the Schwann cells which are responsible for the production of myelin. However, not all organophosphorus inhibitors of butyrylcholinesterase cause neurotoxicity, and inhibition of the enzyme does not appear to be the direct cause of the lesion. In the formation of the phosphoryl enzyme, the group denoted as X (in the general formula given on page 716) is hydrolysed off and may act as a toxophore which is therefore liberated at the site of myelin formation. For example, the fluoride ion, which is released in this way from dyflos, is particularly toxic. No drug is effective in the treatment of neurotoxicity; treatment consists simply of physiotherapy.

Passive permeability and active transport. There is evidence that acetylcholine, acting as a local hormone, and acetylcholinesterase together may control passive permeability or active ion transport in some excitable membranes. Anticholinesterase drugs inhibit active sodium transport across isolated frog skin, across the membrane of frog muscle cells, and through the isolated gills of a variety of crab, but no evidence of a similar action has yet been demonstrated in mammalian tissues.

Inhibition of enzymes other than cholinesterase. The reversible inhibitors such as neostigmine and physostigmine are relatively specific for the cholinesterases; very large doses of physostigmine have been shown to inhibit choline acetyltransferase *in vitro*.

Although their main pharmacological and toxic effects are due to cholinesterase inhibition, organophosphorus inhibitors are not specific for the cholinesterases and inhibit a wide variety of enzymes; most of these are esterases (including proteases) but a few are oxidases or dehydrogenases. Esterases have been divided into three classes—A, B and C—according to their reaction with organophosphorus compounds. Most esterases other than cholinesterase are believed to possess only an esteratic site. A-esterases are present in the liver, kidney and serum; they combine with organophosphorus compounds but the phosphorylated enzyme is then rapidly hydrolysed, so that the compounds act as substrates and not as inhibitors of these enzymes; they largely account for the rapid disappearance of free organophosphorus compounds from the extracellular fluid. B-esterases include the cholinesterases, chymotrypsin, trypsin, thrombin and many others. In this case the phosphorylated enzyme is stable and the enzyme is therefore inhibited. C-esterases do not react with organophosphorus compounds in any way.

Drugs Which Block the Muscarinic Actions of Acetylcholine

These drugs are believed to act by combining reversibly with muscarinic receptors on the effector cells; most of them block the muscarinic actions of acetylcholine and related drugs by competition. The responses of most effector cells to nerve impulses in the postganglionic cholinergic nerves of the autonomic nervous system are also blocked, although the doses required to block the effects of nerve stimulation are greater than those which block the effects of injected acetylcholine.

Atropine and hyoscine. Preparations of the solanaceous plants, *Atropa belladonna* (deadly nightshade), *Hyoscyamus niger* (black henbane) and *Datura stramonium* (thornapple), have been used in medicine since ancient times. The main alkaloids they contain are hyoscyamine and hyoscine.

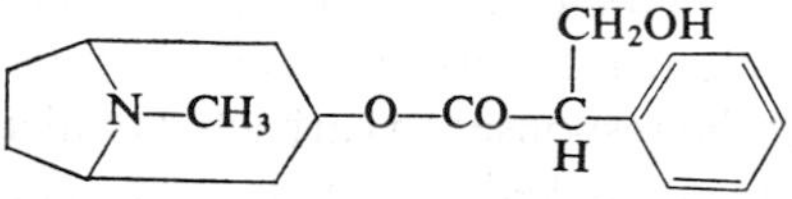

Hyoscyamine 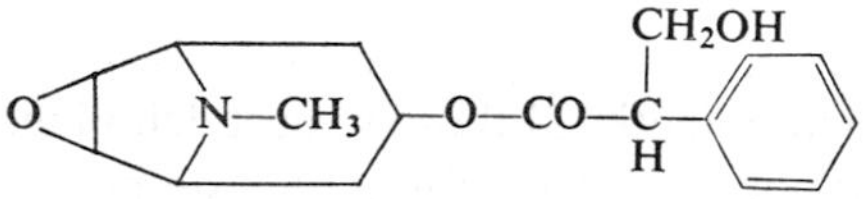   Hyoscine

These alkaloids are optically active, the laevo isomers being much more potent than the dextro isomers which are almost inert. Atropine is racemic hyoscyamine and, although the (−)-isomer is more potent, the racemic form is preferred because it is more stable chemically. The pharmacopoeal form of hyoscine is the (−)-isomer, which is also known as *scopolamine*.

Atropine was first isolated in 1831 by Mein. In 1867, von Bezold and Bloebaum found that the drug prevented the slowing of the heart produced by vagal stimulation and shortly afterwards Schmiedeberg and Adamück demonstrated, by experiments on the frog heart and on the eye, that the site of action was peripheral to the postganglionic nerve endings. In 1914, Dale showed that atropine antagonized all of the muscarinic actions of acetylcholine. The peripheral actions of hyoscine are closely similar to those of atropine.

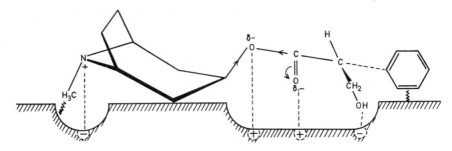

FIG. 28.6. Hypothetical depiction of the attachment of (−)-S-hyoscyamine to the muscarinic receptor. At the pH of the body fluids, the nitrogen atom is ionized and combines with the anionic site of the receptor. The hydroxyl group may be bound to a negatively charged site, and here hydrogen bonding is probably important. (Cf. Fig. 28.1.)

The combination of (−)-hyoscyamine with the muscarinic receptor may be pictured as in Fig. 28.6. At plasma pH values, the nitrogen atom is ionized and is believed to combine with an anionic site of the receptor.

The effects of atropine on the longitudinal smooth muscle of the isolated innervated oesophagus of a chick are illustrated in Fig. 28.7. Acetylcholine, carbachol or stimulation of the vagus nerve produced contraction of the oesophagus. Atropine abolished the responses to acetylcholine and carbachol and depressed those to nerve stimulation. Physostigmine, added in the continued presence of atropine, restored the responses to nerve stimulation and restored and potentiated those to acetylcholine, but the responses to carbachol (which is not a substrate for cholinesterase) remained blocked by the atropine. This antagonistic action of anticholinesterase drugs against atropine in smooth muscle may be compared with their antagonistic action against tubocurarine block in striated muscle (Fig. 26.2b, page 666).

Both atropine and hyoscine block the central actions of anticholinesterase drugs but they also exert actions on the CNS which may not be related to their antimuscarinic effects. The latter central actions are not antagonized by anticholinesterase or parasympathomimetic drugs. Furthermore, although (−)-hyoscyamine is more potent than atropine in its antimuscarinic actions, it is less powerful in some of its actions on the CNS.

The central actions of atropine and hyoscine differ, atropine being stimulant and then depressant while hyoscine is usually only depressant.

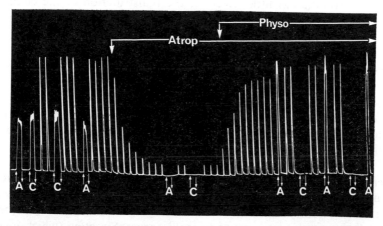

FIG. 28.7. Contractions of the isolated oesophagus of the chick produced by acetylcholine (0·1 μg/ml) at A, by carbachol (0·05 μg/ml) at C, and by stimulation of the right parasympathetic nerve at a frequency of 10/sec for 2 sec (unlabelled contractions). The times of addition and removal of acetylcholine and carbachol are indicated by the small arrows. Atropine (Atrop, 0·01 μg/ml) and physostigmine (Physo, 0·2 μg/ml) were added to the reservoir of Krebs' solution and remained in contact with the tissue throughout the periods indicated. For further explanation see text. This figure was supplied by Dr. S. D. Everett.

Pharmacological effects of atropine. The effects of atropine can be largely deduced from a knowledge of the functions of the autonomic nervous system. They may be summarized as follows:

Cardiovascular system. Small doses of atropine (0·5 to 1 mg in man) may temporarily decrease the rate of the heart beat as a result of a slight stimulant action of the drug on the vagal centres in the medulla. The main effect of large doses (about 2 mg) is to produce tachycardia by blocking the effect of the vagus; this is most marked in young adults in whom vagal tone is at its height. Blood pressure and cardiac output are not usually affected because of compensatory circulatory mechanisms. In children and in old people, vagal tone is slight and atropine produces little acceleration of the heart. Doses of atropine greatly in excess of those required to block the effects of the vagus on the heart prevent cardiac arrhythmias produced by adrenaline in the presence of cyclopropane anaesthesia.

Few blood vessels receive parasympathetic innervation, although blood vessels in skeletal muscle receive a cholinergic innervation from sympathetic fibres. These fibres are vasodilator and are active mainly during exercise. However, atropine has little effect on the redistribution of the circulation during exercise; this is because vasodilatation occurs in exercised muscles chiefly through the action of metabolites released by the active tissue.

Large doses of atropine cause vasodilatation of the skin blood vessels which is unconnected with its antimuscarinic effect, and which may be due to a direct dilator action of atropine or to histamine release.

Motility of the gastrointestinal tract. Atropine causes a prolonged reduction in tone and movements of the gut from the stomach to the rectum. It also reduces the stimulant effects of parasympathomimetic drugs.

Secretions. Atropine prevents the secretions of glands that are stimulated by cholinergic nerves. Thus, the flow of saliva and of mucus from the glands lining the respiratory tract is reduced and drying of the mucous membranes of the mouth, nose, pharynx and bronchi occurs. Sweating (which involves cholinergic sympathetic nerve fibres) is suppressed and the skin becomes hot and dry; after large doses of atropine the body temperature rises. Lacrimation is reduced by atropine. Acid-secreting cells of the gastric mucosa are largely under hormonal rather than vagal control (pages 311–312) and atropine does not significantly alter acid production in the doses usually employed in man. In fact, the concentration of HCl may rise because of the reduced volume of the secretion, and atropine is therefore of little value in the treatment of peptic ulcer. However, large doses of atropine reduce the volume and the total acid content of gastric secretion. Secretion of pancreatic juice is also largely under hormonal control and is little affected by atropine.

Atropine does not affect the secretion of milk, urine or bile. However, it inhibits contractions of the urinary bladder and the gall bladder.

The eye. Atropine applied to the conjunctiva causes a prolonged blockade (several days) of the contractions of the parasympathetically innervated circular muscle of the iris and of the ciliary muscle of the lens, and therefore dilates the pupil (the mydriatic action) and paralyses accommodation (the cycloplegic action) so that the lens is focused for distant vision. Unlike the mydriasis caused by sympathomimetic amines, that produced by atropine is accompanied by block of the light and accommodation reflexes. Intraocular pressure is not much affected in young adults with normal eyes. However, when the intra-ocular pressure is already above normal, and in people over 40, the contraction of the iris into the angle of the anterior chamber blocks the drainage of intra-ocular fluids. An attack of glaucoma may be precipitated and this constitutes a serious hazard, particularly in the use of atropine in older patients.

Other smooth muscles. The smooth muscles of the bronchi and bronchioles are relaxed, and a widening of the airway results. Tone and contractions of the ureter are decreased. The detrusor muscle of the bladder is relaxed. The bile ducts and gall bladder are slightly relaxed but not sufficiently to justify the use of atropine alone in the treatment of biliary spasm.

Central nervous system. In the doses usually used in man (0·5 to 1 mg), central stimulation is slight. With large doses, central effects are more pronounced and give rise to restlessness, irritability, disorientation, hallucinations and delirium. Stimulation is followed by depression, and respiratory paralysis is the cause of death in atropine poisoning. The mechanism of these central actions is un-known but does not appear to be related to antimuscarine activity.

Atropine is useful in suppressing the rigidity in Parkinsonism, and this may be an 'antiacetylcholine' effect exerted in the brain stem. It is also useful in abating motion sickness. The use of atropine in abolishing the central actions of anticholinesterase drugs and of drugs with muscarinic action has already been described.

Resistance to atropine. Even in large doses atropine fails to abolish completely: (i) vasodilatation in the salivary glands produced by stimulation of the chorda tympani, (ii) contraction of the dog uterus produced by stimulation of cholin-ergic fibres in the hypogastric nerve, (iii) contraction of the bladder produced by stimulation of the pelvic nerves and (iv) hyperactivity of the gastro-intestinal tract produced by stimulation of the vagus. The reason for this resistance is not known except in the salivary glands where vasodilatation is not entirely due to acetylcholine (see 'bradykinin', page 181). Atropine completely prevents the effects produced by injected acetylcholine on these structures.

Some species of animals, including rodents and marsupials, possess an enzyme known as atropinesterase which is present in the liver and serum and which is capable of rapidly hydrolysing atropine. In rabbits, the enzyme is genetically determined and some rabbits can exist on a diet of belladonna leaves without showing signs of atropine poisoning.

Other actions of atropine. Large doses of atropine exert a weak local anaes-thetic action; its chemical structure is similar to that of cocaine (page 657). Cocaine, however, is practically devoid of antimuscarinic activity. Atropine also exerts a weak antihistaminic activity in doses slightly greater than those necessary to block muscarine-like actions. These side-effects are important in experimental pharmacology. When atropine is used as a tool to test for muscarinic activity of another compound, the dose of atropine used must be small enough to avoid the possibility of producing actions other than the anti-muscarinic action. Very large doses of atropine, greatly in excess of those used clinically, may block the nicotinic actions of acetylcholine at ganglia and in skeletal muscle, particularly in amphibian skeletal muscle. Very small concentrations of atropine, below those needed to block muscarinic receptors, have been shown to stimulate muscarinic receptors and cause contraction of isolated gut, showing that atropine may act as a partial agonist.

Hyoscine (Scopolamine). The peripheral antimuscarinic actions of hyoscine are similar to those of atropine but it is more potent in its actions on the eye and on secretions. Unlike atropine, hyoscine is a CNS depressant and is used as a sedative and minor tranquillizer. The depressant actions of hyoscine occur with the doses used in medicine. As with atropine, death through overdosage is due to depression of the respiratory centre.

Dosage, absorption and excretion of atropine and hyoscine. The alkaloids are readily absorbed from the alimentary tract and may also be injected. Most of the alkaloids are metabolized and rendered inactive in the liver, only about 14% of atropine and 1% of hyoscine being excreted unchanged in the urine. The usual dose of atropine sulphate is 0·5 to 1 mg, and of hyoscine hydrochloride, 0·3 to 0·6 mg; these drugs are given subcutaneously, intravenously or orally.

Uses of atropine and hyoscine

Premedication before surgical operations. Atropine or hyoscine is given to dry up bronchial secretions and supposedly to protect the heart from vagal inhibition; in fact, the dose used is rarely large enough to block the cardiac vagus. The sedative action of hyoscine is partularly useful to soothe patients before operations. Hyoscine is often given together with morphine in obstetrics to produce a soporific state known as 'twilight sleep'.

In ophthalmic practice. The drugs are applied to the conjunctiva to dilate the pupil thereby aiding the examination of the retina. For this purpose atropine is used as a 1% solution and hyoscine as a 0·1 to 0·5% solution.

Antispasmodic action. Spasm of smooth muscle of the intestinal and urinary tract causes pain known as colic. These spasms are relieved by atropine and hyoscine.

Bronchodilatation. In asthma the bronchi are dilated by atropine or hyoscine which may be injected or inhaled. For the latter purpose cigarettes made of stramonium leaves and potassium nitrate are smoked. However, the alkaloids are not of great value as bronchodilators.

Antidotes to poisoning. The toxicity of muscarine-like drugs and anticholin-esterases is decreased by atropine or hyoscine.

Prevention of motion sickness. Hyoscine, but not atropine, is used for this purpose.

Control of rigidity in parkinsonism. Useful results are produced only with very large doses; newer drugs are more commonly used nowadays.

Synthetic atropine-like drugs

Numerous synthetic compounds, as well as derivatives of the natural alkaloids, have been prepared in an attempt to produce drugs with a more selective action than atropine and hyoscine, particularly on the gut. A drug free of anti-cholinergic side-effects but capable of reducing peptic activity by depressing the secretion of hydrochloric acid would be valuable in the treatment of peptic ulcer. The naturally-occurring solanaceous alkaloids depress gastric secretion only in the largest tolerable doses and, despite many claims to the contrary, few of the synthetic compounds are much better. The best that can be said for the most active ones is that they permit a less rigid diet, and antacid treatment is more effective. However, side-effects such as dry mouth, blurred vision, constipation, and difficulty in micturition may still be produced. Although of restricted use in peptic ulcer, many atropine-like drugs are useful antispas-modics and are used to prevent spasm, hypermotility and colic of the gut and of the urino-genital tract. Some are used for their mydriatic action which, being relatively short-lasting, is less likely to give rise to raised intra-ocular tension.

Most of the atropine-like drugs conform to the general structure shown below:

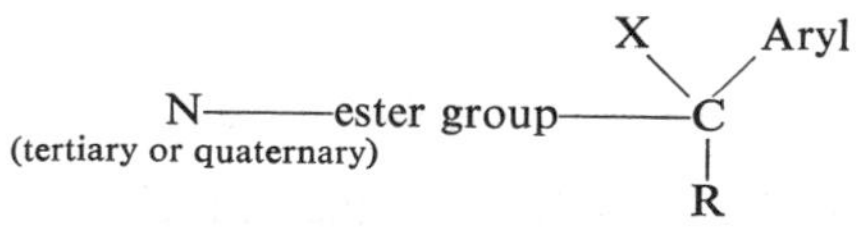

$$\underset{\text{(tertiary or quaternary)}}{N} \!\!-\!\!-\!\!-\text{ester group}\!\!-\!\!-\!\!\overset{\displaystyle X \diagdown \quad \diagup \text{Aryl}}{\underset{\displaystyle R}{\overset{\displaystyle |}{C}}}$$

where the aryl group is usually phenyl or a polycyclic group containing phenyl. R may range in size from hydroxymethyl to cyclohexyl and phenyl. X may be H, OH, CN, CO_2R, $CONH_2$ or alkyl.

TERTIARY AMINES. These include *homatropine* and *eucatropine* which are used for their relatively short-lasting mydriatic and cycloplegic action. Tertiary atropine substitutes used largely for their antispasmodic action include *amprotropine* (Syntropan), *adiphenine* (Trasentin) and *adiphenine 6-H, caramiphen, carbofluorene aminoester hydrochloride* (Paratrine) and *dactil*. In addition to their antimuscarinic activity, most of these compounds possess a non-specific relaxant action of the papaverine-like type, together with some local anaesthetic action; both of these contribute to their antispasmodic action. Many of them are said to be without significant atropine-like action on structures other than the gut and urino-genital tract.

QUATERNARY AMMONIUM COMPOUNDS. This group includes *homatropine methylbromide* (Novatropine), *oxyphenonium* (Antrenyl), *penthienate* (Monodral), *cantil*, *diphemanil* (Diphenatil, Diphenmethanil), *tricyclamol* (Lergine, Elorine), *dibutoline* and *hexocyclium*. The quaternized derivatives of the natural alkaloids may also be included in this group. Those available for use are *atropine methonitrate* (Eumydrin), *hyoscine methonitrate*, *hyoscine methobromide* (Pamine bromide) and *hyoscine* n-*butylbromide* (Buscopan).

In general, quaternization of an atropine-like compound results in increased antimuscarinic activity on the intestine relative to other actions, so that fewer side-effects are produced; antispasmodic action of the papaverine-like type is reduced. Quaternization also imparts ganglion-blocking activity to the compound and this probably contributes to their action on the gut. With a few of the compounds, some inhibition of acid secretion may be produced without the production of severe side-effects. The quaternary drugs may be administered orally, but their absorption from the gut is less efficient than for the corresponding tertiary amine. They do not readily penetrate to the CNS; consequently they have little or no central action.

All of the quaternary compounds are used as antispasmodics. Those most effective in the treatment of peptic ulcer are *propantheline* and the quaternary derivatives of *hyoscine*. *Atropine methonitrate*, *lachesine* and *dibutoline* are also used as short-acting mydriatics and cycloplegics; they are applied to the conjunctiva for this purpose.

Anti-Parkinsonian drugs

Lesions of the basal ganglia, the substantia nigra, their interconnecting fibres and the extrapyramidal pathways cause abnormalities in muscular movement, tone and posture. The commonest clinical syndrome is *parkinsonism* in which there is rigidity, tremor and akinesia. In *athetosis*, there are writhing movements and hypotonia, and in *chorea* there are sudden jerky movements and hypotonia. The clinical picture depends on the tracts or nuclei involved, some of which are excitatory and some inhibitory. Destructive surgical lesions in selected parts of the basal ganglia often remove the symptoms arising from a lesion in some other part of the extra-pyramidal system.

It has been reported that brain dopamine levels are abnormally low in patients with Parkinson's disease, and it is possible that the reduced dopamine content of the corpus striatum (in which the concentration of this amine is normally high) and the substantia nigra may in some way give rise to the akinesia. There is also evidence that the 5-hydroxytryptamine levels are low. The deficiency of these amines does not appear to be the result of a deficiency in the decarboxylase enzymes which form them, as the levels of these enzymes have been found to be within normal limits on post mortem examination of Parkinsonian patients. It is of interest that prolonged dosage with reserpine, which depletes the brain of these amines produces Parkinsonian-like symptoms.

The rigidity characteristic of parkinsonism appears to be the result of overactivity of the γ-efferents which innervate the muscle spindles (page 114). Destruction of the globus pallidus in animals produces rigidity, probably by removing inhibitory control from the γ-efferents (see Fig. 4.10) and this may be analogous to the rigidity of Parkinson's disease. Tremor can be produced in animals by destruction of part of the reticular formation of the brain stem. Whatever the site of the lesions giving rise to rigidity and tremor in Parkinson's disease, it seems that the disordered nervous activity is relayed through the reticular formation where many of the synapses appear to be cholinergic.

Most of the drugs used for the treatment of parkinsonism possess atropine-like activity, and their development and use followed from the observation in 1901 that belladonna alkaloids may produce beneficial effects. The chief atropine-like drugs used in the treatment of parkinsonism are given in Fig. 28.8. They are believed to act by blocking muscarinic receptor sites on neurones in the reticular formation. They are of limited use and several of them are usually tried before the patient can be stabilized on the best regime. The dose is gradually increased to the maximum the patient can tolerate. Sudden withdrawal, even of a partially effective drug, often results in severe rigidity. The principal side-effects are those characteristic of atropine and the drugs are therefore contraindicated in glaucoma and when there is a possibility of urinary retention. Some (e.g. *benzhexol, procyclidine* and *cycrimine*) may cause mental confusion, and several of them possess antihistaminic activity (e.g. *benzhexol, diethazine, orphenadrine, chlorophenoxamine* and *benztropine*). *Orphenadrine* is also used for its antidepressant action. The drugs are chiefly effective against the rigidity of Parkinson's disease. Muscarinic sites do not appear to be involved in the production of akinesia, and this symptom is resistant to treatment with the atropine-like anti-Parkinson drugs. However, the catecholamine precursor *dihydroxyphenylalanine* (dopa) has been found to diminish the akinesia in Parkinsonian patients, and this has particular

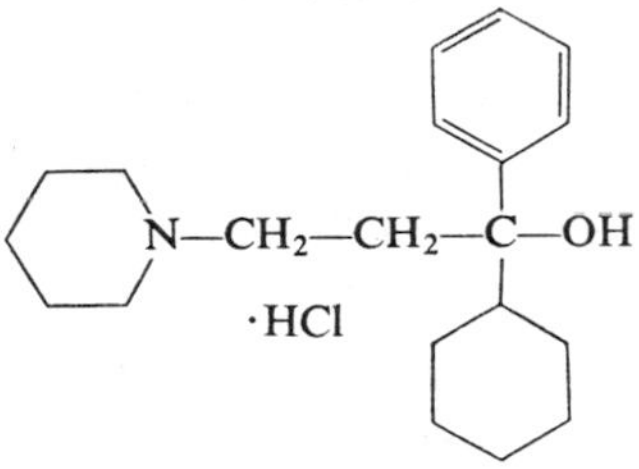

Benzhexol

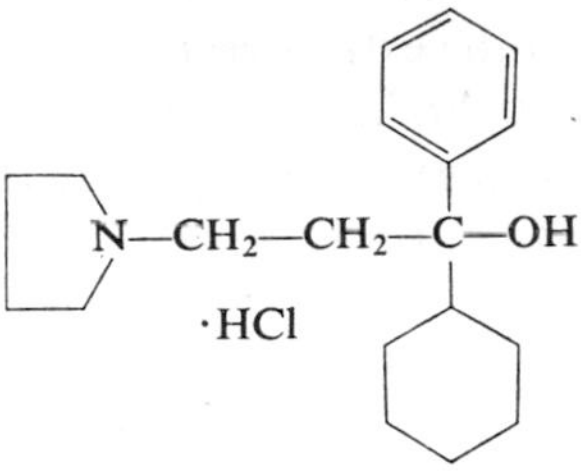

Procyclidine

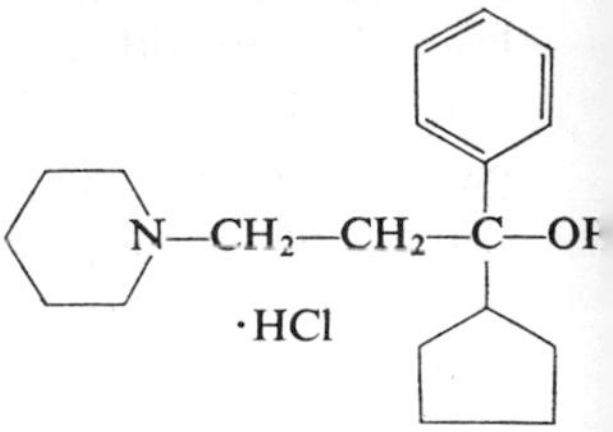

Cycrimine

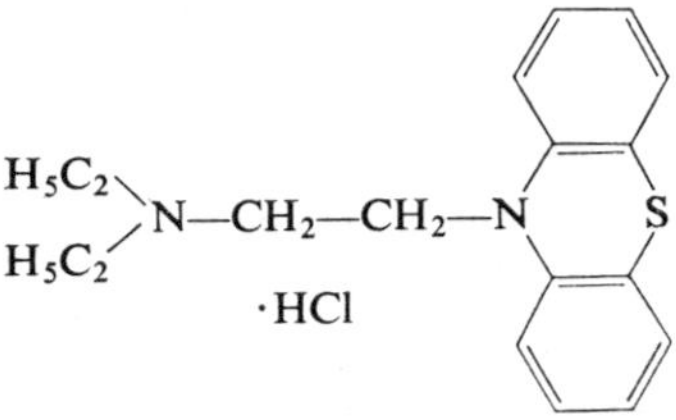

Diethazine

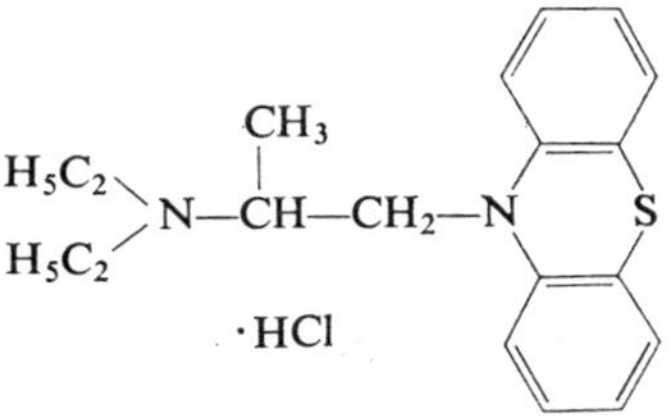

Ethopropazine

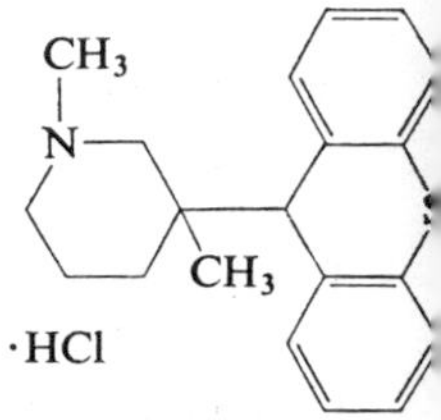

Methixene

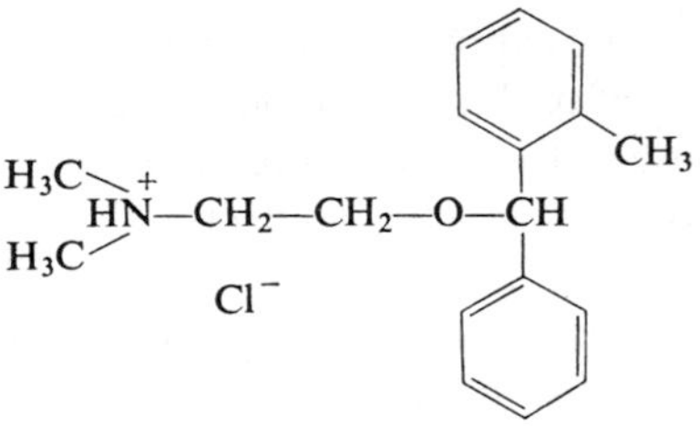

Orphenadrine
(cf. diphenhydramine, page 782)

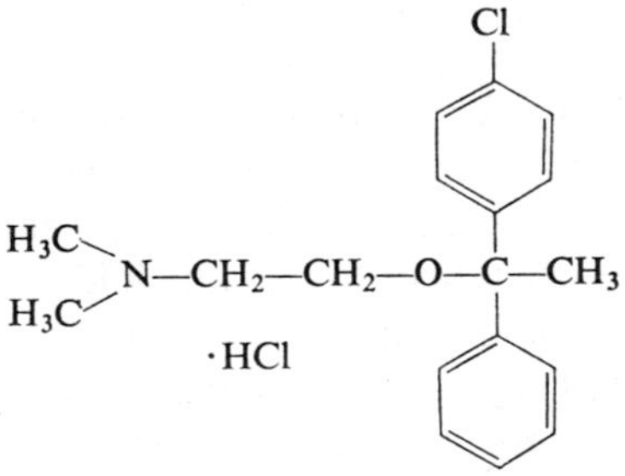

Chlorphenoxamine

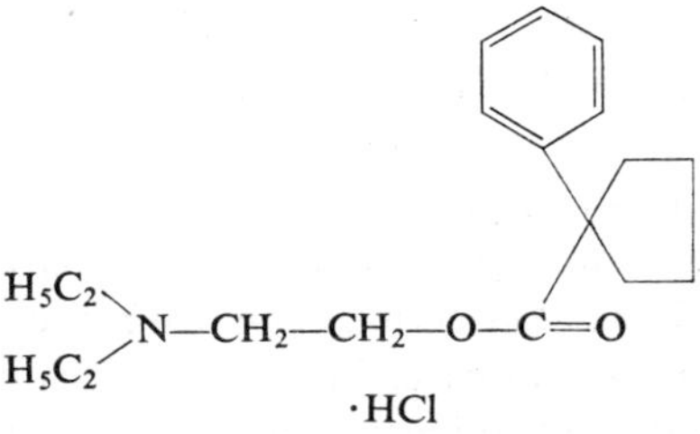

Caramiphen

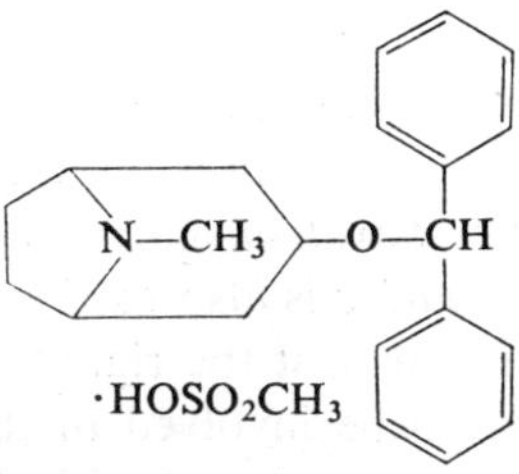

Benztropine

FIG. 28.8. Chemical formulae of some anti-Parkinson drugs.

relevance to the possibility that this symptom may arise from deficiency of dopamine.

Other drugs with a limited use in parkinsonism include amphetamine, pipradol and methylphenidate (page 618). These drugs are partly of value because they improve mood, but they also exert a more direct effect which is not understood, although it may be related to the disturbed central catecholamine metabolism believed to be present in the disease.

The drug tremorine (1:4-dipyrrolidinobut-2-yne) produces tremor, akinesia and parasympathetic symptoms resembling those of Parkinson's disease, and this provides a useful means of detecting anti-Parkinson activity. Most agents effective in the disease are also active in antagonizing the effects of tremorine in animals. Tremorine has been shown to stimulate the activity of choline acetyltransferase and this effect occurring in the brain stem may be the basis of its mechanism of action. Tremorine owes its action to a metabolite, *oxotremorine*, formed in the liver. Inhibitors of liver microsome enzymes prevent the production of oxotremorine and activity is abolished. Pretreatment of mice with 5-hydroxytryptophan and a monoamine oxidase inhibitor, causes an increase in brain 5-hydroxytryptamine levels, and markedly delays the action of tremorine. Another experimental method sometimes used for the detection of new anti-Parkinson agents involves the production of tremor in monkeys by inducing *electrolytic* lesions in the brain stem; other lesions may remove the tremor.

CHAPTER 29

Sympathomimetics and Drugs Modifying
Their Action

The growth of knowledge about noradrenaline as the transmitter at sympathetic adrenergic nerve endings is described in Chapter 5. The present chapter deals firstly with the pharmacology of sympathomimetics, that is, substances having actions which mimic the effects of sympathetic nerve stimulation, and secondly with the pharmacology of drugs which modify the effects of sympathomimetics and of sympathetic nerve stimulation. The term 'sympathomimetic' was proposed by Dale to indicate that a compound produced effects similar to those of sympathetic nerve stimulation; however, he stated that this involved no preconception as to the precise mechanism of action. Two concepts about the mode of action of sympathomimetics have been introduced in recent years. (i) There are at least two types of receptors, these being designated α-receptors and β-receptors. Sympathomimetics which act by combining with the receptors are termed 'directly acting'. (ii) The actions of sympathomimetics depend not only on these receptors, but also on the presence of the storage sites for noradrenaline in the adrenergic neurones. In addition to acting on the receptors, noradrenaline and some other sympathomimetics are taken up at these storage sites. Some sympathomimetics have little action on the receptors, but in being taken up at the storage sites they displace noradrenaline which then stimulates the receptors; these drugs are designated 'indirectly acting'.

Sympathomimetic drugs

Catecholamine sympathomimetics. The formulae of the catecholamines of major interest in medicine and pharmacology are given in Fig. 29.1. The compounds that are natural constituents of the tissues are noradrenaline, adrenaline, dopamine, epinine and dimethyl-noradrenaline; their relationships in the biosynthesis of catecholamines are shown in Fig. 5.9 (page 162).

NORADRENALINE. All the responses to stimulation of adrenergic sympathetic nerves are reproducible by injections of noradrenaline. The responses to sympathetic nerve stimulation listed in Table 4.1 (pages 123 to 124) include some that are mediated by acetylcholine released from cholinergic sympathetic nerves, the main effector tissues so innervated being the eccrine sweat glands

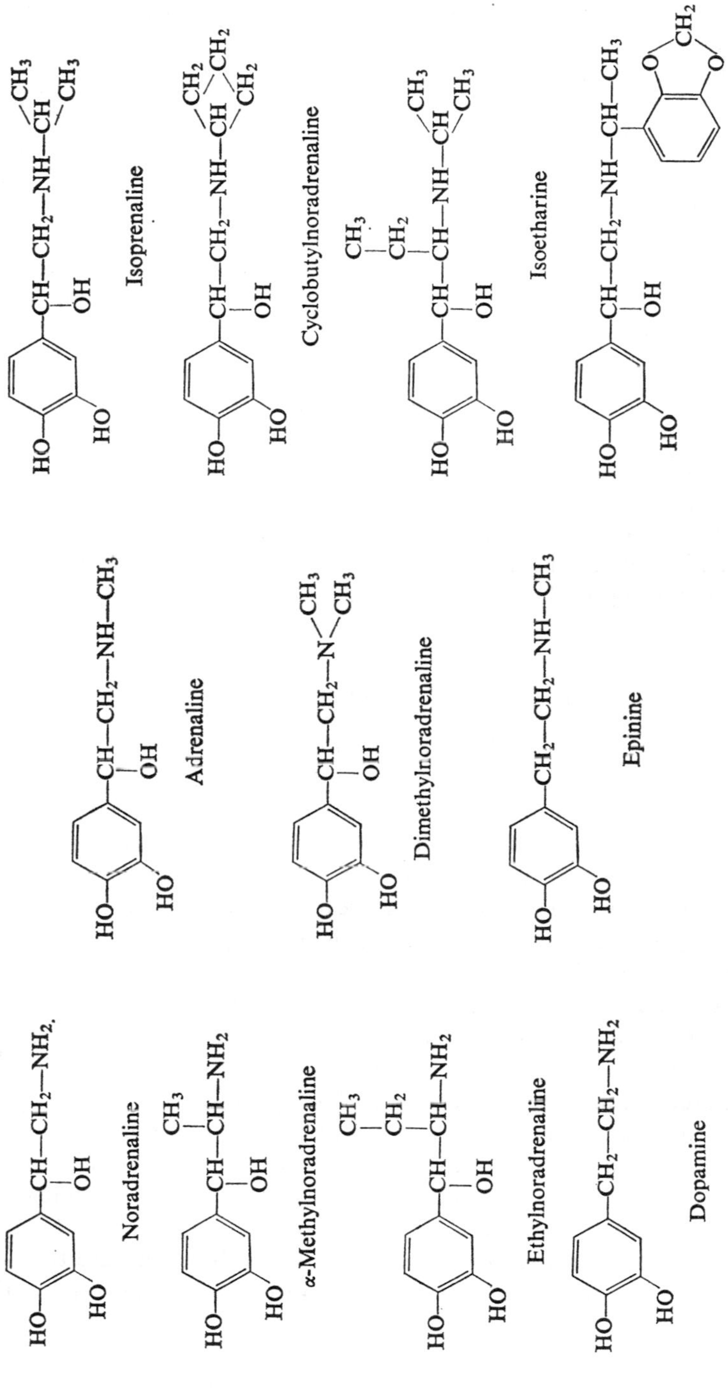

FIG. 29.1. Formulae of some catecholamine sympathomimetic drugs.

and those blood vessels of skeletal muscle that respond to nerve stimulation with vasodilatation. The remainder of the postganglionic sympathetic nerves are adrenergic, and the responses to stimulation are mediated by noradrenaline. The biosynthesis, storage and release of noradrenaline in adrenergic neurones is dealt with on pages 158–166.

The pharmacopoeal preparation (B.P. and U.S.P.) of noradrenaline is the laevo-isomer. In the U.S.A. it has the official name of *levarterenol* and is usually known as *norepinephrine*. The prefix *nor-* as used by organic chemists signifies the homologue with one methyl or methylene group less than the named compounds (adrenaline), although it has been suggested that *nor* is an abbreviation of the German '*N ohne Radikal*', meaning N without the radical (i.e., methyl group).

ADRENALINE. The occurrence of adrenaline in the body is dealt with on pages 161–163. The pharmacopoeal preparation is the *laevo*-isomer, which is the naturally occurring form. In the U.S.A., the drug is known as *epinephrine*. Adrenaline is prepared synthetically, or is obtained by extraction from the adrenal glands of cattle. Preparations obtained from adrenal glands are permitted to contain up to 4% of noradrenaline, although they usually contain less.

The uses and actions of noradrenaline and adrenaline

CARDIOVASCULAR SYSTEM. The actions of sympathetic stimulation on the individual effector organs of the cardiovascular system that are indicated in Table 4.1 (pages 123–124) are not identical with the effects produced when noradrenaline is administered to the intact organism because of homeostatic mechanisms which counteract the changes produced. The injection of noradrenaline produces a rise in blood pressure due to vasoconstriction, both systolic and diastolic pressure being increased. The rise in blood pressure activates the baroreceptors so that the cardio-inhibitory centre is stimulated and the heart is slowed through increased activity of the vagus nerves. When this reflex mechanism is operating, noradrenaline produces bradycardia, although the action of noradrenaline on the heart itself is to produce tachycardia. The effect of noradrenaline on the coronary blood flow is complex, being the resultant of at least four factors: (i) A direct vasoconstrictor action in larger arteries tending to diminish flow. (ii) A direct vasodilator action in smaller arteries tending to increase flow. (iii) The rise of systemic blood pressure which tends to increase the flow. (iv) Vasodilatation, produced by metabolites released during the increased cardiac work, also tends to increase the flow. (The increase in cardiac work is due partly to the positive inotropic action of noradrenaline and partly to the increased peripheral resistance.) The net effect is usually an increased flow. The main medicinal use of noradrenaline is to maintain the blood pressure in hypotensive conditions (but see pages 845–850). It is given by intravenous infusion at a rate which produces a suitable response, usually between 5 and 25 μg/min.

Adrenaline constricts blood vessels in splanchnic viscera and the skin, but dilates blood vessels in striated muscle. In animal experiments, adrenaline, like noradrenaline, is pressor when the blood pressure is low (as it is in spinal animals). However, when the pressure is high (e.g. in light anaesthesia with ether), small doses of adrenaline may have a depressor action owing to the predominance of vasodilatation in striated muscle vessels. In man, adrenaline causes an increase in systolic pressure and a decrease in diastolic pressure, thus the pulse pressure is increased; the mean pressure may rise or fall slightly. Intravenous adrenaline may produce feelings of anxiety or panic, a state of restlessness, dizziness and headache. Adrenaline has a more pronounced action than noradrenaline on the heart, and the cardio-inhibitory reflexes are not stimulated to the same extent: the heart rate and the cardiac output are therefore increased. The effect of adrenaline on the coronary blood flow resembles that of noradrenaline. In patients predisposed to angina, adrenaline may induce an attack. There is a risk of precipitating cardiac arrhythmias with adrenaline and this risk is high in patients under chloroform, trichloro-ethylene or cyclopropane anaesthesia (pages 575-579), and in hyperthyroid patients.

At one time adrenaline was used as a pressor agent in hypotension, but as it is prone to cause cardiac arrhythmias, it has been largely superseded by noradrenaline and other pressor amines. Subcutaneous injections of adrenaline produce local blanching of the skin due to constriction of arterioles. Adrenaline is often added to preparations of local anaesthetics to delay their absorption from the site of injection by constricting the blood vessels locally; the concentration of adrenaline used is about 10 μg/ml, stronger solutions causing such extreme ischaemia that necrosis occurs. On topical application to the skin (in creams), less than 0·1% is absorbed. However, on abraded skin or on mucosal surfaces, topical adrenaline reduces capillary bleeding. Adreno-chrome, which is an oxidation product of adrenaline (page 166), is available as the monosemicarbazone for use as a haemostatic in the control of capillary bleeding, and in diseases with increased capillary permeability and fragility.

ACTIONS ON SMOOTH MUSCLE. Of all the actions of noradrenaline on smooth muscle, only the vascular effects are exploited in medicine. Adrenaline is more powerful than noradrenaline in causing relaxation of smooth muscle. In the relief of asthmatic bronchospasm, adrenaline may be administered in a

24

spray or aerosol; by this means, the effects are largely confined to a local action on the smooth muscle of the bronchi, but cardiovascular disturbances often occur as a result of absorption through the alveolar membranes into the blood.

METABOLIC ACTIONS OF NORADRENALINE AND ADRENALINE. Both compounds cause an increase in the rate of glycolysis in liver and muscle, adrenaline being the more potent. There is a rise in blood glucose level, and adrenaline has been used to counteract hypoglycaemia in insulin overdosage. There is an increase in glucose utilization, and an increase in lactic acid production despite an increase in oxygen consumption. The plasma K^+ concentration increases, the liver being the chief source of the potassium. The blood level of free fatty acids is increased as a result of activation of lipase in adipose tissue.

　　The first step that leads to the increased breakdown of glycogen is the formation of cyclic-3′,5′-adenosine monophosphate (cyclic-AMP) from ATP, by activation of an enzyme known as *adenyl cyclase*.

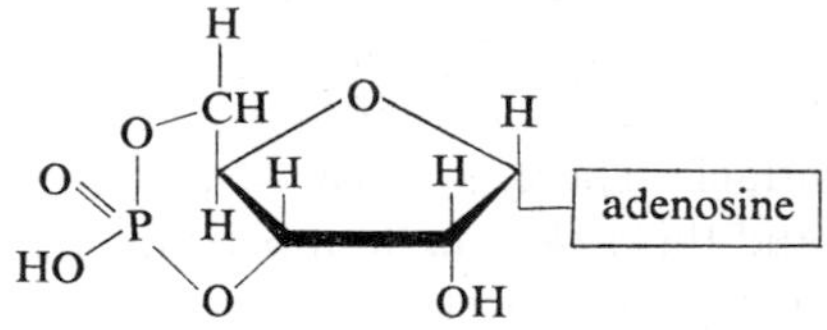

The following reactions are concerned with the formation and destruction of cyclic-AMP.

$$\text{ATP} \xrightarrow{\text{adenylcyclase}} \text{Cyclic-3′,5′-AMP} + 2 \text{ phosphates} \xrightarrow{\text{phosphodiesterase}} \text{5-AMP}$$

Cyclic-AMP stimulates the activity of a *kinase* which converts an inactive phosphorylase to an active form known as *phosphorylase a*.

$$\text{Phosphorylase } b \xrightarrow[\text{kinase}+\text{ATP}]{\text{Cyclic-AMP}} \text{Phosphorylase } a$$
$$\text{(inactive)} \qquad\qquad\qquad \text{(active form)}$$

The active phosphorylase then catalyses the following reaction:

$$\text{Glycogen} + \text{Phosphate} \xrightarrow{\text{phosphorylase } a} \text{Glucose-1-phosphate}$$

Glucose-1-phosphate is converted by phosphoglucomutase to glucose-6-phosphate; this is converted to glucose in liver cells (as shown in Fig. 2.8, page 46) and to lactic acid in muscle cells (as shown in Fig. 2.9, page 48). Cyclic-AMP is also involved in the lipolytic action of catecholamines, the lipase being activated.

Stimulation of adenyl cyclase is believed to occur with a number of hormones, in addition to the catecholamines. These hormones include glucagon, ACTH, luteinizing hormone and vasopressin. The structure of the enzyme is thought to vary from tissue to tissue so that different hormones act specifically in certain tissues.

ISOPRENALINE. The name is derived from isopropylnoradrenaline. The pharmacopoeal preparation is the racemic compound. In the U.S.A., it is known as *isoproterenol*. The principal medical use of isoprenaline is in the relief of bronchospasm in asthma, when it is administered sublingually or by inhalation of a spray or aerosol. Isoprenaline is more potent than adrenaline in increasing the rate and force of the heart beat. It produces vasodilatation in all blood vessels and causes a fall in blood pressure with a marked increase in heart rate. The tachycardia is due to the action of isoprenaline directly on the heart, and it is reinforced by stimulation of the cardio-accelerator reflex induced by the fall in blood pressure. Isoprenaline is considerably more active than noradrenaline in its relaxing action on smooth muscle, in stimulating the heart, and in some of its metabolic actions. On the other hand, it is considerably weaker than noradrenaline in its contracting action on smooth muscle. These differences are due to differences in the affinity of the drugs for the two types of catecholamine receptors.

Catecholamine receptors.—The steps that led to the development of the current concepts about catecholamine receptors are summarized under the following headings.

VASOMOTOR REVERSAL. In 1913, Dale found that the pressor action of adrenaline in the spinal cat was abolished after injections of ergotoxine (page 760), and then adrenaline had a depressor action. The interpretation of this reversal is that the pressor effect is due to the predominance of vasoconstriction over vasodilatation, and that ergotoxine specifically blocks the vasoconstrictor component of the response, thus allowing the vasodilatation to be manifested as a fall in blood pressure.

SYMPATHIN E AND SYMPATHIN I. Stimulation of sympathetic nerves produces effects which are classified on the one hand as excitatory, stimulant or motor, and on the other hand as inhibitory or relaxant. Cannon and Rosenblueth (1933–37) suggested that transmitters released by excitatory nerves and by inhibitory nerves combined with a 'receptive' substance to form substances that were termed *sympathin E* (excitatory) and *sympathin I* (inhibitory). However, when it was discovered that noradrenaline was the transmitter for all adrenergic nerves, regardless of the nature of the response, it was realized that the differences in response lay in the effector cells.

DIFFERENCES BETWEEN TISSUES IN THEIR SENSITIVITY TO VARIOUS CATECHOLAMINES. In 1948, Ahlquist compared the relative potency on different tissues of a number of sympathomimetics including noradrenaline, adrenaline and isoprenaline. He found that the order of potency on smooth muscles that responded with contraction was adrenaline > noradrenaline > isoprenaline, whereas on smooth muscle that responded with relaxation the order of potency was isoprenaline > adrenaline > noradrenaline. The order of potency for stimulation of the heart was similar to that for relaxation of smooth muscle. In order to explain these findings, he postulated that there were two types of receptor which were designated α-receptors and β-receptors. Effector cells with α-receptors (or α-adrenoreceptors) have a high sensitivity to adrenaline and noradrenaline and a very low sensitivity to isoprenaline, whereas those with β-receptors have a higher sensitivity to isoprenaline than to other

TABLE 29.1. Comparison of actions of noradrenaline and isoprenaline, and the types of catecholamine receptors in various tissues.

Tissues	Actions of Noradrenaline (N)	Actions of Isoprenaline (I)	Receptors
Pilomotor muscles	Contraction	No contraction	α
Vas deferens	Contraction	Inhibition of contractions	α, β
Dilator pupillae	Contraction	No contraction	α
Nictitating membrane	Contraction	Inhibition of contractions	α, β
Blood vessels	Constriction	Dilatation	α, β
Intestinal smooth muscle	Relaxation	Relaxation (I > N)	α, β
Uterus, rabbit and human	Contraction	Relaxation	α, β
Uterus, rat and non-pregnant cat	Relaxation	Relaxation (I > N)	$\alpha?, \beta$
Adipose tissue	Fatty acids released	Fatty acids released	$\alpha?, \beta$
Liver	Potassium release.	No potassium release	α
	Glycolysis	Glycolysis	α, β
Muscle	Glycolysis	Glycolysis (I > N)	β
Bronchial smooth muscle	Relaxation	Relaxation (I > N)	β
Heart	Increased rate	Increased rate (I > N)	β
	Increased force	Increased force (I > N)	β

catecholamines and are usually more sensitive to adrenaline than to noradrenaline. Table 29.1 compares the actions of noradrenaline and of isoprenaline, and summarizes the information about the types of receptors in various tissues.

DIFFERENCES IN EFFECTS OF ANTIADRENALINE DRUGS. The explanation for the phenomenon of vasomotor reversal can be restated in terms of α- and β-receptors in the following way: ergotoxine blocks the action of adrenaline on α-receptors and allows its effect on β-receptors to predominate. Drugs that abolish actions of catecholamines exerted *via* the stimulation of α-receptors are now generally known as α-receptor blocking drugs. It is only in recent years that specific β-receptor blocking drugs have become available.

PROBLEMS IN THE CONCEPT OF α- AND β-RECEPTORS. This concept has gained prominence in pharmacology as it summarizes conveniently a considerable amount of information. However, there are a number of observations which do not fit readily into the scheme. Four of these are cited: (1) Ergotamine (a so-called α-blocking drug) antagonizes the action of adrenaline on frog heart (an action said to be due to stimulation of β-receptors). (2) Both α- and β-receptor blocking drugs reduce the inhibitory action of catecholamines on intestinal smooth muscle; it has been proposed that yet another type of adrenoreceptor, designated γ-receptor, may be present in intestinal smooth muscle cells. However, it is more likely that the tissue contains both α- and β-receptors since it has been found that β-receptor blocking drugs are most effective against the inhibitory action of isoprenaline and α-receptor blocking drugs are most effective against the inhibitory action of noradrenaline. (3) The inconsistency of blocking drugs in affecting the metabolic actions of catecholamines led to the proposal that the receptors involved be designated δ-receptors. However, these inconsistencies arise chiefly because of differences between species and tissues. Probably, actions at both α- and β-receptors produce the metabolic effects. (4) The depressor response to isoprenaline is reversed to a pressor response by ergotoxine. The explanation that has been advanced for this finding is that ergotoxine antagonizes the vasodilator effect of isoprenaline, but not the cardiac stimulant action.

Smooth muscle with a low resting tone is incapable of exhibiting relaxation. Tissues containing such smooth muscle are the vas deferens, the seminal vesicles, and the nictitating membrane. The absence of effect of β-receptor agonists on these tissues has in the past led to the supposition that the smooth muscle contains no β-receptors. However, it has been shown that isoprenaline antagonizes the contracting action of other drugs, including α-receptor agonists, and this indicates that β-receptors are present. A problem in discriminating between α-receptor antagonists and β-receptor agonists arises, since the result (i.e. diminution in the response to an α-receptor agonist) is the same in either case. Previously, it had been assumed that certain drugs of the isoprenaline type (i.e., with large substituents on the amino group) were antagonists of noradrenaline because of observations made on tissues with low tone.

In experiments on isolated vascular smooth muscle, isoprenaline has no relaxing action as tone is not present, but in some cases it counteracts the effects of vasoconstrictor drugs. Large doses of isoprenaline are vasoconstrictor, and this indicates that it is weakly active on α-receptors.

OPTICAL ISOMERS OF NORADRENALINE AND ADRENALINE. The laevo-isomers of noradrenaline and adrenaline are 10 to 100 times more potent than the *dextro*-isomers, the potency ratios depending on the preparations on which they are tested. The absolute configurations of the isomers have been recently

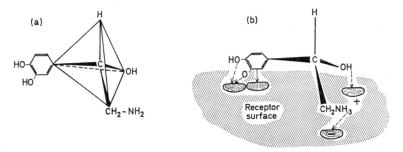

FIG. 29.2. (a). The absolute configuration about the asymmetric C-atom of *l*-noradrenaline with substituents at the apices of a tetrahedron. (b). Schematic diagram of the receptor, showing the relative positions of the 3 points of attachment of *l*-noradrenaline.

elucidated, the *laevo*-isomers having L- or R-configuration. The arrangement of the substituents on the asymmetric C-atom of noradrenaline is shown in Fig. 29.2(a). It has been pointed out that differences in potency between the optical isomers imply a 3-point attachment to the receptor. This has been represented schematically in Fig. 29.2(b). The amino group is mostly ionized at the pH value of the tissues, and this suggests that it forms an ion pair with an anionic site. The alkyl hydroxy group is probably attached by hydrogen bonding. The catechol nucleus is probably bound by chelate formation between an organometallic group and the catechol hydroxyls, and this is strengthened by van der Waals' binding of the aryl ring.

THE NATURE OF THE CATECHOLAMINE RECEPTORS. Belleau proposed a model for a single catecholamine receptor that contains sites for attachment of agonists of both the α- and β-type. The attachment of noradrenaline to the receiver surface in this model is shown in Fig. 29.3. In this case, the positively charged group, —N^+H_3, forms an ionic bond with a negatively charged phosphate group on the surface, and in general, agonists that act on the α-receptor are able to form such a bond. However, a large substituent on the N-atom, as for example, the isopropyl group, impedes the formation of the ionic bond. Nevertheless a catecholamine such as isoprenaline can still be attached by chelation through the phenolic hydroxyls. Belleau suggested that formation of the drug-receptor complex by chelation, without simultaneous formation of an ionic bond, leads to one type of response (β), whereas occupation of both sites leads to another (α).

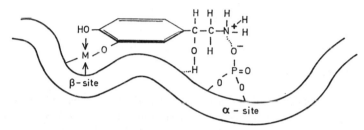

FIG. 29.3. Attachment of noradrenaline to a model of the receptor containing an α-site, which forms an ionic bond, and a β-site, at which chelation occurs. A molecule having a large group on the N-atom would be unable to combine with the α-site.

Other explanations concerning the nature of the β-receptor have been proposed. Some research workers believe that β-receptor effects are mediated by the cyclic-AMP formed in the effector cell, and it has been suggested that the β-receptor is actually located on the enzyme adenyl cyclase. Isoprenaline is the most potent β-receptor agonist and is also the most potent in stimulating the formation of cyclic-AMP. Changes produced by β-receptor activation do not appear to result from glycolysis, since the intestine and heart respond to isoprenaline and adrenaline before sufficient time has elapsed even for phosphorylase to be activated, and the gut is still relaxed by these drugs when rendered glycogen-free and in the absence of glucose from the surrounding medium. It has therefore been concluded that the formation of cyclic-AMP by β-receptor activation is a common step both in muscle glycolysis and in the electrical and mechanical responses of the effector cell, but that the latter are not dependent on the former. According to this theory, cyclic-AMP has actions, in addition to activation of phosphorylase, which result in an increase in the availability of energy-rich phosphate compounds. In the heart, the production of these compounds leads to the positive inotropic and chronotropic responses; in smooth muscle it leads to hyperpolarization of the cell membrane which inhibits any spontaneous propagated electrical activity (upon which the tone of the smooth muscle depends) so that the muscle relaxes.

Lundholm proposed that the vasodilator response to adrenaline was due to the smooth muscle relaxant properties of lactic acid which is formed as the end product of stimulated glycolysis, and it is possible that lactic acid is responsible for the secondary vasodilator response which is often produced by adrenaline. However, the initial vasodilatation occurs long before any lactic acid has been formed.

The α-receptors are believed to be located in the cell membrane. When the response of the cell to α-receptor activation is contraction, it is the result of depolarization of the cell membrane. Thus, the effect of drugs, such as adrenaline, which combine with both α- and β-receptors, depends on the proportion of the two types of receptor present and on the resting tone of the muscle.

Other catecholamines

α-Methylnoradrenaline is also known as *corbasil* or *cobefrine*. The presence of the α-methyl group renders this substance immune from attack by monoamine oxidase; however, it is still subject to metabolism by catechol-O-methyltransferase. Like noradrenaline, the α-methyl derivative is taken up by the adrenergic nerve terminals, and can then be released again from them by nerve impulses or by indirectly-acting sympathomimetics. The actions of α-methylnoradrenaline are qualitatively identical with those of noradrenaline, but the laevo-isomer has one-half to one-tenth the potency of (−)-noradrenaline depending on the tissue used for the comparison. The reduction in activity is probably attributable to steric hinderance by the α-methyl group of the attachment of the amino group to the receptor. The α-methyl derivative of adrenaline, also known as *dihydroxyephedrine*, is again less active than adrenaline, but qualitatively identical in its actions.

α-Ethylnoradrenaline, also known as Butanefrine, has actions resembling those of isoprenaline, except that it has little effect on the heart. It is sometimes used as a bronchodilator in asthma. The influence of the α-ethyl group in reducing agonist activity on α-receptors and enhancing that on β-receptors is probably due to the increase in the effective size of the molecule in the vicinity of the amino group.

Cyclobutylnoradrenaline has only recently been developed. Its structure suggests that it acts predominantly on β-receptors, and, in fact, it is a powerful bronchodilator. Since it has relatively less effect on the heart than isoprenaline, its use in the relief of asthmatic bronchospasm is being tested.

Isoetharine, or Dilabron, is the α-ethyl derivative of isoprenaline. It resembles isoprenaline in producing tachycardia and in relaxing smooth muscle, but has little effect on blood pressure. It is also used as a bronchodilator in asthma.

Protochylol, or Caytine, is used as a bronchodilator, and in general its actions resemble those of isoprenaline.

Dopamine and *epinine* are derivatives of catecholethylamine. Their occurrence as intermediaries in the biosynthesis of noradrenaline and adrenaline is mentioned on page 159 and in Fig. 5.9. Dopamine (also known as 3-*hydroxy-tyramine*) and epinine are considerably weaker than the corresponding ethanolamine compounds. The lack of the alcoholic hydroxyl group on the side chain results in a weaker attachment to the receptor, and they may be compared with the dextro-isomers of noradrenaline and adrenaline. Their sympathomimetic actions are due partly to excitation of the receptors and partly to the release of catecholamines from the adrenergic neurones.

Orciprenaline is a structural analogue of isoprenaline and has similar actions and uses; it is less potent than isoprenaline and its duration of action is longer. It is a resorcinol rather than a catechol derivative, having the aryl hydroxyl groups in the 3 and 5 positions.

Directly- and indirectly-acting sympathomimetics. When noradrenaline is added to a sympathetically innervated structure, part of it acts on the receptors of the

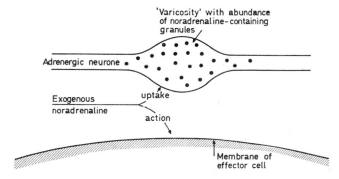

FIG. 29.4. When noradrenaline is administered to an adrenergically-innervated structure, part of it acts on the receptors, and part of it is taken up in the noradrenaline storage sites. These stores are located principally in the granules which pack the swellings or nodules that occur at intervals along the adrenergic axons within the tissue.

effector cells and part is taken up by the noradrenaline storage sites in the adrenergic neurones. This is illustrated diagrammatically in Fig. 29.4. In a tissue

24*

which has been sympathetically denervated, the sites of uptake are absent and the actions of noradrenaline are enhanced. This is the explanation for *denervation supersensitivity*. A number of drugs increase the activity of noradrenaline by decreasing the affinity of the storage site for noradrenaline (reserpine probably acts in this way) or by preventing the access of noradrenaline to the storage site (cocaine is one of several drugs which do this). All of the sympathomimetics which act or have an enhanced action on tissues that have been sympathetically denervated or treated with cocaine (or a related drug) are termed *directly acting*, since they owe their activity to direct excitation of the receptors.

Catecholamines are directly acting but the extent to which they can be taken up in the storage sites differs amongst them. Adrenaline is not taken up as avidly as is noradrenaline, and its actions, therefore, are not enhanced to the same extent as those of noradrenaline by denervation or after giving cocaine. Isoprenaline is not taken up by the stores and its actions are not enhanced by these procedures.

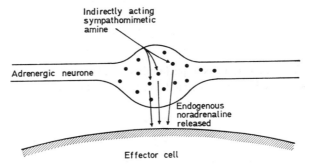

FIG. 29.5. An indirectly-acting sympathomimetic amine displaces noradrenaline from the storage sites in the adrenergic neurone.

The loss of the groups on the noradrenaline molecule that are concerned with attachments to the receptors results in compounds with weaker direct action. However, providing that the basic amino group remains intact, these compounds still have affinity for the noradrenaline storage site, and, in attaching to the storage site, they displace the noradrenaline which is then released and acts on the receptors. Sympathomimetics that act in this way are termed *indirectly acting;* their mode of action is illustrated diagrammatically in Fig. 29.5. They are ineffective in sympathectomized tissues as there is no noradrenaline store for them to act upon. The adrenergic neurones may be depleted of their content of noradrenaline by treatment with reserpine, and this too results in loss of effect of the indirectly acting compounds. However, if an infusion of noradrenaline or of one of its precursors is given, the noradrenaline content is then temporarily increased and the response to an indirectly acting substance is restored.

Derivatives of phenolethanolamine. The formulae of sympathomimetics possessing a single phenolic hydroxyl on the aryl ring and an alcohol hydroxy group on the side chain are illustrated in Fig. 29.6. These compounds have actions which, in general, are like those of the corresponding catecholamines although they are weaker. The following generalizations may be made about the relationships of chemical structure to pharmacological activity: those with large substituents on the amine group act predominantly on β-receptors; those with an unsubstituted amine or a methylamine group act partly directly on α-receptors and partly by releasing noradrenaline; those with a *meta*-hydroxyl group have more powerful direct actions than those with a *para*-hydroxyl group; the presence of an α-methyl group results in prolongation of action as these compounds are not attacked by monoamine oxidase.

The *para*-hydroxyphenylethanolamine compounds, *octopamine* and *synephrine*, occur in tissues of some animals where they are probably concerned in minor pathways of the biosynthesis of catecholamines (Fig. 5.9, page 162).

Metaraminol, known commercially as Aramine, is available as the laevo-isomer. It is used to raise the blood pressure in hypotensive states and as a nasal decongestant. These effects depend on the vasoconstrictor action of metaraminol. The actions of metaraminol are unaffected by depletion of the tissue stores of noradrenaline; it has, therefore, direct actions. In addition, it is one of the most effective compounds known in displacing and replacing noradrenaline from the stores in adrenergic neurones.

Synephrine is found in some tissues as the naturally occurring laevo-isomer. The synthetic pharmaceutical compound, *oxedrine*, is the racemate; it is also known as *sympatol* or *parasympatol*. Its actions and uses are similar to those of phenylephrine, but it is less potent.

Phenylephrine is available as the laevo-isomer, and is known commercially as Neosynephrine or Metasympatol. Its actions resemble those of noradrenaline, but they have a longer duration; it is much less potent than noradrenaline and large doses are needed to achieve an equivalent effect. It is used as a pressor drug in hypotensive states and has the advantage over adrenaline that it has less effect on the heart and is less likely to produce cardiac arrhythmias. The pressor effect of injected phenylephrine is accompanied by reflex bradycardia, in which respect it resembles noradrenaline more than adrenaline. Attacks of paroxysmal atrial or nodal tachycardia may be controlled by evoking the reflex vagal discharge caused by the pressor response to phenylephrine. It is also used as a nasal decongestant by virtue of its vasoconstrictor activity, and is applied

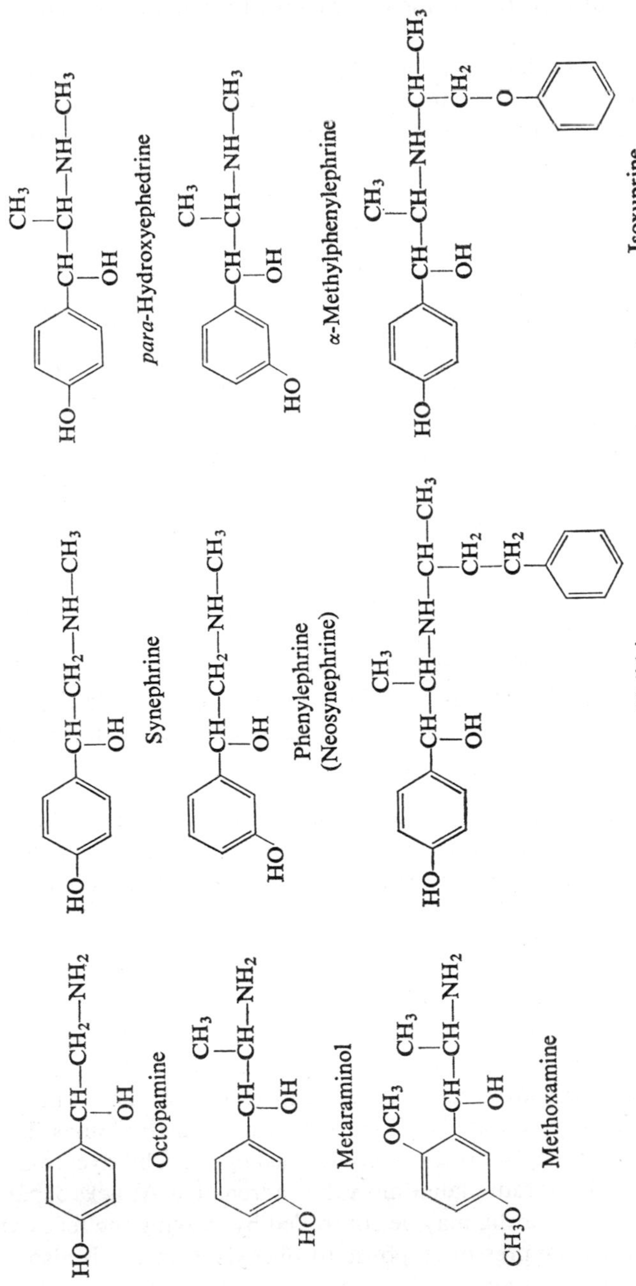

Fig. 29.6. Phenolethanolamine derivatives.

topically. Strong solutions applied to the conjunctiva have a mydriatic action and it is sometimes used for this purpose.

Nylidrin (Arlidin) and *isoxuprine* (Vasodilan, Duvadilan) are α-methyl derivatives of *p*-hydroxyphenylethanolamine with large substituent groups on the nitrogen. They are predominantly isoprenaline-like in their actions, and cause a fall in blood pressure which is due to peripheral vasodilatation. They are used in the treatment of peripheral vascular spasm. Nylidrin is reported to be without effect on the heart rate but to increase cardiac output. Isoxuprine is used to relax the uterus in cases of threatened abortion and in dysmenorrhoea with uterine spasm. Both compounds are effective after oral administration and they have prolonged actions, probably because they are immune from attack by monoamine oxidase and catechol-O-methyltransferase and are not taken up by noradrenaline binding sites.

Methoxamine, commercially known as Vasoxine, has a pressor action due to vasoconstriction. It has little effect on the heart and no bronchodilator action; thus it appears to be devoid of effects due to stimulation of β-receptors and has in fact been shown to possess some β-receptor blocking activity. It is used as a nasal decongestant and in the treatment of hypotensive states. Methoxamine is not a phenolic compound but it contains an ethanolamine chain (Fig. 29.6) and it resembles phenylephrine pharmacologically.

Derivatives of phenolethylamine. The formulae of sympathomimetics possessing a phenolic ring and an alkylamine side chain are shown in Fig. 29.7.

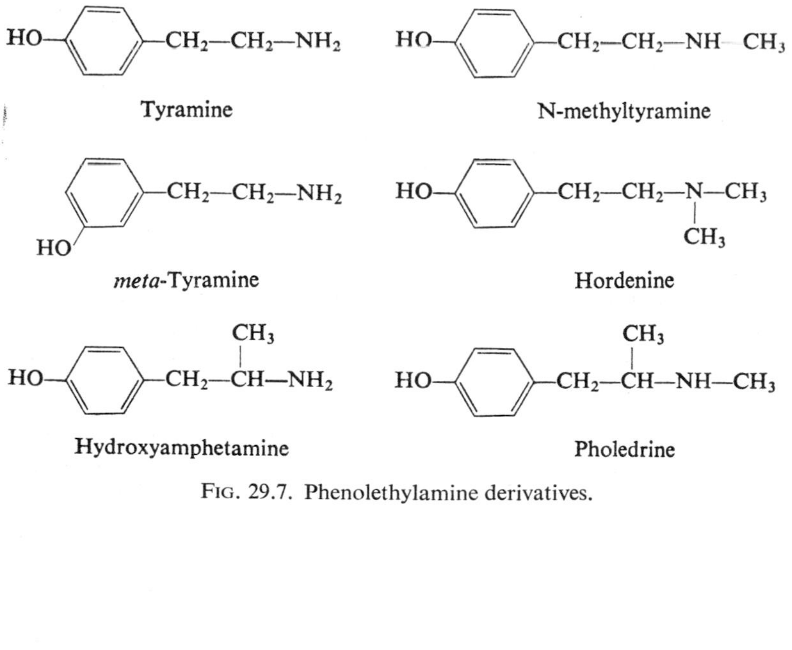

Tyramine	N-methyltyramine
meta-Tyramine	Hordenine
Hydroxyamphetamine	Pholedrine

FIG. 29.7. Phenolethylamine derivatives.

Tyramine is present in various foodstuffs, where it is formed by decarboxylation of tyrosine. Its *N-methyl* and N,N-dimethyl derivative (*hordenine*) occur naturally in certain plants. These compounds have pressor activity and other sympathomimetic properties which are chiefly due to displacement of noradrenaline from stores in adrenergic neurones. The next highest member in the series is a quaternary amine and is also pressor, but its actions are due to nicotinic stimulation of ganglion cells and the adrenal medulla. Tyramine is occasionally used in medicine to test for the integrity of peripheral stores of noradrenaline. It occurs in the CNS and may play a role there (page 185). The tyramine content of foodstuffs may give rise to complications in patients treated with monoamine oxidase inhibitors (pages 625–626 and 775).

Hydroxyamphetamine, the α-methyl derivative of tyramine, is known commercially as Paredrine. It is a pressor agent producing vasoconstriction and stimulation of the heart. It has been used to maintain blood pressure, as a nasal decongestant, and as a mydriatic when applied to the conjunctiva. Its stimulant action on the CNS is less than that of amphetamine, probably because the phenolic hydroxyl group impairs its penetration through the blood-brain barrier.

Pholedrine is known commercially as Paredrinol or Veritol. It increases the blood pressure through vasoconstriction having little effect on the heart rate or cardiac output, and is reported to be without stimulant activity on the CNS. Its main use is to maintain the blood pressure in hypotensive states.

Derivatives of phenylethanolamines. The formulae of the important members of this series of sympathomimetics are shown in Fig. 29.8.

Phenylethanolamine has a predominantly indirect sympathomimetic action. The intensity of the weak direct component of action depends on the isomer used, that of (−)-phenylethanolamine being the greater. The absolute configuration of the laevo-rotatory isomer is the same as in (−)-noradrenaline, and this allows attachment at 2 points of the noradrenaline receptor surface shown in Fig. 29.2b.

Phenylpropanolamine, or *norephedrine*, is known commercially as Propadrine; it resembles ephedrine in its actions except that it has less action on responses mediated through β-receptors and it has less CNS stimulant activity. It is used to relieve congestion of the nasal mucosa and sinuses and is usually administered orally, often in mixtures containing antipyretic analgesics, sedatives or antihistamines.

Ephedrine. The molecule has two asymmetric carbons and there are thus four isomers, (+)- and (−)-ephedrine and (+)- and (−)-pseudoephedrine. The

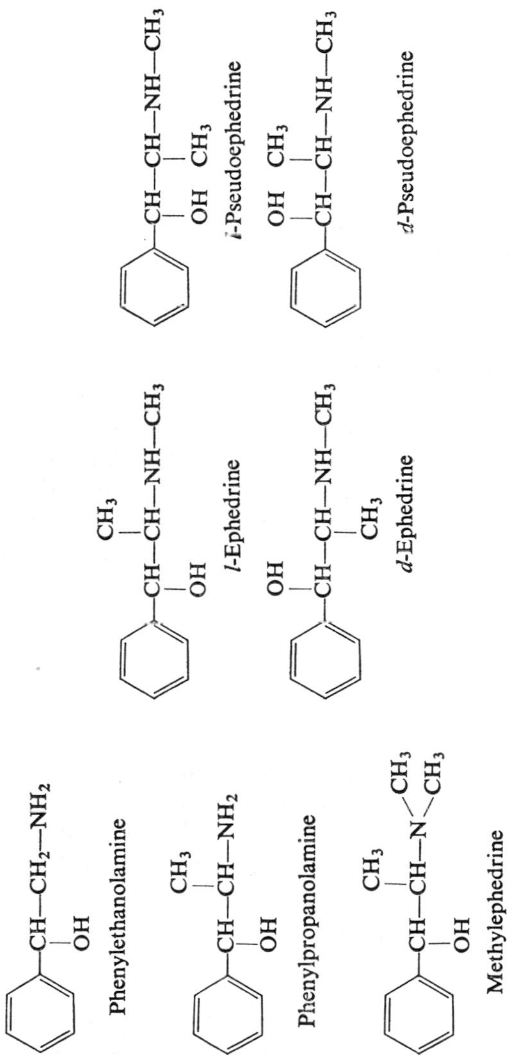

FIG. 29.8. Phenylethanolamine derivatives, including the four isomers of ephedrine.

pharmacopoeal preparation is (−)-ephedrine. The same deoxy derivative, (+)-methylamphetamine, is obtained from (−)-ephedrine and (−)-pseudo-ephedrine, hence the configuration on the α-carbon is identical in these two compounds. The differences between the four isomers are shown diagrammatically in Fig. 29.8. Their absolute configurations are known. The ephedrines have largely an indirect action. The most potent of the group in sympathomimetic activity is (−)-ephedrine. The relative extent of indirect and direct activity differs somewhat amongst the isomers. Ephedrine is an alkaloid obtained from plants of *Ephedra* species, and preparations of these were used in China for centuries under the name *ma-huang*, meaning 'yellow drug'. It was introduced into Western medicine in 1923, and was the first of the sympathomimetics to be used in medicine. Probably for this reason it has been used in a wide variety of conditions. Its main use is as a nasal decongestant in allergic rhinitis and hay fever, in which states it acts by causing vasoconstriction in the mucosa. Its vasoconstrictor action is also employed in the treatment of vascular collapse and local vasodilation in allergic and anaphylactic states. Part of the pressor response to ephedrine is due to cardiac stimulation, and this effect has been used in the treatment of episodes of heart block which may result in a drastic fall of blood pressure and fainting (Stokes-Adams syndrome). Ephedrine has a mydriatic action when applied to the conjunctiva, being readily absorbed. It penetrates to the CNS and has a stimulant action (but less than that of amphetamine). It has been used in the treatment of nocturnal enuresis; this action has been attributed to the sympathomimetic effects of relaxation of the detrusor muscle of the bladder and constriction of the trigone, but it is more likely to be due to a decrease in the depth of sleep so that the patient awakens to empty his bladder. Ephedrine has also been used in the treatment of myasthenia gravis (page 680).

Methylephedrine has considerably less pressor activity than ephedrine and no action on the CNS, but it is more effective as a bronchodilator, for which purpose it is used. Probably, the bulk of the substituents on the amino group endows the molecule with greater agonistic activity on β-receptors.

Derivatives of phenylethylamine. The formulae of the compounds in this class are shown in Fig. 29.9.

Phenylethylamine (or phenethylamine) is the decarboxylation product of phenylalanine. Like tyramine, it occurs in some foodstuffs.

Amphetamine is the α-methyl derivative of phenylethylamine. The pharmacopoeal preparation of amphetamine is the racemic form; its commercial name is Benzedrine. The dextro-isomer, (+)-amphetamine, has the official name of

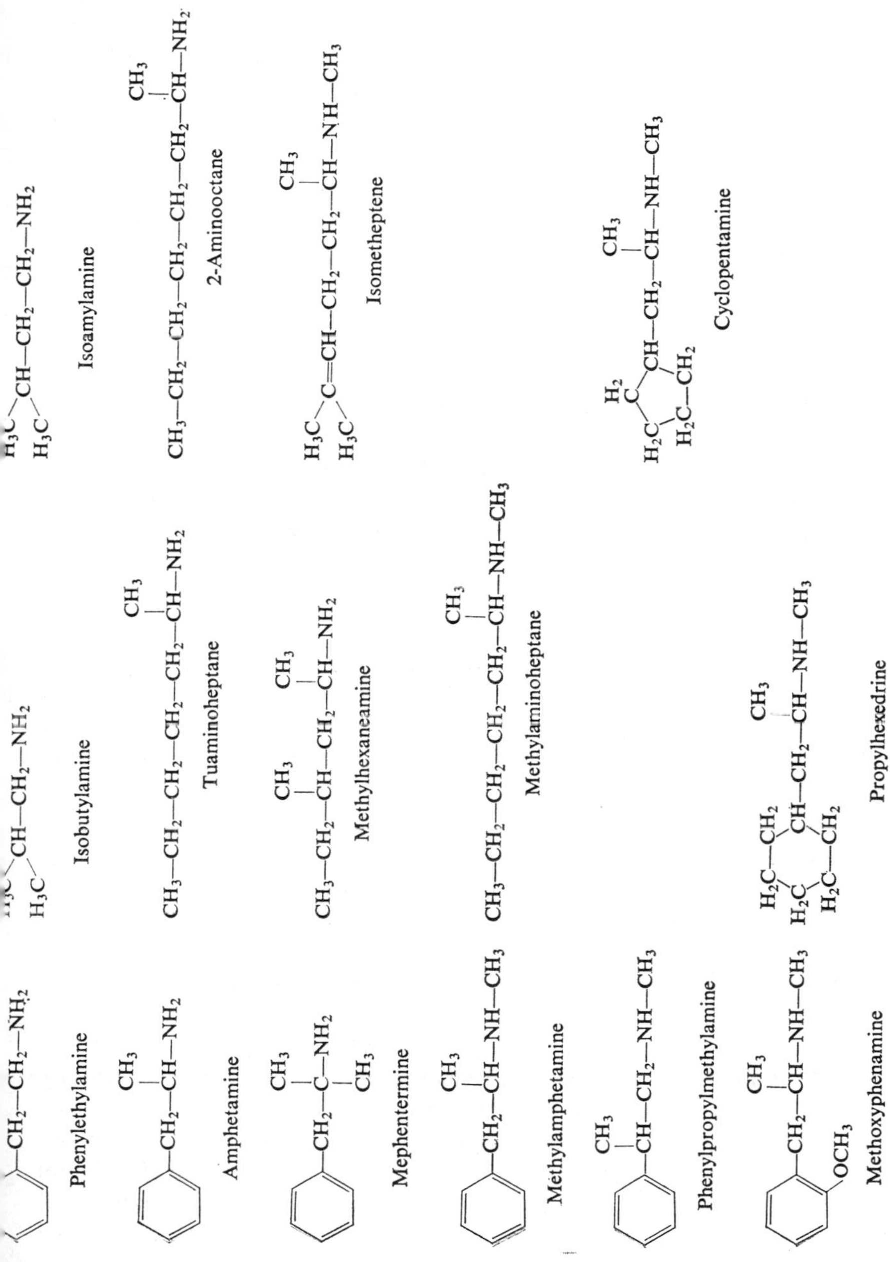

FIG. 29.9. Phenylalkylamines and alkylamines with sympathomimetic actions.

dexamphetamine and the commercial name Dexedrine. All forms of amphet-amine have indirect sympathomimetic actions. The free base is volatile and is administered by inhalation to produce vasoconstriction, hence decongestion, of the nasal mucosa. Salts of amphetamine (usually the sulphate) are employed for oral and parenteral administration, and are used principally for their CNS stimulant effects. The dextro-isomer is the more potent on the CNS. The medicinal use of the CNS stimulation produced by amphetamine is in the maintenance of a wakeful state in fatigue, in the treatment of narcolepsy, and as an analeptic in barbiturate poisoning (page 618). The amphetamines are also of value as appetite suppressants in the treatment of obesity (page 619).

Methylamphetamine, or *desoxyephedrine*, is commercially known as Methe-drine or Pervitin. It has the same actions and uses as amphetamine but is less potent. It is also used as a pressor agent in hypotensive states.

Mephentermine is known commercially as Mephine or Wyamine. It has similar actions and uses to amphetamine. It is said to have less action on the heart than amphetamine, which makes it safer to use as a vasoconstrictor pressor agent in the treatment of hypotensive states.

Phenylpropylmethylamine has a methyl group substituted in the β-position on the ethylamine side chain. The commercial name is Vonedrine. It is like amphetamine in its actions except that CNS excitation is said to be absent. It is used as a nasal decongestant and is reported to have the advantage that the temporary relief of the condition is not followed by a 'rebound' vasodilatation and exacerbation of the congestion.

Methoxyphenamine, commercially known as Orthoxine, is used as a nasal decongestant and also as a bronchodilator in asthma, although it acts pre-dominantly on α-receptors. It has little effect on the CNS.

Aliphatic amines with sympathomimetic actions. Some of these compounds of pharmacological or medical interest are shown in Fig. 29.9. *Isobutylamine* and *isoamylamine* are the decarboxylation products of the amino acids, valine and leucine (Fig. 1.6, page 15); they have weak activity. Sympathomimetic activity is optimal with compounds having 7 or 8 carbon atoms. The sympathomimetic action of *tuaminoheptane*, or *2-aminoheptane*, was first described by Barger and Dale in 1910; its commercial name is Tuamine. *Methylhexaneamine* (Forthane) and *methylaminoheptane* (Octin) have similar actions to tuaminoheptane, all three being used as nasal decongestants; they have no stimulant action on the CNS.

TABLE 29.2. Summary of sympathomimetic amines according to their principal medicinal uses.

Pressor action (in treatment of hypotensive states, see page 846).

Noradrenaline	Pholedrine
Adrenaline	Phenylpropanolamine
Metaraminol	Mephentermine
Methoxamine	Methylaminoheptane
Phenylephrine	

Nasal decongestant action (in treatment of allergic rhinitis, common cold, hay fever)

Phenylpropanolamine	Naphazoline
Propylhexedrine	Tetrahydronaphazoline
Methoxamine	Ephedrine
Phenylpropylmethylamine	Hydroxyamphetamine
Phenylephrine	Amphetamine
Cyclopentamine	Mephentermine
Tuaminoheptane	Methylhexaneamine

Local vasoconstrictor action (to promote haemostasis, page 913; to prolong action of local anaesthetics, page 656)

Adrenaline	Methoxamine

Bronchodilator action (in the treatment of asthma)

Isoprenaline	Isoetharine
Ephedrine	Protochylol
Adrenaline	Methoxyphenamine
Ethylnoradrenaline	Phenylpropanolamine
Orciprenaline	

Relaxation of visceral smooth muscle (in treatment of intestinal or uterine spasm)

Isometheptane	Isoxuprine

Vasodilator action (in the treatment of peripheral vascular disease, page 830)

Nylidrine	Isoxuprine

Mydriatic action (for ophthalmological examination, pages 895–897)

Ephedrine	Hydroxyamphetamine
Phenylephrine	

CNS stimulant action (in the treatment of depression and narcolepsy; to alleviate fatigue; as analeptic. See page 618)

Dexamphetamine	Amphetamine
Methylamphetamine	Ephedrine

Anorexigenic action (in the treatment of obesity. See page 619)

Amphetamine	Methylamphetamine
Dexamphetamine	Phenylpropanolamine

Isometheptene (Oenethyl) has a pressor action when given by injection and a mydriatic action when applied to the conjunctiva. These actions are attributable to stimulation of α-receptors. However, it appears to have considerable activity on β-receptors, and is used as a bronchodilator and to relax visceral smooth muscle.

Cyclopentamine (Clopane) has vasoconstrictor activity and is used as a pressor agent in hypotensive states and as a nasal decongestant. *Propylhexedrine* (Benzedrex) is the cyclohexyl analogue of methylamphetamine, which it resembles in its peripheral actions, although this and other cyclohexyl sympathomimetics are less active than the corresponding phenyl compounds. The free base of propylhexedrine is volatile and is used in inhalers for its nasal decongestant action. It has no stimulant action on the CNS, and was in fact developed for use in inhalers to prevent their misuse by amphetamine addicts.

Sympathomimetics containing an iminazole group. *Naphazoline* (Privine) and *tetrahydrozoline* (Tyzine) have marked vasoconstrictor action and are used as nasal decongestants. These compounds are unusual in that their effect on the CNS is depressant. Their chemical structures are related to that of the anti-adrenaline drugs, tolazoline and phentolamine (cf. Fig. 29.12). Presumably, the iminazole nucleus attaches to the α-receptor and the configuration of the rest of the molecule determines whether there is agonistic or antagonistic activity.

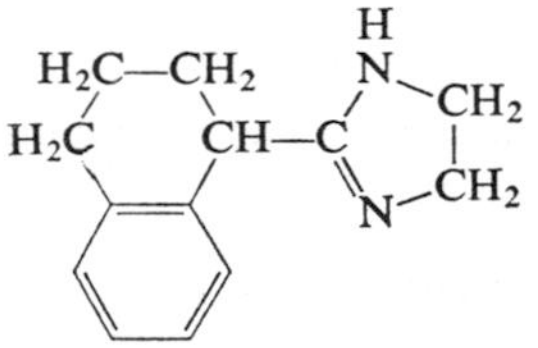

Tetrahydrozoline 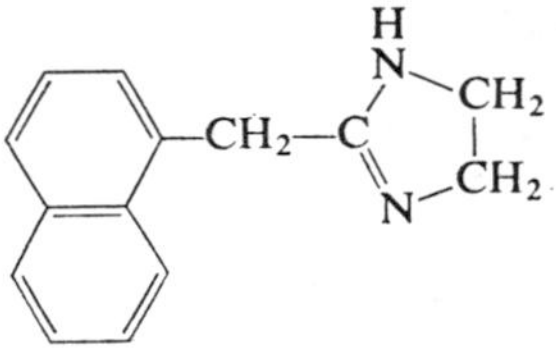   Naphazoline

The medicinal uses of sympathomimetics are summarized in Table 29.2.

Drugs which block the actions of sympathomimetics and the responses to sympathetic nerve stimulation

The term *adrenolytic* was introduced to describe drugs which block the actions of adrenaline and related drugs. Some of these drugs did not block responses to stimulation of sympathetic nerves, whereas others did, and for these the term *sympatholytic* was introduced. Objection has been taken to these terms on the grounds that the suffix '-lytic' should be reserved to convey the sense of destruction. However, the terms are useful for making the distinction which is important for practical reasons in medicine.

Drugs which block the actions of sympathomimetic amines have been termed *adrenergic blocking drugs*. This term would better serve to describe drugs which act on adrenergic nerves to prevent the release of noradrenaline, but it is too much identified with drugs which block receptors. There is no virtue in perpetuating this terminology. Drugs which block the receptors for sympathomimetic amines are here described as *antiadrenaline drugs*, and they are divided into two classes: α-receptor blocking and β-receptor blocking drugs.

Drugs which prevent the release of noradrenaline from sympathetic adrenergic nerve endings by the nerve impulse are classified as *adrenergic neurone-blocking drugs*. Drugs which prevent the release of noradrenaline by indirectly acting sympathomimetic amines have not yet been assigned any generally accepted name for classifying them.

Drugs blocking adrenoreceptors (anti-adrenaline drugs)

Drugs which antagonize the direct actions of sympathomimetics can be broadly classified into α- and β-receptor blocking drugs according to the type of receptor on which they act, and divided again on the basis of their chemical structure. These classifications are summarized in Table 29.3.

TABLE 29.3. Anti-adrenaline drugs

Type of chemical structure	Main compounds in medical use	Type of receptor blocked
Lysergic acid amides	Ergot alkaloids	α (some β)
Haloalkylamines	Phenoxybenzamine	α
Iminazolines	Phentolamine	α
Benzodioxanes	Piperoxane	α
Phenoxyalkylamines	Gravitol	α
Yohimbine-like alkaloids	None	α
Analogues of isoprenaline	Propranolol	β

Ergot alkaloids

Ergot is a fungus which grows on rye. Poisoning by ergot (ergotism) occurs from eating bread made from the fungus-infected grain. At one time ergotism was endemic, and large numbers of people were affected in some areas during famine years when no food was wasted and ergot-infected rye was harvested. Sporadic outbreaks of ergotism still occur occasionally when ergotized-rye is accidentally included in the manufacture of bread.

The symptoms of ergotism include effects on blood vessels and on the CNS; the particular pattern depends on the amounts ingested and the time over which the ergot is eaten. In chronic ergotism, the predominant symptoms are due to prolonged intense vasoconstriction: the skin is dry and cold, and there are intense pains from the ischaemic tissues, particularly in muscles and in the extremities (which gave rise to the old name of the disease—St. Anthony's fire); later, the ischaemic extremities become gangrenous. The effects on the CNS give rise to the symptoms which predominate in acute poisoning: these include vomiting, dizziness, headache, confusion, drowsiness, unconsciousness and convulsions. Ergot causes powerful contractions of the uterus and produces abortion.

Ergot was first used in medicine to hasten childbirth. The study of the pharmacology of ergot by Dale is recognized as one of the most important events in the history of pharmacology. During investigations of methods for the biological assay of the extracts, Dale discovered that ergot alkaloids possessed anti-adrenaline activity. The presence in ergot extracts of histamine, acetylcholine and the sympathomimetic amines, tyramine and isoamylamine, led to the first intensive investigations of the pharmacology of these compounds.

The ergot alkaloids are derivatives of lysergic acid amide (or lysergamide), as shown in Fig. 29.10. The group attached to the lysergamide moiety is propanol in the case of ergometrine and a complex polypeptide group in the case of ergotamine and the other alkaloids. On hydrolysis, the polypeptide group yields *d*-proline and *l*-phenylalanine or *l*-valine or *l*-leucine: these amino acid moieties are indicated in the structural formula. There are twelve naturally occurring alkaloids consisting of six isomeric pairs; the optical activity depends on the lysergamide group. (Methylergometrine and the dihydro derivatives are prepared semi-synthetically). In each pair, the laevo-isomer possesses considerably greater pharmacological activity than the dextro-isomer. Only the laevo-isomers are named in the figure; the names of the dextro-isomers have a terminal -inine instead of -ine.

Ergotamine has marked vasoconstrictor activity and produces the symptoms of ergotism, including the CNS disturbances. It antagonizes the action of drugs that act on α-adrenoreceptors, and has both adrenolytic and sympatholytic activity. It has only weak oxytocic activity. Ergotamine is used principally in the treatment of migraine, but the side-effects are troublesome. It often produces nausea and vomiting, and may have ill-effects during pregnancy or in patients suffering from constriction of blood-vessels in other parts of the body (occlusive vascular disease).

Dihydroergotamine is a synthetic derivative of ergotamine having much less vasoconstrictor and oxytocic activity, but a greater antiadrenaline activity

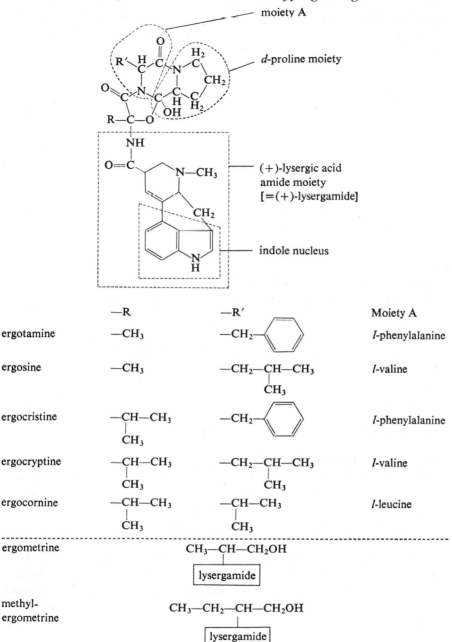

FIG. 29.10. Structural formulae of the ergot alkaloids.

than the parent compound. It is used in the treatment of migraine and produces fewer side-effects than ergotamine. Dihydroergotamine (often abbreviated to DHE) is the best of the adrenaline antagonists in the ergot group. It is a competitive antagonist, combining reversibly with the α-receptors.

Ergometrine (also known as ergonovine, ergobasine, ergostetrine and ergotocine) is the most powerful oxytocic amongst the ergot alkaloids and has completely replaced ergot in obstetrics. It is now used to control post partum bleeding, which it does by contracting the uterus. It has little constrictor activity on blood vessels or other non-uterine smooth muscle and negligible anti-adrenaline activity. It has been used to treat migraine, but is less effective than ergotamine. Ergometrine is rapidly absorbed after oral administration although it is usually given by injection. *Methylergometrine* has a more powerful and prolonged oxytocic action. It is of no value in the treatment of migraine.

Ergotoxine was the name given to the first alkaloid fraction isolated from ergot, but it was later found to be a mixture of three alkaloids: *ergocornine, ergocristine* and *ergocryptine*. Ergotoxine has oxytocic action, causes vascular spasm, and has antiadrenaline activity; it has been used in obstetrics and in the treatment of migraine. The mixture of the dihydro derivatives of the three alkaloids in ergotoxine is known commercially as Hydergine. As with ergotamine, the saturation of the double bond results in compounds with enhanced antiadrenaline activity and less action in contracting smooth muscles. Hydergine produces a fall in blood pressure, flushing of the skin and congestion of mucosal surfaces, and it is used in the treatment of peripheral vascular spasm. Its use in obstetrics to hasten delayed parturition is due to its action in *relaxing* the cervix. It is effective in the relief of migraine.

RATIONALE OF TREATMENT OF MIGRAINE. The effectiveness of ergotamine in the treatment of migraine was once attributed to its vasoconstrictor activity, since the cerebral blood vessels are dilated and have marked pulsation during the attack (page 110). However, dihydroergotamine was also shown to relieve migraine although it was without vasoconstrictor activity. It was then suggested that the antiadrenaline activity of these compounds was implicated, but this hypothesis was in turn rejected with the realization that there was no correlation between antiadrenaline activity of related substances and their effectiveness in the control of migraine. It has recently been suggested that antagonism of 5-hydroxytryptamine, which is an action shared by all the effective ergot derivatives, may be implicated.

HALOALKYLAMINES. The formulae of two well-known haloalkylamines are shown in Fig. 29.11, and many hundreds of related compounds have been prepared. The structural features common to those that are effective in blocking α-adrenoreceptors are a tertiary N-atom to which is attached a β-halogenated alkyl chain (the chloro-compounds are chemically the most stable), and an unsaturated ring system (phenoxyethyl compounds have the highest activity). The β-haloalkylamines undergo cyclization to form an ethylene iminium ion, and it is thought that this ion is first attached to the negatively-charged portion of the receptor by ion pair formation, and then alkylates the receptor by re-arrangement.

The blocking action of the haloalkylamines develops rather slowly after administration but is very persistent and cannot be overcome even by high concentrations of agonists. The initial antagonism is competitive since a high concentration of an agonist administered prior to the haloalkylamine prevents the development of blockade. However, once the blockade is produced by the haloalkylamines, it is irreversible. The effect is explained by the high strength of the covalent bond formed with the receptor compared to the weak ionic linkage formed by an α-receptor agonist.

Haloalkylamines are related to nitrogen mustard [$CH_3N(CH_2CH_2Cl)_2$]; this is a strong alkylating agent used as a cytotoxic drug in the treatment of cancer. Haloalkylamines have many pharmacological action in addition to α-receptor blockade, and these are no doubt due to alkylation of receptors or active centres. They have been shown to have antagonistic actions on histamine, 5-HT and acetylcholine (muscarinic) receptors, and to inhibit cholinesterase. They do not block the β-receptors. As well as acting on α-receptors, they act on the noradrenaline storage site in adrenergic neurones; at first they release some noradrenaline (which is able to act on β-receptors, and causes, for example, acceleration of the heart) and then they prevent the uptake of amines (thereby potentiating noradrenaline and adrenaline on β-receptors and antagonizing the action of drugs which act by displacing noradrenaline from the stores). However, they do not impair the release of noradrenaline by nerve impulses or by acetylcholine acting at the nerve ending. In fact, the amount of noradrenaline that is released into the venous outflow by stimulation of sympathetic nerves at low frequencies is increased by phenoxybenzamine. The explanations that have been advanced for this observation are (i) that the re-uptake of the released noradrenaline is prevented, and (ii) that the inhibition of cholinesterase potentiates acetylcholine in releasing larger amounts of noradrenaline (see page 164). The noradrenaline that is released by nerve impulses has no effect on the blocked α-receptors. In tissues that contain predominantly α-receptors, haloalkylamines are sympatholytic as well as adrenolytic. However, the effects of stimulation of adrenergic nerves that impinge on β-receptors are enhanced.

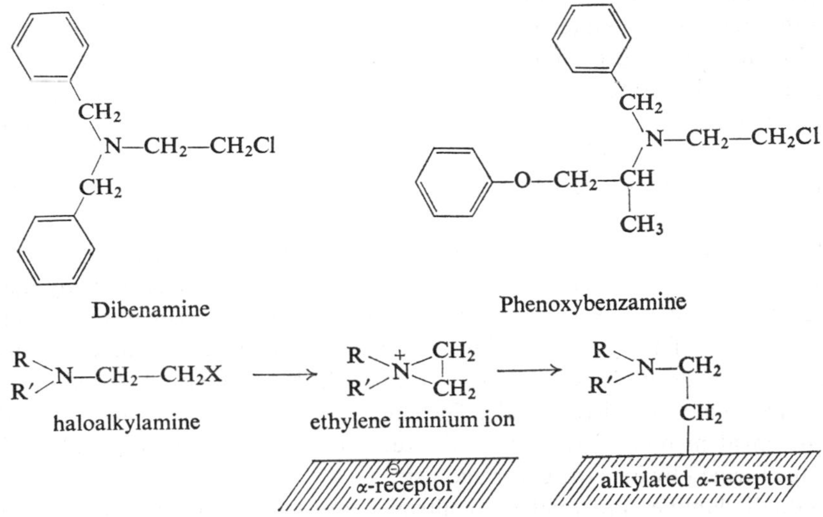

FIG. 29.11. Haloalkylamine antiadrenaline (α-receptor blocking) compounds.

Dibenamine is no longer used in medicine but *phenoxybenzamine* (Dibenyline, Dibenzyline) is used in the treatment of peripheral vascular spasm. Its effect in these disorders may be used to indicate whether sympathectomy of the affected region is likely to give good results. It has no direct vasodilator action, its beneficial effect in vascular spasm being due to blockade of vasoconstriction. It has little effect on the blood pressure in essential hypertension, but it is of value in reducing the blood pressure in patients with phaeochromocytoma (page 832) and is used in the differential diagnosis of this disorder. It has been used to prevent the occurrence of cardiac arrhythmias during cyclopropane and chloroform anaesthesia (page 580), and its effectiveness has been taken as evidence that stimulation of α-receptors by catecholamines is responsible for arrhythmias (stimulation of β-receptors leads to acceleration of the rate and force of the heart beat). However, it is probable that the arrhythmias are due to a combination of direct action of catecholamines on the heart (action on β-receptors) coupled with a reflex slowing of the heart (via the vagi) elicited by the rise in blood pressure produced largely by adrenaline released from the adrenals. The effectiveness of phenoxybenzamine in preventing arrhythmias is then due to prevention of the rise in blood pressure. Patients being treated for bronchial asthma with adrenaline may be given phenoxybenzamine, which prevents the pressor effect of adrenaline but not the bronchodilatation.

Phenoxybenzamine may also be useful in the treatment of shock; the rationale and results are described elsewhere (page 847).

IMINAZOLINE DERIVATIVES. The formulae of the two iminazoline anti-adrenaline drugs of medicinal importance are shown in Fig. 29.12. They are competitive antagonists at α-adrenoreceptors and have no effect on the β-receptors of smooth muscle, although they reduce the actions of agonists acting on cardiac β-receptors. Their sympatholytic activity is considerably less than their adrenolytic activity.

Tolazoline (Priscol) exhibits a wide range of pharmacological activity in addition to its antiadrenaline action. It stimulates the gastric secretion of hydrochloric acid, thus resembling histamine in its actions. Tolazoline stimulates the gastro-intestinal tract producing diarrhoea; it also causes increased sweating and secretion of saliva and pancreatic juice. These effects are blocked by atropine, so presumably a cholinergic mechanism is involved, and this is explained by the finding that tolazoline possesses anticholinesterase activity. Tolazoline produces peripheral vasodilatation; this is not affected by atropine, it is not a histamine-like effect, and it is not due to release of adrenergic vasomotor tone; consequently it is described as a direct vasodilator action: it is exploited clinically in the treatment of peripheral vascular spasm.

Phentolamine (Rogitine, Regitine) has fewer side-effects than tolazoline and is about 10 times more powerful in its α-receptor blocking activity. However, it has direct vasodilator action and intravenous injections cause a fall in blood pressure; there is also tachycardia which is at least partly reflexly induced. Phentolamine is used mainly to treat hypertensive crises that are due to circulating catecholamines (e.g., in phaeochromocytoma, and in case of over-dosage or excessive response with injections of adrenaline or noradrenaline). It is of less use than phenoxybenzamine in the diagnosis of phaeochromocytoma because of its direct depressor effect; however, it has fewer side effects than phenoxybenzamine which gives it an advantage in the control of the disease.

Azapetine (Fig. 29.12) is not an iminazoline derivative but its pharmacological actions closely resemble those of tolazoline.

BENZODIOXANES. Many of these compounds were synthesized by Fourneau (hence the 'F' in the serial number) and were examined pharmacologically by Bovet. The formulae of the benzodioxanes used in medicine are shown in Fig. 29.13. *Piperoxane* is used like phentolamine in the diagnosis of phaeochromocytoma and in the management of hypertensive crises due to circulating cate-

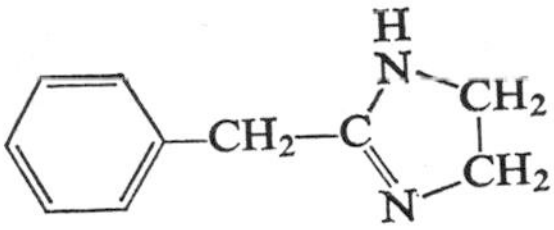

Tolazoline

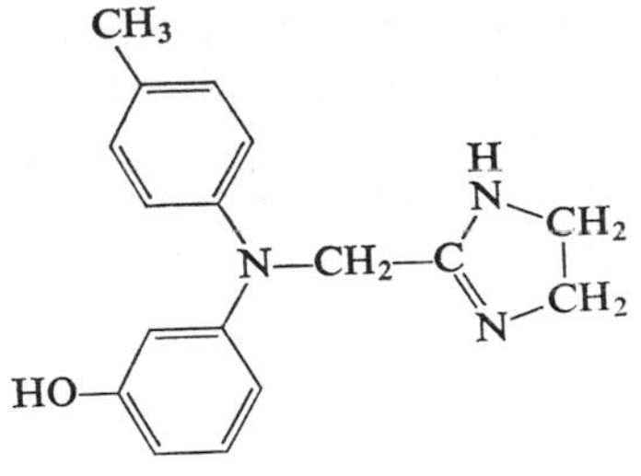

Phentolamine

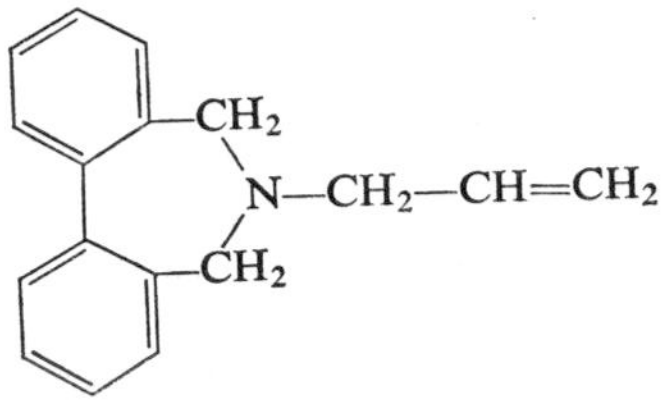

Azapetine

FIG. 29.12. Structural formulae of the iminazoline antiadrenaline compounds, tolazoline and phentolamine, and the pharmacologically related drug azapetine.

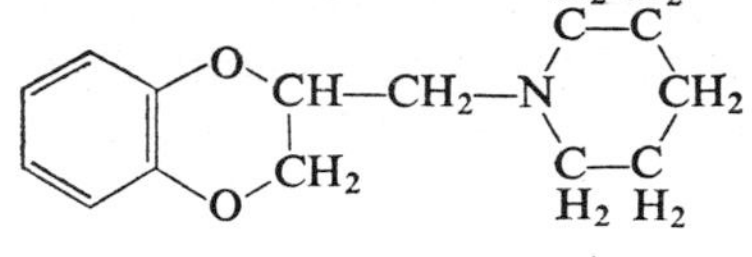

F-883 (Prosympal)

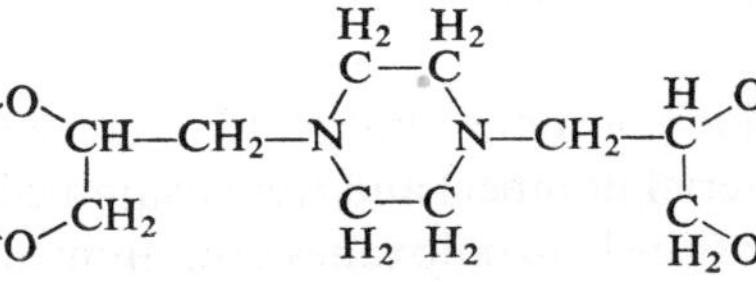

F-933 (Piperoxane)

Dibozane

FIG. 29.13. Benzodioxane antiadrenaline drugs.

cholamines. Piperoxane antagonizes the actions of agonists on α-adreno-receptors, but has no blocking action at β-receptors. It is only weakly sympatholytic, whereas *Prosympal* is both adrenolytic (at α-receptors) and sympatholytic. *Dibozane* is the most recent addition to the group of benzo-dioxane anti-adrenaline drugs and it too acts only on α-receptors.

PHENOXYALKYLAMINES. The formulae of some of these compounds are shown in Fig. 29.14. Phenolic ethers of alkyl tertiary amines have antiadrenaline activity but the position of the phenolic —OH group has a profound

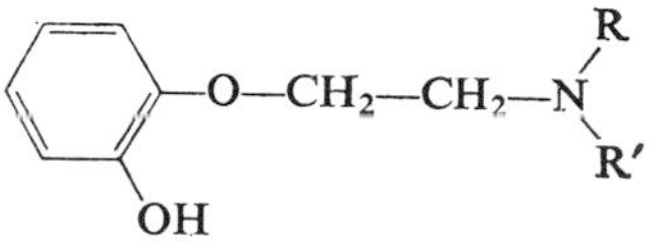

ortho-Hydroxyphenoxyalkylamines

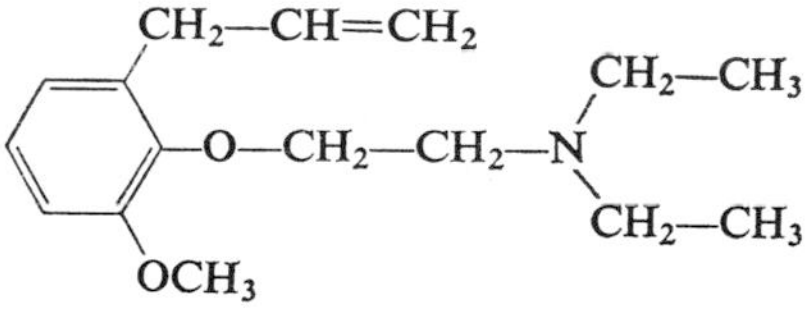

Gravitol

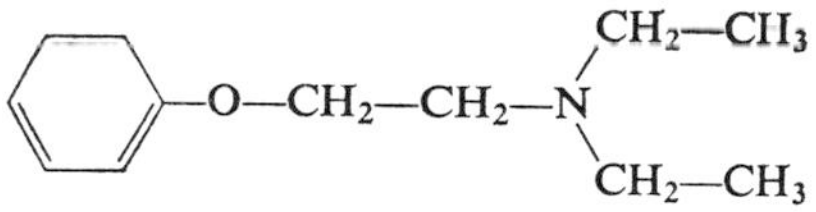

F-928   (Phenoxyethyldiethylamine)

FIG. 29.14. Phenoxyalkylamine derivatives with antiadrenaline activity.

effect on the activity of the compounds. Substitution in the *o*-position yields antiadrenaline drugs, whereas compounds substituted in the *m*-position are pressor; substitution in the *p*-position yields compounds with nicotine-like actions. Increasing the size of the R and R' substituents on the nitrogen gives rise to depressor drugs, resembling isoprenaline. None of these compounds has been developed for therapeutic use, but they have been included because of their chemical resemblance to many other groups of drugs, including adrenergic neurone-blocking drugs (cf. xylocholine, page 769), antihistamines (cf. 929F page 781) and local anaesthetics (cf. procaine, page 657). The compound F-928 has antihistamine activity and was the starting point in the development of a series of these compounds. *Gravitol* has antiadrenaline activity; it also contracts the uterus and has been used in obstetrics as an oxytocic.

YOHIMBINE AND RELATED ALKALOIDS. *Yohimbine* and a number of other naturally occurring alkaloids and their semi-synthetic derivatives have anti-adrenaline activity and are also sympatholytic. Chemically, these compounds resemble the ergot alkaloids in containing an indole grouping as part of a complex molecule. Yohimbine has many other pharmacological actions. It is a vasodilator. It has a reputation as an aphrodisiac, in which respect it is thought to act partly peripherally by causing vasodilatation with congestion of blood in the erectile tissue of the genitalia, and partly centrally in enhancing the reflexes concerned in ejaculation. It is also a local anaesthetic with about the same potency as cocaine. It has the property of releasing ADH from the neurohypophysis.

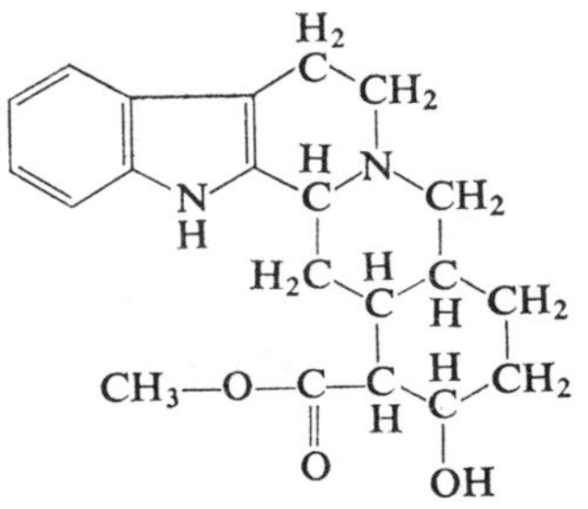

Yohimbine

Analogues of isoprenaline that block β-receptors. Drugs that block β-receptors have been developed only during the last few years. The most potent of them are analogues of isoprenaline, and they have a more obvious chemical relationship to the β-receptor agonists than do the α-receptor blocking drugs to the α-receptor agonists. The chemical formulae of some β-receptor blocking drugs are shown in Fig. 29.15. The β-receptor blocking drugs behave as competitive antagonists.

Dichloroisoprenaline (DCI) is the analogue of isoprenaline with the two phenolic hydroxyl groups replaced by chlorine atoms. DCI was discovered in 1957 and was the first specifically β-receptor blocking drug to be described. It is a partial agonist and is not used clinically because of the intense initial β-receptor agonist activity which is produced by blocking doses. Nevertheless, the discovery of DCI stimulated the search for more powerful blocking drugs with less agonistic activity.

Pronethalol and propranolol are two chemically related compounds with powerful β-receptor blocking activity and with considerably less agonistic activity than has DCI. Propranolol is more potent than pronethalol and has supplanted pronethalol in clinical use, since the latter was shown to produce lymphoid tumours after prolonged administration in mice (though not in dogs or rats).

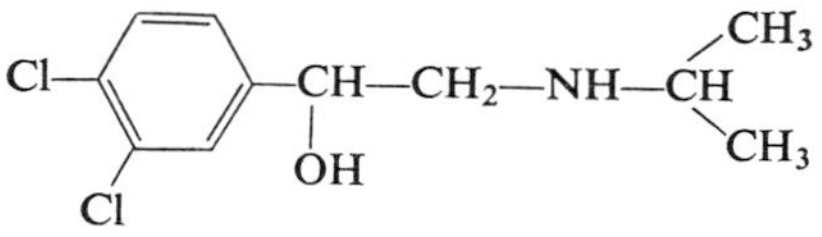

Dichloroisoprenaline (DCI)

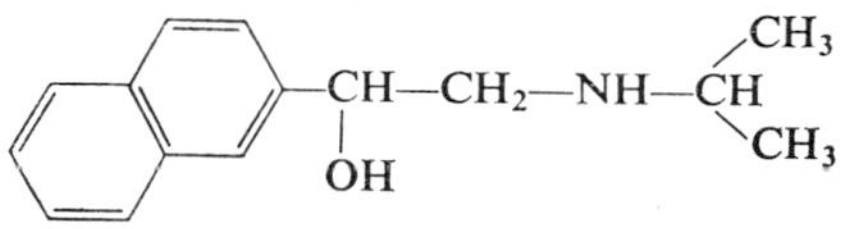

Pronethalol

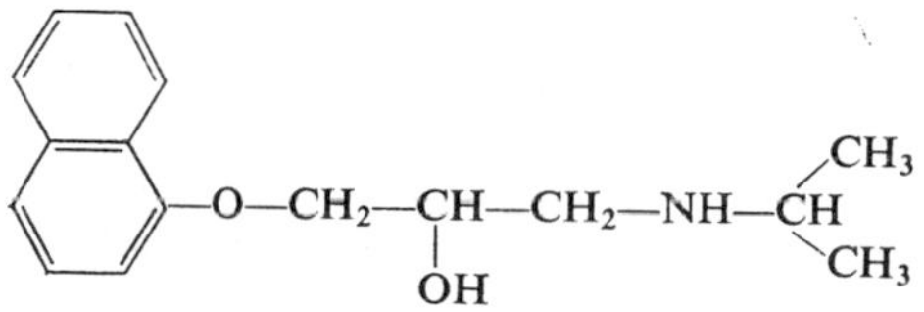

Propranolol

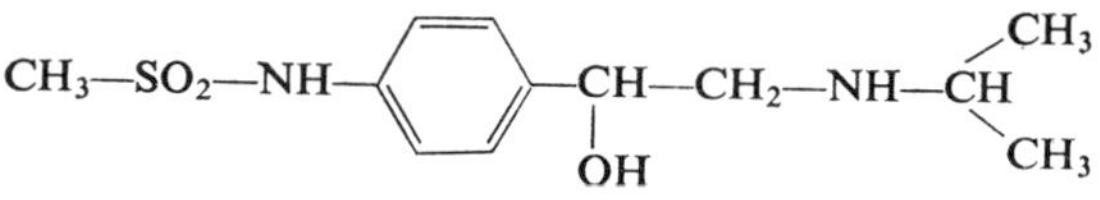

MJ-1999

FIG. 29.15. Drugs that block β-receptors.

Both compounds possess the following actions in addition to β-receptor blocking activity. (1) A powerful local anaesthetic action; they have about twice the potency of procaine. (2) A quinidine-like antiarrhythmic action on the heart. (3) They block the polysynaptic flexor reflex by an action in the spinal cord, but are without effect on the monosynaptic knee-jerk. Pronethalol is more potent than propranolol because it penetrates the blood-brain barrier more readily. This central action of pronethalol is of interest because in a recent clinical trial it was found to reduce the increase in tremor produced by adrenaline in Parkinsonian patients and to be of subjective benefit to the patients.

Pronethalol and propranolol are racemic compounds and the β-receptor blocking activity resides largely in the laevo-isomers. For example, racemic propranolol has about 50 times the β-receptor blocking potency of (+)-propranolol. However, quinidine-like activity is less dependent on steric configuration, the two isomers having approximately equal activity.

The clinical uses of propranolol are still being assessed: they include the following. (1) It has been found effective in some cases of angina (page 824) where it probably acts by preventing the increase in cardiac activity in response to sympathetic activity during exercise. Most patients being treated with propranolol can achieve a greater amount of exercise before anginal pain is experienced. (2) It lowers blood pressure in hypertensive patients (page 844). (3) It may be used to prevent the occurrence of cardiac arrhythmias during anaesthesia or digitalis intoxication, and to reduce the tachycardia associated with phaeochromocytoma. The antiarrhythmic action of propranolol is in part due to its quinidine-like action, but the drug is of especial benefit in arrhythmias associated with sympathetic activity or catecholamine release or administration.

*MJ*1999 is a newer β-receptor blocking drug. It is less potent than propranolol and has much less local anaesthetic, quinidine-like and β-receptor agonist activity.

A number of other drugs of similar structure have been introduced. They have not yet been given official names and include **H** 13/57, **KÖ** 592 and N-isopropyl-1-nitrophenylethanolamine.

The β-receptor blocking activity of methoxamine was mentioned above. This drug, and derivatives of it, have been studied chiefly for their effects in preventing the metabolic actions of catecholamines. They block the rise in plasma free fatty acids, blood glucose and lactic acid induced by catecholamines. Methoxamine also possesses α-agonist activity and its use to produce β-receptor blockade therefore results in hypertension, piloerection and other manifestation of α-receptor activation. N-Isopropylmethoxamine, though itself without α-agonistic activity, produces the same effects as methoxamine because it is dealkylated to methoxamine in the body. However, N-tertiary-butylmethoxamine (butoxamine) is not dealkylated to methoxamine and blocks the metabolic effects of catecholamines without producing signs of α-receptor stimulation. Butoxamine is said to block metabolic responses to catecholamine without producing β-receptor blockade in the heart or smooth muscle.

Adrenergic neurone-blocking drugs

The characteristic feature of this class of drugs is that they abolish the responses to stimulation of postganglionic adrenergic nerves, without abolishing responses to noradrenaline. This property was first discovered in 1956 during pharmacological experiments with xylocholine, and in the 10 years since then many hundreds of other adrenergic neurone-blocking drugs have been prepared. The formulae of the most important of these are shown in Fig. 29.16.

XYLOCHOLINE. This substance is the xylyl ether of choline. It is also known as TM 10, being the tenth in a series of substituted phenyl choline ethers. The first compound in the series, TM 1, is phenylcholine ether, and it has powerful nicotinic activity. Xylocholine has only weak nicotinic activity and then antagonizes the nicotinic actions of acetylcholine. It also has muscarinic activity. Xylocholine has some activity as an antagonist of noradrenaline and adrenaline, and is closely related chemically to the phenoxyalkylamine group of antiadrenaline drugs. It also has local anaesthetic properties and is a weak inhibitor of monoamine oxidase.

β-Methyl TM 10. The potential advantages offered in treating hypertension with a drug possessing the adrenergic neurone-blocking activity of xylocholine were quickly realized. However, the acetylcholine-like activity of xylocholine is sufficiently strong to preclude its use, so congeners have been studied that are less active in terms of these side-effects. One of these, β-methyl TM 10, was found to be effective in lowering high blood pressure in man but it was not exploited commercially.

Parabenzoyl TM 10 (B.W. 172C58). This substance has more powerful adrenergic neurone blocking activity than xylocholine in laboratory experiments and is highly specific, but its action is short lasting and it is not particularly active in man.

BRETYLIUM. Like β-methyl TM 10, bretylium was developed in the search for a drug having fewer side-effects than xylocholine. It was the first of the adrenergic neurone-blocking drugs commercially available for the treatment of hypertension; it is supplied as bretylium tosylate (Darenthin) as this salt was convenient for pharmaceutical reasons. The major disadvantages of bretylium are that the amounts absorbed after oral administration are erratic, and that tolerance develops, necessitating steadily increasing doses. It has now been largely superseded.

GUANETHIDINE. This drug was developed independently of the investigations based on xylocholine, and at one time it was thought that the differences, both in structure (a guanidine instead of a quaternary nitrogen group), and in its spectrum of pharmacological activity, placed this compound in a class of adrenergic neurone-blocking drugs having a different mode of action. In particular, guanethidine causes the depletion of noradrenaline from adrenergically innervated structures; however, this is not the explanation of its adrenergic neurone-blocking activity. The use of guanethidine in the treatment of hypertension is discussed on pages 838–839.

Bethanidine. This is a benzyl guanidine drivative with the proprietory name Esbatal. It has a rapid onset and a short duration of action.

25

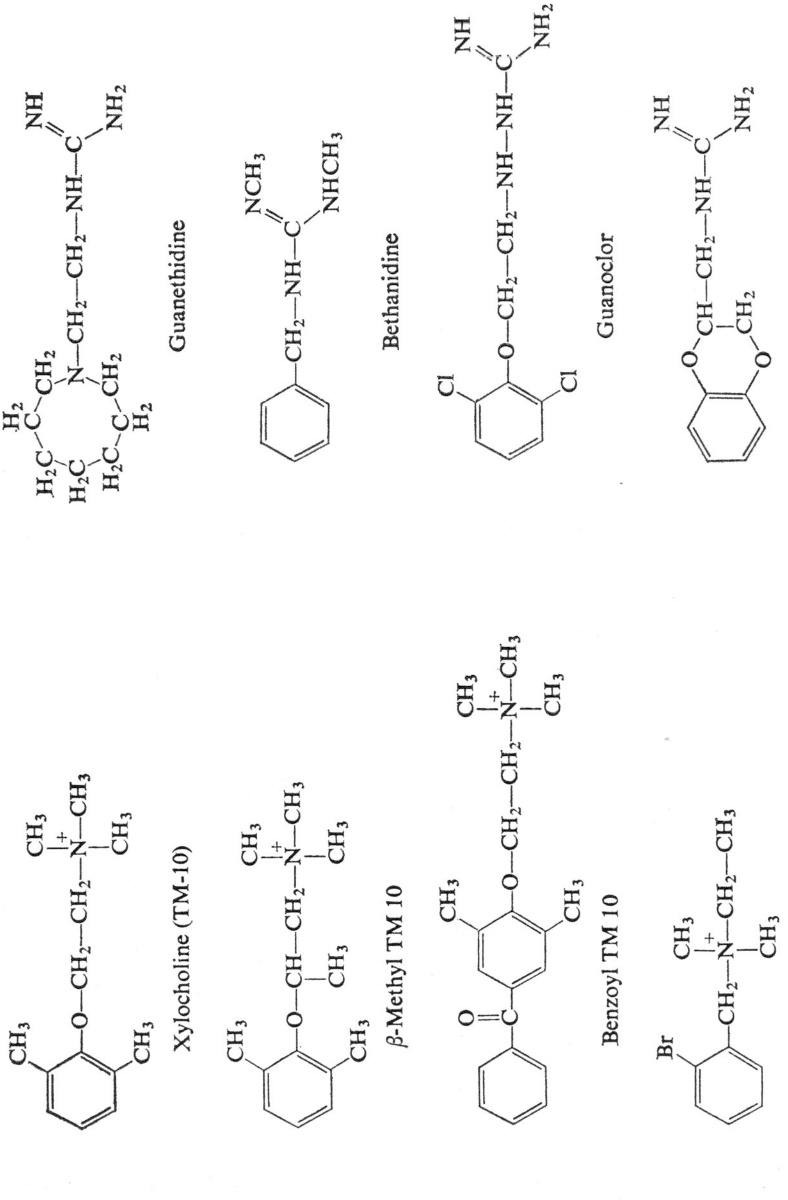

Guanethidine

Bethanidine

Guanoclor

Guanoxan

Xylocholine (TM-10)

β-Methyl TM 10

Benzoyl TM 10

Bretylium

FIG. 29.16. Adrenergic neurone-blocking drugs.

Guanoxan (Envacar) also has a guanidine group and a benzodioxane nucleus. In addition to its adrenergic neurone blocking activity, guanoxan has anti-adrenaline activity which may be attributable to its chemical relationship to the benzodioxane α-receptor blocking drugs. Like guanethidine, this drug depletes peripheral, adrenergic neurones of their noradrenaline content, but in addition it depletes the amine content of the CNS. In these respects, its actions resemble those of reserpine.

Guanoclor (Vatensol) also depletes amines from both peripheral and central neurones. It inhibits ethylamine β-oxidase, the enzyme that catalyses the conversion of dopamine to noradrenaline (page 159).

Actions of adrenergic neurone-blocking drugs. The discovery of this type of drug action in the laboratory was made from the observation that xylocholine abolished the contraction of the cat's nictitating membrane in response to sympathetic nerve stimulation but not to the injection of noradrenaline; in this way, the action differs from that of sympatholytic adreno-receptor blocking drugs. The responses to both pre- and postganglionic nerve stimulation are abolished, and this allows these drugs to be distinguished from ganglion-blocking drugs. Responses to stimulation of cholinergic sympathetic nerves (e.g. sweating in the cat's paw) are not affected, indicating that the action is exerted only on adrenergic neurones.

In the identification of adrenergic neurone-blocking activity, a variety of preparations have been employed. In addition to the nictitating membrane-cervical sympathetic nerve *in situ*, there are many convenient isolated organ preparations. The one most commonly used is the rabbit ileum with lumbar nerves attached; these nerves accompany the mesenteric blood vessels, and this makes for convenience in dissection. In conscious animals, the consequences of blockade of adrenergic neurones may be detected in several ways: in cats, the nictitating membrane, which is usually retracted and only just visible, is relaxed and is clearly seen; in rats, the sympathetically-innervated muscle in the eyelid (page 415) is relaxed, giving rise to the symptom of *ptosis*.

The uses of adrenergic neurone blocking drugs in medicine, and their actions and side-effects in man, are discussed in Chapter 32; their effects on the cardiovascular system in animals are also dealt with there. The diversity of other actions possessed by these drugs is best discussed here, in the context of their mode of action.

Mode of action of adrenergic neurone-blocking drugs

LOCAL ANAESTHETIC ACTIVITY. All of these compounds have local anaesthetic activity, which led to the suggestion that they prevent the release of transmitter from adrenergic neurones by blocking the conduction of the nerve impulse. However, sympathetic blockade is produced without any accompanying local anaesthetic effect on sensory C fibres (adrenergic neurones are also C fibres, page 72). It has been found that some adrenergic neurone-blocking drugs are sequestered in adrenergic nerves (probably this is true for all these drugs), and this finding led to the speculation that the preferential uptake of the drugs in the sympathetic neurones may be responsible for a selective local anaesthetic action. Evidence against this hypothesis is that the action potentials are still propagated in sympathetic nerve trunks, even though the responses to stimulation are abolished. The discoverers of the adrenergic neurone-blocking activity of xylocholine also studied a closely related compound, TE 10, the N-triethyl analogue: this substance is as powerful a local anaesthetic as TM 10, but has no adrenergic neurone-blocking activity.

EFFECTS ON NORADRENALINE STORES. The depletion of noradrenaline by guanethidine and some other adrenergic neurone-blocking drugs has already been mentioned. This effect is also observed with large doses of bretylium and xylocholine, the distinction being in the ratio of doses required for blockade and for depletion. The depletion may be due to the displacement of noradrenaline from the stores or to facilitation of the neuronal process that leads to noradrenaline release. The latter explanation is the more likely, since adrenergic neurone-blocking drugs do not liberate noradrenaline from isolated granules, whereas the indirectly acting sympathomimetic amines do. The release of noradrenaline produces sympathomimetic effects such as a rise in blood pressure in spinal animals or contraction of the nictitating membrane.

The indirectly-acting sympathomimetic amines antagonize adrenergic neurone-blockade; thus, in a cat treated with guanethidine in sufficient amount to block the responses of the nictitating membrane to sympathetic nerve stimulation, amphetamine produces a restoration of the responses to nerve stimulation. There is evidence that this interaction has the characteristics of a competitive antagonism, and this indicates an action on some underlying process that is involved in common by sympathomimetic amines and adrenergic-blocking drugs.

ACTIONS ON CHOLINERGIC TRANSMISSION. In the whole animal, adrenergic neurone-blocking drugs have only a slight and transient effect in blocking ganglionic transmission, but in isolated preparations they are as powerful in this respect as many ganglion-blocking drugs. Furthermore, they impair neuromuscular transmission. These are sites at which acetylcholine has a nicotinic action. Acetylcholine has a nicotinic action on sympathetic nerve endings, causing the release of noradrenaline, and this too may be abolished by adrenergic neurone-blocking drugs. These observations fit into the hypothesis that acetylcholine is concerned as an intermediary in release of noradrenaline at adrenergic junctions (page 164).

STRUCTURE-ACTION RELATIONSHIPS AMONGST THE ADRENERGIC NEURONE-BLOCKING DRUGS. From the structures illustrated in Fig. 29.16, the following generalizations can be made: (1) The molecule has a positively charged group. The guanidine group is as effective as a quaternary nitrogen, and at physiological pH is almost completely ionized (page 491). Interchange between guanidine and quaternary nitrogen groups results in molecules with essentially the same adrenergic neurone-blocking activity, as in the guanidine analogue of xylocholine and the quaternary nitrogen analogue of guanethidine. Other strongly basic groups, such as hydrazinium, $[—N^+(CH_3)_2NH_2]$ are equally effective. (2) The substituents on the basic group are small. As mentioned above, the triethyl analogue of xylocholine is ineffective. (3) The remainder of the molecule consists of a short chain between the basic group and an aryl or alkyl group. (4) There may be an atom carrying a lone pair of electrons at about 4 Å distance from the positively charged group: in xylocholine it is the ether oxygen and in guanethidine it is the tertiary nitrogen.

Drugs with differential effects on directly and indirectly acting sympathomimetics

EFFECTS OF RESERPINE. Changes similar to those produced by chronic denervation occur after treatment with the drug, reserpine. (The formula of reserpine is shown in Fig. 22.1, and its actions as a CNS depressant are described on pages 599–600.) Reserpine does not destroy the neurone, and its effects are slowly reversible. Its mode of action in depleting noradrenaline is not known but it probably weakens the affinity of the binding site for noradrenaline. The release of noradrenaline from adrenergic neurones (and of catecholamines from the adrenal medulla) by reserpine is slow and there is usually no sympathomimetic action due to the released catecholamines. However, under some circumstances, an initial sympathomimetic effect is seen. For example, in animal experiments it is possible to observe a sympathomimetic pressor action when the inactivation of the released catecholamines by COMT is prevented, (e.g. with catechol, page 775), or when the animal is sensitized to circulating catecholamine (e.g. by destroying the CNS).

The consequences of the depletion by reserpine of noradrenaline from adrenergic neurones are (1) an increased response to noradrenaline and adrenaline since the uptake into the neuronal stores is impaired and more is available for action at the receptors, and (2) a loss of response to indirectly-acting sympathomimetic amines since there is no noradrenaline in the store to be released.

EFFECT OF COCAINE. Over 30 years ago, Burn and Tainter observed that cocaine abolished the action of tyramine but potentiated adrenaline. Later it was found that cocaine caused the same change in activity of sympathomimetic amines as did denervation, the actions of some being enhanced and of others being abolished. Then, after observations with reserpine had led to the concept of direct and indirect actions, it was realized that cocaine potentiated the directly-acting and antagonized the indirectly-acting sympathomimetic amines. Cocaine does not deplete noradrenaline from adrenergic neurones, and, in fact, responses to nerve stimulation are enhanced. The explanation for the actions of cocaine is that it prevents the access of amines to the storage sites in the adrenergic neurone. Many other drugs have a substantially similar action; examples include methylphenidate (page 618), imipramine (page 621) and chlorpromazine (page 595). These drugs all have actions on the CNS, and it is possible that an effect on central adrenergic neurones similar to that seen on peripheral neurones may be part of the mechanism contributing to their central action.

EFFECTS OF INDIRECTLY-ACTING SYMPATHOMIMETIC AMINES. Amphetamine, ephedrine and other sympathomimetics with an α-methyl substituent exhibit tachyphylaxis: responses to repeated injections rapidly become smaller. This occurs without appreciable depletion of the noradrenaline stores. The mechanism appears to be that a readily available portion of the store is easily displaced, but then the access to the remainder of the store is impeded. These drugs potentiate noradrenaline by impairing its uptake. The α-methyl group renders these amines immune from attack by monamine oxidase; this enzyme is present within the cytoplasm of the adrenergic neurone.

ANTIADRENALINE DRUGS. Most of the antiadrenaline drugs, both those that block α-receptors and those that block β-receptors, impair the uptake of noradrenaline into the storage sites, and also block the access of indirectly acting amines to the store.

Effects of drugs on monoamine oxidase and catechol-O-methyl transferase. The actions of these enzymes, MAO and COMT, were described on pages 165 to 166.

MAO INHIBITORS. The mechanism for terminating the effects of transmitter at adrenergic junctions differs considerably from that at cholinergic junctions. The importance of cholinesterase at cholinergic junctions and the marked effects of anticholinesterase drugs has been stressed. At adrenergic junctions, the effects of released transmitter are terminated largely by re-uptake into the neurone, and by diffusion away from the tissue: inactivation of monamine oxidase has little effect on responses to nerve stimulation or to catecholamines. However, the effects of some indirectly-acting sympathomimetic amines are greatly increased; in particular, these are the ones without an α-methyl substituent. They are rapidly metabolized by monoamine oxidase: consequently they are inactive when given by mouth, short acting when given intravenously, do not readily display tachyphylaxis, and have little or no action on the CNS. Treatment with monoamine oxidase inhibitors reverses all these properties. The effect of eating foodstuffs containing sympathomimetic amines in patients being treated with monoamine oxidase inhibitors is described on pages 625–626. The amines are formed by bacterial decarboxylation of amino acids: they include tyramine and phenylethylamine (from tyrosine and phenylalanine respectively) and possibly isobutylamine and isoamylamine (from valine and leucine respectively).

Many monoamine oxidase inhibitors have sympathomimetic activity of the indirect type. The structural resemblance of phenelzine, pheniprazine and tranylcypromine to the phenylalkylamines is obvious (cf. Fig. 23.1, page 622, with Fig. 29.9). Cocaine has monoamine oxidase inhibitory activity, as do the α-methylated sympathomimetic amines, but this has little to do with their pharmacological effects.

COMT INHIBITORS. It has been known for many years that catechols potentiate catecholamines, and that this effect is due to inhibition of COMT. Substances with this action include catechol itself, pyrogallol, quercetin, β-methyltropolone and rutin. These substances are used for various purposes in medicine, none of which is related to inhibition of COMT. No medical indication for a COMT inhibitor has been proposed, nor is there a drug available that would be suitable for this purpose in man. The substance formed from adrenaline by COMT, 3-methoxymetanephrine, has no effect itself on receptors, but sensitizes them to the effect of adrenaline.

CHAPTER 30

Histamine, 5–Hydroxytryptamine and Polypeptides Acting on Smooth Muscle

Histamine

Histamine is formed in the body by decarboxylation of the essential amino-acid, histidine (see page 175). It may also be manufactured synthetically. The free base is a light brown, unstable solid and the hydrochloride or acid phosphate is usually used. The following are the chief pharmacological actions of histamine.

ACTION ON BRONCHIOLAR SMOOTH MUSCLE. Histamine causes contraction of the smooth muscle of the bronchioles of most species. This is very marked in the lungs of the guinea-pig and an asthma-like effect results; large doses produce lethal asphyxia.

ACTION ON VASCULAR SMOOTH MUSCLE. The intravenous injection of a small dose of histamine causes a short-lasting fall in blood pressure which is due to dilatation of arterioles. The depressor effect is often followed by a secondary rise in pressure due to liberation of adrenaline from the adrenal medulla. Larger doses of histamine produce a profound fall in blood pressure and blood accumulates in the capillaries. Capillary permeability is increased and fluid is lost from the circulation into the tissues, the volume of the circulating blood thereby being decreased. The vasodilatation and loss of circulatory volume result in shock and circulatory collapse. When histamine is injected intradermally, the triple response occurs (see page 177); dilatation of the skin blood capillaries is followed by an increase in their permeability and the surrounding arterioles dilate and produce the flare which is probably due to an axon reflex.

In the dog, histamine contracts the muscular tissue around the hepatic veins; the liver, portal veins and mesenteric veins become engorged with blood. The intense haemorrhagic congestion in the mucosa of the small intestine is most marked in the duodenum; the capillaries in the villi become distended with blood and there is increased capillary permeability. Finally, the blood vessels rupture and the resulting petechiae (blood spots) and bleeding may be so severe that death follows. In the rabbit, the smooth muscle in the walls of the pulmonary arteries is constricted by histamine; the blood is dammed back in the right side of the heart and failure of the circulation may follow.

ACTION ON SMOOTH MUSCLE OF THE GASTRO-INTESTINAL TRACT. Histamine contracts the smooth muscle of the intestine. Strips of ileum of the guinea-pig are very sensitive, rabbit tissues are not nearly so sensitive, and rat and mouse tissues are insensitive to histamine.

ACTION ON SMOOTH MUSCLE OF THE REPRODUCTIVE TRACT. As with the muscle of the gastro-intestinal tract; the uterus of the guinea-pig is contracted by histamine but that of the rat and mouse is unaffected or even relaxed.

ACTION ON GASTRIC SECRETION. Histamine stimulates acid gastric secretion, probably by acting directly upon the glandular secretory cells of the gastric mucosa, and this may be a physiological function of histamine. The action of histamine in increasing the acid secretion is not antagonized by antihistamine drugs.

ACTION ON THE HEART. Histamine increases the rate and force of beating of isolated hearts through a direct action on cardiac tissue. In the whole animal an intravenous injection of histamine causes an increase in heart rate and cardiac output but these effects are mainly reflexly induced by the fall in arterial pressure and rise in venous pressure produced by the vascular actions of histamine.

ACTION ON CEREBRO-SPINAL FLUID PRESSURE. Histamine produces an increase in the cerebro-spinal fluid pressure and this has been stated to be a cause of some headaches. The characteristic throbbing headache which occurs in man after a histamine injection is due to stretching of pain-sensitive structures in the dura mater by the alterations in the pressure of both cerebro-spinal fluid and blood vessels.

ACTION IN GROWTH, DEVELOPMENT AND REPAIR. There is some evidence to show that histamine may be connected with the metabolic machinery related to the anabolic processes of growth and development. For example, some tumours are very active in decarboxylating histidine during their periods of active growth and histamine can stimulate their growth. The foetuses of some species are capable of forming large amounts of histamine during periods of active growth and histamine can augment development. During regeneration in animals (as after partial hepatectomy) and after wounding (as during the healing of skin incisions), histamine is capable of stimulating anabolic processes.

ACTION ON SENSORY NERVE ENDINGS IN THE SKIN. The intradermal injection of histamine causes an itching sensation and histamine is thought to be one of the agents involved in the production of itch. When injected into the skin more deeply, a burning sensation is felt.

HISTAMINE AND ITS RELATION TO ALLERGY AND ANAPHYLAXIS. After the injection of foreign protein (antigen) into an animal, the reticulo-endothelial system responds by forming specific antibodies. The antibodies circulate and are later absorbed by the tissues. When a fairly large dose of the same protein is injected intravenously three or more weeks later, it combines with the antibodies. The antigen-antibody reaction damages the tissue mast cells so that their constituents (which include histamine) are released. The animal is thrown into a shock-like state termed anaphylaxis. The effects are similar in many respects to those produced by histamine. If the animal survives, it is insensitive to further doses of the antigen. Some drugs can be converted into antigens by being attached to proteins of the body to form what are in effect foreign proteins; the subsequent injection of the drug may then produce anaphylactic shock.

The main symptom of anaphylaxis in the guinea-pig is broncho-constriction, resembling that occurring in asthma; this may be severe enough to cause death by asphyxia. In the dog, venous engorgement of the liver occurs, and this may be followed by intestinal haemorrhage; heparin is released along with the histamine, the two substances being liberated from the tissue mast cells in the liver, from which they pass via the lymph through the thoracic duct to the blood stream. In the rabbit, constriction of the pulmonary arteries may result in right-sided heart failure. In all three species, these effects are similar to those produced by injections of large doses of histamine. In some species (for example, the rat), the main symptoms of anaphylaxis are intense intestinal haemorrhage and the production of severe petechiae in the heart and lungs; however, histamine is not the only mediator responsible for these effects in these species. Bradykinin (see page 181) is also capable of producing these changes and may be formed from plasma globulin by proteolytic enzymes during anaphylaxis. A slow-reacting substance (SRS-A, page 183) is released from the lungs of guinea-pigs during anaphylactic shock and may augment the broncho-constrictor action of histamine. SRS-A may be separated from histamine and partly purified by treating the perfusate from guinea-pig lungs during anaphylaxis with activated charcoal (which absorbs SRS-A) and then eluting it with butanol.

Anaphylaxis may occur in man after the ingestion of some foods or after treatment with drugs such as penicillin. A shock-like state develops or skin rashes appear; occasionally there are blood and liver dyscrasias. Allergy and asthma are related to anaphylaxis in that there is a release of histamine and this causes the allergic and asthmatic phenomena which include urticaria, hay fever, paroxysmal rhinitis and angioneurotic oedema. In asthma, human lungs release histamine and SRS-A. Drug allergy not involving antibody reactions is also known. If it is accepted that histamine plays a major role in allergic conditions, then it might be assumed that its removal from allergic patients will cure or reduce the severity of the symptoms; this is precisely what does occur, though the means whereby the histamine is removed from the tissues are still too drastic and treacherous for general use. Injections of histamine increase phagocytosis in some species and there may be a relation between allergy and resistance to infection; removal of histamine may then cure the allergy but increase the risk of infection. The problem of allergy remains unsolved. There may be a genetic factor since the disposition to asthma is partly familial.

HISTAMINE-LIBERATORS. Certain chemical compounds are capable of releasing histamine from the tissue stores. Release of histamine may be effected by displacing it from the molecular site of binding by rupture of the histamine-containing cytoplasmic granules, or by damage to the histamine-containing cells (especially mast cells). Recently it has been shown that granules containing the histamine may pass through small pores in the cell membrane and appear outside the cell, still carrying the histamine.

Susbstances which release histamine may be classified as follows: (1) snake and wasp venoms, (2) trypsin and other proteolytic enzymes, (3) detergents and other surface active agents, and (4) a large group of basic substances such as amines, amidines and guanidines. Many drugs contain such basic groups and are histamine liberators, which often constitutes a serious disadvantage and may be responsible for the side-effects of certain drugs amongst which are morphine, codeine, atropine and tubocurarine. An animal may be depleted

General structure
of Compound
48/80,
a polymer

of its histamine by using a powerful histamine-liberator such as Compound 48/80, and studies on such histamine-depleted animals may reveal the importance of histamine in physiological functions. The release of histamine may also follow the ingestion of certain foodstuffs and various types of allergic phenomena result. Potent histamine-liberators have been found, for example, in fresh egg-white, strawberry extracts and shell-fish.

QUANTITATIVE ESTIMATION OF HISTAMINE. The most popular isolated tissue for the bioassay of histamine is the terminal ileum of the guinea-pig; the tissue is suspended in Tyrode's solution containing atropine ($10^7\,\mu g/ml$). Of the other bioassay methods available, the depressor effect on the blood pressure of the anaesthetized atropinized cat or dog is often used. Chemically, histamine can be assayed spectrophotofluorimetrically after condensation with 2:4-dinitrofluorobenzene or isotopically after reaction with *p*-iodobenzene-sulphonyl chloride.

Antihistamines

Antihistamines selectively antagonise the pharmacological effects of histamine, with the exception of its effect on gastric acid secretion. Since histamine is a factor involved in the production of some of the symptoms exhibited in allergy and anaphylaxis, antihistamines may be of value in the treatment of these disorders. Most antihistamines also possess other properties that are unrelated to antagonism of histamine.

The development of antihistamines very largely began in 1937 when French workers discovered compounds which protected guinea-pigs against both the lethal effects of histamine and those of anaphylactic shock. The first compound to be tried clinically was thymoxyethyldiethylamine (Fig. 30.1); this was designated F929, after Fourneau the chemist who prepared it. A number of aniline derivatives were then prepared and they were more potent and more specific in their action but too toxic for clinical use. However, in 1942, N-diethyl-aminoethyl-N-benzyl-aniline or *Antergan* (designated RP2339 after Rhone-Poulone, a French pharmaceutical company) was prepared and this became the first aniline derivative to be used in medicine as an antihistamine (see Fig. 30.1). More potent, more specific and less toxic compounds were then prepared, and among these was *mepyramine* (also called Neoantergan and Anthisan). Mepyramine (Fig. 30.1) has retained its position among the drugs used in the treatment of allergies since 1944 when it was first prepared. At about the same time, another potent compound allied to mepyramine was prepared in the U.S.A. This was *tripelennamine* (Pyribenzamine) and this too has remained a popular anti-histamine drug in clinical use (Fig. 30.1). *Antazoline* is another compound allied to Antergan but slightly less potent; it is benzyl-N-methyli-midazolineaniline and contains the imidazoline grouping as in histamine (Fig. 30.2)

Other types of drugs have been prepared and used for their antihistamine activity. For example, the best known of the benzhydryl ethers in clinical use today is *diphenhydramine* (Benadryl) wh:ch is widely used to reduce motion-sickness (Fig. 30.2). The most important of the phenothiazine derivatives possessing antihistaminic properties is *promethazine* (Phenergan), the formula of which is shown in Fig. 30.2; some of these phenothiazines are, in addition, antagonists of 5-HT, adrenaline and acetylcholine, as well as depressants of the central nervous system. In the piperazine series, the most important is *chlor-cyclizine* (Histantin). Recent additions to the list of potent and safe antihistamines are *pheniramine* and *chlorpheniramine* (Piriton), two derivatives of pyridine which are usually used in the form of more stable and long acting organic salts. *Thenophenopiperidine*, which is a sulphur-containing molecule

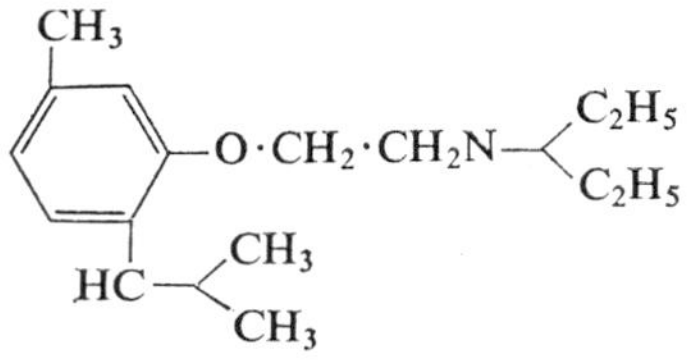

F 929

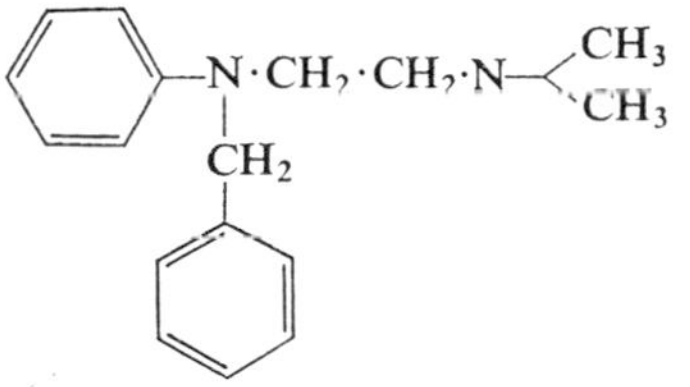

Antergan (RP2339)

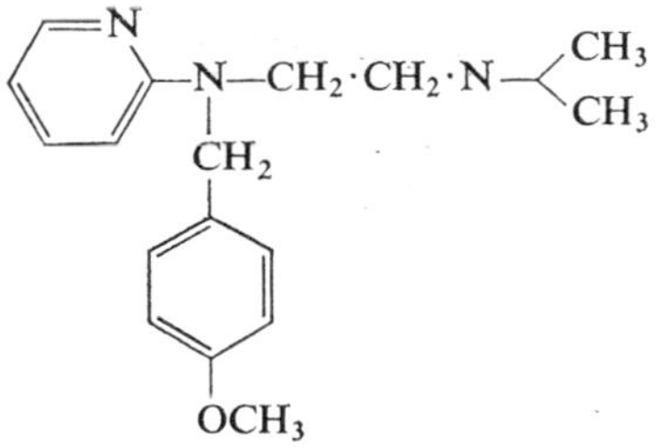

Mepyramine

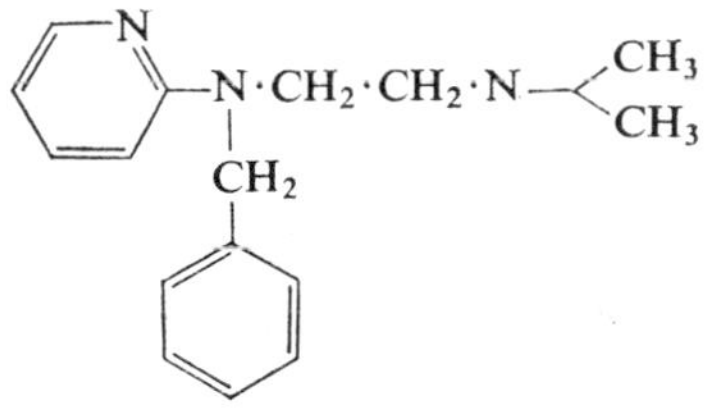

Tripelennamine

Fig. 30.1. Examples of antihistamines.

(see Fig. 30.2) was reported to produce agranulocytosis and is no longer used. Clinicians differ in their opinions as to the value of so many antihistamines; some maintain that each drug has its advantages whereas others believe that there is an unnecessary replication of drugs having substantially similar actions.

Chemically, antihistamines are a diverse group of compounds although many are substituted ethylamines. The aromatic nucleus (which is electropositive) is joined to the basic side-chain usually by an oxygen or a nitrogen atom, and this type of structure is reminiscent of the structure of many anti-adrenaline and anti-5-HT drugs. Antihistamines act by preventing histamine from reaching its site of action, that is, by competition for the receptors.

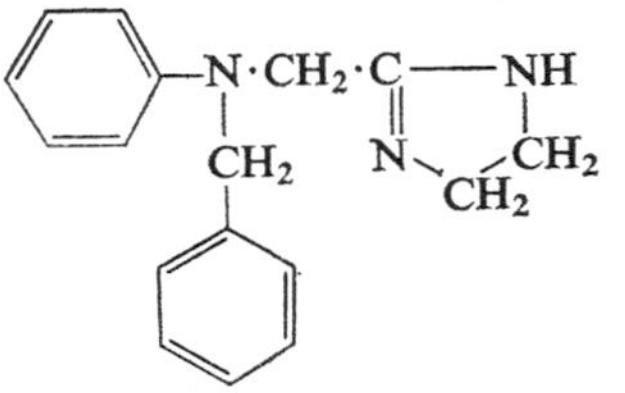

Antazoline

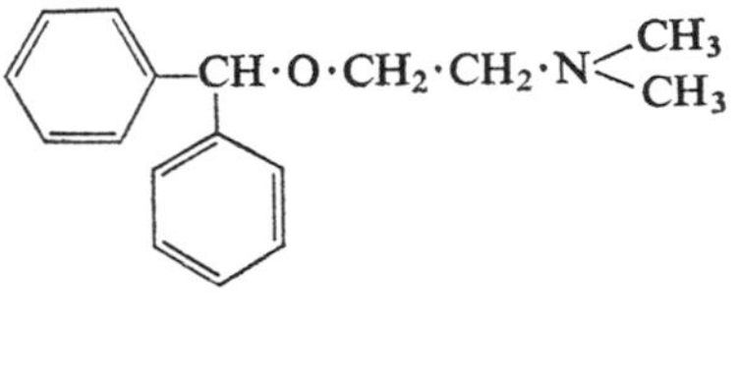

Diphenhydramine

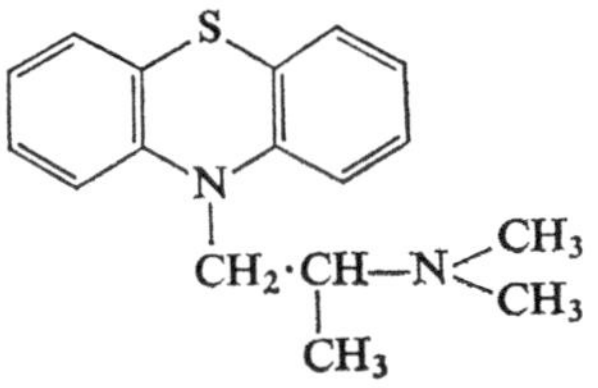

Promethazine

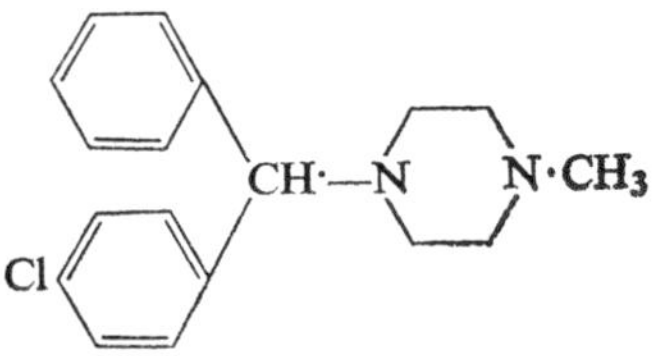

Chlorcyclizine

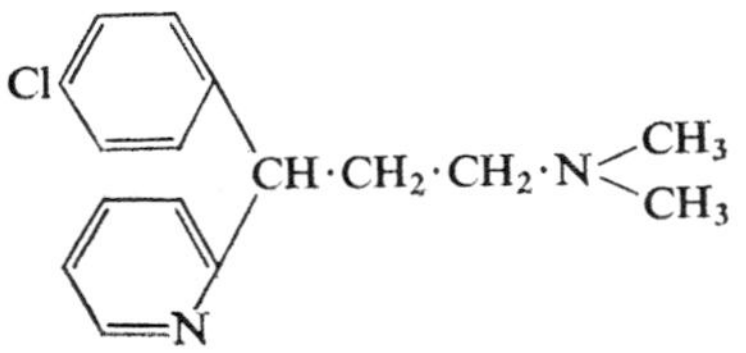

Chlorpheniramine

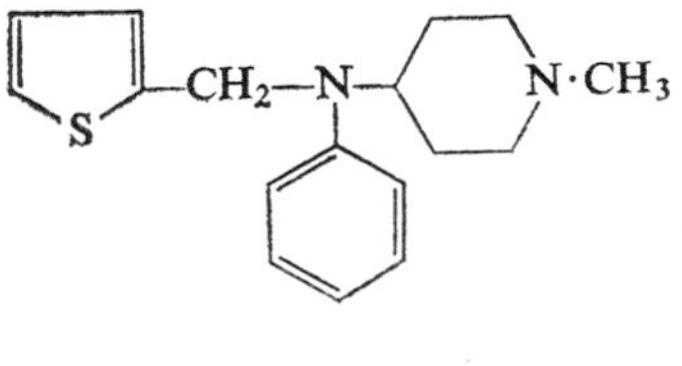

Thenophenopiperidine (withdrawn)

FIG. 30.2. Further examples of antihistamines.

Antihistamines also affect the central nervous system, usually causing depression but sometimes stimulation. The clinically useful antihistamines are readily absorbed; they are mostly metabolized in the liver.

ESTIMATION OF ANTIHISTAMINE POTENCY. The standard methods by which antihistaminic activity is measured are (1) protection of guinea-pigs from the lethal effects of intravenous injections of histamine, (2) protection of guinea-pigs from the toxic effects of a histamine aerosol, (3) antagonism of histamine-induced contractions of the isolated guinea-pig ileum, (4) antagonism of the vasodilator effect of histamine in cats and dogs, and (5) the ability to abolish the wheal produced by the intradermal injection of histamine in man. Antihistamines also protect many animals against anaphylactic shock although they are relatively ineffective in protecting rats and mice.

CLINICAL USES OF ANTIHISTAMINES. Acute urticaria and angioneurotic oedema usually respond well to antihistamines although severe cases are often relieved more quickly by adrenaline. Seasonal hay fever responds well but nasal sprays containing vasoconstrictor drugs are also useful. Any relief obtained from antihistamines in the common cold is due to a reduction of secretions. Perennial vasomotor rhinitis and non-urticarial rashes are less often helped. Asthma responds poorly or not at all to antihistamines although their atropine-like effect on the bronchi may be useful. Relief of itching is probably due to their sedative or local anaesthetic effect. Prolonged local application is to be avoided as the drugs are liable to cause senstitivity reactions. They may be used systemically against bee or wasp stings which contain histamine and cause histamine release in the tissues. Antihistamines are used as anti-emetics and in Parkinsonism. It is not known whether these central actions involve blockade of histamine present in the CNS.

SIDE-EFFECTS OF ANTIHISTAMINES. These are qualitatively similar in almost all of the antihistamines but vary in intensity from drug to drug. Sedation is the commonest effect; diphenhydramine and tripelennamine are particularly prone to cause sedation. Accidents may be caused if the patient is in charge of a car while under antihistamine treatment; besides, there is synergism with alcohol and other central nervous system depressants. Other toxic side-effects include dryness of the mouth and throat, dizziness, fatigue, insomnia, nervousness, and gastric upsets. Dermatitis and agranulocytosis can occur. Severe poisoning due to overdose results in coma and sometimes in convulsions.

5-Hydroxytryptamine.

5-Hydroxytryptamine (5-HT) is formed in the body by decarboxylation of the amino-acid, 5-hydroxytryptophan(5-HTP, see page 178). 5-HT stimulates many smooth muscles, ganglion cells (page 700), and sensory nerve endings (page 183) and so produces a wide range of responses which vary between species and between tissues of the same species. The variability may be largely explained by the extent to which the smooth muscle stimulant action and the neuronal components of action contribute to the effects produced. Tachyphylaxis in the responses to 5-HT is usually evident when large doses are frequently administered, and then sensitivity to other agonists is not affected; one method of selectively blocking the actions of 5-HT is therefore to administer one or more large doses of 5-HT itself.

ACTION ON VASCULAR SMOOTH MUSCLE. 5-HT produces complex effects on the cardiovascular system. Vasoconstriction due to a direct action on the smooth muscle in the skin and splanchnic vessels is the predominant response in animals in which the nervous control of the blood vessels has been interrupted (as in pithed animals). Renal vessels are constricted by 5-HT and this effect in some species may be sufficient to cause necrosis of the cortex of the kidney. 5-HT exerts an antidiuretic effect, especially in rats, and this is largely the result of constriction of the afferent glomerular arteries. Veins are also powerfully constricted by 5-HT. The coronary vessels and the vessels in skeletal muscle are however dilated. In rodents (but not in most other species), small doses of 5-HT increase capillary permeability.

5-HT exerts a direct action on the heart and the rate and force of beat are increased. However, it also stimulates afferent nerve endings and so initiates reflex changes in cardiac activity. In particular, stimulation of chemoreceptors elicits the Jarisch-Bezold reflex (page 274) in which there is bradycardia and peripheral vasodilatation.

An intravenous injection of 5-HT into an intact mammal usually produces a triphasic response. An initial short-lasting depressor response (due to reflexly-induced bradycardia) is followed by a rise in blood pressure (due to the direct vasoconstrictor action) and later there may be another depressor response (due to vasodilatation in skeletal muscle).

ACTION ON SMOOTH MUSCLE OF THE GASTRO-INTESTINAL TRACT. 5-HT increases the tone and motility of most divisions of the gastro-intestinal tract and facilitates the peristaltic reflex. An intravenous infusion of 5-HT or of its precursor, 5-HTP, produces intestinal colic in man and evacuation of the bowels.

5-HT stimulates the longitudinal muscle of the isolated ileum of the guinea-pig through two mechanisms. It exerts a direct stimulant action on the smooth muscle which is blocked by dibenamine, phenoxybenzamine and lysergic acid diethylamide, and it also stimulates ganglion cells causing the post-ganglionic neurones to release acetylcholine. This indirect neuronal action of 5-HT is prevented by cocaine which anaesthetizes the nerve fibres, by atropine which blocks the action of the released acetylcholine, and by morphine which acts both on the ganglion cells to antagonize the action of 5-HT and on the post-ganglionic nerve endings to prevent the release of acetylcholine. The receptors involved in the direct action of 5-HT on the smooth muscle cells are known as D receptors (dibenamine-sensitive) and those in the ganglion cells are known as M receptors (morphine-sensitive). Other tissues have been shown to possess similar receptors.

In the dog, 5-HT increases the secretion of mucus from the gastric glands but antagonizes the action of histamine in increasing the volume and acidity of the gastric juice. These effects on secretions are mainly reflex in origin and are prevented by vagotomy.

ACTION ON RESPIRATORY SYSTEM. 5-HT usually produces a brief increase in respiratory minute volume in the dog and in man as a result of stimulation of carotid and aortic chemoreceptors. It also causes a powerful broncho-constriction in many species which is due to a direct action on the bronchiolar smooth muscle.

MALIGNANT CARCINOID SYNDROME. Carcinoid tumours develop from argentaffin cells located in the gastro-intestinal tract. The syndrome consists of watery diarrhoea, colic, flushing of the skin and attacks of bronchocon-striction; the attacks may be provoked by various stimuli such as food and drink. The tumour produces large quantities of 5-HT which raises the blood 5-HT level and increases the urinary excretion of both 5-HT and its metabolite 5-HIAA. The estimation of the latter substance provides one of the means of confirming the diagnosis. In cases of malignant carcinoid the excretion is increased to at least 5 times the normal value. Surgical removal of the tumour is possible.

Antagonists of 5-hydroxytryptamine. The action of 5-HT on many smooth muscles is antagonized by lysergide (lysergic acid diethylamide, LSD) but

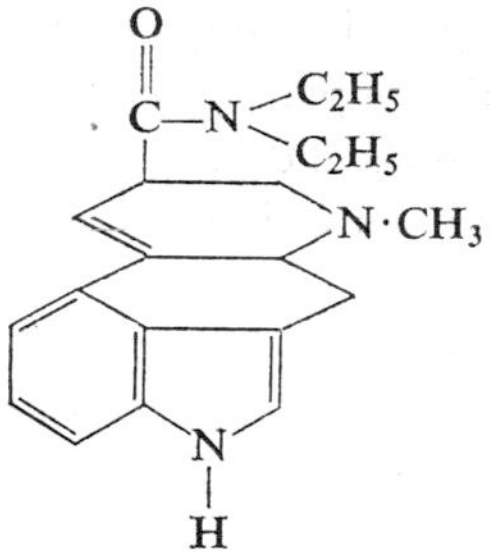

Lysergide
Lysergic acid diethylamide
(LSD)

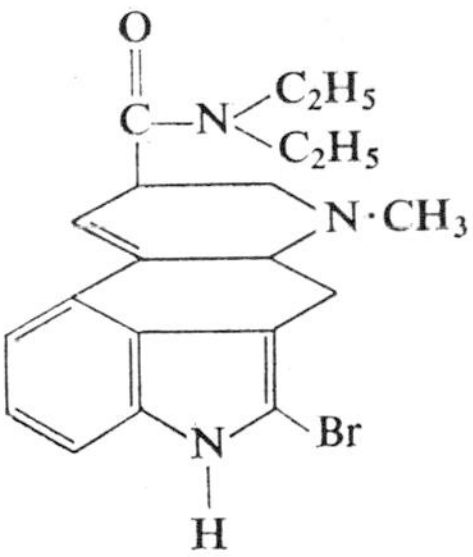

2-Bromo-lysergic acid
diethylamide (BOL)

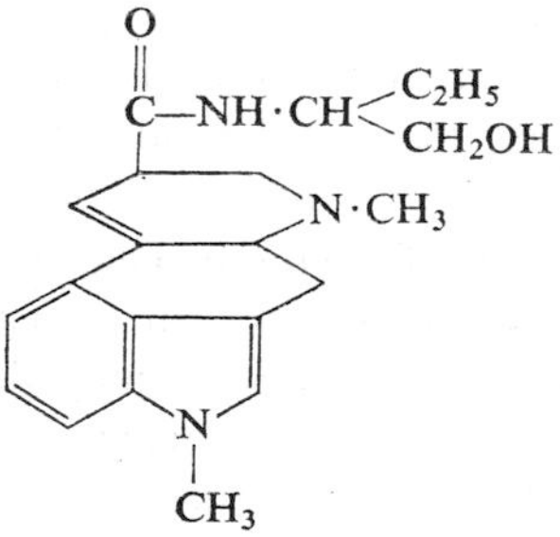

Methysergide

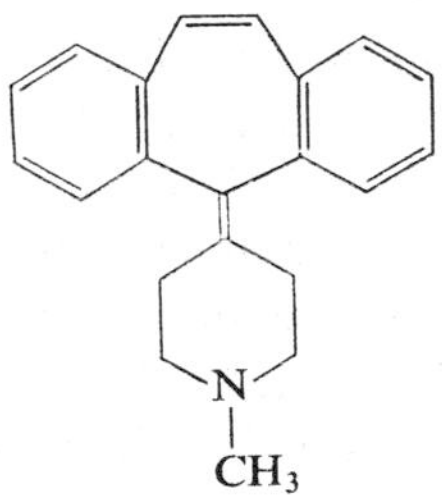

Cyproheptadine

FIG. 30.3. Examples of antagonists of 5-HT.

contractions produced by other smooth muscle stimulants are not. The 2-bromoderivative of LSD (Fig. 30.3) is equally active and has less tendency to stimulate the tissues. Methysergide (1-methyl-lysergic acid butanolamide, UML-491) is about 4 times as active and has been used in the symptomatic treatment of patients with the malignant carcinoid syndrome. Dihydroergotamine is also a 5-HT antagonist. Another potent antagonist of the actions of 5-HT on the rat uterus, on the bronchial muscles of the guinea-pig, and in increasing capillary permeability in the rat, is cyproheptadine (Periactin).

5-HT antagonists sometimes produce effects on the central nervous system such as hallucinations and convulsions. It is possible that these are the result of antagonism of endogenous 5-HT but the evidence is not clear.

Methysergide is used in the treatment of migraine. Its actions and side effects resemble those of ergot alkaloids (pages 757–760).

Polypeptides acting on smooth muscle

OXYTOCIN AND VASOPRESSIN. Oxytocin and vasopressin (see pages 365–368) are octapeptide amides, both having a 20 membered ring of 5 amino acids and a side-chain of 3 amino acids. Vasopressin differs from oxytocin only in two of its amino acids: it has phenylalanine in place of isoleucine in the ring structure, and arginine in place of leucine in the side-chain. Vasopressin from hog pituitary is called lysine-vasopressin since it contains lysine in place of arginine in the side-chain. Both polypeptides are secreted by neurones in the anterior hypothalamus and are stored in the neurohypophysis in the form of dense granules. Their release occurs under many conditions and, although both are released together, their relative concentrations differ according to the stimulus.

Oxytocin plays a physiological role in parturition and in milk ejection during nursing. This is illustrated by the close similarity between the uterine contractions occurring naturally in pregnancy and those produced by injections of oxytocin. There is a marked increase in the sensitivity of the uterus to oxytocin at term. During breast feeding, sucking extracts milk from the large ducts of the lactating mammary glands but the greater part of the milk in the alveoli and finer ducts is ejected by the contractile action of the special myoepithelial cells which are stimulated by minute quantities of oxytocin. The latent period for the milk-ejection reaction is only a few seconds and this suggests that oxytocin is secreted reflexly in response to sucking. Oxytocin may also have a lactogenic effect since it can delay involution of the mammary gland. There is some evidence that calcium ions are involved in these effects.

Vasopressin (also called antidiuretic hormone) is released during dehydration and other conditions and acts to regulate water balance. The injection of hypertonic saline into the carotid artery produces antidiuresis, associated with the release of both oxytocin and vasopressin. The antidiuretic response of the mammalian kidney is effected by an increase in the permeability of the distal tubule to water (see page 347).

Oxytocin and vasopressin have a number of pharmacological activities of unknown significance. For example, the pressor activity of vasopressin in mammals (which is about 100 times that of oxytocin) is of doubtful physiological significance. The ability of oxytocin to increase the excretion of sodium and potassium is likewise only of pharmacological interest. Oxytocin is more than 10 times as potent as vasopressin in stimulating the rat uterus *in vitro*, and about 5 times as potent in producing a depressor response in birds and in evoking the milk ejection response in the rabbit.

SUBSTANCE P. Substance P (see also pages 182 and 188) is a potent smooth muscle stimulant obtained from alcoholic extracts of brain and intestine. It stimulates most smooth muscle preparations including the isolated rat duodenum and the hen rectal caecum, which allows it to be distinguished from bradykinin. Its actions are unaffected by ganglion blocking drugs, atropine, antihistamines or 5-HT antagonists.

KININS. Kinins (see also pages 181–182) are polypeptides that are released from plasma protein precursors (α-globulins) by proteolytic enzymes which have trypsin-like activity. Kinins have pharmacological activity in minute amounts; they cause contraction most of smooth muscles, although vascular smooth muscle is relaxed and they cause vasodilatation; they increase capillary permeability.

Bradykinin is a nonapeptide with the amino acid sequence shown below:

H–Arg–Pro–Pro–Gly–Phe–Ser–Pro–Phe–Arg–OH

It is formed from its globulin precursor, bradykininogen, by plasmin (fibrinolysin), by enzymes in sweat and saliva, and by trypsin. It was first discovered in plasma incubated with snake venom; a substance which caused a slow contraction of the isolated guinea pig ileum appeared in plasma treated in this way, and the name bradykinin was coined to describe this slow contraction-producing effect. The action of bradykinin on the guinea-pig ileum is antagonised by some derivatives of phenothiazine, dihydrodibenzazepine and dibenzocycloheptane. Bradykinin can also be liberated by various physical processes, including contact with hydrophilic surfaces and dilution of plasma with Tyrode's solution. It can be distinguished from most other stimulants of intestinal smooth muscle in that it causes relaxation of the rat duodenum. The isolated rat uterus is one of the most sensitive tissues to the contracting action of bradykinin and may be used for bioassay. However, the uterus *in situ* is but little affected.

The bronchoconstrictor action of bradykinin in the guinea-pig *in vivo* is specifically antagonized by acetylsalicylic acid, phenylbutazone and amidopyrine. Intravenous injections of bradykinin produce a fall of blood pressure due to vasodilatation, and this may be followed by a rise in blood pressure due to the action of catecholamines released from the adrenal glands by the kinin. Bradykinin produces vasoconstriction in perfused isolated veins and this effect is antagonized by some anti-inflammatory agents, notably *pyridinolcarbamate*.

Kallidin is a decapeptide, the lysine-homologue of bradykinin:—

H–Lys–Arg–Pro–Pro–Gly–Phe–Ser–Pro–Phe–Arg–OH

It is converted to bradykinin by amidopeptidases and trypsin. Like bradykinin it is released from an α-globulin precursor. The enzyme that releases kallidin is known as *kallikrein*. This occurs in an inactive form, known as *kallikreinogen*, in the blood, and in pancreatic and intestinal secretions. The active enzyme is found in saliva and urine: it is formed by changes in pH and by the action of proteolytic enzymes. The pharmacological actions of kallidin resemble those of bradykinin.

The effects of bradykinin and kallidin *in vivo* are ephemeral as they are rapidly inactivated by enzymes which split off a portion of the peptide necessary for pharmacological activity. A related polypeptide, *eledoisin*, isolated from the posterior salivary glands of certain molluscan species, is resistant to the destructive enzymes and consequently has longer-lasting effects. Its structure is shown below:

Pyroglutamyl–Pro–Ser–Lys–Asp(OH)–Ala–Phe–Ileu–Gly–Leu–Met–NH_2

ANGIOTENSIN. Angiotensin (see also pages 182, 276 and 378–380), at one time called hypertensin or angiotonin, is a polypeptide derived from an inactive precursor (angiotensinogen) belonging to the α_2-globulin fraction of plasma. The enzyme, *renin*, which releases angiotensin from angiotensinogen occurs in extracts of kidney. It is located in the juxta glomerular apparatus from where it is released by various physiological stimuli. The release of angiotensin takes place in two stages. First a decapeptide (angiotensin I) is released, and from it an octapeptide (angiotensin II) is formed. The amino acid sequence of angiotensin II is shown below:

Asp–Arg–Val–Tyr–Ileu–His–Pro–Phe

In man, angiotensin produces a sharp rise in blood pressure, which is unaffected by ganglion blocking drugs or anti-adrenaline drugs. It is about ten times as active as adrenaline on a weight basis. Angiotensin also has marked renal effects, reducing urinary flow (page 339). The physiological and pathological significance of angiotensin is highly controversial.

CHAPTER 31

Drugs Acting on the Gastro-intestinal Tract

Many drugs are used to correct or alleviate the symptoms of disorders of the gastro-intestinal tract; those such as the parasympathomimetics and the atropine-like drugs have actions at many other sites and are described elsewhere. The substances described in this chapter are mainly those used specifically for their effects on the alimentary canal and its associated structures.

Bitters. Bitters are substances taken before a meal to stimulate appetite. They act by stimulating the taste buds in the tongue, thereby reflexly causing the secretion of saliva and gastric juice. Substances used include *simple bitters* such as *strychnine* or *tincture of nux vomica, quinine* or *tincture of cinchona,* and *extracts of quassia, gentian* and *calumba,* as well as *aromatic* bitters such as *tincture of orange or lemon,* which contain a volatile oil as well as a bitter principle. In addition to their medical use, many of these substances are contained in alcoholic aperitifs.

Tonics. Tonics are usually mixtures intended to restore appetite and a feeling of well-being. They often contain bitters, the glycerophosphates of sodium, potassium and calcium, iron salts, haemoglobin, vitamins (e.g. in the form of yeast) and liver extracts. Apart from the action of bitters in stimulating appetite, any beneficial effect they have is as a placebo.

Carminatives. Carminatives are substances used to assist in expelling gas from the intestines. Their mechanism of action is unknown although most of them contain volatile oils which possess an irritant action and which possibly act by reflexly stimulating movements of the alimentary canal and relaxing sphincters. Their irritant action on the gut also reflexly produces a transient increase in respiration, blood pressure and in the action of the heart, and they have some use as reflex restoratives in syncope. They include, preparations of *cardamom, ginger, peppermint, dill, aniseed, fennel, coriander, cloves, nutmeg* and *cinnamon,* as well as alcoholic solutions of *ether* and *chloroform.* The volatile oils in certain liqueurs may have carminative value.

Adsorbents. Adsorbents are used to remove gases and poisonous substances from the intestine. They are also sometimes applied externally to ulcerating surfaces. Medicinally useful adsorbents include *activated charcoal* (also used in gas masks), *kaolin* and *magnesium trisilicate.*

789

Demulcents. Demulcents are colloidal solutions of a gum or a protein which are used to coat mucous membranes. They are effective to some extent in protecting membranes against mild irritation and are used in conditions of sore throat, gastritis, or after ingestion of irritant poisons. They are prepared from *starch, acacia, tragacanth, mucin* or *egg albumin.*

Astringents. Astringent substances cause precipitation of proteins and form an insoluble protective layer of coagulated protein on mucous membranes or inflamed skin. They are used to protect the tissue from irritant substances and to inhibit exudations including the secretions of mucous glands and small haemorrhages. In the intestine, they exert an action in checking diarrhoea.

Substances used as astringents include the salts of metals such as *lead, zinc, copper* and *aluminium* which are usually used for external application to the skin, and the vegetable astringents consisting of preparations which liberate *tannic acid.* Tannic acid precipitates proteins and is present in *oak-galls, eucalyptus gum, krameria root, witch-hazel* and *catechu,* all of which have been used medicinally. Preparations containing tannic acid are used in throat lozenges and in the treatment of burns. When taken internally, it is important that the tannic acid be liberated slowly as it is irritant to the mucous membrane of the stomach. Tannic acid also has the property of precipitating alkaloids and has been used in the treatment of alkaloidal poisoning.

Emetics. The mechanism of vomiting is described on page 313. Afferent fibres from the stomach, intestine and heart reach the vomiting centre in the medulla by way of the vagus and sympathetic nerves. Irritation or distension of the stomach, intestine or gall-bladder, or occlusion of the coronary vessels, results in a discharge of impulses to the vomiting centre which in turn discharges impulses along the efferent nerves to the respiratory and abdominal muscles. A complex series of contractions of these skeletal muscles compresses the stomach, starting at the pyloric end, and forces the contents along the oesophagus into the mouth. In addition to the vomiting centre, there is a chemoreceptor trigger zone in the reticular formation of the medulla which may be stimulated by certain chemical agents present in the blood-stream. This in turn excites the vomiting centre. The nervous connections with the vomiting centre are complex and vomiting may also rise from various unrelated phenomena, such as feelings of disgust, severe pain, increased intra-cranial pressure and disturbance to the labyrinth apparatus (the cause of most cases of motion-sickness). Prolonged vomiting may be dangerous to life as fluid and more particularly hydrogen and sodium ions are lost from the body.

Emetics are drugs which cause vomiting. On rare occasions, they are used to remove poisons from the stomach when the use of a stomach pump is impracticable.

REFLEX EMETICS cause vomiting by irritating the stomach. They are rapidly effective when given by mouth but are inactive when injected. Reflex emetics include strong suspensions of *mustard* or strong solutions of *common salt*, 1 % solutions of *zinc* or *copper sulphate* and *ipecacuanha* or its main alkaloid, *emetine*. Emetine is also used in the treatment of amoebic dysentery where it is given intravenously to avoid vomiting. The safest way of producing vomiting is for the patient to stimulate his throat with his own fingers.

CENTRAL EMETICS cause vomiting by stimulating the chemoreceptor trigger zone in the brain stem and are therefore active after systemic administration. *Morphine* and allied drugs possess this action, the most potent being the partly synthetic compound, *apomorphine* which is injected subcutaneously. However, apomorphine retains all the other actions of morphine and is therefore rarely used nowadays. Numerous other drugs, such as the tetracyclines and the cardiac glycosides, cause vomiting as an unwanted side-effect.

Anti-emetics. Vomiting may arise from a number of causes such as irritation of the gastric mucosa, motion sickness, radiation sickness and pregnancy, and as a side-effect of certain drugs. The best treatment is to remove the cause, but this is not always possible or, in the case of pregnancy, may not be desirable.

Most of the drugs used against motion sickness possess a weak sedative action and some atropine-like action; their effect may be due to blockade of synaptic transmission at some central cholinergic site. Some of them are also antihistaminic (although an antihistaminic action by itself does not prevent motion sickness). In clinical trials, *hyoscine* has usually been found most effective; other drugs used include *atropine, meclozine, promethazine, diphenhydramine, dimenhydrinate* and *cyclizine. Chlorpromazine*, although effective against other forms of sickness, has no action against motion sickness.

Meclozine is probably the most useful drug in vomiting of pregnancy but chlorpromazine and *pyridoxine* are also used. The mechanism of action of pyridoxine is unknown.

Radiation sickness, post-anaesthetic vomiting, and vomiting as a side-effect of drug therapy, are usually treated with chlorpromazine, meclozine or pyridoxine.

Expectorants. Expectorants are drugs used in the treatment of certain types of cough to increase the secretions of the respiratory tract, the mucus then acting as a demulcent serving to protect the inflamed surfaces. The reason for including expectorants in this chapter is that some of them are closely related to the emetics, small doses of which act as expectorants. Expectorants act in one of two ways:

1. REFLEX EXPECTORANTS. These stimulate bronchial secretion by a reflex action initiated in the stomach and small intestine. They include *creosote, ipecacuanha, squill, guiacols* and the *chloride, bicarbonate* and *acetate* of *ammonia* and the *iodides* of *sodium, potassium* and *calcium*.

2. DIRECT STIMULANTS. These directly stimulate the bronchial secretory cells to increase production. *Volatile oils* act in this way and *guiacols, creosote* and *iodides* probably also exert this effect.

The choice of drug for the treatment of cough depends upon the type of cough and the desired effect. For depression of useless cough, codeine, pholcodeine and methadone, among many others, are used to depress the cough centre in the medulla. These drugs are dealt with in Chapter 24.

Gastric antacids. Gastric antacids are substances used to reduce gastric acidity and to relieve the pain that occurs in hyperchlorhydria and peptic ulcer. The protection of ulcers from the acid gastric juice may also aid healing.

The gastric juice has a pH of 1 to 2 and this is necessary for gastric digestion to take place. The transfer of H^+ and Cl^- ions into the lumen of the stomach leaves the concentration of sodium in the blood unchanged; to compensate for the loss of chloride, the plasma bicarbonate is increased to balance the sodium. The intestinal secretions, however, are alkaline because sodium and bicarbonate ions are secreted into the intestine. The blood concentration of $NaHCO_3$ is therefore lowered as a result of intestinal secretion. The net effect of both gastric and intestinal secretions on the blood is therefore a loss of Na^+ and Cl^- ions. However, the imbalance is only temporary as much of the sodium and chloride is reabsorbed in the intestines.

The indiscriminate use of antacids is inadvisable and may be deleterious since excessive neutralization of the gastric contents inhibits the digestive enzymes, and interference with the acid-base balance in patients whose kidney function is inadequate may call for special treatment to restore fluid and electrolyte balance.

Substances used as gastric antacids may be divided into two groups, the systemic antacids and the non-systemic antacids.

SYSTEMIC ANTACIDS are mildly alkaline substances which, after absorption, are capable of altering the acid-base balance of the body. The chief ones are *sodium* and *potassium bicarbonate* which are rapid but short-lived in their action. When these substances are taken by mouth, the gastric contents are neutralized in the stomach and CO_2 is formed. Any excess of the bicarbonate remains unchanged. On entering the intestine, no further neutralization is required and the excess bicarbonate, together with the bicarbonate from the intestinal juice is reabsorbed. The concentration of blood buffers is therefore increased (alkalosis) and the kidneys excrete an alkaline urine to restore the balance.

NON-SYSTEMIC ANTACIDS act in two ways, both of which are less likely to result in systemic alkalosis. One type neutralizes the gastric acid with the production of an insoluble salt which is not absorbed, while the other type simply acts as a physical adsorbent of the gastric acid. Examples of non-systemic antacids are: (1) *aluminium hydroxide* which reacts with gastric acid to form aluminium chloride, and this in turn reacts with the intestinal secretions to form insoluble salts, the chloride being reabsorbed: (2) *magnesium trisilicate* which neutralizes the acid with the formation of magnesium chloride; in the intestine, the soluble magnesium carbonate is formed and the chloride is reabsorbed: (3) *magnesium oxide:* (4) *magnesium carbonate:* (5) *calcium carbonate*: and (6) *calcium hydroxide*. Aluminium hydroxide and magnesium trisilicate also act as physical adsorbents. Magnesium salts have an additional action in causing diarrhoea by acting as bulk purgatives, whereas calcium and aluminium salts cause constipation. By combining these salts, it is possible to neutralize acidity without much affecting the activity of the gut.

The ion exchange resin, *polyaminostyrene*, has also been used to reduce gastric acidity but it is not sufficiently effective for use in peptic ulcer. In the treatment of peptic ulcer, the aim is to raise the pH of the stomach contents to a level at which the proteolytic enzyme pepsin is inhibited (about pH 4) and no longer capable of acting on the ulcerous area of the gastric mucosa. The use of atropine-like drugs in peptic ulcer is described on page 726.

Purgatives. Purgatives are drugs taken by mouth to stimulate defaecation. They are also sometimes described as laxatives, cathartics, evacuants or aperients. Although used regularly by a large proportion of the population, their indiscriminate use is unnecessary and may be harmful. Constipation may arise from a number of causes: (1) It may follow an acute illness, especially if associated with lack of exercise and a reduced food intake so that insufficient food residues reach the colon. The rational treatment of this type of constipation is to increase the quantity of water and of non-absorbable food residues of the diet such as cellulose which is present in fruit and vegetables. (2) It may arise from inactivity or spasmodic contraction of the colon; the former condition is often overcome by increasing the non-absorbable residue of the diet: spasm of the colon may be relieved by small doses of atropine. (3) It may arise from insensitivity of the rectum (dyschezia) so that the defaecation reflex is not initiated. Haemorrhoids or other anal lesions may depress the sensitivity of the rectum and pain associated with the act of defaecation may cause the patient to postpone it as long as possible. Postponement of defaecation itself leads to dyschezia. (4) Psychosomatic factors may also play an important role as placebos to which a purgative action is attributed have a purgative action in many patients who claim to be constipated.

Normal defaecation empties only the descending colon whereas the powerful purgatives empty the whole colon. Thus, after the successful use of a purgative, a few days may elapse while material collects in the colon before natural defaecation occurs again. During these few days the patient may believe that he is again constipated and take more purgative so that a cycle is built up which is difficult to break. This often occurs in individuals who have the mistaken belief that daily defaecation is necessary to maintain health. The headache and discomfort associated with mild constipation is not, as was commonly believed, the result of absorption of toxins from the colon. It probably arises reflexly as a result of increased tension in the rectum, since it has been shown that cotton wool inserted into the rectum produces similar symptoms.

Constipation is also a side-effect of treatment with drugs such as morphine, codeine, ephedrine and amphetamine, and it may be necessary to administer purgatives during treatment with them. Purgatives are also given to remove poisons from the alimentary canal, to prepare patients for X-ray examination of the abdomen, and to remove parasites from the gut after treatment with anthelmintic drugs.

Constipation is one of the symptoms arising from obstruction of the bowel and in this case the use of purgatives is dangerous. Treatment is then to remove the obstruction.

Purgatives are usually classified, according to their mechanism of action, into bulk purgatives, irritant purgatives and lubricant purgatives.

BULK PURGATIVES. Bulk purgatives increase the volume of the non-absorbable intestinal contents and, by stretching the wall of the intestine, initiate reflex bowel activity. They produce purgation within 1–3 h and are therefore usually taken in the morning. The bulk purgatives are of two types: (i) *Hydrophilic colloid purgatives* and (ii) *Saline purgatives.*

Hydrophilic colloid purgatives are usually of plant origin. They are indigestible and not absorbed. In the intestine they absorb water and swell, promoting a soft but solid stool. The hydrophilic colloids include *agar* and *sodium alginate*, both of which are obtained from sea-weeds, *psyllium seeds* which contain a large amount of mucilage, *methyl cellulose* which is a partially depolymerized form of cellulose, and *sodium carboxymethylcellulose*. Bran, dried fruits (prunes, dried apples and figs) and vegetables contain a large amount of non-absorbable matter, most of which is cellulose, and these too may be used as bulk purgatives. Prunes and figs also contain mildly irritant organic substances.

Saline purgatives are soluble inorganic salts (or the salts of inorganic cations) which are absorbed only slightly or not at all from the gastro-intestinal tract. Their osmotic effect increases the bulk of the intestinal contents by retaining water in the intestine and, when given as hypertonic solutions, by absorbing it from the tissues. They promote a fluid stool and may cause considerable loss of water from the body. All soluble salts of magnesium, and the sulphate, phosphate and tartrate of sodium act as saline purgatives. The commonly used saline purgatives are *magnesium sulphate* (Epsom salts), *sodium sulphate* (Glauber's salt) and *sodium potassium tartrate* (Rochelle salt). Rochelle salt mixed before drinking with tartaric acid and sodium bicarbonate forms an effervescent drink called Seidlitz powder or Compound Effervescent Powder.

When taken with too little water, the saline purgatives produce vomiting. Magnesium salts injected intravenously do not produce purgation but cause anaesthesia. Small children have occasionally absorbed sufficient magnesium sulphate from the gut to produce unconsciousness, and this may also occur in patients with renal failure.

IRRITANT PURGATIVES. The irritant purgatives reflexly increase peristalsis in the colon by irritating the sensory nerve endings in the mucosa of the gut (the peristaltic reflex is described on page 322). Some act first on the intestinal mucosa, the increased motility of the intestine produced then reflexly increasing peristalsis in the colon.

Castor Oil. Castor oil is usually given on an empty stomach. The oil itself is non-irritant and is used in eye-drops as a bland lubricant or vehicle. It is a glycoside and in the small intestine it is hydrolysed with the production of the irritant *ricinoleic acid* which stimulates the intestine. Ricinoleic acid is absorbed in the intestine so that little reaches the colon. The purgation produced by castor oil is powerful and a period of constipation usually follows its use. It should not be used regularly and is usually reserved for occasions when a single purgation is all that is required. Its irritant effect is powerful enough to bring on labour in pregnant women.

Phenolphthalein. Phenolphthalein stimulates the colon directly. Some is absorbed in the small intestine and excreted in the urine and bile. Its re-entry into the intestines with the bile causes further purgation so that its action is prolonged. It is a relatively safe drug, and is incorporated into many proprietary purgatives. Its use is often followed by a period of constipation. Very occasionally, phenophthalein causes a skin rash. Its indicator properties impart a red colour to alkaline urine. *Acetophenylisatin* is similar to phenolphthalein but is about fifteen times more powerful.

Bisacodyl is a synthetic substance administered in the form of pills or supossitories; it exerts its purgative action by stimulating the colon directly.

Anthraquinone Purgatives. The anthraquinone purgatives are vegetable in origin and include senna, cascara, rhubarb, aloes and frangula. Of these, senna is probably the best, and biologically standardized preparations are available. The biological standardization is based on the number of wet faeces produced after oral administration to mice. All of the drugs in this class, and particularly senna, are liable to cause griping. This may be prevented by the administration of belladonna or the oils of peppermint or clove.

Aloes and aloin (a mixture of the active principles of aloes) are ingredients of many proprietary laxatives but are rarely prescribed. They stimulate the uterus as well as the colon and are contraindicated in pregnancy. Rhubarb contains tannin as well as anthraquinones and the astringent action of the tannin often leads to constipation after the purgation. Cascara is a popular laxative and is less liable to cause griping than aloes or senna. Frangula has an action similar to that of cascara.

The anthraquinone purgatives contain the active principle *emodin* (tri-hydroxy-methyl-anthraquinone) and most contain *chrysophanic acid* (di-hydroxy-methyl-anthraquinone) in addition. These substances produce purgation in about half an hour when injected. However, the crude drugs taken orally require 8–10 h to act. This is because the active principles in the crude drug are combined with sugars to form inactive glycosides. The glycosides are believed to be absorbed in the small intestine and hydrolysed in the body. The active principle is then thought to be excreted into the colon where it stimulates motility. Some of the emodin and chrysophanic acid are excreted by the kidneys. The latter substance, having indicator properties, turns acid urine yellow and alkaline urine red. Emodin is also excreted in the milk in quantities which are sometimes sufficient to affect an infant.

There are a number of other irritant purgatives, most of which are now obsolete for one reason or another. These include croton oil and the resins of jalop, ipomoea, elaterin, colocynth, podophyllum and gamboge, all of which are too drastic in their action. They are sometimes referred to as hydrogogue purgatives because they cause a profuse watery stool. Sulphur is a mild irritant purgative and is an ingredient of a number of preparations. Its irritant action is due to the formation of sulphides, the offensive smell of which may be detected in the breath. Compounds of mercury act as irritant purgatives; mercurous chloride (calomel) and metallic mercury, finely divided with chalk (grey powder) were at one time widely used to produce purgation in children. However, the possibility of producing mercury poisoning is a hazard and has led to their abandonment.

LUBRICANT PURGATIVES. The most important lubricant purgative is medicinal *liquid paraffin* which is a colourless and tasteless mixture of aliphatic hydrocarbons. It is not digested and only very small amounts are absorbed. It softens the stools and eases defaecation when it has been taken for 2 or 3 days; it is often given to patients in whom straining is to be avoided (e.g. patients with haemorrhoids). The oil may be taken by itself, or in the form of an emulsion, or combined with phenolphthalein or magnesium oxide. Its regular use is to be discouraged since it is not without dangers. It may impede absorption of fat soluble vitamins and of calcium and phosphate from the diet, and a few cases of chronic lipoid pneumonia have been reported to follow its prolonged use. Habitual use may be a contributory cause of some cases of cancer of the bowel.

Dioctyl sodium sulphosuccinate is an anionic surface active agent which is occasionally used as a lubricant purgative. It is believed to soften the stools by lowering the surface tension of the faecal mass thereby facilitating the penetration of water.

Drugs used to control diarrhoea. The drugs used for the symptomatic treatment of diarrhoea are of three types. (1) *Adsorbent powders* including *kaolin, chalk* and *bismuth subgallate* help to solidify the stools by absorbing water. (2) *Morphine-like drugs* including the alkaloids of opium and some other morphine-like drugs (but not pethidine), which depress the motility of the gut (see page 635), are often used together with an adsorbent powder. (3) *Atropine-like drugs* are sometimes used in chronic diarrhoea when the continued use of opium alkaloids is undesirable.

CHAPTER 32

Drugs Acting on the Cardiovascular System

This chapter is concerned with drugs used principally in the treatment of disorders of the heart and circulation. The basis of classification is therefore in terms of medicinal use, and this is the only justification for including such a heterogeneous group of drugs in one chapter (cf. pages 447–449).

Cardiovascular disease is the most common cause of death in technically advanced countries where infectious diseases are well controlled by public health measures and can usually be cured by chemotherapy. The incidence of death from cardiovascular disease in the United Kingdom rose from 20% of all deaths in 1900 to more than 40% in 1960.

Cardiac glycosides

The term *cardiac glycosides* refers to a number of chemically related substances that have qualitatively the same actions on the heart. They contain a *genin* or *aglycone* portion consisting of a steroid nucleus to which is attached a lactone ring, and a carbohydrate portion consisting of sugar residues linked to the genin by an ether bond. The effects of cardiac glycosides on the heart depend on the dose. In low doses they increase the force of myocardial contraction, and this is the basis of their use in medicine for the treatment of heart failure. In higher doses, they have toxic effects on the heart. The stimulant effect of cardiac glycosides on the heart differs from that of the sympathomimetic amines in that it is not accompanied by a corresponding increase in oxygen utilization; that is, the cardiac glycosides increase the force and the efficiency of myocardial contraction, whereas sympathomimetic amines increase the force but decrease the efficiency of contraction.

The chemical structure of naturally occurring cardiac glycosides. The general structural formula of the cardiac glycosides is shown in Fig. 32.1. All genins of the cardio-active glycosides have hydroxyl groups attached at C-3 and C-14, methyl groups attached at C-10 and C-13, and an unsaturated lactone ring at C-17. These are the minimum substituents, but in addition, methyl, hydroxyl or aldehyde groups are attached at various positions in the more complex genins. The configuration of the junction between the A and B rings is usually *cis;* that is, the methyl group on C-10 and the hydrogen on C-5 are both on the same side of the junction. The junction of the B and C rings is *trans*, as it is in all steroids. The C and D rings are in *cis*-configuration in all cardio-active steroids, but in no other naturally occurring steroids. The lactone ring may be 5- or

6-membered. The methyl substituents, the 14-OH and the lactone ring are all in the β-configuration; that is, they are orientated above the planes of the steroid rings to which they are attached. The 3-OH of the A ring is also usually β-orientated.

Fɪɢ. 32.1. The general structure of cardiac glycosides. The steroid nucleus, cyclopentanophenanthrene, contains A, B, C and D rings; the systematic numbering of the carbon skeleton is shown. The glycosidal link is at C-3, and the unsaturated lactone ring is attached at C-17.

The carbohydrate portion of the glycoside may consist of one to four sugar residues. Some 16 different sugars have been isolated as hydrolytic products of cardiac glycosides; of these, only glucose, rhamnose and fucose are widely distributed in nature. The remaining sugars are of rare occurrence, although they are not confined to cardiac glycosides; they are aldohexoses and have a 3-methoxy substituent and/or are 2-deoxy (cf. pages 9–10). Where more than one sugar residue is present, the rarer sugars are usually attached to the genin. The terminal sugar may be combined with a formyl or an acetyl group.

Sources of cardiac glycosides. The cardiac glycosides commonly used in medicine in the United Kingdom and in the U.S.A. are obtained from species of *Digitalis*. For this reason *digitalis* is sometimes applied as a generic name to the various drugs and preparations containing cardiac glycosides, and a number of terms are derived from it; thus, a patient under treatment is said to be *digitalized*, and one showing the toxic signs of an excessive dose is *over-digitalized*.

Cardiac glycosides are obtained from many other plant sources, including species of *Strophanthus*, *Urginea* (squill) and *Convallaria*. The various glycosides obtained from these sources may have occasional use in the United Kingdom, but are more widely used in Continental Europe. The venom of the skin glands of toads of the genus *Bufo* contain cardio-active genins, and dried toad skin has been used in traditional Chinese medicine.

Digitalis. The purple and the white foxglove (*Digitalis purpurea, D. lanata*) were used in folk medicine in Europe for centuries. In 1775, the English physician William Withering identified foxglove leaves (*D. purpurea*) as the active ingredient of a family remedy containing 20 or more herbs which was effective in curing dropsy (oedema). He subsequently made a careful study of the medicinal properties of digitalis and published his observations in 1785. Withering recognized that digitalis 'has a power over the motion of the heart to a degree yet unobserved in any other medicine, and that this power may be converted to salutary ends'. In the succeeding 150 years or so digitalis was used indiscriminately and fell into disrepute as a result of its severe toxic effects when used in excessive doses. At the beginning of the present century, its importance in the treatment of atrial fibrillation was established, and a few years later it was realized that its main value is in the treatment of congestive heart failure.

Pharmacopoeial preparations of digitalis are obtained from the whole dried leaf of *D.purpurea* which is either powdered and incorporated into tablets, or extracted in the form of a tincture. The preparations are standardized by biological assay. Their use is now almost obsolete, the crude preparations having been replaced with pure glycosides.

The relationships between the glycosides and genins obtained from digitalis are shown in Fig. 32.2.

The fresh leaves of *D. purpurea* contain desacetyl-lanatosides A and B; these are also known as purpurea glycosides A and B. During drying, a glucose residue is split off to yield the secondary glycosides *digitoxin* and *gitoxin*. An amorphous mixture of glycosides known as *gitalin* is extracted from either the fresh or dried leaves. A similar mixture extracted from the seeds is known as *digitalin*. Digitoxin is the most active of the glycosides and is present in the highest concentration. Acid hydrolysis of digitoxin and gitoxin splits off the digitoxose residues to yield the aglycones *digitoxigenin* and *gitoxigenin;* the mixture of genins obtained by hydrolysis of gitalin is known as gitaligenin.

The fresh leaves of *Digitalis lanata* contain lanatosides A, B and C. On mild alkaline and enzymatic hydrolysis, which may take place during drying of the leaf, a glucose and an acetic acid molecule are split off to yield the secondary glycosides digitoxin and gitoxin (as in *D. purpurea*), and also *digoxin*. The aglycone produced on acid hydrolysis of digoxin is *digoxigenin.*

The pure crystalline digitalis glycosides used in medicine are digoxin, digitoxin, lanatoside C, desacetyl-lanatoside C and acetyldigitoxin.

Strophanthus. Preparations of the seeds and other parts of strophanthus species were used as arrow poisons in Africa and strophanthus glycosides were

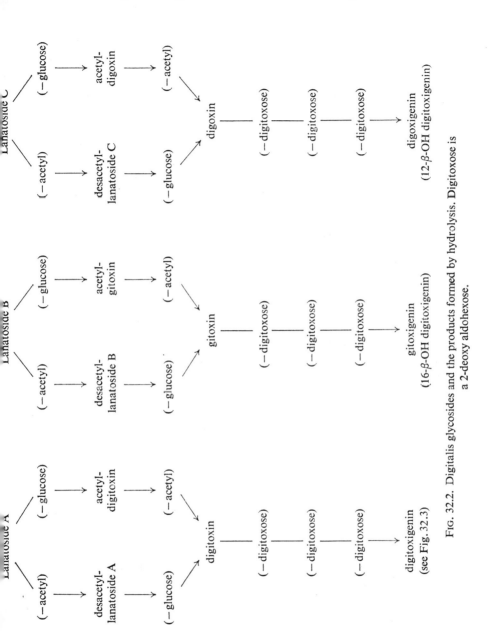

Fig. 32.2. Digitalis glycosides and the products formed by hydrolysis. Digitoxose is a 2-deoxy aldohexose.

26

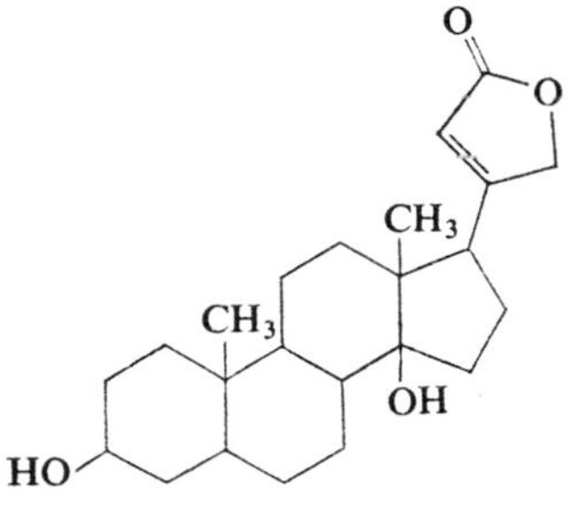

Digitoxigenin

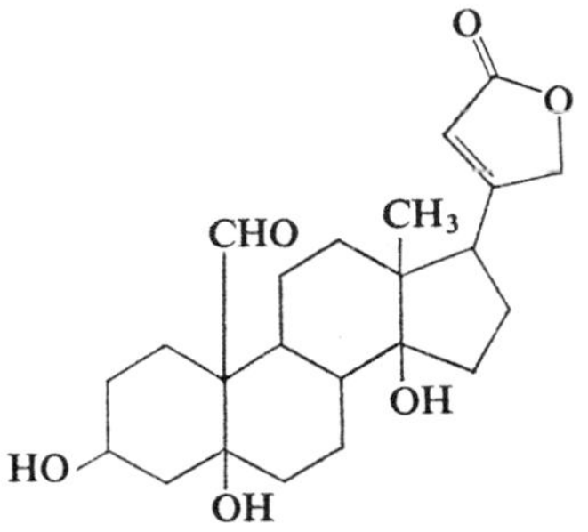

Strophanthidin

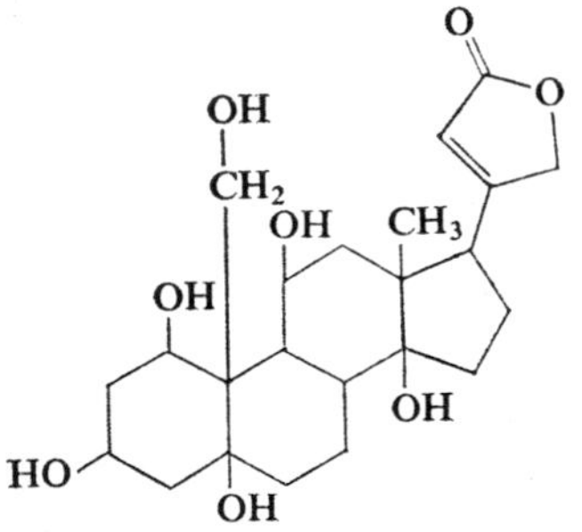

Ouabagenin

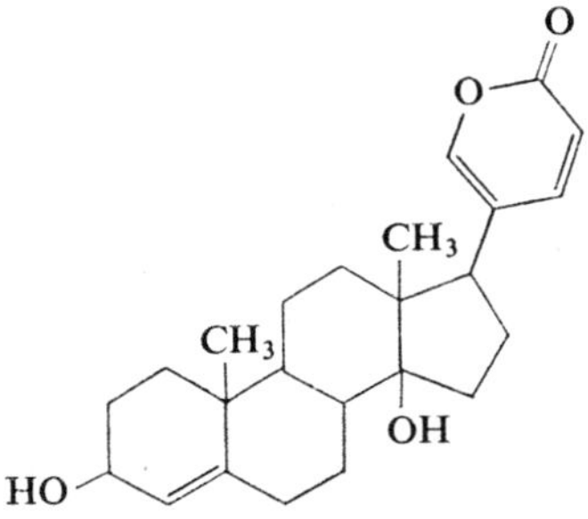

Scilliroside

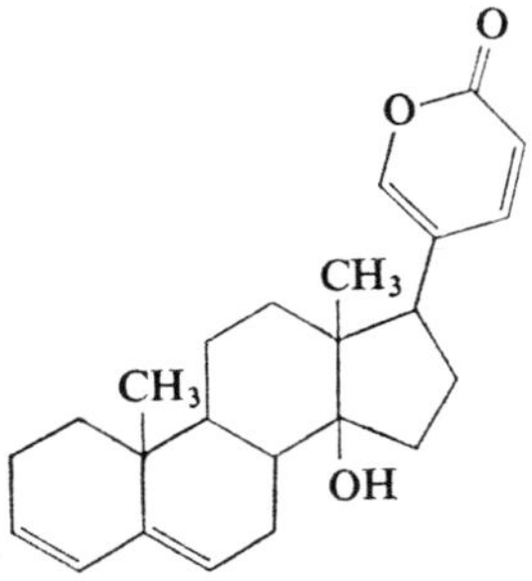

Scillaridin A
This is derived from scilliroside, the 3-OH and the 5-H being lost during hydrolysis.

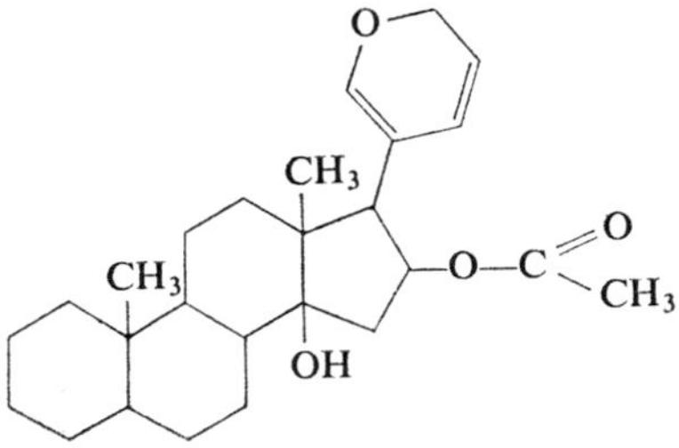

Bufotalin

FIG. 32.3. Formulae of some genins of cardio-active glycosides.

introduced into medicine in 1890 because of their digitalis-like action. One group of glycosides derived from the genin *strophanthidin* (Fig. 32.3) have been extracted from the seeds of *Strophanthus kombé*. The relationship of these glycosides is as follows:

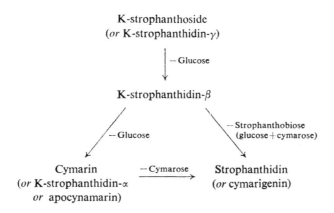

K-strophanthoside
(*or* K-strophanthidin-γ)

— Glucose

K-strophanthidin-β

— Glucose

— Strophanthobiose
(glucose + cymarose)

Cymarin
(*or* K-strophanthidin-α
or apocynamarin)

— Cymarose

Strophanthidin
(*or* cymarigenin)

Pharmacopoeial preparations are *strophanthus*, the dried ripe seeds of *S. kombé*, and *strophanthin-K*, a mixture of strophanthus glycosides.

The seeds of another species, *S. gratus*, contain the glycoside *ouabain* (or G-strophanthin). It is composed of the sugar rhamnose and the aglycone *ouabagenin* (Fig. 32.3). Ouabain is the most water-soluble of the cardiac glycosides.

Squill. The dried bulb of *Urginea* (*Scilla*) *maritima* is called squill; it was used as a medicine by the ancient Egyptians. Squill contains the glycosides *scillaren A* and *scilliroside;* the products of hydrolysis are as follows:

scillaren A $\xrightarrow{\text{— glucose}}$ proscillaridin A $\xrightarrow{\text{— rhamnose}}$ scillaridin A

scilliroside $\xrightarrow{\text{— glucose}}$ scillirosidin

The formulae of the aglycones are shown in Fig. 32.3. Although the squill glycosides exert the typical effects of the cardio-active glycosides, they are rarely used for treating heart failure. Squill is used mainly as a rodenticide. Squill extracts are also used in expectorants.

Convallaria. The lily-of-the-valley (*Convallaria majalis*) is a member of the Liliaceae, as is squill. The principal glycoside it contains is *convallatoxin*, which is a glycoside of rhamnose and the aglycone strophanthidin. Extracts of convallaria (and its glycosides) are extensively employed for the treatment of heart failure in Russia, where they have been used traditionally.

Oleander. The decorative shrub *Nerium oleander* contains a glycoside consisting of oleandrose and oleandrigenin (16-acetyl-gitoxigenin). It is not used medicinally, but cases of poisoning by *N. oleander* which have occurred exhibit the typical signs of toxicity of cardiac glycosides.

Adonis venalis. The chief glycoside in this plant is cymarin; extracts of the plant are used medicinally.

Helleborus species, like adonis, are in the Rananculaceae family; the principal glycosides are formed from the aglycone hellebrigenin which differs from strophanthidin only in that it has a 6-membered lactone ring.

Thevita glycosides occur in plants of various species of the Apocynaceae family (which also includes strophanthus); the principal glycosides are formed with digitoxigenin and various rare sugars.

Toad poisons. The steroidal constituents of the skin glands are known as *bufagins;* they are partly free and partly conjugated bufotalin (Fig. 32.3).

Therapeutic effects of cardiac glycosides

The two principal uses of cardiac glycosides are (a) in the treatment of heart failure, and (b) in the treatment of atrial arrhythmias.

Action of cardiac glycosides in heart failure

THE PATHOLOGICAL PHYSIOLOGY OF HEART FAILURE. In heart failure the capacity of the ventricles to do work is diminished so that the ejection of blood during systole (the stroke volume, page 259) is reduced. Failure is due either to coronary insufficiency or to prolonged overwork of the myocardium. Thus, coronary thrombosis may cause a sudden onset of failure, and the relative coronary insufficiency occurring in thyrotoxicosis may ultimately lead to failure. Myocardial overwork causes, in the first place, hypertrophy of the cardiac muscle; if the overwork is maintained, failure gradually supervenes. Failure of the left ventricle may follow from the overwork occurring in hypertension, aortic stenosis, or defect of the aortic valves. Right ventricular failure may be caused by mitral valve disease, pulmonary artery stenosis or pulmonary embolism. Heart failure may be divided into left or right ventricular failure; however, as the disorder progresses, both ventricles become involved.

The cardiac output in heart failure is insufficient to maintain an adequate circulation of blood through the tissues. This leads to a number of symptoms by which the disorder may be recognized. The usual symptoms are oedema (the disorder is termed *congestive heart failure* when this is marked), raised venous pressure, dyspnoea, cyanosis, tachycardia and weakness. In left ventricular failure of sudden onset, the reduced output results in an increase in pulmonary venous pressure and pulmonary oedema is marked: this condition is sometimes referred to as *cardiac asthma.*

Many of the disturbances that occur in the cardiovascular system during heart failure begin as homeostatic responses that are tending to reverse the deleterious consequences of the impaired circulation. However, if these homeostatic mechanisms do not successfully restore the circulation, they tend to make the condition worse, thereby establishing a vicious cycle. For example,

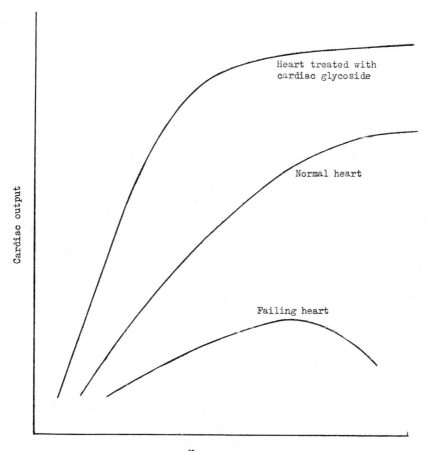

FIG. 32.4. The difference of function of the normal and failing heart expressed in terms of Starling's law of the heart. The scales are arbitary and the axes of the graph could be labelled stroke volume (ordinate) *versus* diastolic filling, *or*, force of systolic contraction *versus* fibre length in diastole. The myocardium of the failing heart is less well able to respond to increased filling by increasing its output, and the point at which increased filling leads to *decreased* output is lower than with the normal heart.

the decrease in blood flow through the kidneys results in the release of renin from the juxta-glomerular apparatus (page 276). The renin activates angiotensin from its plasma precursor (page 182), and angiotensin stimulates the adrenal secretion of aldosterone (page 378) which acts on the renal tubules to increase the re-absorption of sodium (pages 344–345). Hence, there is an increase in body sodium chloride and retention of body water, with a consequent rise in blood volume and an increased formation of tissue fluid. The poor flow of blood through the kidney also contributes to the retention of body fluid. The venous pressure rises because of the increased blood volume, and this in turn causes a greater formation of tissue fluid (see Fig. 8.5, page 245). The formation of oedema in the lungs hinders gaseous exchange leading to dyspnoea. The peripheral tissues are cyanosed because of the inadequate oxygenation of the blood and the poor peripheral circulation, and the cyanosis results in increased capillary permeability causing a still further accumulation of tissue fluid.

In the normal heart the raised venous pressure gives an increase in cardiac output according to Starling's law of the heart (pages 213 and 261). However, in heart failure the ability of the heart to increase its output is impaired. The differences in the function of the normal and the failure heart are illustrated in Fig. 32.4. In the failing heart, increases in venous pressure soon lead to a progressive diminution in output, which, in turn results in a further increase in venous pressure: when failure reaches the point of diminution of output with increasing venous pressure it is described as *uncompensated*. Experimentally, it has been found that reduction of venous pressure in patients with uncompensated heart failure causes an increase in cardiac output; however, the procedures used were not practical as therapeutic measures, as they involved venesection or the application of tourniquets to the limbs.

The volume of the heart is increased in heart failure owing to the increase in end-systolic volume and the increase in diastolic filling from the raised venous pressure: this enlargement can be observed in X-ray examination. The fall in arterial blood pressure which tends to arise from the diminished stroke volume is partly compensated by reflex circulatory adjustments. Thus, there is an increase in heart rate (tachycardia) and constriction of arterioles which tends to produce peripheral ischaemia, which in addition to the anoxia, results in a further formation of tissue fluid.

TREATMENT OF HEART FAILURE WITH CARDIAC GLYCOSIDES. (The term digitalis is here used generically.) Digitalis increases the force of myocardial contraction, and this single effect can account for the relief of all of the symptoms of heart failure, although other effects of digitalis may be contributory. The curve expressing the law of the heart during failure in Fig. 32.4 is shifted upwards; hence the cardiac output is increased. The increase in force of contraction provides for more complete emptying of the heart at each stroke, which decreases the diastolic volume. The blood pressure and circulation are improved as a result of the increased cardiac output, and the venous congestion is reduced. The improvement in renal blood flow results in more rapid excretion of water, both directly, and indirectly by removing the stimulus for the release of renin. Angiotensin production ceases, aldosterone secretion is no longer stimulated, and this facilitates the excretion of sodium. The improved pulmonary blood flow results in increased oxygenation of the blood and the improved peripheral circulation mobilizes the oedema fluid. This fluid is rapidly eliminated from the blood through the kidneys. The reflex drive that has maintained the tachycardia is diminished and the slower beat of the heart enables more efficient emptying of the ventricles.

The other actions of digitalis which may contribute to alleviation of the symptoms of heart failure, but probably only to a minor extent, are (a) a direct diuretic action exerted on the renal tubule, and (b) slowing of the heart by facilitation of vagal impulses.

METHODS OF INVESTIGATING THE ACTIONS OF CARDIAC GLYCOSIDES. Convincing evidence that the effect of cardiac glycosides in relieving the signs of heart failure were due to an effect on the heart was first obtained with the heart-lung preparation. It was observed that cardiac glycosides increased the cardiac output, and this was due to increased ventricular work since there were increases in the maximum intraventricular systolic pressure and in the rate of rise of systolic pressure. In this preparation, venous pressure, peripheral resistance and blood volume may be kept constant, and the heart is not influenced by autonomic nerve impulses. A similar cardio-tonic effect may be seen with isolated perfused hearts and also with excised strips of ventricular muscle.

An increase in dose of the cardiac glycoside beyond that producing the maximum tonic effect leads to the appearance of the typical toxic effects in these preparations.

The action of the cardiac glycosides on the normal heart is similar to its action in the failing heart. However, when the cardiac output is adequate, it is usually not significantly altered by therapeutic doses of the glycosides because reflex compensatory mechanisms partly counteract the effect. An intravenous injection of a glycoside produces a rise in blood pressure which is due partly to increased cardiac output, partly to a direct action on the peripheral arterioles, and partly to an action on the central nervous system. When sufficient is injected to produce arrhythmia, the blood pressure decreases, and falls to zero with the onset of ventricular fibrillation.

OTHER DRUGS USED IN HEART FAILURE. The conditions underlying the myocardial failure are treated as far as possible; those which respond favourably to drug treatment are hypertension (pages 831–845) and thyrotoxicosis (pages 851–853).

Diuretics are valuable adjuncts to digitalis in decreasing the oedema. The mercurial diuretics (e.g. mersalyl, pages 875–878) are used, but intravenous injection is avoided as they may cause cardiac arrhythmia when given by this route. Chlorothiazide (page 881) is given together with a potassium supplement, otherwise the potassium depletion potentiates digitalis to the extent that toxic actions become pronounced giving the signs of digitalis overdosage (see page 809). Spironolactone is useful, particularly as it antagonizes aldosterone and aids in breaking the vicious cycle of events that occurs as a result of heart failure (see page 885).

Oxygen helps in overcoming the diminished oxygenation of the blood, and is particularly useful when cyanosis and dyspnoea are pronounced.

Action of cardiac glycosides in atrial flutter and fibrillation. In flutter, the rate of the atrial beat is 200 to 300 per min. These beats usually originate from an ectopic focus in the atria which has been caused by a disorder such as rheumatic heart disease, hypertension or coronary insufficiency. The atrio-ventricular bundle is unable to conduct impulses at this high rate, and hence there is some degree of heart block; ventricular beating is somewhat irregular since it depends on the arrival of the next atrial impulse after the end of the refractory period following the previous conducted impulse. The erratic rhythm itself tends to upset patients. There may be sudden changes in rhythm as the degree of vagal tone changes: increased vagal activity lengthens the refractory period of the A-V bundle. There are usually some signs of diminished cardiac output associated with atrial flutter.

Digitalis strengthens the heart beat, and thereby corrects the state of failure, as it does in heart failure without arrhythmia. In addition, the flutter is converted to fibrillation. This is probably due to a decrease in the refractory period of the atrial muscle and is allied to the toxic effect of digitalis, but in this disorder it is a beneficial effect. The atrio-ventricular conduction time is prolonged, and this slows the rate of ventricular beating. With many patients, the atrial rhythm returns to normal when the digitalis is stopped.

Atrial fibrillation is more common than flutter. There are no co-ordinated atrial beats; the atrial myocardial fibres contract asynchronously, each at a rate of 400 to 500 per min. The ventricle rate is rapid and it is irregular as the strength of stimulation of the A-V node by atrial impulses is erratic, and weak stimuli may be subthreshold even though they do not fall in a refractory period. Treatment may consist of controlling the atrial arrhythmia, as described below (pages 817–820). However, if there is evidence of heart failure, digitalis is indicated. A dose sufficient to raise the threshold of excitability of the A-V node and to prolong the refractory period is used, and this slows the rate. There is some evidence that slowing the rate is itself useful in increasing the cardiac output.

Toxic effects of cardiac glycosides. The infusion of cardiac glycosides into experimental animals produces a characteristic sequence of cardiac arrhythmias which may be detected in the electrocardiograph (refer to pages 253–257). The first change in the ECG is an alteration in the configuration of the T-wave, which reflects the increased rate of repolarization of the action potential of heart cells. The P-R interval may be prolonged, reflecting an increase in atrio-ventricular conduction time. Then the pacemaker shifts from the sino-atrial node, usually to the atrio-ventricular node, which causes the P-wave to be fused with the QRS (ventricular) complex. Occasional ventricular extrasystoles occur, in which the QRS complexes are broader and may be inverted; then there are runs of extrasystoles; this is followed by continuous ventricular ectopic beating. Finally, the ventricular complexes degenerate and give way to fibrillation. Similar effects are observed with over-digitalization in man, where the first sign of toxicity may be atrial fibrillation or ventricular extrasystoles. Cardiac glycosides increase the excitability of the myocardium, and consequently there is a tendency for the development of ectopic foci from which the extrasystoles arise. The lethal effect of cardiac glycosides is due to ventricular fibrillation. The tendency of cardiac glycosides to produce fibrillation follows from the changes they produce in the myocardial action potential (cf. Fig. 7.10 page 215). The rate of repolarization is increased; that is, the duration of the action potential is reduced, and hence the refractory period of the myocardial fibres is reduced (cf. page 214). Impulses arising from ectopic foci in the hyper-excitable myocardium have a much greater chance of propagating than usual, and the rapid re-entry of impulses which is allowed by the short refractory period culminates in the complete disintegration of the rhythmic pattern of impulse propagation; in other words, fibrillation occurs. Cardiac glycosides are contraindicated in patients with ventricular arrhythmias. The lethal dose of cardiac glycosides in animals is 5 to 10 times the smallest dose which exerts a positive inotropic effect and about twice the dose which produces the first sign of arrhythmia. Consequently the margin of safety, or 'therapeutic index' is small, particularly if the dose is raised to produce the maximal therapeutic effect. Overdosage is usually the result of the cumulative effect of maintenance doses (see pages 529–530).

The toxic effects of cardiac glycosides on the heart are increased by raising the calcium concentration or decreasing the potassium concentration; conversely, they are reduced by decreasing calcium or raising potassium concentrations (see pages 810 and 812).

26*

Cardiac arrhythmias occurring as a result of overdigitalization may be treated with antifibrillatory drugs, such as quinidine or procaine amide (pages 817–820). Recent clinical trials indicate that the β-receptor anti-adrenaline drugs described on pages 766–768 are particularly valuable in correcting arrhythmias arising from cardiac glycoside toxicity. The β-receptor blocking drugs possess anti-arrhythmic activity which is especially effective when a sympathetic component contributes to the arrhythmia; however, only those that possess a quinidine-like action are effective in controlling digitalis arrhythmias.

In addition to the effects on the heart, cardiac glycosides have so-called extra-cardiac toxic actions. The chief of these are diarrhoea, vomiting and disturbances of vision. The diarrhoea is probably due to an increase in excitability of intestinal smooth muscle; this effect of cardiac glycosides may be observed with isolated intestinal preparations. The emetic action of cardiac glycosides is mainly due to stimulation of the chemoreceptor trigger zone of the brain-stem and is preceded by nausea and salivation. Anorexia may also occur. The effects on vision, which include blurring and the appearance of a yellow or green cast to objects, are probably also due to effects on the CNS. Dizziness, headache, disorientation, and mental confusion are further effects attributable to actions on the brain. In man, the doses of cardiac glycosides which produce these effects also have pronounced toxic actions on the heart. However, in certain animals, particularly in rodents, the heart is relatively resistant to the effects of cardiac glycosides and the effects on the central nervous system are much more pronounced. Thus in rats, cardiac glycosides have little effect on the heart but produce fatal convulsions. This is the basis of the use of squill as a rodenticide. The bait is eaten, and rats, being unable to vomit, retain the full dose, whereas domestic pets such as dogs and cats eliminate the poisoned food by vomiting.

Mechanisms of action of cardiac glycosides. The mechanism underlying the actions of the cardiac glycosides of the heart have not been fully elucidated. However, some possible explanations have been put forward on the basis of their effects on the distribution of ions across cell membranes and on contractile proteins.

SODIUM AND POTASSIUM. The activity of cardiac glycosides is modified by altering the potassium concentration in the plasma or the extracellular fluid of cardiac muscle preparations. A decrease in potassium leads to an increase in the toxic action of cardiac glycosides on the heart, and the depletion of plasma K^+ concentration by chlorothiazide diuretics may precipitate toxic signs in digitalized patients. Arrhythmias resulting from overdosage with cardiac glycosides can be counteracted by increasing the plasma K+ concentration.

Toxic doses of cardiac glycosides cause a loss of potassium from the heart and a gain in sodium. This effect may be understood by considering the processes concerned with the distributions of ions across the cell membrane. Sodium ions are expelled from cells by an active transport system (the 'sodium pump', page 74) and potassium ions are taken up; this involves an enzyme system using energy supplied by the breakdown of ATP to ADP. One theory explaining the working of the enzyme system, described as *transport ATP-ase*, is as follows. The energy-rich phosphate groups from intra-cellular ATP are transferred to phosphoprotein molecules in the inner surface of the cell membrane. This reaction occurs only if intracellular sodium and magnesium ions are present. The phosphorylated phosphoprotein binds sodium but not potassium ions; in the dephosphorylated form, the reverse is true. Thus at the inner surface of the membrane:

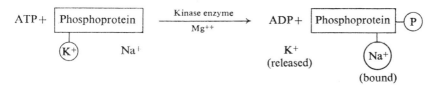

At the external surface of the cell membrane, the complex is dephosphorylated and, if potassium ions are present, sodium ions are released, potassium ions being bound in their place. Thus at the external surface:

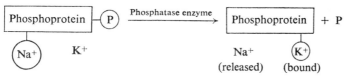

The dephosphorylated phosphoprotein-potassium complex is then available to repeat the cycle. The overall reaction is the utilization of the high energy terminal phosphate of ATP to transfer Na+ to the outside and K+ to the inside of the membrane. The reaction that occurs at the external surface is blocked by cardiac glycosides; since the two reactions are coupled, the transfer of both sodium and potassium by the ATP-ase system is inhibited. Cardiac glycosides act only on transport ATP-ases of cell membranes; they do not inhibit the ATP-ase activity associated with myosin or other ATP-ases.

The molecular features of cardiac glycosides that are essential for their toxicity to the heart and for their positive inotropic action are the same as those for inhibition of the transport ATP-ase of red blood cells, and variation between species to the cardiac activity of cardiac glycosides is reflected in varying sensitivities of erythrocyte transport ATP-ase. It is generally accepted that the toxic actions of cardiac glycosides are due to inhibition of transport ATP-ase. These are four observations in accord with this: (i) There is a good correlation between the toxicity of various cardiac glycosides and their ability to inhibit cardiac transport ATP-ase. (ii) An increase in concentration of potassium protects against inhibition of transport ATP-ase and against toxicity. (iii) Magnesium ions enhance the activity of transport ATP-ase and decrease the toxic effects of the glycosides. (iv) Calcium ions inhibit enzyme activity and increase the toxic effects of the glycosides. However, it is doubtful whether the concentrations of the glycosides produced by therapeutic doses are high enough to block the cardiac transport ATP-ase system. In fact, recent evidence indicates that low concentrations of the glycosides have the opposite effect; that is, they stimulate rather than inhibit cardiac transport ATP-ase. It is possible that the positive inotropic action of the cardiac glycosides is the result of an increase of ATP-ase activity, but adequate experimental evidence in support of this is lacking as yet.

CALCIUM. The concentration of extracellular calcium has a marked effect on the activity of cardiac glycosides. An increase in calcium concentration potentiates the toxic actions of cardiac glycosides on the heart, and a decrease in calcium diminishes their toxicity. Cardiac arrhythmias and deaths from ventricular fibrillation have been precipitated by the administration of calcium-containing compounds to patients on digitalis; conversely, injection of sodium edetate (Fig. 18.10, pages 468 to 469) reduces plasma calcium ion concentration by chelation and counteracts the toxic signs of over-digitalization.

Calcium is of considerable importance in muscle activity; when the external Ca^{++} concentration is low, the force of myocardial contraction is weak. The role of calcium in excitation-contraction coupling is mentioned on pages 198–199. Calcium moves into the muscle cells during depolarization of the cell membrane and the calcium ions initiate shortening of the contractile system. Binding of these intracellular calcium ions terminates the excitation, and relaxation follows. It has been shown that an increase in the amount of calcium entering the myocardial cells, which is produced by procedures such as reduction of the external Na^+ or an increase in K^+ concentrations, results in a proportional increase in the tension developed in contraction. Ouabain produces an increase in uptake of calcium into beating heart muscle, and it has been suggested that this is the basis of the positive inotropic effect. However, another suggestion is that the intracellular binding of calcium ions is prevented by cardiac glycosides. There is general agreement that cardiac glycosides owe their positive inotropic action to an increase in intracellular calcium ions, thereby facilitating the contractile process, but it is uncertain whether this is due to an increase in movement of calcium ions into the myocardial cells or a decrease in binding of the intracellular calcium.

EFFECTS ON CONTRACTILE PROTEINS. Cardiac glycosides have been shown to increase the viscosity of actin solutions and to decrease the thixotrophy of actomyosin. These effects may follow from an increase in the binding of potassium (and possible other ions) to the proteins. Artificial fibres of actomyosin from heart muscle contract in the presence of ATP (see page 193) and the rate and force of contraction is increased in the presence of cardiac glycosides. These observations suggest that the inotropic action of the drugs may be the result of a direct action on the contractile proteins. However, there is again some doubt whether therapeutic doses produce concentrations large enough to give these effects.

Bioassay of cardiac glycosides. Bioassay methods are still officially required for plant extracts and preparations which contain mixtures of cardio-active principles but not for the purified substances. Although these methods are of waning importance in the standardization of crude preparations, they are still of use in the study of structure–activity relationships among the cardiac glycosides and genins.

There are considerable species differences in sensitivity to cardiac glycosides. These drugs are particularly potent in man, cat and dog and slightly less active in the guinea-pig. Bioassay methods commonly employ the cat and the guinea-pig. Rabbits are about one-half as sensitive and rats are about one-hundredth as sensitive as cats. Frogs (species of *Rana*) are sensitive enough for them to have been used for bioassay, but toads (species of *Bufo*) are almost completely unaffected. These differences in sensitivity are not due entirely to differences in rate of metabolism, since isolated hearts and other organs such as intestine and uterus also exhibit similar species variability in responsiveness.

The first methods that were employed for the bioassay of digitalis preparations utilized the lethal dose in the frog after injection into the dorsal lymph sac. This was replaced by methods using the lethal dose in cats or guinea-pigs, which were given intravenous infusions at rates which produced fibrillation within a defined time limit (usually between 20 and 40 min); when too long a time is taken, as with weak infusions, much of the drug is eliminated before the animal dies, and when too short a time is taken (with strong infusions) an excessive dose is given before the effect is manifested: in either case, the lethal dose is higher than that found with the optimum rate of infusion. The theoretical objection to the use of toxic activity in animals as a basis for determining the therapeutic dose in man has been met by standardizing batches of digitalis by observing their potency in altering the T-wave in human volunteers (see page 550).

Another bioassay method with animals depends on the production of emesis in pigeons, and yet another on cardio-toxicity in pigeons. A particularly sensitive method employs the isolated embryo chick heart which is dissected from eggs after about 48 hr of incubation. As little as 0·2 μg of digoxin/ml in a chamber of 0·05 ml containing the embryo heart produces characteristic arrhythmias followed by cardiac arrest.

Relationship between structure and cardiac activity of glycosides and genins. The sugar moiety of the glycosides confers greater aqueous solubility than possessed by the genin alone, and this facilitates transport through the tissues. The sugar is not essential to cardio-activity, although the potency of a monoside is usually greater than that of the corresponding genin; diosides and triosides are usually less potent than monosides. Of the monosides, those formed with glucose or rhamnose are usually more potent than those formed with other sugars.

The essential features of cardio-active genins were mentioned above in connection with their general chemical structure. Reduction of the lactone ring to form the saturated structure results in considerable loss of activity. Opening of the lactone ring, or cross-linking it to the D-ring leads to complete loss of activity. Epimerization of the lactone ring (i.e., alteration of its attachment to the D-ring from β to α) abolishes activity. Genins with a 6-membered lactone ring are more active than those with a 5-membered ring having an identical steroidal structure. Cardiac activity is lost after alteration of the configuration of the C/D ring junction, whether this is produced by removal or epimerization of the 14-OH or the 13-CH$_3$ groups. A change in configuration of the A/B ring junction from *cis* to *trans* considerably reduces activity, as does epimerization of the 3-OH from β to α. Acetylation of the 3-OH reduces activity, and oxidation to the corresponding 3-keto derivative leads to further loss of activity.

The changes in activity following various chemical changes do not significantly alter the ratio of cardio-tonic to toxic activity. It seems probable that these two effects are inherent, arising necessarily from the mechanisms of action. This may explain why it is that the cardio-active glycosides and genins are unique among the major groups of drugs in that there are no synthetic analogues or substitutes.

Absorption, distribution, metabolism and excretion. Consideration of these factors explains the differences in routes of administration that are used in practice with various cardiac glycosides, and accounts for the differences in rate of onset and persistence of effect. Digitoxin is one of the least water soluble and most lipid soluble glycosides; it is well absorbed after oral administration, the onset of action is slow but the duration of action is long. The more water soluble glycosides may be administered by intravenous injection. Ouabain is invariably given in this way, lanatoside C is frequently given by injection, and digoxin injections are occasionally used. The rates of onset of their action are in the order: ouabain > lanatoside C > digoxin, but the effects of the most rapidly acting glycosides are the shortest lasting. Digitoxin and digoxin are strongly bound to plasma albumin, lanatoside C is weakly bound and ouabain is not bound.

Digitoxin is metabolized in the liver, one of the metabolites being digoxin. The metabolites and a small percentage of unchanged digitoxin are excreted in the urine. Digoxin, lanatoside C and ouabain are excreted largely unchanged.

In galenical preparations the absorption of glycosides may be facilitated by the surface-active saponins that are present.

Anti-arrhythmic drugs

Types of arrhythmia. Atrial fibrillation is a common and important cardiac arrhythmia. The nature of this disorder and the use of digitalis in its treatment, is described above. Digitalis is also used to treat atrial flutter (page 808). An atrial arrhythmia of less degree, *atrial tachycardia*, may be due to a rapid rate of discharge of impulses from the sino-atrial node with a regular heart rate of up to 150 beats/min or to discharges from an ectopic focus. If the ectopic focus discharges rapidly, a regular heart rate of up to 200 beats/min may be produced during an attack; this condition is described as *supraventricular paroxysmal tachycardia*. If the atrial ectopic focus discharges occasionally, an additional heart beat is inserted. The next normal impulse after an extrasystole may not be propagated if it falls within the refractory period of the aberrant beat. The occasional occurrence of atrial extrasystoles is not uncommon and is of no great pathological significance.

Conduction of the cardiac impulse from the atria to the ventricles may be impaired or completely blocked. In one type of disorder, the P-R interval gradually increases until one ventricular beat is lost and then the cycle starts again. A longer delay in atrio-ventricular conduction with the ventricles failing to beat results in a sudden fall of blood pressure and unconsciousness from cerebral anoxia: these are termed *Stokes-Adams attacks*.

Ventricular arrhythmias follow the same pattern as the atrial arrhythmias, but are more serious in their consequences. *Ventricular extrasystoles* often accompany or signify a defect in the coronary circulation, and they may progress into a more severe arrhythmia. In *ventricular tachycardia*, the beats arise from an ectopic focus in the ventricles and the heart rate may increase to over 200 beats/min. Ventricular tachycardia is usually associated with a history of serious heart disease such as coronary thrombosis. It may progress into *ventricular fibrillation*, in which there are no co-ordinated beats and the circulation ceases.

DRUG-INDUCED ARRHYTHMIAS. The arrhythmias produced by cardiac glycosides have been discussed above. Sympathomimetic amines also have a tendency to produce arrhythmias. Certain anaesthetics, particularly chloroform and cyclopropane, are liable to precipitate arrhythmia during induction; this tendency is enhanced when there is excitation of cardiac sympathetic nerves, release of catecholamines from the adrenal medulla, or administration of sympathomimetic amines. Some hydrocarbon solvents (e.g. benzene) have a similar effect to chloroform.

Aconitine, an alkaloid from *Aconitum napellus* (monkshood or wolfsbane), has a minor use in the treatment of neuralgia, in which it is applied topically: it is extremely toxic owing to its tendency to produce fibrillation. The application of a drop of aconitine solution to the surface of the atrial myocardium is sufficient to set up fibrillation. The mechanism of this action is that aconitine depresses the rate of conduction of the cardiac impulse at the site of application. When impulses from the sinus pacemaker sweep through the syncytium in normal atria, impulses travelling by different paths to the same point arrive sufficiently close together for the second impulse to occur during the refractory period following the first impulse. However, an impulse that has been slowed by passing through the region affected by aconitine may arrive at a portion of the atrial syncytium that has completely recovered from the more rapidly travelling impulse in the surrounding normal myocardium; in this case the tissue is re-excited and an aberrant wave of excitation passes through the myocardium. When this arrives again at the region affected by aconitine, the same process occurs again. In this way, the rhythmic beating is completely disorganized and fibrillation occurs. The region affected by aconitine acts as a focus for re-entry of excitation, and differs therefore from a spontaneously discharging ectopic focus. Aconitine does not produce arrhythmia if it is applied to an atrial appendage into which propagation of impulses have been prevented by clamping it off from the remainder of the atrium. Removal of the clamp momentarily to allow one wave of excitation to enter the appendage, or initiation of an impulse in the appendage by electrical stimulation, results in the establishment of arrhythmia. Aconitine has similar effects on the ventricular myocardium.

Choline esters applied to the atrial surface produce arrhythmia, but have no effect on the ventricular myocardium.

The efficacy of anti-fibrillatory drugs is evaluated by studying their effects in experimentally produced arrhythmias. Drugs used to produce fibrillation for this purpose include ouabain, aconitine, chloroform, benzene and choline esters. Electrical stimulation of the heart is often used to precipitate fibrillation in the presence of amounts of these drugs that are ineffective by themselves.

Other methods of assessing anti-fibrillatory potential depend on observations on the effective refractory period: one of these is mentioned in Table 18.1 (page 448).

The drug treatment of arrhythmias. The less severe forms of atrial arrhythmia may often be corrected by reflexly eliciting efferent discharges of the vagus nerves, or by injection of methacholine (page 704), carbachol (page 705) or neostigmine (page 715). These manoeuvres decrease the rate of impulse formation in the atrial pacemaker and depress atrio-ventricular conduction (page 263). In some patients, the awareness of the arrhythmia may be disturbing even though it is not indicative of major disease, in which case sedation with amylobarbitone or a similar drug is helpful.

The impaired atrio-ventricular conduction responsible for Stokes-Adams attacks has been treated with ephedrine. The mechanism of action is obscure: it may be facilitation of conduction, or it may be that the increased excitability of the myocardium favours a rapid establishment of a ventricular pacemaker which maintains the blood pressure.

Ventricular fibrillation requires immediate treatment for there to be any hope of successful recovery, since cessation of the circulation rapidly results in irreversible damage from cerebral anoxia. Restoration of circulation by massage of the heart is often a practical procedure for fibrillation occurring during surgery. Techniques have been developed recently for maintaining the circulation by exerting rhythmic pressure on the sternum, thereby compressing the heart. Defibrillation may be accomplished by passage of electric shocks through the heart from electrodes applied to the chest. The excitation from the electrical pulses tends to regularize the heart since all parts of the myocardium except those in an absolute refractory period are stimulated synchronously; subsequent shocks, spaced at appropriate intervals, recruit still more of the myocardial fibres to a synchronized beat.

The major drug used in treating arrhythmia, particularly atrial fibrillation, is quinidine: its action, in general terms, is to depress the excitability of the heart. Other anti-arrhythmic drugs with a similar action are procaine amide, lignocaine, and certain antihistamines (diphenhydramine and antazoline). Recently, the β-adrenoreceptor blocking drugs have been found effective. An anti-epileptic drug, phenytoin, is also used.

QUINIDINE. The formula of quinidine is shown in Fig. 32.5. It is the dextro-isomer of the anti-malarial drug quinine. The discovery of the effectiveness of quinine in suppressing atrial fibrillation was made by a Dutch merchant who observed it empirically by treating himself and then convinced his physician of the truth of the claim. His case was published in 1914, and by 1918 it had

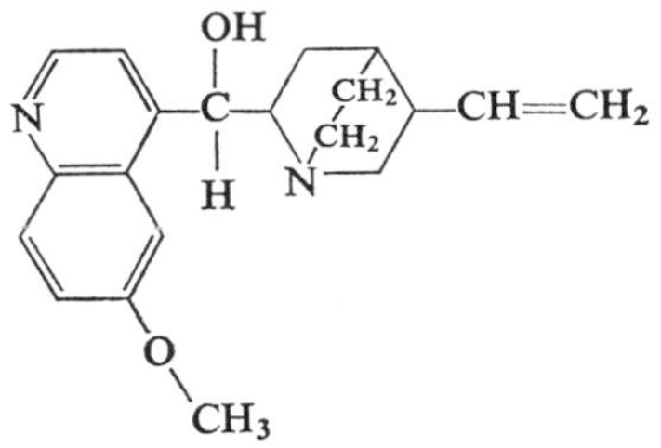

Quinidine

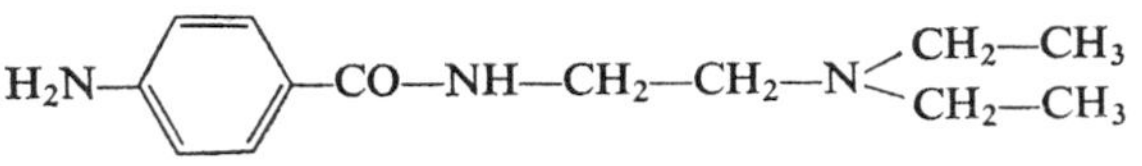

Procainamide

Fig. 32.5. The formulae of the commonest antifibrillatory drugs.

been established that quinidine was the most effective of the cinchona alkaloids for the treatment of atrial fibrillation.

The pharmacological effects of quinidine have been extensively explored. Those which are thought to explain its beneficial action in the treatment of arrhythmias are (a) prolongation of the refractory period of myocardial and conducting tissues, (b) reduction of the velocity of conduction of cardiac impulses, and (c) reduction of excitability of pacemaker, myocardial and conducting tissues. All of these follow from the one effect of quinidine on the cell membrane, namely, that it decreases the permeability to sodium. The de-polarization phase of the action potential is due to a sudden increase in per-meability of the cell membrane to sodium (see pages 77–78). After giving quinidine in therapeutic concentrations, the rate of depolarization is slowed by about 60%. The consequences, in terms of the three actions listed above, are as follows: (a) The action potentials, having a slower rate of depolarization, are unable to cause excitation of adjacent tissue that is in the relative refractory period (cf. page 216). In fibrillation, an action potential is propagated into any continguous portion of the myocardium that has passed out of the absolute refractory period of the preceding impulse. That is, one impulse follows immediately on the wake of another, and depolarizes the membrane in the relative refractory period before it is fully repolarized. (b) The rate of rise of the action potential being slower, the rate of current change through the membrane in the path of the action potential is slower and the conduction velocity decreases. Quinidine prolongs the P-R interval by slowing atrio-ventricular conduction and the QRS complexes are broader because conduction through the ventricular conducting system and myocardium is slowed. (c) The resting potential is rendered more stable, a greater stimulus being required to initiate an action potential.

Many of the side effects of quinidine are an extension of its therapeutically useful action. Thus, by prolonging the duration of ventricular systole to the extent that some parts of the myocardium have relaxed before others have fully contracted, it reduces the stroke volume. Any tendency towards impaired A-V conduction may be exacerbated by quinidine. Although quinidine generally supresses arrhythmias, it may precipitate ventricular fibrillation in large doses.

During atrial fibrillation, the blood in atrial appendages is relatively static and has a tendency to clot. In the treatment of long-standing atrial fibrillation with quinidine, there is a danger that the restoration of effective rhythmic contractions may discharge a thrombus from the atria into the circulation so that pulmonary embolism, cerebral embolism or coronary thrombosis results. Treatment with anti-coagulants before attempting to restore the rhythm has been advocated.

Other toxic effects of quinidine (and of quinine) consist of ringing in the ears, with impaired hearing, dizziness, blurring of vision, nausea and vomiting: these symptoms are termed *cinchonism*. Allergic reactions may occur with the cinchona alkaloids; these include urticaria and asthmatic attacks.

Quinidine is usually administered orally as the sulphate or the gluconate. If it is not well tolerated by this route as a result of gastric irritation or vomiting, the gluconate may be injected intramuscularly.

PROCAINAMIDE. Both procaine and procainamide have local anaesthetic and anti-fibrillatory properties (see Chapter 25); however, the amide is more persistent, being hydrolysed more slowly, and it is less toxic on the CNS. The mechanism of action of procainamide is similar to that of quinidine. It has been extensively used in the treatment and prevention of auricular fibrillation and ventricular tachycardia, and it is used during surgery to prevent or arrest cardiac arrhythmias. It may be given orally, intramuscularly or by slow intravenous injection. The toxic effects of procainamide are similar to those of quinidine. Hydrolysis of procainamide yields aminobenzoic acid, which antagonizes the actions of the sulphonamides and allowance should be made for this in patients being treated with both procainamide and sulphonamides.

Other quinidine-like drugs. The action of quinidine on cardiac muscle which underlies its anti-fibrillatory activity is shared by many other drugs, including certain antihistamines and local anaesthetics. Among the antihistamines, diphenhydramine and antazoline (page 782) have been used; among the local anaesthetics, lignocaine (page 658) has been used, and is said to possess the advantage over quinidine and procainamide that it produces less depression of the circulation.

PROPRANOLOL. The actions and uses of propranolol and other β-adreno-receptor blocking drugs are described on pages 766–768. Recent clinical trials have indicated that propranolol is effective in treating various types of cardiac arrhythmia. Its use in cases of digitalis overdosage is mentioned above (page 810). It appears to be particularly useful in treating the arrhythmias associated with thyrotoxicosis, those occurring during surgery, and those due to sympathetic stimulation or sympathomimetic amines.

PHENYTOIN. The use of this drug in treatment of epilepsy is mentioned on page 610. It has recently been found to have a beneficial action in atrial fibrillation, having advantages over quinidine-like drugs in that it has fewer toxic effects. Its mode of action differs from that of quinidine in that it slows the rate of conduction in the atrial myocardium without any great effect on the rate of depolarization of the action potential.

Anti-anginal drugs

Angina pectoris is a referred pain that results from anoxia of cardiac muscle (see page 262). This anoxia also produces characteristic changes in the T-wave of the ECG (page 256). Myocardial anoxia may be caused in a number of ways (cf. pages 298–299). (a) *Ischaemic anoxia*, in which there is occlusion of coronary vessels, may be caused either by a thrombosis forming on an atheroma, or the lodgement of an embolism, or a spasm of the vessels. Ischaemia resulting from intra-vascular clotting may be treated with anti-coagulant drugs (pages 906–911); that due to coronary arterial spasm (which is said to be of rare occurrence) may be relieved with coronary vasodilator drugs. (b) *Anaemic anoxia* may result in anginal pain and is treated by correcting the anaemia (pages 913–916). (c) *Anoxic anaemia* of the myocardium may occur at high altitudes, in carbon monoxide poisoning, and in methaemoglobinaemia. (d) A *functional anoxia* is usually responsible for the angina of effort. In this disorder, an increase in demand of the myocardium for oxygen is not met by a corresponding increase in coronary blood flow, the coronary vessels having lost their capacity to dilate owing to arteriosclerotic changes in their walls (page 280). The oxygen consumption of the myocardium depends on the work being done by the heart, and increases therefore in exercise, owing to the increased cardiac output (page 275). Myocardial work is also increased by an increase in peripheral resistance, as occurs in hypertension. The increase in cardiac work that is induced by sympathomimetic amines or by sympathetic nerve impulses is accomplished by a disproportionately high increase in cardiac oxygen consumption, because myocardium metabolism becomes less efficient. In anxiety and other emotional states there may be an increase in cardiac sympathetic tone. Myocardial metabolism is also less efficient in hyperthyroid states, and there is a tendency to angina. Loss of function in part of the myocardium, caused, for example, by infarction throws a greater load on the remaining portion, and thereby increases the chance of anoxia. Even a slight imbalance between myocardial work and the coronary blood supply may result in anoxia. The oxygen content of coronary venous blood is about 25 to 30% that of arterial blood, and this is the highest arterio-venous oxygen difference for any organ except severely exercised somatic muscle. Cardiac muscle is unable to accumulate an oxygen debt, therefore any increase in metabolic activity must be met by an increase in coronary flow.

Treatment of angina. In those cases in which the underlying cause of the anginal pain can be identified, it is treated as far as possible. Little can be done to correct arteriosclerotic degeneration of blood vessels, which is the usual underlying cause of angina of effort, and the use of drugs is directed at (i) reducing cardiac work, (ii) increasing the efficiency of myocardial metabolism, (iii) reducing sympathetic excitation of the heart, and (iv) relieving the pain and anxiety that occur in angina.

Nitrites and organic nitrates. The formulae of these drugs are shown in Fig. 32.6.

AMYL NITRITE. Amyl nitrite is a pale yellow liquid. Being very volatile, it is administered by inhalation, for which purpose it is usually dispensed in crushable glass capsules that are wrapped in gauze to protect the fingers and to soak up the liquid. At the first sign of an anginal attack, the vapour released from the crushed capsule is inhaled. The onset of action is rapid (about 30 sec) but the duration of effect is brief (about 5 min). Inhalation of amyl nitrite causes flushing of the face and neck. In some patients there may be headache from cerebral vasodilatation and giddiness and faintness from the hypotension. Nausea, vomiting and sweating may occur. Dilatation of intra-ocular blood vessels may cause glaucoma in susceptible subjects. In addition, smooth muscle of the bronchi, gall bladder, bile duct, and alimentary tract is relaxed. It tends to produce methaemoglobinaemia. Amyl nitrite was the first effective drug to be used in treating angina; its beneficial effect was described in 1897 which was 8 years after the discovery of the substance. The use of amyl nitrite in angina is rare nowadays.

OTHER NITRITES. *Ethyl nitrite* (nitrous ether) has the same actions as amyl nitrite, and has been used in angina. *Octyl nitrite* has been used as substitute for

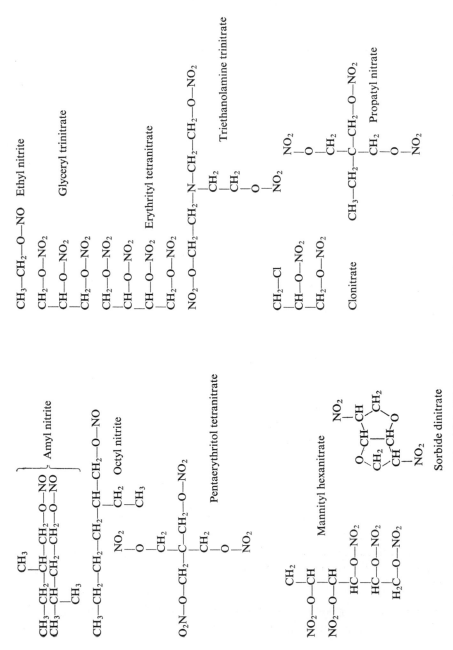

FIG. 32.6. Nitrites and nitrates used in the treatment of angina.

amyl nitrite; being less volatile, the odour is less marked which causes less embarrassment to the user, the onset of action is slower and the duration slightly longer. It is usually administered from an inhaler. *Sodium nitrite* ($NaNO_2$) has similar actions to the organic nitrites. It has been used prophylactically in angina, but its main use is in the treatment of cyanide poisoning; it acts by producing methaemoglobin which has a strong affinity for cyanide and forms the harmless substance cyanomethaemoglobin.

GLYCERYL TRINITRATE. The pure substance, otherwise known as nitroglycerin, is a highly explosive liquid. It is usually adsorbed onto lactose and made into tablets or dissolved in oil and made into capsules, in which forms it is stable. These preparations are chewed and then held under the tongue. The drug is effective when absorbed from the buccal mucosa, but not effective after absorption from the gut, being metabolized in the liver. The actions of glyceryl trinitrate are like those of amyl nitrite, but the onset of action takes about 2 min and the duration of effect is about 30 min. It is taken at the start of pain or prophylactically before beginning any exertion which is likely to produce anginal pain. Glyceryl trinitrate was first tried in cases of angina in 1879, this being stimulated by the similarity between its actions and those of amyl nitrite. It remains the drug of choice in the treatment of angina of effort.

ERYTHRITYL TETRANITRATE. This substance is also explosive when pure and is adsorbed onto an inert medium. Absorption from the gastro-intestinal tract is erratic and the tablets are usually placed sublingually. The onset of its action is relatively slow (about 45 min) but its duration of effect is several hours. It is used prophylactically rather than for treatment of acute anginal attacks.

PENTAERYTHRITOL TETRANITRATE. This is another explosive substance and has the general pharmacological properties of glyceryl trinitrate. It is more effective when taken sub-lingually than when swallowed. The action is fairly rapid in onset (about 10 min) and persists for some hours. It reduces the intensity and frequency of anginal attacks but does not abolish them.

OTHER ORGANIC NITRATES. *Mannityl hexanitrate* is similar in actions and uses to erythrityl tetranitrate. *Triethanolamine trinitrate* is claimed to be less liable to cause methaemoglobinaemia and other toxic effects. It is used prophylactically and has a long lasting effect. *Isosorbide dinitrate, clonitrate* and *propatyl nitrate* have recently been introduced.

Mode of action of nitrites and organic nitrates in angina. These drugs increase coronary blood flow through perfused hearts in which coronary perfusion pressure, heart rate and force of contraction remain constant, and they cause an increase in coronary blood flow in healthy human subjects. Their action in relieving angina due to coronary spasm is by dilating the vessels. However, it is probable that the vessels are not capable of such a dilator response in angina due to sclerosis of coronary vessels. Furthermore, the anoxia, which is responsible for the anginal symptoms, is itself a powerful vasodilator stimulus and produces a maximal vasodilator response, even though this response is not sufficient to remove the symptoms of anoxia; it seems unlikely that a further vasodilator effect could be superimposed upon it. For these reasons it is now generally considered that the main effect of nitrites and nitrates in relieving angina is due to peripheral vasodilatation. The decrease in systemic vascular resistance reduces the amount of work done in systole, therefore, the oxygen requirement of the myocardium is reduced. The reduced resistance to flow allows the ventricles to empty more completely, hence stroke volume increases. The fall in blood pressure reflexly evokes tachycardia. Cardiac output is increased owing to the increase in rate and stroke volume. The greater volume of blood ejected into the aorta maintains the diastolic pressure, and provides for adequate perfusion of the coronary vessels in diastole when the tension in the walls of the heart is low.

The mechanism of the vasodilator action of nitrites is not fully understood, but it has been demonstrated they inhibit an ATP-ase concerned with the energy supply of vascular smooth muscle.

Relief of angina may also be accomplished by depressing the appreciation of pain, that is, by an analgesic action. In this connection, it is interesting that glyceryl trinitrate was first used in medicine against toothache.

The main piece of evidence that the nitrites and nitrates relieve angina by correcting the functional anoxia is that they prevent the changes in the ECG and the pain that are produced by exercise in susceptible subjects.

Patients suffering from angina frequently respond to placebos, and this complicates the evaluation of the efficacy of anti-anginal drugs. Since many of the newly introduced drugs have not been adequately evaluated in controlled trials, some doubts have been raised about their effectiveness. Tolerance develops to the anti-anginal effects of the nitrates, and this raises a further problem in evaluating their efficacy. The mechanism of the tolerance has not been adequately explained. A few days abstinence from treatment usually restores the beneficial effects.

Propranolol. This drug blocks β-adrenoreceptors (see pages 766–768), and consequently prevents the responses of the heart to sympathetic nerve stimulation. It has been found effective in the prophylactic treatment of angina, and it prevents the ECG changes on exercise in patients predisposed to angina. The failure of the heart to respond to reflex sympathetic stimulation by an increase in work may produce an impairment of the circulation resembling that occurring in heart failure, in which case digitalis is used to strengthen the heart beat.

Monamine oxidase inhibitors (see also pages 623–626). During the early trials on the antidepressant activity of iproniazid, it was noticed that anginal patients experienced remission of symptoms. However, many controlled trials with this and other monamine oxidase inhibitors failed to demonstrate their superiority over a placebo; there is still controversy over this. Whether or not the mono-amine oxidase inhibitors relieve anginal pain, it seems clear that they do not prevent the ECG changes in exercise. It is suggested therefore that their main action is in the relief of anxiety and as mild analgesics.

Ethyl alcohol. Advocacy of the use of alcoholic drinks in angina on the grounds that ethyl alcohol dilates coronary vessels has no factual basis. Any relief of angina they produce is probably due to lessening of anxiety.

Recently introduced anti-anginal drugs. The formulae of some drugs that have been recently introduced are shown in Fig. 32.7.

DIPYRIDAMOLE. This drug is a vasodilator and causes relaxation of most smooth muscles; it is particularly effective as a dilator of coronary vessels, and relieves experimentally produced coronary spasm. Dipyridamole decreases the arterio-venous oxygen difference of coronary blood, which suggests that it reduces the oxygen consumption of the myocardium. It increases the myocardial content of adenyl compounds.

The status of dipyridamole for the treatment of angina of effort is still undecided. In some trials it has been shown to be little better than a placebo, and to have no effect on the ECG in exercise.

The mechanism of the vasodilator action of dipyridamole is of some interest. It causes marked potentiation of adenosine (page 180), which is believed to be due to blockade of the uptake of adenosine into cells so that they exert their pharmacological effects more intensely. The vasodilator action exerted by dipyridamole itself may be brought about by inhibition of re-uptake of adenosine released from cells.

Dipyridamole decreases the adhesiveness of platelets, probably by potentiation of this action of adenosine, and thereby diminishes the risk of thrombosis. Long term administration of dipyridamole leads to an increase in development of collateral coronary vessels. These two actions may be beneficial in the treatment of myocardial infarction.

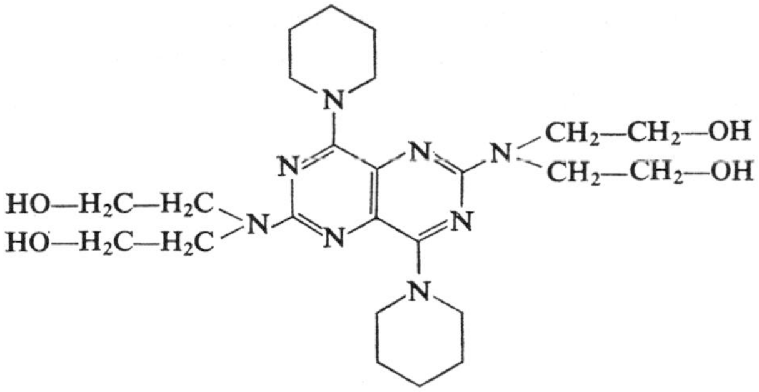

Dipyridamole

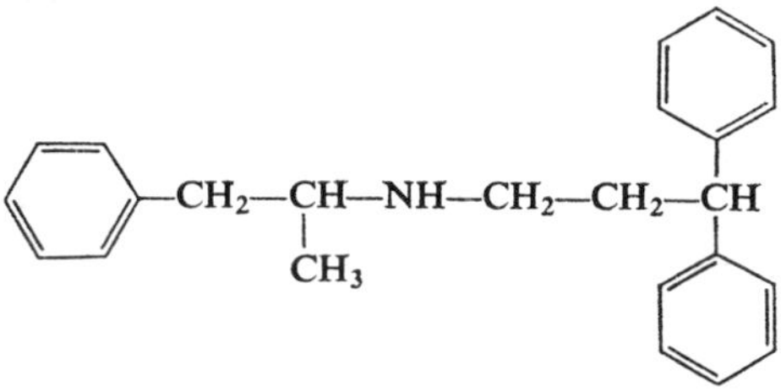

Prenylamine

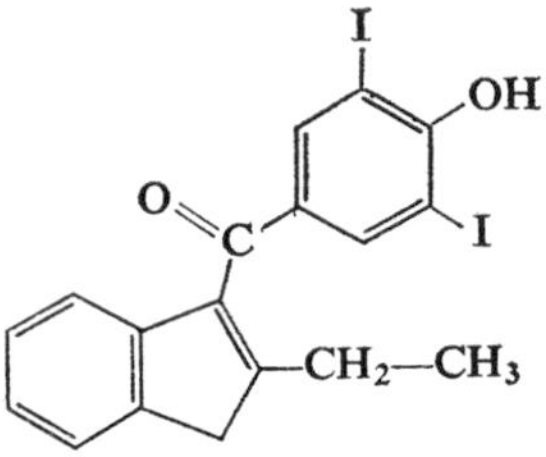

Benziodarone

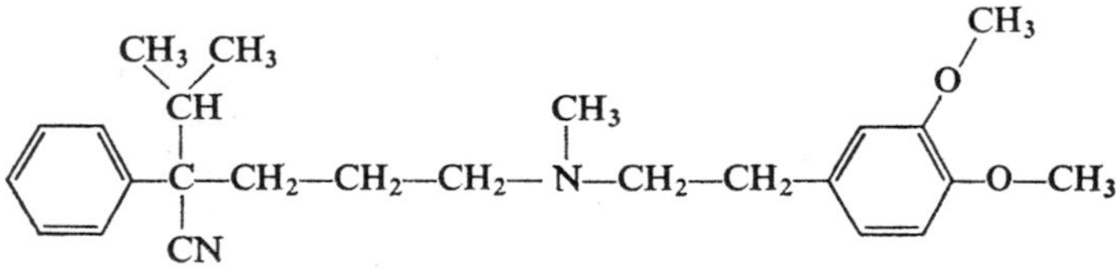

Iproveratril

FIG. 32.7. Some anti-anginal drugs that have been recently introduced into therapeutics.

BENZIODARONE. This drug causes relaxation of smooth muscles and dilatation of coronary arteries. Its usefulness in angina has not been firmly established as yet. Its side effects include hypoprothrombinaemia and suppression of thyroid activity.

PRENYLAMINE. This drug produces a transient increase in coronary blood flow. Its other pharmacological actions include adrenergic neurone blockade and sedation. It does not affect the ECG changes of anginal patients on exercise, nor the appearance of pain. However, spontaneously occurring anginal attacks are fewer and less severe. It is thought to owe its effect chiefly to sedation, although blockade of responses to cardiac sympathetic impulse may be a contributory factor.

IPROVERATRIL. Iproveratril has marked coronary vasodilator activity, being 100 times more potent than papaverine (see below). It reduces the coronary arterio-venous oxygen difference, as does dipyridamole, but its mechanism of action differs since it has no effect on metabolism of adenyl compounds. In some respects iproveratril resembles propranolol; for example, it has anti-arrhythmic activity resembling that of quinidine, and it blocks β-receptors. Its value in the treatment of angina is still under investigation.

Older (and almost obsolete) drugs used in angina. The formulae of these drugs are given in Fig. 32.8.

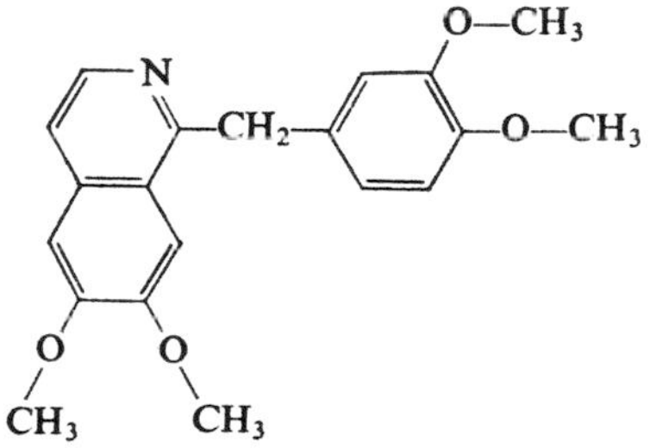

Papaverine

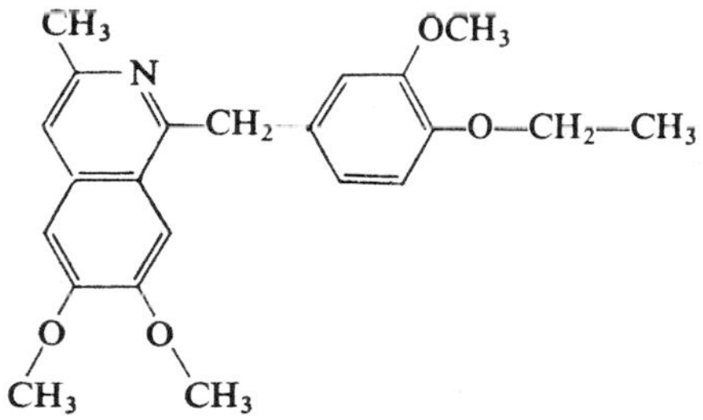

Dioxyline

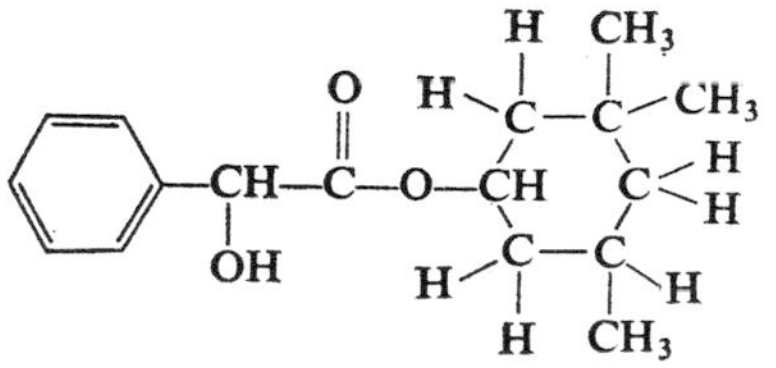

·Cyclandelate

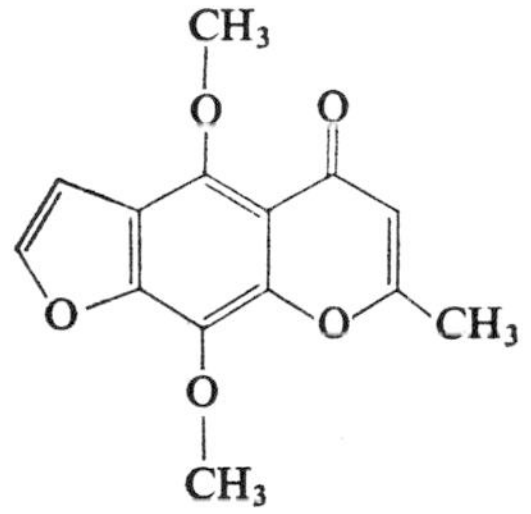

Khellin

FIG. 32.8. Drugs once used in angina, but now almost entirely discarded.

PAPAVERINE. This alkaloid is found in opium (page 631). It is a potent coronary vasodilator with a prolonged action. It also dilates pulmonary and peripheral arteries and is often used in the treatment of embolism of pulmonary, cerebral and other peripheral vessels. Papaverine reduces tone and motility of smooth muscle generally, this action being most pronounced when the tone is high or the smooth muscle is in spasm due to the action of drugs or to nervous activity. This antispasmodic action is exerted on blood vessels, the bile duct, ureters and intestines, and hence papaverine has been used in the treatment of peripheral vascular spasm, in ureteral or biliary colic and in spasm of the gastro-intestinal tract. The mechanism of the relaxant activity of papaverine is not known beyond the fact that it is exerted directly on the smooth muscle. Apart from its action on coronary vessels, papaverine also affects the myocardium, depressing conduction and irritability, and increasing the refractory period. Although these effects tend to protect against arrhythmia, large doses cause arrhythmias.

The precise evaluation of the anti-anginal effects of papaverine has given equivocal results, despite the fact that the drug has been used for many years. Its onset of action is too slow for it to be used to abort anginal attacks, and large and frequent doses are necessary to obtain a sustained prophylactic effect. Papaverine affords some protection against the ECG changes occurring in exercise. It is thought that its action in angina is at least partly due to a decrease in cardiac work which results from depression of the myocardium. Papaverine also has mild sedative activity which may also be implicated in its anti-anginal effect. *Dioxyline* and the tetra-ethoxy analogue of papaverine have substantially the same actions and uses as the parent substance.

Cyclandelate and a number of other esters of mandelic acid possess papaverine-like antispasmodic activity. Cyclandelate is more potent and less toxic than papaverine and has been used in the treatment of angina pectoris and also of peripheral vascular disease, and spasm of the bile duct, gall bladder and gastro-intestinal tract.

KHELLIN. This is a naturally-occurring compound obtained from the fruit and seeds of an umbelliferous herb *Ammi visnaga*. It has a papaverine-like anti-spasmodic action, relaxing spasm of the bile duct, gall bladder and ureter. It appears also to have a selective action on the coronary vessels which dilate with doses which do not alter the calibre of peripheral blood vessels; however, it is less potent than the nitrites in this respect. Khellin has bronchodilator activity, which may be due to its antihistamine property, and has been used in the symptomatic treatment of both asthma and whooping cough. Overdosage leads to nausea and vomiting, pain and insomnia. Its use in angina has been discontinued, owing to its lack of efficacy and the high incidence of side-effects.

THEOPHYLLINE PREPARATIONS. Theophylline has been mentioned previously (see page 620). It is generally given in combination with ethylenedi-amine (this preparation being known as aminophylline), choline or sodium glycinate. Theophylline dilates the coronary vessels, has a direct stimulant action on the myocardium, relaxes peripheral blood vessels, has diuretic activity, relaxes bronchial smooth muscle and stimulates the respiratory centre. It has been used as a prophylactic in angina pectoris, in coronary infarction and in the treatment of congestive heart failure and cardiac and bronchial asthma.

It has no effect other than as a placebo in angina, and its usefulness in the other disorder has been questioned.

Drugs used in peripheral vascular disease

Disorders of blood vessels leading to ischaemic anoxia of the tissues of the extremities are collectively known as peripheral vascular diseases (see page 281). Exercise of ischaemic muscle results in the severe pain known as claudication; this is probably allied to the pain of angina (cf. pages 110 and 184).

Peripheral vascular disease that is due to arteriosclerotic degeneration, or to blockade of vessels by thrombus formation or embolism is usually treated with anticoagulant drugs to prevent excessive intravascular clotting. It is clear from the nature of the disorder that vasodilator drugs would be of little avail.

Vasodilator drugs are used in the treatment of spasm of peripheral blood vessels, as occurs in Raynaud's disease, in reactions to cold such as chilblains and frostbite, and as a toxic side-effect of treatment with drugs derived from ergot (particularly ergotamine, page 758 and methysergide, page 786). Drugs that block the vasoconstrictor actions of noradrenaline are also used, particularly in the treatment of vascular spasm that is due to an excessive response to impulses arriving in adrenergic vasoconstrictor nerves (i.e., in Raynaud's disease and chilblains).

Chilblains. Cold provides a stimulus for sympathetic vasoconstriction of the digits. The local ischaemia produces itching and pain, and also results in increased capillary permeability, giving rise to oedema. Treatment may include the use of vitamin K analogues (particularly acetomenaphthone) and members of the P group of vitamins, in addition to vasodilator drugs. The rationale of this treatment is to decrease capillary permeability which is presumed to be defective in those susceptible to chilblains.

Anti-adrenaline drugs used in peripheral vascular disease. *Tolazoline, phentolamine* and *azapetine* (page 763) are antagonists of α-adrenoreceptors and hence they block the vasoconstrictor response to injected noradrenaline; however, these drugs are much less effective in blocking responses to noradrenaline liberated by adrenergic nerve stimulation (i.e., they are adrenolytic rather than sympatholytic). The explanation for any beneficial effect they possess in the treatment of Raynaud's disease is that they have a direct vasodilator action. Another antagonist of α-adrenoreceptors, *phenoxybenzamine* (page 762), is more effective as a sympatholytic. It is used in treating Raynaud's disease, and also as a guide to the possibility of success in relieving the vascular spasm by sympathectomy of the afflicted region. Phenoxybenzamine provides relief in some cases of chilblains. *Hydergine*, the mixture of dihydro-compounds in ergotoxine (page 760), has been used in treating a variety of peripheral vascular diseases. It will be recalled that the hydrogenation of the ergot alkaloids increases their α-adrenoreceptor blocking activity and reduces their vaso-constrictor activity. Hydergine is in fact a vasodilator.

Blockade of sympathetic vasoconstrictor nerve activity offers a theoretical possibility for the treatment of neurogenic local vascular spasm. The ganglion blocking drug hexamethonium has been used for this purpose, but the use of the more recently developed drugs that block ganglionic transmission or that prevent the release of noradrenaline from sympathetic nerve has not been systematically exploited.

Vasodilator drugs used in peripheral vascular disease. Many of the drugs mentioned previously as coronary vasodilators are also used to dilate peripheral blood vessels. In particular, these are papaverine and the papaverine-like drug cyclandelate. Papaverine has been given by intra-arterial injection and applied locally to the vessel in spasm.

The vasodilator action of certain choline esters has been utilized in the treatment of peripheral vascular spasm. Thus *carbachol* and *methacholine* (Table 28.1, page 704) have been used in the treatment of Raynaud's disease; the latter drug has been applied iontophoretically to obtain a maximal local effect. The other actions of choline esters may lead to exacerbation of asthmatic conditions and of gastrointestinal ulcers.

Sympathomimetic vasodilators related to isoprenaline act on β-adreno-receptors to produce relaxation of vascular smooth muscle. *Nylidrin* and *isoxuprine* (page 749) have more powerful vasodilator actions in muscle than in the splanchnic region. Nylidrin increases cardiac output, and this maintains blood flow through the dilated vessels. These drugs are used in the treatment of claudication occurring in Raynaud's disease. They are contra-indicated in angina.

Nicotinic acid, one of the B-group of vitamins (pages 32–33), has powerful vasodilator activity and has been used in the treatment of vasoconstriction occurring in chilblains and frostbite, and in claudication. It produces flushing of the face and neck with unpleasant itching, but has comparatively little effect on the blood vessels of the extremities. Nicotinamide has vitaminic but no vasodilator activity. Two derivatives of nicotinic acid have recently been introduced for the treatment of chilblains: these are *nicotinyl alcohol* and *inositol nicotinate*. (Inositol is another of the B vitamins, page 36.) They slowly release nicotinic acid as a result of metabolic conversions. Thus, it is claimed that they produce a more prolonged vasodilatation but the unpleasant flushing is avoided. The results of clinical trials with these drugs have been disappointing.

Ethyl alcohol has been used traditionally as a vasodilator; however, recent investigations indicate that its direct effect on blood vessels is to constrict them: the flushing of the face that is produced by alcoholic drinks and which gives rise to the feeling of warmth is due to reflex vasodilatation. Tobacco smoking has been traditionally contra-indicated in peripheral vascular disease on the grounds that it worsens or may even be the cause of the vascular spasm; the vasoconstrictor activity of nicotine has been implicated in this. However it has recently been demonstrated that intra-arterial injections of nicotine cause predominantly vasodilatation in normal subjects.

Anti-hypertensive drugs

Hypertension is briefly discussed on page 282. The relationship between blood pressure and age is shown in Fig. 10.3 (page 270). This graph gives the average values, but the blood pressure of healthy individuals in any one age group may extend over a wide range of values. Hypertension, a state of disease characterized by an abnormally high blood pressure, may be reckoned arbitarily to exist when the pressure exceeds 140 mm Hg systolic and 90 mm Hg diastolic. Since this is within the normal range for older subjects, the diagnosis of hypertension may then rest on the findings of abnormality of the urine or of the retinal blood vessels. The retinal vessels, which may be observed directly with the ophthalmoscope, reflect the state of blood vessels generally and observations of them are used to grade the severity of the disease: in grade I, the retinal arteries are narrower and more tortuous than normally; in grade II, the arteries, being under tension, partly occlude the veins by compression at crossings of these vessels; in grade III, there are points of haemorrhage or exudate formation; and in Grade IV, there is general oedema of the retina (*papilloedema*).

Hypertension may be classified on the basis of the cause of the disorder:

Essential hypertension. (Also known as *primary* or *idiopathic hypertension*.) This is the commonest type, accounting for more than 80% of cases of hypertension. In this there is over-activity of the sympathetic vasoconstrictor nerve-vascular smooth muscle complex. However, the exact site, the nature and the underlying cause of the defect is not known. There is some evidence indicating a defect in adrenergic neurones which results in abnormally small stores of noradrenaline; it appears that the storage mechanism, rather than the synthesis of noradrenaline, is defective. It is postulated that less of the noradrenaline released by nerve impulses is taken up again into the neuronal storage site, so that more noradrenaline is available to produce vasoconstriction (see pages 745–746). This may be one of the factors accounting for the increased vasoconstrictor response to injected noradrenaline observed in some vascular beds of hypertensive patients. The vasoconstrictor action of angiotensin has also been reported to be greater than normal in hypertensive patients. The concentration of sodium ions in the body fluids of patients with essential hypertension has been found to be abnormally high. Constriction of vascular smooth muscle itself increases the sodium concentration of the smooth muscle cells and this in turn enhances the vasoconstrictor action of pressor agents.

Secondary hypertension. These can be further subdivided according to the underlying cause: these include *renal hypertension* (page 276), *phaeochromocytoma* (page 166), and *aldosterone-producing tumour*.

Hypertensive attacks may also be caused by drugs, or occur as a result of interaction between one drug and another, or a drug and a dietary constituent.

The main causes of secondary hypertension, and the factors involved in both essential and secondary hypertension are shown in a schematic form in Fig. 32.9.

In normotensive animals and men, *acute* elevation of the blood pressure reflexly inhibits the discharge of impulses in the sympathetic vasoconstrictor nerves (page 275). However, in hypertensive patients the baroreceptors and the vasomotor centre adapt to the *chronic* abnormally high level of blood pressure, and the discharge of impulses in the sympathetic vasomotor nerves is normal. The carotid sinus reflexes are still operative, but they act to maintain the blood pressure at the hypertensive level. After a sustained anti-hypertensive effect, the vasomotor reflexes become reset at a lower level so that the pressure may become easier to control.

The relationship between blood pressure, cardiac output and total peripheral resistance may be expressed in the form, blood pressure = cardiac output × peripheral resistance (see page 269), and reduction either of cardiac output or of peripheral resistance (or of both) will therefore lower blood pressure. Essential hypertension is characterized by an increased total peripheral resistance coupled with a normal cardiac output. Ideally, the drugs used should selectively lower total peripheral resistance; that is, they should decrease blood pressure without affecting cardiac output, but in fact, most of the potent antihypertensive drugs (ganglion blocking drugs and adrenergic neurone blocking drugs) reduce cardiac output as well as peripheral resistance.

At one time, radical sympathetic ganglionectomy was undertaken surgically to arrest malignant hypertension. This was an extreme measure that was justified on the grounds that the rapid increase in symptoms in malignant hypertension caused an early death. The relief was only temporary, probably because the denervated blood vessels became supersensitive to circulating catecholamines (page 746). The development of drugs that interrupt sympathetic nerve

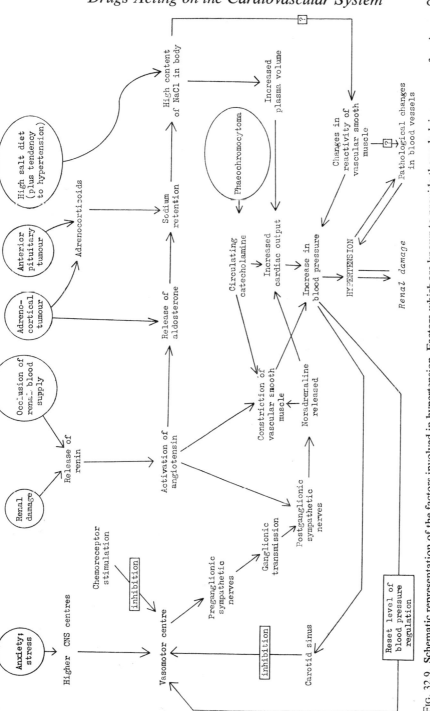

Fig. 32.9. **Schematic representation of the factors involved in hypertension.** Factors which are known to provide the underlying causes of various types of secondary hypertension are encircled. The various points at which drugs used in the treatment of hypertension may act are also included in the scheme.

pathways has rendered the surgical procedure obsolete. However, tolerance develops to many of these drugs; one reason for this is increased sensitivity to circulating catecholamines.

Blockade of peripheral sympathetic nerve function decreases the effectiveness of the vasoconstrictor and cardiac nerves, thereby lowering the blood pressure. The hypotension is slight in patients lying at rest but it is pronounced on changing to a sitting or standing position; such an effect is termed *orthostatic hypotension*. Circulatory adjustments to changes in posture, for example, a shift from a lying to a standing position, involve redistribution of the blood which is brought about by sympathetic nerve activity. Without this adjustment, there is pooling of blood in the lower parts of the body, and a marked fall in systemic blood pressure. This effect, which is termed *postural hypotension*, is a direct consequence of anti-hypertensive action produced by interference with sympathetic function. When it is excessive, it constitutes an unwanted effect and is objectionable to patients. Similarly, in exercise there is failure of the cardiac and the vascular components of circulatory adjustment, giving an excessive fall in pressure termed *exertional hypotension*. If the hypotension is severe, the venous return may be inadequate to maintain the cardiac output, and the decrease in the cerebral blood supply results in syncope (fainting). Impairment of sympathetic vasoconstrictor tone in the nasal mucosa leads to congestion and complaints of 'stuffy nose' which are common in patients on antihypertensive therapy.

There are many sites at which drugs may act to lower the blood pressure in hypertension. They may be roughly divided into three major categories, and further subdivided according to the particular action as shown below. (Question marks indicate that there is some doubt or controversy about the mechanism of action.)

1. Decreased sympathetic activity

    (*a*) DECREASED OUTPUT FROM VASOMOTOR CENTRE
     (i) *Direct depression* (Rauwolfia alkaloids (?), Hydrallazine (?))
    (ii) *Decreased drive from higher centres* (Sedatives, Monoamine oxidase inhibitors (?)
   (iii) *Reflex inhibition* (Veratrum alkaloids)

    (*b*) DECREASED GANGLIONIC TRANSMISSION
     (i) *Blockade of transmission* ('Antinicotinic' ganglion blocking drugs)
    (ii) *Increased inhibition by catecholamines* (Monoamine oxidase inhibitors (?))

(*c*) DECREASED RELEASE OF NORADRENALINE

(i) *Prevention of release* (Adrenergic neurone blocking drugs)

(ii) *Depletion of noradrenaline* (Rauwolfia alkaloids)

(iii) *Replacement of noradrenaline by weaker transmitter* (Methyldopa, Monoamine oxidase inhibitors (?))

(*d*) DECREASED ACTION OF CATECHOLAMINES

(i) *Blockade of vasoconstriction* (α-Receptor blocking drugs)

(ii) *Decreased reactivity of vascular smooth muscle* (Sodium-depleting diuretics (?))

(iii) *Blockade of cardiac stimulation* (β-Receptor blocking drugs)

2. Direct vasodilatation

Vasodilator drugs (Hydrallazine (?), Thiocyanate)

3. Reduction in blood volume

Diuretics (Thiazides, Aldosterone antagonists)

The drugs used to lower arterial blood pressure in a particular patient depend partly on the severity of the hypertension, as the maximum tolerable dose of some drugs is inadequate when the hypertension is severe. In many cases, a combination of drugs gives more effective control than a single drug, and the necessity for only relatively small doses of each drug then reduces side effects to a minimum. Restricted dietary sodium in conjunction with drug therapy is also commonly employed.

Maintained adequate control of the blood pressure of hypertensive patients significantly prolongs life, prevents the development of renal failure, congestive heart failure and retinal damage, and slows the progression of atherosclerosis in the cerebral and coronary arteries. Mild renal or retinal damage, if already developed, may be arrested or reversed.

Antihypertensive drugs acting wholly or partly on the central nervous system. *Sedatives*, particularly barbiturates (pages 588–592) lower blood pressure in many subjects with benign hypertension. *Phenobarbitone* was preferred for this use at one time, but now it has been largely supplanted by *amylobarbitone*.

Chlorpromazine (pages 595–598) has occasional use as an antihypertensive drug. Its tranquillizing action diminishes the excitation of the vasomotor centre that occurs in anxiety and in stressful situations; it also directly depresses the vasomotor centre. In addition to these central actions, chlorpromazine is a fairly powerful antagonist of sympathomimetic amines, it impairs the release of noradrenaline from adrenergic neurones and has slight ganglion blocking activity. The many side effects of chlorpromazine limit its usefulness in the treatment of essential hypertension, but it is the drug of choice in the treatment of hypertensive crises that may occur in patients under treatment with mono-amine oxidase inhibitors who are given sympathomimetic amines or who take in sympathomimetic amines in the diet (see pages 625–626, 750, 775).

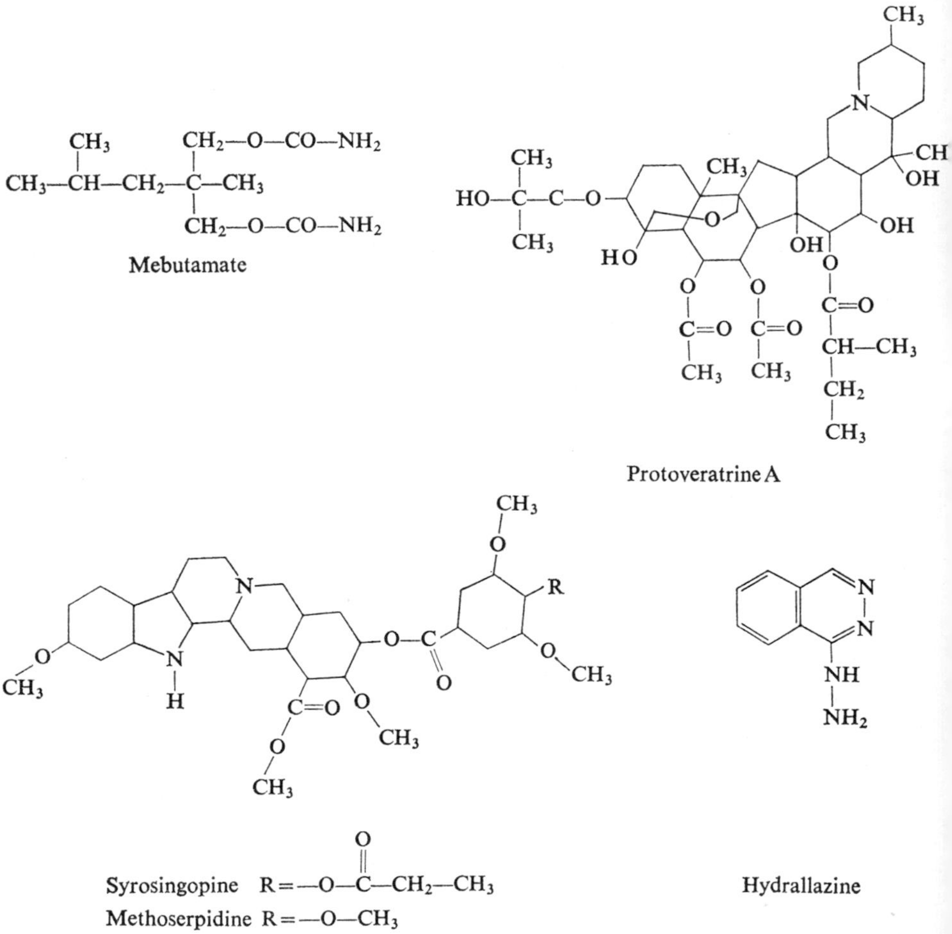

FIG. 32.10. Some antihypertensive drugs.

Mebutamate is a derivative of meprobamate (page 603). Its formula is given in Fig. 32.10. Mebutamate was developed as a centrally acting antihypertensive as a result of incidental observations of hypotension made on patients being treated with meprobamate. The actions of the two substances are closely similar, but mebutamate is reported to have fewer side effects. The hypotensive effect is due to depression of the vasomotor centre and also impairment of spinal sympathetic pathways.

Hydrallazine (also spelt hydralazine) produces a fall of blood pressure in which there is peripheral vasodilation accompanied by tachycardia of reflex origin. The vasodilatation is thought to arise partly from depression of the vasomotor centre and partly from direct vasodilatation. It has slight anti-adrenaline activity. It is claimed that hydrallazine increases renal blood flow, which confers an advantage in that renal function is well maintained. Hydrallazine has occasional use in moderately severe hypertension. The hypotensive effect is produced about 2 h after oral administration and persists for 6 to 8 h. The chemical structure of hydrallazine is shown in Fig. 32.10.

VERATRUM ALKALOIDS. These are alkaloids occurring in species of hellebore, particularly *Veratrum viride* and *V. album*. Pharmacopoeal preparations consist usually of more or less purified extracts. Various alkaloids have been isolated, the main ones being veratridine, protoveratrine A and B and germerine; they have complex structures, as illustrated for protoveratrine A in Fig. 32.10.

The hypotensive action of veratrum alkaloids is due to depression of the vasomotor centre by reflexes evoked by excitation of sensory nerve endings in the heart, its neighbouring blood vessels and the lung, and by excitation of the carotid sinus nerves (see Fig. 32.9). The sensory nerves that are stimulated in the thoracic region are contained in the vagus nerves and convey impulses from baroreceptors and chemoreceptors: the depressor reflexes evoked by their stimulation are discussed on page 274. The hypotensive action of veratrine is completely abolished by vagotomy; in order to abolish the action of protoveratrine, the carotid sinus nerves must be divided as well as the vagus nerves.

All excitable cell membranes are affected by the veratrum alkaloids but there are wide differences in the sensitivity of different tissues, the sensory receptors giving rise to the depressor reflex generally being the most sensitive. However, the use of these drugs is severely limited by the incidence of retching and vomiting.

The effect of veratrine on the action potential is mentioned on page 83. Veratrum alkaloids increase the negative after-potential and cause repetitive responses to single stimuli. The alkaloids have been shown to disrupt a monolayer of stearic acid by reacting with the carboxyl groups. This occurs with concentrations that affect cell membranes, and, like the action on the cell membrane, it is antagonized by excess calcium ions or by procaine. A similar disruption of the lipid layer of the cell membrane may explain the increased ion fluxes that are responsible for the repetitive activity in response to a single stimulus.

Antihypertensive drugs that impair peripheral sympathetic nerve function

GANGLION BLOCKING DRUGS. These are described on pages 690–695. They have been useful in the past in the control of severe hypertension but their numerous disadvantages have led to their being supplanted by guanethidine and other adrenergic neurone blocking drugs. A brief synopsis of their use in hypertension will suffice here. The quaternary compounds suffer from the disadvantage that they are poorly and erratically absorbed after oral administration, necessitating the inconvenience of frequent injections. The development of non-quaternary ganglion blocking drugs that are well absorbed constituted a considerable advance in antihypertensive therapy. However, all ganglion blocking drugs suffer from the disadvantages that they impair transmission in both sympathetic and parasympathetic ganglion. The major unwanted effects of these drugs are due to blockade of parasympathetic ganglia (pages 693–694). Ganglion blocking drugs such as *pentolinium, mecamylamine, pempidine* and *trimethaphan* (Fig. 27.2, page 691) find a limited use in some hypertensive emergencies when it is necessary to lower the blood pressure rapidly, and in malignant hypertension when the effect of other drugs may be too slow in onset. They are also used in combination with other drugs, in which case the incidence of unwanted effects is minimal.

ADRENERGIC NEURONE BLOCKING DRUGS. These are described on pages 768 to 773. *Bretylium* was the first of these drugs to be widely used for the treatment of hypertension, but it is rarely used now. The absorption of bretylium is erratic and tolerance to its effect develops rapidly. Bretylium commonly produces intense pain in the parotid glands which is sometimes precipitated by chewing. It is due to an excessive hyperaemia which is produced partly by stimulation of the gland and partly by blockade of the sympathetic vasoconstrictor nerves. Parotid pain occurs, but only rarely, with other adrenergic neurone blocking drugs.

The main adrenergic neurone blocking drugs currently used in antihypertensive therapy are *guanethidine* and *bethanidine*. These drugs, being guanidines rather than quaternary amines, are somewhat less highly ionized and are better absorbed than bretylium (see page 491). Bethanidine has a more rapid onset of action and a shorter duration of action than is the case with guanethidine. *Guanoclor*, a more recently introduced adrenergic neurone blocking drug has substantially the same actions as guanethidine; another, *guanoxan*, is reported to cause a high incidence of liver disorders.

The antihypertensive effect on the adrenergic neurone blocking drugs is due entirely to the impairment of release of noradrenaline from adrenergic nerve junctions with vascular smooth muscle, resulting in release of vasoconstrictor tone. They produce orthostatic hypotension. The main unwanted effects of these drugs are a direct consequence of this action. These are postural hypotension, particularly on first arising from bed, exertional hypotension, and an excessive hypotension in hot environments: in each case hypotension is due to failure of circulatory control by sympathetic readjustment of regional blood vessels. Loss of vasoconstrictor tone in the nasal mucosa leads to congestion and stuffiness. Impairment of the sympathetic cardiac nerves may lead to heart failure. Impairment of the sympathetic hypogastric nerve activity results in failure of ejaculation.

Attempts to correct an excessive hypotension produced by adrenergic neurone blocking drugs by injection of pressor catecholamines may be dangerous, since the catecholamines are markedly potentiated because of impairment of their uptake into the neuronal storage sites. For the same reason, the administration of adrenergic blocking drugs in patients with phaeochromocytoma is contra-indicated; they cause a further rise in blood pressure by potentiating the actions of the circulating catecholamines.

Adrenergic neurone blocking drugs may be displaced from their attachment to the adrenergic neurone by indirectly acting sympathomimetic amines (page 745), and this displacement terminates their neurone blocking action. This has important implications for antihypertensive therapy in that the concurrent administration of guanethidine (or related drugs) and drugs having indirect sympathomimetic actions (such as amphetamine) will completely nullify the antihypertensive effect. The administration of such mixtures of drugs is not uncommon, and may be responsible for many reports of failure to produce adequate hypotension. Reasons for unwittingly prescribing drugs that antagonize the action of guanethidine include the following. 1. Reduction of body weight improves the prognosis for hypertensives, but amphetamine and many other anorexigenic drugs (page 619) prevent the action of adrenergic neurone blocking drugs and their use is contra-indicated. 2. The common occurrence of nasal congestion has been mentioned previously; attempts to treat it symptomatically with the sympathomimetic amines mentioned in Table 29.2 (page 755) may also prevent the control of hypertension. 3. Hypertensive patients are frequently worried and anxious, but many antidepressant drugs, including amphetamine and its derivatives, ephedrine, and monoamine oxidase inhibitors prevent adrenergic neurone blockade. 4. Combinations of antihypertensive drugs are frequently useful; this applies to combinations of adrenergic neurone blocking drugs with ganglion blockers, hydrallazine, reserpine and diuretics, but *not* to combination with antihypertensive monoamine oxidase inhibitors.

RAUWOLFIA ALKALOIDS. The chemical structures and properties of the Rauwolfia alkaloids are described on pages 599–600 in connection with their use as tranquillizers. Their tranquillizing action may contribute to their anti-hypertensive effect, but it is mainly due to impairment of sympathetic nerve function. Reserpine, the principal Rauwolfia alkaloid, interferes with the binding of catecholamines in adrenergic neurones and chromaffin cells, and hence it causes depletion from storage sites (see pages 163, 600, 773–774). Complete depletion of catecholamines may be produced by reserpine in all tissues, but the doses and duration of treatment required for this vary widely from tissue to tissue. Noradrenaline levels in the heart are readily depleted by reserpine; after large doses of reserpine in experimental animals, depletion of cardiac noradrenaline is detectable within 1 h and is maximal after 24 h. Doses as small as 5 μg/kg will also cause maximal depletion if given daily for several days. Depletion of adrenaline from the adrenal medulla is slower and requires high doses of reserpine.

Impairment of transmission at adrenergic neuroeffector junctions by reserpine is the result of depletion of noradrenaline from the nerve endings. Transmission failure occurs when the noradrenaline content falls below about 80% of normal. Once depleted, the stores regain catecholamines very slowly so that repeated doses of reserpine have a cumulative effect even when given at intervals of a week or more.

The fall in blood pressure produced by reserpine is chiefly the result of transmission failure at adrenergic nerve endings but it is unlikely that this is the sole mechanism involved, since the antihypertensive effect is much longer lasting than the effect of surgical sympathectomy. Furthermore, intra-arterial injection of reserpine produces vasodilatation in both normal and sympathectomized limbs of man, and in some tissues responses to acetylcholine, 5-HT, vasopressin, barium and potassium are non-specifically depressed.

When catecholamine depletion is produced rapidly by large doses of reserpine, the responses of tissues to noradrenaline, including isolated blood vessels, are enhanced. This effect resembles the increased sensitivity after denervation and may be the result of a similar mechanism (pages 745–746). Reserpine may precipitate acute cardiac insufficiency if the heart is subjected to additional stress such as heavy exercise, hypoxia or anaesthesia.

The usual dose of reserpine when used as an antihypertensive in man is 0·25–0·5 mg per day by mouth. The hypertensive action of reserpine takes a considerable time to develop with the usual doses given in human patients. The effect can be accelerated by giving larger doses, and by administering it parenterally. However, the risk of precipitating the unwanted effects of marked depression of the CNS and gastro-intestinal disturbance is disproportionately increased. This limits the amount that can be given to lower the blood pressure and consequently reserpine is chiefly of value only in cases in which a small hypotensive effect is required.

Many of the side effects of reserpine are dealt with on page 600. The main side effects that are disadvantages in antihypertensive therapy are the following: (1) Nasal congestion, flushing and shivering (from the greater heat loss incurred with peripheral vasodilation): these are all a direct consequence of the hypotensive action. (2) Stimulation of appetite and gain in weight: overweight and obesity tend to exaggerate hypertensive conditions. (3) Retention of fluid: the adverse effect of this in hypertension is illustrated in Fig. 32.9. Combination of reserpine with diuretic drugs corrects the fault, and gives improved control of hypertension.

The powdered root and alkaloidal extracts of *Rauwolfia serpentina* are sometimes used in place of reserpine in the treatment of hypertension. Their actions are qualitatively similar to that of reserpine and most of the activity is probably due to this alkaloid. *Deserpidine* and *rescinnamine*, which are also alkaloids from Rauwolfia (page 599), possess similar actions to reserpine but are less powerful. *Syrosingopine* and *methoserpidine* (see Fig. 32.10) deplete peripheral tissues of catecholamines but are relatively inactive in depleting the catecholamine stores in the central nervous system. They possess antihypertensive action but very little sedative action. Both are less active antihypertensive drugs than is reserpine.

METHYLDOPA. The chemical name of this substance is α-methyl-3,4-dihydroxy-L-phenylalanine: it is a synthetic analogue of the amino acid, dopa, which is an intermediary in the biosynthesis of the catecholamines as shown in Fig. 5.8 (page 160).

Methyldopa is effective in the treatment of most cases of hypertension. The original reason for using methyldopa was based on the observation that it competitively inhibits dopa decarboxylase *in vitro*, thereby preventing the conversion of dopa to dopamine. It was thought that this would lead to decreased production of noradrenaline, hence transmission failure in adrenergic nerves, decrease of sympathetic vasoconstriction, and relief of hypertension. However, a number of observations indicate that the mechanism of its hypertensive action is more complicated. Thus methyldopa produces a prolonged depression in the levels of noradrenaline despite the fact that decarboxylase inhibition is relatively transient and dopamine levels quickly return to normal. Furthermore, the antihypertensive effect is not enhanced when additional inhibition of decarboxylase enzymes is produced by another inhibitor, methyldopa hydrazine.

Methyldopa is a substrate for dopa decarboxylase, although it is metabolized slowly compared with dopa. The product of decarboxylation is α-methyldopamine, which is in turn metabolized to α-methylnoradrenaline. These reactions are summarized in Fig. 32.11. The presence of the α-methyl

27*

group renders the amines immune from attack by monoamine oxidase, hence they tend to accumulate in the adrenergic neurone where they are formed. They compete with dopamine and noradrenaline for the storage sites in adrenergic neurones, until finally there is almost complete loss of noradrenaline, its place being taken by α-methylnoradrenaline. This substance is released by nerve impulses, just as noradrenaline is, and acts on the effector cells. Thus it serves as a false transmitter. However, its action on the receptor is less than that of noradrenaline (see page 744), consequently the effectiveness of sympathetic stimulation is impaired.

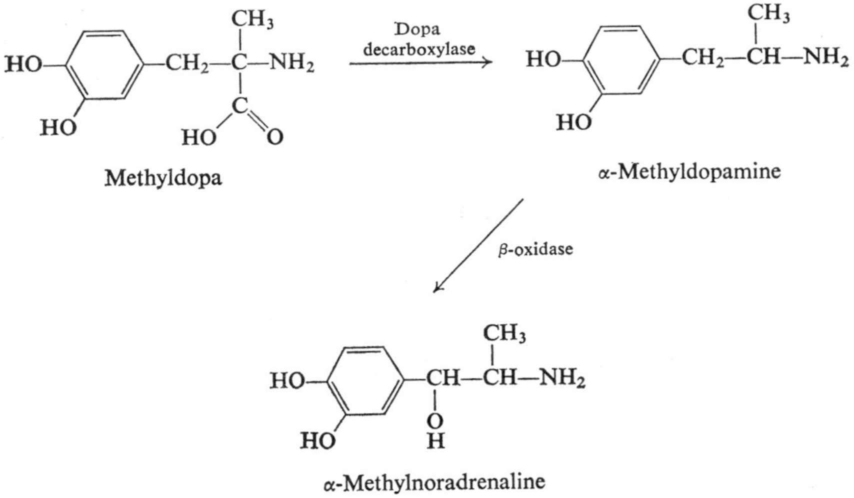

FIG. 32.11. Metabolic conversion of methyldopa to the false transmitter, α-methylnoradrenaline.

The antihypertensive effect of methyldopa is slow in onset, the full effect requires some days of treatment. The hypotensive effect of methyldopa is considerably greater in hypertensive than in normotensive subjects, but it is not pronounced, and is usually insufficient for control of acute and malignant hypertension. Methyldopa lowers the blood pressure in the supine as well as the standing position; as may be expected from this finding, postural hypotension is not troublesome. The reason for the retention of sufficient sympathetic function to achieve circulatory adjustment is that a maximal discharge of sympathetic impulses may release enough of the false transmitter to produce the full response of the vascular smooth muscle.

Methyldopa may produce drowsiness and sedation, but these effects usually disappear with continued treatment and may be replaced by mild euphoria. The actions of methyldopa on the CNS may be due to the formation of α-methylnoradrenaline which at first displaces, then replaces noradrenaline.

A gain in weight and retention of fluid may occur in patients on methyldopa, therefore it is commonly supplemented with diuretics.

Haemolytic anaemia may occasionally occur as a side effect during treatment with α-methyldopa. The haemolysis is due to the production of an auto-immune antibody to the patients own red cells. Prednisone (page 857) corrects the anaemia by suppressing antibody formation.

MONOAMINE OXIDASE INHIBITORS. The use of monamine oxidase inhibitors as antidepressive agents is described on pages 623–626. Several of them were observed to produce a hypotensive effect and one of the non-hydrazine inhibitors, *pargyline,* has some use in antihypertensive therapy. The antihypertensive effect commences several days after the beginning of treatment and persists for several weeks after it is discontinued. The fall in blood pressure is intermediate in extent between that produced by methyldopa and that produced by guanethidine. There is an orthostatic hypotension, suggesting that sympathetic function is impaired, but the mechanism of the antihypertensive effect is obscure. Two explanations have been proposed; they are (i) that ganglionic transmission is impaired, and (ii) that false transmitters are released. (i) Ganglionic transmission is inhibited by catecholamines (pages 700–701). Monoamine oxidase inhibitors increase the content and availability of catecholamines in tissues. Noradrenaline is present in ganglia and may act physiologically to modulate transmission. An increase in this effect, resulting from increased release of noradrenaline, would tend to inhibit ganglionic transmission. (ii) There are a number of alternative pathways in the biosynthesis of catecholamines in which various amines are formed that are less potent than noradrenaline on the effector cells; such amines include octopamine and synephrine (Fig. 5.9, page 162). These amines, and dopamine, all compete with noradrenaline for the storage site in adrenergic neurones. The role of monoamine oxidase in the neurone may be to limit the extent to which these amines accumulate, and inhibition of monoamine oxidase allows their accumulation. The nerve impulse then liberates a mixture of amines, including some that are less potent than noradrenaline, these amines serving as false transmitters. The resultant is that sympathetic impulses are less effective in maintaining vasoconstriction, the net effect being vasodilatation.

The side effects of treatment with monoamine oxidase inhibitors have been described elsewhere (pages 623–626).

ANTI-ADRENALINE DRUGS. The anti-adrenaline drugs are described in pages 757–768. The α-receptor blocking drugs are of no value in essential hypertension although they may be of use in the secondary hypertension due to phaeochromocytoma. They are also of use in treating hypertensive crises produced by sympathomimetic amines. They do not affect the cardiac responses to catecholamines, therefore there may be an excessive tachycardia which can be relieved by blockade of β-receptors with propranolol.

It has been shown clinically that propranolol reduces the blood pressure in essential hypertension. It is thought that the effect is due to a reduction in cardiac output resulting from blockade of cardiac sympathetic nerves. Peripheral resistance is actually higher, and this constitutes a theoretical disadvantage to its use.

Vasodilator drugs in hypertension. The possibility of using drugs that lower blood pressure by a direct vasodilator action has not been realized in practice. As mentioned above, hydrallazine may have a component of direct vasodilator activity, but this drug is not widely used.

Before the introduction of the ganglion blocking drugs, one of the few drugs available for treating hypertension was *thiocyanate* (as the sodium or potassium salt). The antihypertensive effect of thiocyanate is attributed to dilatation of small blood vessels owing to a direct relaxant action on vascular smooth muscle resembling that of the nitrites. There is a narrow margin between the plasma concentration necessary for an effective action (8 mg %) and that causing severe toxic effects (14 mg %). The toxic effects resemble those occurring in brominism and iodism; these are skin eruptions, symptoms resembling the common cold, thyroid dysfunction, and disturbance of the CNS.

A direct vasodilator action is probably responsible for the antihypertensive effect of *Hydergine* (page 760), but in addition, diminution of vasoconstriction by blockade of α-receptors may contribute. The drug may be given orally, or by injection if a rapid effect is desired in a hypertensive crisis.

Use of diuretic drugs in the treatment of hypertension. The value of reducing the circulatory blood volume in hypertension can be judged from the scheme presented in Fig. 32.9.

Mercurial diuretics (page 875) produce a small but significant lowering of blood pressure in hypertensive subjects. Diuretics that act by inhibition of carbonic anhydrase (page 879) and the xanthine diuretics (page 873) also have only slight antihypertensive activity. However, the thiazide diuretics (page 881) have good antihypertensive activity and potentiate the actions of other antihypertensive drugs. They act by decreasing the reabsorption of sodium from the renal tubules, thereby increasing the elimination of sodium. Recent clinical trials with diuretics that antagonize the sodium retaining action of aldosterone, such as spironolactone (page 885), indicate that they too are useful in antihypertensive therapy. Therefore two factors appear to be involved, one is the reduction in body fluids, the other is reduction in the sodium content of the tissues. The beneficial effect of restriction of intake of dietary salt (sodium chloride) in hypertensives also suggests that reduction of tissue sodium may assist in controlling hypertension. Although hypertension is aggravated by salt, the ingestion of salt, even in large amounts is not itself sufficient to cause hypertension. Restriction of dietary salt allays the progress of hypertension in experimental animals and in patients. A rice diet is especially effective on account of its low sodium content.

Drugs used in hypotensive states and in shock

The nature of shock and circulatory collapse is described briefly on page 281. There are three primary factors which may result in an impairment of the circulation that culminates in circulatory collapse. (1) *Peripheral vasodilatation.* This may be caused by reduced activity of the vasomotor centre, vasodilator toxins or drugs. (2) *Decreased cardiac output.* This may be caused by myocardial damage, pulmonary embolism or excessive acidosis. (3) *Decreased circulating fluid volume.* This may be caused by loss of blood, by haemorrhage, or loss of plasma through damaged or excessively permeable capillary walls.

The impairment of the circulation then brings into play a number of secondary factors which react upon each other and lead to a further deterioration of the circulation. The tissues become anoxic, having insufficient blood flowing through them, and the capillary permeability increases, which results in increased formation of tissue fluid and a decreased circulating volume. Anoxia of the tissues and the poor circulation through the lungs produce acidosis, which impairs the action of the heart. The pooling of blood in the dilated capillaries together with the loss of fluid into the tissues results in a reduction in venous return and a decreased cardiac output. The fall in blood pressure results in inadequate coronary perfusion, and eventually to heart failure. The impairment of renal blood flow results in anuria and accumulation of toxic metabolites, and in hyperkalaemia, which depresses the myocardium. When the state of shock is fully established, the progressive deterioration of the circulation leads to cardiac arrest and death.

Profound hypotension is the striking feature of shock, and because of this vasoconstrictor drugs are used to elevate the blood pressure. However, it is now recognized that the hypotension may exist despite a maximal sympathetic vasoconstrictor drive, which constitutes the homeostatic reflex response to a fall in blood pressure. It follows that the prevailing hypotensive state in shock represents the inadequacy of the homeostatic mechanisms to maintain blood pressure. In fact, a further vasoconstriction produced by drugs may worsen the peripheral ischaemia, and tighten the vicious cycle of the interlocking secondary factors. This consideration led to the trial in shock of vasodilator drugs and of drugs which prevent sympathetic vasoconstriction. Encouraging results have been obtained.

Pressor drugs. Sympathomimetic amines that are used to raise the blood pressure in hypotensive states are listed in Table 29.2 (page 755). Their use is based on the following general considerations: (i) They constrict the peripheral blood vessels, which forces blood back into circulation. (ii) Their vasoconstrictor action is most marked in the splanchnic and skin vessels, and blood mobilized from these regions is then available for the perfusion of more essential organs. (iii) They cause an increase in blood pressure which provides for better perfusion of coronary and renal vessels. (iv) They constrict the veins which forces more blood into the heart and increases cardiac output. (v) They stimulate the heart, which further increases cardiac output. Special considerations apply to particular drugs. *Adrenaline* exerts a pressor action mainly by increasing the cardiac output; however it is liable to cause arrhythmias. *Noradrenaline* produces marked peripheral vasoconstriction and has a relatively weak action on the heart, so that the rise in blood pressure it produces is accompanied by reflex bradycardia. The effects of adrenaline and noradrenaline are ephemeral, and they must be given by continuous intravenous infusion. If these drugs are inadvertently injected into the tissues, the local vasoconstriction and ischaemia may be severe enough to produce necrosis. The main disadvantage of the catecholamines is that tachyphylaxis develops to their pressor action and the concentration infused must be continually increased in order to maintain the blood pressure. When the infusion is stopped, the blood pressure may collapse rapidly. Sympathomimetic amines with an α-methyl group are less rapidly destroyed and may be given in single intravenous injections, or intramuscularly. The indirectly acting sympathomimetic amines suffer from the disadvantage that tachyphylaxis develops to them (see page 774). *Metaraminol* (page 747) and *methoxamine* (page 749) are the sympathomimetic amines most commonly used for the treatment of hypotension. Metaraminol is the least liable to produce tachyphylaxis. Methoxamine does not stimulate the heart.

Angiotensin. This vasoconstrictor polypeptide (page 182) was first used clinically to replace sympathomimetic amines as a pressor agent in hypotensive states because it has no stimulant effect on the heart. In fact, the rise in blood pressure produced by angiotensin causes reflex bradycardia and a decrease in cardiac output. There is little indication for counteracting hypotension or shock with a combination of peripheral vasoconstriction and decreased cardiac output, and the main place of angiotensin is the maintenance of vasoconstriction tone when tachyphylaxis has developed after prolonged infusion of noradrenaline. Tachyphylaxis also develops with angiotensin.

Drugs which block sympathetic vasoconstriction and vasodilator drugs. The rationale for the use of these drugs in shock depends on the following considerations: (i) The arterioles that are thrown into constriction by sympathetic impulses are relaxed. (ii) The perfusion of the ischaemic tissue is improved. (iii) Relaxation of precapillary sphincters tends to divert blood from the arterio-venous anastomoses into the capillary beds. (iv) The blood that has been trapped in the capillaries is brought back into the circulation. (v) The decrease in peripheral resistance lessens the work load of the heart.

The vasodilatation increases the capacity of the vascular bed, and the circulating fluid volume must be increased by intravenous administration of blood or fluids in order to maintain an adequate venous return to the heart.

The following drugs have been used successfully in the treatment of shock.

Phenoxybenzamine. This drug blocks α-adrenoreceptors; its actions are described on pages 761–763. The blockade of the effects of noradrenaline released from sympathetic vasoconstrictor nerves results in a decrease in peripheral vascular resistance in shock, particularly in the splanchnic viscera. Phenoxybenzamine does not block the effects of sympathetic impulses on the heart, consequently cardiac output is not impaired and may even increase. Additional actions of phenoxybenzamine which may contribute to its beneficial effects in shock are antagonism of the actions of histamine and of 5-hydroxytryptamine.

Chlorpromazine. The vasodilator actions of chlorpromazine are due to depression of the vasomotor centre, impairment of sympathetic nerve activity and blockade of noradrenaline. In addition it is a powerful antagonist of histamine and 5-hydroxytryptamine.

Ganglion blocking and adrenergic neurone blocking drugs have only recently been used in shock, apparently with promising results.

Isoprenaline. This drug increases the cardiac output by a direct effect on the heart and decreases the peripheral resistance (page 739). The sympathetically induced vasoconstriction is antagonized physiologically by isoprenaline (see page 467); that is, isoprenaline exerts the contrary effect of vasodilatation by an action on the β-adrenoreceptors of vascular smooth muscle. Although isoprenaline has a depressor effect on the normal cardiovascular system, in shock its actions result in a rise of blood pressure. The renal blood flow is increased and pulmonary vascular resistance is decreased by isoprenaline.

Hydrallazine and other vasodilator drugs have also been used in the treatment of shock.

The use of analgesic drugs in shock. Pain, which may be present in many types of shock, tends to intensify the condition. Morphine and other powerful analgesics are therefore useful adjuncts to the treatment of shock, but large doses may increase the circulatory collapse.

Treatment of particular types of shock

ANAPHYLACTIC SHOCK. Hypotension is due primarily to peripheral vaso-dilatation which is mediated by the release of a number of pharmacologically active substances from the tissues; these include histamine, bradykinin and 5-hydroxytryptamine. The capillary permeability is increased, and the excessive formation of tissue fluid may result in a considerable reduction of circulating volume. Sympathomimetic amines, particularly adrenaline, are mainly used in the treatment of anaphylactic shock.

HYPOTENSION DUE TO VASOVAGAL SYNDROME. In certain individuals, various stimuli may precipitate vasovagal attacks in which there is bradycardia and vasodilatation, syncope usually occurs. The hypotension is orthostatic, and the fainting attack usually limits the condition. Otherwise, sympathomimetic pressor amines are indicated.

HYPOTENSION IN SPINAL ANAESTHESIA. A profound hypotension may occur as a result of blockade of sympathetic pathways in the spinal cord. The blood pressure may be maintained with sympathomimetic amines.

HYPOTENSION DUE TO DRUGS. Overdoses of barbiturates, morphine and its congeners, chlorpromazine, nitrites and organic nitrates, and organic arseni-cals (the 'nitroid' crisis) may give rise to an excessive fall in blood pressure. Symptomatic treatment may be adequately achieved with sympathomimetic pressor amines.

TRAUMATIC SHOCK OR WOUND SHOCK. The following primary factors are involved: (i) Loss of blood volume by haemorrhage. (ii) Release of vasodilator substances from the damaged tissues. (iii) Pain. Provided prompt measures are taken to remedy these, the development of the secondary factors is prevented. The measures are (i) giving blood or plasma transfusions or other intravenous fluids, (ii) excluding the damaged region from the general circulation (as far as possible), and (iii) alleviating pain with analgesic drugs. When the secondary factors come into play, the use of vasodilator drugs is indicated.

BURN SHOCK. The main factor involved is loss of fluid from the blood vessels that are damaged by the burn; administration of intravenous fluids makes this good. Pain and the release of vasodilator substances from the damaged tissue may contribute to the shock.

SURGICAL SHOCK. In prolonged surgery, in which the blood pressure is purposely kept at a low level to reduce bleeding, there is a risk that the second-ary factors responsible for shock may set in. Manipulation of abdominal viscera may result in the release of vasodilator substances. Reflex stimulation may also result in vasodilation and vagal slowing of the heart. Obstruction of the venous return during surgery may impair the cardiac output. Pain, as an aftermath of surgery, contributes to the development of shock. Adrenaline and other sympathomimetic pressor amines were once commonly used to treat surgical shock. Metaraminol is the one which gives the least tachyphylaxis. Methox-amine puts least strain on the heart. The incidence of surgical shock is diminish-ing as surgical techniques have improved.

HYPOTENSION AFTER REMOVAL OF PHAEOCHROMOCYTOMA. In patients with phaeochromocytoma, the blood pressure is maintained by the circulating catecholamines, sympathetic vasoconstrictor activity being reflexly depressed. Probably the vasomotor centre is adapted to these conditions. Removal of the tumour is sometimes followed by excessive hypotension, but the blood pressure may be maintained at an adequate level with noradrenaline infusions until vasomotor activity re-adapts.

SHOCK PRODUCED BY BACTERIAL ENDOTOXINS. The endotoxins elabora-ted by many Gram-negative organisms produce dilatation of peripheral vessels and constriction of pulmonary vessels. These effects are probably mediated by histamine, 5-hydroxytryptamine and vasoactive kinins liberated by the toxins from blood and tissues. Drugs with glucocorticoid or mineralocorticoid activity (page 378) are of benefit; their action is probably due to the prevention of release of vasodilator substances from the tissues. The secondary factor of sympathetic vasoconstriction increases the peripheral pooling of blood in endotoxin shock. Blockade of this vasoconstriction improves recovery.

PANCREATITIS. In this condition, the blood pressure may fall to a critically low level and there is much pain. Trypsin from the pancreas activates plasma precursors to produce the kinins bradykinin and kallidin (pages 181–182); these may be responsible for the pain (page 183) and vasodilatation. The forma-tion of the kinins may be prevented by a substance known as *Trasylol*. This is a protein which was first obtained from the lungs, and then found to occur in ox parotid glands which is the present commercial source. Trasylol is an inhibitor of trypsin and trypsin-like enzymes (including plasmin or thrombokinase, kallikrein and pepsin). Trasylol differs from other trypsin inhibitors in that it is not antigenic, and can therefore be used without risk of producing sensitization. Trasylol, in large doses, is reported to have beneficial effects in pancreatitis, and it may be of prophylactic value in preventing shock that sometimes occurs after surgery involving the pancreas.

MYOCARDIAL INFARCTION. The sudden occlusion of a coronary vessel by a thrombus may occur in arteriosclerotic disease, an atheroma serving as a site for the initiation of clotting. Occlusion of a large vessel is immediately fatal. However, if the region of the ischaemic area, or infarct, is not too large, the remainder of the myocardium continues to work. However, there may be considerable hypotension which is due primarily to a decrease in cardiac output; this hypotension rapidly progresses into shock. There may be severe anginal pain, which contributed to the shock; it is treated with powerful analgesics, such as morphine. Failure of the functional portion of the myocardium is treated with digitalis (pages 806–807). Anti-anginal drugs may be given to decrease the work load on the heart (pages 820–825). Pressor drugs have been used to correct excessive hypotension; the rationale for their use is that an increased blood pressure allows a greater perfusion of the remaining coronary vessels. However, this must be balanced against the increase in cardiac work. Methoxamine offers the advantage that it increases the blood pressure without having a sympathomimetic stimulant action on the heart.

PULMONARY EMBOLISM. The hypotensive state is due to decreased output. Pressor amines are used to improve the coronary perfusion, particularly of the vessels in the overworked right ventricle.

PERICARDIAL TAMPONADE. The accumulation of fluid in the pericardium decreases the diastolic filling of the heart, the pericardium being an indistensible structure composed of fibrous connective tissue; hence there is a decrease in stroke volume, and the fall in cardiac output may lead to hypotension. The fluid may be blood from haemorrhage or plasma exudate. The condition is corrected by draining the fluid, but meanwhile, sympathomimetic amines may be of value since they decrease the end diastolic volume, thereby increasing the stroke volume.

CHAPTER 33

Drugs Acting on the Endocrine System

Substances considered in this chapter may be divided conveniently into three principal categories: (1) Those used in substitution or replacement therapy when endogenous secretion fails or after surgical removal of an endocrine gland, examples being the use of thyroxine in myxoedema or of hydrocortisone after bilateral adrenalectomy. (2) Those used in suppressive therapy when an endocrine organ is producing an excess of its natural product or when normal hormonal secretion may be having adverse effects, examples being the use of propylthiouracil in the treatment of hyperthyroidism or of stilboestrol in cases of androgen-dependent prostatic tumour. (3) Stimulant substances which enhance the secretion of individual endocrine glands, an example being the use of tolbutamide in non-insulin-dependent diabetes mellitus. In addition, there are many conditions in which endocrine drugs are useful although the rationale is not obvious, examples being the use of ACTH and cortisone in rheumatoid arthritis and of topical hydrocortisone in many dermatoses.

There are many disadvantages in the use of the natural hormone in therapeutics. Most hormones have to be extracted from animal tissues which contain low concentrations or they are obtained by synthesis, and both procedures are usually extremely expensive. Naturally occurring hormones also tend to possess a range of activities, and only one activity often appears to be required in the treatment of individual conditions. Furthermore, many hormones are inactive orally, and so have to be injected. Considerable effort has therefore been devoted to the production of specific, potent, synthetic hormonal substitutes, many of which are orally effective.

Anti-thyroid drugs

Excessive production of the thyroid hormones may be countered either by surgical removal of part of the thyroid gland, or by treatment with drugs which inhibit synthesis, or by local irradiation of the gland. Even in cases where surgery is indicated, it is often desirable to use anti-thyroid agents beforehand. Iodide is selectively concentrated by the thyroid gland where subsequent synthesis of the iodine-containing thyroid hormones takes place. The hormones are stored in the colloid of the acinus, and all processes, from the uptake of iodide to the release of thyroxine, are under control of pituitary thyrotrophin. In turn, the output of thyrotrophin is regulated, at least in part, by the blood level of thyroid hormones.

851

The development of hypothyroidism after periods of low iodine intake is well understood. However, the paradox of the successful treatment of hyperthyroidism with excessive amounts of iodide has not yet been satisfactorily explained. In the hyperactive thyroid gland, iodide promotes involution of the hypertrophied glandular tissue with an increase in the storage of colloid. The response is often dramatic and may be obvious within 24 h of administration; the maximum effect is obtained in 10 to 15 days, after which time the condition may relapse. The large amounts of iodide have no effect upon the peripheral actions of the thyroid hormones nor do they permanently depress hormonal synthesis. It is attractive to speculate that excess iodide in some way inhibits the production of TSH in the pituitary but as yet there is no conclusive proof of this hypothesis. One difficulty is that the pituitary is unresponsive to changes in iodide level in euthyroid subjects.

The discovery of the goitrogen class of anti-thyroid agents dates from 1928 when it was found that rabbits fed on a cabbage diet developed hyperplastic thyroid glands. It was shown later that patients treated for hypertension with *thiocyanates* also developed goitre. Further work established that other anions such as *perchlorate* and *nitrate* also decrease thyroid hormone synthesis. The active goitrogen in cabbage plants was then found to be a derivative of thiourea and intensive study of structure–activity relationships in drugs of this type has led to the development of modern anti-thyroid agents.

Both the anions and the thio-ureas produce goitre as a result of the release of excess TSH following block of thyroxine synthesis. Their mode of action differs, however, for whereas the action of perchlorate is antagonized by increased iodide, that of thio-urea is not. The anions interfere with the ability of the thyroid to maintain the iodide concentration gradient, but the thio-ureas prevent the organic combination of iodide within the thyroid cell.

Thio-urea itself is too toxic for clinical use, but many compounds containing a thioureylene radical have been tried including sulphur-substituted uracils and imidazoles (Fig. 33.1). Some sulphonamides (for example, sulphaguanidine) also exhibit anti-thyroid activity. Clinically-used compounds are *methyl-* and *propyl-thiouracil, methimazole* and *carbimazole*. Carbimazole is converted to methimazole in the body. As with thyroid hormones, the anti-thyroid drugs are all orally active. The major hazard of prolonged therapy is the risk of blood dyscrasias.

In cases of exophthalmic goitre, there are difficulties in performing surgery because the elevated basal metabolic rate incurs an increased risk of anaesthetic accidents, the heart has a tendency to arrhythmia and the highly vascular, hypertrophied thyroid tissue is prone to excessive bleeding. It is standard practice to correct the hyperthyroidism prior to operation by treatment with carbimazole for 4 to 6 weeks, adding iodide in the last 10 days. The two

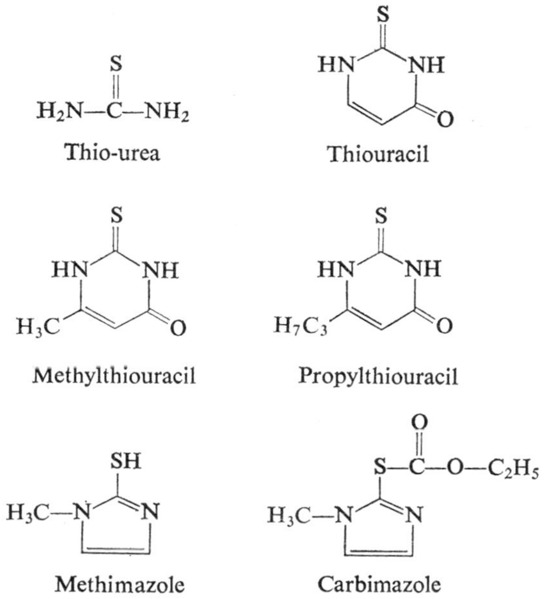

Fig. 33.1. Structural formulae of some anti-thyroid drugs.

agents together inhibit thyroxine synthesis and reduce thyroid size and vascularity.

Radioactive iodine, ^{131}I, has been used recently with great success in thyroid clinics. Diagnostically, its γ-ray emission may be used to determine the ability of the thyroid to take up and store iodine. Therapeutically, larger amounts are given so that highly localized emission of its β-rays destroys the overactive thyroid tissue.

Hypoglycaemic agents

There is no substitute for *insulin*. Many compounds share its ability to lower the blood sugar level but none possess the full range of its actions. Furthermore, hyperglycaemia is a symptom of a disease, not a disease in itself, and reduction of blood sugar levels *per se* only affords symptomatic relief.

Insulin is inactive orally and has to be injected. Since it is only short-acting, it has to be given frequently, and various insulin preparations have been devised to prolong the effectiveness of a single injection. Initially, insulin–protein complexes were used, but under controlled precipitating conditions it is now possible to prepare insulin-zinc complexes which have varying durations of action. These range from 12 to 40 h.

In cases of insulin-dependent diabetes where there is an absence of β-cell pancreatic function, insulin is the only effective form of treatment. However, in non-insulin-dependent diabetes where there is still some functional pancreatic β-cell tissue, it may be possible to control the patient without the use of exogenous insulin.

The hypoglycaemic activity of some sulphonamide derivatives was first noted by Loubatieres in 1942. The compounds he studied were thiodiazole sulphonamides of the type illustrated by RP 2254 in Fig. 33.2. No immediate clinical use was made of this discovery, partly because of the high toxicity of the compounds. In 1955, *carbutamide* (BZ 55), a straight chain, substituted sulphonylurea, was shown to be clinically useful in the control of some diabetics. Subsequently, *tolbutamide, chlorpropamide, metahexamide* and *acetohexamide* have displaced carbutamide in the clinic because they have fewer side-effects.

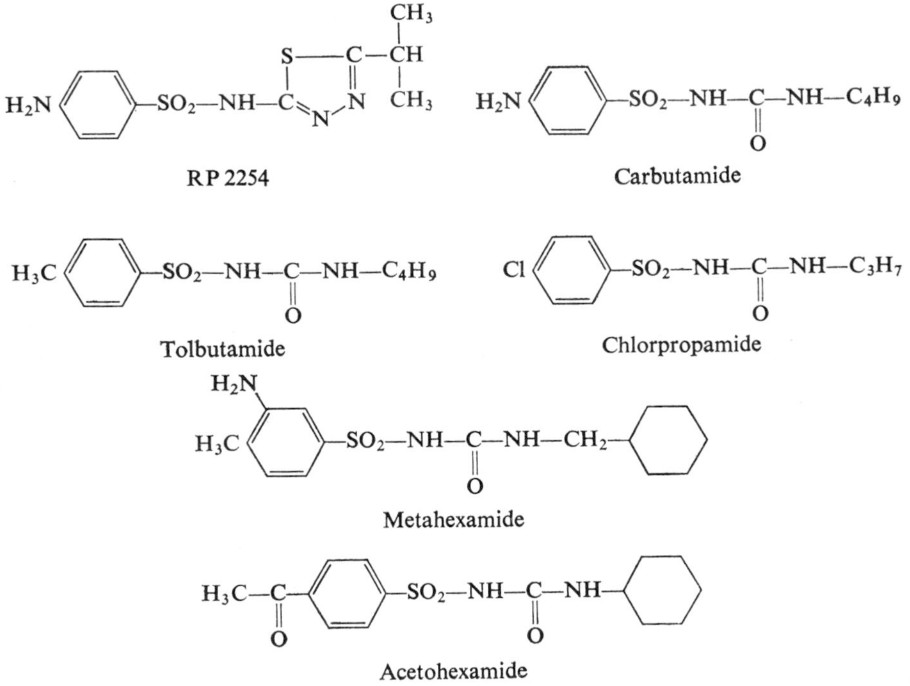

Fig. 33.2. Structural formulae of some hypoglycaemic sulphonamides.

The pancreas plays a vital role in the mechanism of the hypoglycaemic action of all these substances and the sulphonylureas are uniformly inactive after total removal of the pancreas, However, hypoglycaemia may still be produced in an experimental animal when only 10% of its pancreas remains. It is believed that these substances act by stimulation of insulin secretion by the pancreas.

Thus, in experimental alloxan diabetes, the severity of diabetes is inversely related to the hypoglycaemic response to the sulphonylureas.

The hypoglycaemic sulphonylureas produce extensive degranulation of the pancreatic β-cells as shown by electron microscopy; the changes are associated with an active secretory process. Similar changes may be seen in response to naturally induced insulin secretion after large doses of glucose. The prolonged administration of tolbutamide leads to hyperplasia of the islets of Langerhans and the formation of new β-cells. The sulphonylureas reduce the hepatic output of glucose but this is probably a secondary effect of insulin release. Other proposed mechanisms of hypoglycaemic action include an inhibition of insulinase and the displacement of insulin from a protein-binding site where it is held in an inactive form.

The side-effects of the oral hypoglycaemic sulphonylureas are principally agranulocytosis and skin rashes. Severe liver damage is rare and there is little danger of hypoglycaemic coma (possibly because of adrenaline release after higher doses). Tolbutamide is probably the safest agent but its duration of action is relatively short (6 to 8 h); it is metabolized to the inactive *p*-carboxylic acid. Tolbutamide has been used intravenously as a diagnostic aid in diabetes. When there is no fall in blood sugar level within 15 min, the patient is unlikely to respond to oral therapy and requires insulin. Chlorpropamide is not metabolized and is excreted unchanged; this accounts for its longer duration of action (16 to 20 h).

Another chemical class of orally active hypoglycaemic agents is the biguanides. As early as 1918, the hypoglycaemic activity of guanidine was discovered and in 1926 several naturally occurring guanidine derivatives (synthalins) were tried clinically. They fell into disrepute as they had toxic side-effects but only recently interest has been revived with the introduction of *phenformin* (phenethylbiguanide). This compound is hypoglycaemic in the absence of functional islet cells. It does not affect the actions of insulin but inhibits cellular respiration whilst stimulating anaerobic glycolysis; how these findings relate to hypoglycaemia is unknown. Phenformin is of limited clinical use.

Phenformin

Adrenocortical hormones

The adrenal cortex secretes a variety of steroid hormones of which the most important are hydrocortisone, corticosterone and aldosterone; they play a vital role in the regulation of carbohydrate and electrolyte metabolism. More than thirty steroids have been obtained from the adrenal cortex but only seven possess the ability to maintain life in adrenalectomized animals. The most potent life-maintaining steroid is aldosterone.

The first attempts at replacement therapy in cases of adrenocortical insufficiency were made in 1930 with extracts of adrenal tissue. The first synthetic corticosteroid, 11-*deoxycorticosterone*, became available in 1937 and this provided a major advance in substitution therapy, although it was only active parenterally. It was another 10 years before the synthesis of *cortisone* became possible on the commercial scale. This major success was followed by the synthesis of *hydrocortisone* in 1950 and the elucidation of the structure of aldosterone in 1954, followed by its synthesis in 1957.

Apart from their use in adrenocortical failure, cortisone and hydrocortisone were found to have dramatic effects in ameliorating the symptoms of rheumatoid arthritis and rheumatic fever. This discovery revolutionized medical thought in relation to organic disease of many types. When given in amounts in excess of normal requirements, hydrocortisone suppresses the inflammatory reaction, both to known and unknown toxins, and it also suppresses allergic reactions such as asthma. In addition, hydrocortisone reduces the formation of antibodies and causes a shrinkage of lymphatic tissue. Finally, by inhibiting the release of ACTH from the pituitary, prolonged dosage leads to adrenocortical atrophy.

Although great benefit as regards symptomatic relief follows cortisone or hydrocortisone treatment in arthritis, the possible side-effects and complications of the high level of dosage required must be understood. Most important is the potential suppression of the normal reaction to infections, which may exhibit no symptoms until they are far advanced. Their gluconeogenic activity may lead to excessive protein breakdown, resulting in muscle weakness and osteoporosis. Prior to increased glycogen deposition, there is marked hyperglycaemia and this may lead to excessive stimulation of insulin release and may provoke incipient diabetes mellitus. A serious side-effect, without obvious rationale, is an increased risk of peptic ulcer, and hydrocortisone is contraindicated in patients with a history of ulceration. Electrolyte disturbances may occur as hydrocortisone has some sodium-retaining activity; the commonest reactions are oedema and potassium deficiency. Chronic treatment with high doses of hydrocortisone abolishes the pituitary-adrenal response to stress, and such patients must receive extra steroid before surgical operation; like diabetics, they should always carry a card stating their daily dosage. When continued treatment of arthritis results in clinical remission, therapy should be discontinued tradually to enable the chronically suppressed adrenal gland to regain its function without an intervening period of cortical hypofunction.

The complications of cortisone and hydrocortisone therapy stimulated the search for an anti-inflammatory steroid which did not have strong salt-retaining and gluconeogenic activity. Hydrocortisone is more potent than cortisone but it is now known that cortisone is converted to the former in the body. Increase in anti-inflammatory potency *per se* is of little value unless accompanied by dissociation of other activities.

One of the first synthetic derivatives to come into clinical use was 9-α-*fluorohydrocortisone* (fludrocortisone). Its gluco-corticoid activity is about 12 times greater than that of hydrocortisone but its salt-retaining effect is increased by 75 times (see Table 33.1). It is used in cases of adrenal insufficiency to control electrolyte metabolism; its oral activity confers on it a distinct advantage over the naturally-occurring hormone deoxycortone (deoxycorticosterone) which had to be given by injection.

TABLE 33.1. Comparison of biological activity of synthetic adrenocortical hormones, taking the potency of hydrocortisone as unity

Compound	Animal experiments			Anti-rheumatic in man
	Sodium retention	Anti-inflammatory	Glycogen deposition	
Cortisone	0·6	0·6	0·6	0·6
Hydrocortisone	1	1	1	1
Prednisone	0·6	4	4	4
Prednisolone	1	4	4	4
Fludrocortisone	75	6	12	10
Dexamethasone	0·1	200	20	30
Betamethasone	0·1	70	11	28
Paramethasone	0·1	50	150	12
Methylprednisolone	0·1	6	11	6
Triamcinolone	0·1	7	7	5
Deoxycortone	25	—	0·006	—
Aldosterone	2500	—	1	—

Later, it was found that the introduction of a double bond in the C_1–C_2 position in ring A ($\varDelta^1$-dehydrogenation, see Fig. 33.3) of cortisone or hydrocortisone increased the anti-inflammatory and glycogenic activity four-fold, without change in salt-retention activity. These synthetic steroids, *prednisone* and *prednisolone*, have been considered the agents of choice in systemic corticoid therapy.

Triamcinolone, introduced in 1957, is a modification of fludrocortisone and prednisolone. The anti-inflammatory activity is enhanced by both the 9-α-fluro substitution and the Δ^1-dehydrogenation, but salt-retention is eliminated by substitution in the 16-position of an hydroxyl group. However, the advantages of triamcinolone are counter-balanced by side-effects including anorexia, headaches and muscular weakness. More recent additions include 6-*methyl-prednisolone, dexamethasone, betamethasone* and *paramethasone*, all of which have minimal salt-retaining activity. Dexamethasone and betamethasone show the greatest potency in inflammatory diseases but they offer little significant advantage in the reduction of unwanted glucocorticoid properties. The relative potencies of various steroids are compared in Table 33.1, and their chemical formulae are shown in Fig. 33.3.

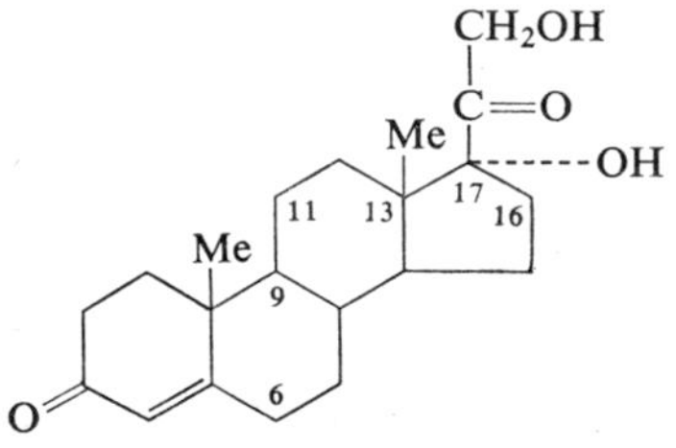

Type A 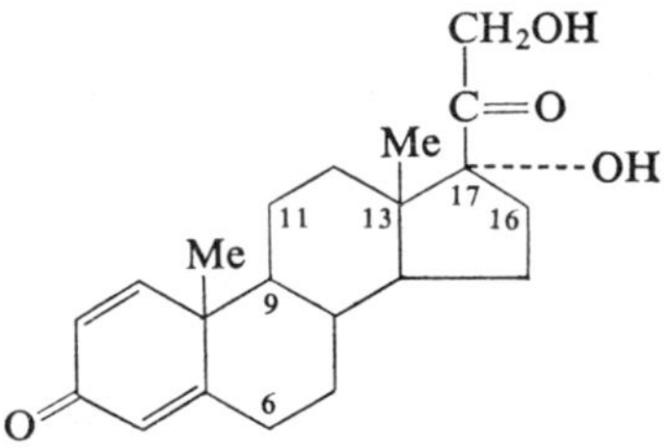   Type B

| Approved name | Type | Structure | | | | | |
| | | Substituent and position | | | | | |
		6	9	11	13	16	17
Cortisone	A	—	—	=O	CH$_3$	—	OH
Hydrocortisone (cortisol)	A	—	—	β—OH	CH$_3$	—	OH
Fludrocortisone	A	—	α—F	β—OH	CH$_3$	—	OH
Prednisone	B	—	—	=O	CH$_3$	—	OH
Prednisolone	B	—	—	β—OH	CH$_3$	—	OH
Methylprednisolone	B	α—CH$_3$	—	β—OH	CH$_3$	—	OH
Triamcinolone	B	—	α—F	β—OH	CH$_3$	α—OH	OH
Dexamethasone	B	—	α—F	β—OH	CH$_3$	α—CH$_3$	OH
Betamethasone	B	—	α—F	β—OH	CH$_3$	β—CH$_3$	OH
Paramethasone	B	α—F	—	β—OH	CH$_3$	α—CH$_3$	OH
Fluocinolone	B	α—F	α—F	β—OH	CH$_3$	α—CH	OH
Corticosterone	A	—	—	β—OH	CH$_3$	—	[No OH]
Aldosterone	A	—	—	β—OH	CHO	—	[No OH]
Deoxycortone	A	—	—	—	CH$_3$	—	[No OH]

FIG. 33.3. Structural formulae of some corticosteroids.

Considerable benefit may be obtained in many skin diseases by the topical application of adrenocortical hormones. Although they seldom effect a cure, the symptomatic relief is often extensive. At first it was thought that systemic absorption would be low and that there would be no side-effects. However, when a large area of skin is affected, systemic effects have been observed after topical application. The most useful agent appears to be *fluocinolone* which has about 100 times the activity of hydrocortisone.

Corticotrophin. In certain conditions, e.g. rheumatoid arthritis, ACTH has been used clinically to increase the production of corticosteroids by the patient's own adrenal gland. The main advantages of this form of therapy are the avoidance of pituitary-adrenal suppression which invariably occurs with exogenous corticosteroid and the production of a balanced level of the different adrenal hormones. However, ACTH has to be given by injection, making it less convenient than oral medication for the patient.

Adrenocortical antagonists. During the examination of potential synthetic oestrogens, some compounds were found to cause adrenal hypertrophy coupled with suppression of the secretion of 17-hydroxycorticosteroids. One of the most potent of these adrenal inhibitors was *amphenone B* (Fig. 33.4) but it proved too toxic for clinical use. However, a more recent analogue, *metyrapone*, possesses similar activity and is much less toxic. This class of compound inhibits hydroxylation in the 11β position, and so decreases the

Amphenone B

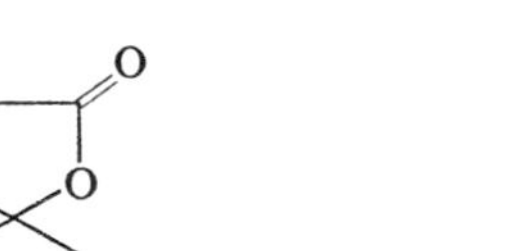

Metyrapone

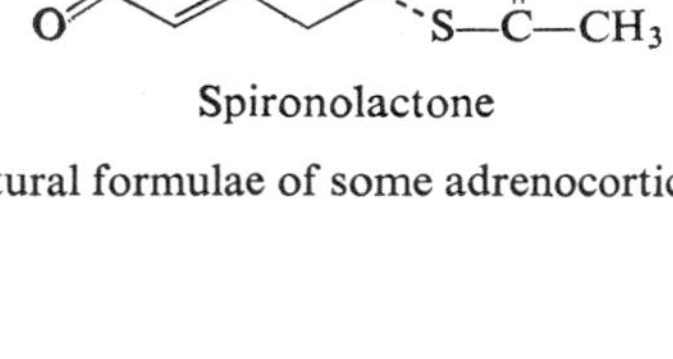

Spironolactone

FIG. 33.4. Structural formulae of some adrenocortical antagonists.

synthesis of hydrocortisone, corticosterone and aldosterone in the adrenal cortex. Metyrapone acts as a diuretic in cases of water retention resulting from aldosterone hypersecretion and may be used to diagnose pituitary ACTH deficiency. As it decreases the output of glucocorticoids, the rate of ACTH release increases with consequent adrenocortical stimulation. In the presence of metyrapone, the adrenal secretes large quantities of 11-deoxysteroids which appear in the urine, provided pituitary ACTH reserves are adequate.

Spironolactone (page 885) antagonizes the action of aldosterone on the distal renal tubules. Since it decreases the renal re-absorption of sodium, it has an advantageous diuretic action without loss of potassium.

Oestrogens

The naturally occurring ovarian steroids are, in ascending order of potency, *oestriol, oestrone* and *oestradiol*. They are active orally but only at 20 times the parenteral dose. Rapid absorption, metabolism and excretion necessitates frequent oral administration, and parenteral dosage is often inconvenient for the patient. Chemical modifications have consequently been made to the oestrogen nucleus in an attempt to prolong activity and increase potency. The most useful semi-synthetic oestrogen, 17-*ethinyloestradiol*, is as effective orally as is intramuscular oestradiol. (*Mestranol* is the 3-methylether of ethinyloestradiol.) Other semi-synthetic derivatives include *oestradiol benzoate* and *diproprionate* which are more slowly absorbed from the injection site than is oestradiol.

A number of synthetic chemicals of a less complex nature than the steroids also possess marked oestrogenic activity. Dodds and his associates studied the structure–activity relationships in a series of diphenylethylene derivatives, the most active of which was *stilboestrol* which has only about one-tenth the activity of ethinyloestradiol. Other active compounds of this type include *dienoestrol, hexoestrol, chlorotrianisene* and *methallenoestril* (see Fig. 33.5). At first sight, the structural configurations of the synthetic oestrogens do not closely resemble that of oestradiol. However, it is only the trans-isomer of stilboestrol which is markedly oestrogenic and this fact, together with other findings, has stimulated much work into structure-activity relationships. The relation between the configuration of the synthetic and natural oestrogens is shown in Fig. 33.5. Despite this knowledge, little or no significant therapeutic advantage has been found in these synthetic oestrogens when compared with ethinyloestradiol.

Chlorotrianisene is unusual in that it is stored in body fat and released slowly. It is subsequently converted to an oestrogen of much greater activity than the parent compound and for this reason has been termed a pro-oestrogen.

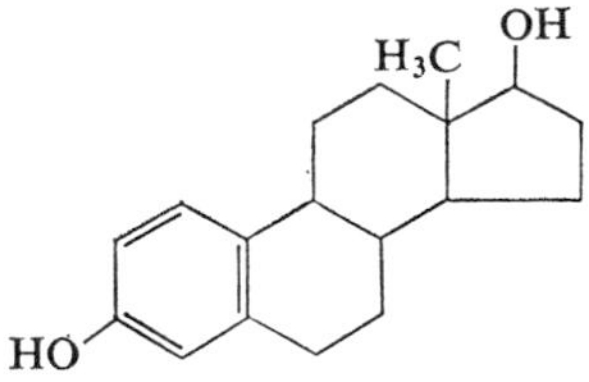

Oestradiol

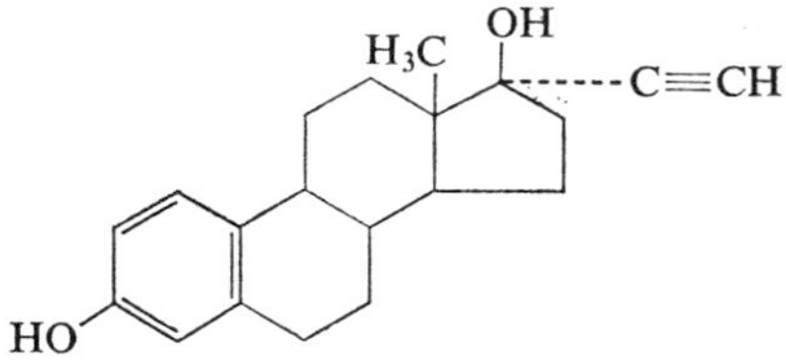

17-α-Ethinyloestradiol

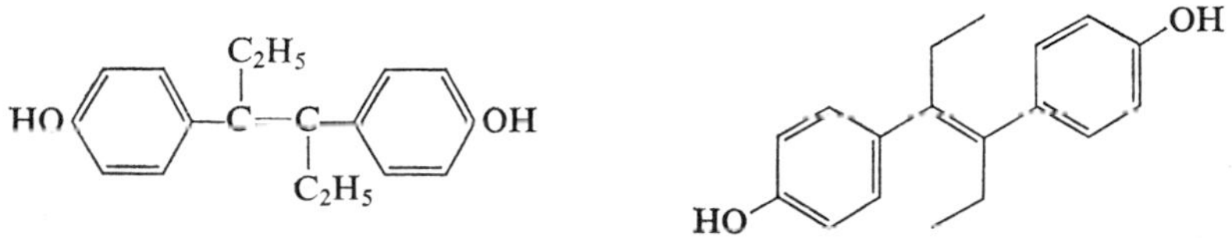

Stilboestrol

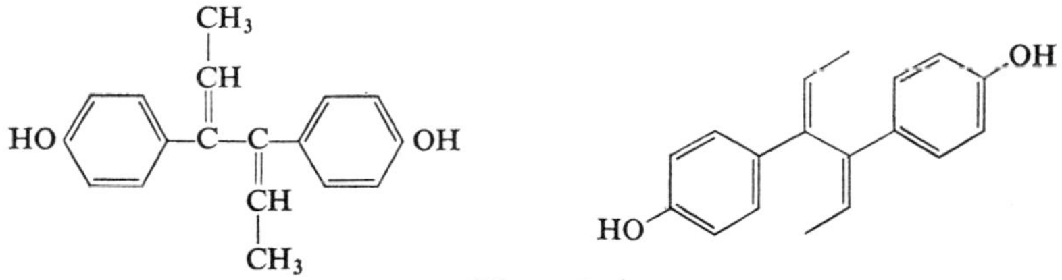

Dienoestrol

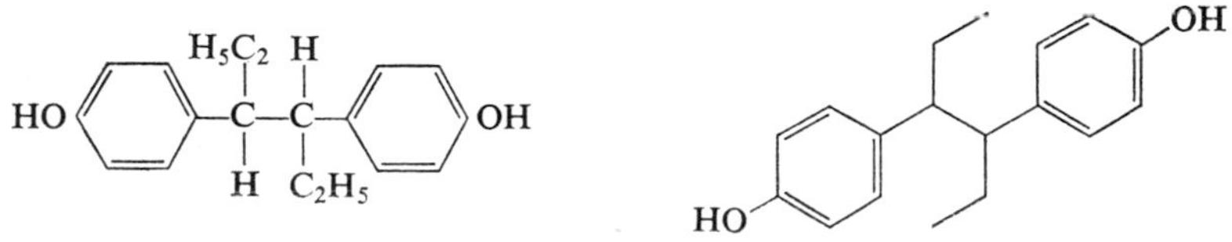

Hexoestrol

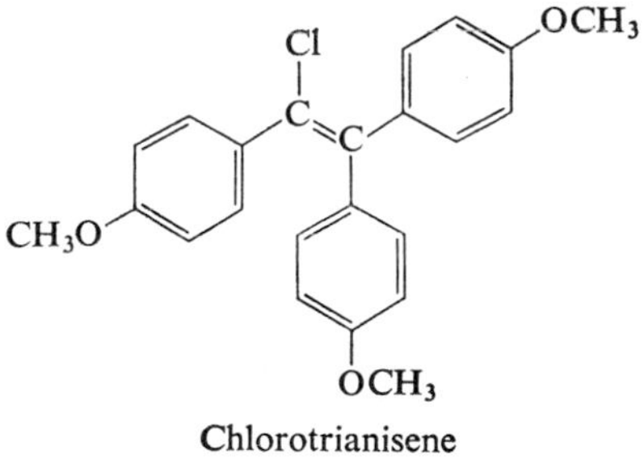

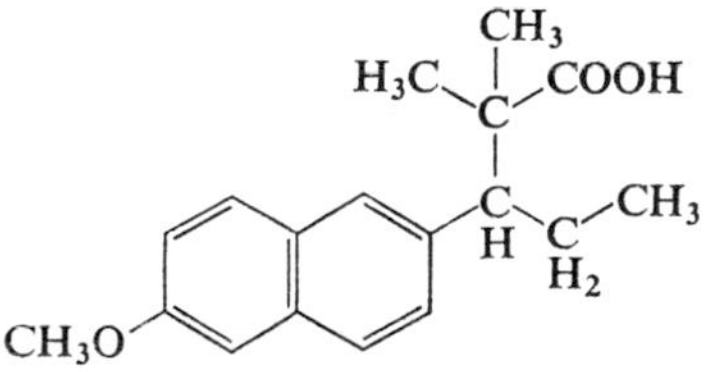

Chlorotrianisene

Methallenoestril

FIG. 33.5. Structural formulae of some oestrogens. The formulae of stilboestrol, dienoestrol and hexoestrol are drawn in two ways: on the left-hand side in the conventional manner, and on the right-hand side in such a way as to show their resemblance to the steroids.

The oestrogens principally affect the reproductive system. Oestrogens initiate and maintain the changes which occur at puberty and participate in the cyclic control of menstruation. At high blood levels, they suppress pituitary FSH release and inhibit lactation. The symptoms at the menopause are mainly due to a fall in oestrogen production. Oestrogen therapy is aimed at correction of natural oestrogen production or at suppression of gonadotrophic hormone release.

Unfortunately, the success of oestrogen treatment is often marred by disturbing side-effects. These include nausea, vomiting, anorexia, general malaise, dizziness and mild diarrhoea. In larger doses, oestrogens enhance reabsorption of sodium leading to water retention, oedema and possible cardiac embarrassment. Furthermore, oestrogenic agents have been implicated in the development of malignant disease of the genital tract. Although a causal relationship has not been established, an element of doubt about potential carcinogenicity merits limitation of oestrogen therapy to specific indications.

The primary indications of oestrogen treatment are given below:

(1) *Menopause:* The unpleasant effects at this time include hot flushes, nausea and insomnia. Frequently there are severe emotional disturbances and a tendency to become obese. Oestrogen treatment is usually beneficial.

(2) *Amenorrhoea.* Large doses of oestrogen cause hyperplasia of the endometrium and when dosing is stopped, menstruation or 'withdrawal bleeding' follows. It must be emphasized that oestrogen has no effect on the ovary and does not cause ovulation. When the amenorrhoea is of psychological origin, several artificially induced cycles may restore the normal menstrual pattern.

(3) *Other menstrual disorders* may be improved by cyclic oestrogen therapy. Prolonged menstrual bleeding may be stopped by oestrogens but relief of dysmenorrhoea is not often achieved.

(4) *Suppression of lactation.* Oestrogens suppress lactation, provided that it has not become established. This activity may be due to inhibition of LTH release or to an increase in the threshold of alveolar sensitivity to the pituitary hormone.

(5) *Malignant disease.* Carcinoma of the prostate is an androgen-dependent tumour which frequently regresses under oestrogen treatment. The site of oestrogen action is not known but is probably peripheral rather than at the pituitary level. Oestrogens may also produce remission in recurrent mammary carcinoma.

(6) *Miscellaneous.* Oestrogens are used in cases of post-menopausal vaginitis and by topical application as a cosmetic aid to under-developed breasts. There is less evidence in favour of their use in the treatment of acne.

Stilboestrol implants are used in cockerels to antagonize androgen, thus reducing aggressiveness and improving the edible quality of the carcass.

Anti-oestrogens. Certain substances appear to have an anti-oestrogenic action. For example, *clomiphene*, a relative of chlorotrianisene, has been used clinically in cases of chronic abnormal production of oestrogens (Stein-Lerenthal syndrome). It appears to act at both a peripheral and at the pituitary levels, but its precise mode of action is unknown.

Progestogens

Until recently, progestational therapy has not been practicable. *Progesterone* is not active after oral adminstration, and its sparing solubility in oil has meant that daily injections of large volumes must be given. Furthermore, dosage has usually been inadequate since it is now known that much larger quantities of progesterone are produced than had been originally suspected. Extended chemical effort has not yielded any progestins of non-steroidal structure. Synthesis of progesterone analogues is complicated and costly, and only recently have orally-active progestational agents become freely available. The first orally active progestin was anhydrohydroxyprogesterone or *ethisterone* (see Fig. 33.6), formed by the loss of a molecule of water from the C-17 side chain and the addition of a hydroxyl group. This compound is therefore a derivative of testosterone and may be called 17-ethinyl-testosterone.

Currently available progestational agents are all derivatives of progesterone or testosterone. The simplest modification is *isopregnenone*, an isomer of progesterone in which the C_{10} angular methyl group is alpha instead of beta and with the addition of another double bond in the 6 position. The caproic acid ester of 17-hydroxyprogesterone is not used orally but its high solubility in oil affords a good parenteral preparation. Other derivatives of 17-hydroxyprogesterone which are orally active include *medroxyprogesterone*, *megestrol* and *chlormadinone* (Fig. 33.6). In addition to ethisterone, another active testosterone derivative is *dimethisterone*. However, a most important discovery was the oral progestational activity of testosterone derivatives from which the 10-methyl group had been removed. The first such compound was *norethynodrel*, and this was followed by *norethisterone*, *lynoestrenol*, *allyloestrenol* and *ethynodiol diacetate*.

With the exception of progesterone cyclopentyl-3-enol ether (enol luteovis), none of the synthetic progestational agents is metabolized to pregnanediol, the normal metabolite of progesterone. This suggests that the synthetic compounds possess intrinsic progestational activity and do not need to be converted to progesterone *in vivo* to exert their effects.

In the normal individual, progesterone stimulates the secretory changes in the oestrogen-primed uterine endometrium which are associated with the luteal phase of the menstrual cycle. These changes are essential for implantation. Continued secretion of large amounts of progesterone is necessary for the

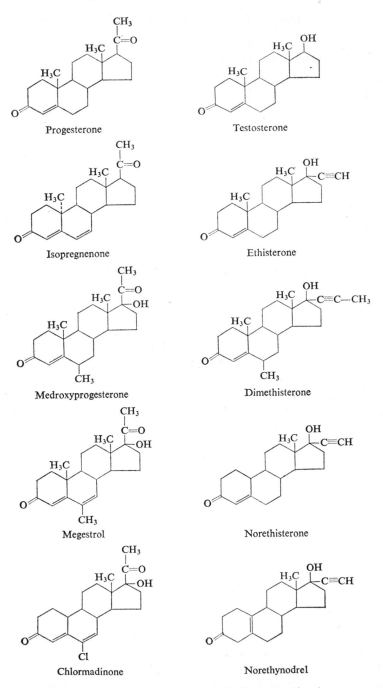

FIG. 33.6. Structural formulae of some synthetic progestational agents.

maintenance of pregnancy. Progesterone also facilitates alveolar development in the mammary gland.

The effects of exogenous progestogens are largely confined to the uterus and therefore there are few unwanted side-effects. However, because of the central position of progesterone in steroid bio-synthesis, repeated doses of progestational agents may lead to the formation of abnormal amounts of oestrogens, androgens and adrenocorticosteroids (Fig. 33.7). The most serious side-effect is virilization or masculinization of a female foetus when the mother requires progestational therapy during pregnancy. This risk occurs both with progesterone itself and with the synthetic agents, especially the testosterone derivatives. In pregnancy, it is best to use injections of 17-hydroxy-progesterone caproate. Mcdroxyprogesterone causes some suppression of ACTH release which is not surprising when the structure is compared with that of corticosterone.

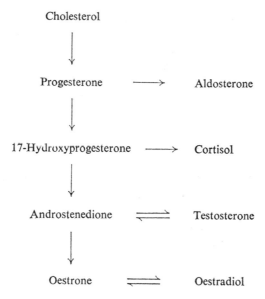

Fig. 33.7. Diagrammatic representation of known pathways of steroid biosynthesis from progesterone.

Indications for the therapeutic use of progestational agents include the following:

(1) *Threatened and habitual abortion.* During pregnancy, the daily output of progesterone varies between 100 and 400 mg per day. Cases of threatened abortion due to progesterone deficiency may respond well but beneficial effects in habitual abortion are rare.

28

(2) *Pre-menstrual tension.* The administration of progestational agents during the second half of the menstrual cycle often provides relief in this state.

(3) *Dysfunctional uterine bleeding.* In this condition, there is loss of fresh blood from the uterine endometrium, as opposed to the sloughing of mucus and blood at normal menstruation. The fact that haemostasis usually follows progestin treatment indicates that it is due to progesterone deficiency. The endometrium shows excessive glandular development without the secretory changes of the luteal phase. When progestin treatment is stopped, withdrawal bleeding occurs, akin to a normal menstruation.

(4) *Amenorrhoea.* Addition of progestogens to oestrogen therapy from day 15 to 25 of cyclic treatment usually induces menstruation. The value of treatment is dependent upon the cause of the amenorrhoea.

Oral concentraception

Ovulation does not occur during pregnancy, because of high blood levels of ovarian hormones. In animal experiments, ovulation can be suppressed by the exogenous administration of either oestrogen or progesterone. Clinical exploitation of these findings was delayed for many years for two main reasons. Firstly, although periodic administration of an oestrogen successfully inhibited ovulation in women, the side-effects were unpleasant; foremost was the production of a non-secretory endometrium which often bled profusely on withdrawal of therapy, and there was also water retention, weight gain and breast pain. Secondly, the oral inefficacy of progesterone coupled with the high cost of synthetic ethisterone made continued use prohibitively expensive.

Djerassi and co-workers announced their synthesis of orally active progestins in 1954 and 3 years later Rock, Garcia and Pincus published the first account of successful oral contraception in women. The first compound subjected to an exhaustive field-trial was norethynodrel. During the synthesis of norethynodrel, traces of ethinyloestradiol-3-methyl ether (mestranol) appear and the final tablet ('Enovid, or Enavid in Britain') contained 1·5% of the oestrogen.

The method of dosage to ensure success is important. The tablets must be started on day 5 of the cycle (taking onset of menstruation as day 1) and continued with absolute regularity until day 24. Then within 2 or 3 days, 'normal' menstruation occurs, as adequate amounts of progestogen have ensured the development of a secretory endometrium. The treatment is not without side-effects. Most frequent is the complaint of nausea, especially during the first cycle of treatment, and headache, fluid retention and weight gain. More serious is the stimulation of the growth of existing uterine fibroids. The suspicion of an increased incidence of peripheral thromboembolism has not been confirmed beyond doubt. The most inconvenient, and distressing side-effect is so-called 'breakthrough bleeding' or 'spotting' which is due to premature breakdown of the uterine endometrium.

Norethisterone in combination with ethinyloestradiol has proved as reliable as Enavid and has rather fewer side-effects. Both norethynodrel and norethisterone are C-19 nor-steroids or testosterone derivatives and thus have certain intrinsic androgenic potential. Attention is now turning to the 17-hydroxy progesterone derivatives, *chlormadinone* and *megestrol*, in the hope that they may prove more acceptable.

The mode of action of the oral contraceptives is not perfectly understood. Initially, it was thought that the progestin component suppressed the ovulation-stimulating release of LH at mid-cycle. However, studies with the non-oestrogenic 17-hydroxy progesterones suggest that much higher doses than those provided in oral contraceptive pills are required to suppress LH release in the human. There is much evidence to support the view that it is the oestrogen component which is responsible for inhibiting follicular development by suppressing release of FSH. It is known that endogenous oestrogen production is severely curtailed whilst oral contraceptive mixtures are being taken and that it is vital to commence dosage as early as day 5. A further point to this argument is given by the successful clinical trial of a sequential treatment in which pure oestrogen (mestranol) was given for days 5 to 19 and oestrogen plus progestogen (mestranol and chlormadinone) for days 20 to 24. In this case, it appears that oestrogen suppressed both follicular development and ovulation—stimulated endometrial growth. The final addition of progestogen converted the endometrium to a fully secretory state, which was followed by a menstruation closely resembling the normal.

Androgens

The natural androgen produced by the interstitial cells of the testis is *testosterone*. Small amounts of another androgen, *androsterone*, are produced in the adrenal cortex. It is many times less active than testosterone and its physiological significance is unknown.

Testosterone is inactive orally and is usually used as subcutaneous implants which provide slow release over several months. Esters of testosterone are given as oily intramuscular injections as an alternative. There are two orally active androgens, 17-*methyltestosterone* and *fluoxymesterone* (9-α-fluor-11β-hydroxy-17-methyl testosterone) Methyltestosterone is given sub-lingually as this route avoids rapid conjugation and inactivation by the liver.

The androgens initiate and maintain the male sexual characters and facilitate spermatogenesis. In addition, they have an anabolic action associated with nitrogen retention and protein deposition. The only side-effects are occasional

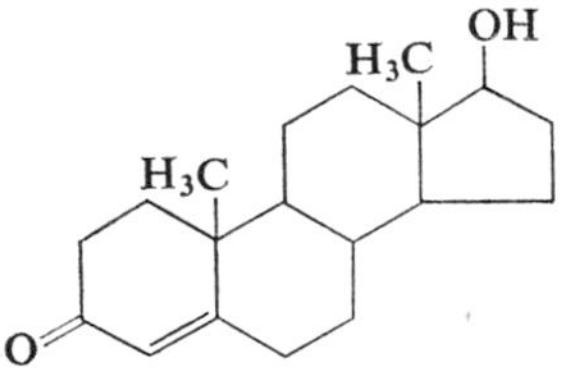

FIG. 33.8. Structural formulae of some androgenic and anabolic agents.

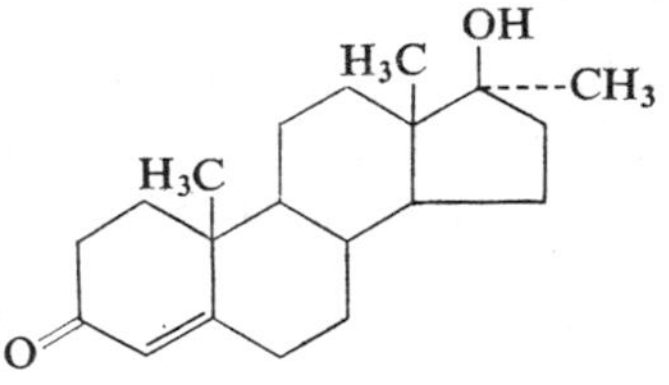

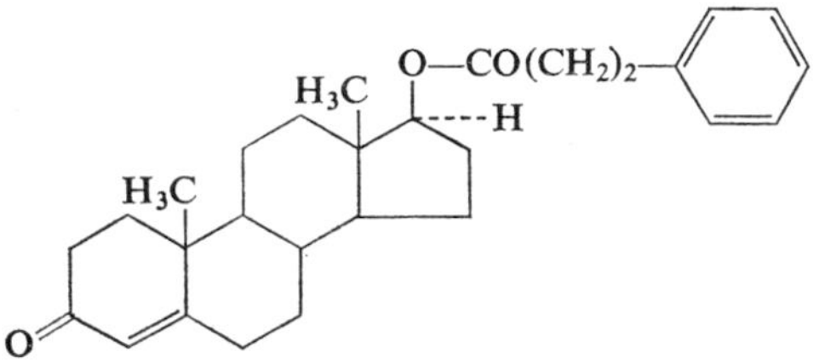

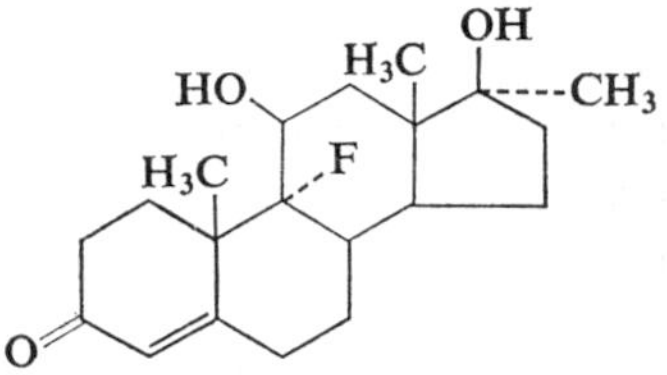

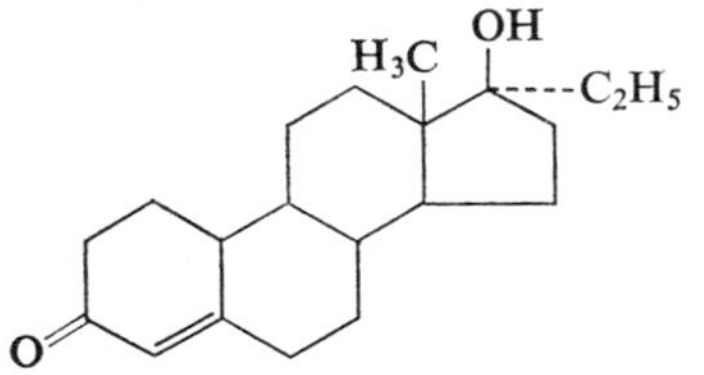

jaundice and salt and water retention, with the risk of virilization in the female. Androgens exert a depressive action upon gonadotrophin release but only in relatively high dosage. They may therefore lead to reduced spermatogenesis or menstrual disorders.

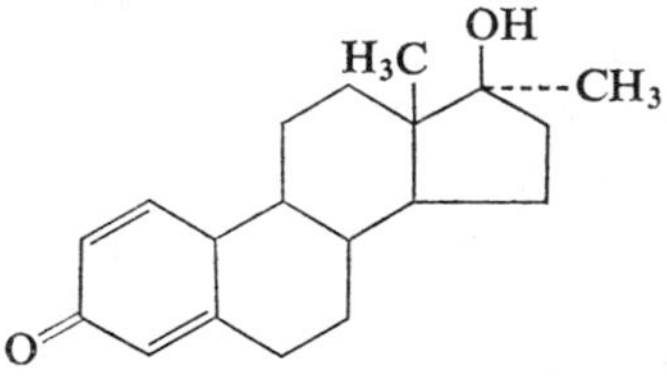

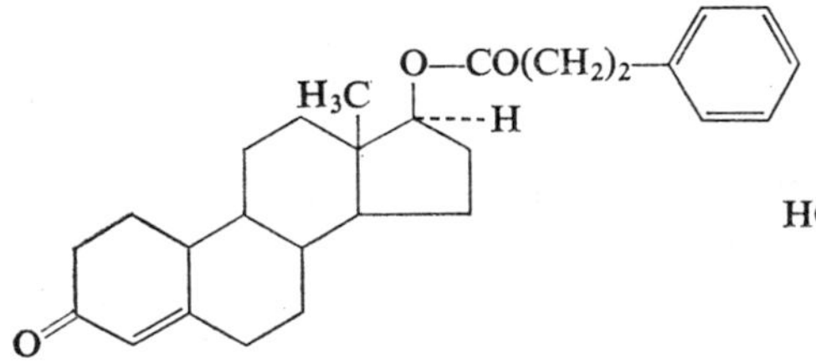

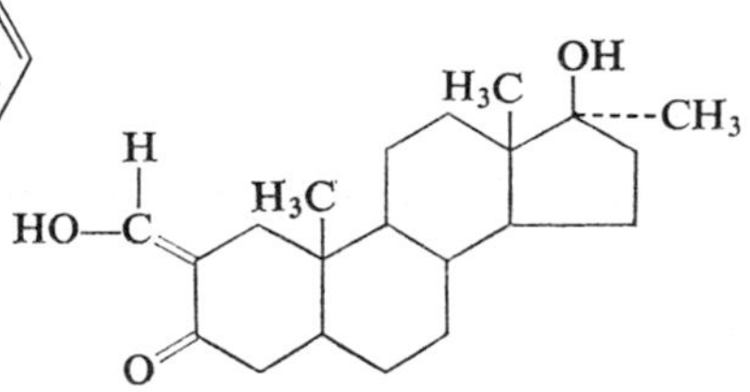

Androgen treatment has only limited applications. Pre-pubertal or adult testicular insufficiency may often be successfully treated by substitution therapy and remission may be produced in some cases of mammary cancer. Androgens may improve protein deposition in debilitating conditions.

Because of the risk of virilization, attempts have been made to dissociate androgenic and anabolic activity. The relative activities are determined in the immature castrated rat. After 2 weeks of dosing, the secondary sex glands and the levator ani muscle are removed and weighed. An ideal anabolic agent promotes muscle growth without influencing the prostate or seminal vesicles. The ratio of myotrophic to androgenic activity aids the comparison of different anabolic agents.

The most important compounds examined so far are *norethandrolone, methandienone, nandrolone phenylpropionate* and *oxymetholone* (Fig. 33.8). They appear to have a useful role in osteoporosis, acute renal failure and long-term glucocorticoid therapy. In osteoporosis, there is gradual decalcification and both urinary and faecal losses of calcium are antagonized by anabolic steroids. The checking action on protein break-down reduces blood urea levels, giving a useful short-term effect in renal failure. Similarly, the catabolic gluconeogenetic effect of prolonged glucocorticoid therapy may be antagonized by anabolic agents.

Hypocholesterolaemic agents

There is an increased incidence of ischaemic heart disease in otherwise healthy individuals who show elevated serum cholesterol levels. Many patients suffering from angina pectoris or a recent coronary thrombosis also have high blood cholesterol figures. It has been widely assumed, although not proved, that hypercholesterolaemia predisposes towards atherosclerosis in all its forms.

Serum cholesterol levels can be effectively reduced either by dietary or by drug treatment but it remains to be seen whether or not such treatment significantly affects the prognosis. Many workers have suggested that abnormal lipid patterns result from some hormonal inadequacy. Certainly, oestrogens produce marked and sustained falls in cholesterol and triglycerides but only in doses sufficiently large to have feminizing effects in males. It has not been possible to dissociate oestrogenic from hypocholesterolaemic activity but for a while *triparanol* (Fig. 33.9), a non-oestrogenic compound resembling chlorotrianisone, achieved clinical popularity. However, its mode of action is to inhibit cholesterol synthesis at its penultimate stage, and the resultant accumulation of desmosterol produces toxic effects without compensating clinical benefit.

Thyroxine and androsterone have also been shown to possess hypocholesterolaemic activity, but in ischaemic heart disease thyroxine administration is fraught with hazard. Recent work has demonstrated the hypocholesterolaemic

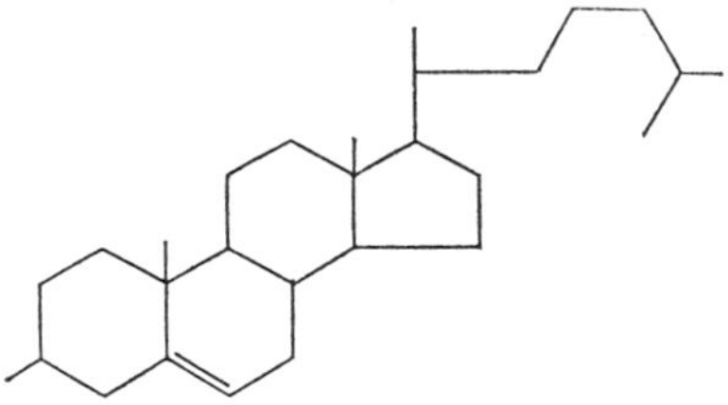

Cholesterol

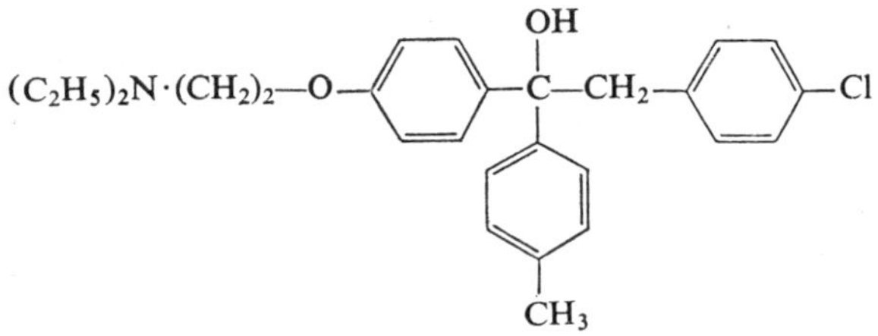

Triparanol

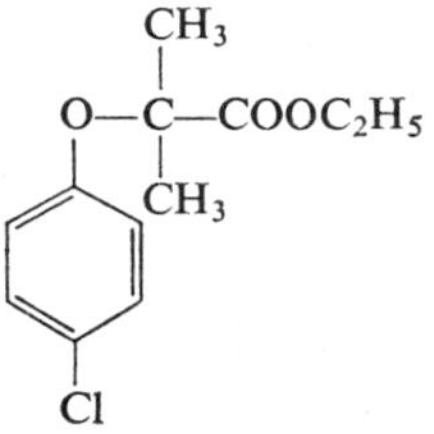

Clofibrate

FIG. 33.9. Structural formulae of cholesterol and some hypocholesterolaemic agents.

activity of a series of simple branched chain acids of which the most effective was the ethyl ester of parachlorophenoxy-isobutyric acid (clofibrate). Its activity was found to be dependent upon the addition of androsterone in the monkey but, in man, clofibrate itself appears to have a dramatic effect upon elevated serum lipids without toxicity. Clofibrate is strongly bound to plasma albumen and prevents protein binding of serum lipids. It also increases thyroxine uptake by the liver. Both factors serve to decrease hepatic lipid synthesis.

CHAPTER 34

Drugs Acting on the Urinary System

The renal mechanisms which maintain within narrow limits the volume, pH and ionic composition of the body fluids are described in Chapter 13. These mechanisms may be modified by drugs.

Diuretics

Diuretics are drugs used to increase urine flow; their chief medical application is the removal of excess extracellular fluid (oedema) in disease. They act by increasing the quantity of sodium ion in the urine, the increased salt excretion being accompanied by an increased water excretion as a result of the osmotic imbalance produced. Diuretics achieve this effect by one of the following means—(1) They inhibit the reabsorption of sodium ions by a direct action in the kidney tubules. Compounds in this class include *xanthines, aminouracils, triazines, mercurials, inhibitors of carbonic anhydrase, benzothiadiazines, benzenesulphonamides, sulphamoyl-benzophenone derivatives, frusemide, ethacrynic acid, aldosterone antagonists, triamterene* and *potassium salts*. (2) They inhibit tubular reabsorption of sodium ions by an indirect mechanism. *Osmotic diuretics* and *inhibitors of aldosterone secretion* act in this way. (3) They increase the filtered load of sodium ions in the glomeruli. *Acidifying salts, glucocorticoids* and *corticotrophin* and *plasma expanders* are examples of drugs acting by this process.

An increased urine flow may also be produced by suppressing the secretion of antidiuretic hormone (ADH) from the neurohypophysis. Both water and ethyl alcohol produce this effect: absorption of water lowers the blood osmotic pressure and the osmoreceptors (page 368) are no longer stimulated so that the reflexly-induced secretion of ADH dimishes: alcohol suppresses the secretion of ADH by a direct action on the neurohypophysis. The permeability of the collecting tubules to water is dependent on the presence of ADH (page 347); in its absence, water remains within the lumen of the tubules and the volume of urine is increased. However, water and alcohol do not increase the excretion of electrolytes and they are therefore of no value in the relief of oedema. With water, there is little difference between the extra volume excreted and that imbibed. An increase in the intake of water may be a desirable means for increasing urine formation during treatment with either urinary antiseptics, when the amount flowing through the kidneys needs to be increased, or with drugs (or their metabolites) which are sparingly soluble in water and which may therefore precipitate in the kidney tubules and block them (as may occur with sulphamerazine).

Oedema. The choice of a diuretic depends in part on the aetiology of the oedema being treated. Transport of fluid from the blood to the tissues (that is, oedema formation, page 247) is favoured by (i) an increase in capillary blood pressure, (ii) a decrease in plasma colloid osmotic pressure, (iii) an increase in the protein content of tissue fluid, as in inflammatory conditions (page 248), and (iv) changes in renal function arising, for example, from an increased secretion of aldosterone by the adrenal cortex. Increased secretion of aldosterone (secondary aldosteronism), occurs in response to raised levels of angiotensin (pages 182 and 833). This results whenever the blood pressure or colloid osmotic pressure in the afferent arterioles of the kidney is low, and under these conditions there is increased distal sodium reabsorption. Severe oedema may occur in kidney disease (nephrotic oedema), in cirrhosis of the liver, in congestive heart failure (cardiac oedema), in some endocrine disorders, in dietary deficiencies (nutritional oedema, and in some disorders of pregnancy (pages 407–408).

CARDIAC OEDEMA. In congestive heart failure, venous pressure in the kidneys is increased and renal blood flow reduced so that there is a fall in glomerular filtration rate and in the excretion of water and solutes. In addition, the generalized increase in venous pressure results in an increased filtration pressure in the capillaries of the tissues. Both of these factors tend to shift water and electrolyte from the blood to the tissue spaces. Treatment of the cardiac disorder by cardiac glycosides (pages 806–807) increases the urine volume by increasing cardiac output, so that renal blood flow and glomerular filtration rate are increased, and venous pressure in the kidneys and elsewhere is reduced. In addition, digitalis and ouabain have been shown, in animal experiments, to depress the active reabsorption of sodium in the kidney tubules, probably as a result of ATP-ase inhibition (see pages 810–812). However, it is not yet known to what extent this action contributes to their diuretic effect in congestive heart failure. The cardiac glycosides alone usually do not adequately mobilize accumulated oedema fluid, and diuretic therapy is also necessary.

HEPATIC CIRRHOSIS. This condition involves atrophy of liver cells and an increase in fibrous tissue giving rise to an increased capillary pressure within the portal venous system (portal hypertension). Impaired protein synthesis by the damaged liver cells results in a fall in plasma protein concentration and this may be further lowered as a result of gastro-intestinal haemorrhage resulting from the portal hypertension. Water and electrolytes pass from the blood not only into the tissue spaces (oedema) but also into the peritoneal cavity (ascites). The fall in the circulating blood volume reduces renal blood flow and stimulates the secretion of aldosterone, which, because of the liver cell damage, is not metabolized and accumulates. These factors augment the oedema by further reducing sodium and water excretion.

NEPHROTIC OEDEMA. In chronic nephrosis (a disease of childhood and young adults), there is a reduction in the effective filtering surface of the glomeruli and an increased glomerular permeability to protein. The decreased filtration rate is therefore accompanied by loss of plasma protein into the urine. The resulting decrease in plasma colloid osmotic pressure stimulates aldosterone secretion so that sodium reabsorption is enhanced. Cellular proteins are metabolized to replace the plasma proteins and intracellular potassium ions, normally held in association with the cellular proteins, are released into the circulation and into the oedema fluid.

NUTRITIONAL OEDEMA. Oedema due to nutritional deficiency may arise during starvation when the diet is low in calories, or, as in many tropical countries, when the caloric intake is adequate but there is a marked deficiency in protein intake (protein deficiency oedema or kwashiorkor). The former condition is the result of a general deficiency of plasma solutes; the latter is due to a low plasma colloid osmotic pressure, and to this extent it resembles nephrotic oedema.

OEDEMA OF PREGNANCY. Some degree of oedema in pregnancy occurs normally, but sometimes it is excessive and is associated with other toxaemic symptoms (page 407). In the oedema associated with pre-eclampsia, aldosterone secretion is usually not increased and may even be lower than normal.

CYCLICAL OEDEMA. Oestrogens and progesterone may impair sodium excretion, and women with endocrine disturbance sometimes suffer from a cyclical formation of oedema which is associated with the menstrual cycle. Aldosterone secretion is also increased. Treatment usually consists of restriction of dietary sodium or the administration of mild diuretics.

Drugs acting directly on the renal tubules

1. Xanthines. Some actions of the xanthines—*caffeine, theobromine* and *theophylline*—are described on page 620. All three possess diuretic action but this is most marked with theophylline, which is the only one now used clinically as a diuretic. The free bases are well absorbed from the gastro-intestinal tract but they are often conjugated with other compounds to improve their water solubility for parenteral injection. Theophylline ethylenediamine (aminophylline), theophylline sodium acetate and theophylline methylglucamine are the conjugates usually used for systemic administration.

The xanthines produce their diuretic effect in three ways: (i) They inhibit the

28*

tubular reabsorption of sodium and chloride, this effect being most pronounced with theophylline. Potassium excretion also increases but this is a non-specific effect which occurs when there is a general increase in solute excretion. (ii) Caffeine increases the number of functioning glomeruli and this finding (in frogs) led to the suggestion that the xanthines raise filtration pressure by dilating the afferent arterioles to a greater extent than the efferent arterioles. Total renal blood flow is increased by caffeine and theobromine but it is usually decreased by theophylline. (iii) The direct actions of the drugs on kidney blood flow are augmented by their stimulant action on the heart which results in an increased cardiac output. Theophylline is used as a diuretic mainly in oedema of cardiac origin, especially when other drugs have proved ineffective. The xanthines are contra-indicated when there is renal insufficiency. Tolerance to their action develops with repeated dosage and may be already present in habitual tea and coffee drinkers. Theophylline is often combined with mercurial diuretics, the potencies of which are increased; so they are effective in lower doses and hence less toxic.

2. Aminouracils. Derivatives of aminouracil are intermediates in the synthesis of xanthines and some of them are at least as potent in their diuretic action and are better tolerated. The 1,3-disubstituted derivatives of 6-aminouracil possess diuretic action but the monosubstituted compounds do not. The compounds which have been used clinically as orally active diuretics are *aminometradine* and *amisometradine*. Amisometridine is about half as potent as aminometridine

Aminometradine   Amisometradine

by weight, but gastro-intestinal side effects (nausea, vomiting and diarrhoea) occur less frequently and so higher dosage may be tolerated. Their action appears to be solely due to inhibition of tubular reabsorption of sodium. They lose their effectiveness when the plasma sodium level falls—usually after about five consecutive days of treatment. These compounds have been employed to control oedema in patients with mild congestive heart failure, but they have largely dropped out of use.

3. Triazines. The diuretic action of some members of this series has been known for some time but most are too toxic to the kidney for use. However, *chlorazanil* is one of the most active and least toxic members. It appears to act by inhibiting tubular reabsorption of sodium. In rats it produces a powerful diuretic effect when a sodium chloride load is given, but it is antidiuretic when a water load is given. The effects of deoxycorticosterone and chlorazanil on

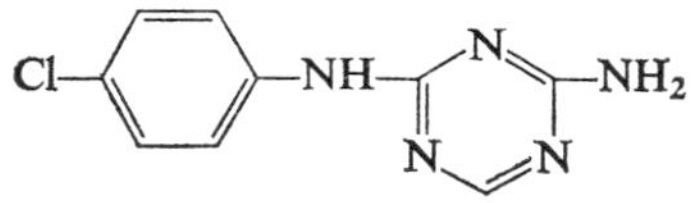

Chlorazanil

sodium and potassium excretion have been shown to be mutually antagonistic, suggesting that the action of chlorazanil on sodium reabsorption is exerted in the distal tubules.

Tolerance to the action of chlorazanil does not develop. It is contra-indicated in patients with renal insufficiency. Chlorazanil has been used with some success in the treatment of hypertension. Side-effects include nausea, vomiting, loss of appetite and muscle weakness.

4. Mercurials. The organic mercurial diuretics produce a powerful and dependable diuresis, especially in oedema resulting from severe congestive heart failure. The diuretic properties of mercury compounds have been known for centuries. Most organic mercurials are less potent than ionizable mercury salts, but the organic mercurials are considerably less toxic and do not precipitate protein at the site of injection. The mercurials used clinically are usually injected intramuscularly, being too irritant for subcutaneous injection (except for mercaptomerin) and too toxic for intravenous injection. Sudden death due to ventricular fibrillation has followed intravenous injection. They may be given orally, but absorption is slow and erratic and gastro-intestinal irritation gives rise to nausea, vomiting and diarrhoea. *Chlormerodrin* is an exception and is better tolerated when given by mouth than are other mercurials, although gastro-intestinal disturbances do sometimes occur.

All the mercurials used as diuretics (Table 34.1) are derivatives of mercuripropanol:

$$R-CH_2-CH-CH_2-HgX$$
$$|$$
$$O(H \text{ or } CH_3)$$

R is a polar hydrophilic radical; in most cases it contains a carboxyl group and is linked to the rest of the molecule through a carbamyl group. When R is attached to the rest of the molecule by an ester or ether linkage, diuretic activity is weak except in the case of the mannitol derivative, *diglucomethoxane*,

TABLE 34.1. Some mercurial diuretics. Chlormerodrin is used orally; all others are injected intramuscularly.

Mercurial	R	CH_2——$\underset{\underset{Y}{|}}{CH}$—$CH_2$—Hg $\diagdown$ X	Y	X
Mersalyl	benzene ring with –CO—NH– and –O—CH₂—COONa		—OCH₃	—OH + Theophylline
Mercurophylline	NaOOC— (cyclopentane) —CO—NH— , —CH₃ , CH₃ CH₃		—OCH₃	—OH + Theophylline
Mercaptomerin	NaOOC— (cyclopentane) —CO—NH— , —CH₃ , CH₃ CH₃		—OCH₃	—S—CH₂—COONa
Mercumatilin	NaOOC (coumarin ring) O, O		—OCH₃	—OH + Theophylline
Digluco-methoxane	CH₂OH — H—C—OH — H—C—O— — (HOCH)₂ — CH₂OH		—OH	—S—CH₂ (CHOH)₄ CH₂OH
Meralluride	CH₂—CO—NH—CO—NH— , CH₂—COONa		—OCH₃	—OH + Theophylline
Chlormerodrin	NH₂—CO—NH—		—OCH₃	—Cl

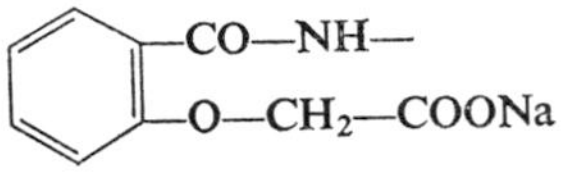

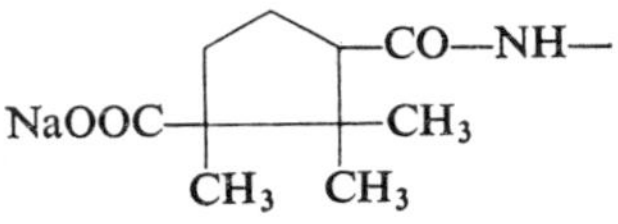

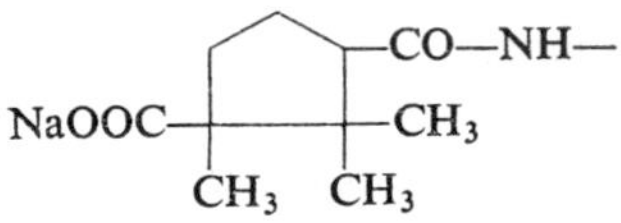

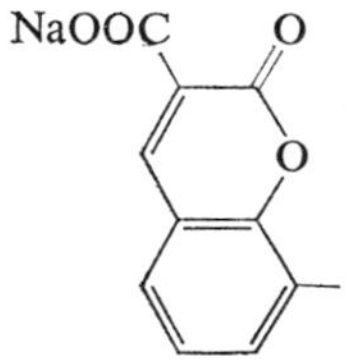

which is one of the most potent mercurials tested in clinical trial. The function of the X substituent, which is usually theophylline, a halogen or a thiol derivative, is to reduce toxicity and to increase the rate of absorption from the intramuscular site of injection. Theophylline also diminishes local irritant effects and hastens the appearance of the drug in the urine. The amount of theophylline included is too small to exert a diuretic action by itself. When X is a monothiol, such as cysteine or glutathione, cardiac toxicity is reduced while diuretic effect is unimpaired. When X is mercaptoacetic acid, as in *mercaptomerin* (Table 34.1), the compound is rapidly absorbed, less toxic to the heart and sufficiently non-irritant to be given subcutaneously, although about 20% of patients complain of some discomfort when injected by this route.

Mercurial diuretics increase the excretion of sodium and chloride ions, the increase of chloride being greater than that of sodium. The excess chloride is accompanied in the urine by other cations such as potassium, although diuresis produced by mercurials is accompanied by less potassium loss than that following the use of many other diuretics. Excretion of ammonium ion, titratable acid and bicarbonate ion is not affected by the mercurials. After prolonged use of mercurials, the loss of chloride in excess of sodium, coupled with the unimpaired reabsorption of bicarbonate, results in an alkalosis (i.e. an excess of blood buffers). When this occurs the diuretic effect diminishes, but it may be restored by the administration of acid-forming salts such as ammonium chloride or nitrate. Experiments using the technique of stop-flow analysis (page 341) have shown that the site of action of the mercurials is in the proximal tubules. Glucose reabsorption, which occurs in the proximal tubules, is also inhibited to some extent by mercurials. Pathological and biochemical studies also indicate that the proximal tubules are the site of action since the necrotic effects of overdosage are first exerted there, and enzyme inhibition is confined to this region.

There have been conflicting views as to whether the primary effect of mercurials is on sodium or on chloride reabsorption. However, sodium reabsorption is the active process, chloride passively following the electro-chemical gradient created by the movement of the cation (page 342). If the primary effect is inhibition of proximal sodium reabsorption, both sodium and chloride will be retained in the proximal tubular urine. The excessive chloride excretion in the final urine might then be explained if the exchange of sodium for potassium or hydrogen in the distal segments is not impaired; some of the sodium will be reabsorbed there in exchange for other cations so that chloride excretion exceeds that of sodium. A possible explanation of the action of organic mercurials which fits most of the experimental data is as follows. When mercury is incorporated into a suitable organic molecule, its penetration into cells is facilitated. Within the cells, small amounts of mercuric ion are liberated, and these ions impair the active reabsorption of sodium in the proximal tubules. The liberation of mercuric ions may be facilitated by an intra-cellular acidosis and this would explain the diminishing diuretic effect which accompanies the production of alkalosis, and the restorative and potentiating effects of acid-forming salts.

Mercurial diuretics provide an example of drugs which are preferentially taken up by the tissue on which they exert their main action. Studies with radioactive tracers have shown that most of the mercury bound by the kidneys is located in the cortex where the concentration may be over a hundred times that in the plasma. The heart and skeletal muscle contain very little. Like most heavy metals, mercury has a strong affinity for sulphydryl (—SH) groups; this appears to be the mechanism of binding in the kidney and the selective uptake by the renal cortex may be the result of the large number of—SH binding groups there, coupled with the rich renal blood supply. The dithiol, *dimercaprol* (BAL, page 468), forms a stable complex with mercury and abolishes the diuretic effect of the organic mercurials. There appears to be a connection between the rate of tubular secretion of mercurials and their diuretic action. Although fixed in the kidney, mercurials which do not possess diuretic action are only slowly excreted, and in species of animal in which mercurial diuretics have been found to be relatively inactive (e.g. rats), excretion has been found to be correspondingly slow. Most of the organic mercurial present in the plasma is bound to protein and cannot therefore be filtered into the glomerulus. Mercurials do not alter filtration rate and do not affect renal blood flow. They are secreted into the urine chiefly by the proximal tubular cells and it appears to be at some stage during their temporary fixation in the tubular cells that they exert the action which gives rise to the diuresis. Mercurials inhibit the —SH containing enzymes, *ATP-ase* and *succinic dehydrogenase*, in kidney slices and this may be the basis of their diuretic action. Inhibition of succinic dehydrogenase in the tubules has been studied histochemically and found to be greatest in the proximal portion of the tubules. No connection between succinic dehydrogenase and active sodium transport in the tubules is known, but ATP-ases are known to be involved in active sodium transport in other tissues. Mercurials are eliminated in the urine in complexes with the monothiol radicals of cysteine or acetylcysteine.

A decade ago, the mercurials were the most powerful and widely used diuretics, but the introduction of newer orally-active drugs has limited their use. They are used primarily in oedema of cardiac origin and in ascites due to liver disease. Ammonium chloride is often used simultaneously to enhance their action. Toxic side-effects of mercurials include kidney damage, gastric disturbance, skin eruptions and fever. They should not be used in acute nephritis.

5. Carbonic anhydrase inhibitors. The metabolites of some of the anti-bacterial sulphonamides are sparingly soluble in acid media and are liable to precipitate in the kidney tubules causing renal damage. Urine analysis was therefore routinely carried out when using these drugs. The use of *sulphanilamide* was found to be associated with the production of a metabolic acidosis and a large volume of alkaline urine containing bicarbonate ions. This effect of sulphanilamide was later shown to be the result of inhibition of the enzyme, carbonic anhydrase. Carbonic anhydrase accelerates the attainment of equilibrium in the reaction $CO_2 + H_2O \rightleftharpoons H_2CO_3$ and its role in the tubular secretion of hydrogen ions and the acidification of the urine is described on pages 343–345. Other sulphonamides with unsubstituted sulphonamido groups ($-SO_2NH_2$) were also found to inhibit the enzyme, but this action is lost with substitution on the sulphonamido nitrogen as in most of the bacteriostatic sulphonamides. The first sulphonamide to be used clinically as

Acetazolamide

5-*n*-butyramide-1,3,4-thiadiazole-2-sulphonamide

Ethoxzolamide

a diuretic was *acetazolamide*, a highly potent and specific inhibitor of carbonic anhydrase, which is well absorbed after oral administration. Kinetic studies indicate that the enzyme inhibition is non-competitive in nature. Inhibition of carbonic anhydrase depresses the reabsorption of bicarbonate in the proximal tubule, prevents the acidification of the urine, promotes potassium excretion by reducing the supply of hydrogen ions taking part in the coupled exchange of hydrogen and potassium for sodium in the distal tubules, and inhibits the ammonium mechanism which is normally brought into play when the pH of the urine falls to about 6 (see page 346) .The increased bicarbonate excretion is accompanied by increased excretion of both sodium and potassium so retaining water in the tubules, and diuresis results.

The response to acetazolamide is rapid in onset and of relatively short duration. With repeated dosage the action is self-limiting. One of the factors responsible for the development of refractoriness is the loss of bicarbonate from the extra-cellular fluid (bicarbonate and its accompaning cation represent only about 20% of the extra-cellular electrolytes). Another factor is the development of acidosis. In acidosis, the blood buffers are acidified and sufficient hydrogen ion is available without the action of carbonic anhydrase.

The self-limiting action of acetazolamide restricts its use to the treatment of mild oedema. It is particularly useful in cyclical oedema of pregnancy, but is of little value in severe congestive heart failure where prolonged action is necessary. Acetazolamide is not useful in the treatment of nephrotic oedema or oedema associated with hepatic cirrhosis or with therapy with adrenocortical steroids, since in those conditions there is a susceptibility to potassium loss and this is augmented by the diuretic.

Other carbonic anhydrase inhibitors which have been used clinically are *ethoxzolamide* and the butyramido derivative shown on the previous page. They are about equipotent with acetazolamide but are more likely to produce

TABLE 34.2. Some benzothiadiazine diuretics

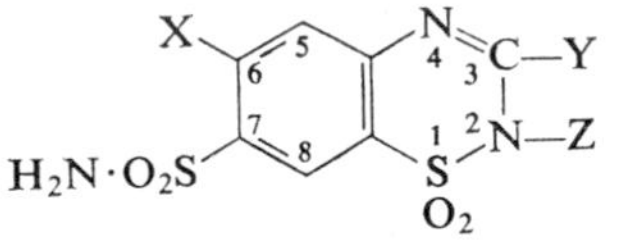

Compound	X	3:4 bond	Y	Z	Approx. daily dose (mg)
Chlorothiazide	—Cl	unsaturated	H	H	1000
Flumethiazide	—CF$_3$	unsaturated	H	H	1000
Hydrochlorothiazide	—Cl	saturated	H	H	100
Hydroflumethiazide	—CF$_3$	saturated	H	H	100
Benzthiazide	—Cl	unsaturated	—CH$_2$·S·CH$_2$— 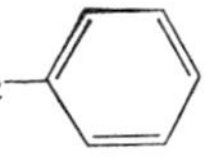	H	100
Trichlormethiazide	—Cl	saturated	—CHCl$_2$	H	10
Bendrofluazide	—CF$_3$	saturated	—CH$_2$— 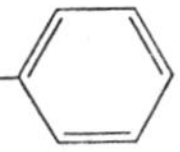	H	10
Methyclothiazide	—Cl	saturated	—CHCl$_2$	CH$_3$	5
Cyclopenthiazide	—Cl	saturated	—CH$_2$— 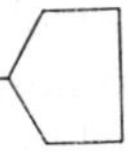	H	1
Polythiazide	—Cl	saturated	—CH$_2$·S·CH$_2$·CF$_3$	CH$_3$	1

untoward side-effects which include nausea, lethargy, a tingling sensation, and muscular weakness.

Acetazolamide is also useful in the treatment of glaucoma (page 895) and epilepsy (page 610). Presumably the catalyzed reaction $H_2CO_3 \rightleftharpoons H_2O + CO_2$, is involved in the production of aqueous humour, and inhibition of the enzyme therefore slows down the rate of aqueous formation so that intraocular pressure is lowered. The anti-convulsant action of acetazolamide in both *grand* and *petit mal* is not understood. The drug is believed to inhibit discharges from epileptic focal cells, presumably by an action on neuronal enzymes. Unlike its action on the kidney, and unlike the action of other anti-convulsant drugs (page 608), the anti-convulsant action of acetazolamide shows little tachyphylaxis. Methylation of one of the two acidic centres in acetazolamide produces compounds which penetrate the eye and the blood-brain barrier more efficiently, and which possess enhanced *in vitro* enzyme inhibitory potency. Such compounds may therefore be useful as anticonvulsants and in the treatment of glaucoma.

6. Benzothiadiazines (thiazides). The discovery of compounds in this group, like that of acetazolamide, began with the observation that sulphonamides inhibit carbonic anhydrase. However, although these compounds do inhibit this enzyme, this is not their main mechanism of action in producing diuresis.

Chlorothiazide is the prototype of the class and may be regarded as being formed from a sulphonamide by ring closure:

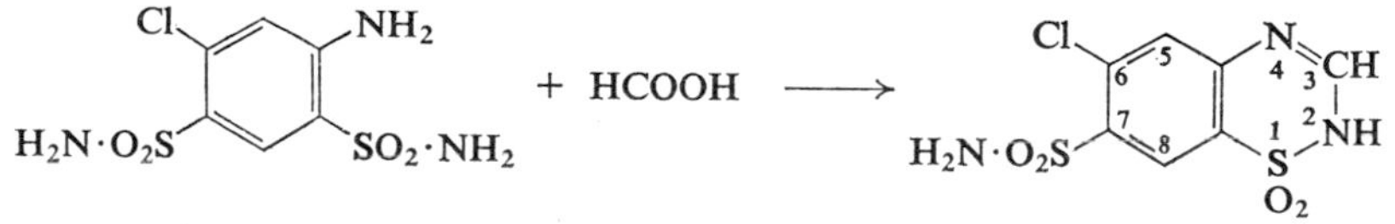

| 6-Chlorodisulphamyl aniline | Formic acid | Chlorothiazide |

In some related drugs, the Cl at position 6 is replaced by CF_3. Saturation of the 3:4 double bond in the heterocyclic ring increases diuretic potency although such compounds are less effective as carbonic anhydrase inhibitors. Substitution in the 3 position of the heterocyclic ring further increases diuretic potency and again carbonic anhydrase inhibiting potency is reduced. The formulae of the clinically useful compounds in this group are shown in Table 34.2.

All the benzothiadiazine diuretics have qualitatively similar properties but differ quantitatively. They also differ in the relative importance of carbonic anhydrase inhibition for their diuretic effect. They act directly on the tubules to decrease the reabsorption of sodium, potassium, chloride and bicarbonate. Increased amounts of these ions therefore remain in the urine and are accompanied by a corresponding increase in water excretion. The more potent members of the group have relatively less effect on carbonic anhydrase and therefore cause relatively less elimination of bicarbonate. The tubular enzymes, other than carbonic anhydrase, which are acted upon by these drugs are not known, but experiments using stop flow analysis have shown that inhibition of sodium and chloride reabsorption takes place in the proximal tubule. Potassium loss is probably an indirect effect arising from the fact that increased concentrations of sodium reach the distal tubules, where its exchange for potassium is enhanced.

The development of the benzothiadiazines constitutes the greatest advance in diuretic therapy since the discovery of the organic mercurials. They are well tolerated and potent when given by mouth, and are effective in both acidosis (when acetazolamide is inactive) and in alkalosis (when mercurials are inactive). Refractoriness on prolonged use is slow to develop and they have no serious effects on damaged kidneys. They are useful in cardiac oedema as well as other oedematous conditions, although they must be used with care in patients with hepatic cirrhosis who are especially sensitive to the effects of potassium loss. The main toxic side-effects of the drugs are those resulting from excessive potassium loss. Severe hypokalaemia sensitizes the heart to the action of digitalis (page 810), which is important in patients with congestive heart failure, produces muscular weakness with eventual impairment of respiration, leads to severe damage of the renal tubules, and may precipitate hepatic coma in patients with cirrhosis of the liver. Excessive depletion of potassium during therapy with the benzothiadiazines is prevented by giving the appropriate quantity of potassium chloride. The formerly popular enteric-coated potassium chloride tablets have now been found to produce intestinal ulcers in a few patients; this effect is due to the release of a high local concentration of potassium chloride. Furthermore, absorption is irregular, and for these reasons this type of preparation is best avoided. When potassium supplements are necessary in diuretic therapy, slow-release preparations are preferable.

The more potent benzothiadiazines are more lipid soluble than is chlorothiazide and are more efficiently absorbed from the gastro-intestinal tract. The compounds are eliminated both by glomerular filtration and by secretion in the tubules, although some of the more potent ones are reabsorbed to some extent. Increased absorption from the gut and reabsorption from the kidney tubules contribute to the high potency of these compounds.

Except in very large doses, the benzothiadiazines have little ganglion blocking or anti-adrenaline action, and yet they all possess a mild antihypertensive action in hypertensive patients. This effect is probably due to increased sodium and chloride excretion, thereby diminishing the plasma volume and removing oedema fluid from the walls of the arterioles. Restricted dietary sodium chloride also lowers blood pressure in hypertensive patients. Diuretics are often used to augment the action of antihypertensive drugs (page 844). In this way, the dose of antihypertensive drug may be reduced and the incidence of side-effects is thereby diminished.

7. Benzenesulphonamides and sulphamoyl benzophenones. Compounds in this group include 6-amino-4-chloro-benzene-1,3-disulphonamide, *disulphamide* and *chlorthalidone*. They are chemically, related to the benzothiadiazines

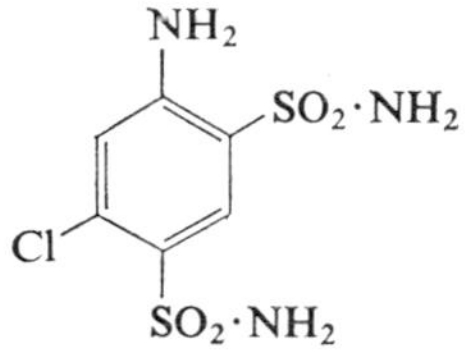

6-amino-4-chloro-benzene-
1,3-disulphonamide

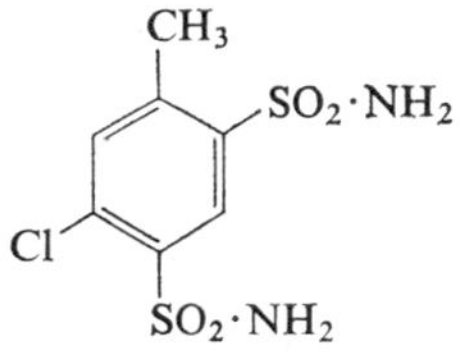

Disulphamide

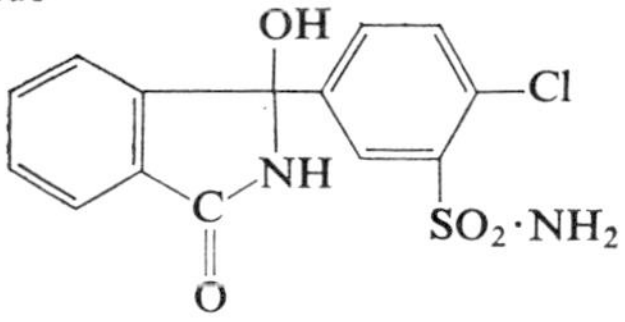

Chlorthalidone

and have similar actions, being intermediate in potency between chlorothiazide and hydrochlorothiazide. Benzothiadiazines substituted with an organic radical in the 3 position (e.g. bendrofluazide and trichlormethiazide, Table 34.2) spontaneously hydrolyse within the body fluids, with the production of a non-toxic aldehyde and 6-amino-4-chloro-benzene-1,3-disulphonamide. Both the parent compound and the metabolite are active diuretics.

Chlorthalidone is slowly absorbed from the gut and a single dose produces a prolonged diuretic effect lasting for 2 or 3 days. Carbonic anhydrase inhibition does not appear to be important in its action and potassium excretion is only slightly raised, the increased urine flow being accompanied chiefly by increased sodium and chloride excretion. The diuretic effect is not influenced by acidosis.

8. Frusemide. This substance is chemically related to the thiazides and to chlorthalidone. It produces a diuresis of very rapid onset but its action lasts for only about 4 h; it is active orally, intravenously or intramuscularly. Frusemide may be useful, under close supervision, when a rapid powerful action is required. The drug inhibits the reabsorption of sodium ions in the proximal tubule and in the ascending limb of the loop of Henle, but not in the distal tubule. High doses have been found, in animal experiments, to produce some inhibition of carbonic anhydrase, but this effect is probably not important with therapeutic doses. Potassium loss occurs and potassium supplements are necessary with long term treatment. The drug is excreted in both urine and faeces even after intravenous injection.

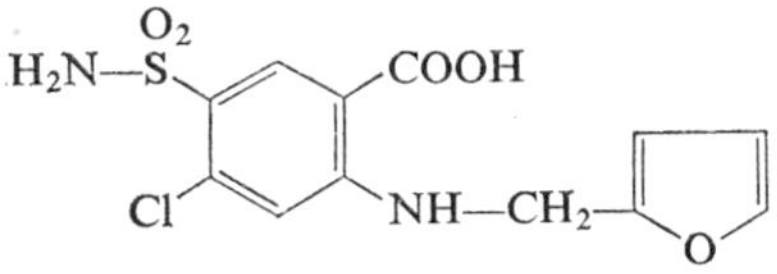

Frusemide

9. Ethacrynic acid. This substance is a very powerful diuretic which is active after oral or intravenous injection. It is especially useful in severely oedematous patients who do not respond well to other diuretics.

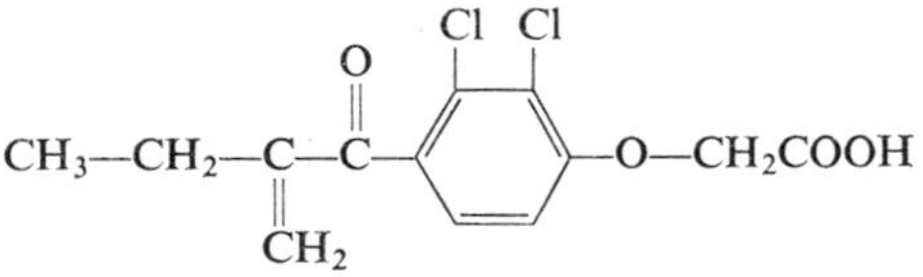

Ethacrynic acid

It is believed to act, like the mercurials, by inhibiting the sulphydryl groups of renal enzymes involved in the reabsorption of sodium ions. Unlike the mercurials, ethacrynic acid inhibits sodium reabsorption throughout the nephron including the ascending limb of the loop of Henle, and it is active in acidosis and in alkalosis. Chloride is the main anion accompanying the excess sodium ion loss and this is so whatever the acid-base balance. Unlike the thiazides, ethacrynic acid does not increase bicarbonate excretion during alkalosis. Potassium loss is variable but long-term use demands potassium replacement.

It is excreted in the bile and in the urine. Side-effects include electrolyte imbalance, hypotension, gastro-intestinal disturbances and possibly blood disorders.

10. Aldosterone antagonists. Some steroid lactones have been found to antagonize the action of aldosterone, and a spirolactone known as *spirono-*

lactone is used for this purpose in man. The effects of aldosterone on the distal tubules (page 345) are blocked by spironolactone so that sodium and chloride excretion are increased and water accompanies these ions; potassium, hydrogen and ammonium excretion are decreased. This is an unusual effect as most other diuretics increase potassium loss to some extent. The effect of spironolactone is determined by the extent to which sodium reabsorption is controlled by aldosterone. It is therefore ineffective in patients with untreated Addison's disease (page 380), and is of little value in oedema associated with pre-eclampsia of pregnancy in which aldosterone secretion is low. Spirono-lactone has been found useful in cases of primary aldosteronism, in nephrotic

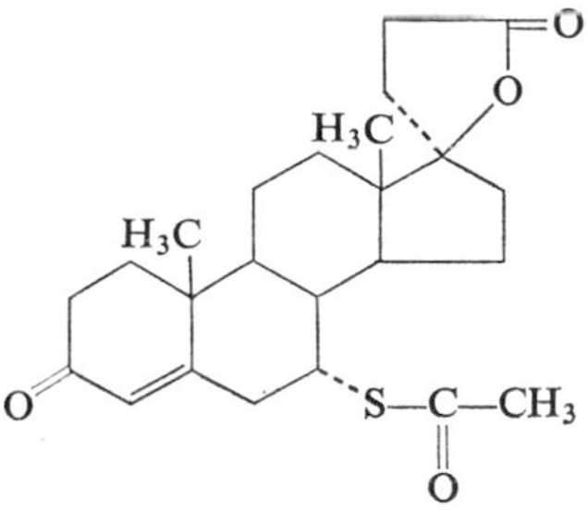

Spironolactone

oedema, and in hepatic cirrhosis, but it is of little benefit in cardiac oedema. It may be used in conjunction with other diuretics (e.g. benzothiadiazides and mercurials) to reduce excessive potassium loss. In the presence of spirono-lactone, the unrestricted loss of sodium ion in the distal tubule provokes a compensatory increase in aldosterone secretion from the adrenal cortex and this is accompanied by increased aldosterone excretion in the urine.

A steroid ($3\beta,16\alpha$-dihydroxy-allo-pregnan-20-one) isolated from the adrenal cortex of the pig has been shown to enhance sodium excretion and therefore opposes the action of aldosterone. The steroid, which has been synthesized, may provide the prototype for a new type of diuretic drug.

11. Triamterene. This compound is administered only by the oral route. It is not a very powerful diuretic and is usually used in conjunction with other diuretics. It inhibits the reabsorption of sodium ions probably by a direct action on the tubular enzymes, and the urine contains increased amounts of sodium and chloride ions. It remains effective in adrenalectomized animals and its mechanism of action is therefore independent of aldosterone, although it was originally thought to be an aldosterone antagonist. Unlike most other diuretics, it does not cause potassium loss and in some conditions may reduce it by an action in the distal tubule. Triamterene contains a pteridine nucleus and may therefore interfere with the actions of folic acid which also contains pteridine (page 35).

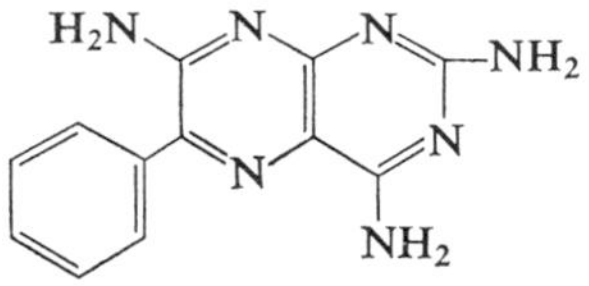

Triamterene

It is especially useful when administered in conjunction with the thiazide diuretics because it diminishes the excessive potassium loss produced by these agents alone.

12. Potassium salts. Although they act as osmotic diuretics (see below), potassium salts also act by more specific mechanisms. In the distal tubule, potassium competes with hydrogen to exchange for sodium which is reabsorbed (page 345). When excess potassium is available, acidification of the urine is diminished and an alkaline urine is produced. Some of the administered potassium ion exchanges for sodium ion in the oedema fluid and the urine contains increased quantities of sodium. In addition, administration of potassium salts appears to dilate renal blood vessels thereby increasing kidney blood flow. Potassium salts administered to man include the chloride, bicarbonate, nitrate, citrate and acetate but they are rarely used as diuretics.

Drugs decreasing sodium reabsorption by indirect mechanisms

1. Osmotic diuretics. The intravenous administration of a hypertonic solution of any solute filtered by the glomerulus may produce an osmotic diuresis when the amount delivered to the tubules exceeds their reabsorptive capacity. The dissolved compound in the tubular fluid exerts an osmotic pressure which is additive with that of the solutes already present. Water reabsorption in the proximal tubules is therefore reduced and sodium and chloride reabsorption retarded. The high rate of tubular urine flow interferes in some way with the distal concentrating mechanisms, anti-diuretic hormone being inactive under these conditions, and this further increases the urine volume. Similar effects are produced by solutes reaching the blood from the gastro-intestinal tract, and to be clinically useful an osmotic diuretic should be orally active. The diuresis associated with diabetes mellitus is the result of the osmotic effect of the high blood glucose.

Osmotic diuretics are rarely used nowadays. Compounds which have been used in the past include urea, mannitol and glucose. Glucose is still occasionally used to dehydrate the tissues in cerebral oedema, and mannitol is sometimes used to measure glomerular filtration rate. Intramuscular injection of hypertonic magnesium sulphate solutions has been recommended for use in eclampsia of pregnancy. Magnesium salts exert an anticonvulsant action as well as an osmotic diuretic effect.

2. Inhibitors of aldosterone secretion. The compounds amphenone B and metyrapone are referred to on pages 859–860. Amphenone B inhibits a number of enzymes concerned with steroid synthesis but is too toxic for clinical use. Metyrapone has been found to be more specific and less toxic. Metyrapone inhibits the enzyme concerned with 11-hydroxylation of the steroid nucleus so that secretion of cortisol, corticosterone and aldosterone is inhibited while that of the 11-deoxysteroids is increased (pages 377–378 and 859). Diminished sodium reabsorption and diuresis accompanies the diminished secretion of aldosterone. However, the effect is short-lived because diminished cortisol secretion stimulates the production of pituitary ACTH which then increases the liberation of the 11-deoxysteroids from the adrenal. In high concentration, one of these (deoxycorticosterone) has the same effect on sodium reabsorption as has aldosterone, and therefore the diuretic effect is reduced unless pituitary ACTH secretion is inhibited by simultaneous administration of prednisolone. Metyrapone is still in the experimental stage but in the future drugs of this type may have a limited use in the treatment of severe oedemas associated with excessive aldosterone secretion. Metyrapone is mainly used as a diagnostic aid in the determination of pituitary function.

Drugs which increase the filtered load of sodium chloride

1. Acidifying salts. Acidifying salts which have been used as oral diuretics include ammonium chloride, ammonium nitrate and calcium chloride. After absorption of ammonium chloride, the liver converts the ammonium ion to urea which is partly excreted (exerting an osmotic diuretic effect) and partly reabsorbed. The chloride ion displaces bicarbonate ion which is converted first to carbonic acid and then to carbon dioxide and water. The carbon dioxide is eliminated in the lungs. Thus there is a loss of blood buffer in exchange for chloride; that is, an acidosis is produced. Since ammonium ions are converted to urea and chloride replaces bicarbonate, there is no change in total ion content but only a change in the proportion of chloride. Increased chloride ion, with accompanying cation (mainly sodium) is therefore filtered in the glomeruli and an appreciably greater amount escapes reabsorption with an osmotic equivalent of water. Thus sodium ion and oedema water are mobilized and excreted. However, the diuresis lasts only for a short time and is greatest on the first day of treatment. During the second and third days of treatment, sodium loss is restricted by the removal of potassium from cells and calcium from bone, these cations replacing the sodium. During the fourth and fifth days, the tubules secrete hydrogen ion in exchange for sodium ion which is reabsorbed. As the pH of the urine falls, the ammonium mechanism of the tubular cells comes into play (page 346) and by the sixth day the ammonium chloride excreted begins to equal the amount absorbed, and the diuretic effect is lost. A similar mechanism accounts for the diuresis produced by ammonium nitrate; eventually the amount excreted equals the amount absorbed. After administration of calcium chloride, some of the calcium is removed in the faeces as phosphate or carbonate and some is absorbed and incorporated into bone. The absorbed chloride ion displaces bicarbonate and the situation is then similar to that produced by ammonium chloride.

Acidifying diuretics should be used only in cycles and discontinued when compensation is achieved. Their main use is in conjunction with mercurials. They should not be used when there is kidney damage as the kidneys may be incapable of compensating for the acidosis, and acidaemia and death may result.

2. Glucocorticoids and corticotrophin. The glucocorticoids (page 378) and corticotrophin (page 362) influence renal mechanisms in a number of ways, and may be used partly to restore water and electrolyte balance in certain pathological conditions including Addison's disease, protein deficiency oedema, and nephrosis. Cortisol-like steroids increase glomerular filtration rate and renal blood flow, thereby augmenting urine flow. There is also evidence that they depress the release of antidiuretic hormone from the neurohypophysis and hasten its disappearance from the circulation. In Addison's disease and in protein deficiency oedema, there is an abnormal delay in the elimination of imbibed water, probably because there is an excessive transfer of water from the extracellular to the intracellular compartment. Glucocorticoids counteract this tendency, maintaining the extracellular fluid volume.

In nephrotic patients, glucocorticoids and corticotrophin decrease the renal protein loss and increase the plasma albumin, thereby mobilizing oedema fluid and augmenting the diuresis. It has been suggested that the nephrotic syndrome is the result of an auto-immune reaction. Glucocorticoids and corticotrophin probably depress the formation of some antibodies and may benefit nephrotic patients by interfering with the antigen–antibody reaction.

In large doses, the glucocorticoids exert mineralocorticoid action and treatment of nephrotic oedema with these steroids may therefore result in sodium retention and excessive potassium loss. Some of the synthetic analogues (prednisone, prednisolone, triamcinolone and dexamethasone) possess relatively more pronounced glucocorticoid activity, and their use may therefore be preferable to that of the naturally occurring glucocorticoids and corticotrophin.

3. Plasma expanders. These are high molecular weight substances which act as substitutes for plasma proteins. They include *human serum albumin, dextran* and *methylcellulose.* By increasing plasma colloid osmotic pressure in conditions such as cirrhosis of the liver, nephrotic oedema and kwashiorkor, they should mobilize oedema fluid and promote diuresis. However, in these conditions, the cell protein stores are frequently so low that huge amounts of albumin or dextran are required. In cirrhosis, much of the plasma expander is lost into the ascitic fluid, and in nephrosis it rapidly passes through the damaged glomeruli so that the diuretic effect is transient. In general, treatment with the newer diuretic drugs is more successful.

Cation exchange resins

Although not diuretics, cation exchange resins may be used as adjuncts in the treatment of oedema. They are either carboxylic acid or sulphonic acid resins and they are administered by mouth to reduce the absorption of sodium from the intestine. Sodium ions in the ingested food are taken up by the resin, in exchange for ammonium or hydrogen ions, and are eliminated in the faeces. The ammonium or hydrogen ions, along with anion, are absorbed into the blood-stream so that the overall effect resembles that of acidifying salts such as ammonium chloride. An acidosis is produced and a strongly acid urine is excreted. Cation exchange resins, usually combined with mercurial diuretics, have been used in cardiac oedema, nephrosis and cirrhosis. They should not be used in cases where the kidney may be unable to compensate for the acidosis produced. The most serious side-effects usually arise from excessive depletion of sodium, potassium and calcium, and the administration of salts of these cations may be necessary to restore ionic balance.

Tests for diuretic action in animals

Animal tests have proved useful in the detection of potentially useful diuretics and in determining their mechanism of action, but they are of little value for assessing relative therapeutic potency in man. Final assessment must therefore be carried out in clinical trials on patients.

The species usually used are rats or dogs previously loaded with water or saline. Mercurials are relatively inactive in rats, and dogs are therefore more suitable when studying this type of diuretic. The effects of the drugs on the volume and ionic composition of the urine are determined. Experimental oedema may be produced in dogs by administering mineralocorticoids and the chlorides of sodium and potassium along with the water load. Experimental ascites in dogs and protein deficiency oedema in weanling rats have also been produced, and the effects of potential diuretics in relieving these conditions assessed. Tests to determine the mechanism of action include biochemical studies on enzymes in kidney slices, histochemical staining of tubular enzymes, and the technique of stop-flow analysis (page 341).

Antidiuretics

Drugs which reduce urine output are of little therapeutic value but several drugs used for other purposes may produce this effect. The antidiuretic hormone (vasopressin) is used in the treatment of diabetes insipidus. This is an example of hormonal replacement therapy and is described on page 368.

Drugs which produce an antidiuretic effect may act (1) by stimulating the release of ADH from the posterior lobe of the pituitary (e.g. nicotine, acetylcholine and morphine), (2) by reducing renal blood flow either through lowering the systemic arterial pressure (e.g. hexamethonium or isoprenaline) or by constricting the renal blood vessels (e.g. adrenaline or noradrenaline), (3) by delaying the absorption of water from the gut (e.g. ether) and (4) by reducing thirst and water intake (e.g. amphetamine).

CHAPTER 35

Drugs Acting on the Eye

Those aspects of the structure and the physiology of the eye which are important for understanding the actions of drugs are described on pages 412–424. The effects of drugs on the eye may be considered from two points of view. Firstly, the eye and the orbit contain autonomically innervated effector systems which are amenable to observation and which have thus proved useful in studying the mechanism of action of drugs. Secondly, there are the practical aspects of the use of drugs for the treatment of organic and infectious diseases of the eye, and for ophthalmological examination of the eye.

Administration of drugs to produce local effects on the eye. Most of the drugs which are given to facilitate ophthalmological examination of the eye, or for the treatment of diseases of the eye have marked effects elsewhere in the body when they are given systemically. However, drugs can be applied topically to the conjunctival surfaces, from which they may be absorbed through the cornea. Since it is required to achieve maximum absorption through the cornea relative to absorption into the blood vessels of the conjunctiva, the drug solution is placed in the lower conjunctival fornix and the patient is instructed to close his eyes and look downward. Drainage of the solution through the lacrimal ducts can be prevented by pressing with a finger on the inner canthus of the eye.

The cornea is penetrated more readily by non-polar drugs and by undissociated drug molecules than by ionized molecules. As long ago as 1884, Köller observed that the action of cocaine in anaesthetizing the rabbit's cornea was enhanced in alkaline solutions. Drugs which are partly dissociated in the range of pH of solvents which can be applied to the eye have their effects enhanced if the pH is adjusted to produce more of the undissociated form. Surface active compounds penetrate the cornea and enhance the penetration of drugs. The distribution of the drug between the vehicle and the cornea also affects penetration; this is one of the reasons for applying some drugs topically to the eye in oily solutions.

Solutions intended for application to the conjunctiva are called collyria. They should be sterile and isotonic. Hypotonic solutions cause some oedema of the cornea with the result that it may become turbid and impair vision. Absorption of drugs dissolved in hypertonic solution is impaired and the solution tends to withdraw water from the surface of the eye. The pH should be within the range 6·6 to 9 to avoid irritation. Aqueous solutions intended as vehicles for drugs may be made with sodium chloride, often with sodium phosphate as a pH buffer, or tonicity and pH may be adjusted simply by using sodium borate or sodium bicarbonate solutions. Drugs may also be introduced into the conjunctival sac by impregnating them onto thin gelatin discs called lamellae.

Parasympathomimetic and anticholinesterase drugs (Chapter 28). Acetylcholine, injected intravenously, contracts the smooth muscle of the constrictor pupillae and the ciliary body, thus diminishing the pupil diameter and allowing the lens to bulge so that it is focused for near vision. However, these changes occur only when doses of acetylcholine large enough to produce marked changes in blood pressure are given. Section and degeneration of the parasympathetic nerves to the eye leads to a large increase in sensitivity of the pupil and ciliary muscle to injected acetylcholine. The effect of injected acetylcholine on the intra-ocular pressure is complicated. The increase in filtration angle caused by contraction of the pupil has little consequence for the normal eye; dilatation of blood vessels within the eyeball tends to increase intra-ocular pressure, but the fall in systemic blood pressure tends to diminish it.

Other structures of the orbit which respond to acetylcholine are the lacrimal glands, from which secretion is induced, and the nictitating membrane, which is contracted. The effect on the nictitating membrane is interesting because its smooth mucle is believed not to be innervated by cholinergic nerve fibres. These actions of acetylcholine are potentiated by physostigmine and blocked by atropine.

The actions of injected acetylcholine on the eye are of academic interest but have no application in medicine. Similar effects are produced by the other parasympathomimetic drugs.

Acetylcholine applied to the conjunctiva has no miotic action because it is so rapidly destroyed by cholinesterase. It is poorly absorbed through the cornea because of its ionized quaternary nitrogen group. *Carbachol* (page 705), being immune from destruction by cholinesterases, does have a miotic action after conjunctival instillation. Solutions or ointments containing 1 % carbachol may be used for reducing intra-ocular pressure in glaucoma. *Furtrethonium* (page 705) acts like carbachol in relieving glaucoma, but it is reported to cause damage to the eye if used continually. *Pilocarpine* (page 703) is a tertiary amine, and is readily absorbed through the cornea. It is given in a 1% solution, or in a lamella. It produces miosis and cycloplegia, and, in patients with glaucoma, it causes a decrease in intra-ocular pressure.

Anticholinesterase drugs constrict the pupil. They act by preventing the destruction of acetylcholine liberated from the parasympathetic nerve endings. When conduction through the ciliary ganglia and along the ciliary nerves has been blocked by an injection of procaine behind the eyeball, the anticholinesterases are not miotic, although carbachol and pilocarpine, which act directly on the smooth muscle, retain their activity. The miotic action of *physostigmine* (page 714) was discovered by Fraser in 1863, long before it was established that it acted to prevent hydrolysis of acetylcholine.

Anticholinesterase drugs are used in the treatment of glaucoma and to reverse the effects of atropine and related drugs which have been given as mydriatics for ophthalmological examination. In glaucoma they reduce the intra-ocular pressure by widening the filtration angle, thus allowing easier access of the aqueous humour into the canal of Schlemm where it is resorbed. After the use of atropine-like drugs, they correct the dilatation of the pupil and reduce the rise in intra-ocular pressure should this have occurred. It has been found that physostigmine is much better for this purpose than carbachol or pilocarpine. The basis for this is that carbachol and pilocarpine can produce miosis in the presence of atropine only when in a sufficient concentration to overcome the competitive blockade of receptors by atropine. However, acetylcholine liberated from the parasympathetic nerve endings, when its destruction is prevented by physostigmine, can readily accumulate in sufficient quantities because the changes produced by atropine (dilatation of the pupil and inability to focus on near objects) reflexly induce a rapid rate of discharge of acetylcholine from the nerves. Physostigmine is instilled into conjunctiva as a 0·5 to 1% solution, or in a lamella containing 0·065 mg. Its miotic action begins within 5 min and persists for about 12 h. *Neostigmine* (in a 3·5% solution) has actions and uses similar to those of physostigmine. The stronger solution of neostigmine is necessary because, being a quaternary ammonium compound, it is less readily absorbed than physostigmine.

Dyflos (page 719) has a longer lasting action in inhibiting cholinesterase. It is unstable in aqueous solution and is given in arachis oil as a 0·1% solution. Usually only one drop is given daily and the effects of a single application may persist for more than 2 weeks. Because of its persistence of action and the occasional unpleasant side-effects it may cause, dyflos is used only in severe cases which are not adequately treated by other drugs. *Echothiophate* is another organophosphorus anticholinesterase (a phosphostigmine, page 716) which is occasionally used in the treatment of glaucoma. It has the advantage over dyflos that it is relatively stable in aqueous solution. A 0·1–0·25% solution is instilled once or twice weekly.

$$C_2H_5O \diagdown \underset{C_2H_5O \diagup}{\overset{\diagup O}{P}} \diagdown SCH_2CH_2\overset{+}{N}(CH_3)_3 \qquad I^-$$

Echothiophate

The side effects of anticholinesterases used locally to treat glaucoma include the following: twitching of the eyelids and the extraocular muscles; blurred distant vision, since they produce spasm of the ciliary muscle; pain, probably arising from the smooth muscle thrown into spasm; and headache.

A combination of a parasympathomimetic drug and an anticholinesterase drug is often used in the treatment of glaucoma. Anticholinesterases are more active than the parasympathomimetics in causing contraction of the ciliary muscle relative to miosis.

Atropine and related drugs (pages 723–730). *Atropine* blocks the actions of acetylcholine on the smooth muscle of the constrictor pupillae and the ciliary body. These muscles are innervated by parasympathetic nerves, hence atropine paralyses them, producing a passive mydriasis and cycloplegia (the pupil is fully dilated and the lens focused for distant vision). The filtration angle in the anterior chamber is narrowed and this causes a rise in intra-ocular pressure by hindering absorption of aqueous humour from the canal of Schlemm. In patients with glaucoma, or a predisposition to glaucoma (which includes all patients over 40 years of age), the rise in intra-ocular pressure may cause severe damage. Drugs which are both mydriatic and cycloplegic are used not only to dilate the pupil and relax the lens to facilitate ophthalmological examination, but also to break up adhesions between the iris and the lens in inflammatory conditions. The passive mydriasis produced by atropine-like drugs may be potentiated by giving them together with mydriatics such as cocaine or ephedrine, which actively contract the dilator pupillae.

Atropine solutions containing 0·5 to 2% of the drug are instilled into the conjunctiva. The effects are fully developed in about an hour, and they then persist for several days. The long-lasting disturbance of vision is a disadvantage. Sufficient atropine may be absorbed through the mucous membranes of the conjunctiva and the nose (after passage through the naso-lacrimal ducts) to produce systemic effects.

Homatropine is more usually used for ophthalmological investigation of the eye since the persistence of its effect is much less than with atropine. It has qualitatively the same actions as atropine, but it is less potent. Children are often resistant to the cycloplegic action of homatropine. *Eucatropine* is about as potent as homatropine as a mydriatic, but it is only weakly cycloplegic. Its persistence is less than that of homatropine. *Lachesine* (1% solution) produces a slowly developing mydriasis persisting from 5 to 6 h. It does not give rise to irritation of the conjunctiva and is used to replace atropine, homatropine and hyoscine should patients develop idiosyncrasy to these drugs. *Dibutoline* is both mydriatic and cycloplegic. Its persistence is similar to that of homatropine. It is surface active and this results in promotion of absorption into the anterior chamber and also confers antiseptic properties. However, it is slightly irritant. *Cyclopentolate* rapidly produces mydriasis and cycloplegia. Its effects wear off rather more rapidly than do those of homatropine. *Hyoscine* is more potent than atropine as a mydriatic and cycloplegic after systemic administration and has about 6 times the potency of atropine in causing mydriasis with relatively less cycloplegia. Its effects do not last as long as those of atropine.

Intra-ocular pressure. Drugs which act to alter the calibre of blood vessels produce changes in the intra-ocular pressure through their effect on blood vessels. However, the effect on the eye also depends on the change in systemic blood pressure that the drug may produce. Thus, *noradrenaline* applied locally constricts the blood vessels inside the eyeball and reduces intra-ocular pressure, but noradrenaline given systemically has little effect on the blood vessels of the eye and the rise in blood pressure results in an increase in intra-ocular pressure. *Amyl nitrite* dilates blood vessels and causes a fall in systemic pressure, however the blood vessels of the eye are particularly sensitive to amyl nitrite and their dilatation results in a rise in intra-ocular pressure despite the fall in systemic blood pressure.

Although the vascular effects of drugs are important in affecting intra-ocular pressure, other effects, such as alteration of the filtration angle or spasm of the striated or smooth muscle of the orbit, usually dominate in determining intra-ocular pressure.

Recently glaucoma has been treated with *carbonic anhydrase inhibitors*. The reduction of intra-ocular pressure is due to a reduced formation of aqueous humour. This observation strongly supports the evidence that at least part of the formation of aqueous humour can be accounted for by active secretion. *Acetazolamide* (page 879) was the first of this group to be used in the treatment of glaucoma. *Ethoxzolamide*, *dichlorphenamide* and *methazolamide* have also been found useful. They are given systemically as they are ineffective when applied to the conjunctiva.

Neuromuscular blocking drugs. During surgery of the extra-ocular muscles (to correct squint), tubocurarine is used as a relaxant. The fibres of the extra-ocular muscles are multiply-innervated (see page 207) and are contracted by neuromuscular blocking drugs of the depolarizing type such as decamethonium and suxamethonium: they share this property with other multiply innervated striated muscles such as the frog's rectus abdominis and certain avian muscles (page 674). Suxamethonium may produce an increase in intra-ocular pressure as a result of this action.

Sympathomimetic drugs. Injections of noradrenaline and other sympatho-mimetic amines produce the following effects on the eye and its associated structures. Mydriasis is produced as a result of contraction of the dilator pupillae. The nictitating membrane is retracted. The smooth muscle of the eyelids is contracted, resulting in widening of the palpebral fissure. The effects on intra-ocular pressure depend on the relative changes in systemic blood pressure and vasoconstriction in the eyeball. Solutions of sympathomimetic amines applied topically to the eye constrict the blood vessels resulting in blanching of the conjunctiva. This reduces the absorption of drugs from the conjunctival sac into the blood and so limits the systemic actions. Sympathomimetics which penetrate the cornea act within the eyeball to cause mydriasis and a reduction in intra-ocular pressure by constricting the blood vessels, thus reducing the rate of formation of aqueous humour.

The actions of noradrenaline and adrenaline on the eye are potentiated in the presence of *cocaine*. Cocaine alone instilled into the conjunctiva has a mydriatic action and constricts the blood vessels of the conjunctiva, probably by potentiating the effects of noradrenaline released from the sympathetic nerve endings (see also page 774 for discussion of relationship between cocaine and sympathomimetic amines). In addition, cocaine acts as a local anaesthetic on the sensory nerves of the conjunctival surfaces (see below).

The actions of noradrenaline and adrenaline are also enhanced in animals pretreated with reserpine (see page 774) and in the eye which has been sympathetically denervated by removal of the superior cervical ganglion. Noradrenaline is potentiated more than adrenaline by cocaine, by reserpine treatment and by sympathetic denervation. Indirectly-acting sympathomimetic amines such as amphetamine and ephedrine have their actions diminished by these three procedures.

All of the actions of sympathomimetic amines on the eye can be blocked by anti-adrenaline drugs of the α-receptor blocking group. For example, ergotamine and ergotoxine may be absorbed through the cornea in sufficient concentrations to block the mydriatic response to sympathomimetic amines and to stimulation of the sympathetic nerves. Conjunctival instillation of ergotamine produces contraction of the pupil.

The mydriasis caused by sympathomimetics can be abolished by stimulating the opposing smooth muscle, the constrictor pupillae, with miotic drugs. In ophthalmological practice the mydriasis produced by ephedrine to facilitate examination of the eye is counteracted and terminated by instilling 1% pilocarpine solution.

Mydriasis can be produced by sympathomimetic amines and by cocaine which act by contracting the dilator pupillae, and by atropine and related drugs which have an anti-muscarinic action and which act by preventing the contraction of the constrictor pupillae. The differences in the actions of a typical drug from each group are summarized in Table 35.1.

TABLE 35.1. Differences between types of mydriatic drugs.

Phenylephrine	Homatropine
Contraction of dilator pupillae	Paralysis of constrictor pupillae
Mimics response to stimulation of sympathetic nerves	Blocks response to stimulation of parasympathetic nerves
Pupillary light reflex persists	Pupillary light reflex absent
No effect on ciliary muscle	Blockade of response of ciliary muscle to parasympathetic nerves. Cycloplegia
Intra-ocular pressure not raised, but may be lowered because of constriction of blood vessels in eyeball	Intra-ocular pressure may be raised because the filtration angle is narrowed
Moderate dilation of pupil, usually not sufficient for refraction in children but safe in adults over 40 years old	Marked dilation of pupil, which may be further enhanced by addition of a sympathomimetic amine or cocaine for refraction in children. Risk of dangerous increase in intraocular pressure where tendency to glaucoma exists, e.g. in adults over 40

A 1% solution of *adrenaline* applied to the conjunctiva helps to control bleeding in eye surgery. It causes mydriasis of a few hours duration. Eyedrops containing adrenaline and zinc sulphate are used to treat inflammation of the conjunctiva. *Phenylephrine* instilled into the conjunctiva in solutions containing 0·5 to 10% is used to dilate the pupils and to produce a temporary lowering of the intraocular pressure. Solutions over 2% in strength are irritant and a local anaesthetic is used to protect against this. *Ephedrine* (2 to 5% solution) produces mydriasis in 15 to 30 min and its actions persist for 4 to 12 h. Ephedrine is ineffective as a mydriatic when the iris is inflamed, and it is less effective on heavily pigmented than on lightly pigmented eyes. It has been reported to be virtually inactive as a mydriatic in negroes and asiatics. Observations on this difference in response are mentioned on pages 542–543. *Amphetamine* instilled into the conjunctiva in a 1% solution is effective as a mydriatic, but it is seldom used. A derivative, hydroxyamphetamine, is used as a 1 to 4% solution; it gives a mydriasis lasting 3 to 4 hr. *Naphazoline* is a sympathomimetic drug which is a derivative of imidazoline. It is used in a 0·1% solution as a conjunctival decongestant and mild mydriatic.

Cocaine in solutions containing 1 to 4% is used as a mydriatic especially when there is an advantage in producing anaesthesia of the conjunctiva.

29

Drugs acting on ganglion cells

GANGLIONIC STIMULANTS. The effects of systemically administered *nicotine* on the pupil vary among different species. The response observed probably depends on the balance between the actions of nicotine on the central nervous system, on the ciliary and superior cervical ganglia, on the iris itself, and in increasing circulating catecholamines. In man, there is at first constriction, followed by dilatation. Nicotine also causes contraction of the ciliary muscle, retraction of the nictitating membrane and of the eyelids, contraction of the extra-ocular muscles and lacrimation. All of these effects can be ascribed to stimulation of autonomic ganglion cells. Nicotine applied topically causes first miosis and then mydriasis in most species of animal. Tobacco amblyopia is a rather rare disease in which the field of vision is constricted and colour vision is disturbed. It is thought to be due to the constriction of retinal blood vessels by nicotine, and the symptoms are said to be relieved by giving vasodilator drugs, such as the nitrites. There is some doubt whether tobacco is concerned in the production of this disease, since the incidence has diminished although tobacco consumption has increased.

GANGLIONIC BLOCKING DRUGS. In patients treated with ganglion blocking drugs to relieve hypertension, transmission through the ciliary ganglia is blocked so that accommodation is paralysed (near objects cannot be focused). The pupil is usually slightly dilated because blockade of the relatively greater parasympathetic tone has a greater consequence than blockade of the sympathetic tone.

In animals, ganglion blocking drugs produce mydriasis and relaxation of the nictitating membrane.

Adrenergic neurone-blocking drugs. In animals these drugs produce relaxation of the nictitating membrane, but do not change, or reduce, the pupil diameter. The palpebral fissure is narrowed. Patients being treated with these drugs for hypertension do not suffer from defects in vision as a side-effect. Topically applied guanethidine has been used successfully in the treatment of glaucoma.

Local anaesthetics. Blockade of the sensory nerve endings in the conjunctiva and the anterior chamber of the eye is required to relieve the irritation and pain of local infections and inflammation, to facilitate the removal of foreign bodies, for surgery and during ophthalmological examinations, particularly tonometry (measurement of the intra-ocular pressure) which is a painful procedure. Small amounts of a local anaesthetic on the cornea help people to become accustomed to wearing contact lenses.

The anaesthesia of the cornea produced by instillation of cocaine into the conjunctival sac was first reported by Köller in Vienna in 1884. One drop of a

2 % solution of cocaine rapidly produces complete insensibility of the cornea. In addition, the local application of cocaine produces mydriasis (see above) and constriction of conjunctival blood vessels. The surface of the eye becomes dry and this may result in damage to the corneal surface. The intra-ocular pressure is slightly reduced, probably because the blood vessels inside the eyeball are constricted. The palpebral fissure may be widened.

Instillation of a solution containing 0·5 to 4 % of cocaine produces anaesthesia of the cornea in 5 to 10 min and which persists for 1 or 2 h.

The local anaesthetic drugs that are not used by instillation into the conjunctiva are those that do not penetrate well into mucous membranes (e.g. procaine), and those that are too irritant to the conjunctiva (e.g. amylocaine). Procaine is given by infiltration into the conjunctiva, or is injected into the orbital cavity to block the nerves supplying the eyeball.

The corneal anaesthetics that are most commonly used are the following. They all differ from cocaine in that they do not cause mydriasis or blanching of the conjunctiva. *Amethocaine* (0·25 to 1 %), produces almost immediate anaesthesia persisting for 2 to 3 h: *butacaine* (1 to 2 %) acts in a few minutes and its effect persists for about 2 h; it may cause congestion of the conjunctiva; *cinchocaine* (0·1 to 0·2 %) has a slow onset of action which persists for 3 to 4 h: *phenacaine* (1 %) acts in 1 to 10 min and persists for about 1 h; it causes some congestion of the conjunctiva, but it has the advantage of possessing a bactericidal action: *oxybuprocaine* (0·4 %) which acts in 1 min and persists for ½ to 1 h, also has a bactericidal action and does not irritate the conjunctiva: *proxymetacaine* (0·5 %) acts immediately and its effects wear off in 10 to 20 min.

Morphine and related analgesics. A well-known symptom of morphine intoxication in man is pin-point pupils and the intra-ocular pressure is lowered in both normal and glaucomatous eyes. Constriction of the pupil does not occur when morphine is instilled into the conjunctival sac; the effect is due to an action on the central nervous system, and it is abolished by cutting the ciliary nerve or by atropine applied locally or systemically. The miotic action of morphine is partly the result of enhancement of the pupillary light reflex but some additional effect is produced even in complete darkness. The effect is believed to be produced by stimulation of the cell bodies in the nucleus of the IIIrd cranial nerve (the oculomotor, page 93, which includes the cell bodies of the parasympathetic neurones innervating the eye) in the midbrain. However, the stimulant effect on the IIIrd nucleus may be an indirect one arising from depression of inhibitory fibres which arise in the cortex and synapse in the IIIrd nucleus (i.e. a dis-inhibition rather than a direct stimulation). This conclusion is based on the finding that removal of the cerebral cortex in dogs abolishes the miotic effect of morphine. The miotic action of morphine is shared by most of the potent analgesics which can be used to replace morphine, with the exception of those in the pethidine group. These exceptions may be explained by the atropine-like activity of pethidine and its congeners. The effects of morphine on the pupil vary with species. For example, in cats and monkeys, morphine produces mydriasis.

Conjunctival irritants. *Ethylmorphine* has, in general, the same actions as codeine (page 636). However it has an especial use in ophthalmological practice. Application of ethylmorphine to the conjunctiva causes at first a sharp burning sensation. This irritation induces dilatation of vascular and lymphatic channels, marked oedema of the conjunctiva and swelling of the eyelids. There is complete recovery from these effects. They are induced in order to speed up the healing of corneal ulcers, to clear corneal keratinization and to treat infections of the cornea and anterior chamber.

Ether has an irritant action on the conjunctiva. Instillation of oil into the conjunctiva gives protection against this during anaesthesia.

Tear gases cause irritation of the conjunctiva and produce a reflex secretion of tears and spasm of the eyelid. They are known as lacrimators.

The tear gas most commonly used in police actions to break up civil disturbances is chloroacetophenone (CAP).

It produces lacrimation in a concentration of 0·5 mg per cubic metre of air. The lacrimation clears up in an hour or so and within 12 h the signs of irritation have worn off. It may cause permanent damage if high concentrations are used.

Other war gases which have pronounced lacrimator activity relative to their other actions are bromobenzylcyanide (BBC) and phenylcarbylamine chloride (PCC).

Bromobenzylcyanide   Phenylcarbylamine chloride

Organic chemicals with marked lacrimator actions include: bromo- and chloro- derivatives of benzene, xylene, acetone and other ketones; chlorosulphonates; bromoacetic and iodoacetic ether; acrolein, which is formed from fats decomposed by excessive heat, for example, during cooking. Some of these chemicals, including acrolein, have been employed in warfare. The conjunctival irritation caused by vapours from onion and garlic is due to volatile oils containing organic sulphides.

Treatment of eye infections. Antibiotics are the newest of the drugs used to treat infections of the eye. Despite their efficacy in treating infectious diseases, many of the older forms of treatment are more suitable for certain eye conditions.

ANTIBIOTICS. In infections confined to the conjunctiva of the eyelids or cornea, antibiotics are applied topically. Frequent applications are necessary to maintain effective concentrations because the antibiotics are diluted and washed out of the eye by lacrimal secretion, particularly since some antibiotics are prone to cause irritation. The presence of pus or inflammatory exudates render the antibiotics less effective, and these should be removed first. The antibiotics are comparatively ineffective against deep infections of the orbit or infections inside the eyeball. Local injections of antibiotics are given into the conjunctiva, behind the bulb, or even into the eyeball. Systemic administration of anti-antibiotics requires large doses since they do not readily penetrate the eye tissues.

Penicillin is used in eye-drops or ointments containing 20,000 to 100,000 units per ml (or per g). A disadvantage in using penicillin for local, topical administration is that it frequently results in a sensitization with dangerous consequences should penicillin be injected subsequently. There is also the risk of establishing penicillin resistant strains of bacteria.

Chloramphenicol in concentrations of 1 to 10 mg/ml is used topically for treating superficial infections of the eye with organisms resistant to other antibiotics. Chloramphenicol has the additional advantage that it penetrates into the bulb better than do other antibiotics, although less well than does sulphacetamide.

Streptomycin in eye-drops containing 0·25% may be used for treating infections caused by penicillin-resistant forms. It is not absorbed through the cornea, except when there has been extensive abrading. Its use may lead to contact sensitivity of the conjunctiva.

Tetracyclines. Chlortetracycline or oxytetracycline in drops or ointments containing 0·5 to 1% are used in eye infections; they are particularly useful because of their broad spectrum of activity. Bacitracin is applied topically in concentrations of 250 to 1000 units per ml or per g in drops and ointments. Its advantages are that its antibiotic activity is not diminished in the presence of pus or exudates, and it does not readily cause sensitization.

SULPHONAMIDES. Certain sulphonamides are administered systemically or topically for the treatment of eye infections.

Those sulphonamides that are given by injection or that are well absorbed after oral administration diffuse from the blood-stream into the aqueous humour. Absorption through the cornea after topical application to the conjunctiva is less efficient. The limitation of the sulphonamides for topical application in the treatment of eye infections is that few of them are sufficiently soluble to achieve a strength adequate to effect absorption of significant quantities. Solutions of the more soluble sodium salts usually have a pH above that which can be tolerated on the cornea. The sulphonamides are prone to cause sensitivity, particularly when given locally and some of them actually impair tissue healing. However *sulphacetamide sodium* is valuable for use on the eye. It is readily soluble and the solution can be buffered; sometimes sulphacetamide, as the acid, is used to buffer the solution. A solution containing 3·5% is isotonic, and up to 5% does not cause pain. Stronger solutions, up to 30%, cause burning and stinging, but this can usually be tolerated.

Maphenide (*p*-amino-methylbenzenesulphonamide hydrochloride) is very soluble, not irritant, and does not impair wound healing. It is used in eye-drops as a 5% solution.

ANTISEPTICS. Organic chemicals used as antiseptics for ophthalmological application include chlorbutol, proflavine, organic mercurials (phenylmercuric salts, thimersal, nitromersal and mercurochrome). Benzalkonium chloride is also used, it has an additional advantage in that it is surface active and promotes the penetration of drugs through the cornea.

Fluorescein has a special application in ophthalmological examination. It does not stain undamaged corneal epithelium, but if the surface is ulcerated or scarred by foreign bodies the damaged regions stain green. Two of the coloured antiseptics, proflavine and mercurochrome, have also been used to detect corneal damage.

Inorganic antiseptics. Silver nitrate solutions (0·2 to 1%) and colloidal preparations containing silver complexes were formerly used extensively for the treatment of conjunctivitis. In some states of the U.S.A. it was compulsory by law to bathe the eyes of new-born infants with silver nitrate as prophylaxis against *ophthalmia neonatorum*. The use of sulphonamides and antibiotics has rendered obsolete the use of silver in ophthalmological practice.

Compounds of mercury are used as antiseptics in the treatment of conjunctivitis and blepharitis (inflammation of the margins of the eye-lids). They have an irritant action: the most strongly irritant, the red mercuric oxide, is not used, but the milder irritant action of others such as the yellow allotrope of mercuric oxide is exploited to promote healing of corneal ulcers. They are also used as disinfectants in ophthalmological solutions.

Boric acid, sodium borate and sodium propionate are mild antiseptics used for preparing eye lotions.

ANTI-INFLAMMATORY DRUGS. The property of glucocorticoids in suppressing inflammation and allergic reactions is of value in the symptomatic treatment of some diseases of the eye. However, the underlying cause of the disease must also be treated, otherwise serious and permanent damage may be done in return for the temporary relief of the symptoms. The glucocorticoids are especially valuable when the symptoms of the disease cause loss of visual acuity, such as the keratinization of the cornea in syphilitic infections of the eye, and the opacities of the lens and of the vitreous body which arise from infection by various pathogens.

Inflammatory exudates from the structures within the bulb may cause a rise in intra-ocular pressure: this form of glaucoma can be controlled with the glucocorticoids. In other forms of glaucoma, the corticosteroids cause an increase in intra-ocular pressure.

Injury to one eye, whether accidental or as the result of ophthalmological surgery, often has as its sequel inflammatory changes in the other eye which may be so severe as to cause blindness. This condition is known as sympathetic ophthalmia. The explanation of this condition may be provided by an experiment reported by Dale. Extracts of the lens taken from the eye of a guinea-pig were injected into the same animal. Some weeks later an extract of the lens from the other eye was injected and the guinea-pig died with the symptoms of anaphylactic shock. Translating this experiment to the condition of sympathetic ophthalmia, injury to one eye may result in the appearance of antigens from the structures in that eye entering the bloodstream and stimulating the production of specific antibodies. In turn, these antibodies may pass into the other eye and there produce an anaphylactic inflammation. At one time sympathetic ophthalmia was prevented by promptly removing the injured eye if it seemed likely that the damage would result in loss of sight; in this way the sight of the uninjured eye was preserved. Removal of the injured eye after the beginning of sympathetic ophthalmia was useless—both eyes lost their sight. Now, the inflammatory and allergic changes are controlled with the glucocorticoids.

The glucocorticoids that are used in ophthalmological applications may be applied topically, injected into the conjunctiva, or given systemically. For topical applications, cortisone or hydrocortisone in concentrations of 0·5 to 2·5% or prednisone or prednisolone in concentration of 0·25 to 0·5% are used in drops or ointments.

Antihistamines. Relief of the symptoms of allergic conjunctivitis may be obtained with antihistamines given systemically or topically. Antazoline is the one most usually used for local application. Its advantages are that it is less irritating to the tissues than most of the others. It also produces local anaesthesia of the cornea. It is sometimes used together with a vasoconstrictor drug such as naphazoline to give enhanced clearing of the inflammation.

Astringents. Zinc sulphate is used in eye-drops to relieve conjunctivitis by its astringent action. It is sometimes used in conjunction with adrenaline, which assists by constricting the blood vessels. Silver nitrate has an astringent action, as well as being an antiseptic. Copper sulphate is used in eye-drops as an astringent; in addition it has a fungicidal action. Borax (sodium borate) solutions are used as conjunctival astringents; they have a mild antiseptic action.

Sodium bicarbonate solutions are used to dissolve mucus and clean the surface of the cornea.

Drugs affecting vision. *Cardiac glycosides*, in doses sufficient to cause other signs of toxicity (page 810), may affect vision. The patient sees as if through a yellow haze, and irregular areas of other colours sometimes appear. These effects seem to be due to an action of the drugs on the parts of the brain concerned with vision, since no changes can be detected in the retina. These disturbances disappear after stopping the drugs.

Nitrites. When the nitrites produce a profound fall in blood pressure, some people experience the sensation of coloured bands around objects. This is apparently due to changes in the retinal circulation.

Strychnine has a curious effect on the retina. It increases the ability to discriminate colours and intensities of illumination and particularly increases the area of the blue visual field. These effects can be produced by systemic administration or by instillation of strychnine into the conjunctiva. These effects of strychnine may be comparable to its effects on the spinal cord; it should be remembered that the retina is formed as an outgrowth of the brain. It seems likely that a similar mechanism of increased irradiation of impulses from sensory receptors explains its actions in the retina and in the cord. Strychnine has been used to treat amblyopia.

Methyl alcohol has a toxic effect on the optic nerve and the retinal cells. The ingestion of methyl alcohol, for example by drinking methylated spirits, can cause blindness. Its actions are probably due to the metabolic formation of formaldehyde, which cannot be detoxified in the eye.

Oxygen treatment may cause blindness in babies, but not in adults. When new-born and premature babies are anoxic they are treated by exposing them to a high oxygen tension in an incubator or oxygen tent. When the oxygen concentration is more than about 40% and particularly when its use is suddenly stopped, rather than gradually terminated, the aftermath of the treatment may be a condition known as retrolental fibroplasia. The following changes have been observed: the retinal blood vessels are at first constricted, then there is outgrowth of new blood vessels which penetrate the vitreous body, the retina detaches and fibrous tissue is produced behind the lens. These reactions are seen only in the developing retina.

Quinine and quinidine in high doses contract retinal blood vessels to the point where they are obliterated. The retinal nerve cells and the optic nerve fibres then degenerate and atrophy. In smaller doses colour vision may be temporarily affected.

Sodium aminoarsonate was once used in the treatment of trypanosomiasis, syphilis and malaria, but its use has now been abandoned because it causes changes in the central nervous system and atrophy of the optic nerve leading to blindness. It was once known under the optimistic name, *atoxyl*.

Santonin is used against roundworm infestations. It causes defects in colour vision, producing at first a violet and then a yellow cast on white objects.

Male fern is used to treat tapeworm infestations. Overdoses may produce damage to the optic nerve leading to temporary impairing of vision or even permanent blindness.

29*

CHAPTER 36

Drugs Affecting Blood and Blood Formation

Drugs affecting coagulation of blood

The processes of blood coagulation are described on pages 230–234. Blood coagulation can be delayed or prevented by anticoagulant drugs. These are of two types: (a) those that inhibit clotting in shed blood, the so-called *in vitro* anticoagulants, and (b) those that reduce the coagulability of the blood only when they are administered *in vivo*. A recent advance in the pharmacology of blood coagulation has been the introduction of both fibrinolytic agents which accelerate the removal of blood clots that have formed in the vessels and of drugs which inhibit the action of fibrinolysin (see page 231). Finally, blood coagulation may be facilitated, particularly as an aid to haemostasis, by coagulant drugs.

Anticoagulant drugs

The prevention of coagulation of shed blood is required for three main purposes: (i) the collection of samples of blood for various diagnostic tests, (ii) the collection from donors of blood which is to be used for transfusion, and (iii) the establishment of extracorporeal circulations, as for example the passage of the blood through heart–lung machines in cardiac surgery and through artificial kidneys in renal failure.

Compounds which remove calcium ions. The participation of calcium ions in coagulation is described on page 230. Removal of the calcium ions by precipitation or by the formation of calcium chelates prevents coagulation. Precipitation of the calcium as the insoluble fluoride, sulphate or oxalate is suitable for the collection of samples for certain diagnostic tests. Chelation of the calcium with sodium edetate (ethylenediaminetetra-acetate, EDTA) removes it into a soluble but non-ionized form; the mechanism is given in Fig. 18.10 (page 469). Sodium citrate is also used as an anticoagulant calcium-chelating agent, mainly in the collection of blood for transfusion. The blood from the donor is withdrawn into a flask containing ACD solution; this is a mixture of citric acid (A) sodium citrate (C) and glucose (dextrose, D). The advantage of citrate is that it is completely metabolized in the Krebs cycle (Fig. 2.5, page 43) by the recipient. Inhibition of coagulation by removal of calcium ions is not feasible for reducing the coagulability of blood *in vivo*, as calcium ions possess many other roles in physiological processes (see Table 1.4, page 30).

Heparin. The anticoagulant action of heparin is described on page 231. Heparin is a strongly acidic substance, owing to the presence of sulphate groups in the molecule (Fig. 36.1). The anti-coagulant activity of heparin is lost when these groups are removed by hydrolysis and the action is prevented when the groups are neutralized by combination with strongly basic molecules such as protamine (page 19), the dyestuff toluidine blue (also known as tolonium chloride), or the amine-containing polymer hexadimethrine. Probably, the anticoagulant action of heparin is due to its combination with basic groups of enzymes, and this

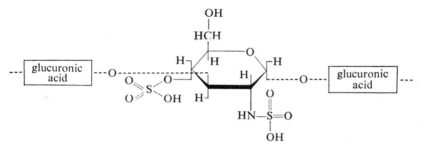

FIG. 36.1. Sulphated glucosamine unit alternating with glucuronic acid moieties in the heparin chain which comprises at least 16 such units.

results in their inhibition. These enzymes are responsible for the formation of the clot; in particular they are the enzymes involved in thromboplastin synthesis and in the action of thromboplastin and thrombin. The antithrombin action of heparin requires the presence of a heparin cofactor. This is believed to be an α-globulin occurring in the plasma.

As the name implies, heparin was first found in the liver. Subsequently, heparin was obtained from lungs and more recently from intestinal mucosa. It is present in these tissues in mast cells. Heparin is released when mast cells disrupt, as they do during anaphylactic shock or peptone shock in some species (page 778), and the blood may thereby be rendered incoagulable. Extracted heparin is prepared as the soluble sodium salt.

The potency of heparin preparations is determined by bioassay (see Table 20.5, page 553). The International Unit is defined as 1/130 mg of a sample of pure heparin from beef lung.

For the collection of blood samples for diagnostic tests, the concentration used is 10 units/ml. It is usually supplied for this purpose as 100 units dried on to the surface of a 10 ml container. Heparin is also used to inhibit blood coagulation *in vivo*, particularly when a rapid but short-lasting effect is required, as in extracorporeal circulations. Heparin is rapidly destroyed in the body, but only slowly destroyed in blood *in vitro*. The effect of heparin may be prolonged by administration of an intravenous drip or by repeated injections. A depot preparation for intramuscular injection is available. Heparin is ineffective by mouth. Thrombo-embolic disease may be treated with heparin to obtain an immediate anticoagulant effect, but for long-term treatment the more slowly acting anticoagulants of the coumarin or phenindione type are preferred. The main danger in the use of heparin is the risk of promoting bleeding, and it is contra-indicated in patients with ulcers or other disorders in which there is a predisposition to haemorrhage.

HEPARIN-LIKE SUBSTANCES. A number of other strongly acidic substances have a heparin-like anticoagulant effect. *Dextran sulphate* is a sulphated poly-saccharide having a molecular weight of 7500, which is slightly less than that of heparin. The effects and uses of dextran sulphate are as for heparin. The azo-sulphonic dyestuffs, *chlorazol fast pink* and *chlorazol sky blue* have a heparin-like action but are not used as anticoagulants. The prolonged bleeding that may follow from removal of a leech from the skin is due to the anticoagulant activity of *hirudin*, a buccal secretion that renders incoagulable the blood withdrawn by the leech.

Coumarin and indanedione anticoagulants

These substances decrease the synthesis of prothrombin, factor VII and other clotting factors in the liver by interfering with vitamin K; consequently they reduce the rate of coagulation of the blood (see Fig. 8.3, page 233 and page 234).

The discovery of drugs of the coumarin type followed from the observations in the early 1920s that cattle feeding on spoiled sweet clover hay were prone to suffer from prolonged bleeding after operations such as de-horning or castration, and many developed spontaneous haemorrhages which were frequently lethal. About 20 years of research on this haemorrhagic disease culminated in the identification of dicoumarol (Fig. 36.2) as the agent responsible, and soon after dicoumarol was used in medicine as an anticoagulant.

DICOUMAROL. The effect of dicoumarol on coagulation is not fully seen until the reserves of prothrombin and other factors in the blood have been largely depleted by being utilized. This latent period is of the order of 1 to 3 days. The dicoumarol is stored in the liver and its effect may persist for 5 days or more after the cessation of treatment. The persistence varies considerably in different individuals, being particularly prolonged in patients with inefficient kidney or liver function. Its most important and dangerous side-effect is haemorrhage which occurs when insufficient care has been taken to maintain the prothrombin times at safe values (35 to 60 sec), but this is difficult owing to the slow onset of action and its persistence. For this reason, the use of this drug has been largely discontinued. Haemorrhage resulting from over-dosage may be treated promptly by transfusion of blood or plasma to make good the deficit of clotting factors. Administration of vitamin K or synthetic analogues of vitamin K

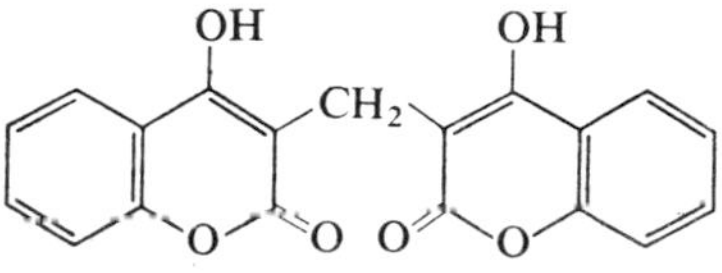

Dicoumarol

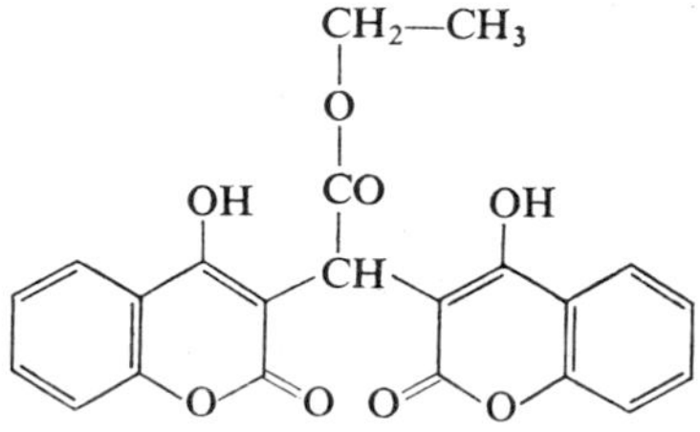

Ethyl biscoumacetate

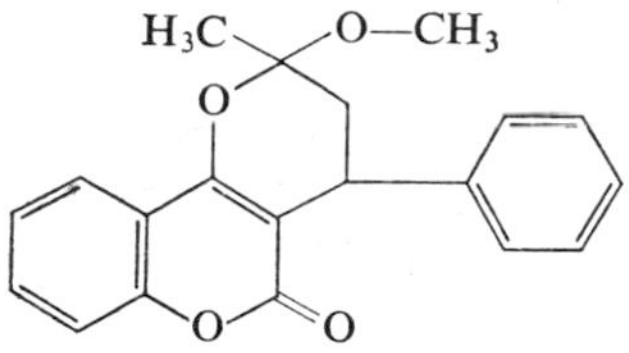

Cyclocoumarol

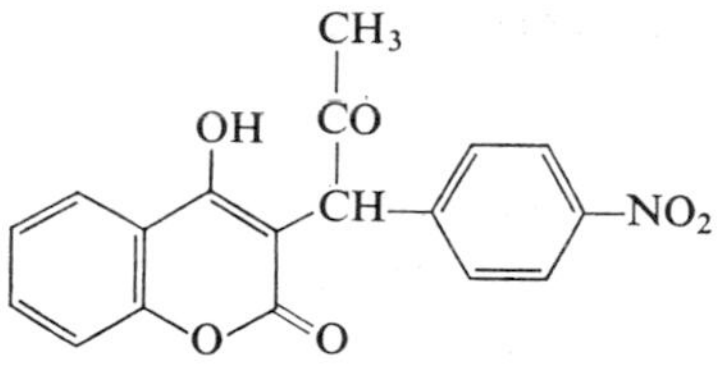

Nicoumalone

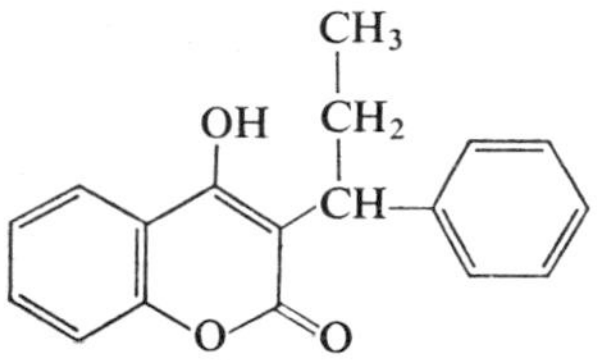

Phenylpropylhydroxycoumarin

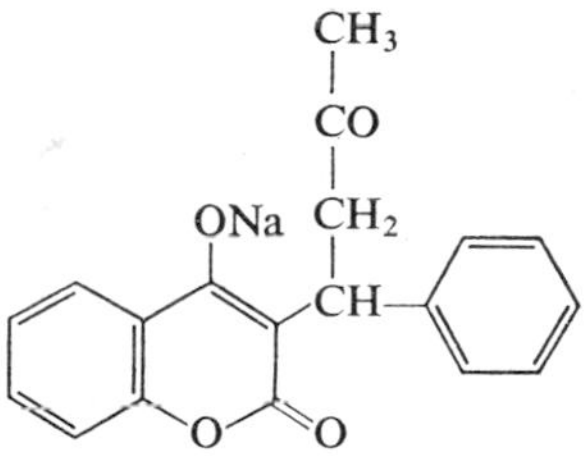

Warfarin sodium

FIG. 36.2. Structural formulae of some coumarin derivatives.

competitively overcomes the effects of dicoumarol, but it takes 1 to 3 days before the prothrombin levels are increased.

The conditions in which dicoumarol has been used as a prophylactic against intravascular clotting include coronary thrombosis, cerebral thrombosis, post-operative venous thrombosis and pulmonary embolism.

Many hundreds of compounds chemically related to dicoumarol have been tested for their anticoagulant activity. Only a few of these are used in medicine; the formulae of the most common are given in Fig. 36.2.

ETHYL BISCOUMACETATE. This substance acts more rapidly than dicoumarol, being more rapidly absorbed. It is not stored in the liver and its effects are transient. It is therefore easier to stabilize the prothrombin time.

Cyclocoumarol, nicoumalone and phenylpropylhydroxycoumarin resemble dicoumarol in latent period and persistence, but are less liable to cause gastrointestinal upset.

WARFARIN SODIUM. The coumarin derivatives mentioned above are insoluble in water and are administered by mouth. Warfarin is also orally active, being completely absorbed from the gut, but it is water-soluble and may be given by intravenous injection. This is a particular advantage in patients who exhibit vomiting or gastro-intestinal disorders with coumarin anti-coagulants. The onset of action is more rapid and the duration less than with other coumarins except ethyl biscoumacetate.

Warfarin as a rodenticide. Warfarin is extensively used for poisoning rats and mice. It is readily accepted in bait where it is used in low concentration (0·25 mg/g bait). Its effectiveness depends on the fact that it is cumulative. When the deficiency of the clotting factors becomes pronounced, death occurs as a result of internal haemorrhage. Non-rodent species are less suceptible to the poison and are unlikely to consume the bait in large enough quantities for the several days necessary to accumulate a toxic dose. Should accidental poisoning occur, it can be readily treated with vitamin K. Recently, there has appeared a mutant strain of rats which are resistant to warfarin. These rats are resistant to both injected as well as ingested warfarin, which indicates that the resistance is not due to impaired absorption of warfarin from the gut. The clotting system in the resistant rats is slightly affected by large doses of warfarin, but the impairment of coagulation is not sufficient to cause death. Research into the mechanism of the resistance has thrown some light on the nature of the genetic control of production of the clotting factors. In addition to the genes that control and stimulate synthesis of the clotting factors, there is a regulator gene which determines the production of a suppressor substance that inhibits synthesis. When the suppressor is combined with vitamin K, it loses its inhibitory action and synthesis proceeds. However, in normal rats the inhibitor action is not affected by the combination of suppressor with warfarin. It is thought that the nature of the suppressor manufactured by the mutant rats is such that it combines less readily with warfarin.

PHENINDIONE AND DIPHENADIONE. These substances are indanediones. Their formulae are given in Fig. 36.3. They are similar in mode of action, therapeutic uses, and in the precautions necessary during use, to the coumarin derivatives to which they are chemically related. They are more potent than dicoumarol and when given by mouth they are rapidly and completely absorbed. Their onset of action is rapid, taking 1 to 2 days to reach the full effect. The duration of effect of phenindione is about 24 h, but diphenadione has a prolonged action extending for some weeks after the drug has been withdrawn. Phenindione produces a reddish colour in the urine which is due to a metabolite of the drug. It was thought that this was of no practical significance, but more recently, an increased incidence of renal damage has been reported following the prolonged use of phenindione.

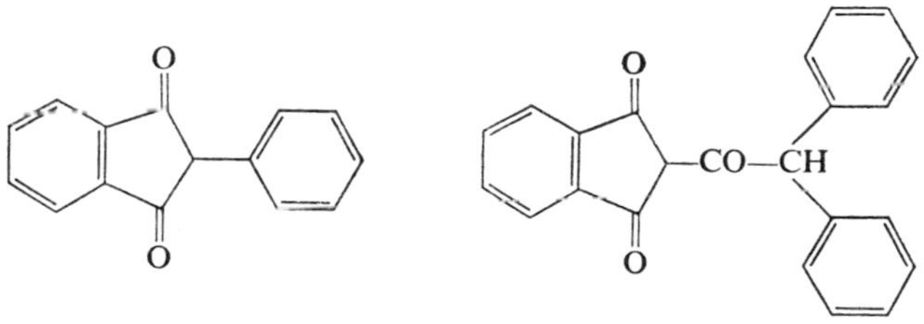

Phenindione   Diphenadione

FIG. 36.3. Structural formulae of some indanedione anticoagulants.

Two other indanediones, *anisindione* and *chlorphenindione*, have been introduced. In general they resemble phenindione in activity.

Vitamin K and its analogues. The chief natural source of vitamin K is from that synthesized by intestinal bacteria; a nutritional deficiency is unlikely to occur except when the intestinal flora are severely disturbed as in chronic diarrhoea or after sterilization of the gut contents. However, there may be a deficiency of the vitamin in obstructive jaundice and certain diseases of the intestinal tract in which there is interference with the absorption of vitamin K. In these conditions there may be hypoprothrombinaemia. The pharmacological importance of vitamin K and its analogues is mainly to reverse the anticoagulant activity of the coumarin and indanedione anticoagulants, and also the hypoprothrombinaemia caused by salicylates (page 646). The naturally occurring forms of vitamin K (pages 37 and 234) are fat-soluble. Some of the synthetic analogues are fat soluble (*menaphthone* and *acetomenaphthone*) whereas others are water soluble (*menadiol sodium phosphate*). These are shown in Fig. 36.4.

The water-soluble compounds are given by intravenous injection or by mouth; they are too slowly acting to be of benefit in preventing haemorrhage caused by overdosage of anticoagulants. The fat-soluble forms are given by the intramuscular or intravenous routes. Parenteral preparations of the fat-soluble drugs, including vitamin K (phytomenadione), consist of colloidal solutions or emulsions with surfactants. Their main use is in those conditions in which hypoprothrombinaemia is due to impaired absorption of vitamin K. The

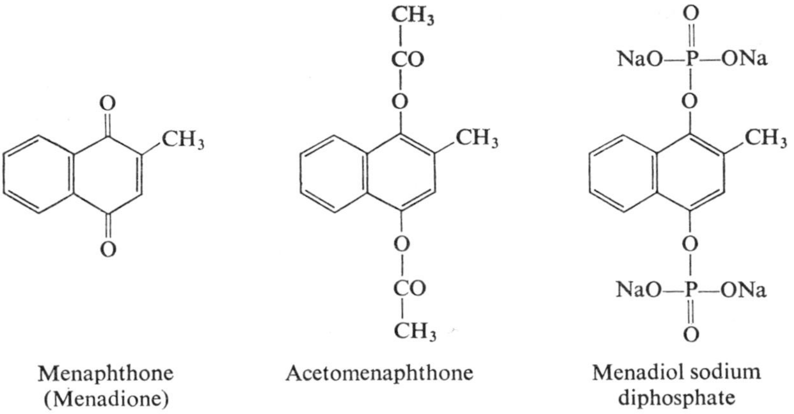

| Menaphthone (Menadione) | Acetomenaphthone | Menadiol sodium diphosphate |

FIG. 36.4. Formulae of some structural analogues of vitamin K (compare with formula of vitamin K, page 234).

actions of these compounds are very prolonged and antagonism to the anti-coagulants may last for several weeks, therefore the dosage must be carefully adjusted and frequent determinations of prothrombin times are necessary.

Fibrinolytic agents and antifibrinolysins

The *in vitro* coagulants are used to prevent a tendency to intravascular clotting. Fibrinolytic agents are used to remove a clot that has already formed. Fibrinolysin, or plasmin, is an enzyme that breaks down fibrin; it is described on page 231. It is formed from a globulin precursor known as plasminogen by various activators, the natural activator being released by the clotting process. The fibrinolytic activity of plasmin is held in check by an anti-plasmin substance in the blood stream. The dissolution of a thrombus or embolus may be achieved by infusion of plasmin or a plasmin activator, the main activators being the enzymes, *streptokinase* and *urokinase*. Streptokinase is extracted from a strain of haemolytic streptococcus. It occurs together with *streptodornase*, an enzyme that attacks DNA and DNA-proteins. The enzymes are given together to aid the removal of blood and purulent masses from body cavities. A mixture of beef blood fibrinolysin and beef pancreas desoxyribonuclease is also used for this purpose. The intravenous administration of streptokinase for intravascular clotting often produces febrile reactions, and the substance is antigenic, which thereby limits its use. Urokinase, which is extracted from urine, is not pyrogenic nor is it antigenic. The plasmin activators are standardized by an assay procedure which depends on the rate of liquefaction of a blood clot *in vitro*.

The main risk of fibrinolytic therapy is that fibrinogen and other coagulation factors may be used up in maintaining the clot, and this entails the risk of haemorrhage. The plasmin that is liberated naturally by extensive intravascular clotting, which may be a sequel to severe trauma, surgery, or disease with severe tissue damage, may also exhaust the fibrinogen reserves. The haemorrhagic tendency that is caused by excessive plasmin production may be counteracted with antifibrinolytic drugs. *Aminocaproic acid* inhibits the formation of plasmin and in higher concentrations it inhibits the action of plasmin. *Aminomethylcyclohexane carboxylic acid* has a similar action. A trypsin inhibitor, *Trasylol*, which is extracted from lungs, is a potent inhibitor of plasmin. It was first used as an inhibitor of the enzyme that converts bradykininogen to bradykinin. (See also page 849.)

Haemostatic agents

These are substances that are applied locally to arrest bleeding. *Alum* is still used for this purpose in the form of sticks or pencils; it acts by precipitating the blood proteins. Solutions of *adrenaline* may be applied to mucosal surfaces and exposed tissues. It produces local vasoconstriction which facilitates clotting by slowing the blood flow. *Absorbable gelatin sponge* is used in surgery to arrest capillary bleeding, and since it is absorbable it can be left in the wound after closure. The spongy mass takes up many times its own weight of blood and acts as a matrix in which clotting occurs: the whole mass adheres to the wounded surface. *Human fibrin foam* is prepared by treating a solution of fibrinogen with thrombin; it is used particularly to prevent bleeding during surgery of the brain and the lung. *Human thrombin*, prepared by allowing prothrombin to react with thromboplastin in the presence of calcium ions, is used as a local haemostatic in general surgery and as an adhesive in plastic surgery. It has been used orally to arrest bleeding in gastric haemorrhage. *Oxidized cellulose* is a special type of surgical gauze which reacts with blood to form a coagulated mass which has been termed an artificial clot. The whole mass is gradually absorbed. *Russell's viper venom* has been used by local application to control dental bleeding in haemophiliacs and as a haemostatic after tonsillectomy and adenoidectomy.

Drugs used in the treatment of the anaemias

Iron-deficiency anaemia. In this condition, the red cells are *hypochromic* and *microcytic*; that is, they contain less haemoglobin and are smaller than normal. Anaemic patients are pale and experience lassitude. Long-standing anaemia may result in physical changes in the nails and other epithelial tissues. Deficiency may be due to an inadequate dietary intake of iron, but this is now unusual on standard Western diets except when there is an increased demand for iron, as in growing children, during pregnancy, or as a result of chronic haemorrhage.

Iron is absorbed as the ferrous ion from the upper part of the duodenum. The formation of extremely insoluble iron salts, such as the phosphate, after admixture with pancreatic secretions, prevents absorption in more distal parts of the intestines. The ferrous ion is oxidized to ferric in the mucosal cell and is bound to a protein, *apoferritin* to form *ferritin*. It is thought that saturation of mucosal apoferritin limits iron absorption. The iron is slowly released from the ferritin stores in the ferrous form, and passes into the blood stream where it combines with a β-globulin to form *transferrin*, being converted again into the ferric form in this complex. The circulating iron is largely transported to the bone marrow, where it is first bound as ferritin and as another protein complex known as *haemosiderin*, and then it enters into haemoglobin synthesis. Part of the circulating iron is removed and bound as ferritin and haemosiderin in iron stores which are mainly in the liver, spleen, kidney and gut. Iron released during erythrocyte destruction in the reticulo-endothelial system is also redistributed in the body as transferrin: this amounts to about 25 mg of iron per day, and may be considerably more in haemolytic anaemias. Normally, circulating iron takes up about one-third of the plasma transferrin. An excess of iron leads to considerable depositions in the iron-storage tissues, a condition known as haemochromatosis.

Iron has been regarded in the past as a tonic, and it was used in a rather unspecific way to treat lassitude. However, it is potentially dangerous because of its acute toxicity in large doses and a chronic toxicity due to overloading of the iron stores with continued treatment. The modern tendency is to determine that an iron-deficiency anaemia does actually exist before prescribing iron. The main sign of a hypochromic, microcytic anaemia may also occur with haemolytic anaemias (pages 240–241). Since the iron stores are high in this disorder, further tests may be necessary. These include determinations of plasma iron and bone marrow iron.

The most common iron preparations consist of simple ferrous salts made up in tablets, pills or capsules. *Ferrous sulphate* is widely used; it is usually dispensed as pills or tablets coated to protect them from moisture, as ferrous sulphate rapidly oxidizes in air to form ferric sulphate. The presence of a reducing agent aids absorption and for this reason ascorbic acid is sometimes given in iron-containing mixtures. *Ferrous carbonate* (as Blaud's Pills) was introduced into medicine more than a century ago; these pills must be fresh or they may pass through the intestinal tract unabsorbed. In severe anaemia, ferrous carbonate may be dispensed in capsules so that larger amounts may be administered. Ferrous salts of organic acids are claimed to be less likely to cause gastro-intestinal irritation than the older salts of inorganic acids. Of these, *ferrous succinate* is said to offer the best absorbable form of iron. *Ferrous gluconate, fumarate, glycine sulphate* and *glutamate* have also been used successfully in treating anaemia. Iron given as *ferrous citrate* and *tartrate* is less well absorbed, probably because it is held in chelate form in these compounds. The chelate compounds, *ferric versenate* and *ferric ammonium citrate* have been used with the intention of reducing the toxic actions of iron. The rationale is that iron is slowly released, thus avoiding the build up of an irritant concentration, and the slow conversion to the ferrous form prevents too rapid an absorption. These preparations are commonly given as solutions, in which form they are preferred to solutions of ferrous sulphate, since the latter compound stains the teeth (but this can be avoided by drinking it through a straw). *Colloidal ferric hydroxide* has been used orally and is said to be attended by a minimum of gastro-intestinal complaints. *Reduced iron* occurs as a grey powder and is insoluble in water: it is thus dispensed in capsules or compressed tablets.

Many of the iron containing tablets are presented with a brightly-coloured sugar coating. They have caused fatal poisoning in children who thought them to be sweets, so care must be taken in the storage of such tablets. The toxic effects of orally administered iron include diarrhoea, gastro-intestinal upsets, vomiting and haematuria.

In patients who are intolerant of oral iron preparations, and in those in whom a satisfactory response cannot be obtained with oral iron due to inadequate absorption, iron preparations may be given parenterally. Iron in parenteral preparations must be in a non-ionized form. *Iron sorbitol* injection is a low molecular weight complex of iron with sorbitol and citric acid. It is rapidly absorbed and about one-third of the dose is then excreted by the kidneys. The remainder of the iron is taken up by transferrin. The injection is given intramuscularly by inserting the needle in two stages along a Z-shaped track so as to seal the mass deep within the muscle, otherwise some leaks back and produces an unsightly staining of the skin. *Iron dextran* is a high molecular weight complex and is slowly absorbed. It is taken up by reticulo-endothelial cells from which iron is slowly released. Iron dextran may also be given intravenously by slow infusion. *Saccharated iron oxide* is a preparation of ferric oxide and sucrose that may be given intravenously; it is more toxic than iron dextran.

Some of the toxic effects of iron have been mentioned. Overdosage taken by mouth irritates the gastro-intestinal mucosa, causing pain, vomiting and diarrhoea, and it may produce necrosis of the mucosa with bleeding. Excessive levels of circulating iron, whether absorbed or injected, result in cardiovascular collapse, nausea and vomiting. The toxic effects of iron can be treated with *desferrioxamine B*. This is a polyhydroxamic acid that is found as a complex with iron (ferrioxamine) in certain micro-organisms. Desferrioxamine has a great affinity for iron, exceeding that of transferrin. Injections of desferrioxamine are given to treat systemic iron poisoning, the ferrioxamine being excreted in the urine. Oral desferrioxamine binds iron in the gut and prevents absorption.

Vitamin-deficiency anaemias

Anaemia due to deficiency of cyanocobalamin, folic acid or ascorbic acid is discussed on pages 238–240. In these conditions, red blood cells are macrocytic and the count is low.

Cyanocobalamin. The structural formula is given on page 34. The commercial source of the vitamin is now from various strains of streptomyces grown in large-scale cultures. The increase in availability and reduction in cost has led to the treatment of pernicious anaemia with cyanocobalamin given by mouth in extremely large doses, in which case some is absorbed despite the lack of intrinsic factor. Cyanocobalamin in the blood stream is bound to a plasma protein, but when the binding capacity of the plasma is exceeded, the excess of cyanocobalamin passes into the glomerular filtrate and appears in the urine, none being reabsorbed by the tubular cells. This has been utilized for the determination of glomerular filtration rate (see pages 349–350) using the following procedure. The plasma binding capacity is first saturated with cyanocobalamin, then an injection of radiocobalt-labelled cyanocobalamin is given, and the concentrations of this in the blood and urine are measured.

Hydroxocobalamin is more strongly bound to plasma protein and has a longer duration of action than cyanocobalamin.

Folic acid and folinic acid. The formula of folic acid is given on page 35. In the body, it is converted to folinic acid, which is the agent required for thymine synthesis (see page 239). In the treatment of pernicious anaemia, folic acid is sometimes given together with cyanocobalamin. Folic acid is never given alone in this disorder, since it improves the blood picture but has no effect on the associated neurological lesions. Folic acid is sometimes given with iron preparations when the response to iron alone in hypochromic anaemias is inadequate.

The symptoms of folic-acid deficiency may be produced by certain drugs. The folic acid antagonists, aminopterin and amethopterin, which are used in the treatment of leukaemia, block the conversion of folic to folinic acid. Should a macrocytic anaemia develop, this may be treated with folinic acid. The action of folinic acid may be interfered with by sulphonamides and by some anticonvulsant drugs (primidone, phenytoin and phenobarbitone). The side-effect of macrocytic anaemia produced by these drugs may be counteracted by folic acid.

Blood plasma substitutes

Blood loss from wounds is ideally made good by blood or plasma transfusion. This is not always practicable, and much attention has been paid to the provision of alternative fluids to expand the plasma volume, and thereby to prevent the development of haemorrhage shock. The theoretical considerations are that the electrolyte constituents should be approximately those of plasma, which poses no great difficulty, and that the plasma albumin should be replaced by a substance having a similar molecular weight (approximately 70,000). This substance should be non-toxic, not too rapidly eliminated or metabolized, non-antigenic and stable during storage.

Dextran. This is a glucose polymer. It is prepared commercially from sucrose by bacterial action. Partial hydrolysis yields fractions with varying molecular weights. Those in the range of 40,000 to 200,000 are used in 6 to 10 per cent solutions in saline or glucose solution. The smaller dextran molecules are lost in the urine in a few hours. The larger molecules are taken up the reticulo-endothelial cells and may produce sensitization by acting antigenically. Dextrans, particularly those with high molecular weights, tend to cause clumping of the erythrocytes. This may interfere with the interpretation of blood-grouping tests and cause difficulties for the subsequent transfer of the patient to blood transfusion. Therefore a sample of blood for matching is taken before giving dextran, whenever this is possible.

Polyvidone. This is a polymer of vinylpyrrolidone (PVP). The unit structure is:

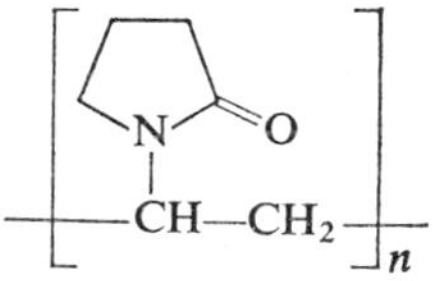

$$\left[\begin{array}{c} \underset{\underset{\displaystyle CH-CH_2}{|}}{N} \diagdown O \end{array} \right]_n$$

The molecular weight of the polymers used as plasma substitutes is 20,000 to 40,000. It has no acute toxicity, but it is known to cause sarcomas in rats. Polyvidone is excreted in the urine. It does not interfere with blood matching tests.

Gelatin. A non-antigenic preparation with a molecular weight of about 33,000 has been used as a plasma substitute. About half is excreted in the urine, and the remainder enters into the body's amino acid pool. Gelatin may interfere with blood matching.

Drugs affecting plasma lipids

It is thought that the development of arteriosclerotic disease is favoured by high-circulating levels of lipid. Consequently, considerable attention has been paid to antilipaemic drugs and procedures as a prophylactic measure against the formation of atheroma.

The plasma lipids include glycerides, phospholipids and cholesterol (both free and esterified). These lipids are associated with plasma proteins. In the

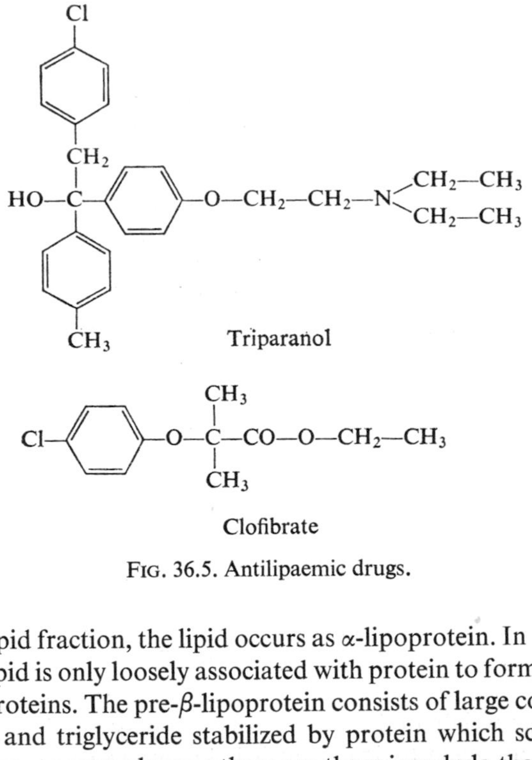

Triparanol

Clofibrate

FIG. 36.5. Antilipaemic drugs.

high-density lipid fraction, the lipid occurs as α-lipoprotein. In the low-density fraction, the lipid is only loosely associated with protein to form β-lipoproteins or pre-β-lipoproteins. The pre-β-lipoprotein consists of large conglomerations of cholesterol and triglyceride stabilized by protein which scatter light and produce a milky, opaque plasma; these are the microchyla that are present in blood after a fatty meal.

Heparin. The antilipaemic action of heparin is due to the liberation of a lipase which acts particularly on triglycerides in microchyla.

Poly-unsaturated fatty acids. The substitution of saturated animal fat in the diet (in items such as cream, butter, cheese and fatty meats) by unsaturated vegetable oils results in a reduction of plasma cholesterol and β-lipoprotein. The oils are obtained from cottonseed, soya, safflower and corn and contain a high content of glycerol esters of linolenic and linoleic acid. It is thought that arachidonic acid, an unsaturated acid metabolite of these dietary acids, is concerned in cholesterol transport and favours the formation of α-lipoprotein.

Oestrogens decrease the plasma α-, β-, and pre-β-lipoprotein.

Thyroxine and some of its derivatives lower plasma cholesterol concentrations: this effect is unrelated to their action of increasing metabolic rate.

Sitosterols interfere with the absorption of cholesterol.

Nicotinic acid lowers blood cholesterol, mainly that in the β-lipoprotein fraction. The side-effect of flushing (see page 830) militates against its use.

Triparanol inhibits the synthesis of cholesterol in the liver. It has been withdrawn from clinical use on account of its toxic effects, which include nausea and vomiting, albuminuria, baldness, cataract and skin lesions. The formula of triparanol is given in Fig. 36.5.

Clofibrate reduces the plasma triglyceride and cholesterol levels, mainly those in the pre-β-lipoprotein fraction. It also reduces the plasma uric acid level and has been used in the treatment of xanthomas. Its formula is given in Fig. 36.5.

CHAPTER 37

Chemotherapy of Infection and Cancer

Drugs used in bacterial chemotherapy

The sulphonamides. From the early studies of Ehrlich and others, certain dye-stuffs were found to be selectively absorbed by pathogenic protozoal parasites. These dyes not only stained cells but frequently killed them. Then, in 1935, Domagk showed that some azo dyestuffs containing the sulphanilamide residue (*p*-aminobenzenesulphonamide) had *in vivo* anti-streptococcal activity in mice, and *Prontosil Red* became the first sulphonamide to be successfully introduced into clinical medicine.

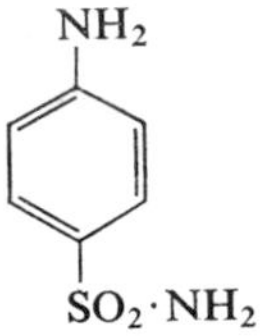

Sulphanilamide

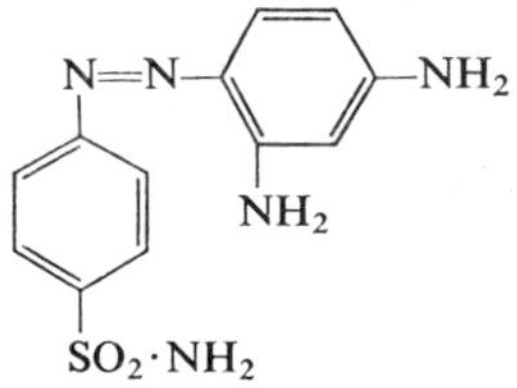

Prontosil Red

Since only those dyestuffs which contained the sulphanilamide residue were active, Trefouel and his co-workers suggested that the tissues broke down the compounds to yield *sulphanilamide* and this was responsible for the anti-bacterial activity (see also page 508). Sulphanilamide was found to be effective in the treatment of gonorrhoea and meningococcal meningitis but to be of little value in pneumonia. Many derivatives were then rapidly introduced into medicine, an important one being *sulphapyridine* (also termed M & B 693

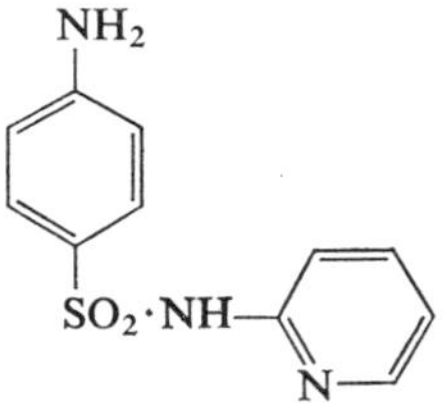

Sulphapyridine

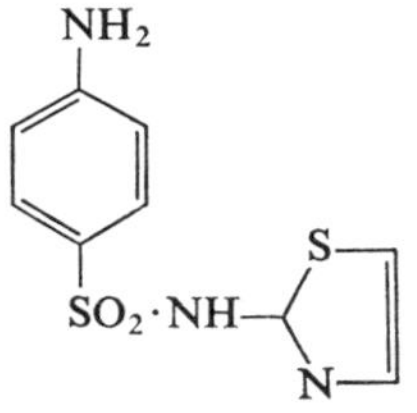

Sulphathiazole

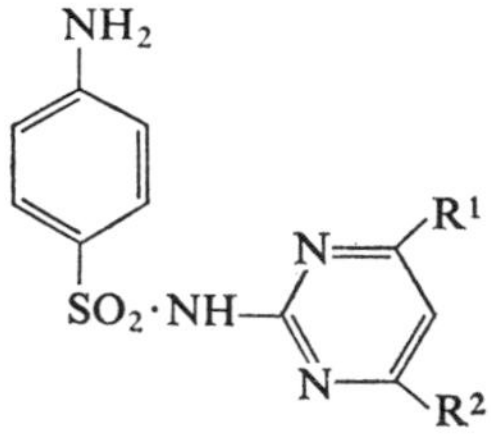

Sulphadiazine
($R^1 = R^2 = H$)

[Sulphadimidine has $R^1 = R^2 = CH_3$, whereas sulphamerazine has $R^1 = CH_3$ and $R^2 = H$]

920

after the name of the pharmaceutical firm of May & Baker). Sulphapyridine is active against pathogenic streptococci, gonococci, meningococci and pneumococci, and has been successfully used in treating lobar pneumonia. Other derivatives of clinical importance are *sulphathiazole, sulphadiazine, sulphadimidine* and *sulphamerazine*.

During the 1939–45 war, *sulphaguanidine* was widely and successfully used to treat bacillary dysentery. *Succinylsulphathiazole* is now also used for this purpose. More recently, sulphonamides with a much more prolonged effect have been synthesized, an example being *sulphamethoxypyridazine*. There is evidence that the long-acting sulphonamides are absorbed on to serum proteins and therefore they are not excreted or metabolized very rapidly; however, the protein binding lowers their antibacterial activity.

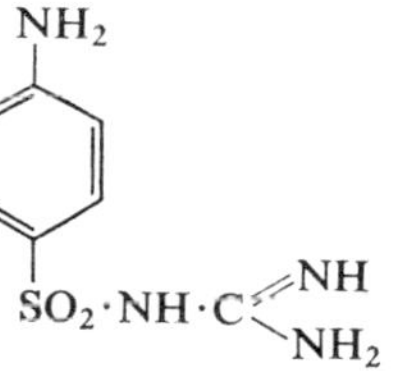

Sulphaguanidine 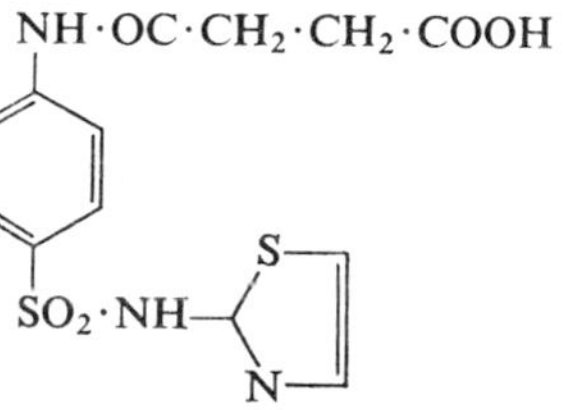   Succinylsulphathiazole 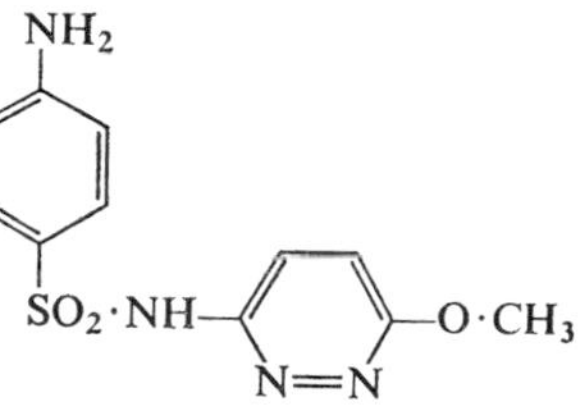   Sulphamethoxypyridazine

USES. Sulphonamides do not kill the infecting agent but help the body to overcome and deal with infection. They are used in the following ways:

(*a*) *Systemic injection*. This is particularly useful in the treatment of urinary infections because some sulphonamides (e.g. sulphanilamide) are secreted at a high concentration into the urine. Sulphonamides are also used for infections of the blood, meninges and lungs (that is, septicaemia, meningitis and pneumonia).

(*b*) *Local application* is used in the treatment of infections of the eye or the throat. Sulphonamides which are water-soluble such as *sulphacetamide* are used for this purpose.

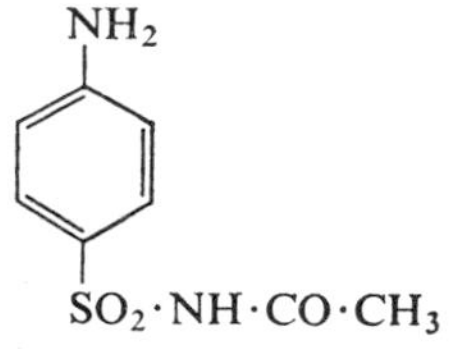

Sulphacetamide

(*c*) *Oral use*. High concentrations of the sulphonamides must be maintained in the gut for effective treatment of intestinal infections, particularly bacillary dysentery. The three compounds commonly employed are (1) sulphaguanidine, a fairly soluble compound which is but poorly absorbed because the molecule is highly ionized (page 491), (2) succinylsulphathiazole, and (3) *phthalylsulpathiazole*. The last two compounds are poorly absorbed because they are insoluble. Sulphathiazole is slowly released from them by the action of bacterial enzymes (page 509). They may be used to render the large bowel sterile before surgery.

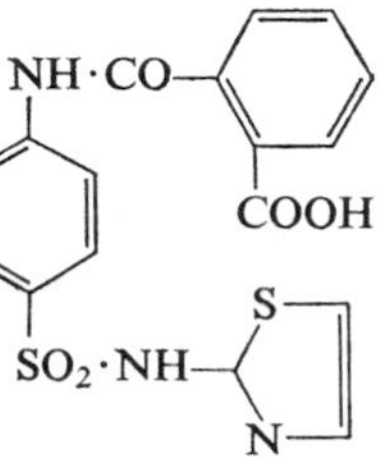

Phthalylsulphathiazole

Mode of action. Sulphonamides act on invading pathogenic bacteria by inhibiting their growth. They interfere with the uptake and utilization by bacteria of the essential metabolite, *p*-aminobenzoic acid.

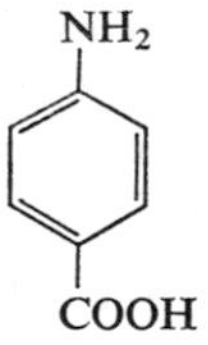

p-Aminobenzoic acid

Sulphonamides and *p*-aminobenzoic acid compete with one another for bacterial enzyme receptors, and filtrates from bacterial cultures contain substances which inhibit the action of sulphonamides by binding them. Sulphonamides cannot be utilized by the cell as metabolites, and growth and reproduction are consequently slowed down and then stopped. Methionine and folic acid also antagonize the actions of the sulphonamides. Bacteria that are sensitive to sulphonamides, unlike the tissues of the animal host, cannot take up preformed folic acid and are dependent on synthesizing it and it seems likely that the sulphonamides prevent cellular synthesis of folic acid by inhibiting *p*-aminobenzoic acid utilization. Folic acid contains the *p*-aminobenzoic acid moiety in its structure as shown on page 35.

Structure–action relationships. For activity, the amino group must be in the para position to the sulphonamide group, and when it is not free the activity is generally much reduced. For maximal activity, the —SO_2NH_2 group is also necessary and it may be substituted. Sulphathiazole is considered to be one of the most potent of the sulphonamides in general use, with sulphadiazine, sulphapyridine and sulphanilamide next in that order. Potency is generally related to the ability of the compound to ionize.

Administration and absorption. The sulphonamides are usually given by mouth and they produce persistent blood levels. During the first 2 or 3 days of serious infection, absorption may be poor and sulphanilamide then is often given intravenously as the sodium salt, which is very soluble but alkaline in solution. Doses are administered every 6 h to maintain high blood concentrations.

Distribution. The sulphonamides after administration are found in nearly all secretions and particularly in the urine. It is usual to continue to give the sulphonamide for a few days after the infection has been cleared to be sure that all bacteria have been eliminated. Many sulphonamides are partly acetylated by the body, and these acetylated derivatives are usually inactive. They are less soluble in acid media than the free sulphonamide and tend to precipitate in the urine.

Toxic actions. Kidney damage may result from the less soluble acetyl derivatives of the sulphonamides being precipitated in the renal tubules and ureters. The urine must therefore be kept alkaline and large quantities of fluid should be administered by mouth. Another serious side-effect of the sulphonamides is agranulocytosis when treatment is continued beyond 10 days. Sometimes, allergic reactions are produced, and the temperature is raised and skin rashes appear. In these cases, it is advisable to try another sulphonamide. In other patients, methaemoglobinaemia and acute haemolytic anaemia may result but these toxic effects are rare.

Drug resistance. Some strains of streptococci, pneumococci, meningococci and gonococci acquire resistance to the action of the sulphonamides, and this cross-resistance is shown to other sulphonamides (although not to antibiotics). The mechanism of development of the resistance probably involves a change either in the needs of the organism for *p*-aminobenzoic acid, or in its use of sulphonamide which may become converted into a utilizable metabolite. It is thus best to avoid long periods of treatment and to use high doses of sulphonamides for short periods. Recently, many new derivatives of sulphonamide have been introduced and these have a much more prolonged effect. However, they may bind to plasma proteins more extensively and this increases their liability to produce toxic effects.

The sulphones. These compounds are closely related to the sulphonamides both in structure and in therapeutic action. Their effects are similarly antagonized by *p*-aminobenzoic acid. They possess potent *in vivo* activity against the causative organism of leprosy and tuberculosis. Leprosy is due to infection with *Mycobacterium leprae*, an organism which cannot as yet be cultivated *in vitro*. The sulphones cause the organism to undergo changes in shape, but this is a slow process and generally the drugs must be used for periods up to 5 years. The best known sulphone is *dapsone*, a compound with high antibacterial potency but also high toxicity. It is rapidly and completely absorbed from the intestinal tract. Recently, derivatives of dapsone have been used; these are said to be converted *in vivo* into the parent compound. The toxic actions of the sulphones are similar to those of the sulphonamides.

The sulphones are not always tolerable and other compounds must then be used in the treatment of leprosy. Among these compounds is *thiambutosine*, a phenylthiourea derivative, related to the antithyroid drugs. This type of compound is commonly used in the early stages of treatment and then dapsone is gradually introduced.

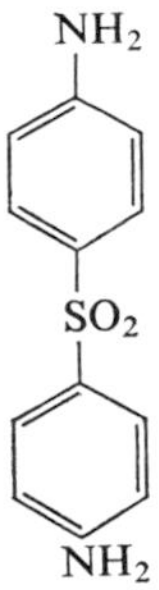

NH$_2$

SO$_2$

NH$_2$

Dapsone

Antibiotics

An antibiotic is defined as a chemical substance which is produced by micro-organisms and is capable at a high dilution of either inhibiting the growth of or destroying another micro-organism. Antibiotics are produced by moulds, actinomycetes and bacteria, and some are now synthesized. Their action is probably due to an effect on vital enzyme systems connected with metabolism or reproduction.

Penicillin. In 1929, Fleming noted that a plate culture of staphylococci growing in his laboratory had been contaminated by a mould and lysis of the staphylococcal colonies had occurred around the area of growth of the mould. It was then shown that the mould had produced a potent antibacterial substance which inhibited the growth of streptococci, staphylococci, pneumococci and gonococci, as well as that of the causative organism of diphtheria. This observation led to the isolation of *penicillin* by Chain, Florey, Abraham and others. Penicillin was the first of the clinically-useful antibiotics. Its lack of toxicity, high antibacterial potency and activity in the presence of pus, particularly against staphylococci, were unique advantages, and penicillin is still the most important antibiotic in use today. It does not, however, inhibit organisms belonging to the coliform-typhoid group.

Production and chemistry. The organism originally used for the production of penicillin was *Penicillin notatum*, but the one now cultivated and which gives better yields is *P. chrysogenum*. Penicillins are β-lactam thiazolidine derivatives. Antibacterial activity varies with the nature of group R (see the general formula in Fig. 37.1), which is altered by using different acids in the culture medium. For example, in the presence of phenylacetic acid, *P. chrysogenum* synthesizes *benzylpenicillin* (or penicillin G); with phenoxyacetic acid, it is *phenoxymethylpenicillin* (or penicillin V).

The general method of producing penicillins has been a microbiological one, leaving the mould to incorporate the chemical grouping into the penicillin molecule. Penicillin G was synthesized in 1946 and more recently the total synthesis of penicillin V has been achieved. In 1959, 6-*aminopenicillanic acid* was obtained from a culture of *P. chrysogenum*. This compound possesses a low antibacterial activity but its rate of destruction by penicillinase is much slower than that of penicillin G. The newly isolated substance has proved the starting-point for the chemical production of several new penicillins and important advances have been made, notably the production of a form of penicillin (*methicillin*) effective against staphylococci which are resistant to the conventional form of penicillin, and of another form of penicillin (*ampicillin*) effective against many Gram-negative organisms. Some staphylococci are able to synthesise *penicillinase* which is an enzyme that inactivates penicillin by removing the carboxyl group from the lactam ring: staphylococci which produce this enzyme are penicillin resistant. The introduction of side groups into the penicillin molecule prevents the action of penicillinase. Although these substituted derivatives are less active than penicillin G (benzylpenicillin) on penicillin-sensitive staphylococci, they are invaluable in that they are active on resistant staphylococci, being unaffected by the penicillinase produced by them.

Penicillin G is hydrolysed by acid with the loss of antibiotic activity. This may occur at the pH of gastric contents. Parenteral administration is therefore more effective for producing adequate plasma levels. In buffered preparations the rate of hydrolysis of penicillin is reduced, but there is also a decrease in the rate of absorption (cf. pages 488–492). Some of the derivatives of penicillin which are not subject to acid hydrolysis are active orally. New forms of penicillin have been produced which are claimed to be more suitable for oral administration than penicillin V (such as *phenethicillin* and *propicillin*). A recent development is the production of isoxazolyl penicillin (*cloxacillin*) which is effective against benzylpenicillin-resistant staphylococci and is reasonably well absorbed when given orally.

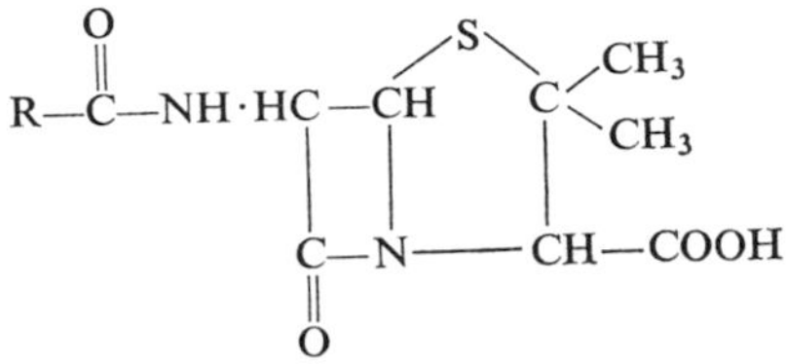

$$R—\overset{\overset{\displaystyle O}{\|}}{C}—NH\cdot HC—CH \quad \overset{\displaystyle S}{\underset{\underset{C—N}{\|}{O}}{}} \quad C\overset{\displaystyle CH_3}{\underset{CH_3}{}}$$

In Penicillin G or benzylpenicillin, $R = —CH_2 \cdot C_6H_5$.
In Penicillin V or phenoxymethylpenicillin, $R = —CH_2 \cdot O \cdot C_6H_5$.

Methicillin
(Cebenin, BRL 1241)

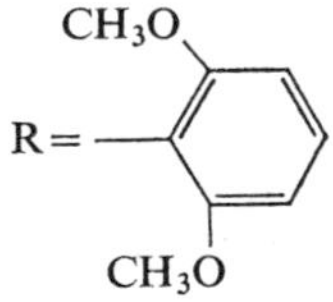

$R = $ (dimethoxyphenyl with CH_3O groups)

Ampicillin
(Penbritin, BRL 1341)

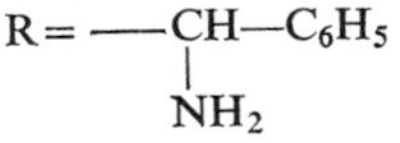

$R = —\underset{NH_2}{CH}—C_6H_5$

Phenethicillin
(Broxil)

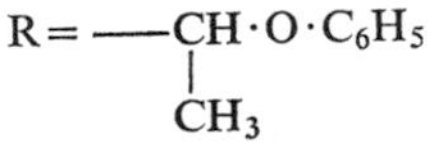

$R = —\underset{CH_3}{CH}\cdot O \cdot C_6H_5$

Propicillin
(Brocillin, Ultrapen)

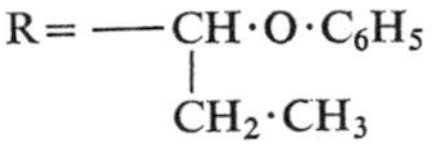

$R = —\underset{CH_2 \cdot CH_3}{CH}\cdot O \cdot C_6H_5$

Cloxacillin

$R = —\overset{\|}{C}\overset{}{—}\overset{\|}{C}\cdot C_6H_5$ (isoxazolyl ring with H_3C, C, O, N)

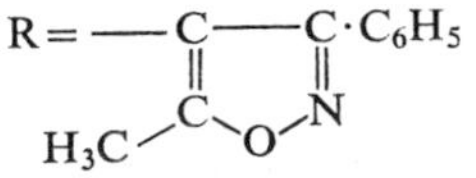

Fig. 37.1. Structural formulae of some penicillins

Penicillin G is generally prepared as the calcium, sodium or potassium salt. Activity is measured in terms of the International Standard crystalline penicillin G (1 unit = 0·6 μg), a preparation which is stable only in the dry form. Penicillin G is administered usually by intramuscular injection in acute infections, high blood levels being maintained for several hours. Injections are given several times a day.

Procaine penicillin G is the salt formed by combining penicillin with the local anaesthetic, procaine. It is sparingly soluble in water and is usually formulated as a suspension in oil. It is given daily by intramuscular injection and has a more prolonged action than penicillin G but with correspondingly lower blood concentrations. It is thus not the preparation of choice in severe infections. It has been widely used in the treatment of gonorrhoea and syphilis.

Penicillin V is suitable for oral administration as it is stable in the presence of acid; consequently, it is not destroyed in the stomach. It is as effective though not always as reliable as intramuscular benzylpenicillin.

Benzathine penicillin is N,N'-dibenzylethylenediamine dipenicillin G. It has a comparatively low solubility but a very prolonged effect when given intramuscularly. It is useless for acute infections as the blood levels are only very low. The injection is liable to be rather painful, but the dose may be given by mouth. It is not used extensively.

Methicillin was one of the first of the synthetic penicillins generally available for clinical use. It is a white crystalline solid, extremely soluble in water but unstable in acid solution. Cultures of *Staphylococcus pyogenes* are sensitive to methicillin, regardless of their resistance to other antibiotics. Methicillin is not affected by staphylococcal penicillinase and few methicillin-resistant staphylococci have so far been encountered. It is usually given by deep intramuscular injection. It does not penetrate well into the cerebrospinal fluid.

Ampicillin is active against a wide range of Gram-negative as well as Gram-positive organisms. It is stable in acid solution and is well absorbed when given orally. It is destroyed by staphylococcal penicillinase.

Phenethicillin is better absorbed than penicillin V when given orally and high blood levels are maintained for longer periods. Staphylococci which are resistant to penicillin are also resistant to phenethicillin.

Propicillin is active orally and is considered to be particularly suitable for the treatment of streptococcal infections.

Cloxacillin is considerably more active than methicillin against a variety of penicillin-resistant staphylococci. It is active orally and diffuses well into most body fluids.

INHIBITION OF EXCRETION OF PENICILLIN. Probenecid inhibits the excretion of penicillin by the renal tubules, and therefore the blood concentration of penicillin is maintained longer. It competes with penicillin for a transport mechanism in the cells of the renal tubules (see page 524).

Mode of action of penicillin. The visible effect of penicillin on sensitive micro-organisms is to cause them to increase in size and become misshapen. It is thought that penicillin acts by inhibiting the synthesis of a mucopeptide that forms parts of the bacterial cell wall. N-acetylmuramic acid, one of the constituents of the mucopeptide, has a structure resembling that of penicillin. In the presence of penicillin the incorporation of the acetylmuramic acid into the peptide is prevented. Thus the cell wall is faulty and it rapidly ruptures owing to the high intracellular osmotic pressure (which is about 25 atmospheres).

Resistance of staphylococci to penicillin appears to be of three types: (1) an inherent capacity to tolerate penicillin, (2) an ability to destroy it through penicillinase (giving penicilloic acid as the product), and (3) an ability to destroy it through an amidase (giving 6-aminopenicillanic acid as one of the products). Cross-resistance between penicillin and the sulphonamides does not occur.

Toxicity of penicillin. Penicillin is non-toxic to all mammalian species except guinea-pigs, although in some patients it produces rashes and anaphylactic shock.

STREPTOMYCIN. Streptomycin (or N-methyl-1-glucosamido-streptosido-streptidine) is an antibiotic obtained from the soil-dwelling organism, *Streptomyces griseus*, an actinomycete. Whereas penicillin is an acid, streptomycin is a basic compound containing three ionizable amino groups. The importance of streptomycin lies in its activity against *Myco. tuberculosis*; it is also used in some forms of dysentery and brucellosis and is effective against the plague bacillus.

The antibiotic is not absorbed (although it is not inactivated) when given by mouth and it is therefore usually given in divided doses by intramuscular injection. The main toxic risk of streptomycin consists of damage to the vestibular division of the 8th cranial nerve which leads to vertigo and sometimes to tinnitus. The auditory portion of the nerve is also affected in a small number of patients. Streptomycin may be given intrathecally in small repeated doses in tubercular meningitis. For the treatment of tuberculosis, streptomycin should always be used in conjunction with para-aminosalicylic acid or with isoniazid to obviate drug resistance.

Dihydrostreptomycin has the same activity as streptomycin against microorganisms. It has a weaker effect than streptomycin on the vestibular portion of the 8th cranial nerve but a much more serious effect on the auditory portion and this may lead to permanent deafness. For this reason the use of dihydrostreptomycin has been abandoned.

Para-aminosalicylic acid (PAS) is a relatively weak tuberculostatic agent. Its action was discovered when benzoic and salicylic acids were shown to increase the oxygen uptake of *Myco. tuberculosis* and PAS inhibited this effect.

Large doses of PAS, up to 20 grams a day by mouth, are required and this is a disadvantage as PAS is rather unpleasant to take. Nevertheless it has proved invaluable as an adjunct to streptomycin to prevent the emergence of streptomycin-resistant strains of *Myco. tuberculosis*. Its mode of action is still not fully understood, but its effect is antagonized by *p*-aminobenzoic acid.

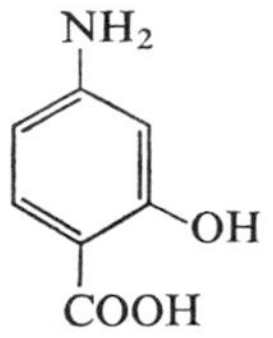

p-Amino-
salicylic acid

Isoniazid (isonicotinic acid hydrazide) is a more pleasant drug to take than is PAS and it is given in smaller doses by mouth or injection. It is a potent tuberculostatic drug but when used alone it leads to the development of resistant strains. Consequently it is given with PAS in the treatment of pulmonary tuberculosis, tuberculous meningitis, and miliary tuberculosis. Isoniazid may cause symptoms of headache, constipation and occasionally convulsions. Its mode of action is still not known but it may act as an antimetabolite.

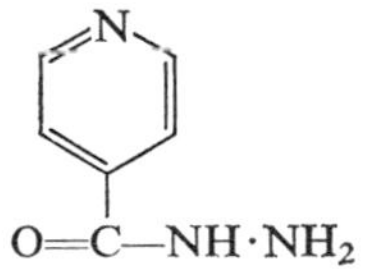

Isoniazid

The mycobacterium of tuberculosis appears to develop a resistance when one drug is given alone in the course of about 6 weeks of treatment. When treatment with streptomycin was first tried, the lives of patients with acute miliary tuberculosis were extended, but the common and more chronic forms of pulmonary tuberculosis were little affected as resistant strains of the organism developed. The simultaneous use of two antitubercular agents obviated this resistance in most cases as cross-resistance did not occur. The compound, *ethambutol*, is fully active against strains of *Myco. tuberculosis* resistant to streptomycin or isoniazid, and may be useful in the future. Clinical data is scanty, and there are reports of visual disturbances and peripheral neuritis.

30

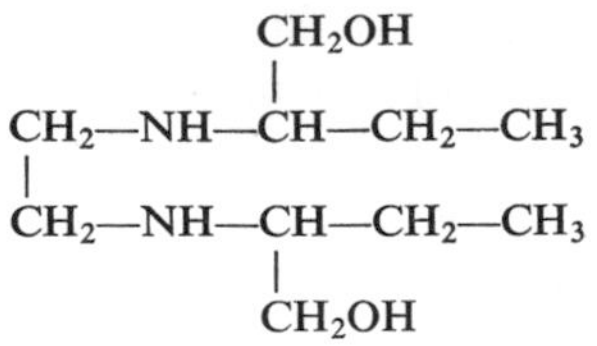

$$CH_2OH$$
$$|$$
$$CH_2-NH-CH-CH_2-CH_3$$
$$|$$
$$CH_2-NH-CH-CH_2-CH_3$$ Ethambutol
$$|$$
$$CH_2OH$$

NEOMYCIN. In 1949, neomycin, another water-soluble, basic antibiotic, was isolated from cultures of the soil-dwelling actinomycete, *Str. fradiae*. It is chemically related to streptomycin and its antibacterial spectrum is similar. It also may damage the 8th cranial nerve. Neomycin is active against gastro-intestinal infections; it has also been used in urinary tract infections, in chronic bronchitis, and in treating infections of the eyes and skin.

CHLORAMPHENICOL. This is produced by the soil-dwelling organism *Str. venezuelae*. It was the first clinically important antibiotic to be synthesized. It is a stable compound, and active orally. The absorption and metabolism of chloramphenicol is described in Fig. 19.5 (page 514). It penetrates the blood-brain barrier.

It is a bacteriostatic agent of outstanding value in the treatment of typhoid fever. It has also been used in the treatment of chronic respiratory and intestinal infections. Toxic side-reactions in man include inflammation of the mouth and gastric upsets. Aplastic anaemia and other blood dyscrasias may follow its prolonged administration, and the use of chloramphenicol should be restricted to infections in which the causative organisms have first been shown to be highly sensitive to it, and resistant to other antibiotics.

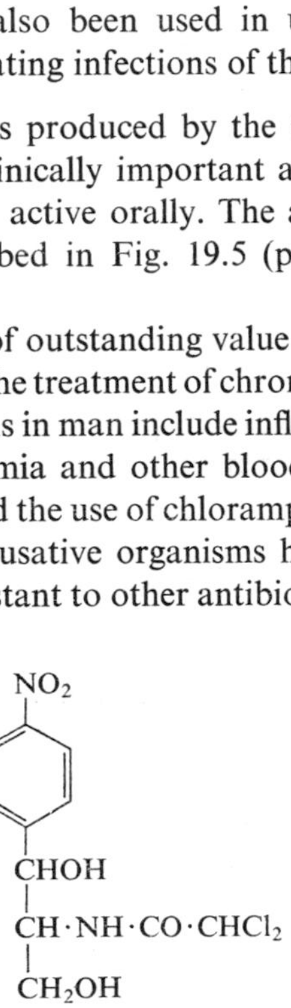

$$NO_2$$

$$CHOH$$
$$|$$
$$CH \cdot NH \cdot CO \cdot CHCl_2$$
$$|$$
$$CH_2OH$$

Chloramphenicol

THE TETRACYCLINES. The tetracyclines are a group of four chemically related antibiotics. *Chlortetracycline* was the first to be discovered and it was followed by *oxytetracycline*, then by *tetracycline* and recently by *dimethyl-chlortetracycline*. All four possess similar antimicrobial spectra, being effective against a wide range of bacteria and against rickettsia and large viruses. There is complete cross-resistance, that is, organisms resistant to one tetracycline are resistant to the others. The mode of action of the tetracycline is not known, although it is thought that they inhibit protein synthesis.

Chlortetracycline was discovered in 1948. It is produced by an actinomycete, the soil-dwelling organism *Str. aureofaciens*. It is a weak base, insoluble in water but fairly stable. Its main indications are in infections due to rickettsiae. It is rapidly and well absorbed from the gastro-intestinal tract.

Oxytetracycline was obtained in 1950 from *Str. rimosus*. It is absorbed more efficiently and excreted in greater quantity in the urine and faeces than is chlortetracycline and is of considerable value in the treatment of amoebic dysentery.

Tetracycline is a stable soluble compound obtained by the catalytic hydrogenation of chlortetracycline. It is stated to be less toxic with less frequent side-effects. It has been widely used in treating pulmonary and genito-urinary infections.

Dimethylchlortetracycline (Ledermycin) was discovered in 1957 when it was found in the culture of a mutant of the original strain of *Str. aureofaciens*. It is very stable and more slowly eliminated than the other tetracylines. After a single oral dose a chemotherapeutic level is maintained in the blood for about twice as long as with the other compounds. Large doses produce gastro-intestinal disturbances.

Dimethylchlortetracycline

ERYTHROMYCIN. This is the best known of a group of antibiotics that consist of large lactone rings linked glycosidically to sugars or diethylamino sugars; they are produced by streptomyces. *Oleandomycin* and *spiramycin* belong to the same group and have properties similar to those of erythromycin. They are all effective against infections with most Gram-positive organisms.

KANAMYCIN. This is derived from strains of *Str. kanamyceticus* and is chemically related to neomycin. It is absorbed rapidly from intramuscular sites and excreted in the urine by glomerular filtration. The antibacterial activity of kanamycin is identical with that of neomycin and there is complete cross-resistance between the two drugs. Kanamycin should be reserved for serious systemic infections caused by staphylococci that are resistant to safer antibiotics and for urinary tract infections in which it is the only antibiotic to which the organism is sensitive. It has been reported to cause kidney damage.

NOVOBIOCIN (Albamycin). This antibiotic is produced from cultures of *Str. spheroides* and *Str. niveus*. It is used primarily to treat infections due to penicillin-resistant strains of *Staph. aureus* and infections of the urinary tract caused by *Proteus vulgaris*.

ANTIFUNGAL ANTIBIOTICS. *Griseofulvin* was originally isolated in 1939 from *P. griseofulvum* but it is in fact produced by several species of *Penicillium*.

It is absorbed after oral administration in man to reach a peak serum level in about 6 h. The main clinical uses of the drug are in the treatment of ringworm of the scalp, fungal infections of the skin, and of fungal infections of finger- and toe-nails. The drug is remarkably non-toxic. It is fungistatic and not fungicidal. Germination of the spores is not inhibited but there is a

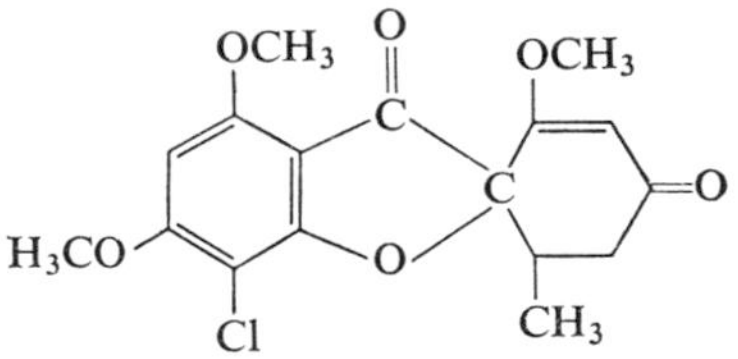

Griseofulvin

marked effect upon the shape and growth of the germ tubes and hyphae. The hyphae are stunted and distorted and characteristically curl into the form of a helix. The inhibition of growth of *Myco. canis* by griseofulvin is partially reversed by various purines, suggesting that its effect is at least partly due to inhibition of nucleic acid synthesis.

Amphotericin B is antibiotic produced by streptomyces, which is used for deep fungus diseases.

Nystatin is produced by streptomyces, and is used locally for infections of mucous membranes.

Undecylenic acid. It was originally found that sweat was antiseptic, and contained a derivative of undecylenic acid. This is an unsaturated fatty acid with an 11-carbon-chain. This and its zinc salt are used in ointments to treat ringworm of the feet and body.

$$CH_2{=}CH(CH_2)_8 \cdot COOH$$

Undecylenic acid

Drugs used in protozoal chemotherapy

Chemotherapy of malaria

Malaria is a disease of the tropics and sub-tropics, its distribution being wide-spread, with the highest incidence in warm, wet and marshy regions. It is characterized by periodic bouts of fever. Malaria is due to infection with proto-zoan parasites of the genus *Plasmodium*. Four species infect man: these are *P. malariae, P. vivax, P. falciparum* and *P. ovale*. The parasite is transmitted to man by the bite of an infected anopheles mosquito. Recently malaria has become an eradicable disease in most areas of the world as a result of advances in the treatment of the disease and in the control of the mosquito vectors.

The life-cycle of the malaria parasite (see Fig. 37.2). The small ring-form of the parasite penetrates the human erythrocyte and grows inside the red blood cell. It then divides asexually to form a *schizont*. The infected cell bursts, and more red blood cells become infected. A small number of parasites however grow into male or female *gametocytes* which are free in the blood. When this blood is ingested by a mosquito, the female gamete is fertilized by the male and the motile *zygote* burrows into the wall of the mosquito's stomach. Here the *oocyst* develops, and produces numerous *sporozoites* which migrate to the salivary glands. When the mosquito feeds again, the sporozoites in the saliva of the insect are injected into the new human host. They find their way to the parenchymal cells of the liver where they develop into large *exoerythrocytic schizonts* which, when mature, release the small ring-forms of the parasite. These then infect the red cells of the blood, and the cycle is complete. The exoerythrocytic forms of *P. vivax* may infect other liver cells. *P. vivax* may therefore persist in the liver for considerable periods and unless the parasite is completely eradicated relapses may occur.

Antimalarial drugs may act at various points in the life cycle of the parasite. Schizonticides are drugs which act upon the asexual parasites in the erythro-cytes. Rapidly acting, efficient drugs of this type are used in the treatment of malarial fever. *Quinine* and *mepacrine* have now been almost entirely superseded by the less toxic 4-aminoquinoline derivatives, *chloroquine* and *amodiaquine* (Fig. 37.3). Such drugs do not affect exoerythrocytic stages of *P. vivax* in the liver.

Drugs that kill exoerythrocytic parasites are termed *tissue schizonticides*. These include 8-aminoquinoline compounds such as *primaquine*, and also *proguanil, chlorproguanil* and *pyrimethamine*. Such drugs are useful in treating patients who have left malarious areas. These drugs also kill gametocytes and hence are also called *sporonticides* (see Fig. 37.3). They act slowly on asexual parasites, although they are effective prophylactics when taken regularly. There is as yet no drug which is very effective against sporozoites, and when

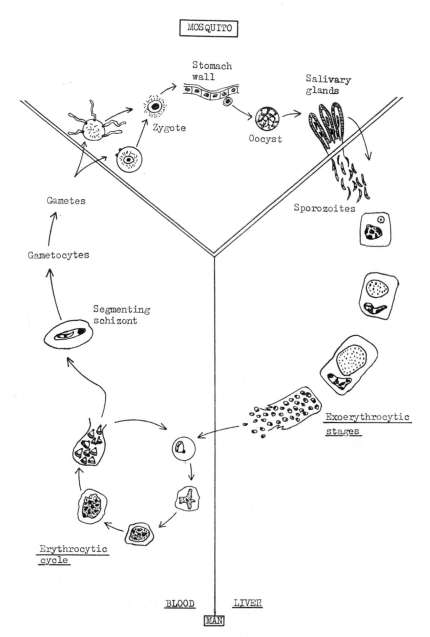

FIG. 37.2. The life-cycle of the malaria parasite.

such a drug is discovered it will be possible to prevent malarial infection from the outset. Table 37.1 summarizes the relative activity of antimalarial drugs at different stages in the life cycle of the parasite.

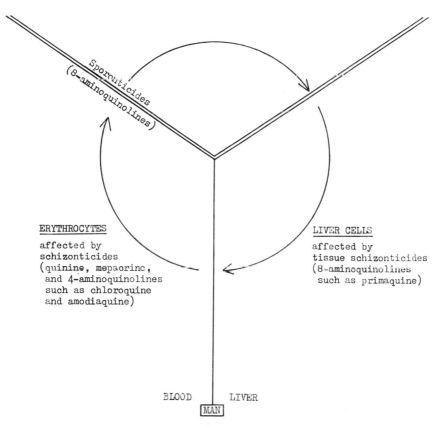

Fig. 37.3. Points of attack of drugs on the malaria parasite.

Quinine. This is the oldest of the antimalarial drugs. The difficulty of obtaining it from its natural source and the development of effective synthetic drugs led to its largely being replaced, except for an occasional use in the treatment of cerebral malaria in which the hydrochloride is injected intravenously. However, the demand for quinine is now increasing again owing to the development of parasites which are resistant to other drugs.

Mepacrine (atebrine, quinacrine). This was one of the first of the synthetic antimalarial drugs. Its main use now is as an anthelmintic (page 947).

Mepacrine

4-Aminoquinoline derivatives. These are the most extensively used and most efficient schizonticides. *Chloroquine* in a single dose usually cures malarial fever in patients who have some immunity to the infection. More doses are needed when the patient has no acquired immunity. *Amodiaquine* is as active as chloroquine. To suppress malaria, doses are given once weekly. Toxic side-effects are few but the drugs have a bitter taste. Chloroquine is concentrated and stored in the liver and although it has no action against exoerythrocytic malaria parasites it is effective in amoebic hepatitis. Very little is known of the mode of action of these 4-aminoquinoline derivatives.

Chloroquine   Amodiaquine

Proguanil, chlorproguanil and pyrimethamine. These three drugs have similar modes of action but differ in potency. Pyrimethamine is the most persistent of the three and is effective as a prophylactic even when given at intervals of three to four weeks.

Proguanil (Paludrine) was found in 1948 to be effective against the malarial parasite *in vivo*. However, it is without activity in tissue culture indicating that its *in vivo* activity is due to a metabolite. This active metabolite was isolated and found to be chemically similar to pyrimethamine which was being tested in the chemotherapy of cancer. The high activity of pyrimethamine in human malaria was then discovered and the drug is now widely used for prophylaxis.

Pyrimethamine acts by depriving the malaria parasite of folinic acid at the point in its life history when this metabolite is most in demand, that is, during division of the nucleus. Its action in acute malaria may be slow unless the

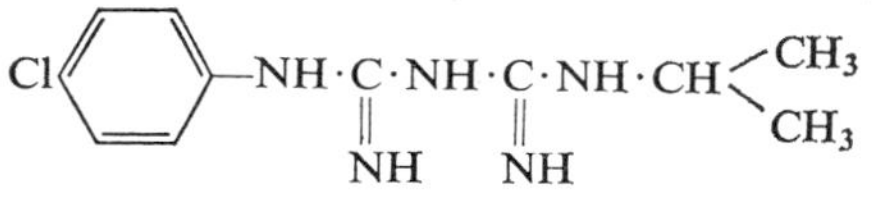

Proguanil

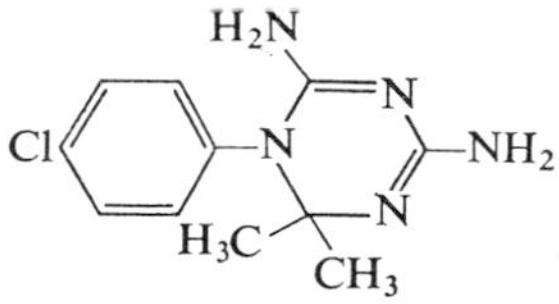

Metabolite of proguanil

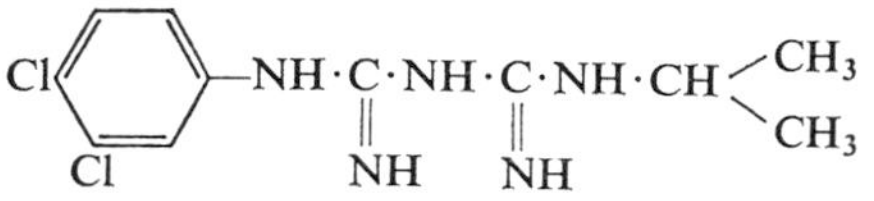

Chlorproguanil

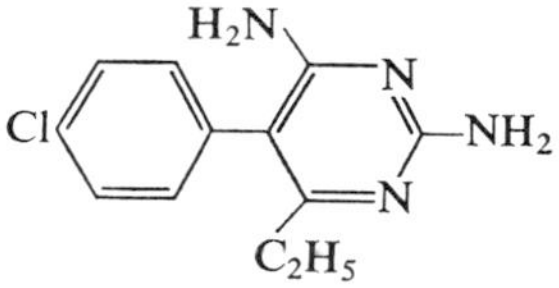

Pyrimethamine

schizonts are maturing rapidly. Pyrimethamine has a selective toxicity to the parasite because the plasmodium relies upon the synthesis of folic and folinic acids from *p*-aminobenzoate, whereas the host makes use of pre-formed folic and folinic acids absorbed from the gut. Sulphonamides and sulphones are also active antimalarials as they compete with *p*-aminobenzoate and so they may potentiate the action of pyrimethamine.

8-*Aminoquinoline derivatives*. The first synthetic antimalarial was introduced in 1926 under the name of *pamaquin*. Its activity against gametocytes was high but it also had a high toxicity to human erythrocytes. Recently, other 8-aminoquinoline derivatives have been found to be active and less toxic, the main one being *primaquine*, the primary amine corresponding to pamaquin. It is widely used in combination with chloroquine for the treatment of *P. vivax* malaria.

The chief dangers associated with the use of 8-aminoquinoline derivatives are intravascular haemolysis and methaemoglobinaemia. Sensitivity to the haemolytic action of primaquine occurs in patients with an inherited abnormality of their erythrocytes in which the activity of glucose 6-phosphate dehydrogenase is deficient. This enzyme utilizes reduced glutathione (page 25) as a cofactor. When primaquine is metabolized, the methyl group is removed and the resulting 6-hydroxy compound has powerful oxidizing activity, and it may affect erythrocytes deficient in reduced glutathione.

Combinations of antimalarial drugs have been successfully used. For example, primaquine once weekly, together with chloroquine to kill erythrocytic parasites, provides adequate protection against *P. vivax* infection. Such an association of an 8-aminoquinoline with a 4-aminoquinoline compound may in the future afford a suppressive and curative effect against all

30*

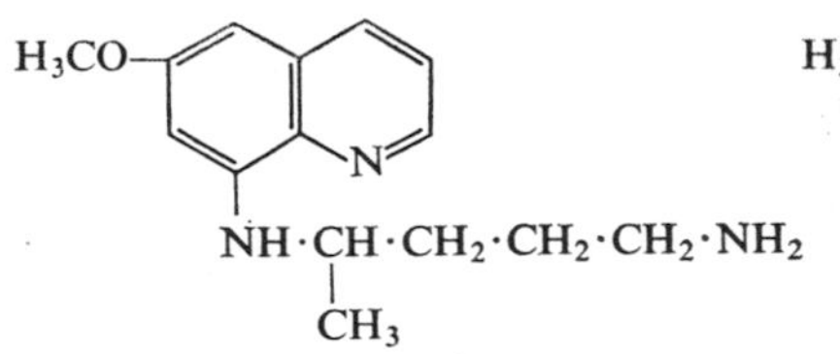

Primaquine

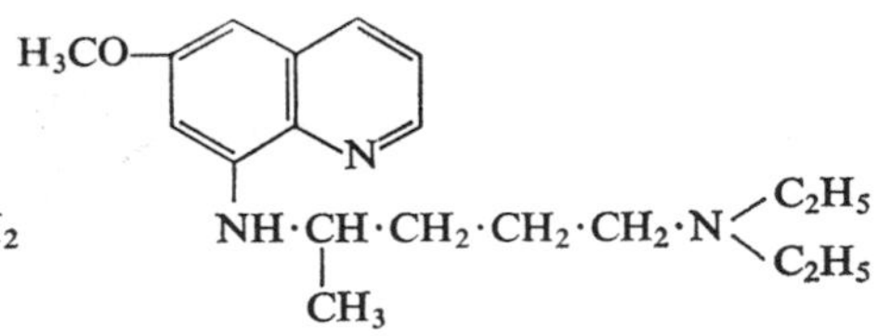

Pamaquin

forms of malaria. The combination of chlorproguanil or pyrimethamine with chloroquine exerts effects on the asexual blood parasites, on the tissue forms in the liver, and on the gametocytes.

TABLE 37.1. Activity of antimalarial drugs on the malarial parasite
in various stages of its life-cycle.

Drug	Asexual blood parasites	Gametocytes—sexual erythrocytic forms	Exoerythrocytic parasites in the liver	Sporozoites
Quinine, mepacrine	Good	No effect	No effect	No effect
Chloroquine, amodiaquine	Good	No effect	No effect	No effect
Primaquine	Good but very slow	Very good	Very good	No effect
Proguanil, chlorproguanil, pyrimethamine	Good but slow	Good	Good	No effect

There are some strains of the malaria parasite which are resistant to proguanil or pyrimethamine, but fortunately these strains are sensitive to the 4-aminoquinolines. Resistance to chloroquine has previously been encountered only rarely in human malaria although several cases have recently been described in South America and it is a particular problem in Vietnam.

Chemotherapy of amoebiasis

Amoebiasis is caused by infection with the protozoan parasite, *Entamoeba histolytica*. The disease is widespread in tropical and subtropical areas, but it also occurs in temperate regions. About 10% of the population of the United

States harbour the parasite, although these people are free from symptoms. The incidence of amoebiasis in Britain is less.

The life-cycle of *E. histolytica* is shown in Fig. 37.4. Infection is caused by the ingestion of viable cysts after contamination of food, drink or hands

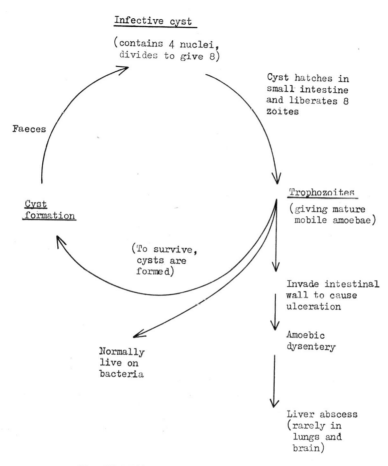

Infective cyst

(contains 4 nuclei, divides to give 8)

Cyst hatches in small intestine and liberates 8 zoites

Faeces

Cyst formation

Trophozoites

(giving mature mobile amoebae)

(To survive, cysts are formed)

Invade intestinal wall to cause ulceration

Amoebic dysentery

Normally live on bacteria

Liver abscess (rarely in lungs and brain)

FIG. 37.4. Life-cycle of *Entamoeba histolytica*.

with infected faeces. Symptom-free carriers of *E. histolytica* may pass cysts in the stools. In patients with symptoms of amoebic dysentery there are motile amoebae in the stools, and there may be inflammation and abscesses of the liver as a result of the infection spreading from the intestine (amoebic hepatitis).

Drugs used in amoebiasis. *Emetine* is an alkaloid present in the dried roots of *Cephaelis ipecacuanha*. It is used by subcutaneous or intramuscular injection in the form of emetine hydrochloride, and by mouth in enteric-coated capsules as emetine bismuth iodide. Emetine hydrochloride is the drug of choice for treatment of acute cases of amoebic dysentery, daily injections being given for up to 7 days. Since it is concentrated in the liver and lungs, it is of great value in treating amoebic abscesses. The amoebae are killed but not the cysts. Emetine bismuth iodide is used for the oral treatment of amoebiasis, since it effectively destroys the intestinal infection. It is usually used after the dysentery has been controlled with emetine hydrochloride. Emetine bismuth iodide is insoluble in acids and liberates emetine only in the intestine. Emetine is a toxic substance, and muscle pain, weakness and fever are common side-effects. The most dangerous effects are upon the heart, where emetine has a direct toxic action upon the myocardium. The patient must therefore be confined to bed.

Chloroquine (see page 936). This is useful for hepatic amoebiasis as it is concentrated in the liver, but it is not effective against intestinal amoebiasis.

Di-iodohydroxyquinoline. This is frequently used as a prophylactic to treat symptom-free carriers. It may be combined with emetine for treatment of chronic intestinal amoebiasis. It is ineffective in amoebic abscess of the liver.

Di-iodohydroxyquinoline　　　7-Iodo-8-hydroxyquinoline-5-sulphonic acid

Chiniofon. This is a mixture of 7-iodo-8-hydroxyquinoline-5-sulphonic acid with sodium bicarbonate. It is used in the treatment of chronic intestinal amoebic dysentery but is of no value in hepatic forms of the disease.

Organic arsenicals. Carbasone is effective in treatment of the intestinal

Carbasone　　　　　　　　　　Acetarsone

infection in chronic amoebic dysentery. It inhibits thiol-enzymes. Acetarsone is also used but it is more toxic than carbasone.

Antibiotics. These are used to treat secondary infections of amoebic abscesses. It is possible that they destroy the bacterial flora in the intestine which produce the metabolites for the amoebae.

Diloxanide. This drug is used in treatment of chronic amoebiasis, as it has a specific action on the cysts of *E. histolytica.* Its toxicity is very low.

Diloxanide (Entamide)

Chemotherapy of trypanosomiasis

Trypanosomes are motile, flagellate, protozoal parasites of vertebrates including man and cattle. The parasite is transmitted by insect vectors. Trypanosomiasis in cattle reduces the economic yield from the land and causes severe loss of livestock. In man it gives rise to chronic disease, debility and death. *Sleeping sickness* is the human disease caused by *Trypanosoma gambiense* and *T. rhodesiense.* The symptoms are due to the presence of trypanosomes in the central nervous system. Patients are drowsy, lethargic and apathetic and sleep for long periods; they become weak and emaciated.

Trypanosomiasis is best treated in its early stages before the parasites have entered the tissues of the central nervous system. Eradication of the disease is being attempted by the use of prophylactic drugs, by destroying the insect vector (the tsetse fly) and its breeding places, and by destruction of game which may act as reservoirs of the pathogenic trypanosomes.

Many compounds of arsenic possess trypanocidal activity, but they are not effective against all pathogenic trypanosomes. Usually arsenicals are effective only in the early stages of trypanosomiasis, the exceptions being tryparsamide and melarsoprol. Trypanocidal activity is confined to compounds containing trivalent arsenic; the pentavalent compounds are pro-drugs being reduced *in vivo* to the active trivalent form.

Tryparsamide. This pentavalent arsenic compound is water-soluble. As it crosses the blood-brain barrier, it is effective in the treatment of the more advanced cases of infection with *T. gambiense* and *T. rhodesiense.* It possesses some toxic side-effects, the most important being optic nerve atrophy, skin rashes and diarrhoea, and these effects are usually controlled by removing the arsenic with dimercaprol (page 468). Tryparsamide-resistant strains of trypanosomes have appeared.

Sodium para-aminophenylarsonate. This was the first pentavalent arsenical widely used for the treatment of trypanosomiasis. It gives good results in early cases but it is toxic and may cause blindness. It has now been replaced by less toxic drugs.

Sodium para-aminophenylarsonate Tryparsamide Butarsen

Melarsoprol. This is a complex of melarsen oxide (which contains trivalent arsenic) with dimercaprol, and it is effective in infections due to tryparsamide-resistant organisms. Its great value lies in its ability to cure trypanosomiasis in which the central nervous system is involved and in which there is a concurrent meningitis or encephalitis. There are frequent side-effects, including abdominal pain, dermatitis, and allergic reactions.

Butarsen. This trivalent arsenical is effective in early cases of African trypanosomiasis.

Trypanosomes sensitive to arsenic take it up from the surrounding medium and bind it firmly. The organic arsenicals are believed to release trivalent arsenic which combines with and inactivates vital enzymes by reacting with free thiol groups. One of these enzymes is hexokinase which catalyses the conversion of glucose to glucose 6-phosphate. The trypanosomes have a high metabolic rate and oxidize large amounts of glucose, so that compounds which inhibit or prevent glucose uptake or utilization are likely to lead to death of the organisms. It is possible that the arsenic resistant species of trypanosomes contain large amounts of protective substances such as glutathione which react with and inactivate the drug.

Diamidines. Diamidines are effective trypanocides *in vitro* and the aromatic derivatives are effective *in vivo*. Pentamidine is widely used as a prophylactic aid for the treatment of early cases of African trypanosomiasis. Stilbamidine and propamidine are also effective in early cases but are more toxic than pentamidine. Pentamidine appears to be the best available prophylactic drug for mass use. The exact point of attack of diamidines on the organism is still not certain. It was first thought that diamidines prevented glucose uptake, but later studies showed that this is not the full story.

Suramin. A number of dyestuffs were shown many years ago to be capable of curing experimental trypanosome infections in mice, but these were ineffective in man. Colourless compounds based upon the structure of the active dyestuffs

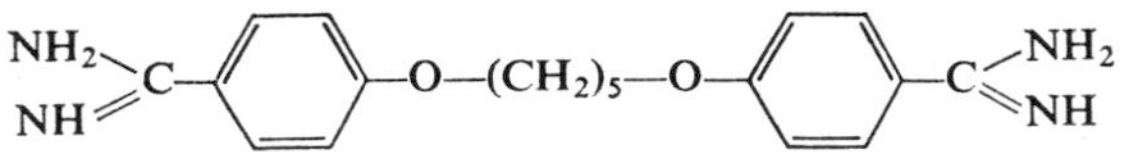

Pentamidine

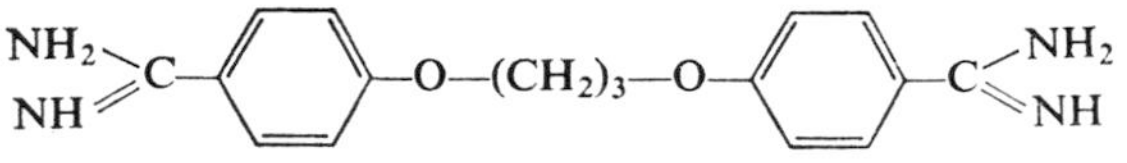

Propamidine

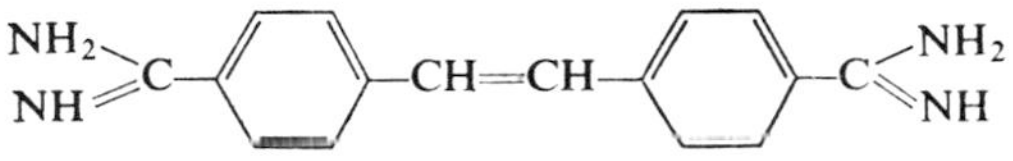

Stilbamidine

(trypan red, trypan blue and afridol violet) were later prepared and one of these is suramin, a complex derivative of urea. It probably binds to tissue proteins and to the organisms, and this may be the first step in its lethal action. It has been suggested that it inhibits anaerobic glycolysis. Suramin is a long-acting drug and is particularly useful as a prophylactic. It is effective in early African trypanosomiasis but is of no use in the advanced form of the disease as it fails to penetrate nervous tissues. The drug is given by intramuscular injection. Side-effects are numerous and include nausea, vomiting and diarrhoea.

Chemotherapy of leishmaniasis

Kala-azar is the name given to visceral leishmaniasis caused by *Leishmania donovani*, a type of trypanosome. Infection is transmitted by the bite of a sand fly which is the insect vector. It is believed that the main vertebrate reservoir is the dog. The leishmanias are taken up by the cells of the reticulo-endothelial system which swell and burst so that more cells become infected. Symptoms therefore are due to heavy parasitization of the reticulo-endothelial system. Organic antimonials containing pentavalent antimony remain the most widely used and effective drugs in the treatment of kala-azar. A large number of

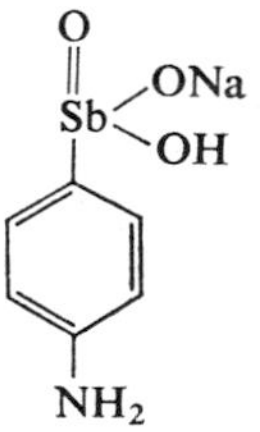

Stibamine

compounds including stibamine are derivatives of para-aminophenylstibonic acid. Amongst the newer compounds of antimony, *glucantime* (N-methyl-glucamine antimoniate), appears to be safe and effective and it may be given by intravenous injection. The mode of action of these compounds is not certain; they probably inhibit essential enzymes by reacting with free thiol groups.

Stilbamidine, an aromatic diamidine (see page 943), is also very effective in the treatment of kala-azar, but it is a toxic substance, damage to the trigeminal nerve often being observed after prolonged treatment. Pentamidine is now used instead of stilbamidine.

Chemotherapy of helminthiasis

Infestation with parasitic worms (helminthiasis) is the cause of much chronic ill-health and inefficiency, and its control by drugs and other measures remains an urgent problem in the tropics. Although helminths cause severe damage in the human tissues, very few infect laboratory animals which poses a problem in setting up suitable systems for testing new drugs. Drugs which are used to destroy and eliminate parasitic worms are known as *anthelmintics*. A wide range of compounds of different types have anthelmintic activity and there is no obvious relationship between structure and activity.

The parasitic helminths of man include nematodes (threadworms, round-worms, hookworms, whipworms and filarial worms), trematodes (schisto-somes), and cestodes (tapeworms).

Drugs effective against nematodes. Piperazine, which was introduced for the treatment of gout and rheumatism is absorbed from the intestine of man and excreted in the urine. It was later found to be effective against roundworms which inhabit the lower part of the bowel. It blocks neuromuscular trans-mission in the worms and they become flaccid and unable to maintain their position in the small intestine. In consequence, they are swept onwards by the peristaltic waves of the gut and expelled. The action of acetylcholine on muscle from the worm is blocked by piperazine, but the mechanism of neuro-muscular transmission differs from that in higher animals which are not

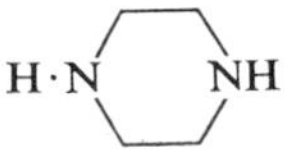

$$H \cdot N \diagup \diagdown NH$$

Piperazine

paralysed by piperazine. *Diethylcarbamazine* is a derivative of piperazine with a potent action on certain nematodes. Its chief value is in the treatment of filarial infections. The surfaces of the larvae of the worms become modified in such a way that they are devoured by histiocytes in the capillaries of the lung and liver. *Bephenium* is also effective in treating infestation with round-worms and hookworms. It has low toxicity but it is a bitter substance. It is poorly absorbed by the host and is therefore likely to act by contact with the cuticle of the worm. The chemical structure of the drug suggests that it acts on the neuromuscular system but little is known of its mode of action. It is usually used as the hydroxynaphthoate.

$$H_3C—N\overbrace{\quad\quad}N—CO\cdot N\underset{C_2H_5}{\overset{C_2H_5}{\diagup}}$$

Diethylcarbamazine

$$\bigcirc—O\cdot CH_2\cdot CH_2\cdot \underset{\overset{|}{CH_3}}{N}—CH_2—\bigcirc$$

Bephenium

It is inconvenient to use deeply-coloured substances in human medicine but the disadvantages of dyes are sometimes overshadowed by their usefulness in the treatment of otherwise intractable infections. *Gentian violet* was for many years the drug of choice in the treatment of threadworm infections. Later the red dye, *pyrvinium*, and the blue cyanine dye, *dithiazanine*, were used for the treatment of roundworms and hookworms. It is possible that the mode of action of all these dyes is concerned with inhibition of the carbohydrate meta-bolism of helminths.

Drugs effective against trematodes. The most important trematode parasites of man are the schistosomes, and the disease, schistosomiasis (*bilharziasis*), is widespread in Africa, South America, China and Japan. There are millions of cases of the disease in the Nile Valley. The intermediate host of the helminth is a freshwater snail, and the infection is contracted by bathing in, or drinking, the water into which the infective forms of the parasite have emerged from the tissues of the snail. The adult flukes live within the blood vessels of the gut or bladder of man. Chronic illness and severe damage to tissues is caused by the passage of the eggs shed by the females through all the tissues. Eggs which enter the portal systems lodge in the liver and cause fibrosis. The life cycle of the parasite involves the passage of eggs into the bladder and intestine from which they are excreted with the urine and faeces. The eggs hatch in water to form miracidia which are motile larvae. These pene-trate the tissues of the snail in which they finally develop into cercariae. The cercariae liberated from the snail live an independent existence in the water until they infect a human host. The organism penetrates the skin and makes its way via the lymphatics to the blood vessels in which it finally lodges.

Trivalent organic antimony compounds were amongst the earliest remedies for schistosomiasis and they are still in use today. Both *sodium antimony tartrate* and *potassium antimony tartrate* (tartar emetic) are effective in killing the adult schistosomes. The side-effects are often serious and coughing, vomiting and pains in the abdomen are common. *Sodium antimonyl gluconate* is less toxic but no antimonial is completely free from toxic effects upon the heart muscle. *Stibophen* (sodium antimony pyrocatechol disulphonate) has also been used. Trivalent antimony is a powerful inhibitor of schistosome phosphofructo-kinase, the enzyme which catalyses the phosphorylation of fructose-6-phos-phate by adenosine triphosphate. Mammalian phosphofructokinase is much less sensitive to inhibition and the chemotherapeutic action of antimony in schistosomiasis may depend upon this difference in sensitivity of the host and parasite enzymes.

The drug, *lucanthone*, is active by mouth and also kills the adult worms with-out producing severe toxic side-effects. Abdominal discomfort is sometimes produced. Treatment is usually continued for up to 6 days. A new approach has recently been made by combining lucanthone with a synthetic resin from which it is slowly released to maintain a steady concentration in the blood.

Lucanthone

The discovery of the high activity of phenoxyalkane derivatives against schistosome infections in mice opened yet another avenue of research in this field. These compounds prevent the uptake of glucose by the schistosomes but have no direct action upon the enzymes involved in carbohydrate metabolism. Unfortunately, they have a specific toxic effect on the pigment layer of the retina in many animal species and have been found to affect vision in man.

Drugs effective against cestodes. Tapeworms are found in the small intestine of man. When pigs or cattle feed on land contaminated with human faeces, they ingest the eggs of the worm. The eggs hatch in the gut and larvae migrate to the skeletal muscles where they encyst. If the meat is insufficiently cooked, the parasites survive and the life-cycle is completed. Little advance has been made in recent years in the chemotherapy of tapeworm infection in man. *Extract of male fern* is still widely used. *Mepacrine* (page 936) is effective. *Dichlorophen* is a new compound for this infection; worms affected by it are expelled in a partially digested state. Derivatives of dichlorophen are now undergoing clinical trials.

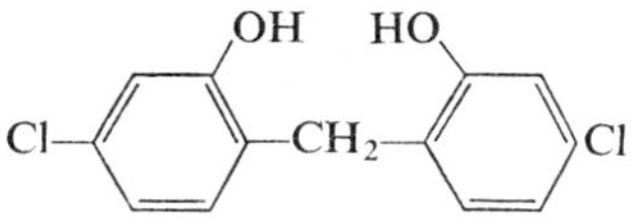

Dichlorophen

Drugs used in the treatment of cancer

Drugs used in the treatment of malignant disease include: (1) radiomimetic drugs, (2) antimetabolites, (3) alkaloids, (4) urethane, (5) antibiotics, (6) hormones and (7) radioactive isotopes.

Radiomimetic drugs. Mustard gas was used as a poison gas during the First World War, and nitrogen mustards possess similar properties. Their effects

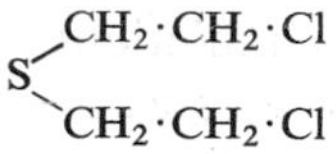

Mustard gas

upon proliferating tissues led to their trial in the treatment of neoplastic disease. They do not specifically or selectively damage malignant cells but also damage normal ones, particularly rapidly-growing normal cells such as those of the bone marrow. Their pharmacological activity is due to the formation of cyclic etheylenimmonium derivatives which are very unstable and highly reactive and which combine with many chemical groupings found in the tissue proteins. Nucleic acids react very readily with the nitrogen mustards and the cytotoxic actions of these drugs may be due to their ability to form cross-linkages between the protein molecules of the chromosomes and so to alter their properties. The di-2-haloethyl structure appears to be essential, and for activity there must be not less than two haloethyl groups, the halogens being in the position β to the sulphur or nitrogen atom. *Mustine* is a simple nitrogen mustard which has been in use in cancer chemotherapy for about 18 years. The drug solution is made up immediately before use, and it must

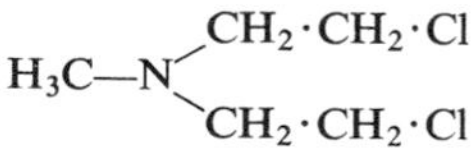

Mustine

be given by the intravenous route. Mustine is used to treat Hodgkin's disease (cancer of lymphatic tissue) and chronic myeloid leukaemia. Chronic lymphatic leukaemia is usually treated with other nitrogen mustards.

Antimetabolites. Folic-acid deficiency is accompanied by leucopenia, and hence antimetabolites of folic acid were synthesized with the object of using them to inhibit the growth of neoplasms in the white blood cell-forming tissues of the body. Other antimetabolites used in the treatment of acute leukaemia in both children and adults include *mercaptopurine* and various amino acid analogues.

Hormones. Oestrogens are employed in the treatment of cancer of the prostate gland. They antagonize the actions of the androgens on the prostate gland, and so may be used in conjunction with surgical removal of the testis.

Both oestrogens and androgens may be used in the treatment of advanced inoperable cases of cancer of the breast in which there are widespread secondary deposits.

Corticotrophin and prednisolone are sometimes used in the treatment of acute leukaemia in children. Both drugs act rapidly and are of value in treating very acute cases of the disease.

Radioactive isotopes. Ionizing radiations destroy both normal and malignant cells and they may therefore be used to irradiate tumours. Radioactive iodine is used for therapeutic and diagnostic purposes in the case of thyroid tumours. Radioactive phosphorus is used in the treatment of cancer of the blood-forming organs.

Suggestions for
Further Reading

Chapter 1 Constituents of Living Matter

BALDWIN E. (1962) *The Nature of Biochemistry*. Cambridge University Press.
BALDWIN E. (1963) *Dynamic Aspects of Biochemistry*. Cambridge University Press.
DIXON M. & WEBB E.C. (1964) *Enzymes*. Longmans, London.
HARRISON K. (1962) *A Guide-book to Biochemistry*. Cambridge University Press.
HUTCHINSON D.W. (1964) *Nucleotides and Coenzymes*. Methuen, London.
NEIL M.W. (1961) *Vertebrate Biochemistry*. Pitman, London.
STEINER R.F. (1965) *The Chemical Foundations of Molecular Biology*. Van Nostrand, Princeton.
WAGNER A.F. & FOLKERS K. (1964) *Vitamins and Coenzymes*. Wiley, London.

Chapter 2 Cells and Tissues

BELL D.J. & GRANT J.K. (ed.) (1963) *The Structure and Functions of the Membranes and Surfaces of Cells*. Cambridge University Press.
BLOOM W. & FAWCETT D.W. (1962) *Textbook of Histology*. Saunders, Philadelphia.
BOURNE G.H. (1962) *Division of Labour in Cells*. Academic Press, New York.
BUTLER J.A.V. (1964) *The Life of the Cell*. Allen and Unwin, London.
CLOWES R.C. (ed.) (1965) Recent research in molecular biology. *Br. med. Bull.*, **21**, 183.
CRICK F.H.C. (1962) The genetic code. *Scient. Am.*, **207**(4), 66.
CSÁKY T.Z. (1965) Transport through biological membranes. *A. Rev. Physiol.*, **27**, 415.
DAVIDSON J.N. (1957) *The Biochemistry of the Nucleic Acids*. Methuen, London.
DICKENS F. (ed.) (1953) Some aspects of enzyme research. *Br. med. Bull.*, **9**, 85.
DUVE C. DE (1963) The lysosome. *Scient. Am.* **208**(5), 64.
GREEN D.E. (1964) The mitochondrion. *Scient. Am.*, **210**(1), 63.
LEHNINGER A.L. (1964) *The Mitochondrion*. Benjamin, New York.
NIRENBERG M.W. (1963) The genetic code, II. *Scient. Am.*, **208**(3), 80.
RAVIN A.W. (1965) *The Evolution of Genetics*. Academic Press, New York.
ROBERTSON J.D. (1962) The membrane of the living cell. *Scient. Am.*, **206**(4), 64.
SINNOTT E.W., DUNN L.C. & DOBZHANSKY T. (1958) *Principles of Genetics*. McGraw-Hill, New York.
SWANSON C.P. (1960) *Cytology and Cytogenetics*. Macmillan, London.
WILSON G.B. & MORRISON J.H. (1966) *Cytology*. Reinhold, New York.

Chapter 3 Properties of Neurones

BAKER P.F. (1966) The nerve axon. *Scient. Am.*, **214**(3), 74.
BOURNE G.H. (1959) Subcellular structure of the neurone. *International Review of Cytology*, vol. 8,

BRAZIER M.A.B. (1960) *The Electrical Activity of the Nervous System*. Pitman, London.

DOUGLAS W.W. & RITCHIE J.M. (1962) Mammalian non-myelinated nerve fibres. *Physiol. Rev.*, **42**, 297.

ECCLES J.C. (1957) *The Physiology of Nerve Cells*. Johns Hopkins Press, Baltimore.

ECCLES J.C. (1964) *The Physiology of the Synapse*. Springer-Verlag, Berlin.

ECCLES J.C. (1965) The synapse. *Scient. Am.*, **212**(1), 56.

FIELD J. (ed.) (1959) *Neurophysiology*, vol. 1, chaps. 2–7. American Physiological Society, Washington.

HODGKIN A. L. (1964) *The Conduction of the Nervous Impulse*. Liverpool University Press.

RUCH T.C., PATTON H.D., WOODBURY J.W. & TOWE A.L. (1965) *Neurophysiology*. Saunders, Philadelphia.

SHANES A.M. (1958) Electrochemical aspects of physiological and pharmacological action in excitable cells. *Pharmac. Rev.*, **10**, 59.

WHITTAKER V.P. & GRAY E.G. (1962) The synapse—biology and morphology. *Br. med. Bull.*, **18**, 223.

Chapter 4   The Nervous System

ANAND B.K. (1961) Nervous regulation of food intake. *Physiol. Rev.*, **41**, 677.

ANDERSSON B. & LARSSON S. (1961) Physiological and pharmacological aspects of the control of hunger and thirst. *Pharmac. Rev.*, **13**, 1.

BRAZIER M.A.B. (1962) The analysis of brain waves. *Scient. Am.*, **206**(6), 142.

BROWN-GRANT K & CROSS B.A. (ed.) (1966) Recent studies on the hypothalamus. *Br. med. Bull.*, **22**, 195.

CAMPBELL H.J. (1966) *Correlative Physiology of the Nervous System*. Academic Press, London.

CANNON W.B. (1929) *Bodily Changes in Pain, Hunger, Fear and Rage*. Reprinted in 1963 by Harper & Row, New York.

CHUSID J.G. & McDONALD J.J. (1964) *Correlative Anatomy and Functional Neurology*. Lange Medical Publications, Los Altos, California.

DOBBING J. (1961) The blood-brain barrier. *Physiol. Rev.*, **41**, 130.

FELDBERG W.S. (ed.) (1957) Autonomic nervous system. *Br. med. Bull.*, **13**, 153.

FELDBERG W.S. (1963) *A Pharmacological Approach to the Brain from its Inner and Outer Surfaces*. Arnold, London.

FIELD J. (ed.) (1960) *Neurophysiology*, vol. 2. American Physiological Society, Washington.

GERARD R.W., FESSARD A. & KONORSKI J. (ed.) (1961). *Brain Mechanisms and Learning*. Davis, Philadelphia.

GRANIT R. (1962) *Receptors and Sensory Perception*. Yale University Press, New Haven.

GREEN J.D. (1964) The hippocampus. *Physiol. Rev.*, **44**, 561.

HUNT C.C. & PERL E.R. (1960) Spinal reflex mechanisms concerned with skeletal muscle. *Physiol. Rev.*, **40**, 538.

JOUVET M. (1967) The states of sleep. *Scient. Am.*, **216**(2), 62.

KLEITMAN N. (1960) Patterns of dreaming. *Scient. Am.*, **203**(5), 82.

KLEITMAN N. (1963) *Sleep and Wakefulness*. Chicago University Press.

MAGOUN H.W. (1963) *The Waking Brain*. Thomas, Springfield.

MATTHEWS P.B.C. (1964) Muscle spindles and their motor control. *Physiol. Rev.*, **44**, 219.

MAYER J. & THOMAS D.W. (1967) Regulation of food intake and obesity. *Science*, **156**, 328.

OLDS J. (1962) Hypothalamic substrates of reward. *Physiol. Rev.*, **42**, 554.

OSWALD I. (1962) *Sleeping and Waking*. Elsevier, New York.

OSWALD I. (1966) *Sleep*. Penguin Books, Middlesex.

PAVLOV I.P. (1963) *Lectures on Conditioned Reflexes* (2 vols.). Translated by Gantt W.H. Lawrence & Wishart, London.

PÉON R.H. (ed.) (1963) *The Physiological Basis of Mental Activity*. Elsevier, Amsterdam.

RANSON S.W. & CLARK S.L. (1958) *Anatomy of the Nervous System*. Saunders, Philadelphia.

SHERRINGTON C. (1961) *The Integrative Action of the Nervous System*. Yale University Press, New Haven.

SIMON A., HERBERT C.C. & STRAUS R. (ed.) (1961) *The Physiology of Emotions*. Thomas, Springfield.

SPERRY R.W. (1964) The great cerebral commissure. *Scient. Am.*, **210**(1), 42.

WALSH E.G. (1964) *Physiology of the Nervous System*. Longmans, London.

WALTER W.G. (1953) *The Living Brain*. Duckworth, London.

WILSON V.J. (1966) Inhibition in the central nervous system. *Scient. Am*, **214**(5), 102.

WOLFF H.G. (1963) *Headache and Other Head Pains*. Oxford University Press, New York.

WOLSTENHOLME G.E.W. & O'CONNOR C.M. (ed.) (1958) *The Cerebrospinal Fluid* (Ciba Foundation symposium). Churchill, London.

WOLSTENHOLME G.E.W. & O'CONNOR C.M. (ed.) (1958) *On the Neurological Basis of Behaviour* (Ciba Foundation symposium). Churchill, London.

WOOLDRIDGE D.E. (1963) *The Machinery of the Brain*. McGraw-Hill, New York.

Chapter 5   Humoral Transmission of Nervous Impulses

ACHESON G.H. (ed.) (1966) Second symposium on catecholamines. *Pharmac. Rev.*, **18**, 1.

BRADLEY P.B. (ed.) (1965) Pharmacology of the central nervous system. *Br. med. Bull.*, **21**, 1.

BURN J.H. & RAND M.J. (1960) Acetylcholine in adrenergic transmission. *A. Rev. Pharmac.*, **5**, 163.

BURN J.H. & RAND M.J. (1962) A new interpretation of the adrenergic nerve fibre. *Adv. Pharmac.*, **1**, 2. Academic Press, New York.

CROSSLAND J. (1960) Chemical transmission in the central nervous system. *J. Pharm. Pharmac.*, **12**, 1.

CURTIS D.R. (1963) The pharmacology of central and peripheral inhibition. *Pharmac. Rev.*, **15**, 333.

DALE H.H. (1954) The beginnings and the prospects of neurohumoral transmission. *Pharmac. Rev.*, **6**, 7.

DALE H.H. (1963) *Adventures in Physiology*. Pergamon, London.

EULER U.S. VON (1956) *Noradrenaline*. Thomas, Springfield.

EULER U.S. VON (1963) Adrenergic neurohormones. *Comparative Endocrinology*, vol. 2. Euler U.S. von & Heller H. (ed.). Academic Press, New York.

FERRY C.B. (1966) Cholinergic link hypothesis in adrenergic neuroeffector transmission. *Physiol. Rev.*, **46**, 420.

FELDBERG W. (ed.) (1957) Autonomic nervous system. *Br. med. Bull.*, **13**, 153.

KOELLE G.B. (ed.) (1962) *Cholinesterase and Anticholinesterase Agents*. Springer-Verlag, Berlin.

KOELLE G.B., DOUGLAS W.W. & CARLSSON A. (ed.) (1965) *Pharmacology of Cholinergic and Adrenergic Transmission*. Pergamon, Oxford.

MARTIN A.R. (1966) Quantal nature of synaptic transmission. *Physiol. Rev.*, **46**, 51.

MCLENNAN H. (1963) *Synaptic Transmission*. Saunders, Philadelphia.

McLennan H. (1965) Synaptic transmission in the central nervous system. *Physiological Pharmacology*, vol. 2. Root W.S. & Hofmann F.G. (ed.). Academic Press, New York.

Triggle D.J. (1965) *Chemical Aspects of the Autonomic Nervous System*. Academic Press, London.

Varley H. & Gowenlock A.H. (ed.) (1963) *The Clinical Chemistry of Monoamines*. Elsevier, Amsterdam.

Vane J.R. (ed.) (1960) *Adrenergic Mechanisms* (Ciba Foundation symposium). Churchill, London.

Whittaker V.P. (1963) Cholinergic neurohormones. *Comparative Endocrinology*, vol. 2. Euler U.S. von & Heller H. (ed.). Academic Press, New York.

Chapter 6   Local Hormones

Ambache N. (1963) Physiologically active lipid anions. *Comparative Endocrinology*, vol. 2. Euler U.S. von & Heller H. (ed.). Academic Press, New York.

Berne R.M. (1964) Regulation of coronary blood flow. *Physiol. Rev.*, **44**, 1.

Bülbring E.(1961) The intrinsic nervous system of the intestine and local effects of 5-hydroxy-tryptamine. *Regional Neurochemistry*. Kety S.S. & Elkes J. (ed.). Pergamon, Oxford.

Burn J.H. (1954) Acetylcholine as a local hormone for ciliary movement and the heart. *Pharmac. Rev.*, **6**, 107.

Erdös F.G. (ed.) (1964) Structure and function of biologically active peptides: bradykinin, kallidin and congeners. *Ann. N.Y. Acad. Sci.*, **104**, 1.

Erspamer V. (1954) Pharmacology of indolealkylamines. *Pharmac. Rev.*, **6**, 425.

Erspamer V. (1961) Pharmacologically active substances of mammalian origin. *A. Rev. Pharmac.*, **1**, 175.

Gaddum J.H. (ed.) (1955) *Polypeptides which Stimulate Plain Muscle*. Livingstone, Edinburgh.

Green H.N. & Stoner H.B. (1950) *Biological Actions of the Adenine Nucleotides*. Lewis, London.

Hornykiewicz O. (1966) Dopamine (3-hydroxytyramine) and brain function. *Pharmac. Rev.*, **18**, 925.

Kahlson G. (1960) A place for histamine in normal physiology. *Lancet*, **1**, 67.

Keele C.A. & Armstrong D. (1964) *Substances Producing Pain and Itch*. Arnold, London.

Lewis G.P. (ed.) (1958) *5-Hydroxytryptamine*. Pergamon, Oxford.

Nachmansohn D. (1959) *Chemical and Molecular Basis of Nerve Activity*. Academic Press, New York.

Peart W.S. (1965) The renin-angiotensin system. *Pharmac. Rev.*, **17**, 143.

Rocha e Silva M. (1963) The physiological significance of bradykinin. *Ann. N.Y. Acad. Sci.*, **104**, 190.

Schachter M. (ed.) (1960) *Polypeptides which Affect Smooth Muscle and Blood Vessels*. Pergamon, Oxford.

Schildkraut J.J. & Kety S.S. (1967) Biogenic amines and emotion. *Science*, **156**, 21.

Stern P. (1963) Substance P as a sensory transmitter and its other central effects. *Ann. N.Y. Acad. Sci.*, **104**, 403.

Vogt W. (1958) Naturally occurring lipid-soluble acids of pharmacological interest. *Pharmac. Rev.*, **10**, 407.

Wolstenholme G.E.W. & O'Connor C.M. (ed.) (1956) *Histamine* (Ciba Foundation symposium). Churchill, London.

Chapter 7 Properties of Muscle

ADOLPH E.F. (1967) The heart's pacemaker. *Scient. Am.*, **216**(3), 32.

BLINKS J.R. & KOCH-WESER J. (1963) Physical factors in the analysis of the actions of drugs on myocardial contractility. *Pharmac. Rev.*, **15**, 531.

BOURNE G.H. (ed.) (1960) *Structure and Function of Muscle*, vols. 1, 2 and 3. Academic Press New York.

BÜLBRING E. (ed.) (1964) *Pharmacology of Smooth Muscle. Proceedings of Second International Pharmacological Meeting*, vol. 6. Pergamon, Oxford.

BURNSTOCK G. & HOLMAN M.E. (1963) Smooth muscle: autonomic nerve transmission. *A. Rev. Physiol.*, **25**, 61.

BURNSTOCK G., HOLMAN E. & PROSSER C.L. (1963) Electrophysiology of smooth muscle. *Physiol. Rev.*, **43**, 482.

CARVALHO A.P. DE, DE MELLO W.C. & HOFFMAN B.F. (ed.) (1961) *The Specialized Tissues of the Heart*. Elsevier, Amsterdam.

CSILLIK B. (1965) *Functional Structure of the Post-synaptic Membrane*. Hungarian Academy of Sciences, Budapest.

GUTMANN E. (ed.) (1962) *The Denervated Muscle*. Czechoslovak Academy of Sciences, Prague.

GUTTMANN E. & HNÍK P. (ed.) (1963) *The Effect of Use and Disuse on Neuromuscular Functions*. Elsevier, Amsterdam.

HOFFMAN B.F. & CRANEFIELD P.F. (1960) *Electrophysiology of the Heart*. McGraw-Hill, New York.

HUXLEY A.F. & HUXLEY H.E. (organizers) (1964) A discussion on the physical and chemical basis of muscular contraction. *Proc. R. Soc. B.*, **160**, 434.

HUXLEY H.E. (1965) The mechanism of muscular contraction. *Scient. Am.*, **213**(6), 18.

KATZ B. (1966) *Nerve, Muscle and Synapse*. McGraw-Hill, London.

KOCH-WESER J. & BLINKS J.R. (1963) The influence of the interval between beats on myocardial contractility. *Pharmac. Rev.*, **15**, 601.

PATON W.D.M. (ed.) (1956) Physiology of voluntary muscle. *Br. med. Bull.*, **12**, 161.

PAUL W.M., DANIEL E.E., KAY C.M. & MONCKTON G. (ed.) (1964) *Muscle*. Pergamon, London.

OLSON R.E. (1962) Physiology of cardiac muscle. *Circulation*, vol. 1. Hamilton W.F. (ed.). American Physiological Society, Washington.

SCHAEFER H. & HAAS H.G. (1962) Electrocardiography. *Circulation*, vol. 1. Hamilton W.F. (ed.). American Physiological Society, Washington.

SCHER A.M. (1962) Excitation of the heart. *Circulation*, vol. 1. Hamilton W.F. (ed.). American Physiological Society, Washington.

TACCARDI B. & MARCHETTI G. (ed.) (1963) *International Symposium on Electrophysiology of the Heart*. Pergamon, Oxford.

WOODBURY J.W. (1962) Cellular electrophysiology of the heart. *Circulation*, vol. 1. Hamilton W.F. (ed.). American Physiological Society, Washington.

Chapter 8 Blood and Tissue Fluids

BIGGS R. & MACFARLANE R.G. (1962) *Human Blood Coagulation and its Disorders*. Blackwell, Oxford.

CLINE M.J. (1965) Metabolism of the circulating leucocyte. *Physiol. Rev.*, **45**, 674.

DOLE V.P. & HAMLIN J.T. (1962) Particulate fat in lymph and blood. *Physiol. Rev.*, **42**, 674.

GUEST M.M. (1965) Circulatory effects of blood clotting, fibrinolysis, and related hemostatic processes. *Circulation*, vol. 3. Hamilton W.F. (ed.). American Physiological Society, Washington.

GALTON D.A.G. (ed.) (1959) Haematology. *Br. med. Bull.*, **15**, 1.

GOLDSMITH K.L.G. (ed.) (1959) Blood groups. *Br. med. Bull.*, **15**, 89.

HARRIS J.W. (1963) *The Red Cell*. Harvard University Press, Massachusetts.

HOLBOROW E.J. (ed.) (1963) Antibodies. *Br. med. Bull.*, **19**, 169.

JACOBSON L.O. & DOYLE M. (ed.) (1962) *Erythropoiesis*. Grune & Stratton, New York.

LAKI K. & GLADNER J.A. (1964) Chemistry and physiology of the fibrinogen-fibrin transition. *Physiol. Rev.*, **44**, 127.

LANDIS E.M. & PAPPENHEIMER J.R. (1963) Exchange of substances through the capillary walls. *Circulation*, vol. 2. Hamilton W.F. (ed.). American Physiological Society, Washington.

LAWSON H.C. (1962) The volume of blood—a critical examination of methods for its measurement. *Circulation*, vol. 1. Hamilton W.F. (ed.). American Physiological Society, Washington.

MAYERSON H.S. (1963) The lymphatic system. *Scient. Am.*, **208**(6), 80.

MAYERSON H.S. (1963) The physiologic importance of lymph. *Circulation*, vol. 2. Hamilton W.F. (ed.). American Physiological Society, Washington.

NOSSAL G.J.V. (1964) How cells make antibodies. *Scient. Am.*, **211**(6), 106.

O'BRIEN J.R. (1966) Platelet stickiness. *A. Rev. Med.*, **17**, 275.

RACE R.R. & SANGER R. (1962) *Blood Groups in Man*. Davis, Philadelphia.

RIGGS A. (1965) Functional properties of hemoglobins. *Physiol. Rev.*, **45**, 619.

SCHROEDER W.A. (1963) The hemoglobins. *A. Rev. Biochem.*, **32**, 301.

SEEGERS W.H. (1962) *Prothrombin*. Harvard University Press, Massachusetts.

STAFFORD J.L. (ed.) (1964) Fibrinolysis. *Br. med. Bull.*, **20**, 171.

WOLSTENHOLME G.E.W. & O'CONNOR C.M. (ed.) (1960) *Haemopoiesis: Cell production and its Regulation* (Ciba Foundation symposium). Churchill, London.

ZUCKER M.B. (1961) Blood platelets. *Scient. Am.*, **204**(2), 58.

Chapter 9 Cardiovascular System: The Heart

BING R.J. (1965) Cardiac metabolism. *Physiol. Rev.*, **45**, 171.

RANDALL W.C. (ed.) (1965) *Nervous Control of the Heart*. Williams & Willkins, Baltimore.

RUSHMER R.R. (1962) Effects of nerve stimulation and hormones on the heart; the role of the heart in general circulatory regulation. *Circulation*, vol. 1. Hamilton W.F. (ed.). American Physiological Society, Washington.

SARNOFF S.J. & MITCHELL J.H. (1962) The control of the function of the heart. *Circulation*, vol. 1. Hamilton W.F. (ed.). American Physiological Society, Washington.

WILLIUS F.A. & KEYS T.E. (1961) *Classics of Cardiology* (2 vols.). Dover, New York.

Chapter 10 Cardiovascular System: Blood Vessels and Circulation

AVIADO D.M. (1960) The pharmacology of the pulmonary circulation. *Pharmac. Rev.*, **12**, 159.

BARCROFT H. (ed.) (1963) Peripheral circulation in man. *Br. med. Bull.*, **19**, 97.

BERNE R.M. (1964) Regulation of coronary blood flow. *Physiol. Rev.*, **44**, 1.

CHAPMAN C.B. & MITCHELL J.H. (1965) The physiology of exercise. *Scient. Am.*, **212**(5), 88.

EICHNA L.W. & McQUARRIE D.G. (ed.) (1960) Symposium on central nervous system control of circulation. *Physiol. Rev.*, Supplement No. 4.

FOLKOW B., HEYMANS C. & NEIL E. (1965) Integrated aspects of cardiovascular regulation. *Circulation*, vol. 3. Hamilton W.F. (ed.). American Physiological Society, Washington.

GREEN H.D. & KEPCHAR J.H. (1959) Control of peripheral resistance in major systemic vascular beds. *Physiol. Rev.*, **39**, 617.

GREGG D.E. (1950) *Coronary Circulation in Health and Disease*. Lea & Febiger, Philadelphia.

GRIGOR'EVA T.A. (1962) *The Innervation of Blood Vessels*. Pergamon, New York.

HAMILTON W.F. (ed.) (1963) *Circulation*, vol. 2. American Physiological Society, Washington.

HERTZMAN A.B. (1959) Vasomotor regulation of cutaneous circulation. *Physiol. Rev.*, **39**, 280.

HEYMANS C. & NEIL E. (1958) *Reflexogenic Areas of the Cardiovascular System*. Little, Brown & Co., Boston.

HOFF E.C., KELL J.F. & CARROL M.N. (1963) Effects of cortical stimulation and lesions on cardiovascular function. *Physiol. Rev.*, **43**, 68.

MCDONALD D.A. (1960) *Blood Flow in Arteries*. Williams & Wilkins, Baltimore.

PAGE I.H. & MCCUBBIN J.W. (1965) The physiology of arterial hypertension. *Circulation*, vol. 3. Hamilton W.F. (ed.). American Physiological Society, Washington.

Chapter 11 The Respiratory System

ANTONINI E. (1965) Interrelationship between structure and function in hemoglobin and myoglobin. *Physiol. Rev.*, **45**, 123.

CAMPBELL E.J.M. (1958) *The Respiratory Muscles and the Mechanics of Breathing*. Year Book, Chicago.

CARO C.G. (ed.) (1966) *Advances in Respiratory Physiology*. Arnold, London.

CLEMENTS J.A. (1962) Surface tension in the lungs. *Scient. Am.*, **207**(6), 120.

COMROE J.H. (1965) *Physiology of Respiration*. Year Book, Chicago.

COMROE J.H. (1966) The lung. *Scient. Am.*, **214**(2), 57.

CUNNINGHAM D.J.C. & LLOYD B.B. (ed.) (1962) *The Regulation of Human Respiration*. Blackwell, Oxford.

DEJOURS P. (1962) Chemoreflexes in breathing. *Physiol. Rev.*, **42**, 335.

FENN W. O. & RAHN H. (ed.) (1964) *Respiration*, vols. 1 and 2. American Physiological Society, Washington.

HUGH-JONES P. & CAMPBELL E.J.M. (ed.) (1963) Respiratory physiology. *Br. med. Bull.*, **19**, 1.

LIERE E.J. VAN & STICKNEY J.C. (1963) *Hypoxia*. University of Chicago Press.

MEAD J. (1961) Mechanical properties of lungs. *Physiol. Rev.*, **41**, 281.

NAHAS G.G. (ed.) (1963) Regulation of respiration. *Ann. N.Y. Acad. Sci.*, **109**, 415.

PATTLE R.E. (1965) Surface lining of lung alveoli. *Physiol. Rev.*, **45**, 48.

REUCK A.S.V. DE & O'CONNER M. (ed.) (1961) *Pulmonary Structure and Function* (Ciba Foundation symposium). Churchill, London.

WIDDICOMBE J.G. (1963) Regulation of tracheobronchial smooth muscle. *Physiol. Rev.*, **43**, 1.

Chapter 12 The Digestive System and the Liver

BABKIN B.P. (1950) *Secretory Mechanism of the Digestive Glands*. Hoeber, New York.

BOOTH C.C. (1963) Absorption from the small intestine. *Lectures on the Scientific Basis of Medicine Annual Reviews*. Athlone Press, University of London.

BOSMA J.F. (1957) Deglutition: pharyngeal stage. *Physiol. Rev.*, **37**, 275.

CRANE R.K. (1960) Intestinal absorption of sugars. *Physiol. Rev.*, **40**, 789.

FARRAR G.E. & BOWER R.J. (1967) Gastric juice and secretion: physiology and variations in disease. *A. Rev. Physiol.*, **29**, 141.

GROSSMAN M.I. (ed.) (1966) *Gastrin.* Butterworths, London.
HUNT J.N. (1959) Gastric emptying and secretion in man. *Physiol. Rev.*, **39**, 491.
INGELFINGER F.J. (1958) Esophageal motility. *Physiol. Rev.*, **38**, 533.
JAMES A.H. (1957) *The Physiology of Gastric Digestion.* Arnold, London.
MAGEE D.F. (1962) *Gastrointestinal Physiology.* Thomas, Springfield.
REUCK A.V.S. DE & CAMERON M.P. (ed.) (1962) *The Exocrine Pancreas: Normal and Abnormal Functions* (Ciba Foundation symposium). Churchill, London.
ROUILLER C. (ed.) (1963–4) The liver. *Morphology, Biochemistry, Physiology*, vols. 1 and 2. Academic Press, New York.
SUN D.C.H. (ed.) (1962) The management of peptic ulcer. Part I. Gastric secretion. *Ann. N.Y. Acad. Sci.*, **99**, 4.
SUN D.C.H. (ed.) (1967) Gastric pepsin, mucus, and clinical secretory studies. *Ann. N.Y. Acad. Sci.*, **140**, 685.
THOMAS J.E. (1957) Mechanics and regulation of gastric emptying. *Physiol. Rev.*, **37**, 453.
WOODWARD E.R. & DRAGSTEDT L.R. (1960) Role of the pyloric antrum in regulation of gastric secretion. *Physiol. Rev.*, **40**, 490.

Chapter 13   The Urinary System

BLACK D.A.K. (1957) *Essentials of Fluid Balance.* Blackwell, Oxford.
CHINARD F.P. (1964) Kidney, water and electrolytes. *A. Rev. Physiol.*, **26**, 187.
CHRISTENSEN H.N. (1964) *Body Fluids and the Acid-base Balance.* Saunders, Philadelphia.
HARTROFT P.M. (1966) The juxtaglomerular complex. *A. Rev. Med.*, **17**, 113.
KURN M. (1965) Nervous control of micturition. *Physiol. Rev.*, **45**, 425.
MERRIL J.P. (1961) The artificial kidney. *Scient. Am.*, **205**(1), 56.
MILLS J.N. (1963) Mechanisms of renal homeostasis. *Recent Advances in Physiology.* Creese R. (ed.). Churchill, London.
MILLS J.N. (1963) Other aspects of renal function. *Recent Advances in Physiology.* Creese R. (ed.). Churchill, London.
O'CONNOR W.J. (1962) *Renal Function.* Arnold, London.
PITTS R.F. (1959) *The Physiological Basis of Diuretic Therapy.* Blackwell, Oxford.
PITTS R.F. (1963) *The Physiology of the Kidney and Body Fluids.* Year Book, Chicago.
ROBINSON J.R. (1962) *Fundamentals of Acid-base Regulation.* Blackwell, Oxford.
SPERBER I. (1959) The secretion of organic anions in the formation of urine and bile. *Pharmac. Rev.*, **11**, 109.
ULLRICH K.J. & MARSH D.J. (1963) Kidney, water and electrolyte metabolism. *A. Rev. Physiol.*, **25**, 91.
WINDHAGER E.E. & GIEBISCH G. (1965) Electrophysiology of the nephron. *Physiol. Rev.*, **45**, 214.

Chapter 14   The Endocrine System

ALBERT A. (ed.) (1961) *Human Pituitary Gonadotropins.* Thomas, Springfield.
COLE H.H. (ed.) (1964) *Gonadotropins: their Chemical and Biological Properties and Secretory Control.* Freeman, San Francisco.
COPE C.L. (1965) *Adrenal Steroids and Disease.* Pitman, London.
COPP D.H. (1964) Parathyroids, calcitonin and control of plasma calcium, *Recent Prog. Horm. Res.*, **20**, 59.

DANOWSKI T.S. (1962) *Clinical Endocrinology* (4 vols.). Williams & Wilkins, Baltimore.

EULER U.S. VON & HELLER H. (ed.) (1963) *Comparative Endocrinology*, vol. 1. Academic Press, New York.

FRASER T.R. (1963) Human growth hormone. *Lectures on the Scientific Basis of Medicine Annual Reviews.* Athlone Press, University of London.

GROLLMAN A. (1964) *Clinical Endocrinology and its Physiologic Basis.* Lippincott, Philadelphia.

HARRISON T.S. (1964) Adrenal medullary and thyroid relationships. *Physiol. Rev.*, **44**, 161.

KNOBIL E. & HOTCHKISS J. (1964) Growth hormone. *A. Rev. Physiol.*, **26**, 47.

KRAHL M.E. (1961) *The Action of Insulin on Cells.* Academic Press, New York.

LERNER A.B. (1962) Hormones and skin color. *Scient. Am.*, **205**(1), 98.

LEVINE R. & MAHLER R. (1964) Production, secretion and availability of insulin. *A. Rev. Med.*, **15**, 413.

LI C.H. (1963) The ACTH molecule. *Scient. Am.*, **209**(1), 46.

LITWACK G. & KRITCHEVSKY D. (1964) *Actions of Hormones on Molecular Processes.* Wiley, New York.

MALOOF F. & SOODAK M. (1963) Intermediary metabolism of thyroid tissue and the action of drugs. *Pharmac. Rev.*, **15**, 43.

MEITES J. & NICOLL C.S. (1966) Adenohypophysis: prolactin. *A. Rev. Physiol.*, **28**, 57.

MOON H.D. (ed.) (1961) *The Adrenal Cortex.* Hoeber, New York.

MYANT N.B. (ed.) (1960) The thyroid gland. *Br. med. Bull.*, **16**, 89.

PITT-RIVERS R. & TATA R. (1959) *The Thyroid Hormones.* Pergamon, Oxford.

PRUNTY F.T.G. (ed.) (1962) The adrenal cortex. *Br. med. Bull.*, **18**, 89.

RASMUSSEN H. (1961) The parathyroid hormone. *Scient. Am.*, **204**(4), 56.

ROSS E.J. (1962) Biological properties of aldosterone. *Br. med. Bull.*, **18**, 164.

SAWYER W.H. (1961) Neurohypophysial hormones. *Pharmac. Rev.*, **13**, 225.

SHARP G.W.G. & LEAF A. (1966) Mechanism of action of aldosterone. *Physiol. Rev.*, **46**, 593.

THORN N.A. (1958) Mammalian antidiuretic hormone. *Physiol. Rev.*, **38**, 169.

TROTTER W.R. (ed.) (1964) *The Thyroid Gland.* Butterworths, London.

WOLFF J. (1964) Transport of iodide and other anions in the thyroid gland. *Physiol. Rev.*, **44**, 45.

WURTMAN R.J. & AXELROD J. (1965) The pineal gland. *Scient. Am.*, **213**(1), 50.

YATES F.E. & URQUHART J. (1962) Control of plasma concentrations of adrenocortical hormones. *Physiol. Rev.*, **42**, 359.

YOUNG F.G. (ed.) (1960) Insulin. *Br. med. Bull.*, **16**, 175.

ZARROW M.X., YOCHIM J.M. & McCARTHY J.L. (1964) *Experimental Endocrinology: a Sourcebook of Basic Techniques.* Academic Press, New York.

Chapter 15 The Reproductive System

AUSTIN C.R. (1961) *The Mammalian Egg.* Davis, Philadelphia.

BISHOP D.W. (1962) Sperm motility. *Physiol. Rev.*, **42**, 1.

CAREY H.M. (1963) *Modern Trends in Human Reproductive Behaviour.* Butterworths, London.

CROSS K.W. & DAWES G.S. (ed.) (1966) The foetus and the new-born. *Br. med. Bull.*, **22**, 1.

EIK-NES K.B. (1964) Effects of gonadotrophins on secretion of steroids by the testis and ovary. *Physiol. Rev.*, **44**, 609.

EVERETT J.W. (1964) Central neural control of reproductive function of the adenohypophysis. *Physiol. Rev.*, **44**, 373.

GRADY H.G. & SMITH D.E. (ed.) (1963) *The Ovary*. Williams & Wilkins, Baltimore.

LLOYD C.W. (1964) *Human Reproduction and Sexual Behaviour*. Lea & Febiger, Philadelphia.

LLOYD C.W. & WEISZ J. (1966) Some aspects of reproductive physiology. *A. Rev. Physiol.*, **28**, 267.

MACLEOD J. (ed.) (1952) Biology of the testes. *Ann. N.Y. Acad. Sci.*, **55**, 543.

MASTERS W.H. & JOHNSON V.E. (1966) *Human Sexual Response*. Little, Brown & Co., Boston.

PARKES A.S. (1963) External factors in mammalian reproduction. *Lectures on the Scientific Basis of Medicine Annual Reviews*. Athlone Press, University of London.

ROTHSCHILD Lord (1962) Spermatozoa. *Br. med. J.*, **2**, 743.

SAWYER C.H. (1960) Reproductive behaviour. *Neurophysiology*, vol. 2. Field J. (ed.). American Physiological Society, Washington.

VILLEE C. (1961) *Control of Ovulation*. Pergamon, New York.

ZUCKERMAN S. (ed.) (1962) *The Ovary* (2 vols.). Academic Press, New York.

Chapter 16   The Special Senses

ADES H.W. (1959) Central auditory mechanisms. *Neurophysiology*, vol. 1. Field J. (ed.). American Physiological Society, Washington.

ADEY W.R. (1959) Sense of smell. *Neurophysiology*, vol. 1. Field J. (ed.). American Physiological Society, Washington.

AMOORE J.E., JOHNSTON J.W. & RUBIN M. (1964) The stereochemical theory of odour. *Scient. Am.*, **210**(2), 42.

BARTLEY H.S. (1959) Central mechanisms of vision. *Neurophysiology*, vol. 1. Field J. (ed.). American Physiological Society, Washington.

BEIDLER L.M. (1961) The chemical senses. *A. Rev. Psychol.*, **12**, 363.

BERGEIJK W.A. VAN, PIERCE J.R. & DAVID E.E. (1961) *Waves and the Ear*. Heinemann, London.

BOTELHO S.Y. (1964) Tears and the lacrimal gland. *Scient. Am.*, **211**(4), 78.

BRINDLEY C.S. (1960) *Physiology of the Retina and Visual Pathway*. Arnold, London.

DAVIS H. (1957) Biophysics and physiology of the inner ear. *Physiol. Rev.*, **37**, 1.

DAVIS H. (1959) Excitation of auditory receptors. *Neurophysiology*, vol. 1. Field J. (ed.). American Physiological Society, Washington.

DAVSON H. (ed.) (1962) *The Eye* (4 vols.). Academic Press, New York.

FENDER D.H. (1964) Control mechanisms of the eye. *Scient. Am.*, **211**(1), 24.

FRY G.A. (1959) The image-forming mechanism of the eye. *Neurophysiology*, vol. 1. Field J. (ed.). American Physiological Society, Washington.

GRANIT R. (1955) *Receptors and Sensory Perception*. Oxford University Press.

GRANIT R. (1959) Neural activity in the retina. *Neurophysiology*, vol. 1. Field J. (ed.). American Physiological Society, Washington.

HODGSON E.S. (1961) Taste receptors. *Scient. Am.*, **204**(5), 135.

KALMUS H. & HUBBARD S.J. (1960) *The Chemical Senses in Health and Disease*. Thomas, Springfield.

KUEHNER R.L. (ed.) (1964) Recent advances in odor: theory, measurement, and control. *Ann. N.Y. Acad. Sci.*, **116**, 357.

MACNICHOL E.F. (1964) Three-pigment color vision. *Scient. Am.*, **211**(6), 48.

MONCRIEFF R.W. (1951) *The Chemical Senses*. Leonard Hill, London.

PFAFFMANN C. (1959) The sense of taste. *Neurophysiology*, vol. 1. Field J. (ed.). American Physiological Society, Washington.

RUSHTON W.A.H. (1962) Visual pigments in man. *Scient. Am.*, **207**(5), 120.

SMELSER G.K. (ed.) (1961) *The Structure of the Eye*. Academic Press, New York.

WALD G. (1959) The photoreceptor process in vision. *Neurophysiology*, vol. 1. Field J. (ed.). American Physiological Society, Washington.

WHITTERIDGE D. (1960) Central control of eye movements. *Neurophysiology*, vol. 2. Field J. (ed.). American Physiological Society, Washington.

ZOTTERMAN Y. (1959) Thermal sensations. *Neurophysiology*, vol. 1. Field J. (ed.). American Physiological Society, Washington.

ZOTTERMAN Y. (ed.) (1963) *Olfaction and Taste*. Macmillan, New York.

Chapter 17 Body Temperature

ATKINS E. (1960) Pathogenesis of fever. *Physiol. Rev.*, **40**, 580.

BENZINGER T.H. (1961) The human thermostat. *Scient. Am.*, **204**(1), 134.

CULVER W.E. (1959) Effects of cold on man. An annotated bibliography, 1938–1951. *Physiol. Rev.*, Supplement 3.

DAWKINS M.J.R. & HULL D. (1965) The production of heat by fat. *Scient. Am.*, **213**(2), 62.

DILL D.B. (ed.) (1964) *Adaptation to the Environment*. American Physiological Society, Washington.

EULER C. VON (1961) Physiology and pharmacology of temperature regulation. *Pharmac. Rev.*, **13**, 361.

HARDY J.D. (1961) The physiology of temperature regulation. *Physiol. Rev.*, **41**, 521.

HEMINGWAY A. (1963) Shivering. *Physiol. Rev.*, **43**, 397.

IRVING L. (1966) Adaptations to cold. *Scient. Am.*, **214**(1), 94.

JOEL C.D. (1965) The physiological role of brown adipose tissue. *Adipose Tissue*. Renold A.E. & Cahill G.F. (ed.). American Physiological Society, Washington.

MASORO E.J. (1966) Effect of cold on metabolic use of lipids. *Physiol. Rev.*, **46**, 67.

PICKERING G. (1961) Fever and pyrogens. *Lectures on the Scientific Basis of Medicine Annual Reviews*. Athlone Press, University of London.

SMITH R.E. & HOIJER D.J. (1962) Metabolism and cellular function in cold acclimation. *Physiol. Rev.*, **42**, 60.

STRÖM G. (1960) Central nervous regulation of body temperature. *Neurophysiology*, vol. 2. Field J. (ed.). American Physiological Society, Washington.

Chapter 18 Principles of Drug Action

ALBERT A. (1965) *Selective Toxicity*. Methuen, London.

ARIËNS E.J. (ed.) (1964) *Molecular Pharmacology* (2 vols.). Academic Press, New York.

ARIËNS E.J. (1966) Receptor theory and structure-action relationships. *Advances in Drug Research*, vol. 3. Harper N.J. & Simmonds A.B. (ed.). Academic Press, London.

ARUNLAKSHANA, O. & SCHILD H.O. (1959) A modification of receptor theory. *Br. J. Pharmac. Chemother.*, **11**, 379.

BARLOW R.B. (1964) *Introduction to Chemical Pharmacology*. Methuen, London.

BELLEAU B. (1965) Conformational perturbation in relation to the regulation of enzyme and receptor behaviour. *Advances in Drug Research*, vol. 2. Harper N.J. & Simmonds A.B. (ed.). Academic Press, London.

COOPER J.R. (1964) Biochemical mechanisms of drug action. *A. Rev. Pharmac.*, **4**, 1.

CUTHBERT A.W. (1967) Membrane lipids and drug action. *Pharmac. Rev.*, **19**, 59.

FASTIER F.N. (1964) Modern concepts in relationship between structure and biological activity. *A. Rev. Pharmac.*, **4**, 51.

FURCHGOTT R.F. (1964) Receptor mechanisms. *A. Rev. Pharmac.*, **4**, 21.

FURCHGOTT R.F. (1966) The use of β-haloalkylamines in the differentiation of receptors and in the determination of dissociation constants of receptor-agonist complexes. *Advances in Drug Research*, vol. 3. Harper N.J. & Simmonds, A.B. (ed.). Academic Press, London.

GADDUM J.H. & SCHILD H.O. (ed.) (1957) Drug antagonism. *Pharmac. Rev.*, **9**, 211.

GILL E.W. (1965) Drug receptor interactions. *Progress in Medicinal Chemistry*, vol. 4. Ellis G.P. & West G.B. (ed.). Butterworths, London.

JONGE H. DE (ed.) (1961) *Quantitative Methods in Pharmacology*. North Holland, Amsterdam.

HOLLAND W.C., KLEIN R.C. & BRIGGS A.H. (1964) *Introduction to Molecular Pharmacology*. Macmillan, New York.

MACKAY D. (1966) A new method for the analysis of drug-receptor interactions. *Advances in Drug Research*, vol. 3. Harper N.J. & Simmonds A.B. (ed.). Academic Press, London.

PATON W.D.M. (1961) A theory of drug action based on the rate of drug-receptor combination. *Proc. R. Soc. B.*, **154**, 21.

PATON W.D.M. & RANG H.P. (1966) A kinetic approach to the mechanism of drug action. *Advances in Drug Research*, vol. 3. Harper N.J. & Simmonds A.B. (ed.). Academic Press, London.

ROSSUM J.M. VAN (1966) Limitations of molecular pharmacology. Some implications of the basic assumptions underlying calculations on drug-receptor interactions and the significance of biological drug parameters. *Advances in Drug Research*, vol. 3. Harper N.J. & Simmonds A.B. (ed.). Academic Press, London.

STEPHENSON R.P. (1956) A modification of receptor theory. *Br. J. Pharmac. Chemother.*, **11**, 379.

Chapter 19   Absorption, Distribution, Metabolism and Excretion of Drugs

ARIËNS E.J. & SIMONIS A.M. (1964) Drug transference: drug metabolism. *Molecular Pharmacology*, vol. 1. Ariëns E.J. (ed.). Academic Press, New York.

BINNS T.B. (ed.) (1964) Absorption and distribution of drugs. Livingstone, Edinburgh.

CONNEY A.H. & BURNS J.J. (1962) Factors influencing drug metabolism. *Adv. Pharmac.*, **1**, 31. Academic Press, New York.

FISHMAN W.H. (1961) *Chemistry of Drug Metabolism*. Thomas, Springfield.

GILLETTE J.R. (1966) Biochemistry of drug oxidation and reduction by enzymes in hepatic endoplasmic reticulum. *Adv. Pharmac.*, **4**, 219. Academic Press, New York.

MONGAR J.L. & DE REUCK A.V.S. (ed.) (1962) *Enzymes and Drug Action* (Ciba Foundation symposium). Churchill, London.

LEVINE R.R. & PELIKAN E.W. (1964) Mechanisms of drug absorption and excretion. *A. Rev. Pharmac.*, **4**, 69.

OS G.A.J. VAN, in cooperation with ARIËNS E.J. & SIMONIS A.M. (1964) Drug transference: distribution of drugs in the organism. *Molecular Pharmacology*, vol. 1. Ariëns, E.J. (ed.). Academic Press, New York.

PETERS L. (1960) Renal tubular excretion of organic bases. *Pharmac. Rev.*, **12**, 1.

RALL D.P. & ZUBROD C.G. (1962) Mechanisms of drug absorption and excretion. Passage of drugs in and out of the central nervous system. *A. Rev. Pharmac.*, **2**, 109.

REMMER H. (1965) The fate of drugs in the organism. *A. Rev. Pharmac.*, **5**, 405.

SCHANKER L.S. (1962) Passage of drugs across body membranes. *Pharmac. Rev.*, **14**, 501.

SCHANKER L.S. (1964) Physiological transport of drugs. *Advances in Drug Research*, vol. 1. Harper N.J. & Simmonds A.B. (ed.). Academic Press, London.

SCHOU J. (1961) Absorption of drugs from subcutaneous connective tissue. *Pharmac. Rev.*, **13**, 441.

WEINER I.M. (1967) Mechanisms of drug absorption and excretion. The renal excretion of drugs and related compounds. *A. Rev. Pharmac.*, **7**, 39.

Chapter 20   Evaluation of Drug Action

ARMITAGE P. (1960) *Sequential Medical Trials*. Oxford University Press.

BAILEY N.T.J. (1959) *Statistical Methods in Biology*. English Universities Press, London.

BARNES J.M. & PAGET G.E. (1965) Mechanisms of toxic action. *Progress in Medicinal Chemistry*, vol. 4. Ellis G.P. & West G.B. (ed.). Butterworths, London.

BEER E.J. DE (ed.) (1950) The place of statistical methods in biological and chemical experimentation. *Ann. N.Y. Acad. Sci.*, **52**, 789.

BERNSTEIN L. & WEATHERALL M. (1952) *Statistics for Medical and other Biological Students*. Livingstone, Edinburgh.

BINNS T.B. (ed.) (1965) Symposium on clinical interaction between drugs. *Proc. R. Soc. Med.*, **58**, 943.

BRADFORD HILL A. (1951) The clinical trial. *Br. med. Bull.*, **7**, 282.

BRADFORD HILL A. (chairman) (1960) *Controlled Clinical Trials*. Blackwell, Oxford.

BROWNLEE K.A. (1948) *Industrial Experimentation*. H.M.S.O., London.

BURN J.H., FINNEY D.J. & GOODWIN L.G. (1950) *Biological Standardization*. Oxford University Press.

BURNS J.J. (chairman) (1965) Evaluation and mechanisms of drug toxicity. *Ann. N.Y. Acad. Sci.*, **123**, 1.

CAHEN R.L. (1966) Experimental and clinical chemoteratogenesis. *Adv. Pharmac.*, **4**, 263. Academic Press, New York.

DAWSON M. & DRYDEN W.F. (1967) Tissue culture in the study of the effects of drugs. *J. Pharm. Sci.*, **56**, 545.

EMMENS C.W. (1948) *Principles of Biological Assay*. Chapman & Hall, London.

EMMENS C.W. (ed.) (1950) *Hormone Assay*. Academic Press, New York.

FINNEY D.J. (1952) *Probit Analysis*. Cambridge Univ. Press.

FINNEY D.J. (1964) *Statistical Method in Biological Assay*. Griffin, London.

FISHER R.A. (1960) *The Design of Experiments*. Oliver & Boyd, Edinburgh.

FISHER R.A. (1948) *Statistical Methods for Research Workers*. Oliver & Boyd, Edinburgh.

LAURENCE D.R. & BACHARACH A.L. (ed.) (1964) *Evaluation of Drug Activities: Pharmacometrics* (2 vols.). Academic Press, New York.

LITCHFIELD J.T. (1962) Evaluation of the safety of new drugs by means of tests in animals. *Clin. Pharmac. Ther.*, **3**, 665.

MEYLER L. (ed.) (1966) *Side Effects of Drugs*. Excerpta Medica Foundation, Amsterdam.

MEYLER L. & PECK H.M. (ed.) (1962) *Drug-induced Diseases*. Thomas, Netherlands.

MODELL W. (1959) Problems in the evaluation of drugs in man. *J. Pharm. Pharmac.*, **11**, 577.

PERRY W.L.M. (1950) *The Design of Toxicity Tests*. Special report series, No. 270. H.M.S.O., London.

SMITH W.G. (1961) Pharmacological screening tests. *Progress in Medicinal Chemistry*, vol. 1. Ellis G.P. & West G.B. (ed.). Butterworths, London.

31

STEWART G.A. & YOUNG P.A. (1963) Statistics as applied to pharmacological and toxicological screening. *Progress in Medicinal Chemistry*, vol. 3. Ellis G.P. & West G.B. (ed.). Butterworths, London.
WALPOLE A.L. & SPINKS A. (ed.) (1958) *The Evaluation of Drug Toxicity*. Churchill, London.
WILSON A. & LORD COHEN (chairmen) (1962) *Clinical Trials*. Pharmaceutical Press, London.
ZAIMIS E. (ed.) (1965) *Evaluation of New Drugs in Man*. Pergamon, Oxford.
ZBINDEN G. (1963) Experimental and clinical aspects of drug toxicity. *Adv. Pharmac.*, **2**, 1. Academic Press, New York.

Chapter 21   General Anaesthetics

ADRIANI J. (1963) General anesthetics. 1. Absorption, distribution and elimination. *Physiological Pharmacology*, vol. 1. Root W.S. & Hofmann F.G. (ed.). Academic Press, New York.
BUNKER J.P. & VANDAM L.D. (chairmen) (1965) Effects of anesthesia on metabolism and cellular functions. *Pharmac. Rev.*, **17**, 183.
FEATHERSTONE R.M. & MUEHLBAECHER C.A. (1963) The current role of inert gases in the search for anesthesia mechanisms. *Pharmac. Rev.*, **15**, 97.
GREISHEIMER E.M. (1965) The circulatory effects of anesthetics. *Circulation*, vol. 3. Hamilton W.F. (ed.). American Physiological Society, Washington.
HOLMSTEDT B. & LILJESTRAND G. (1963) Volatile anaesthetics, hypnotics, alcohol, theory of narcosis. *Readings in Pharmacology*, chap. 3. Macmillan, New York.
JACOBSEN E. (1952) The metabolism of ethyl alcohol. *Pharmac. Rev.*, **4**, 107.
KEYS T.E. (1963) *The History of Surgical Anesthesia*. Dover, New York.
KETY S.S. (1951) The theory and applications of the exchange of inert gas at the lungs and tissues. *Pharmac. Rev.*, **3**, 1.
LIEBER C.S. (1966) Hepatic and metabolic effects of alcohol. *Gastroenterology*, **50**, 119.
LUMB W.V. (1963) *Small Animal Anesthesia*. Lea & Febiger, Philadelphia.
MARDONES J. (1963) The alcohols. *Physiological Pharmacology*, vol. 1. Root W.S. & Hofmann F.G. (ed.). Academic Press, New York.
NGAI S.H. (1963) General anesthetics. 2. Effects upon physiological systems. *Physiological Pharmacology*, vol. 1. Root W.S. & Hofmann F.G. (ed.). Academic Press, New York.
PAPPER E.M. & KATZ R.J. (ed.) (1963) *Uptake and Elimination of Anesthetics*. McGraw-Hill, New York.
PATON W.D.M. & SPEDEN R.N. (ed.) (1965) Anaesthetics and the central nervous system. *Br. med. Bull.*, **21**, 1.
PAULING L. (1961) A molecular theory of general anesthesia. *Science*, **134**, 15.
VANDAM L.D. (1966) Anesthesia. *A. Rev. Pharmac.*, **6**, 379.
WYLIE W.D. & CHURCHILL-DAVIDSON H.C. (1966) *A Practice of Anaesthesia*. Lloyd-Luke, London.

Chapter 22   Hypnotics, Sedatives, Tranquillizers, Anticonvulsants and Centrally Acting Muscle Relaxants

BLAIR D. (1963) *Modern Drugs for the Treatment of Mental Illness*. Staples Press, London.
BRADLEY P.B. (1963) Tranquilizers. 1. Phenothiazine derivatives. *Physiological Pharmacology*, vol. 1. Root W.S. & Hofmann F.G. (ed.). Academic Press, New York.

BUSH M.T. (1963) Sedatives and hypnotics. 1. Absorption, fate and excretion. *Physiological Pharmacology*, Vol. 1. Root W.S. & Hofmann F.G. (ed.). Academic Press, New York.

DOMINO E.F. (1962) Sites of action of some central nervous system depressants. *A. Rev. Pharmac.*, **2**, 215.

GORDON M. (ed.) (1964) *Psychopharmacological Agents*. Academic Press, New York.

HAASE H.J. & JANSSEN P.A.J. (1965) *The Action of Neuroleptic Drugs*. Year Book, Chicago.

LEWIS J.J. (1963) Rauwolfia derivatives. *Physiological Pharmacology*, vol. 1. Root W.S. & Hofmann F.G. (ed.). Academic Press, New York.

LUCAS R.A. (1963) The chemistry and pharmacology of the Rauwolfia alkaloids. *Progress in Medicinal Chemistry*, vol. 3. Ellis G.P. & West G.B. (ed.). Butterworths, London.

MARGOLIN S. (1963) Sedatives and hypnotics. 2. Effects upon physiological systems. b. Non-barbiturates. *Physiological Pharmacology*, vol. 1. Root W.S. & Hofmann F.G. (ed.). Academic Press, New York.

MARKS J. & PARE C.M.B. (ed.) (1965) The scientific basis of drug therapy in psychiatry. Pergamon, Oxford.

MILLICHAP J.G. (1965) Anticonvulsant drugs. *Physiological Pharmacology*, vol. 2. Root W.S. & Hofmann F.G. (ed.). Academic Press, New York.

PARKES M.W. (1961) Tranquillizers. *Progress in Medicinal Chemistry*, vol. 1. Ellis G.P. & West G.B. (ed.). Butterworths, London.

SHERROD T.R. (1963) Tranquilizers. 3. Diphenylmethane derivatives. *Physiological Pharmacology*, vol. 1. Root W.S. & Hofmann F.G. (ed.). Academic Press, New York.

SMITH C.M. (1965) Relaxants of skeletal muscle. *Physiological Pharmacology*, vol. 2. Root W.S. & Hofmann F.G. (ed.). Academic Press, New York.

SPINKS A. & WARING W.S. (1963) Anticonvulsant drugs. *Progress in Medicinal Chemistry*, vol. 3. Ellis G.P. & West G.B. (ed.). Butterworths, London.

Chapter 23   Central Nervous System Stimulant Drugs

BLUM R. (ed.) (1964) *Utopiates: the Use and Users of LSD-25*. Atherton Press, New York.

BARRON F., JARVIK M.E. & BUNNELL S. (1964) The hallucinogenic drugs. *Scient. Am.*, **210**(4), 29.

GARATTINI S. & DUKES M.N.G. (ed.) (1967) *Antidepressant Drugs*. Excerpta Medica Foundation, Amsterdam.

GIARMAN N.J. & FREEDMAN D.X. (1965) Biochemical aspects of the actions of psychotomimetic drugs. *Pharmac. Rev.*, **17**, 1.

GORDON M. (ed.). *Psychopharmacological Agents*, vol. 1. Academic Press, New York.

HOLTZ P. & WESTERMAN E. (1965) Psychic energizers and antidepressant drugs. *Physiological Pharmacology*, vol. 2. Root W.S. & Hofmann F.G. (ed.). Academic Press, New York.

KILLAM E.K. (1962) Drug action on the brain stem reticular formation. *Pharmac. Rev.*, **4**, 175.

KLERMAN G.L. & COLE J.O. (1965) Clinical pharmacology of imipramine and related compounds. *Pharmac. Rev.*, **17**, 71.

MARKS J. & PARE C.M.B. (ed.) (1965) *The Scientific Basis of Drug Therapy in Psychiatry*. Pergamon, Oxford.

MODELL W. (1960) The status and prospect of drugs for overeating. *J. Am. med. Ass.*, **173**, 1131.

POLLARD J.C., UHR L. & STERN E. (1965) *Drugs and Phantasy*. Little, Brown & Co., Boston.

WEISS B. & LATIES V.G. (1962) Enhancement of human performance by caffeine and the amphetamines. *Pharmac. Rev.*, **14**, 1.

Chapter 24   Analgesics

BECKETT A.H. & CASY A.F. (1962) The testing and development of analgesic drugs. *Progress in Medicinal Chemistry*, vol. 2. Ellis G.P. & West G.B. (ed.). Butterworths, London.

BECKETT A.H. & CASY A.F. (1965) Analgesics and their antagonists: biochemical aspects and structure-activity relationships. *Progress in Medicinal Chemistry*, vol. 4. Ellis G.P. & West G.B. (ed.). Butterworths, London.

BEECHER H.K. (1959) *Measurement of Subjective Responses: Quantitative Effects of Drugs*. Oxford University Press, New York.

BUCHER K. (1965) Antitussive drugs. *Physiological Pharmacology*, vol. 2. Root W.S. & Hofmann F.G. (ed.). Academic Press, New York.

BUCHER K. (1958) Pathophysiology and pharmacology of cough. *Pharmac. Rev.*, 10, 43.

CHAPPEL C.I. & VON SEEMANN C. (1963) Antitussive drugs. *Progress in Medicinal Chemistry*, vol. 3. Ellis G.P. & West G.B. (ed.). Butterworths, London.

COLLIER H.O.J. (1963) Aspirin. *Scient. Am.*, 209(5), 96.

DENEAU G.A. & SEEVERS M.H. (1964) Pharmacological aspects of drug dependence. *Adv. Pharmac.*, 3, 267. Academic Press, New York.

DOMENJOZ, R. (1966). Synthetic anti-inflammatory drugs: concepts of their mode of action. *Adv. Pharmac.*, 4, 143. Academic Press, New York.

DOYLE F.P. & MEHTA M.D. (1964) Antitussives. *Advances in Drug Research*. Harper N.J. & Simmonds A.B. (ed.). Academic Press, London.

LASAGNA L. (1964) The clinical evaluation of morphine and its substitutes as analgesics. *Pharmac. Rev.*, 16, 47.

MARTIN W.R. (1963) Analgesic and antipyretic drugs. 1. Strong analgesics. *Physiological Pharmacology*, vol. 1. Root W.S. & Hofmann F.G. (ed.). Academic Press, New York.

RANDALL L.O. (1963) Analgesic and antipyretic drugs. 2. Non-narcotic analgesics. *Physiological Pharmacology*, vol. 1. Root W.S. & Hofmann F.G. (ed.). Academic Press, New York.

SEEVERS M.H. & DENEAU G.A. (1963) Physiological aspects of tolerance and physical dependence. *Physiological Pharmacology*, vol. 1. Root W.S. & Hofmann F.G. (ed.). Academic Press, New York.

STEVENS G. DE (ed.) (1965) *Analgetics*. Academic Press, New York.

WAY E.L. & ADLER T.K. (1960) The pharmacologic implications of the fate of morphine and its surrogates. *Pharmac. Rev.*, 12, 383.

Chapter 25   Local Anaesthetics

ADRIANI J. (1960) The clinical pharmacology of local anesthetics. *Clin. Pharmac. Ther.*, 1, 645.

ADRIANI J., ZEPERNICK R., ARENS J. & AUTHMENT E. (1964) The comparative potency and effectiveness of topical anesthetics in man. *Clin. Pharmac. Ther.*, 5, 49.

JONG R.H. DE & WAGMAN I.H. (1963) Physiological mechanisms of peripheral nerve blocks by local anaesthetics. *Anesthesiology*, 24, 684.

GASSER H.S. & ERLANGER J. (1929) The role of fiber size in the establishment of nerve block by pressure or cocaine. *Am. J. Physiol.*, 88, 581. Reprinted in *Readings in Pharmacology*. Shuster L. (ed.). Little, Brown & Co., Boston.

MATTHEWS, P.B.C. & RUSHWORTH G. (1957) The relative sensitivity of muscle nerve fibres to procaine. *J. Physiol.*, 135, 263.

RITCHIE J.M. & GREENGARD P. (1966) On the mode of action of local anesthetics. *A. Rev. Pharmac.*, 6, 405.

SHANES A.M. (1963) Drugs and nerve conduction. *A. Rev. Pharmac.*, **3**, 185.

SKOU J.C. (1961) The effects of drugs on cell membranes with special reference to local anaesthetics. *J. Pharm. Pharmac.*, **13**, 204.

WATSON P.J. (1960) The mode of action of local anaesthetics. *J. Pharm. Pharmac.*, **12**, 257.

WIEDLING S. & TÉGNER C. (1963) Local anaesthetics. *Progress in Medicinal Chemistry*, vol. 3. Ellis G.P. & West G.B. (ed.). Butterworths, London.

Chapter 26   Drugs Modifying Neuromuscular Transmission

BOVET D., BOVET-NITTI F. & MARINI-BETTOLO G.B. (ed.) (1959) *Curare and Curare-like Agents*. Elsevier, Amsterdam.

BOWMAN W.C. (1964) Neuromuscular blocking agents. *Evaluation of Drug Activities: Pharmacometrics*, vol. 2. Laurence D.R. & Bacharach A.L. (ed.). Academic Press, London.

BOWMAN W.C. & RAPER C. (1967) Adrenotropic receptors in skeletal muscle. *Ann. N.Y. Acad. Sci.*, **139**, 741.

CHEYMOL J. (ed.) (1967) Neuromuscular blocking and stimulating agents. *International Encyclopaedia of Pharmacology and Therapeutics*. Sect. 14. Pergamon, Oxford.

CHURCHILL-DAVIDSON H.C. (1963) Muscle relaxants. *Recent Advances in Anaesthesia and Analgesia*. Hewer C.L. (ed.). Churchill, London.

EHRENPREIS S. (ed.) (1967) Cholinergic mechanisms. *Ann. N.Y. Acad. Sci.*, **144**, 383.

GLASER G.H. (1963) Pharmacological considerations in the treatment of myasthenia gravis. *Adv. Pharmac.*, **2**, 113. Academic Press, New York.

KARCZMAR A.G. (1967) Neuromuscular pharmacology. *A. Rev. Pharmac.*, **7**, 241.

LEWIS J.J. & MUIR T.C. (1967) Drugs acting at nerve-skeletal muscle junctions. *The Peripheral Nervous System*. Chap. 5, Burger A. (ed.). Marcel Dekkar, New York.

REUCK A.V.S. DE (ed.) (1962) *Curare and Curare-like Agents*. Churchill, London.

SCHUELER F.W. (1960) The mechanism of action of the hemicholiniums. *Int. Rev. Neurobiol.*, **2**, 77.

SCHUELER F.W. (ed.) (1961) The hemicholiniums. *Fedn. Proc.*, **20**, 561.

STENLAKE J.B. (1963) Some chemical aspects of neuromuscular block. *Progress in Medicinal Chemistry*, vol. 3. Ellis G.P. & West G.B. (ed.). Butterworths, London.

TAYLOR D.B. & NEDERGAARD O.A. (1965) Relation between structure and action of quaternary ammonium neuromuscular blocking agents. *Physiol. Rev.*, **45**, 523.

THESLEFF S. (1960) Effects of motor innervation on the chemical sensitivity of skeletal muscle. *Physiol. Rev.*, **40**, 734.

WASER P.G. (1966) Autoradiographic investigations of cholinergic and other receptors in the motor end plate. *Advances in Drug Research*, vol. 3. Harper N.J. & Simmonds A.B. (ed.). Academic Press, London.

WERNER G. & KUPERMAN A. (1963) Systematic pharmacology of the anticholinesterase (anti-ChE) agents. Actions at the neuromuscular junction. *Cholinesterases and Anticholinesterase Agents*. Koelle G.B. (ed.). Springer-Verlag, Berlin.

Chapter 27   Drugs Acting at Autonomic Ganglia

MACINTOSH F.C. (1959) Formation, storage, and release of acetylcholine at nerve endings. *Canad. J. Biochem. Physiol.*, **37**, 343.

MOE G.K. & FREYBURGER W.A. (1950) Ganglion blocking agents. *Pharmac. Rev.*, **2**, 61.

PATON W.D.M. (1954) Transmission and block in autonomic ganglia. *Pharmac. Rev.*, 6, 59.
PATON W.D.M. & ZAIMIS E.J. (1952) The methonium compounds. *Pharmac. Rev.*, 4, 219.
PERRY W.L.M. (1957) Transmission in autonomic ganglia. *Br. med. Bull.*, 13, 220.
TRENDELENBURG U. (1961) Pharmacology of autonomic ganglia. *A. Rev. Pharmac.*, 1, 219.
VOLLE R.L. (1966) Modification by drugs of synaptic mechanisms in autonomic ganglia. *Pharmac. Rev.*, 18, 839.
VOLLE R.L. (1966) Muscarinic and nicotinic stimulant actions at autonomic ganglia. *International Encyclopaedia of Pharmacology and Therapeutics*. Karczmar A.G. (ed.). Sect. 12, vol. 1. Pergamon Press, Oxford.
ZAIMIS E. (1963) Systematic pharmacology of the anticholinesterase (anti-ChE) agents. Actions at autonomic ganglia. *Cholinesterases and Anticholinesterase Agents*. Koelle G.B. (ed.). Springer-Verlag, Berlin.

Chapter 28   Parasympathomimetics and Drugs Modifying their Actions:
Anti-Parkinsonian Drugs

AMBACHE N. (1955) The use and limitations of atropine for pharmacological studies on autonomic effectors. *Pharmac. Rev.*, 7, 467.
BARLOW R.B. (1964) *Introduction to Chemical Pharmacology*, chaps. 7 and 8. Methuen, London.
BEBBINGTON A. & BRIMBLECOMBE R.W. (1965) Muscarinic receptors in the peripheral and central nervous systems. *Advances in Drug Research*, vol. 2. Harper N.J. & Simmonds A.B. (ed.). Academic Press, London.
BRAND J.J. & Perry W.L.M. (1966) Drugs used in motion sickness. *Pharmac. Rev.*, 18, 895.
FRIEDMAN A.H. & EVERETT G.M. (1964) Pharmacological aspects of Parkinsonism. *Adv. Pharmac.*, 3, 83. Academic Press, New York.
GLASER E.M. (1959) Prevention and treatment of motion sickness. *Proc. R. Soc. Med.*, 52, 965
HEATH D.F. (1961) *Organophosphorus Poisons*. Pergamon, Oxford.
HERXHEIMER A. (1958) A comparison of some atropine-like drugs in man, with particular reference to their end-organ specificity. *Br. J. Pharmac.*, *Chemother.*, 13, 184.
HOLMSTEDT, B. (1959) Pharmacology of organophosphorus cholinesterase inhibitors. *Pharmac. Rev.*, 11, 567.
KOELLE G.B. (ed.) (1963) *Cholinesterase and Anticholinesterase Agents*. Springer-Verlag, Berlin.
KOSTERLITZ H.W. (1967) Cholinergic drugs. Effects upon smooth muscle and secretions from choline esters. *Physiological Pharmacology*, vol. 3. Root W.S. & Hofmann B.F. (ed.). Academic Press, New York.
LONGO V.G. (1966) Behavioural and electroencephalographic effects of atropine and related substances. *Pharmac. Rev.*, 18, 965.
RAND M.J. & STAFFORD A. (1967) Cholinergic drugs. Cardiovascular actions of choline esters. *Physiological Pharmacology*, vol. 3. Root W.S. & Hofmann B.F. (ed.). Academic Press, New York.
TRIGGLE D.J. (1965) *Chemical Aspects of the Autonomic Nervous System*. Academic Press, London.
WASER P.G. (1961) Chemistry and pharmacology of muscarine, muscarone, and some related compounds. *Pharmac. Rev.*, 13, 465.

Chapter 29 Sympathomimetics and Drugs Modifying their Action

ACHESON G.H. (ed.) (1966) Second symposium on catecholamines. *Pharmac. Rev.*, **18**, 1.

BLOOM B.M. & GOLDMAN I.M. (1966) The nature of catecholamine-adenine mononucleotide interactions in adrenergic mechanisms. *Advances in Drug Research*, vol. 3. Harper N.J. & Simmonds A.B. (ed.). Academic Press, London.

GRAHAM J.D.P. (1962) 2-Halogenoalkylamines. *Progress in Medicinal Chemistry*, vol. 2. Ellis G.P. & West G.B. (ed.). Butterworths, London.

HAUGAARD N. & HESS M.E. (1965) Actions of autonomic drugs on phosphorylase activity and function. *Pharmac. Rev.*, **17**, 1.

HUNTER A.R. & MILLAR R.A. (ed.) (1966) Symposium on adrenergic drugs and their antagonists. *Br. J. Anaesth.*, **38**, 666.

MARLEY E. (1964) The adrenergic system and sympathomimetic amines. *Adv. Pharmac.*, **3**, 168. Academic Press, New York.

MORAN N.C. (ed.) (1967) New adrenergic blocking drugs: their pharmacological, biochemical and clinical actions. *Ann. N.Y. Acad. Sci.*, **139**, 541.

PRATESI P. (1963) Chemical structure and biological activity of catecholamines. *Pharmaceutical Chemistry*. Butterworths, London.

PRATESI P. & GRANA E. (1965) Structure and activity at adrenergic receptors of catecholamines and certain related compounds. *Advances in Drug Research*, vol. 2. Harper N.J. & Simmonds A.B. (ed.). Academic Press, London.

TRIGGLE D.J. (1965) *Chemical Aspects of the Autonomic Nervous System*. Academic Press, London.

TRIGGLE D.J. (1965) 2-Halogenoethylamines and receptor analysis. *Advances in Drug Research*, vol. 2. Harper N.J. & Simmonds A.B. (ed.). Academic Press, London.

Chapter 30 Histamine, 5-Hydroxytryptamine and Polypeptides Acting on Smooth Muscle

COLLIER H.O.J. (1962) Kinins. *Scient. Am.*, **207**(2), 111.

DAVIES G.E. (1962) Anaphylactic reactions. *Progress in Medicinal Chemistry*, vol. 2. Ellis G.P. & West G.B. (ed.). Butterworths, London.

DUNÉR H. & PERNOW B. (1963) Histamine. *Comparative Endocrinology*, vol. 2. Euler U.S von & Heller H. (ed.). Academic Press, New York.

ERDÖS E.G. (1966) Hypotensive peptides: bradykinin, kallidin and eledoisin. *Adv. Pharmac.* **4**, 1. Academic Press, New York.

ERSPAMER V. (1963) 5-Hydroxytryptamine. *Comparative Endocrinology*, vol. 2. Euler U.S. von & Heller H. (ed.). Academic Press, New York.

ERSPAMER V. (1966) *5-Hydroxytryptamine and Related Indolealkylamines*. Springer-Verlag, New York.

GARATTINI S. & VALZELLI L. (1965) *Serotonin*. Elsevier, Amsterdam.

GYERMEK L. (1961) 5-Hydroxytryptamine antagonists. *Pharmac. Rev.*, **13**, 399.

HAVERBACK B.J. & WIRTSCHAFTER S.K. (1962) The gastrointestinal tract and naturally occurring pharmacologically active amines. *Adv. Pharmac.* **1**, 309. Academic Press, New York.

LAW H.D. (1965) Polypeptides of medicinal interest. *Progress in Medicinal Chemistry*, vol. 4. Ellis G.P. & West G.B. (ed.). Butterworths, London.

LEWIS G.P. (1960) Active polypeptides derived from plasma proteins. *Physiol. Rev.*, **40**, 647.

MELDRUM B.S. (1965) The snake venoms on nerve and muscle. The pharmacology of phospholipase A and of polypeptide toxins. *Pharmac. Rev.*, **17**, 393.

MONGAR J.L. & SCHILD H.O. (1962) Cellular mechanisms in anaphylaxis. *Physiol. Rev.*, **42**, 226.

PATON W.D.M. (1957) Histamine release by compounds of simple chemical structure. *Pharmac. Rev.*, **9**, 269.

PERNOW B. (1953) Studies on substance P. Purification, occurrence and other biological actions. *Acta physiol. scand.*, **29**, supplement 105.

PINKERTON J.H.M. (ed.) (1965) *Advances in Oxytocin Research*. Pergamon, Oxford.

ROCHA E SILVA M. (1963) Kinins: bradykinin, angiotensin, substance P. *Comparative Endocrinology*, vol. 2. Euler U.S. von & Heller H. (ed.). Academic Press, New York.

SCHACTER M. (ed.) (1960) *Polypeptides which Affect Smooth Muscles and Blood Vessels*. Pergamon, Oxford.

SCHRÖDER E. & LÜBKE K. (1966) *The Peptides*, vol. 2. Academic Press, New York.

SPENCER P.S.J. & WEST G.B. (1965) Experimental hypersensitivity reactions. *Progress in Medicinal Chemistry*, vol. 4. Butterworths, London.

UNGAR G. (1966) Pharmacologically active peptides. *Anesthesiology*, **27**, 539.

UVNÄS B. (1963) Mechanism of histamine release in mast cells. *Ann. N.Y. Acad. Sci.*, **103**, 278.

YONKMAN F.F. (ed.) (1950) Antihistamine agents in allergy. *Ann. N.Y. Acad. Sci.*, **50**, 1013.

Chapter 31   Drugs Acting on the Gastrointestinal Tract

CLEAVE T.L. (1963) *Peptic Ulcer: Its Cause, Prevention and Arrest*. Williams & Wilkins, Baltimore.

CODE C.F. (1951) The inhibition of gastric secretion. *Pharmac. Rev.*, **3**, 59.

CODE C.F. (1960) The peptic ulcer problem. A physiologic appraisal. *Am. J. dig. Dis.*, **5**, 288.

HOSKINS D.W. & KEAN B.H. (1963) Drugs for travelers. *Clin. Pharmac. Therap.* **4**, 673.

SUN D.C.H. (ed.) (1962) The management of peptic ulcer. Part III. Advances in anticholinergic drug therapy. *Ann. N.Y. Acad. Sci.*, **99**, 131.

TAINTER M.L. (ed.) (1954) The colon: its normal and abnormal physiology and therapeutics. *Ann. N.Y. Acad. Sci.*, **58**, 293.

VAUGHAN WILLIAMS E.M. (1954) The mode of action of drugs upon intestinal motility. *Pharmac. Rev.*, **6**, 159.

WANG S.C. (1965) Emetic and antiemetic drugs. *Physiological Pharmacology*, vol. 2. Root W.S. & Hofmann F.G. (ed.). Academic Press, New York.

Chapter 32   Drugs Acting on the Cardiovascular System

AVIADO D.M. (1960) Hemodynamic effects of ganglion blocking drugs. *Circulation Res.*, **8**, 304.

BLOCK J.H., PIERCE C.H. & LILLEHEI R.C. (1966) Adrenergic blocking agents in the treatment of shock. *A. Rev. Med.*, **17**, 483.

CHARLIER R. (1961) *Coronary Vasodilators*. Pergamon, Oxford.

COPP F.C. (1964) Adrenergic neurone blocking drugs. *Advances in Drug Research*, vol. 1. Harper N.J. & Simmonds A.B. (ed.). Academic Press, London.

DAVIS J.O. (1965) The physiology of congestive heart failure. *Circulation*, vol. 3. Hamilton W.F. (ed.). American Physiological Society, Washington.

DAWES G.S. (1952) Experimental cardiac arrhythmias and quinidine-like drugs. *Pharmac. Rev.*, **4**, 43.

DIMOND E.G. (ed.) (1957) *Digitalis*. Thomas, Springfield.

ESTES J.W. & WHITE P.D. (1965) William Withering and the purple foxglove. *Scient. Am.*, **212**(6), 110.

FINE J. (1965) Shock and peripheral circulatory insufficiency. *Circulation*, vol. 3. Hamilton W.F. (ed.). American Physiological Society, Washington.

GREEN A.F. (1962) Antihypertensive drugs. *Adv. Pharmac.*, **1**, 162. Academic Press, New York.

GROSS F. (ed.) (1966) *Antihypertensive Therapy*. Springer-Verlag, New York.

HAJDU S. & LEONARD E. (1959) The cellular basis of cardiac glycoside action. *Pharmac. Rev.*, **11**, 173.

HARRINGTON M. (1956) *Hypotensive Drugs*. Pergamon, Oxford.

KAVERINA N.V. (1965) *Pharmacology of the Coronary Circulation*. Pergamon, Oxford.

LEONARD E. & HAJDU S. (1962) Actions of electrolytes and drugs on the contractile mechanism of the cardiac muscle cell. *Circulation*, vol. 1. Hamilton W.F. (ed.). American Physiological Society, Washington.

PARDO E.G., VARGAS R. & VIDRIO H. (1965) Antihypertensive drug action. *A. Rev. Pharmac.*, **5**, 77.

TOBIAN L. (1967) Why do thiazide diuretics lower the blood pressure in essential hypertension? *A. Rev. Pharmac.*, **7**, 399.

TRAUTWEIN W. (1963) Generation and conduction of impulses in the heart as affected by drugs. *Pharmac. Rev.*, **15**, 277.

WÉGRIA R. (1951) Pharmacology of the coronary circulation. *Pharmac. Rev.*, **3**, 197.

WEIN R. (1961) Hypotensive agents. *Progress in Medicinal Chemistry*, vol. 1. Ellis G.P. & West G.B. (ed.). Butterworths, London.

WINBURY M.W. (1964) Experimental approaches to the development of antianginal drugs. *Adv. Pharmac.*, **3**, 2. Academic Press, New York.

WITHERING W. (1785) *An Account of the Foxglove and some of its Medical Uses*. Reprinted by The Broomsleigh Press, London.

WRIGHT S.E. (1960) *The Metabolism of Cardiac Glycosides*. Blackwell, Oxford.

Chapter 33 Drugs Acting on the Endocrine System

BARTTER F.C. (ed.) (1960) *The Clinical Use of Aldosterone Antagonists*. Thomas, Springfield.

BUSH I.E. (1962) Chemical and biological factors in the activity of adrenocortical steroids. *Pharmac. Rev.*, **14**, 317.

COPE C.L. (1965) *Adrenal Steroids and Disease*. Pitman, London.

DANOWSKI T.S. (1962) *Clinical Endocrinology* (4 vols.). Williams & Wilkins, Baltimore.

DRILL V.A. & RIEGEL B. (1958) Structural and hormonal activity of some new steroids. *Recent Prog. Horm. Res.*, **14**, 29.

DUNCAN L.J.P. & BAIRD J.D. (1960) Compounds administered orally in the treatment of diabetes mellitus. *Pharmac. Rev.*, **12**, 91.

JACKSON H. (1966) *Antifertility Compounds in the Male and Female*. Thomas, Springfield.

MALOOF F. & SOODAK M. (1963) Intermediary metabolism of thyroid tissue and the action of drugs. *Pharmac. Rev.*, **15**, 43.

PINCUS G. (1965) *The Control of Fertility*. Academic Press, New York.

PINCUS G. (1966) Control of conception by hormonal steroids. *Science*, **153**, 493.

31*

PINCUS G. & BIALY G. (1964) Drugs used in control of reproduction. *Adv. Pharmac.*, **3**, 285. Academic Press, New York.

PLATT LORD (chairman) (1967) Rise of thromboembolic disease in women taking oral contraceptives. *Br. med. J.*, **2**, 355.

SLATER J.D.H. (1961) Oral hypoglycaemic drugs. *Progress in Medicinal Chemistry*, vol. 1. Ellis G.P. & West G.B. (ed.). Butterworths, London.

TYLER E.T. (1967) Antifertility agents. *A. Rev. Pharmac.*, **7**, 381.

VILLEE C.A. (ed.) (1961) *Control of Ovulation.* Pergamon, New York.

WAYNE E.J., KOUTRAS D.A. & ALEXANDER W.D. (1964) *Clinical Aspects of Iodine Metabolism.* Blackwell, Oxford.

Chapter 34   Drugs Acting on the Urinary System

BAER J.E. & BEYER K.H. (1966) Renal pharmacology. *A. Rev. Pharmac.*, **6**, 261.

BERLINER R.W. & ORLOFF J. (1956) Carbonic anhydrase inhibitors. *Pharmac. Rev.*, **8**, 137.

BEYER K.H. & BAER J.E. (1961) Physiological basis for the action of newer diuretic agents. *Pharmac. Rev.*, **13**, 517.

HELLER H. & GINSBURG M. (1961) Diuretic drugs. *Progress in Medicinal Chemistry*, vol. 1. Ellis G.P. & West G.B. (ed.). Butterworths, London.

MUDGE G.H. (1967) Renal pharmacology. *A. Rev. Pharmac.*, **7**, 163.

PITTS R.F. (1959) *The Physiological Basis of Diuretic Therapy.* Blackwell, Oxford.

PITTS R.F. (1961) A comparison of the modes of action of certain diuretic agents. *Prog. cardiovas. Dis.*, **3**, 537.

STEVENS G. DE (1963) *Diuretics.* Academic Press, New York.

Chapter 35   Drugs Acting on the Eye

GRANT W.M. (1955) Physiological and pharmacological influences upon intraocular pressure. *Pharmac. Rev.*, **7**, 143.

PATERSON G., MILLER S.J.H. & PATERSON G. (ed.) (1966) *Drug Mechanisms in Glaucoma.* Churchill, London.

POTTS A.M. (1965) The effects of drugs upon the eye. *Physiological Pharmacology*, vol. 2. Root W.S. & Hofmann F.G. (ed.). Academic Press, New York.

Chapter 36   Drugs Affecting the Blood and Blood Formation

BIGGS R. & MACFARLANE R.G. (ed.) (1966) *Treatment of Haemophilia and other Coagulation Disorders.* Blackwell, Oxford.

BOTHWELL T.H. & FINCH C.A. (1962) *Iron Metabolism.* Little, Brown & Co., Boston.

DOUGLAS A.S. (1962) *Anticoagulant Therapy.* Blackwell, Oxford.

FOWLER N.O. (1962) Plasma substitutes. *Circulation*, vol. 1. Hamilton W.F. (ed.). American Physiological Society, Washington.

GLASS G.B.J. (1963) Gastric intrinsic factor and its function in the metabolism of vitamin B_{12}. *Physiol. Rev.*, **43**, 529.

HARRIS J.W. (1963) *The Red Cell.* Harvard University Press, Massachusetts.

INGRAM G.I.C. (1961) Anticoagulant therapy. *Pharmac. Rev.*, **13**, 279.

INGRAM G.I.C. & RICHARDSON J. (1965) *Anticoagulant Prophylaxis and Treatment.* Thomas, Springfield.

JACOBSON L.O. & DOYLE M. (ed.) (1962) *Erythropoiesis.* Grune & Stratton, New York.

JORPES J.E. (1963) Heparin. *Comparative Endocrinology*, vol. 2. Euler U.S. von and Heller H. (ed.). Academic Press, New York.

MACMILLAN R.L. & MUSTARD J.F. (ed.). *Anticoagulants and Fibrinolysis*. Lea & Febiger, New York.

RABINOWITZ J. (1960) Folic acid. *The Enzymes*. Boyer P.D., Lardy H. & Myrback K. (ed.). Academic Press, New York.

WERNER M. (1962) Pharmacological considerations of antithrombotic therapy. *Adv. Pharmac.*, **1**, 277. Academic Press, New York.

Chapter 37   Chemotherapy of Infection and Cancer

BROWN S.S. (1963) Nitrogen mustards and related alkylating agents. *Adv. Pharmac.*, **2**, 243. Academic Press, New York.

BUEDING E. & SWARTZWELDER C. (1957) Anthelmintics. *Pharmac. Rev.*, **9**, 329.

BUSHBY S.R.M. (1958) Chemotherapy of leprosy. *Pharmac. Rev.*, **10**, 1.

DELMONTE L. & JUKES T.H. (1962) Folic acid antagonists in cancer chemotherapy. *Pharmac. Rev.*, **14**, 91.

DOYLE F.P. & NAYLER J.H.C. (1964) Penicillins and related structures. *Advances in Drug Research*, vol. 1. Harper N.J. & Simmonds A.B. (ed.). Academic Press, London.

DUSTIN P. (1963) New aspects of the pharmacology of antimitotic agents. *Pharmac. Rev.*, **15**, 449.

GALE E.F. (1963) Mechanisms of antibiotic action. *Pharmac. Rev.*, **15**, 481.

HAWKING F. & LAWRENCE J.S. (1951) *The Sulphonamides*. Grune & Stratton, New York.

HENDERSON J.F. & MANDEL H.G. (1963) Purine and pyrimidine antimetabolites in cancer chemotherapy. *Adv. Pharmac.*, **2**, 297. Academic Press, New York.

HEROLD M. & GABRIEL Z. (1966) *Antibiotics—Advances in Research, Production and Clinical Use*. Butterworths, London.

JAWETZ E. & GUNNISON J.B. (1953) Antibiotic synergism and antagonism: an assessment of the problem. *Pharmac. Rev.*, **5**, 175.

ROBSON J.M. & SULLIVAN F.M. (1963) Antituberculous drugs. *Pharmac. Rev.*, **15**, 169.

ROLLO I.M. (1964) Chemotherapy of malaria. *Biochemistry and Physiology of Protozoa*, vol. 3. Hutner S.H. (ed.). Academic Press, New York.

SAZ H.J. & BUEDING E. (1966) Relationships between anthelmintic effects and biochemical and physiological mechanisms. *Pharmac. Rev.*, **18**, 871.

SCHNITZER R.J. & HAWKING F. (ed.) (1963–66) *Experimental Chemotherapy* (4 vols.). Academic Press, New York.

STERNBERG T.H. & NEWCOMER V.D. (ed.) (1955) *Therapy of Fungus Diseases*. Little, Brown & Co., Boston.

STEWART G.T. (1965) *The Penicillin Group of Drugs*. Elsevier, New York.

TAYLOR E.P. & D'ARCY P.F. (1961) Antifungal agents. *Progress in Medicinal Chemistry*, vol. 1. Ellis G.P. & West G.B. (ed.). Butterworths, London.

WALLS L.P. (1963) The chemotherapy of trypanosomiasis. *Progress in Medicinal Chemistry*, vol. 3. Ellis G.P. & West G.B. (ed.). Butterworths, London.

Index

A bands 191–4, 209
Abducens nerve 93
ABO blood grouping 241–2
Abortion 406–7, 865
  drug-induced 626, 758
Abdominal reflex 115
Abductor muscles 191
Absorption, from gastro-intestinal tract 324–5
  of drugs 485–97
Acceleranstoff 140
Accessory nerve 94, 125, 130
Accommodation (in vision) 417–18, 420–1
  effect of drugs on 418, 898
Accommodation (of nerves) 86
Acepromazine 596, 598
Acetaldehyde 50–1, 505, 586
Acetanilide 487, 489, 516, 647–8
Acetarsone 940–1
Acetazolamide 489, 879–82
  in epilepsy 610
  in glaucoma 895
Acetic acid 20
Acetoacetic acid 328, 355
Acetohexamide 854
Acetomenaphthone 829, 911–12
Acetone in urine 349
Acetophenetidine 647
Acetophenylisatin 795
Acetylation, in acetylcholine synthesis 152–3
  in tricarboxylic acid cycle 42–4
  of drugs 511
Acetylcholine, and membrane permeability 149, 195–8, 479, 688
  as local hormone 172–3
  bioassay 150–1, 550, 686, 721
  depolarizing actions 149, 195–8, 479, 688
  effects, on adrenal medulla 148, 163–4
    on adrenergic neurones 164, 773
    on autonomic ganglia 143, 148–50, 686–701
    on cardiac tissue 215–16
    on cardiovascular system 139–40
    on chemoreceptors 289
    on chromaffin cells 148

Acetylcholine—*continued*
  effects—*continued*
    on CNS 169–71, 425, 605, 619
    on denervated muscle 205, 483
    on eye 892–3
    on pituitary 890
    on piloerection 142, 147, 440
    on parasympathetic effectors 140–1
    on sympathetic nerves 164
    on neuromuscular junction 144–9, 195–8, 200–2, 479, 660–77, 681–5
    on smooth muscle 224, 458
    on sweating 142, 147, 440
  hydrolysis of 20, 156–8
  mechanism of action 148–50
  miotic action 417, 892
  muscarinic actions 138–9, 147, 170, 698–702, 710, 723–4, 728
  nicotinic actions 139, 147–8, 686, 688, 695–8, 728, 772
  non-competitive antagonists of 467
  parasympathomimetic actions, *see* muscarinic actions
  pA values of antagonists 477
  potentiation of 483
  receptors 148, 703, 710–13, 664
  release 154–6
    prevention of, by drugs 663–4, 698–90, 694
    increase by drugs 680
  storage 154
  structure of 138, 704
  synthesis 152–3
    inhibition by drugs 660–3
  tachyphylaxis to 479
Acetylcholinesterase 20, 681
  hydrolysis, of acetylcholine 156–8
    of methacholine 706
  presence, in CNS 169
    in ganglia, 149–50
    in motor endplates 194–5
Acetylcoenzyme A 25–6
  in drug acetylation 511
  in metabolism, of amino acids 51
    of fatty acids 45, 328, 382
  in synthesis of acetylcholine 152–3
  in tricarboxylic acid cycle 42–4, 382, 505

972

32*